The APRN's Complete Guide to Prescribing Drug Therapy

2019

Mari J. Wirfs, PhD, MN, RN, APRN, ANP-BC, FNP-BC, CNE, is a nationally certified adult nurse practitioner (ANCC since 1997) and family nurse practitioner (AANP since 1998) and certified nurse educator (NLN since 2008). Her career spans 45 years in collegiate undergraduate and graduate nursing education and clinical practice in critical care, pediatrics, psychiatric–mental health nursing, and advanced practice primary care nursing. Her PhD is in higher education administration and leadership. During her academic career, she has achieved the rank of professor with tenure in two university systems. She is a frequent guest lecturer on a variety of advanced practice topics to professional groups and general health care topics to community groups.

Dr. Wirfs was a member of the original medical staff in the establishment of Baptist Community Health Services, a community-based nonprofit primary care clinic founded post-hurricane Katrina in the New Orleans Lower Ninth Ward. Since 2002, Dr. Wirfs has served as clinical director and primary care provider at the Family Health Care Clinic, serving faculty, staff, students, and their families at New Orleans Baptist Theological Seminary (NOBTS). She is also adjunct graduate faculty, teaching Neuropsychology and Psychopharmacology, in the NOBTS Guidance and Counseling program. She is a long-time member of the National Organization of Nurse Practitioner Faculties (NONPF), Sigma Theta Tau National Honor Society of Nursing, and several other academic honor societies.

Dr. Wirfs has completed, published, and presented six quantitative research studies focusing on academic leadership, nursing education, and clinical practice issues, including one for the Army Medical Department conducted during her 8 years reserve service in the Army Nurse Corps. Dr. Wirfs has co-authored family primary care certification review books and study materials. Her first prescribing guide, *Clinical Guide to Pharmacotherapeutics for the Primary Care Provider,* was published by Advanced Practice Education Associates (APEA) from 1999 to 2014. *The APRN's Complete Guide to Prescribing Drug Therapy* (launched in 2016), *The APRN's Complete Guide to Prescribing Pediatric Drug Therapy* (launched in 2017), and *The PA's Complete Guide to Prescribing Drug Therapy* (launched in 2017) are published annually by Springer Publishing Company. Each is accompanied by an ebook version and quarterly electronic updates.

The APRN's Complete Guide to Prescribing Pediatric Drug Therapy 2018 was awarded 2nd place, **"Book of the Year 2017" in the Child Health Category**, by the *American Journal of Nursing (AJN)*, official publication of the American Nurses Association (ANA). The panel of judges included the founder of the nurse practitioner role and the first nurse practitioner program, Dr. Loretta C. Ford, Professor Emerita. Dr. Wirfs was the recipient of the **"2018 AANP Nurse Practitioner State Award for Excellence"** from Louisiana by the American Association of Nurse Practitioners. This prestigious award is given annually to a dedicated nurse practitioner in each state who demonstrates excellence in their area of practice.

The APRN's Complete Guide to Prescribing Drug Therapy

2019

*Mari J. Wirfs, PhD, MN, RN,
APRN, ANP-BC, FNP-BC, CNE*

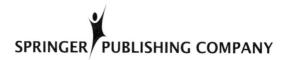

SPRINGER PUBLISHING COMPANY

Springer Publishing Company, LLC
11 West 42nd Street
New York, NY 10036
www.springerpub.com

Acquisitions Editor: Margaret Zuccarini
Composition: Exeter Premedia Services Private Ltd.

ISBN: 978-0-8261-5103-2
e-book ISBN: 978-0-8261-5104-9

19 20 21 22 / 8 7 6 5

This book is a quick reference for health care providers practicing in primary care settings. The information has been extrapolated from a variety of professional sources and is presented in condensed and summary form. It is not intended to replace or substitute for complete and current manufacturer prescribing information, current research, or knowledge and experience of the user. For complete prescribing information, including toxicities, drug interactions, contraindications, and precautions, the reader is directed to the manufacturer's package insert and the published literature. The inclusion of a particular brand name neither implies nor suggests that the author or publisher advises or recommends the use of that particular product or considers it superior to similar products available by other brand names. Neither the author nor the publisher makes any warranty, expressed or implied, with respect to the information, including any errors or omissions, herein.

Library of Congress Cataloging-in-Publication Data
Names: Wirfs, Mari J., author.
Title: The APRN's complete guide to prescribing drug therapy 2018 / Mari J. Wirfs.
Description: New York, NY: Springer Publishing Company, LLC, [2018] |
   Includes bibliographical references and index.
Identifiers: LCCN 2017008900| ISBN 9780826151032 | ISBN 9780826151049 (ebook)
Subjects: | MESH: Drug Therapy—nursing | Advanced Practice Nursing—methods
   | Handbooks
Classification: LCC RM301 | NLM WY 49 | DDC 615.1—dc23
LC record available at https://lccn.loc.gov/2017008900

Contact us to receive discount rates on bulk purchases.
We can also customize our books to meet your needs.
For more information please contact: sales@springerpub.com

Printed in the United States of America.

CONTENTS

SECTION II: APPENDICES

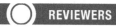
Kelley M. Anderson, PhD, FNP
Assistant Professor of Nursing, Georgetown University School of Nursing and Health Studies, Washington, DC

Kathleen Bradbury-Golas, DNP, RN, FNP-C, ACNS-BC
Associate Clinical Professor, Drexel University, Philadelphia, Pennsylvania; Family Nurse Practitioner, Virtua Medical Group, Hammonton and Linwood, New Jersey

Lori Brien, MS, ACNP-BC
Instructor, Advanced Practice Nursing Department, Georgetown University School of Nursing and Health Studies, Washington, DC

Jill Cash, MSN, APN, CNP
Nurse Practitioner, Logan Primary Care, West Frankfort, Illinois

Catherine M. Concert, DNP, RN, FNP-BC, AOCNP, NE-BC, CNL, CGRN
Nurse Practitioner-Radiation Oncology, Laura and Isaac Perlmutter Cancer Center, New York University Langone Medical Center; Clinical Assistant Professor, Pace University Lienhard School of Nursing, New York, New York

Kate DeMutis, MSN, CRNP
Senior Lecturer, Adult-Gerontology Primary Care Nurse Practitioner Program, Centralized Clinical Site Coordinator-Primary Care, University of Pennsylvania School of Nursing, Philadelphia, Pennsylvania

Gaye M. Douglas, DNP, MEd, APRN-BC
Assistant Professor of Nursing, Francis Marion University, Florence, South Carolina

Brenda Douglass, DNP, APRN, FNP-C, CDE, CTTS
Coordinator of Clinical Faculty, Assistant Clinical Professor, Drexel University College of Nursing and Health Professions, Philadelphia, Pennsylvania

Aileen Fitzpatrick, DNP, RN, FNP-BC
Clinical Assistant Professor, Pace University Lienhard School of Nursing, New York, New York

Nancy M. George, PhD, RN, FNP-BC, FAANP
Director of DNP Program, Associate Clinical Professor, Wayne State University College of Nursing, Detroit, Michigan

Tracy P. George, DNP, APRN-BC, CNE
Assistant Professor of Nursing, Amy V. Cockroft Fellow 2016-2017, Francis Marion University, Florence, South Carolina

Cheryl Glass, MSN, WHNP, RN-BC
Clinical Research Specialist, KePRO, TennCare's Medical Solutions Unit, Nashville, Tennessee

Kathleen Gray, DNP, FNP-C
Assistant Professor, Georgetown School of Nursing and Health Studies, Washington, DC

Norma Stephens Hannigan, DNP, MPH, FNP-BC, DCC, FAANP
Clinical Professor of Nursing, Coordinator, Accelerated Second Degree (A2D) Program/
Sophomore Honors Program, Hunter College, CUNY Hunter-Bellevue School of
Nursing, New York, New York

Ella T. Heitzler, PhD, WHNP, FNP, RNC-OB
Assistant Professor, Georgetown University School of Nursing and Health Studies,
Washington, DC

Mary T. Hickey, EdD, RN
Clinical Professor of Nursing, Hunter College, CUNY Hunter-Bellevue School of
Nursing, New York, New York

Deborah L. Hopla, DNP, APRN-BC
Assistant Professor of Nursing, Director MSN/FNP Track, Amy V. Cockcroft Fellow,
Francis Marion University, Florence, South Carolina

Julia M. Hucks, MN, APRN-BC
Assistant Professor of Nursing, Family Nurse Practitioner, Francis Marion University,
Florence, South Carolina

Honey M. Jones, DNP, ACNP-BC
Acute Care Nurse Practitioner, Duke University Medical Center; Clinical Associate
Faculty, MSN Program, Duke University School of Nursing, Durham, North Carolina

Melissa H. King, DNP, FNP-BC, ENP-BC
Director of Advanced Practice Providers, Director of TelEmergency, Department of
Emergency Medicine, University of Mississippi Medical Center, Jackson, Mississippi

Brittany M. Newberry, PhD, MSN, MPH, APRN, ENP, FNP
Board Certified Emergency and Family Nurse Practitioner; Vice President Education
and Professional Development of HospitalMD; Chair, Practice Committee of American
Academy of Emergency Nurse Practitioners; Adjunct Faculty, Emory University School
of Nursing, Atlanta, Georgia

Andrea Rutherfurd, MS, MPH, FNP-BC
Clinical Faculty Advisor, Adjunct Instructor, FNP Program, Georgetown University
School of Nursing and Health Studies, Washington, DC

Samantha Venable, MSN, RN, FNP
Family Nurse Practitioner, Correctional Nursing, Trabuco Canyon, California

Michael Watson, DNP, APRN, FNP-BC
Lead Family Nurse Practitioner, Wadley Regional Medical Center, Emergency
Department, Texarkana, Texas

*	single-scored tablet
**	cross-scored tablet
***	tri-scored
>	greater than
<	less than
≥	greater than or equal to
≤	less than or equal to
(I), (II), (III), (IV), (V)	Drug Enforcement Agency (DEA) controlled substance schedule
(A), (B), (C), (D), (X)	Federal Drug Agency (FDA) pregnancy categories
AAR	American Academy of Rheumatology
ABSSSI	acute bacterial skin and skin structure infection
ac	before meal
ACEI	angiotensin converting enzyme inhibitor
ACOS	asthma-COPD overlap syndrome
ADA	American Diabetes Association
AF, A-fib	atrial fibrillation
AKI	acute kidney injury
ALP	alkaline phosphatase
ALT	a liver enzyme, alanine transaminase (ALT)
AM	antemeridiem, morning
AMD	age-related macular degeneration
AMI	acute myocardial infarction
APAP	acetaminophen
Apo-B	apolipoprotein B
ARB	angiotensin receptor blocker
ART	antiretroviral treatment
ASA	acetylsalicylic acid, aspirin

ASE	adverse side effect
ASIPP	American Society of Interventional Pain Physicians
AST	a liver enzyme, aspartate transaminase
AVB	atrioventricular heart block
BBW	black box warning
BCG vaccine	*Bacillus Calmette-Guerin* vaccine; tuberculosis vaccine
bid	*bis in die*, twice-a-day
BP	blood pressure
BPH	benign prostatic hyperplasia
BSA	body surface area
BUN	blood urea nitrogen
CAD	coronary artery disease
calib applicator	calibrated applicator
cap	capsule
CAP	community acquired pneumonia
CBC	complete blood count
CCB	calcium channel blocker
CFC	chlorofluorocarbon, inhaler propellant
chew tab	chewable tablet
Child-Pugh A	mild liver disease/dysfunction
Child-Pugh B	moderate liver disease/dysfunction
Child-Pugh C	severe liver disease/dysfunction
CHF	congestive heart failure
CHS	cannabinoid hyperemesis syndrome
CIC	chronic idiopathic constipation
CDAD	*Clostridium difficile*-associated diarrhea
CDC	Centers for Disease Control and Prevention
CK	creatine kinase
CKD	chronic kidney disease
cLN	childhood-onset lupus nephritis
clnsr	Cleanser

Cmax	maximum serum concentration of a drug
CNS	central nervous system
conc	concentrate, concentration
conj estra	conjugated estrogen
cont-rel	controlled-release, continuous-release
COPD	chronic obstructive pulmonary disease
cplt	caplet
Cr	creatinine
CR	controlled-release
CrCl	creatinine clearance measured in mL/min
CRI	chronic renal insufficiency
CRF	chronic renal failure
crm	cream
CSF	cerebral spinal fluid
cSLE	childhood-onset lupus erythematosis
cUTI	complicated urinary tract infection
CVD	cardiovascular disease
CYC	cyclosporine
CYP	cytochrome p
DAA	direct-acting antiviral
DDAVP	desmopressin acetate
dL	deciliter (100 ml)
DM	diabetes mellitus
DMARD	disease modifying anti-rheumatoid drug
DMD	Duchenne muscular dystrophy
DME	diabetic macular edema
DR	diabetic retinopathy
DVT	deep vein thrombosis
ECG	electrocardiogram, EKG
ED	erectile dysfunction

ec	enteric-coat
EDTA	edatate calcium disodium
EE	ethinyl estradiol
eGFR	estimated glomerular filtration rate
EKG	electrocardiogram, ECG
EIA	exercise-induced asthma
EIAED	enzyme-inducing antiepileptic drug
EIB	exercise-induced bronchospasm
ELAR	European League Against Rheumatism
elix	elixir
emol, emol crm	emollient, emollient cream
ent-coat	enteric-coat
EPS	extrapyramidal side effect
ER	extended-release, ext-rel
ESA	erythropoiesis stimulating agent
ESR	erythrocyte sedimentation rate
ESRD	end stage renal disease
est	estradiol
EX, ext-rel	extended-release
FBS	fasting blood sugar
FDA	Federal Drug Administration
film-coat	film-coated
(G)	generic, generic availability
G6PD	glucose-6-phosphate dehydrogenase
GABHS	group a beta-hemolytic streptococcus
GAD	generalized anxiety disorder
GER	gastroesophageal reflux
GERD	gastroesophageal reflux disease
GFR	glomerular filtration rate
GI	gastrointestinal
GLP-1	glucagon peptide-1
gm	gram

gtt, gtts	drop, drops
GU	genitourinary
H_2O_2	hydrogen peroxide
HAART	highly active antiretroviral treatment
HAV	hepatitis A virus
HBV	hepatitis C virus
HCQ	hydroxychloroquine
HCT	hematocrit
HCT, HCTZ	hydrochlorothiazide
HCV	hepatitis C virus
HCQ	hydroxychloroquine
HDL, HDL-C	high density lipoprotein cholesterol
HeFH	heterozygous familial hypercholesterolemia
HF	heart failure
HFA	hydrofluoroalkane (inhaler propellent phasing in)
Hgb	Hemoglobin
HgbA1c	hemoglobin A1c, the standard POC diagnostic test for diabetes
hgc	hard-gel capsule
Hib	*Haemophilus influenzae type b*
HIV	human immunodeficiency virus
HoFH	homozygous familial hypercholesterolemia
HPV	human papillomavirus
Hr	hour
HR	heart rate in beats per minute
HRT	hormone replacement therapy
HS	hour of sleep, bedtime
HSV	herpes simplex virus
HTN	hypertension
Hx	history
HZO	herpes zoster ophthalmicus
IBS-C	irritable bowel syndrome with constipation

IBS-D	irritable bowel syndrome with diarrhea
ID	intradermal
ILD	interstitial lung disease
IM	intramuscular
immed-rel	immediate-release
inhal	inhalation
inj	injection
INR	international normalized ratio
IOP	intraocular pressure
IU	international unit
IUD	intrauterine device
IV	intravenous
JIA	juvenile idiopathic arthritis
JRA	juvenile rheumatoid arthritis
K^+	potassium
kg	kilogram
L	liter (1000 ml)
LAA	long-acting anticholinergic
LABA	long-acting beta agonist
LAR	long-acting release
lb	pound
LDL, LDL-C	low density lipoprotein cholesterol
LFT	liver function test
Liq	liquid
lotn	lotion
LR	lactated ringers IV solution
LVD	left ventricular dysfunction
LVF	left ventricular failure
MAOI	monoamine oxidase inhibitor
max	maximum

mcg	microgram
mCNY	myopic choroidal neovascularization
MDD	major depressive disorder
MDI	metered dose inhaler
MDR-TB	multi-drug resistant tuberculosis
mfr pkg insert	manufacturer package insert
mg	milligram
mg/dL	milligrams per deciliter
mg/kg/day	milligrams per kilogram per day
min	minute
ml, mL	milliliter
MMF	*mycophenolate mofetil*
M-M-R	mumps-measles-rubella
MRSA	methicillin-resistant *Staphylococcus aureus*
MS	multiple sclerosis
MTX	methotrexate
Na^+	Sodium
NaCl	sodium chloride
$NaHCO_3$	sodium bicarbonate
NAMS	North American Menopause Society
NAT	nucleic acid testing
ng	nanogram
ng/dL	nanogram per deciliter
NGU	non-gonococcal urethritis
NMDA	n-methyl-d-aspartate receptor antagonist
NMS	neuroleptic malignant syndrome
NNRTI	nonnucleoside reverse transcriptase inhibitor
NOH	neurogenic orthostatic hypotension
non-HDL-C	non-high density lipoprotein cholesterol
norgest	norgestimate

NOWS	neonatal opioid withdrawal syndrome
nPEP	non-occupational post-exposure prophylaxis
NRTI	nucleoside reverse transcriptase inhibitor
NS	nasal spray; normal saline
NSAID	nonsteroidal anti-inflammatory drug
NTG	nitroglycerine; normal tension glaucoma
N/V	nausea/vomiting
N/V/D	nausea/vomiting/diarrhea
OA	Osteoarthritis
OCD	obsessive compulsive disorder
OCP	oral contraceptive pill
ODT	orally-disintegrating tablet
Oint	ointment
OIT	oral immunotherapy
ophth	ophthalmic, pertaining to the eye
orally-disint	orally-disintegrating
OSAHS	obstructive sleep apnea hypopnea syndrome
OTC	over-the-counter
Otic	pertaining to the ear
OTRP	organ transplant rejection prophylaxis
oz	ounce, 30 ml
PAH	pulmonary arterial hypertension
PBA	pseudobulbar affect
PBC	primary biliary atresia
pc	after meals
PCOS	polycystic ovarian syndrome; Stein-Leventhal disease
PD	Parkinson's disease
PDE5	phosphodiesterase type 5 inhibitor
PE	pulmonary embolus/embolism
PEG	polyethylene glycol

PEP	post-exposure prophylaxis
PID	pelvic inflammatory disease
PIM	potentially inappropriate medication
PJIA	polyarticular juvenile idiopathic arthritis
PLLR	FDA pregnancy and lactation labeling final rule
PLT	platelet
PM	post-meridiem, evening
PMDD	premenstrual Dysphoric Disorder
PMHx	past medical history
PO	per os, per oral, by mouth
$PO4^{3-}$	phosphate
POC	point of care
Post-op	post-operative
PPI	proton pump inhibitor
PR	per rectum
PrEP	pre-exposure prophylaxis
PRN	*pro re nata*, as needed, as required
PSA	prostate-specific antigen
PT	prothrombin time
PTSD	post-traumatic stress disorder
PTT	partial thromboplastin time
PUD	peptic ulcer disease
PVC	premature ventricular contraction
PVD	peripheral vascular disease
PVOD	pulmonary veno-occlusive disease
pwdr	powder
pwdr w. diluent	powder with diluent
q	per, every
qd	once daily
qHS	at hour of sleep, at bedtime

qid	*quater in die*, four times-a-day
RA	rheumatoid arthritis
RAI	reversible anticholinesterase inhibitor
RBC	red blood cell
RDA	recommended daily allowance
RSV	respiratory syncytial virus
RVO	retinal vein occlusion
SC	Subcutaneous
SCII	subcutaneous insulin infusion
sgc	soft-gel capsule
SGOT	serum glutamic-oxaloacetic transaminase
SGPT	serum glutamic-pyruvic transaminase
SL	sublingual, under the tongue
SLE	systemic lupus erythematosis
SMA	spinal muscular atrophy
SNRI	selective serotonin and norepinephrine reuptake inhibitor
soln	solution
SR	sustained-release
SSRI	selective serotonin reuptake inhibitor
STD/STI	sexually transmitted disease/infection
sUA	serum uric acid
supp	suppository
susp	suspension
sust-rel	sustained release
SWSD	shift work sleep disorder
syr	syrup
T1DM	type 1 diabetes mellitus
T2DM	type 2 diabetes mellitus
T3	triiodothyronine
T4	thyroxin, tetraiodothyronine

tab	tablet
tbsp	tablespoon
TCA	tricyclic antidepressant
TG, TRG	triglyceride
TIA	transient ischemic attack
tid	*ter in die*, three times-a-day
TMP/SMX	trimethoprim-sulfamethoxazole
TNF	tumor necrosis factor
trans-sys	transdermal system
TRD	treatment-resistant depression
TSH	thyroid-stimulating hormone
tsp	teaspoon, 4-5 ml
TSSRI	thienobenzodiazepine-selective serotonin reuptake inhibitor
UDT	urine drug test/screen
ULN	upper limit of normal
URI	upper respiratory infection
USPSTF	U.S. Preventive Services Task Force
UTI	urinary tract infection
VLDL	very-low-density-lipoprotein
VMAT2	vesicular monoamine transporter-2
VREF	vancomycin-resistant Enterococcus faecium
VRSA	vancomycin-resistant Staphylococcal aureus
VVC	vulvovaginal candidiasis
w.	with
WBC	white blood cell (leukocyte)
WHO	World Health Organization
XL	extra-long-acting
XOI	xanthine oxidase inhibitor
XR	ext-rel, extended-release

The APRN's Complete Guide to Prescribing Drug Therapy 2018 is a prescribing reference intended for use by health care providers in all clinical practice settings who are involved in the primary care management of patients with acute, episodic, and chronic health problems. It is organized in a concise and easy-to-read format. Comments are interspersed throughout, including such clinically useful information as laboratory values to be monitored, patient teaching points, and safety information.

This reference is divided into two major sections that are organized in a concise and easy-to-read format. **Section I** presents drug treatment regimens for over 500 clinical diagnoses. Each drug is listed alphabetically by generic name, whether the drug is available over the counter (OTC), DEA schedule (I, II, III, IV, V), generic availability (G), adult and pediatric dosing regimens, available dose forms, whether tablets, caplets, or chew tabs are scored (*), cross-scored (**), or tri-scored (***), flavors of chewable, sublingual, buccal, and liquid forms, and information regarding additives (e.g., dye-free, sugar-free, preservative-free or preservative type, and alcohol-free or alcohol content). For drugs initially FDA-approved *prior to June 30, 2015*, the former traditional FDA pregnancy categories still apply (A, B, C, D, or X). Non-pharmaceutical products, and drugs that received *initial FDA-approval on or after June 30, 2015* do not have an FDA pregnancy designation. For information regarding special populations, including pregnant and breastfeeding females, refer to the manufacturer's package insert or visit https://www.accessdata.fda.gov/scripts/cder/daf/ to view the product label online. Visit https://www.drugs.com/pregnancy-categories.html to view the **FDA Pregnancy and Lactation Labeling Final Rule (PLLR)** and new label format.

Section II presents clinically useful information in convenient table format, including: the JNC-8 recommendations for hypertension management, the U.S. schedule of controlled substances and the FDA pregnancy categories, measurement conversions, childhood and adult immunization recommendations, brand-name drugs (with contents) for the management of common respiratory symptoms, anti-infectives by classification, pediatric dosing by weight for liquid forms, glucocorticosteroids by potency and route of administration, and contraceptives by route of administration and estrogen and/or progesterone content. An alphabetical index of drugs by generic and brand name, with FDA pregnancy category and controlled drug schedule, facilitates quick identification of drugs by alternate names, relative safety during pregnancy, and DEA schedule.

Selected diagnoses (e.g., angina, ADHD, growth failure, glaucoma, Parkinson's disease, CMV retinitis, multiple sclerosis, cystic fibrosis) and selected drugs (e.g., anti-neoplastics, antipsychotics, anti-arrhythmics, anti-HIV drugs, and anticoagulants) are included as patients are often referred by surgeons and emergency and urgent care providers to the primary care provider for follow-up monitoring and management.

Safe, efficacious, prescribing and monitoring of drug therapy regimens require adequate knowledge about (a) the pharmacodynamics and pharmacokinetics of drugs, (b) concomitant therapies, and (c) individual characteristics of the patient (e.g., current and past medical history, physical examination findings, hepatic and renal function, and co-morbidities). Users of this clinical guide are encouraged to utilize the manufacturer's package insert, recommendations and guidance of specialists, standard of practice protocols, and the current research literature for more comprehensive information about specific drugs (e.g., special precautions, drug-drug and drug-food interactions, risk versus benefit, age-related considerations, adverse reactions) and appropriate use with individual patients.

ACKNOWLEDGMENTS

This publication, which we consider to be a "must have" for students, academicians, and practicing clinicians with prescriptive authority, represents the culmination of Springer Publishing Company's collaborative team effort. Margaret Zuccarini, Publisher, Nursing, and the Editorial Committee, shared my vision for a handy pocket prescribing reference for new and experienced prescribers in primary care. Joanne Jay, Vice President, Production and Manufacturing, designed the contents for ease and efficiency of user navigation. The production team at Exeter Premedia Services, on behalf of Springer Publishing Company, understood the critical nature of exactness in this prescribing resource, and faithfully managed the complex files as content was updated and cross-paginated for the final product. The work of the reviewers from academia and clinical practice was essential to the process and their contributions are greatly appreciated. I am proud of my association with these dedicated professionals and I thank them on behalf of the medical and advanced practice nursing community worldwide, for supporting the end goal of quality health care for all.

ACE-Is and **ARBs** are contraindicated in the 2nd and 3rd trimesters of pregnancy. Addition of a daily ACE-I or ARB is strongly recommended for renal protection in patients with hypertension and/or diabetes. The "ACE inhibitor cough," a dry cough, is an adverse side effect produced by an accumulation of bradykinins that occurs in 5-10% of the population and resolves within days of discontinuing the drug.

Alcohol is contraindicated with concomitant **narcotic analgesics, benzodiazepines, SSRIs, antihistamines, TCAs,** and other sedating agents due to risk of over-sedation.

Alpha-1 blockers have a potential adverse side effect of sudden hypotension, especially with first dose. Alert the patient regarding this "first-dose effect" and recommend the patient sit or lie down to take the first dose. Usually start at lowest dose and titrate upward.

Antidepressant monotherapy should be avoided until any presence of (hypo) mania or positive family history for bipolar spectrum disorder has been ruled out as antidepressant monotherapy can induce mania in the bipolar patient.

For patients 65 years-of-age and older, consult the **May 2017 Beers Criteria** for Potentially Inappropriate Medication (PIM) Use in Older Adults, to help improve the safety of prescribing medications for older adults, presented in table format at: https://www.priorityhealth.com/provider/clinical-resources/medication-resources/~/media/documents/pharmacy/cms-high-risk-medications.pdf

Aspirin is contraindicated in children and adolescents with *Varicella* or other viral illness, and 3rd trimester of pregnancy.

Beta-blockers, by all routes of administration, are generally contraindicated in severe COPD, history of or current bronchial asthma, sinus bradycardia, and 2nd or 3rd degree AV block. Use a cardio-specific beta blocker where appropriate in these cases.

Biosimilar means the biological product is FDA-approved based on data demonstrating that it is highly similar to an FDA-approved biological product, known as a reference product, and that there are no clinically meaningful differences between the biosimilar product and the reference product (e.g., **Cyltezo** (*adalimumab-adbm*) is biosimilar to **Humira** (*ada-limumab*).

Calcium channel blockers may cause the adverse side effect of pedal edema (feet, ankles, lower legs) that resolves with discontinuation of the drug.

Codeine is known to be excreted in breast milk. <12 years: not recommended; 12-<18: use extreme caution; not recommended for children and adolescents with asthma or other chronic breathing problem. The FDA and the European Medicines Agency (EMA)

are investigating the safety of using **codeine**-containing medications to treat pain, cough, and colds in children 12-<18 years because of the potential for serious side effects, including slowed or difficult breathing.

Corticosteroids increases blood sugar in patients with diabetes and decreases immunity; therefore, consider risk *vs* benefit in susceptible patients, use lowest effective dose, and taper gradually to discontinue.

Check **drug interactions** at https://www.drugs.com/drug_interactions.php

Erythromycin may increase INR with concomitant warfarin, as well as increase serum level of digoxin, benzodiazepines, and statins.

Contraceptives that are estrogen-progesterone combinations and **progesterone-only** are contraindicated in pregnancy (pregnancy category X)

Finasteride, a 5-alpha reductase inhibitor, is associated with low but increased risk of high-grade prostate cancer. Pregnant females should not touch broken tablets.

Fluoroquinolones and **quinolones** are contraindicated <18 years-of-age, pregnancy, and breastfeeding. *Exception:* in the case of anthrax, *ciprofloxacin* is indicated for patients <18 years-of-age and dosed based on mg/kg body weight. Risk of tendonitis or tendon rupture (ex: *ciprofloxacin*, *gemifloxacin*, *levofloxacin*, *moxifloxacin*, *norfloxacin*, *ofloxacin*).

The U.S. Preventive Services Task Force (USPSTF) recommends against using **hormone replacement therapy** (HRT) for primary prevention of chronic conditions among postmenopausal women. The harms associated with combined use of estrogen and a progestin, such as increased risks of invasive breast cancer, venous thromboembolism, and coronary heart disease, far outweigh the benefits.

Ibuprofen is contraindicated in children <6 months of age and in the 3rd trimester of pregnancy.

Live vaccines are contraindicated in patients who are immunosuppressed or receiving immunosuppressive therapy, including immunosuppressive levels of corticosteroid therapy.

Metronidazole and **tinidazole** are contraindicated in the 1st trimester of pregnancy. Alcohol is contraindicated during treatment with oral forms and for 72 hours after therapy due to a possible *disulfiram*-like reaction (nausea, vomiting, flushing, headache).

When prescribing **opioid analgesics**, presumptive urine **drug testing** (UDT) should be performed when opioid therapy for chronic pain is initiated, along with subsequent use as adherence monitoring, using in-office point of service testing, to identify patients who are non-compliant or abusing prescription drugs or illicit drugs. American Society of Interventional Pain Physicians (ASIPP)

Oral **PDE5 inhibitors** are contraindicated in patients taking nitrates due to risk of hypotension or syncope (ex: ***avanafil, sildenafil, tadalafil, vardenafil***).

Proton pump inhibitors (PPIs) should be discontinued, and should not be initiated, in patients with acute kidney injury (AKI) and chronic kidney disease (CKD).

Statins are strongly recommended as adjunctive therapy for patients with diabetes, with **or** without abnormal lipids.

Sulfonamides are not recommended in pregnancy or lactation. CrCl 15-30 mL/min: reduce dose by 1/2; CrCl <15 mL/min: not recommended (ex: ***sulfamethoxazole, trimethoprim***). Contraindicated with G6PD deficiency. A high fluid intake is indicated during sulfonamide therapy to avoid crystallization in the kidneys.

Tetracyclines are contraindicated in children <8 years-of-age, pregnancy, and breastfeeding (discolors developing tooth enamel). A side effect may be photo-sensitivity (photophobia). Do not take with antacids, calcium supplements, milk or other dairy, or 2 hours of taking another drug (ex: ***doxycycline, minocycline, tetracycline***).

Tramadol is known to be excreted in breast milk. The FDA and the European Medicines Agency (EMA) are investigating the safety of using ***tramadol***-containing medications to treat pain in children 12-18 years because of the potential for serious side effects, including slowed or difficult breathing.

The **Transmucosal Immediate Release Fentanyl (TIRF) Risk Evaluation and Mitigation Strategy (REMS)** program is an FDA-required program designed to ensure informed risk-benefit decisions before initiating treatment, and while patients are treated to ensure appropriate use of TIRF medicines. The purpose of the TIRF REMS Access program is to mitigate the risk of misuse, abuse, addiction, overdose, and serious complications due to medication errors with the use of TIRF medicines. You must enroll in the TIRF REMS Access program to prescribe, dispense, **or** distribute TIRF medicines. To register, call the TIRF REMS Access program at 1-866-822-1483 **or** register online at https://www.tirfremsaccess.com/TirfUI/rems/home.action

The APRN's Complete Guide to Prescribing Drug Therapy

2019

SECTION I

DRUG THERAPY BY CLINICAL DIAGNOSIS

ACETAMINOPHEN OVERDOSE

ANTIDOTE/CHELATING AGENT

▶ *acetylcysteine* (B)(G) *Loading Dose:* 150 mg/kg administered over 15 minutes; *Maintenance:* 50 mg/kg administered over 4 hours; then 100 mg/kg administered over 16 hours
Pediatric: same as adult

Acetadote *Vial: soln for IV infusion after dilution:* 200 mg/ml (30 ml; dilute in D5W (preservative-free)

Comment: *acetaminophen* overdose is a medical emergency due to the risk of irreversible hepatic injury. An IV infusion of *acetylcysteine* should be started as soon as possible and within 24 hours if the exact time of ingestion is unknown. Use a serum *acetaminophen* nomogram to determine need for treatment. Extreme caution is needed if used with concomitant hepatotoxic drugs.

ACNE ROSACEA

Comment: All acne rosacea products should be applied sparingly to clean, dry skin as directed. Avoid use of topical corticosteroids.

▶ *ivermectin* (C) apply bid
Soolantra *Crm:* 1% (30 gm)

Comment: **Soolantra** is a macrocyclic lactone. Exactly how it works to treat rosacea is unknown.

TOPICAL ALPHA-1A ADRENOCEPTOR AGONIST

▶ *oxymetazoline hcl* (B) <18 years: not recommended; ≥18 years: apply a pea-sized amount once daily in a thin layer covering the entire face (forehead, nose, cheeks, and chin) avoiding the eyes and lips; wash hands immediately
Rhofade *Crm* 1% (30 gm tube)

Comment: **Rhofade** acts as a vasoconstrictor. Use with caution in patients with cerebral or coronary insufficiency, Raynaud's phenomenon, thromboangiitis obliterans, scleroderma, or Sjögren's syndrome. **Rhofade** may increase the risk of angle closure glaucoma in patients with narrow-angle glaucoma. Advise patients to seek immediate medical care if signs and symptoms of potentiation of vascular insufficiency or acute angle closure glaucoma develop.

TOPICAL ALPHA-2 AGONIST

▶ *brimonidine* (B) apply to affected area once daily
Pediatric: <18 years: not recommended; >18 years: same as adult
Mirvaso
Gel: 0.33% (30, 45 gm tube; 30 gm pump)

Comment: **Mirvaso** is indicated for persistent erythema; *brimonidine* constricts dilated facial blood vessels to reduce redness.

TOPICAL ANTIMICROBIALS

▶ *azelaic acid* (B) apply to affected area bid
Azelex *Crm:* 20% (30, 50 gm)
Finacea *Gel:* 15% (30 gm); *Foam:* 15% (50 gm)
▶ *metronidazole* (B) apply to clean dry skin
MetroCream apply bid
Emol crm: 0.75% (45 gm)
MetroGel apply once daily
Gel: 1% (60 gm tube; 55 gm pump)

MetroLotion apply bid
Lotn: 0.75% (2 oz)
▷ *sodium sulfacetamide* (C)(G) apply 1-3 x daily
Klaron *Lotn:* 10% (2 oz)
▷ *sodium sulfacetamide+sulfur* (C)
Clenia Emollient Cream apply 1-3 x daily
Wash: sod sulfa 10%+sulfur 5% (10 oz)
Clenia Foaming Wash wash affected area once <u>or</u> twice daily
Wash: sod sulfa 10%+sulfur 5% (6, 12 oz)
Rosula Gel apply 1-3 x daily
Gel: sod sulfa 10%+sulfur 5% (45 ml)
Rosula Lotion apply tid
Lotn: sod sulfa 10%+sulfur 5% (45 ml) (alcohol-free)
Rosula Wash wash bid
Clnsr: sod sulfa 10%+sulfur 5% (335 ml)

ORAL ANTIMICROBIALS

▷ *doxycycline* (D)(G) 40-100 mg bid
Pediatric: <8 years: not recommended; ≥8 years, <100 lb: 2 mg/lb on first day in 2
divided doses, followed by 1 mg/lb/day in 1-2 divided doses; ≥8 years, ≥100 lb: same
as adult; *see page 633 for dose by weight*
Acticlate *Tab:* 75, 150**mg
Adoxa *Tab:* 50, 75, 100, 150 mg ent-coat
Doryx *Tab:* 50, 75, 100, 150, 200 mg del-rel
Doxteric *Tab:* 50 mg del-rel
Monodox *Cap:* 50, 75, 100 mg
Oracea *Cap:* 40 mg del-rel
Vibramycin *Tab:* 100 mg; *Cap:* 50, 100 mg; *Syr:* 50 mg/5 ml (raspberry-apple)
(sulfites); *Oral susp:* 25 mg/5 ml (raspberry)
Vibra-Tab *Tab:* 100 mg film-coat
▷ *minocycline* (D)(G) 200 mg on first day; then 100 mg q 12 hours x 9 more days
Pediatric: <8 years: not recommended; ≥8 years, <100 lb: 2 mg/lb on first day in 2
divided doses, followed by 1 mg/lb q 12 hours x 9 more days; ≥8 years, ≥100 lb: same
as adult
Dynacin *Cap:* 50, 100 mg
Minocin *Cap:* 50, 75, 100 mg; *Oral susp:* 50 mg/5 ml (60 ml) (custard) (sulfites,
alcohol 5%)

 ACNE VULGARIS

ORAL CONTRACEPTIVES

see Combined Oral Contraceptives *page 539*
see Progesterone-only Contraceptives (Mini-Pill) *page 550*

Comment: In their 2016 published report, researchers concluded different hormonal
contraceptives have significantly varied effects on acne. Women (n=2,147) who were
using a hormonal contraceptive at the time of their first consultation for acne comprised
the study sample. Participants completed an assessment at baseline to report how the
contraceptive affected their acne. Then the researchers used the Kruskal-Wallis test and
logistic regression analysis to compare the outcomes by contraceptive type. On average,
the vaginal ring and combined oral contraceptives (COCs) improved acne, whereas
depot injections, subdermal implants, and hormonal intrauterine devices worsened

acne. In the COC categories, **drospirenone** was the most helpful in improving acne, followed by **norgestimate** and **desogestrel**, and then **levonorgestrel** and **norethindrone**. Although triphasic progestin dosage had a positive effect on acne, estrogen dosage did not.

REFERENCES

Hui, D., Frisbee-Hume, S., Wilson, A., Dibaj, S. S., Nguyen, T., De La Cruz, M., … Bruera, E. (2017). Effect of Lorazepam With Haloperidol vs Haloperidol Alone on Agitated Delirium in Patients With Advanced Cancer Receiving Palliative Care. *JAMA, 318*(11), 1047. doi:10.1001/jama.2017.11468

Lortscher, D., Admani, S., Satur, N., & Eichenfield, L. F. (2016). Hormonal contraceptives and acne: a retrospective analysis of 2147 patients. *Journal of Drugs in Dermatology, 15*(6), 670–674. http://jddonline.com/articles/dermatology/S1545961616P0670X

TOPICAL ANTIMICROBIALS

Comment: All topical antimicrobials should be applied sparingly to clean, dry skin.
▷ *azelaic acid* (B) apply to affected area bid
    Azelex *Crm:* 20% (30, 50 gm)
    Finacea *Gel:* 15% (30 gm); *Foam:* 15% (50 gm)
▷ *benzoyl peroxide* (C)(G)
  Comment: *benzoyl peroxide* may discolor clothing and linens.
    Benzac-W initially apply to affected area once daily; increase to bid-tid as tolerated
      Gel: 2.5, 5, 10% (60 gm)
    Benzac-W Wash wash affected area bid
      Wash: 5% (4, 8 oz); 10% (8 oz)
    Benzagel apply to affected area one <u>or</u> more x/day
      Gel: 5, 10% (1.5, 3 oz) (alcohol 14%)
    Benzagel Wash wash affected area bid
      Gel: 10% (6 oz)
    Desquam X⁵ wash affected area bid
      Wash: 5% (5 oz)
    Desquam X¹⁰ wash affected area bid
      Wash: 10% (5 oz)
    Triaz apply to affected area daily bid
      Lotn: 3, 6, 9% (bottle), 3% (tube); *Pads:* 3, 6, 9% (jar)
    ZoDerm apply once <u>or</u> twice daily
      Gel: 4.5, 6.5, 8.5% (125 ml); *Crm:* 4.5, 6.5, 8.5% (125 ml); *Clnsr:* 4.5, 6.5, 8.5% (400 ml)
▷ *clindamycin* topical (B) apply to affected area bid
  Pediatric: <12 years: not recommended; ≥12 years: same as adult
    Cleocin T *Pad:* 1% (60/pck; alcohol 50%); *Lotn:* 1% (60 ml); *Gel:* 1% (30, 60 gm);
    Soln w. applicator: 1% (30, 60 ml) (alcohol 50%)
    Clindagel *Gel:* 1% (42, 77 gm)
    Evoclin Foam: 1% (50, 100 gm) (alcohol)
▷ *clindamycin+benzoyl peroxide* topical (C) apply to affected area once daily
  Pediatric: <12 years: not recommended; ≥12 years: same as adult
    Acanya (G) apply to affected area once daily-bid
      Gel: clin 1.2%+benz 2.5% (50 gm)
    BenzaClin (G) apply to affected area bid
      Gel: clin 1%+benz 5% (25, 50 gm)
    Duac apply daily in the evening
      Gel: clin 1%+benz 5% (45 gm)
    Onexton Gel apply to affected area once daily
      Gel: clin 1.2%+benz 3.75% (50 gm pump) (alcohol-free) (preservative-free)

▷ *dapsone* topical **(C)(G)** apply to affected area bid
  Pediatric: <12 years: not recommended; ≥12 years: same as adult
      Aczone *Gel:* 5, 7.5% (30, 60, 90 gm pump)
▷ *erythromycin+benzoyl peroxide* **(C)** initially apply to affected area once daily; increase to
  bid as tolerated
      Benzamycin Topical Gel *Gel:* eryth 3%+benz 5% (46.6 gm/jar)
▷ *sodium sulfacetamide* **(C)(G)** apply tid
      Klaron *Lotn:* 10% (2 oz)

ORAL ANTIMICROBIALS

▷ *doxycycline* **(D)(G)** 100 mg bid
  Pediatric: <8 years: not recommended; ≥8 years, <100 lb: 2 mg/lb on first day in 2
  divided doses, followed by 1 mg/lb/day in 1-2 divided doses; ≥8 years, ≥100 lb: same
  as adult; *see page 633 for dose by weight*
      Acticlate *Tab:* 75, 150**mg
      Adoxa *Tab:* 50, 75, 100, 150 mg ent-coat
      Doryx *Tab:* 50, 75, 100, 150, 200 mg del-rel
      Doxteric *Tab:* 50 mg del-rel
      Monodox *Cap:* 50, 75, 100 mg
      Oracea *Cap:* 40 mg del-rel
      Vibramycin *Tab:* 100 mg; *Cap:* 50, 100 mg; *Syr:* 50 mg/5 ml (raspberry-apple)
      (sulfites); *Oral susp:* 25 mg/5 ml (raspberry)
      Vibra-Tab *Tab:* 100 mg film coat
▷ *erythromycin base* **(B)(G)** 250 mg qid, 333 mg tid or 500 mg bid x 7-10 days; then
  taper to lowest effective dose
  Pediatric: <45 kg: 30-50 mg in 2-4 divided doses x 7-10 days; ≥45 kg: same as adult
      Ery-Tab *Tab:* 250, 333, 500 mg ent-coat
      PCE *Tab:* 333, 500 mg
Comment: *erythromycin* may increase INR with concomitant *warfarin*, as well as
increase serum level of *digoxin, benzodiazepines*, and *statins*.
▷ *erythromycin ethylsuccinate* **(B)(G)** 400 mg qid x 7-10 days
  Pediatric: 30-50 mg/kg/day in 4 divided doses x 7-10 days; may double dose with
  severe infection; max 100 mg/kg/day; *see page 635 for dose by weight*
      EryPed *Oral susp:* 200 mg/5 ml (100, 200 ml) (fruit); 400 mg/5 ml (60, 100,
      200 ml) (banana); *Oral drops:* 200, 400 mg/5 ml (50 ml) (fruit); *Chew tab:* 200 mg
      wafer (fruit)
      E.E.S. *Oral susp:* 200, 400 mg/5 ml (100 ml) (fruit)
      E.E.S. Granules *Oral susp:* 200 mg/5 ml (100, 200 ml) (cherry)
      E.E.S. 400 Tablets *Tab:* 400 mg
Comment: *erythromycin* may increase INR with concomitant *warfarin*, as well as
increase serum level of *digoxin, benzodiazepines*, and *statins*.
▷ *minocycline* **(D)(G)** initially 50-200 mg/day in 2 divided doses; reduce dose to once
  daily after improvement
  Pediatric: <8 years: not recommended; ≥8 years: same as adult
      Dynacin *Cap:* 50, 100 mg
      Minocin *Cap:* 50, 75, 100 mg; *Oral susp:* 50 mg/5 ml (60 ml) (custard) (sulfites,
      alcohol 5%)
      Minolira *Tab:* 105, 135 mg ext-rel
      Solodyn *Tab:* 55, 65, 80, 105, 115 mg ext-rel
Comment: Once-daily dosing of **Minolira** or **Solodyn**, extended-release *minocyclines*,
is approved for inflammatory lesions of non-nodular moderate-to-severe acne
vulgaris for patients ≥12 years-of-age. The recommended dose of **Solodyn** is 1 mg/kg
once daily x 12 weeks.

▷ *tetracycline* (D)(G) initially 1 gm/day in 2-4 divided doses; after improvement, 125-500 mg daily

Pediatric: <8 years: not recommended; ≥8 years, <100 lb: 25-50 mg/kg/day in 2-4 divided doses; ≥8 years, ≥100 lb: same as adult; *see page 646 for dose by weight*

Achromycin V *Cap:* 250, 500 mg

Sumycin *Tab:* 250, 500 mg; *Cap:* 250, 500 mg; *Oral susp:* 125 mg/5 ml (100, 200 ml) (fruit) (sulfites)

Comment: *tetracycline* is contraindicated <8 years-of-age, in pregnancy, and lactation (discolors developing tooth enamel). A side effect may be photo-sensitivity (photophobia). Do not give with antacids, calcium supplements, milk or other dairy, or within two hours of taking another drug.

TOPICAL RETINOIDS

Comment: Wash affected area with a soap-free cleanser; pat dry and wait 20 to 30 minutes; then apply sparingly to affected area; use only once daily in the evening. Avoid applying to eyes, ears, nostrils, and mouth.

▷ *adapalene* (C) apply once daily at HS

Pediatric: <12 years: not recommended; ≥12 years: same as adult

Differin *Crm:* 0.1% (45 gm); *Gel:* 0.1, 0.3% (45 gm) (alcohol-free); *Pad:* 0.1% (30/pck) (alcohol 30%); *Lotn:* 0.1% (2, 4 oz)

▷ *tazarotene* (X)(G) apply to affected area once daily at HS

Pediatric: <12 years: not recommended; ≥12 years: same as adult

Avage Cream *Crm:* 0.1% (30 gm)

Tazorac Cream *Crm:* 0.05, 0.1% (15, 30, 60 gm)

Tazorac Gel *Gel:* 0.05, 0.1% (30, 100 gm)

▷ *tretinoin* (C)(G) apply to affected area once daily at HS

Pediatric: <12 years: not recommended; ≥12 years: same as adult

Atralin Gel *Gel:* 0.05% (45 gm)

Avita *Crm:* 0.025% (20, 45 gm); *Gel:* 0.025% (20, 45 gm)

Retin-A Cream *Crm:* 0.025, 0.05, 0.1% (20, 45 gm)

Retin-A Gel *Gel:* 0.01, 0.025% (15, 45 gm) (alcohol 90%)

Retin-A Liquid *Soln:* 0.05% (alcohol 55%)

Retin-A Micro Gel *Gel:* 0.04, 0.08, 0.1% (20, 45 gm)

Tretin-X Cream *Crm:* 0.075% (35 gm) (parabens-free, alcohol-free, propylene glycol-free)

TOPICAL RETINOID+ANTIMICROBIAL COMBINATIONS

Comment: Wash affected area with a soap-free cleanser; pat dry and wait 20-30 minutes; then apply sparingly to affected area; use only once daily in the evening. Avoid eyes, ears, nostrils, and mouth.

▷ *adapalene+benzoyl peroxide* (C)(G) apply a thin film once daily

Pediatric: <18 years: not recommended

Epiduo Gel *Gel:* adap 0.1%+benz 2.5% (45 gm)

Epiduo Forte Gel *Pump gel:* adap 0.3%+benz 2.5% (15, 30, 45, 60 gm)

▷ *tretinoin+clindamycin* (C)(G) apply a thin film once daily

Pediatric: <18 years: not recommended

Ziana *Gel:* tret 0.025%+*clin* 1.2% (30, 60 gm)

ORAL RETINOID

Comment: Oral retinoids are indicated only for severe recalcitrant nodular acne unresponsive to conventional therapy including systemic antibiotics.

▷ *isotretinoin* (X) initially 0.5-1 mg/kg/day in 2 divided doses; maintenance 0.5-2 mg/kg/day in 2 divided doses x 4-5 months; repeat only if necessary 2 months following cessation of first treatment course
Pediatric: <12 years: not recommended; ≥12 years: same as adult
    Accutane *Cap:* 10, 20, 40 mg (parabens)
    Amnesteem *Cap:* 10, 20, 40 mg (soy)

Comment: *isotretinoin* is highly teratogenic and, therefore, female patients should be counseled prior to initiation of treatment as follows: Two negative pregnancy tests are required prior to initiation of treatment and monthly thereafter. <u>Not</u> for use in females who are <u>or</u> who may become pregnant <u>or</u> who are breastfeeding. Two effective methods of contraception should be used for 1 month prior to, during, and continuing for 1 month following completion of treatment. Low-dose *progestin* (mini-pill) may be an *inadequate* form of contraception. No refills; a new prescription is required every 30 days and prescriptions must be filled within 7 days. Serum lipids should be monitored until response is established (usually initially and again after 4 weeks). Bone growth, serum glucose, ESR, RBCs, WBCs, and liver enzymes should be monitored. Blood should <u>not</u> be donated during, <u>or</u> for 1 month after, completion of treatment. Avoid the sun and artificial UV light. *isotretinoin* should be discontinued if any of the following occurs: visual disturbances, tinnitus, hearing impairment, rectal bleeding, pancreatitis, hepatitis, significant decrease in CBC, hyperlipidemia (particularly hypertriglyceridemia).

 ACROMEGALY

GROWTH HORMONE RECEPTOR ANTAGONIST

▷ *pegvisomant* (B) *Loading dose:* 40 mg SC; *Maintenance:* 10 mg SC daily; titrate by 5 mg (increments <u>or</u> decrements, based on IGF-1 levels) every 4 to 6 weeks; max 30 mg/day
Pediatric: <12 years: not recommended; ≥12 years: same as adult
    Somavert *Inj:* 10, 15, 20 mg

Comment: Prior to initiation of *pegvisomant*, patients should have baseline fasting serum glucose, HgbA1c, serum K^+ and Mg^{++}, liver function tests (LFTs), EKG, and gall bladder ultrasound.

Cyclohexapeptide Somatostatin

▷ *pasireotide* (C) administer SC in the thigh <u>or</u> abdomen; initial dose is 0.6 mg <u>or</u> 0.9 mg bid. Titrate dose based on response and tolerability; for patients with moderate hepatic impairment (Child-Pugh Class B), the recommended initial dosage is 0.3 mg twice daily and max dose 0.6 mg twice daily; avoid use in patients with severe hepatic impairment (Child-Pugh Class C)
Pediatric: <12 years: not recommended; ≥12 years: same as adult
    Signifor LAR *Amp:* 0.3, 0.6, 0.9 mg/ml, single-dose, long-act rel (LAR) susp for inj

 ACTINIC KERATOSIS

Comment: *pasireotide* is also indicated for destroying superficial basal cell carcinoma (sBCC) lesions.
▷ *diclofenac sodium 3%* (C; D ≥30 wks)(G) apply to lesions bid x 60-90 days
Pediatric: <12 years: not established; ≥12 years: same as adult
    Solaraze Gel *Gel:* 3% (50 gm) (benzyl alcohol)

Comment: *diclofenac* is contraindicated with **aspirin** allergy. As with other NSAIDs, **Solaraze Gel** should be avoided in late pregnancy (≥30 weeks) because it may cause premature closure of the ductus arteriosus; may cause premature closure of the ductus arteriosus.

> **Voltaren Gel** apply qid; avoid non-intact skin
> *Gel:* 1% (100 gm)

▶ *fluorouracil* **(X)(G)** apply to lesion(s) daily-bid until erosion occurs, usually 2-4 weeks
  Pediatric: <12 years: not recommended; ≥12 years: same as adult
> **Carac** *Crm:* 0.5% (30 gm)
> **Efudex (G)** *Crm:* 5% (25 gm); *Soln:* 2, 5% (10 ml w. dropper)
> **Fluoroplex** *Crm:* 1% (30 gm); *Soln:* 1% (30 ml w. dropper)

▶ *imiquimod* **(B)**
  Pediatric: <18 years: not recommended; ≥18 years: same as adult
> **Aldara (G)** rub into lesions before bedtime and remove with soap and water
> 8 hours later; treat 2 times per week; max 16 weeks
> *Crm:* 5% (single-use pkts/carton)
> **Zyclara** rub into lesions before bedtime and remove with soap and water 8 hours
> later; treat for 2-week cycles separated by a 2-week no-treatment cycle; max 2
> packs per application; max one treatment course per area
> *Crm:* 3.75% (single-use pkts; 28/carton) (parabens)

▶ *ingenol mebutate* **(C)** limit application to one contiguous skin area of about 25 cm^2 using one unit dose tube; allow treated area to dry for 15 minutes; wash hands immediately after application; may remove with soapy water after 6 hours; *Face and Scalp:* apply 0.015% gel to lesions daily x 3 days; *Trunk and Extremities:* apply 0.05% gel to lesions daily x 2 days
  Pediatric: <18 years: not recommended; ≥18 years: same as adult
> **Picato** *Gel:* 0.015% (3 single-use tubes), 0.05% (2 single-use tubes)

ALCOHOL DEPENDENCE, DETOXIFICATION/ALCOHOL WITHDRAWAL SYNDROME

Comment: Total length of time of a given detoxification regimen <u>and/or</u> length of time of treatment at any dose reduction level may be extended based on patient-specific factors, including potential <u>or</u> actual seizure, hallucinosis, increased sympathetic nervous system activity (severe anxiety, unwanted elevation in vital signs). If any of these symptoms are anticipated <u>or</u> occur, revert to an earlier step in the dosing regimen to stabilize the patient, extend the detoxification timeline and consider appropriate adjunctive drug treatments (e.g., anticonvulsants, antipsychotic agents, antihypertensive agents, sedative hypnotics agents).

▶ *clorazepate* **(D)(IV)(G)** in the following dosage schedule: *Day 1:* 30 mg initially, followed by 30-60 mg in divided doses; *Day 2:* 45-90 mg in divided doses; *Day 3:* 22.5-45 mg in divided doses; *Day 4:* 15-30 mg in divided doses; Thereafter, gradually reduce the daily dose to 7.5-15 mg; then discontinue when patient's condition is stable; max dose 90 mg/day
  Pediatric: <18 years: not recommended; ≥18 years: same as adult
> **Tranxene** *Tab:* 3.75, 7.5, 15 mg
> **Tranxene T-Tab** *Tab:* 3.75*, 7.5*, 15*mg

▶ *chlordiazepoxide* **(D)(IV)(G)**
  Pediatric: <18 years: not recommended; ≥18 years: same as adult
> **Librium** 50-100 mg q 6 hours x 24-72 hours; then q 8 hours x 24-72 hours; then q
> 12 hours x 24-72 hours; then daily x 24-72 hours
> *Cap:* 5, 10, 25 mg

Librium Injectable 50-100 mg IM <u>or</u> IV; then 25-50 mg IM tid-qid prn; max 300 mg/day
Inj: 100 mg

▷ *diazepam* (D)(IV)(G) 2-10 mg q 6 hours x 24-72 hours; then q 8 hours x 24-72 hours; then q 12 hours x 24-72 hours; then daily x 24-72 hours
Pediatric: <18 years: not recommended; ≥18 years: same as adult
Diastat *Rectal gel delivery system:* 2.5 mg
Diastat Acu Dial *Rectal gel delivery system:* 10, 20 mg
Valium *Tab:* 2*, 5*, 10*mg
Valium Injectable *Vial:* 5 mg/ml (10 ml); *Amp:* 5 mg/ml (2 ml); *Prefilled syringe:* 5 mg/ml (5 ml)
Valium Intensol Oral Solution *Conc oral soln:* 5 mg/ml (30 ml w. dropper) (alcohol 19%)
Valium Oral Solution *Oral soln:* 5 mg/5 ml (500 ml) (wintergreen-spice)

▷ *oxazepam* (C) 10-15 mg tid-qid x 24-72 hours; decrease dose <u>and/or</u> frequency every 24-72 hours; total length of therapy 5-14 days; max 120 mg/day
Pediatric: <18 years: not recommended; ≥18 years: same as adult
Cap: 10, 15, 30 mg

ABSTINENCE THERAPY
GABA Taurine Analog

▷ *acamprosate* (C)(G) 666 mg tid; begin therapy during abstinence; continue during relapse; *CrCl 30-50-mL/min:* max 333 mg tid; *CrCl <30 mL/min:* contraindicated
Pediatric: <18 years: not recommended; ≥18 years: same as adult
Campral *Tab:* 333 mg ext-rel

Comment: **Campral** does <u>not</u> eliminate <u>or</u> diminish alcohol withdrawal symptoms.

AVERSION THERAPY

▷ *disulfiram* (X)(G)
Pediatric: <18 years: not recommended; ≥18 years: same as adult
Antabuse 500 mg once daily x 1-2 weeks; then 250 mg once daily
Tab: 250, 500 mg; *Chew tab:* 200, 500 mg

Comment: *disulfiram* use requires informed consent. Contraindications: severe cardiac disease, psychosis, concomitant use of *isoniazid*, *phenytoin*, *paraldehyde*, and topical and systemic alcohol-containing products. Approximately 20% remains in the system for 1 week after discontinuation.

NUTRITIONAL SUPPORT

▷ *thiamine* (A)(G) injectable 50-100 mg IM/IV once daily (<u>or</u> tid if severely deficient)
Pediatric: <18 years: not recommended; ≥18 years: same as adult
Vial: 100 mg/1 ml (1 ml)

 ALLERGIC REACTION: GENERAL

Oral Second Generation Antihistamines *see* Drugs for the Management of Allergy, Cough, and Cold Symptoms page 591
Topical Corticosteroids *see page* 558
Parenteral Corticosteroids *see page* 563
Oral Corticosteroids *see page* 561

FIRST GENERATION PARENTERAL ANTIHISTAMINE

➤ *diphenhydramine* (C)(G) 25-50 mg IM immediately; then q 6 hours prn
Pediatric: <12 years: See mfr pkg insert: 1.25 mg/kg up to 25 mg IM x 1 dose; then q 6 hours prn
Benadryl Injectable *Vial:* 50 mg/ml (1 ml single-use); 50 mg/ml (10 ml multi-dose); *Amp:* 10 mg/ml (1 ml); *Prefilled syringe:* 50 mg/ml (1 ml)

FIRST GENERATION ORAL ANTIHISTAMINES

➤ *diphenhydramine* (B)(G) 25-50 mg q 6-8 hours; max 100 mg/day
Pediatric: <2 years: not recommended; *2-6 years:* 6.25 mg q 4-6 hours; max 37.5 mg/day; *>6-12 years:* 12.5-25 mg q 4-6 hours; max 150 mg/day; *>12 years:* same as adult
Benadryl (OTC) *Chew tab:* 12.5 mg (grape) (phenylalanine); *Liq:* 12.5 mg/5 ml (4, 8 oz); *Cap:* 25 mg; *Tab:* 25 mg; *Dye-free soft gel:* 25 mg; *Dye-free liq:* 12.5 mg/5 ml (4, 8 oz)

➤ *hydroxyzine* (C)(G) 50-100 mg qid; max 600 mg/day
Pediatric: <6 years: 50 mg/day divided qid; *≥6 years:* 50-100 mg/day divided qid
Atarax *Tab:* 10, 25, 50, 100 mg; *Syr:* 10 mg/5 ml (alcohol 0.5%)
Vistaril *Cap:* 25, 50, 100 mg; *Oral susp:* 25 mg/5 ml (4 oz) (lemon)

⬤ ALLERGIES: MULTI-FOOD

Comment: Eight food-types cause about 90% of food allergy reactions: ***Milk*** (mostly in children), ***Eggs, Peanuts, Tree nuts***, (e.g., walnuts, almonds, pine nuts, brazil nuts, and pecans), ***Soy, Wheat*** (and other grains with gluten, including barley, rye, and oats), ***Fish*** (mostly in adults), ***Shellfish*** (mostly in adults). Combining *omalizumab* with oral immunotherapy (OIT) significantly improves the effectiveness of OIT in children with multiple food allergies, according to the results of a recent study. Researchers conducted a blinded, phase 2 clinical trial including children aged 4 to 15 years who had multi-food allergies validated by double-blind, placebo-controlled food challenges. Participants were randomly assigned (3:1) to either receive *omalizumab* with multi-food oral immunotherapy or placebo. *omalizumab* and placebo were administered for 16 weeks, with oral immunotherapy beginning at 8 weeks. Overall, at week 36, a significantly greater proportion of the *omalizumab*-treated participants passed double-blind, placebo-controlled food challenges, compared with placebo (83% vs 33%). No serious or severe adverse events were reported. In multi-food allergic patients, *omalizumab* improves the efficacy of multi-food oral immunotherapy and enables safe and rapid desensitisation.

REFERENCE
Andorf, S., Purington, N., Block, W. M., Long, A. J., Tupa, D., Brittain, E., ... Chinthrajah, R. S. (2017). Anti-IgE treatment with oral immunotherapy in multifood allergic participants: a double-blind, randomised, controlled trial. *The Lancet Gastroenterology & Hepatology*. doi:10.1016/s2468-1253(17)30392-8

IGE BLOCKER (IGG1K MONOCLONAL ANTIBODY)

➤ *omalizumab* (B) 150-375 mg SC every 2-4 weeks based on body weight and pre-treatment serum total IgE level; max 150 mg/injection site
Pediatric: <12 years: not recommended; 30-90 kg + IgE >30-100 IU/ml 150 mg q 4 weeks; 90-150 kg + IgE >30-100 IU/ml or 30-90 kg + IgE >100-200 IU/ml or 30-60 kg + IgE >200-300 IU/ml 300 mg q 4 hours; >90-150 kg + IgE >100-200 IU/ml or >60-90 kg + IgE >200-300 IU/ml or 30-70 kg + IgE >300-400 IU/ml 225 mg q 2

weeks; >90-150 kg + IgE >200-300 IU/ml or >70-90 kg + IgE >300-400 IU/ml or
30-70 kg + IgE >400-500 IU/ml or 30-60 kg + IgE >500-600 IU/ml or 30-60 kg + IgE
>600-700 IU/ml 375 mg q 2 weeks; ≥12 years: same as adult

Xolair *Vial:* 150 mg pwdr for SC injection after reconstitution (preservative-free)

⬤ ALZHEIMER'S DISEASE

NUTRITIONAL SUPPLEMENT

▷ *l-methylfolate calcium (as metafolin)+methylcobalamin+n-acetyl cysteine* take 1 cap
once daily

Cerefolin *Cap: metafo* 5.6 mg+*methyl* 2 mg+n-ace cys 600 mg (gluten-free, yeast-
free, lactose-free)

Comment: Cerefolin is indicated in the dietary management of patients treated
for early memory loss, with emphasis on those at risk for neurovascular oxidative
stress, hyperhomocysteinemia, mild to moderate cognitive impairment with or
without vitamin B12 deficiency, vascular dementia, or Alzheimer's disease.

REVERSIBLE ANTICHOLINESTERASE INHIBITORS (RAIs)

Comment: The RAI drugs do not halt disease progression. They are indicated for early-
stage disease; not effective for severe dementia. If treatment is stopped for more than
several days, re-titrate from lowest dose. Side effects include nausea, anorexia, dyspepsia,
diarrhea, headache, and dizziness. Side effects tend to resolve with continued treatment.
Peak cognitive improvements are seen 12 weeks into therapy (increased spontaneity,
reduced apathy, lessened confusion, and improved attention, conversational language,
and performance of daily routines).

▷ *donepezil* (C)(G) initially 5 mg q HS, increase to 10 mg after 4-6 weeks as needed;
max 23 mg/day

Aricept *Tab:* 5, 10, 23 mg
Aricept ODT *ODT tab:* 5, 10 mg orally-disint

▷ *galantamine* (B) initially 4 mg bid x at least 4 weeks; usual maintenance 8 mg bid;
max 16 mg bid

Razadyne *Tab:* 4, 8, 12 mg
Razadyne ER *Tab:* 8, 16, 24 mg ext-rel
Razadyne Oral Solution *Oral soln:* 4 mg/ml (100 ml w. calib pipette)

▷ *rivastigmine* (B)(G)

Exelon initially 1.5 mg bid, increase every 2 weeks as needed; max 12 mg/day;
take with food

Cap: 1.5, 3, 4.5, 6 mg

Excelon Oral Solution initially 1.5 mg bid; may increase by 1.5 mg bid at intervals
of at least 2 weeks; usual range 6-12 mg/day; max 12 mg/day; if stopped, restart at
lowest dose and re-titrate; may take directly from syringe or mix with water, fruit
juice, or cola

Oral soln: 2 mg/ml (120 ml w. dose syringe)

Excelon Patch initially apply 4.6 mg/24 hr patch; if tolerated, may increase to 9.5
mg/24 hr patch after 4 weeks; max 13.3 mg/24 hr; change patch daily; apply to
clean, dry, hairless, intact skin; rotate application site; allow 14 days before applying new patch to same site

Patch: 4.6, 9.5, 13.3 mg/24 hr trans-sys (30/carton)

▷ *tacrine* (C) initially 10 mg qid, increase 40 mg/day q 4 weeks as needed; max 160 mg/day

Cognex *Cap:* 10, 20, 30, 40 mg

Comment: Transaminase levels should be checked every 3 months.

N-METHYL-D-ASPARTATE (NMDA) RECEPTOR ANTAGONIST

▷ *memantine* (B)(G)

Namenda initially 5 mg once daily; titrate weekly in 5 mg/day increments; *Week 2*: 5 mg bid; *Week 3*: 5 mg AM and 10 mg PM; *Week 4*: 10 mg bid; *CrCl 5-29 mL/min*: max 5 mg bid

Tab: 5, 10 mg

Namenda Oral Solution initially 5 mg once daily; titrate weekly in 5 mg increments administered bid

Oral soln: 2 mg/ml (360 ml) (peppermint) (sugar-free, alcohol-free)

Namenda Titration Pak

Cap: 7 x 7 mg, 7 x 14 mg, 7 x 21 mg, 7 x 28 mg/pck

Namenda XR initially 7 mg once daily; titrate in 7 mg increments weekly; max 28 mg once daily; do not divide doses

Cap: 7, 14, 21, 28 mg ext-rel

Comment: *memantine* does <u>not</u> halt disease progression. It is indicated for moderate to severe dementia.

N-METHYL-D-ASPARTATE (NMDA) RECEPTOR ANTAGONIST+ACETYLCHOLIN-ESTERASE INHIBITOR COMBINATION

▷ *memantine+donepezil* (C)(G) initiate one 28/10 dose daily in the evening after stabilized on *memantine* and *donepezil* separately; start the day after the last dose of *memantine* and *donepezil* taken separately; swallow whole <u>or</u> open cap and sprinkle on applesauce; *CrCl 5-29 mL/min*: take one 14/10 dose once daily in the evening

Namzaric

Cap: **Namzaric 7/10** mem 7 mg+done 10 mg
Namzaric 14/10 mem 14 mg+done 10 mg
Namzaric 21/10 mem 21 mg+done 10 mg
Namzaric 28/10 mem 28 mg+done 10 mg

ERGOT ALKALOID (DOPAMINE AGONIST)

▷ *ergoloid mesylate* (C) 1 mg tid

Hydergine *Tab*: 1 mg
Hydergine LC *Cap*: 1 mg
Hydergine Liquid *Liq*: 1 mg/ml (100 ml w. calib dropper) (alcohol 28.5%)

 AMEBIASIS

AMEBIASIS (INTESTINAL)

▷ *diiodohydroxyquin (iodoquinol)* (C)(G) 650 mg tid pc x 20 days
Pediatric: <6 years: 40 mg/kg/day in 3 divided doses pc x 20 days; max 1.95 gm; 6-12 years: 420 mg tid pc x 20 days
Tab: 210, 650 mg

▷ *metronidazole* (**not for use in 1st; B in 2nd, 3rd**)(G) 750 mg tid x 5-10 days
Pediatric: 35-50 mg/kg/day in 3 divided doses x 10 days
Flagyl *Tab*: 250*, 500*mg
Flagyl 375 *Cap*: 375 mg
Flagyl ER *Tab*: 750 mg ext-rel

▷ *tinidazole* (**not for use in 1st; B in 2nd, 3rd**) 2 gm daily x 3 days; take with food
Pediatric: <3 years: not recommended; ≥3 years: 50 mg/kg daily x 3 days; take with food; max 2 gm/day

Tindamax *Tab:* 250*, 500*mg
▷ *paromomycin* 25-35 mg/kg/day in 3 divided doses x 5-10 days
Pediatric: same as adult
Humatin *Cap:* 250 mg

AMEBIASIS (EXTRA-INTESTINAL)

▷ *chloroquine phosphate* (C)(G) 1 gm PO daily x 2 days; then 500 mg daily x 2 to 3
weeks <u>or</u> 200-250 mg IM daily x 10-12 days (when oral therapy is impossible); use
with intestinal amebicide
Pediatric: see mfr pkg insert
Aralen *Tab:* 500 mg; *Amp:* 50 mg/ml (5 ml)

AMEBIC LIVER ABSCESS

ANTI-INFECTIVES

▷ *metronidazole* (not for use in 1st; B in 2nd, 3rd)(G) 250 mg tid <u>or</u> 500 mg bid <u>or</u>
750 mg daily x 7 days
Pediatric: <12 years: not recommended; ≥12 years: same as adult
Flagyl *Tab:* 250*, 500*mg
Flagyl 375 *Cap:* 375 mg
Flagyl ER *Tab:* 750 mg ext-rel
Comment: Alcohol is contraindicated during treatment with oral *metronidazole* and
for 72 hours after therapy due to a possible *disulfiram*-like reaction (nausea, vomiting,
flushing, headache).
▷ *tinidazole* (not for use in 1st; B in 2nd, 3rd) 2 gm once daily x 3-5 days; take with food
Pediatric: <3 years: not recommended; ≥3 years: 50 mg/kg once daily x 3-5 days; take
with food; max 2 gm/day
Tindamax *Tab:* 250*, 500*mg

AMENORRHEA: SECONDARY

▷ *estrogen+progesterone* (X)
Premarin (*estrogen*) 0.625 mg daily x 25 days; then 5 days off; repeat monthly
Provera (*progesterone*) 5-10 mg last 10 days of cycle; repeat monthly
▷ *estrogen replacement* (X)
see **Menopause** page 295
▷ *human chorionic gonadotropin* 5,000-10,000 units IM x 1 dose following last dose of
menotropins
Pregnyl *Vial:* 10,000 units (10 ml) w. diluent (10 ml)
▷ *medroxyprogesterone* (X) *Monthly:* 5-10 mg last 5-10 days of cycle; begin on the 16th
<u>or</u> 21st day of cycle; repeat monthly; *One-time only:* 10 mg once daily x 10 days
Amen *Tab:* 10 mg
Provera *Tab:* 2.5, 5, 10 mg
▷ *norethindrone* (X) 2.5-10 mg daily x 5-10 days
Aygestin *Tab:* 5 mg
▷ *progesterone, micronized* (X)(G) 400 mg q HS x 10 days
Prometrium *Cap:* 100, 200 mg
Comment: Administration of *progesterone* induces optimum secretory
transformation of the *estrogen*-primed endometrium. Administration of *progesterone*
is contraindicated with breast cancer, undiagnosed vaginal bleeding, genital
cancer, severe liver dysfunction <u>or</u> disease, missed abortion, thrombophlebitis,
thromboembolic disorders, cerebral apoplexy, and pregnancy.

AMYOTROPHIC LATERAL SCLEROSIS (ALS, LOU GEHRIG DISEASE)

PYRAZOLONE FREE RADICAL SCAVENGER

➤ *edaravone* recommended dosage is 60 mg as an IV infusion administered over 60 minutes; Initial treatment cycle: daily dosing for 14 days followed by a 14-day drug-free period; Subsequent treatment cycles: daily dosing for 10 days out of 14-day periods, followed by 14-day drug-free periods

Radicava IV soln: 30 mg/100 ml single-dose polypropylene bag for IV infusion (sodium bisulfite)

Comment: Most common adverse reactions (at least 10%) are confusion, gait disturbance, and headache. There are no adequate data on the developmental risk associated with the use of **Radicava** in pregnancy. There are no data on the presence of *edaravone* in human milk <u>or</u> the effects on the breastfed infant. However, based on animal data, may cause fetal harm. To report suspected adverse reactions, contact MT Pharma America at 1-888-292-0058 <u>or</u> FDA at 800-FDA-1088 <u>or</u> www.fda.gov/medwatch

 ## ANAPHYLAXIS

Parenteral Corticosteroids *see page* 570
Oral Corticosteroids *see page* 569

➤ *epinephrine* (C)(G) 0.3-0.5 mg (0.3-0.5 ml of a 1:1000 soln) SC q 20-30 minutes as needed up to 3 doses
Pediatric: <2 years: 0.05-0.1 ml; 2-6 years: 0.1 ml; ≥6-12 years: 0.2 ml; All: q 20-30 minutes as needed up to 3 doses; ≥12 years: same as adult

ANAPHYLAXIS EMERGENCY TREATMENT KITS

➤ *epinephrine* (C) 0.3 ml IM <u>or</u> SC in thigh; may repeat if needed
Pediatric: 0.01 mg/kg SC <u>or</u> IM in thigh; may repeat if needed; <15 kg: not established; 15-30 kg: 0.15 mg; >30 kg: same as adult

Adrenaclick *Auto-injector:* 0.15, 0.3 mg (1 mg/ml; 1, 2/carton) (sulfites)
Auvi-Q *Auto-injector:* 0.15, 0.3 mg (1 mg/ml; 1/pck w. 1 non-active training device) (sulfites)
EpiPen *Auto-injector: 0.3 mg* (epi 1:1000, 0.3 ml (1, 2/carton) (sulfites)
EpiPen Jr *Auto-injector: 0.15 mg* (epi 1:2000, 0.3 ml) (1, 2/carton) (sulfites)
Symjepi *Prefilled syringe:* 0.3 mg (0.3 ml) single-dose for manual injection
Comment: **Symjepi** is intended for patient's weighing ≥30 kg only. Each syringe is overfilled for stability purposes. More than half the solution remains in the syringe after use (and the syringe cannot be re-used).
Twinject *Auto-injector: 0.15, 0.3 mg* (epi 1:1000) (1, 2/carton) (sulfites)
➤ *epinephrine+chlorpheniramine* (C) *epinephrine* 0.3 ml SC <u>or</u> IM *plus* 4 tabs *chlorpheniramine* by mouth
Pediatric: infants to 2 years: 0.05-0.1 ml SC <u>or</u> IM; ≥2-6 years: 0.15 ml SC <u>or</u> IM plus 1 tab *chlor;* ≥6-12 years: 0.2 ml SC <u>or</u> IM plus 2 tabs *chlor;* ≥12 years: same as adult
Ana-Kit: *Prefilled injector:* 0.3 ml epi 1:1000 for self-injection plus 4 x chlor 2 mg chew tabs

 ## ANEMIA OF CHRONIC KIDNEY DISEASE (CKD) AND CHRONIC RENAL FAILURE (CRF)

ERYTHROPOIESIS STIMULATING AGENTS (ESAs)

➤ *darbepoetin alpha* (erythropoiesis stimulating protein) (C) administer IV <u>or</u> SC q 1-2 weeks; do not increase more frequently than once per month; *Not currently receiving epoetin alpha:* initially 0.75 mcg/kg once weekly; adjust based on Hgb levels (target <u>not</u> to exceed 12 gm/dL); reduce dose if Hgb increases more than 1 gm/dL in any 2-week period; suspend therapy if polycythemia occurs; *Converting from **epoetin alpha** and for dose titration:* see mfr pkg insert

Pediatric: <12 years: not recommended; ≥12 years: same as adult

> **Aranesp** *Vial:* 25, 40, 60, 100, 150, 200, 300, 500 mcg/ml (single-dose) for IV <u>or</u> SC administration (preservative-free, albumin [human] <u>or</u> polysorbate 80)
> **Aranesp Singleject, Aranesp Sureclick Singleject** *Prefilled syringe:* 25, 40, 60, 100, 150, 200, 300, 500 mcg (single-dose) for IV <u>or</u> SC administration (preservative-free, albumin [human] <u>or</u> polysorbate 80)

▷ *peginesatide* (C) use lowest effective dose; initiate when Hgb <10 gm/dL; do <u>not</u> increase dose more often than every 4 weeks; if Hgb rises rapidly (i.e., >1 gm/dL in 2 weeks <u>or</u> >2 gm/dL in 4 weeks), reduce dose by 25% <u>or</u> more; if Hgb approaches <u>or</u> exceeds 11 gm/dL, reduce <u>or</u> interrupt dose and then when Hgb decreases, resume dose at approximately 25% below previous dose; if Hgb does <u>not</u> increase by >1 gm/dL after 4 weeks, increase dose by 25%; if response inadequate after a 12-week escalation period, use lowest dose that will maintain Hgb sufficient to reduce need for RBC transfusion; discontinue if response does <u>not</u> improve; *Not currently on ESA:* initially 0.04 mg/kg as a single IV <u>or</u> SC dose once monthly; *Converting from **epoetin alfa**:* administer first dose 1 week after last ***epoetin alfa***; *Converting from **darbepoetin alfa**:* administer first dose at next scheduled dose of ***darbepoetin alfa***

Pediatric: <12 years: not established; ≥12 years: use lowest effective dose

> **Omontys** *Vial, single-use:* 2, 3, 4, 5, 6 mg (0.5 ml) (preservative-free); *Vial, multiuse:* 10, 20 mg (2 ml) (preservatives); *Prefilled syringe:* 2, 3, 4, 5, 6 mg (0.5 ml) (preservative-free)

ERYTHROPOIETIN HUMAN, RECOMBINANT

▷ *epoetin alpha* (C) individualize; initially 50-100 units/kg 3 x/week; IV (dialysis <u>or</u> nondialysis) <u>or</u> SC (nondialysis); usual max 200 units/kg 3 x/week (dialysis) <u>or</u> 150 units/kg 3 x/week (non-dialysis); target Hct 30-36%

Pediatric: <1 month: not recommended; ≥1 month: individualize; *Dialysis:* initially 50 units/kg 3 x/week IV <u>or</u> SC; target Hct 30-36%

> **Epogen** *Vial:* 2,000, 3,000, 4,000, 10,000, 40,000 units/ml (1 ml) single-use for IV <u>or</u> SC administration (albumin [human]; preservative-free)
> **Epogen Multidose** *Vial:* 10,000 units/ml (2 ml); 20,000 units/ml, (1 ml) for IV <u>or</u> SC administration (albumin [human]; benzoyl alcohol)
> **Procrit** *Vial:* 2,000, 3,000, 4,000, 10,000, 40,000 units/ml (1 ml) single-use for IV <u>or</u> SC administration (albumin [human]) (preservative-free)
> **Procrit Multidose** *Vial:* 10,000 units/ml (2 ml); 20,000 units/ml, (1 ml) for IV <u>or</u> SC administration (albumin [human]; benzoyl alcohol)

 ANEMIA: FOLIC ACID DEFICIENCY

▷ *folic acid* (A)(OTC) 0.4-1 mg once daily

Comment: *folic acid (vitamin B9)* 400 mcg daily is recommended during pregnancy to prevent neural tube defects. Women who have had a baby with a neural tube defect should take 400 mcg every day, even when not planning to become pregnant, and if planning to become pregnant should take 4 mg daily during the month before becoming pregnant until at least the 12th week of pregnancy.

ANEMIA: IRON DEFICIENCY

Comment: Hemochromatosis and hemosiderosis are contraindications to iron therapy. **Iron** supplements are best absorbed when taken between meals and with **vitamin C-rich foods**. Excessive *iron* may be extremely hazardous to infants and young children. All vitamin and mineral supplements should be kept out of the reach of children.

IRON PREPARATIONS

▷ *ferrous gluconate* **(A)(G)** 1 tab once daily
  Pediatric: <12 years: not recommended; ≥12 years: same as adult
  Fergon (OTC)
  Tab: iron 27 mg (240 mg as gluconate)
▷ *ferrous sulfate* **(A)(G)**
  Feosol Tablets (OTC) 1 tab tid-qid pc and HS
  Pediatric: <6 years: use elixir; ≥6-12 years: 1 tab tid pc
  Tab: iron 65 mg (200 mg as sulfate)
  Feosol Capsules (OTC) 1-2 caps daily
  Pediatric: not recommended
  Cap: iron 50 mg (169 mg as sulfate) sust-rel
  Feosol Elixir (OTC) 5-10 ml tid between meals
  Pediatric: <1 year: not recommended; >1-11 year: 2.5-5 ml tid between meals; ≥12 years: same as adult
  Elix: iron 44 mg (220 mg as sulfate) per 5 ml
  Fer-In-Sol (OTC) 5 ml daily
  Pediatric: <4 years, use drops; ≥4 years: 5 ml once daily
  Syr: iron 18 mg (90 mg as sulfate) per 5 ml (480 ml)
  Fer-In-Sol Drops (OTC)
  Pediatric: <4 years: 0.6 ml daily; ≥4 years: use syrup
  Oral drops: iron 15 mg (75 mg as sulfate) per 5 ml (50 ml)

 ANEMIA: PERNICIOUS, MEGALOBLASTIC

Comment: Signs of **vitamin B12** deficiency include megaloblastic anemia, glossitis, paresthesias, ataxia, spastic motor weakness, and reduced mentation.
▷ *vitamin B12 (cyanocobalamin)* **(A)(G)** 500 mcg intranasally once a week; may increase dose if serum B-12 levels decline; adjust dose in 500 mcg increments
  Nascobal Nasal Spray
  Intranasal gel: 500 mcg/0.1 ml (1.3 ml, 4 doses) (citric acid, benzalkonium chloride)
Comment: **Nascobal Nasal Spray** is indicated for maintenance of hematologic remission following IM B-12 therapy without nervous system involvement. Must be primed before each use.

 ANGINA PECTORIS: STABLE

▷ *aspirin* **(D)** 325 mg (range 75-325 mg) once daily
  Comment: Daily *aspirin* dose is contingent upon whether the patient is also taking an anticoagulant <u>or</u> antiplatelet agent.

CALCIUM ANTAGONISTS

Comment: Calcium antagonists are contraindicated with history of ventricular arrhythmias, sick sinus syndrome, 2nd or 3rd degree heart block, cardiogenic shock, acute myocardial infarction, and pulmonary congestion.

▷ *amlodipine* (C)(G) 5-10 mg daily
Pediatric: <12 years: not recommended; ≥12 years: same as adult
    Norvasc *Tab:* 2.5, 5, 10 mg

▷ *diltiazem* (C)(G)
Pediatric: <12 years: not recommended; ≥12 years: same as adult
    Cardizem initially 30 mg qid; may increase gradually every 1-2 days; max 360 mg/day in divided doses
      Tab: 30, 60, 90, 120 mg
    Cardizem CD initially 120-180 mg daily; adjust at 1- to 2-week intervals; max 480 mg/day
      Cap: 120, 180, 240, 300, 360 mg ext-rel
    Cardizem LA initially 180-240 mg daily; titrate at 2 week intervals; max 540 mg/day
      Tab: 120, 180, 240, 300, 360, 420 mg ext-rel
    Cartia XT initially 180 mg or 240 mg once daily; max 540 mg once daily
      Cap: 120, 180, 240, 300 mg ext-rel
    Dilacor XR initially 180 mg or 240 mg once daily; max 540 mg once daily
      Cap: 180, 240 mg ext-rel
    Tiazac initially 120-180 mg daily; max 540 mg/day
      Cap: 120, 180, 240, 300, 360, 420 mg ext-rel

▷ *nicardipine* (C)(G) initially 20 mg tid; adjust q 3 days; max 120 mg/day
Pediatric: not recommended
    Cardene *Cap:* 20, 30 mg

▷ *nifedipine* (C)(G)
Pediatric: <12 years: not recommended; ≥12 years: same as adult
    Adalat CC initially 30 mg once daily; usual range 30-60 mg tid; max 90 mg/day
      Tab: 30, 60, 90 mg ext-rel
    Procardia initially 10 mg tid; titrate over 7-14 days: max 30 mg/dose and 180 mg/day in divided doses
      Cap: 10, 20 mg
    Procardia XL initially 30-60 mg daily; titrate over 7-14 days; max dose 90 mg/day
      Tab: 30, 60, 90 mg ext-rel

▷ *verapamil* (C)(G)
Pediatric: <12 years: not recommended; ≥12 years: same as adult
    Calan 80-120 mg tid; increase daily or weekly if needed
      Tab: 40, 80*, 120*mg
    Calan SR initially 120 mg once daily; increase weekly if needed
      Tab: 120, 180, 240 mg
    Covera HS initially 180 mg q HS; titrate in steps to 240 mg; then to 360 mg; then to 480 mg if needed
      Tab: 180, 240 mg ext-rel
    Isoptin SR initially 120-180 mg in the AM; may increase to 240 mg in the AM; then 180 mg q 12 hours or 240 mg in the AM and 120 mg in the PM; then 240 mg q 12 hours
      Tab: 120, 180*, 240*mg sust-rel

BETA-BLOCKERS

Comment: Beta-blockers are contraindicated with history of sick sinus syndrome (SSS), 2nd or 3rd degree heart block, cardiogenic shock, pulmonary congestion, asthma, moderate to severe COPD with FEV1 <50% predicted, patients with chronic bronchodilator treatment.

▷ *atenolol* (D)(G) initially 25-50 mg daily; increase weekly if needed; max 200 mg daily

Pediatric: <12 years: not recommended; ≥12 years: same as adult

Tenormin *Tab:* 25, 50, 100 mg

▷ *metoprolol succinate* (C)

Pediatric: <12 years: not recommended; ≥12 years: same as adult

Toprol-XL initially 100 mg in a single dose once daily; increase weekly if needed; max 400 mg/day

Tab: 25*, 50*, 100*, 200*mg ext-rel

▷ *metoprolol tartrate* (C)

Pediatric: <12 years: not recommended; ≥12 years: same as adult

Lopressor (G) initially 25-50 mg bid; increase weekly if needed; max 400 mg/day

Tab: 25, 37.5, 50, 75, 100 mg

▷ *nadolol* (C)(G) initially 40 mg daily; increase q 3-7 days; max 240 mg/day

Pediatric: not recommended

Corgard *Tab:* 20*, 40*, 80*, 120*, 160*mg

▷ *propranolol* (C)(G)

Pediatric: <12 years: not recommended; ≥12 years: same as adult

Inderal LA initially 80 mg daily in a single dose; increase q 3-7 days; usual range 120-160 mg/day; max 320 mg/day in a single dose

Cap: 60, 80, 120, 160 mg sust-rel

InnoPran XL initially 80 mg q HS; max 120 mg/day

Cap: 80, 120 mg ext-rel

NITRATES

Comment: Use a daily nitrate dosing schedule that provides a dose-free period of 14 hours <u>or</u> more to prevent tolerance. *aspirin* and *acetaminophen* may relieve nitrate-induced headache. *Isosorbide* is <u>not</u> recommended for use in MI <u>and/or</u> CHF. Nitrate use is a contraindication for using phosphodiesterase type 5 inhibitors: *sildenafil* (**Viagra**), *tadalafil* (**Cialis**), *vardenafil* (**Levitra**).

▷ *isosorbide dinitrate* (C)

Pediatric: <12 years: not recommended; ≥12 years: same as adult

Dilatrate-SR 40 mg once daily; max 160 mg/day

Cap: 40 mg sust-rel

Isordil Titradose initially 5-20 mg q 6 hours; maintenance 10-40 mg q 6 hours

Tab: 5, 10, 20, 30, 40 mg

▷ *isosorbide mononitrate* (C)

Pediatric: <12 years: not recommended; ≥12 years: same as adult

Imdur initially 30-60 mg q AM; may increase to 120 mg daily; max 240 mg/day

Tab: 30*, 60*, 120 mg ext-rel

Ismo 20 mg upon awakening; then 20 mg 7 hours later

Tab: 20*mg

▷ *nitroglycerin* (C)(G)

Pediatric: <12 years: not recommended; ≥12 years: same as adult

Nitro-Bid Ointment initially 1/2 inch q 8 hours; titrate in 1/2 inch increments

Oint: 2% (20, 60 gm)

Nitrodisc initially one 0.2-0.4 mg/Hr patch for 12-14 hours/day

Transdermal disc: 0.2, 0.3, 0.4 mg/hour (30, 100/carton)

Nitrolingual Pump Spray 1-2 sprays on or under tongue; max 3 sprays/15 minutes
> *Spray:* 0.4 mg/dose (14.5 gm, 200 doses)

Nitromist 1-2 sprays at onset of attack, on or under the tongue while sitting; may repeat q 5 minutes as needed; max 3 sprays/15 minutes; may use prophylactically 5-10 minutes prior to exertion; do not inhale spray; do not rinse mouth for 5-10 minutes after use
> *Lingual aerosol spray:* 0.4 mg/actuation (230 metered sprays)

Nitrostat 1 tab SL; may repeat q 5 minutes x 3
> *SL tab:* 0.3 (1/100 gr), 0.4 (1/150 gr), 0.6 (1/4 gr) mg

Transderm-Nitro initially one 0.2 mg/hour or 0.4 mg/hour patch for 12-14 hours/day
> *Transdermal patch:* 0.1, 0.2, 0.4, 0.6, 0.8 mg/hour

NON-NITRATE PERIPHERAL VASODILATOR

▷ *hydralazine* (C)(G) initially 10 mg qid x 2-4 days; then increase to 25 mg qid for remainder of first week; then increase to 50 mg qid; max 300 mg/day
Pediatric: <12 years: not recommended; ≥12 years: same as adult
> *Tab:* 10, 25, 50, 100 mg

NITRATE+PERIPHERAL VASODILATOR COMBINATION

▷ *isosorbide+hydralazine HCl* (C) initially 1 tab tid; max 2 tabs tid
Pediatric: <12 years: not established; ≥12 years: same as adult
> **Bidil** *Tab:* isosorb 20 mg+hydral 37.5 mg

NON-NITRATE ANTI-ANGINAL

▷ *ranolazine* (C) initially 500 mg bid; may increase to max 1 gm bid
Pediatric: <12 years: not recommended; ≥12 years: same as adult
> **Ranexa** *Tab:* 500, 1000 mg ext-rel

> **Comment:** **Ranexa** is indicated for the treatment chronic angina that is inadequately controlled with other antianginals. Use with amlodipine, beta-blocker, or nitrate.

◯ ANOREXIA/CACHEXIA

APPETITE STIMULANTS

▷ *cyproheptadine* (B)(G) initially 4 mg tid prn; then adjust as needed; usual range 12-16 mg/day; max 32 mg/day
Pediatric: <2 years: not recommended; ≥2-6 years: 2 mg bid-tid prn; max 12 mg/day; 7-14 years: 4 mg bid-tid prn; max 16 mg/day; >14 years: same as adult
> **Periactin** *Tab:* cypro 4*mg; *Syr:* cypro 2 mg/5 ml

▷ *dronabinol* (cannabinoid) (B)(III) initially 2.5 mg bid before lunch and dinner; may reduce to 2.5 mg q HS or increase to 2.5 mg before lunch and 5 mg before dinner; max 20 mg/day in divided doses
Pediatric: <12 years: not recommended; ≥12 years: same as adult
> **Marinol** *Cap:* 2.5, 5, 10 mg (sesame oil)

▷ *megestrol* (progestin) (X)(G) 40 mg qid
Pediatric: <12 years: not recommended; ≥12 years: same as adult
> **Megace** *Tab:* 20*, 40*mg
> **Megace ES** *Oral susp (concentrate):* 125 mg/ml; 625 mg/5 ml (5 oz) (lemon-lime)
> **Megace Oral Suspension** *Oral susp:* 40 mg/ml (8 oz); 820 mg/20 ml) (lemon-lime)
> **Megestrol Acetate Oral Suspension** (G) 125 mg/ml

Comment: *megestrol* is indicated for the treatment of anorexia, cachexia, or an unexplained, significant weight loss in patients with a diagnosis of AIDS.

ANTHRAX (*BACILLUS ANTHRACIS*)

POST-EXPOSURE PROPHYLAXIS OF INHALATIONAL ANTHRAX AND TREATMENT OF INHALED AND CUTANEOUS ANTHRAX INFECTION

Comment: *B anthracis* spores are resistant to destruction, are easily spread by release into the air, and cause irreversible tissue damage and death. The most lethal form is inhalational anthrax. Even with the most aggressive treatment, the mortality rate is about 45%. People at risk are those who work in slaughterhouses, tanneries, and wood mills who are exposed to infected animals.

Immune globulin

➢ *bacillus anthracis immune globulin intravenous (human)* administer via IV infusion at a maximum rate of 2 ml/min; dose is weight-based as follows, but may be doubled in severe cases if weight >5 kg:
Pediatric: <16 years: not established; 5-<10 kg: 1 vial; 10-<18 kg: 2 vials; 18-<25 kg: 3 vials; 25-<35 kg: 4 vials; 35-<50 kg: 5 vials; 50-<60 kg: 6 vials; ≥60 kg: 7 vials
 Anthrasil *Vial:* (60 units) sterile solution of purified human immune globulin gm (IgG) containing polyclonal antibodies that target the anthrax toxins of *Bacillus anthracis* for IV infusion
 Comment: **Anthrasil** is indicated for the emergent treatment of inhaled anthrax in combination with appropriate antibacterial agents

MONOCLONAL ANTIBODIES

Comment: *obiltoxaximab* and *raxibacumab* have no antibacterial activity; rather, they are monoclonal antibodies that neutralize toxins produced by *B. anthracis* by binding to the bacterium's protective antigen, preventing intracellular entry of key enzymatic toxin components. *obiltoxaximab* (**Anthim**) and *raxibacumab* are indicated for treatment of inhalational anthrax in combination with appropriate antibacterial drugs and for prophylaxis of inhalational anthrax when alternative therapies are unavailable or inappropriate. Vials must be refrigerated and protected from light. Do not shake the vials. Pre-medicate the patient with *diphenhydramine*.

➢ *obiltoxaximab* 16 mg/kg diluted in 0.9%NS via IV infusion over 90 minutes
Pediatric: see mfr pkg insert for dosing based on kilograms body weight
 Anthim *Vial:* 600 mg in 6 ml (100 mg/ml) single-use, for dilution in 0.9% NS and IV infusion

➢ *raxibacumab* (B) 40 mg/kg diluted in 0.45%NS or 0.9% NS via IV infusion over 2 hours and 15 minutes; see mfr pkg insert for recommended volume of dilution according to weight-based dose
Pediatric: ≤15 kg: 80 mg/kg; >15-50 kg: 60 mg/kg; >50 kg: same as adult
 Vial: 1700 mg/34 ml (50 mg/ml), single-use, for dilution and IV infusion

ANTIBACTERIAL AGENTS

➢ *ciprofloxacin* (C) 500 mg (or 10-15 mg/kg/day) q 12 hours for 60 days (start as soon as possible after exposure)
Pediatric: <18 years: 20-40 mg/kg/day divided q 12 hours; ≥18 years: same as adult
 Cipro (G) *Tab:* 250, 500, 750 mg; *Oral susp:* 250, 500 mg/5 ml (100 ml) (strawberry)
 Cipro XR *Tab:* 500, 1000 mg ext-rel
 ProQuin XR *Tab:* 500 mg ext-rel
Comment: *ciprofloxacin* is usually contraindicated <18 years-of-age, and during pregnancy and lactation. Risk of tendonitis or tendon rupture. Risk/ benefit must be assessed in the case of anthrax.

▷ *doxycycline* (D)(G) 100 mg daily bid
  Pediatric: <8 years: usually contraindicated ≥8 years, <100 lb: 2 mg/lb on first day in 2 divided doses, followed by 1 mg/lb/day in a single or divided doses; ≥8 years, ≥100 lb: same as adult; *see page 633 for dose by weight*
     Acticlate *Tab:* 75, 150**mg
     Adoxa *Tab:* 50, 75, 100, 150 mg ent-coat
     Doryx *Tab:* 50, 75, 100, 150, 200 mg del-rel
     Doxteric *Tab:* 50 mg del-rel
     Monodox *Cap:* 50, 75, 100 mg
     Oracea *Cap:* 40 mg del-rel
     Vibramycin *Tab:* 100 mg; *Cap:* 50, 100 mg; *Syr:* 50 mg/5 ml (raspberry-apple) (sulfites); *Oral susp:* 25 mg/5 ml (raspberry)
     Vibra-Tab *Tab:* 100 mg film-coat

Comment: *doxycycline* is usually contraindicated <8 years-of-age, in pregnancy, and lactation (discolors developing tooth enamel). Risk/ benefit must be assessed in the case of anthrax. A side effect may be photosensitivity (photophobia). Do not take with antacids, calcium supplements, milk or other dairy, or within 2 hours of taking another drug.

▷ *minocycline* (D)(G) 2 mg/lb on first day in 2 divided doses, followed by 1 mg/lb q 12 hours x 9 more days; ≥8 years, >100 mg: 100 mg q 12 hours
  Pediatric: <8 years: usually not recommended; ≥8 years, <100 lb:
     Dynacin *Cap:* 50, 100 mg
     Minocin *Cap:* 50, 75, 100 mg; *Oral susp:* 50 mg/5 ml (60 ml) (custard) (sulfites, alcohol 5%)

Comment: *minocycline* is usually contraindicated <8 years-of-age, in pregnancy, and lactation (discolors developing tooth enamel). A side effect may be photosensitivity (photophobia). Do not give with antacids, calcium supplements, milk or other dairy, or within two hours of taking another drug.

TREATMENT OF GI AND OROPHARYNGEAL ANTHRAX

▷ *ciprofloxacin* (C) 400 mg IV q 12 hours (start as soon as possible); then, switch to 500 mg PO q 12 hours for total 60 days; infuse dose over 60 minutes
  Pediatric: <18 years: usually not recommended; 10-15 mg/kg IV q 12 hours (start as soon as possible); then switch to 10-15 mg/kg PO q 12 hours for 60 days
     Cipro (G) *Tab:* 250, 500, 750 mg; *Oral susp:* 250, 500 mg/5 ml (100 ml) (strawberry); *IV conc:* 10 mg/ml after dilution (20, 40 ml); *IV premix:* 2 mg/ml (100, 200 ml)
     Cipro XR *Tab:* 500, 1000 mg ext-rel
     ProQuin XR *Tab:* 500 mg ext-rel

Comment: *ciprofloxacin* is usually contraindicated <18 years-of-age, and during pregnancy and lactation. Risk of tendonitis or tendon rupture. Risk/ benefit must be assessed in the case of anthrax. Infuse IV *ciprofloxacin* over 60 minutes.

▷ *doxycycline* (D)(G) 100 mg daily bid
  Pediatric: <8 years: not recommended ≥8 years, <100 lb: 2 mg/lb on first day in 2 divided doses, followed by 1 mg/lb/day in a single or divided doses; ≥8 years, ≥100 lb: same as adult; *see page 633 for dose by weight*
     Acticlate *Tab:* 75, 150**mg
     Adoxa *Tab:* 50, 75, 100, 150 mg ent-coat
     Doryx *Tab:* 50, 75, 100, 150, 200 mg del-rel
     Doxteric *Tab:* 50 mg del-rel
     Monodox *Cap:* 50, 75, 100 mg
     Oracea *Cap:* 40 mg del-rel

Vibramycin *Tab:* 100 mg; *Cap:* 50, 100 mg; *Syr:* 50 mg/5 ml (raspberry-apple) (sulfites); *Oral susp:* 25 mg/ml (raspberry)
Vibra-Tab *Tab:* 100 mg film-coat

Comment: *doxycycline* is usually contraindicated <8 years-of-age, in pregnancy, and lactation (discolors developing tooth enamel). Risk/ benefit must be assessed in the case of anthrax. A side effect may be photosensitivity (photophobia). Do not take with antacids, calcium supplements, milk or other dairy, or within 2 hours of taking another drug.

▶ *minocycline* (D)(G) 100 mg q 12 hours
   Pediatric: <8 years: usually not recommended; ≥8 years, <100 lb: 2 mg/lb on first day in 2 divided doses, followed by 1 mg/lb q 12 hours x 9 more days; ≥8 years, ≥100 lb: same as adult
      Dynacin *Cap:* 50, 100 mg
      Minocin *Cap:* 50, 75, 100 mg; *Oral susp:* 50 mg/5 ml (60 ml) (custard) (sulfites, alcohol 5%)

Comment: *minocycline* is usually contraindicated <8 years-of-age, in pregnancy, and lactation (discolors developing tooth enamel). Risk/ benefit must be assessed in the case of anthrax. A side effect may be photosensitivity (photophobia). Do not give with antacids, calcium supplements, milk or other dairy, or within two hours of taking another drug.

ANXIETY DISORDER: GENERALIZED (GAD)/ ANXIETY DISORDER: SOCIAL (SAD)

FIRST GENERATION ORAL ANTIHISTAMINE

▶ *diphenhydramine* (B)(G) 25-50 mg q 6-8 hours; max 100 mg/day
   Pediatric: <2 years: not recommended; 2-6 years: 6.25 mg q 4-6 hours; max 37.5 mg/day; >6-12 years: 12.5-25 mg q 4-6 hours; max 150 mg/day; ≥12 years: same as adult
      Benadryl (OTC) *Chew tab:* 12.5 mg (grape) (phenylalanine); *Liq:* 12.5 mg/5 ml (4, 8 oz); *Cap:* 25 mg; *Tab:* 25 mg; *Dye-free soft gel:* 25 mg; *Dye-free liq:* 12.5 mg/5 ml (4, 8 oz)

▶ *hydroxyzine* (C)(G) 50-100 mg qid; max 600 mg/day
   Pediatric: <6 years: 50 mg/day divided qid; ≥6 years: 50-100 mg/day divided qid
      Atarax *Tab:* 10, 25, 50, 100 mg; *Syr:* 10 mg/5 ml (alcohol 0.5%)
      Vistaril *Cap:* 25, 50, 100 mg; *Oral susp:* 25 mg/5 ml (4 oz) (lemon)

Comment: *hydroxyzine* is contraindicated in early pregnancy and in patients with a prolonged QT interval. It is not known whether this drug is excreted in human milk; therefore, *hydroxyzine* should not be given to nursing mothers.

AZAPIRONE

▶ *buspirone* (B) initially 7.5 mg bid; may increase by 5 mg/day q 2-3 days; max 60 mg/day
   Pediatric: <6 years: not recommended; ≥6 years: same as adult
      BuSpar *Tab:* 5, 10, 15*, 30*mg

BENZODIAZEPINES

Comment: If possible when considering a benzodiazepine to treat anxiety, a short-acting benzodiazepines should be used only prn to avert intense anxiety and panic for the least time necessary while a different non-addictive antianxiety regimen (e.g., SSRI, SNRI, TCA, *buspirone*, beta-blocker) is established and effective treatment goals achieved. Benzodiazepines have a high addiction potential when they are chronically used and are common drugs of abuse. *Benzodiazepine withdrawal syndrome* may include restlessness, agitation, anxiety, insomnia, tachycardia, tachypnea, diaphoresis, and may be potentially life threatening depending on the benzodiazepine and the length of use. Symptoms of withdrawal from short-acting benzodiazepines, such as *alprazolam* (**Xanax**), *oxazepam, lorazepam* (**Ativan**), *triazolam* (**Halcion**), usually appear within 6-8 hours after the last dose and may continue 10-14 days. Symptoms of withdrawal from long-acting benzodiazepines, such as *diazepam* (**Valium**), *clonazepam* (**Klonopin**), *chlordiazepoxide* (**Librium**), usually appear within 24-96 hours after the last dose and may continue from 3-4 weeks to 3 months. People who are heavily dependent on benzodiazepines may experience *protracted withdrawal syndrome* (PAWS), random periods of sharp withdrawal symptoms months after quitting. A closely monitored medical detoxification regimen may be required for a safe withdrawal and to prevent PAWS. Detoxification includes gradual tapering of the benzodiazepine along with other medications to manage the withdrawal symptoms.

Short-Acting Benzodiazepines

▷ *alprazolam* (D)(IV)(G)
    Pediatric: <18 years: not recommended; ≥18 years:
        Niravam initially 0.25-0.5 mg tid; may titrate every 3-4 days; max 4 mg/day
          Tab: 0.25*, 0.5*, 1*, 2*mg orally-disint
        Xanax initially 0.25-0.5 mg tid; may titrate every 3-4 days; max 4 mg/day
          Tab: 0.25*, 0.5*, 1*, 2*mg
        Xanax XR initially 0.5-1 mg once daily, preferably in the AM; increase at intervals of at least 3-4 days by up to 1 mg/day. Taper no faster than 0.5 mg every 3 days; max 10 mg/day. When switching from immediate-release *alprazolam*, give total daily dose of immediate-release once daily.
          Tab: 0.5, 1, 2, 3 mg ext-rel
▷ *oxazepam* (C)(IV)(G) 10-15 mg tid-qid for moderate symptoms; 15-30 mg tid-qid for severe symptoms
    Pediatric: <12 years: not recommended; ≥12 years: same as adult
    Cap: 10, 15, 30 mg

Intermediate-Acting Benzodiazepines

▷ *lorazepam* (D)(IV)(G) 1-10 mg/day in 2-3 divided doses
    Pediatric: <12 years: not recommended; ≥12 years: same as adult
        Ativan *Tab:* 0.5, 1*, 2*mg
        Lorazepam Intensol *Oral conc:* 2 mg/ml (30 ml w. graduated dropper)

Long-Acting Benzodiazepines

▷ *chlordiazepoxide* (D)(IV)(G)
    Pediatric: <6 years: not recommended; ≥6 years: 5 mg bid-qid; increase to 10 mg bid-tid
        Librium 5-10 mg tid-qid for moderate symptoms; 20-25 mg tid-qid for severe symptoms
          Cap: 5, 10, 25 mg
        Librium Injectable 50-100 mg IM <u>or</u> IV; then 25-50 mg IM tid-qid prn; max 300 mg/day
          Inj: 100 mg
▷ *chlordiazepoxide+clidinium* (D)(IV) 1-2 caps tid-qid: max 8 caps/day
    Pediatric: not recommended
        Librax *Cap: chlor* 5 mg+*clid* 2.5 mg
▷ *clonazepam* (D)(IV)(G) initially 0.25 mg bid; increase to 1 mg/day after 3 days
    Pediatric: <18 years: not recommended; ≥18 years: same as adult

Klonopin *Tab:* 0.5*, 1, 2 mg
Klonopin Wafers dissolve in mouth with <u>or</u> without water
    Wafer: 0.125, 0.25, 0.5, 1, 2 mg orally-disint
▷ *clorazepate* (D)(IV)(G) 30 mg/day in divided doses; max 60 mg/day
  Pediatric: <9 years: not recommended; ≥9 years: same as adult
    Tranxene *Tab:* 3.75, 7.5, 15 mg
    Tranxene SD do not use for initial therapy
      Tab: 22.5 mg ext-rel
    Tranxene SD Half Strength do not use for initial therapy
      Tab: 11.25 mg ext-rel
    Tranxene T-Tab *Tab:* 3.75*, 7.5*, 15*mg
▷ *diazepam* (D)(IV)(G) 2-10 mg bid to qid
  Pediatric: <12 years: not recommended; ≥12 years: same as adult
    Diastat *Rectal gel delivery system:* 2.5 mg
    Diastat AcuDial *Rectal gel delivery system:* 10, 20 mg
    Valium *Tab:* 2*, 5*, 10*mg
    Valium Injectable *Vial:* 5 mg/ml (10 ml); *Amp:* 5 mg/ml (2 ml); *Prefilled syringe:*
    5 mg/ml (5 ml)
    Valium Intensol Oral Solution *Conc oral soln:* 5 mg/ml (30 ml w. dropper)
    (alcohol 19%)
    Valium Oral Solution *Oral soln:* 5 mg/5 ml (500 ml) (wintergreen spice)

TRICYCLIC ANTIDEPRESSANTS (TCAs)

Comment: Co-administration of TCAs with SSRIs requires extreme caution.
▷ *doxepin* (C)(G) usual optimum dose 75-150 mg/day; elderly lower initial dose and
therapeutic dose; max single dose 150 mg; max 300 mg/day in divided doses
  Pediatric: <12 years: not recommended; ≥12 years: same as adult
    Sinequan
    Cap: 10, 25, 50, 75, 100, 150 mg; *Oral conc:* 10 mg/ml (4 oz w. dropper)
Comment: Glaucoma, urinary retention, and bipolar disorder are contraindications
to *doxepin*. Separate from MAOIs by at least 14 days. Separate from *fluoxetine* by at
least 5 weeks. Avoid abrupt cessation. *doxepin* is potentiated by CYP2D6 inhibitors
(e.g., *cimetidine*, SSRIs, phenothiazines, type 1C antiarrhythmics).

PHENOTHIAZINES

▷ *prochlorperazine* (C)(G)
  Pediatric: <12 years: not recommended; ≥12 years: same as adult
    Compazine 5 mg tid-qid
      Tab: 5 mg; *Syr:* 5 mg/5 ml (4 oz) (fruit); *Rectal supp:* 2.5, 5, 25 mg
    Compazine Spansule 15 mg q AM <u>or</u> 10 mg q 12 hours
      Spansule: 10, 15 mg sust-rel
▷ *trifluoperazine* (C)(G) 1-2 mg bid; max 6 mg/day; max 12 weeks
  Pediatric: <12 years: not recommended; ≥12 years: same as adult
    Stelazine *Tab:* 1, 2, 5, 10 mg

SELECTIVE SEROTONIN REUPTAKE INHIBITORS (SSRIs)

Comment: Co-administration of SSRIs with TCAs requires extreme caution.
Concomitant use of MAOIs and SSRIs is absolutely contraindicated. Avoid St. John's
wort and other serotonergic agents. A potentially fatal adverse event is *serotonin
syndrome*, caused by serotonin excess. Milder symptoms require HCP intervention
to avert severe symptoms that can be rapidly fatal without urgent/emergent medical
care. Symptoms include restlessness, agitation, confusion, tachycardia, hypertension,
dilated pupils, muscle twitching, muscle rigidity, loss of muscle coordination,

diaphoresis, diarrhea, headache, shivering, piloerection, hyperpyrexia, cardiac arrhythmias, seizures, loss of consciousness, coma, death. Common symptoms of the *serotonin discontinuation syndrome* include flu-like symptoms (nausea, vomiting, diarrhea, headaches, diaphoresis); sleep disturbances (insomnia, nightmares, constant sleepiness); mood disturbances (dysphoria, anxiety, agitation); cognitive disturbances (mental confusion, hyperarousal); and sensory and movement disturbances (imbalance, tremors, vertigo, dizziness, electric-shock-like sensations in the brain often described by sufferers as "brain zaps").

➤ *escitalopram* (C)(G) initially 10 mg daily; may increase to 20 mg daily after 1 week; Elderly or hepatic impairment, 10 mg once daily
  Pediatric: <12 years: not recommended; 12-17 years: initially 10 mg once daily; may increase to 20 mg once daily after 3 weeks
    Lexapro *Tab:* 5, 10*, 20*mg
    Lexapro Oral Solution *Oral soln:* 1 mg/ml (240 ml) (peppermint) (parabens)
➤ *fluoxetine* (C)(G)
    Prozac initially 20 mg daily; may increase after 1 week; doses >20 mg/day may be divided into AM and noon doses; max 80 mg/day
    Pediatric: <8 years: not recommended; 8-17 years: initially 10-20 mg once daily; start lower weight children at 10 mg once daily; if starting at 10 mg once daily, may increase after 1 week to 20 mg once daily
      Cap: 10, 20, 40 mg; *Tab:* 30*, 60*mg; *Oral soln:* 20 mg/5 ml (4 oz) (mint)
    Prozac Weekly following daily *fluoxetine* therapy at 20 mg/day x 13 weeks, may initiate **Prozac Weekly** 7 days after the last 20 mg *fluoxetine* dose
    Pediatric: <12 years: not recommended; ≥12 years: same as adult
      Cap: 90 mg ent-coat del-rel pellets
➤ *paroxetine maleate* (D)(G)
  Pediatric: <12 years: not recommended; ≥12 years: same as adult
    Paxil initially 10-20 mg daily in AM; may increase by 10 mg/day at weekly intervals as needed; max 60 mg/day
      Tab: 10*, 20*, 30, 40 mg
    Paxil CR initially 12.5-25 mg daily in AM; may increase by 12.5 mg at weekly intervals as needed; max 62.5 mg/day
      Tab: 12.5, 25, 37.5 mg ent-coat cont-rel
    Paxil Suspension initially 10-20 mg daily in AM; may increase by 10 mg/day at weekly intervals as needed; max 60 mg/day
      Oral susp: 10 mg/5 ml (250 ml) (orange)
➤ *paroxetine mesylate* (D)(G) initially 7.5 mg daily in AM; may increase by 10 mg/day at weekly intervals as needed; max 60 mg/day
  Pediatric: <12 years: not recommended; ≥12 years: same as adult
    Brisdelle *Cap:* 7.5 mg
➤ *sertraline* (C) initially 50 mg daily; increase at 1 week intervals if needed; max 200 mg daily
  Pediatric: <6 years: not recommended; 6-12 years: initially 25 mg daily; max 200 mg/day; 13-17 years: initially 50 mg daily; max 200 mg/day
    Zoloft *Tab:* 15*, 50*, 100*mg; *Oral conc:* 20 mg per ml (60 ml [dilute just before administering in 4 oz water, ginger ale, lemon-lime soda, lemonade, or orange juice]) (alcohol 12%)

SEROTONIN-NOREPINEPHRINE REUPTAKE INHIBITORS (SNRIs)

➤ *desvenlafaxine* (C)(G) swallow whole; initially 50 mg once daily; max 120 mg/day
  Pediatric: <18 years: not recommended; ≥18 years: same as adult
    Pristiq *Tab:* 50, 100 mg ext-rel

▷ *duloxetine* (C)(G) swallow whole; initially 30 mg once daily x 1 week; then, increase to
  60 mg once daily; max 120 mg/day
  Pediatric: <12 years: not recommended; ≥12 years: same as adult
    Cymbalta *Cap:* 20, 30, 40, 60 mg del-rel
▷ *venlafaxine* (C)(G)
    Effexor initially 75 mg/day in 2-3 divided doses; may increase at 4 day intervals in
    75 mg increments to 150 mg/day; max 225 mg/day
    Pediatric: <18 years: not recommended; ≥18 years: same as adult
      Tab: 37.5, 75, 150, 225 mg
    Effexor XR initially 75 mg q AM; may start at 37.5 mg daily x 4-7 days; then
    increase by increments of up to 75 mg/day at intervals of at least 4 days; usual
    max 375 mg/day
    Pediatric: <18 years: not recommended; ≥18 years: same as adult
      Tab: Cap: 37.5, 75, 150 mg ext-rel

COMBINATION AGENTS
▷ *chlordiazepoxide+amitriptyline* (D)(G)
  Pediatric: <12 years: not recommended; ≥12 years: same as adult
    Limbitrol 3-4 tabs/day in divided doses
      Tab: chlor 5 mg+*amit* 12.5 mg
    Limbitrol DS 3-4 tabs/day in divided doses; max 6 tabs/day
      Tab: chlor 10 mg+*amit* 25 mg
▷ *perphenazine+amitriptyline* (C)(G) 1 tab bid-qid
  Pediatric: <12 years: not recommended; ≥12 years: same as adult
    Tab: **Etrafon 2-10** *perph* 2 mg+*amit* 10 mg
      Etrafon 2-25 *perph* 2 mg+*amit* 25 mg
      Etrafon 4-25 *perph* 4 mg+*amit* 25 mg

 APHASIA: EXPRESSIVE, STROKE-INDUCED

Comment: In a case report published in NEJM, a 52-year-old right-handed woman
who sustained an ischemic stroke 3 years prior, the areas of infarction included the
left insula, putamen, and superior temporal gyrus. Her stroke resulted in expressive
aphasia, leaving her with no intelligible words, but with intact full language
comprehension. *zolpidem* 10 mg was prescribed for insomnia. In repeated measures,
it was found that the patient consistently demonstrated dramatic speech improvement,
durable until HS, and return of the expressive aphasia in the AM. Subsequent single-
photon-emission computed tomography (SPECT) scanning of this patient indicated
that *zolpidem* increases flow in the Broca area of the brain, an area intimately involved
with speech. From these observations, the authors concluded that a select subgroup of
patients with aphasia, perhaps with subcortical lesions and spared but hypometabolic
cortical structures, might benefit from this treatment. It may be worth trying *zolpidem*
in patients who have been labeled with otherwise refractory chronic expressive aphasia.
This finding raises the questions, could this intervention help patients earlier in the
course, patients with milder disease, or patients with other ischemic central nervous
system syndromes?

REFERENCE
Cohen, L., Chaaban, B., & Habert, M.-O. (2004). Transient improvement of aphasia with zolpidem. *New
England Journal of Medicine, 350*(9), 949–950.

▷ **zolpidem** oral solution spray **(C)(IV)(G)** (imidazopyridine hypnotic) 2 actuations (10 mg) immediately before bedtime; *Elderly, debilitated, or hepatic impairment:* 2 actuations (5 mg); max 2 actuations (10 mg)
   Pediatric: <18 years: not recommended; ≥18 years: same adult
      ZolpiMist *Oral soln spray:* 5 mg/actuation (60 metered actuations) (cherry)
Comment: The lowest dose of *zolpidem* in all forms is recommended for persons >50 years-of-age and women as drug elimination is slower than in men.

▷ **zolpidem** tabs **(B)(IV)(G)** (pyrazolopyrimidine hypnotic) 5-10 mg or 6.25-12.5 extrel q HS prn; max 12.5 mg/day x 1 month; do not take if unable to sleep for at least 8 hours before required to be active again; delayed effect if taken with a meal
   Pediatric: <18 years: not recommended; ≥18 years: same adult
      Ambien *Tab:* 5, 10 mg
      Ambien CR *Tab:* 6.25, 12.5 mg ext-rel
Comment: The lowest dose of *zolpidem* in all forms is recommended for persons >50 years-of-age and women as drug elimination is slower than in men.

▷ **zolpidem** sublingual tabs **(C)(IV)** (imidazopyridine hypnotic) dissolve 1 tab under the tongue; allow to disintegrate completely before swallowing; take only once per night and only if at least 4 hours of bedtime remain before planned time for awakening
   Pediatric: <18 years: not recommended; ≥18 years: same adult
      Edluar *SL Tab:* 5, 10 mg
      Intermezzo *SL Tab:* 1.75, 3.5 mg
Comment: **Edular** is indicated for the treatment of insomnia when a middle-of-the-night awakening is followed by difficulty returning to sleep. The lowest dose of *zolpidem* in all forms is recommended for persons >50 years-of-age and women as drug elimination is slower than in men.

APHTHOUS STOMATITIS (MOUTH ULCER, CANKER SORE)

Comment: Aphthous ulcers are very painful sores with an inflamed base and non-viable tissue in the center that appears bacterial or viral. Although the sores are usually neither bacterial nor viral, herpetiform ulcers are most prevalent among the elderly). The sores may be single round/ovoid or several may be coalesced to form larger lesions, and located under the lip, on the buccal membrane, and/or on the tongue. Poor oral hygiene or an underlying immunity impairment can predispose the patient to ulcer formation (e.g., chronic illness, chemotherapy, poor nutrition, vitamin and mineral deficiencies, allergies, local trauma, stress, tobacco use, inflammatory bowel disease). They are frequently the result of local trauma (e.g., orthodontic-ware, chipped tooth) or allergy/irritation to a toothpaste or mouthwash ingredient (e.g. sodium lauryl sulfate). Changing toothpaste and applying dental wax to sharp edges are recommended until dental care is accessed. Debridement of the nonviable tissue by the direct application of salt (osmotic pulling pressure) for a few minutes, thus leaving a healthy tissue crater, speeds healing. Relief of the offending source of tissue trauma and application of a 5 mg prednisone tablet directly to the debrided ulcer are other remedies with reported success. These sores usually first appear in childhood or adolescence. Family history may have a role in the formation of recurrent aphthous stomatitis (RAS). When cases tend to occur in the same family (est 25-40% of the time), the ulcers earlier and with greater severity.

ANTI-INFLAMMATORY AGENTS

▷ **dexamethasone** elixir **(B)** 5 ml swish and spit q 12 hours
   Pediatric: <12 years: not recommended; ≥12 years: same as adult
      Elix: 0.5 mg/ml

▷ *triamcinolone acetonide* 0.1% dental paste **(G)** press (do <u>not</u> rub) thin film onto lesion at bedtime and, if needed, 2-3 x daily after meals; re-evaluate if no improvement in 7 days

Pediatric: <12 years: not recommended; ≥12 years: same as adult

    Oralone *Dental paste:* 0.1% (5 gm)

▷ *triamcinolone* 1% in **Orabase (B)** apply 1/4 inch to each ulcer bid-qid until ulcer heals

Pediatric: <12 years: not recommended; ≥12 years: same as adult

    Kenalog in Orabase *Crm:* 1% (15, 60, 80 gm)

TOPICAL ANESTHETICS

▷ *benzocaine* topical gel **(C)(G)** apply tid-qid

▷ *benzocaine* topical spray **(C)(G)** 1 spray to painful area every 2 hours as needed; retain for 15 seconds, then spit

    Cepacol Spray (OTC), Chloraseptic Spray (OTC)

▷ *lidocaine* viscous soln **(B)(G)** 15 ml gargle <u>or</u> swish, then spit; repeat after 3 hours; max 8 doses/day

Pediatric: <3 years: not recommended; 3-11 years: 1.25 ml; apply with cotton-tipped applicator; may repeat after 3 hours; max 8 doses/day; ≥12 years: same as adult

    Xylocaine Viscous Solution *Viscous soln:* 2% (20, 100, 450 ml)

▷ *triamcinolone* (**Kenalog**) in **Orabase (C)** apply with swab

DEBRIDING AGENT/CLEANSER

▷ *carbamide peroxide 10%* **(OTC)** apply 10 drops to affected area; swish x 2-3 minutes, then spit; do not rinse; repeat treatment qid

Pediatric: <3 years: not recommended; ≥3 years: same as adult

    Gly-Oxide *Liq:* 10% (50, 60 ml squeeze bottle w. applicator)

ANTI-INFECTIVES

▷ *minocycline* **(D)(G)** swish and spit 10 ml susp (50 mg/5 ml) <u>or</u> 1 x 100 mg cap <u>or</u> 2 x 50 mg caps dissolved in 180 ml water, bid x 4-5 days

Pediatric: <8 years: not recommended; ≥8 years: same as adult

    Dynacin *Cap:* 50, 100 mg

    Minocin *Cap:* 50, 75, 100 mg; *Oral susp:* 50 mg/5 ml (60 ml) (custard) (sulfites, alcohol 5%)

▷ *tetracycline* **(D)** swish and spit 10 ml susp (125 mg/5 ml) <u>or</u> one 250 mg tab/cap dissolved in 180 ml water qid x 4-5 days

Pediatric: <8 years: not recommended; ≥8 years: same as adult; *see page* 646 *for dose by weight*

    Achromycin V *Cap:* 250, 500 mg

    Sumycin *Tab:* 250, 500 mg; *Cap:* 250, 500 mg; *Oral susp:* 125 mg/5 ml (100, 200 ml) (fruit) (sulfites)

ASPERGILLOSIS (*SCEDOSPORIUM APIOSPERMUM, FUSARIUM* SPP.)

INVASIVE INFECTION

▷ *isavuconazonium* **(C)** swallow cap whole; *Loading dose:* 372 mg q 8 hours x 6 doses (48 hours); *Maintenance:* 372 mg once daily starting 12-24 hours after last loading dose

Pediatric: <18 years: not established; ≥18 years: same as adult

    Cresemba *Cap:* 186 mg; *Vial:* 372 mg pwdr for reconstitution (7/blister pck) (preservative-free)

Comment: Cresemba is indicated for the treatment of invasive aspergillus and mucor-mycosis in patients >18-years-old who are at high risk due to being severely compromised.

▷ **posaconazole (D)** take with food; swallow tab whole; *Day 1:* 300 mg bid; then 300 mg once daily for duration of treatment (e.g., resolution of neutropenia <u>or</u> immunosuppression)
Pediatric: <13 years: not recommended; ≥13 years: same as adult
    Noxafil *Tab:* 100 mg del-rel; *Oral susp:* 40 mg/ml (105 oz w. dosing spoon) (cherry)

Comment: Noxafil is indicated as prophylaxis for invasive aspergillus and candida infections in patients >13-years-old who are at high risk due to being severely compromised.

▷ **voriconazole (D)(G)** *PO:* <40 kg: 100 mg q 12 hours; may increase to 150 mg q 12 hours if inadequate response; >40 kg: 200 mg q 12 hours; may increase to 300 mg q 12 hours if inadequate response; *IV:* 6 mg/kg q 12 hours x 2 doses; then 4 mg/kg q 12 hours; max rate 3 mg/kg/hour over 1-2 hours
Pediatric: <12 years: not recommended; ≥12 years: same as adult
Vfend *Tab:* 50, 200 mg
    Vfend I.V. for Injection *Vial:* 200 mg pwdr for reconstitution (preservative-free)
    Vfend *Oral susp:* 40 mg/ml pwdr for reconstitution (75 ml) (orange)

 ASTHMA

Parenteral Corticosteroids *see page* 570
Oral Corticosteroids *see page* 569

INHALED RACEPINEPHRINE (BRONCHODILATOR)

Comment: Inhalation racemic epinephrine is indicated for urgent/emergent acute bronchospasm rescue (e.g., acute asthma attack, laryngospasm, croup, epiglottitis, acute inflammation causing airway obstruction) Inhalational racemic epinephrine is only recommended for use during pregnancy when there are no alternatives and benefit outweighs risk.

▷ **racepinephrine (C)(OTC)(G)** for atomized (nebulizer) treatment.
Pediatric: <4 years: not recommended; ≥4 years: same as adult
    Asthmanefrin *Starter kit:* 10 x 0.5 ml vials 2.25% solution for atomized inhalation w. EZ Breathe Atomizer; *Refills:* 30 x 0.5 ml vials 2.25% solution for atomized inhalation

INHALED BETA-2 AGONISTS (BRONCHODILATORS)

▷ **albuterol sulfate (C)(G)**
    AccuNeb Inhalation Solution 1 unit-dose vial tid-qid prn by nebulizer; ages 2-12 years only; not for adult
Pediatric: <2 years: not recommended; 2-12 years: initially 0.63 mg <u>or</u> 1.25 mg tid-qid; 6-12 years: with severe asthma, <u>or</u> >40 kg, <u>or</u> 11-12 years: initially 1.25 mg tid-qid
    Inhal soln: 0.63, 1.25 mg/3 ml (3 ml, 25/carton) (preservative-free)
    Albuterol Inhalation Solution (G) not recommended for adults
Pediatric: <2 years: not recommended; ≥2 years: 1 vial via nebulizer over 5-15 minutes
    Inhal soln: 0.63 mg/3 ml (0.021%); 1.25 mg/3 ml (0.042%) (25/carton)
    Albuterol Inhalation Solution 0.5% (G) not recommended
Pediatric: <4 years: not recommended; ≥4 years: same as adult
    Inhal soln: 0.083% (25/carton)

Albuterol Nebules (G) 2.5 mg (0.5 ml of 5% diluted to 3 ml with sterile NS or 3 ml of 0.083%) tid-qid
Pediatric: use <12 years: other forms; ≥12 years: same as adult
   Inhal soln: 0.083% (25/carton)
Proair HFA Inhaler 1-2 inhalations q 4-6 hours prn; 2 inhalations 15 minutes before exercise as prophylaxis for exercise-induced asthma (EIA)
Pediatric: <4 years: not established; ≥4 years: same as adult
   Inhaler: 90 mcg/actuation (0.65 gm, 200 inh) (CFC-free)
Proair RespiClick 1-2 inhalations q 4-6 hours prn; 2 inhalations 15-30 minutes before exercise as prophylaxis for exercise-induced asthma (EIA)
Pediatric: <12 years: not established; ≥12 years: same as adult
   Inhaler: 90 mcg/actuation (8.5 gm, 200 inh)
Proventil HFA Inhaler 1-2 inhalations q 4-6 hours prn; 2 inhalations 15 minutes before exercise as prophylaxis for exercise-induced asthma (EIA)
Pediatric: <4 years: use syrup; ≥4 years: same as adult
   Inhaler: 90 mcg/actuation with a dose counter (6.7 gm, 200 inh)
Proventil Inhalation Solution 2.5 mg diluted to 3 ml with normal saline tid-qid prn by nebulizer
Pediatric: use syrup
   Inhal soln: 0.5% (20 ml w. dropper); 0.083% (3 ml; 25/carton)
Ventolin Inhaler 2 inhalations q 4-6 hours prn; 2 inhalations 15 minutes before exercise as prophylaxis for exercise-induced asthma
Pediatric: <2 years: not recommended; 2-4 years: use syrup; ≥4 years: same as adult
   Inhaler: 90 mcg/actuation (17 gm, 220 inh)
Ventolin Rotacaps 1-2 cap inhalations q 4-6 hours prn; 2 inhalations 15 minutes before exercise as prophylaxis for exercise-induced asthma (EIA)
Pediatric: <4 years: not recommended; ≥4 years 1-2 caps q 4-6 hours prn
   Rotacaps: 200 mcg/Rotacaps (100 doses/Rotacaps)
Ventolin 0.5% Inhalation Solution
Pediatric: <2 years: not recommended; ≥2 years: initially 0.1-0.15 mg/kg/dose tid-qid prn; 10-15 kg: 0.25 ml diluted to 3 ml with normal saline by nebulizer tid-qid prn; >15 kg: 0.5 ml diluted to 3 ml with normal saline by nebulizer tid-qid prn
   Inhal soln: 20 ml w. dropper
Ventolin Nebules
Pediatric: <2 years: not recommended; ≥2 years: initially 0.1-0.15 mg/kg/ dose tid-qid prn; 10-15 kg: 1.25 mg or 1/2 nebule tid-qid prn; >15 kg: 2.5 mg or 1 nebule tid-qid prn
   Inhal soln: 0.083% (3 ml; 25/carton)
▷ *isoproterenol* **(B)** *Rescue:* 1 inhalation prn; repeat if no relief in 2-5 minutes;
Maintenance: 1-2 inhalations q 4-6 hours
Pediatric: <12 years: not recommended; ≥12 years: same as adult
   Medihaler-1SO *Inhaler:* 80 mcg/actuation (15 ml, 30 inh)
▷ *levalbuterol tartrate* **(C)(G)** initially 0.63 mg tid q 6-8 hours prn by nebulizer; may increase to 1.25 mg tid at 6-8 hour intervals as needed
Pediatric: <12 years: not recommended; ≥12 years: same as adult
   Xopenex *Inhal soln:* 0.31, 0.63, 1.25 mg/3 ml (24/carton) (preservative-free)
   Xopenex HFA *Inh:* 45 mg (15 gm, 200 inh) (preservative-free)
   Xopenex Concentrate *Vial:* 1.25 mg/0.5 ml (30/carton) (preservative-free)
▷ *metaproterenol* **(C)(G)**
   Alupent 2-3 inhalations tid-qid prn; max 12 inhalations/day
   Pediatric: <6 years: use syrup; ≥6 years: via nebulizer 0.1-0.2 ml diluted with normal saline to 3 ml, up to q 4 hours prn

Inhaler: 0.65 mg/actuation (14 gm, 200 doses)

Alupent Inhalation Solution 5-15 inhalations tid-qid prn; q 4 hours prn for acute attack

Pediatric: <6 years: use syrup ≥6 years: via nebulizer 0.1-0.2 ml diluted with normal saline to 3 ml, up to q 4 hours prn

Inhal soln: 5% (10, 30 ml w. dropper)

▷ *pirbuterol* (C) 1-2 inhalations q 4-6 hours prn; max 12 inhalations/day

Pediatric: <12 years: not recommended; ≥12 years: same as adult

Maxair *Autohaler:* 200 mcg/actuation (14 gm, 400 inh); *Inhaler:* 200 mcg/actuation (25.6 gm, 300 inh)

▷ *terbutaline* (B) 2 inhalations q 4-6 hours prn

Pediatric: <12 years: not recommended; ≥12 years: same as adult

Inhaler: 0.2 mg/actuation (10.5 gm, 300 inh)

INHALED ANTICHOLINERGICS

▷ *ipratropium bromide* (C)(G)

Pediatric: <12 years: not established; ≥12 years: same as adult

Atrovent 2 inhalations qid; additional inhalations as required; max 12 inhalations/day

Inhaler: 18 mcg/actuation (14 gm, 200 inh)

Atrovent Inhalation Solution 500 mcg tid-qid prn by nebulizer

Inhal soln: 0.02% (500 mcg in 2.5 ml; 25/carton)

INHALED CORTICOSTEROIDS

Comment: Inhaled corticosteroids are <u>not</u> for primary (rescue) treatment of acute asthma attack. After every inhalation of a steroid <u>or</u> steroid-containing medication treatment, rinse mouth to reduce risk of oral candidiasis. Inhaled corticosteroids are not for primary (rescue) treatment of acute asthma attack. For twice daily dosing, allow 12 hours between doses.

▷ *beclomethasone dipropionate* (C)(G) *Previously using only bronchodilators:* initiate 40-80 mcg bid; max 320 mcg bid; *Previously using inhaled corticosteroid:* initiate 40-160 mcg bid; max 320 mcg/day; *Previously taking a systemic corticosteroid:* attempt to wean off the systemic drug after approximately 1 week after initiating; rinse mouth after use

Pediatric: <12 years: not recommended; ≥12 years: same as adult

Qvar *Inhal aerosol:* 40, 80 mcg/metered dose actuation (8.7 gm, 120 inh) metered dose inhaler (chlorofluorocarbon [CFC]-free)

▷ *budesonide* (B)

Pulmicort Flexhaler initially 180-360 mcg bid; max 360 mcg bid; rinse mouth after use

Pediatric: <6 years: not recommended; ≥6 years: 1-2 inhalations bid

Flexhaler: 90 mcg/actuation (60 inh); 180 mcg/actuation (120 inh)

Pulmicort Respules (G) adults and ≥8 years: use flexhaler

Pediatric: <12 months: not recommended; 12 months-8 years: *Previously using only bronchodilators:* initiate 0.5 mg/day once daily <u>or</u> in 2 divided doses; may start at 0.25 mg daily; *Previously using inhaled corticosteroids:* initiate 0.5 mg once daily <u>or</u> in 2 divided doses; max 1 mg/day; *Previously taking oral corticosteroids:* initiate 1 mg/day daily <u>or</u> in 2 divided doses; ≥8 years: use flexhaler; rinse mouth after use

Inhal susp: 0.25, 0.5, 1 mg/2 ml (30/carton)

▷ *ciclesonide* (C) initially 80 mcg bid; max 320 mcg/day; rinse mouth after use; *Previously on inhaled corticosteroid:* initially 80 mcg bid; *Previously on oral steroid:* 320 mg bid

Pediatric: <12 years: not recommended; ≥12 years: same as adult

Alvesco *Inhal aerosol:* 80, 160 mcg/actuation (6.1 gm, 60 inh)

➤ *flunisolide* (C) rinse mouth after use

AeroBid, AeroBid-M initially 2 inhalations bid; max 8 inhalations/day; rinse mouth after use
Pediatric: <6 years: not recommended; 6-15 years: 2 inhalations bid; ≥15 years: same as adult
Inhaler: 250 mcg/actuation (7 gm, 100 inh)
Aerospan HFA initially 160 mcg bid; max 320 mcg bid
Pediatric: <6 years: not recommended; 6-11 years: 80 mcg bid; max 160 mcg bid; ≥12 years: same as adult
Inhaler: 80 mcg (5.1 gm, 60 doses; 80 mcg, 120 doses)

➤ *fluticasone furoate* (C) *currently not on inhaled corticosteroid:* usually initiate at 100 mcg once daily at the same time each day; may increase to 200 mcg once daily if inadequate response after 2 weeks; max 200 mcg/day; rinse mouth after use
Pediatric: <12 years: not established; ≥12 years: same as adult
Arnuity Ellipta *Inhal:* 100, 200 mcg/dry pwdr per inhalation (30 doses)
Comment: **Arnuity Ellipta** is not for primary treatment of status asthmaticus or acute asthma episodes. **Arnuity Ellipta** is contraindicated with severe hypersensitivity to milk proteins.

➤ *fluticasone propionate* (C)

ArmorAir 1 inhalation bid (12 hours apart); initially 55 mcg bid; *Previously using an inhaled corticosteroid:* see mfr pkg insert; if insufficient response after 2 weeks, may increase the bid dose; max 232 mcg bid; after stability achieved, titrate to lowest effective dose; do not use with spacer or volume-holding chamber
Pediatric: <12 years: not established; ≥12 years: same as adult
Inhaler: 55, 113, 232 mcg/actuation (60 inh)
Flovent, Flovent HFA initially 88 mcg bid; *Previously using an inhaled corticosteroid:* initially 88-220 mcg bid; *Previously taking an oral corticosteroid:* 880 mcg bid; rinse mouth after use
Pediatric: <11 years: use **Flovent Diskus** ≥12 years: same as adult
Inhaler: 44 mcg/actuation (7.9 gm, 60 inh; 13 gm, 120 inh); 110 mcg/actuation (13 gm, 120 inh); 220 mcg/actuation (13 gm, 120 inh)
Flovent Diskus initially 100 mcg bid; max 500 mcg bid; *Previously using an inhaled corticosteroid:* initially 100-250 mcg bid; max 500 mcg bid; *Previously taking an oral corticosteroid:* 1000 mcg bid
Pediatric: <4 years: not recommended; 4-11 years: initially 50 mcg bid; max 100 mcg bid; rinse mouth after use; ≥12 years: same as adult
Diskus: 50, 100, 250 mcg/inh dry pwdr (60 blisters w. diskus)

➤ *mometasone furoate* (C) 220-440 mcg once daily or bid; max 880 mcg/day; rinse mouth after use
Asmanex HFA *Inhaler:* 100, 200 mcg/actuation (13 gm, 120 inh)
Pediatric: <12 years: not established; ≥12 years: same as adult
Asmanex Twisthaler *Inhaler:* 110 mcg/actuation (30 inh), 220 mcg/actuation (30, 60, 120 inh)
Pediatric: <4 years: not recommended; 4-11 years: 110 mcg once daily in the PM; >12 years: may use **Asmanex HFA**; rinse mouth after use

➤ *triamcinolone* (C)

Azmacort 2 inhalations tid-qid or 4 inhalations bid; rinse mouth after use
Pediatric: <6 years: not recommended; 6-12 years: 1-2 inhalations tid or 2-4 inhalations bid; >12 years: same as adult
Inhaler: 100 mcg/actuation (20 gm, 240 inh)

LEUKOTRIENE RECEPTOR ANTAGONISTS (LRAS)

Comment: The LRAs are indicated for prophylaxis and chronic treatment, only. Not for primary (rescue) treatment of acute asthma attack.

▷ *montelukast* (B)(G) 10 mg once daily in the PM; for EIB, take at least 2 hours before exercise; max 1 dose/day
Pediatric: <12 months: not recommended; 12-23 months: one 4 mg granule pkt daily; 2-5 years: one 4 mg chew tab or granule pkt daily; 6-14 years: one 5 mg chew tab daily; ≥15 years: same as adult
  Singulair *Tab:* 10 mg
  Singulair Chewable *Chew tab:* 4, 5 mg (cherry) (phenylalanine)
  Singulair Oral Granules *Granules:* 4 mg/pkt; take within 15 minutes of opening pkt; may mix with applesauce, carrots, rice, or ice cream
▷ *zafirlukast* (B) 20 mg bid, 1 hour ac or 2 hours pc
Pediatric: <7 years: not recommended; 7-11 years: 10 mg bid 1 hour ac or 2 hours pc; ≥12 years: same as adult
  Accolate *Tab:* 10, 20 mg
▷ *zileuton* (C)(G)
Pediatric: <12 years: not recommended; ≥12 years: same as adult
  Zyflo 1 tab qid (total 2400 mg/day)
    Tab: 600 mg
  Zyflo CR 2 tabs bid (total 2400 mg/day)
    Tab: 600 mg ext-rel

IGE BLOCKER (IGG1K MONOCLONAL ANTIBODY)

▷ *omalizumab* (B) 150-375 mg SC every 2-4 weeks based on body weight and pre-treatment serum total IgE level; max 150 mg/injection site
Pediatric: <12 years: not recommended; 30-90 kg + IgE >30-100 IU/ml 150 mg q 4 weeks; 90-150 kg + IgE >30-100 IU/ml or 30-90 kg + IgE >100-200 IU/ml or 30-60 kg + IgE >200-300 IU/ml 300 mg q 4 hours; >90-150 kg + IgE >100-200 IU/ml or >60-90 kg + IgE >200-300 IU/ml or 30-70 kg + IgE >300-400 IU/ml 225 mg q 2 weeks; >90-150 kg + IgE >200-300 IU/ml or >70-90 kg + IgE >300-400 IU/ml or 30-70 kg + IgE >400-500 IU/ml or 30-60 kg + IgE >500-600 IU/ml or 30-60 kg + IgE >600-700 IU/ml 375 mg q 2 weeks
  Xolair *Vial:* 150 mg pwdr for SC injection after reconstitution (preservative-free)

INHALED MAST CELL STABILIZERS (PROPHYLAXIS)

Comment: IMCSs are for prophylaxis and chronic treatment, only. Not for primary (rescue) treatment of acute asthma attack.
▷ *cromolyn sodium* (B)(G)
  Intal 2 inhalations qid; 2 inhalations up to 10-60 minutes before precipitant as prophylaxis; rinse mouth after use
  Pediatric: <2 years: not recommended; 2-5 years: use inhal soln via nebulizer; >5 years: 2 inhalations qid via inhaler
    Inhaler: 0.8 mg/actuation (8.1, 14.2 gm; 112, 200 inh)
  Intal Inhalation Solution 20 mg by nebulizer qid; 20 mg up to 10-60 minutes before precipitant as prophylaxis
  Pediatric: <2 years: not recommended; ≥2 years: same as adult
    Inhal soln: 20 mg/2 ml (60, 120/carton)
▷ *nedocromil sodium* (B)
  Tilade 2 sprays qid; rinse mouth after use
    Pediatric: <6 years: not recommended; ≥6 years: 2 sprays qid
    Inhaler: 1.75 mg/spray (16.2 gm; 104 sprays)
  Tilade Nebulizer Solution 0.5% 1 amp qid by nebulizer
    Pediatric: <2 years: not recommended; ≥2 years: initially 1 amp qid by nebulizer; 2-5 years: initially 1 amp tid by nebulizer; ≥5 years: same as adult
    Inhal soln: 11 mg/2.2 ml (2 ml; 60, 120/carton)

INHALED LONG-ACTING ANTICHOLINERGIC

▷ *tiotropium (as bromide monohydrate)* (C) 2 inhalations once daily using inhalation device; do not swallow caps

Pediatric: <12 years: not recommended; ≥12 years: same as adult

    Spiriva HandiHaler *Inhal device:* 18 mcg/cap pwdr for inhalation (5, 30, 90 caps w. inhalation device)

    Spiriva Respimat *Inhal device:* 1.25, 2.5 mcg/actuation cartridge w. inhalation device (4 gm, 60 metered actuations) (benzylkonian chloride)

Comment: *tiotropium* is for prophylaxis and chronic treatment, only. Not for primary (rescue) treatment of acute attack. Avoid getting powder in eyes. Caution with narrow-angle glaucoma, BPH, bladder neck obstruction, and pregnancy. Contraindicated with allergy to *atropine* or its derivatives (e.g., *ipratropium*).

INHALED ANTICHOLINERGIC+BETA-2 AGONIST

▷ *ipratropium bromide+albuterol sulfate* (C) 2 inhalations qid

Pediatric: <12 years: not recommended; ≥12 years: same as adult

    Combivent 2 inhalations qid; additional inhalations as required; max 12 inhalations/day

      Inhaler: ipra 18 mcg+albu 90 mcg/actuation (14.7 gm, 200 inh)

    Duoneb 1 vial via nebulizer 4-6 times daily prn

      Inhal soln: ipra 0.5 mg (0.017%)+albu 2.5 mg (0.083%) per 3 ml (23/carton)

INHALED LONG-ACTING BETA-2 AGONIST (LABA)

Comment: LABA agents are not for primary (rescue) treatment of acute asthma attack. For twice daily dosing, allow 12 hours between doses.

▷ *arformoterol* (C) 15 mcg bid via nebulizer

Pediatric: <12 years: not recommended; ≥12 years: same as adult

    Brovana *Inhal soln:* 15 mcg/2 ml (2 ml; 30/carton)

Comment: *arformoterol* is indicated for the treatment of COPD but is used off-label for the treatment of asthma. It is used for prophylaxis and chronic treatment, only. Not for primary (rescue) treatment of acute attack.

▷ *formoterol fumarate* (C)

    Foradil Aerolizer 12 mcg q 12 hours

Pediatric: <5 years: not recommended; ≥5 years: same as adult

      Inhaler: 12 mcg/cap (12, 60 caps w. device)

    Perforomist 20 mcg q 12 hours

Pediatric: <12 years: not recommended; ≥12 years: same as adult

      Inhal soln: 20 mcg/2 ml (60/carton)

Comment: *formoterol* is for prophylaxis and chronic treatment, only. Not for primary (rescue) treatment of acute attack. Do not mix *formoterol* with other drugs. Use of *formoterol* is off-label for asthma.

▷ *olodaterol* (C) 12 mcg q 12 hours

Pediatric: <12 years: not established; ≥12 years: same as adult

    Striverdi Respimat

      Inhal soln: 2.5 mcg/cartridge (metered actuation) (40 gm, 60 metered actuations) (benzalkonium chloride)

Comment: **Striverdi Respimat** is contraindicated in persons with asthma without concomitant use of long-term control medication.

▷ *salmeterol* (C)(G) 2 inhalations q 12 hours prn; 2 inhalations at least 30-60 minutes before exercise as prophylaxis for exercise-induced asthma; do not use extra doses for exercise-induced bronchospasm if already using regular dose

Pediatric: <4 years: not recommended; ≥4 years: 1 inhalation q 12 hours prn; 1
inhalation at least 30-60 minutes before exercise as prophylaxis for exercise-induced
asthma; do not use extra doses for exercise-induced bronchospasm if already using
regular drug
> **Serevent Diskus**
> *Diskus (pwdr):* 50 mcg/actuation (60 doses/disk)

INHALED CORTICOSTEROID+LONG-ACTING BETA-2 AGONIST (LABA)

Comment: Inhaled corticosteroids and LABA agents are not for primary (rescue)
treatment of acute asthma attack. For twice daily dosing, allow 12 hours between doses.
After every inhalation of a steroid or steroid-containing medication treatment, rinse
mouth to reduce risk of oral candidiasis.

▷ *budesonide+formoterol* **(C)** 1 inhalation bid; rinse mouth after use
   Pediatric: <12 years: not established; ≥12 years: same as adult
> **Symbicort 80/4.5**
> *Inhaler:* bud 80 mcg+for 4.5 mcg
> **Symbicort 160/4.5**
> *Inhaler:* bud 160 mcg+for 4.5 mcg

▷ *fluticasone propionate+salmeterol* **(C)**
   Advair HFA *Not previously using inhaled steroid:* start with 2 inh 45/21 or 115/21 bid;
   if insufficient response after 2 weeks, use next higher strength; max 2 inh 230/50 bid;
   allow 12 hours between doses; *Already using inhaled steroid;* see mfr pkg insert
> **Advair HFA 45/21** 1 inhalation bid; rinse mouth after use
> *Pediatric:* <12 years: not recommended; ≥12 years: same as adult
>> *Inhaler:* flu pro 45 mcg+sal 21 mcg/actuation (CFC-free)
> **Advair HFA 115/21** 1 inhalation bid; rinse mouth after use
> *Pediatric:* <12 years: not established; ≥12 years: same as adult
>> *Inhaler:* flu pro 115 mcg+sal 21 mcg/actuation (CFC-free)
> **Advair HFA 230/21** 1 inhalation bid; rinse mouth after use
> *Pediatric:* <12 years: not established; ≥12 years: same as adult
>> *Inhaler:* flu pro 230 mcg+sal 21 mcg/actuation (CFC-free)
> **Advair Diskus** *Not previously using inhaled steroid:* start with 1 inh 100/50 bid;
> *Already using inhaled steroid:* see mfr pkg insert; rinse mouth after use
> **Advair Diskus 100/50** 1 inhalation bid; rinse mouth after use
> *Pediatric:* <4 years: not recommended; 4-11 years: 1 bid; >11 years: 1 inhalation
> bid
>> *Diskus:* flu pro 100 mcg+sal 50 mcg/actuation (60 blisters)
> **Advair Diskus 250/50** 1 inhalation bid; rinse mouth after use
> *Pediatric:* <4 years: not recommended; 4-12 years: use 100/50 strength; >12 years:
> same as adult
>> *Diskus:* flu pro 250 mcg+sal 50 mcg/actuation (60 blisters)
> **Advair Diskus 500/50** 1 inhalation bid; rinse mouth after use
> *Pediatric:* <4 years: not recommended; 4-12 years: use 100/50 strength; >12 years:
> same as adult
>> *Diskus:* flu pro 500 mcg+sal 50 mcg/actuation (60 blisters)
> **AirDuo RespiClick** pwdr for oral inhalation; *Not previously using an inhaled*
> *steroid:* 1 inh 55/14 bid; *Already using an inhaled steroid:* see mfr pkg insert; if insuf-
> ficient response after 2 weeks, titrate with a higher strength; max inh 232/14 bid
> *Pediatric:* <12 years: not established; ≥12 years: same as adult
>> **AirDuo RespiClick 55/14** flu pro 55 mcg+sal (as xinafoate) 14 mcg dry pwdr/
>> actuation (60 actuations)
>> **AirDuo RespiClick 113/14** flu pro 113 mcg+sal (as xinafoate) 14 mcg dry pwdr/
>> actuation (60 actuations)

AirDuo RespiClick 232/14 flu pro 232 mcg+sal (as xinafoate) 14 mcg dry pwdr/
actuation (60 actuations)

▷ *fluticasone furoate+vilanterol* (C) 1 inhalation 100/25 once daily at the same time
each day
Pediatric: <17 years: not established; ≥17 years: same as adult
  Breo Ellipta
    Breo Ellipta 100/25 flu 100 mcg+vil 25 mcg dry pwdr per inhalation (30 doses)
    Breo Ellipta 200/25 flu 200 mcg+vil 25 mcg dry pwdr per inhalation (30 doses)
Comment: **Breo Ellipta** is contraindicated with severe hypersensitivity to milk proteins.

▷ *mometasone furoate+formoterol fumarate* (C) 2 inhalations bid; rinse mouth after
use
Pediatric: <12 years: not established; ≥12 years: same as adult
  Dulera
    Dulera 100/5 *Inhaler:* mom 100 mcg/for 5 mcg (HFA)
    Dulera 200/5 *Inhaler:* mom 200 mcg/for 5 mcg (HFA)
Comment: **Dulera** is not a rescue inhaler.

INHALED ANTICHOLINERGIC+LONG-ACTING BETA-2 AGONIST (LABA)

▷ *glycopyrrolate+formoterol fumarate* (C) 2 inhalations bid (AM & PM)
Pediatric: <18 years: not established; ≥18 years: same as adult
    Bevespi Aerosphere 9/4.8 *Metered dose inhaler:* gly 9 mcg+for 4.8 mcg/inhalation
    (10.7 gm, 120 inh)

ORAL BETA-2 AGONISTS (BRONCHODILATORS)

▷ *albuterol* (C)
    Albuterol Syrup (G) *Adult:* 2-4 mg tid-qid; may increase gradually; max 8 mg qid;
    Elderly: initially 2-3 mg tid-qid; may increase gradually; max 8 mg qid
    Pediatric: <2 years: not recommended; ≥2-6 years: 0.1 mg/kg tid; initially max 2
    mg tid; may increase gradually to 0.2 mg/kg tid; max 4 mg tid; >6-12 years: 2 mg
    tid-qid; may increase gradually; max 6 mg qid; ≥12 years: same as adult
      Syr: 2 mg/5 ml
    Proventil 2-4 mg tid-qid prn
    Pediatric: <6 years: not recommended; ≥6 years: same as adult
      Tab: 2, 4 mg
    Proventil Repetabs 4-8 mg q 12 hours prn
    Pediatric: use syrup
      Repetab: 4 mg sust-rel
    Proventil Syrup 5-10 ml tid-qid prn; may increase gradually; max 20 ml qid prn
    Pediatric: <2 years: not recommended; ≥2-6 years: 0.1 mg/kg tid prn; max initially
    5 ml tid prn; may increase gradually to 0.2 mg/kg tid prn; max 10 ml tid; >6-14
    years: 5 ml tid-qid prn; may increase gradually; max 60 ml/day in divided doses;
    >14 years: same as adult
      Syr: 2 mg/5 ml
    Ventolin 2-4 mg tid-qid prn; may increase gradually; max 8 mg qid
    Pediatric: <2 years: not recommended; ≥2-6 years: 0.1 mg/kg tid prn; max initially
    2 mg tid prn; may increase gradually to 0.2 mg/kg tid; max 4 mg tid; >6-14 years:
    2 mg tid-qid prn; may increase gradually; max 6 mg tid
      Tab: 2, 4 mg; *Syr:* 2 mg/5 ml (strawberry)
    VoSpire ER 4-8 mg q 12 hours prn; max 32 mg/day divided q 12 hours; swallow
    whole; do <u>not</u> crush or chew
    Pediatric: <6 years: not recommended; ≥6-12 years: 4 mg q 12 hours; max 24 mg/
    day q 12 hours; >12 years: same as adult
      Tab: 4, 8 mg ext-rel

▷ *metaproterenol* (C) 20 mg tid-qid prn
  Pediatric: <6 years: not recommended (doses of 1.3-2.6 mg/kg/day have been used);
  ≥6-9 years (<60 lb): 10 mg tid-qid prn; >9-12 years (>60 lb): 20 mg tid-qid prn; >12
  years: same as adult
    Alupent *Tab:* 10, 20 mg; *Syr:* 10 mg/5 ml

METHYLXANTHINES

Comment: Check serum theophylline level just before 5th dose is administered.
Therapeutic theophylline level: 10-20 mcg/ml.
▷ *theophylline* (C)(G)
    Theo-24 initially 300-400 mg once daily at HS; after 3 days, increase to 400-600
    mg once daily at HS; max 600 mg/day
    Pediatric: <45 kg: initially 12-14 mg/kg/day; max 300 mg/day; increase after 3
    days to 16 mg/kg/day to max 400 mg; after 3 more days increase to 30 mg/kg/day
    to max 600 mg/day; ≥45 kg: same as adult
      Cap: 100, 200, 300, 400 mg ext-rel
    Theo-Dur initially 150 mg bid; increase to 200 mg bid after 3 days; then to 300 mg
    bid after 3 more days
    Pediatric: <6 years: not recommended; 6-15 years: initially 12-14 mg/kg/day in
    2 divided doses; max 300 mg/day; then increase to 16 mg/kg in 2 divided doses;
    max 400 mg/day; then to 20 mg/kg/day in 2 divided doses; max 600 mg/day; ≥15
    years: same as adult
      Tab: 100, 200, 300 mg ext-rel
    Theolair-SR
    Pediatric: not recommended
      Tab: 200, 250, 300, 500 mg sust-rel
    Uniphyl 400-600 mg daily with meals
    Pediatric: not recommended
      Tab: 400*, 600*mg cont-rel

METHYLXANTHINE+EXPECTORANT COMBINATION

▷ *dyphylline+guaifenesin* (C) 1 tab qid
    Lufyllin GG *Tab:* *dyphy* 200 mg+*guaif* 200 mg; *Elix:* *dyphy* 100 mg+*guaif* 100 mg
    per 15 ml

HUMANIZED INTERLEUKIN-5 ANTAGONIST MONOCLONAL ANTIBODY

▷ *mepolizumab* 100 mg SC once every 4 weeks in upper arm, abdomen, or thigh
  Pediatric: <12 years: not recommended; ≥12 years: same as adult
    Nucala *Vial:* 100 mg pwdr for reconstitution, single-use (preservative-free)
    Comment: **Nucala** is an add-on maintenance treatment for severe asthma. There
    is a pregnancy exposure registry that monitors pregnancy outcomes in women
    exposed to **Nucala** during pregnancy. Healthcare providers can enroll patients
    or encourage patients to enroll themselves by calling 1-877-311-8972 or visiting
    www.mothertobaby.org/asthma.

 ASTHMA-COPD OVERLAP SYNDROME (ACOS)

Comment: An estimated 16% of patients with asthma or COPD have asthma- COPD
overlap syndrome (ACOS), a poorly understood disease with an increasing morbidity
and mortality. PROSPRO (Prospective Study to Evaluate Predictors of Clinical
Effectiveness in Response to Omalizumab), a 48-week, prospective, multicenter,

observational study, included patients (n= 806) who were 12 years-of-age and older who were initiating *omalizumab* treatment for moderate to severe allergic asthma, including patient with co-morbid COPD (n=78). Researchers reported that *omalizumab* (**Xolair**) decreased asthma exacerbations and improved symptom control to a similar extent in patients with ACOS as seen in patients with asthma but no COPD. While patients with COPD typically experience annual declines in lung function, at least some of the ACOS patients in this study, which included one of the largest observational cohorts to date of patients with ACOS, showed preserved lung function after 48 weeks of *omalizumab* treatment (as demonstrated by improved post-bronchodilator FEV$_1$ at end of stud and asthma exacerbations numbers reduced from baseline though month 12, from 3 or more exacerbations in both ACOS and non-ACOS groups to 1.1 or less

REFERENCE

Hanania, N. (2017, November). *Omalizumab helps asthma COPD overlap patients.* Presented at the 2017 CHEST Annual Meeting in Toronto, Canada, as reported by Beck, DL. Family Practice News. http://www.mdedge.com/familypracticenews/article/151778/copd/omalizumab-helps-asthma-copd-overlap-patients?channel=41038&utm_source=News_FPN_eNL_111617_F&utm_medium=email&utm_content=Omalizumab for asthma COPD overlap patients

IGE BLOCKER (IGG1K MONOCLONAL ANTIBODY)

▷ *omalizumab* (B) 150-375 mg SC every 2-4 weeks based on body weight and pre-treatment serum total IgE level; max 150 mg/injection site
Pediatric: <12 years: not recommended; 30-90 kg + IgE >30-100 IU/ml 150 mg q 4 weeks; 90-150 kg + IgE >30-100 IU/ml or 30-90 kg + IgE >100-200 IU/ml or 30-60 kg + IgE >200-300 IU/ml 300 mg q 4 hours; >90-150 kg + IgE >100-200 IU/ml or >60-90 kg + IgE >200-300 IU/ml or 30-70 kg + IgE >300-400 IU/ml 225 mg q 2 weeks; >90-150 kg + IgE >200-300 IU/ml or >70-90 kg + IgE >300-400 IU/ml or 30-70 kg + IgE >400-500 IU/ml or 30-60 kg + IgE >500-600 IU/ml or 30-60 kg + IgE >600-700 IU/ml 375 mg q 2 weeks
  Xolair *Vial:* 150 mg pwdr for SC injection after reconstitution (preservative-free)

ASTHMA, SEVERE EOSINOPHILIA

Comment: *tezepelumab* is a human IgG2 monoclonal antibody that binds to thymic stromal lymphopoietin (TSLP), which is a cytokine produced in response to environmental and pro-inflammatory stimuli. It is an important potential mechanism because it works high up in the inflammatory cascade appears to have a beneficial effect in patients across different asthma phenotypes. Currently available therapies for patients with severe asthma include anti-IgE therapy (*omalizumab*), and anti-interleukin-5 monoclonal antibodies (*mepolizumab* and *reslizumab*, which are FDA approved, and *benralizumab* which is currently being evaluated by the FDA).

HUMANIZED INTERLEUKIN-5 ANTAGONIST MONOCLONAL ANTIBODY

▷ *mepolizumab* 100 mg SC once every 4 weeks in upper arm, abdomen, or thigh
Pediatric: <12 years: not recommended; ≥12 years: same as adult
  Nucala *Vial:* 100 mg pwdr for reconstitution, single-use (preservative-free)
Comment: **Nucala** is an add-on maintenance treatment for severe asthma. There is a pregnancy exposure registry that monitors pregnancy outcomes in women exposed to **Nucala** during pregnancy. Healthcare providers can enroll patients or encourage patients to enroll themselves by calling 1-877-311-8972 or visiting www.mothertobaby.org/asthma.

IGE BLOCKER (IGG1K MONOCLONAL ANTIBODY)

▷ *omalizumab* (B) 150-375 mg SC every 2-4 weeks based on body weight and pre-treatment serum total IgE level; max 150 mg/injection site
Pediatric: <12 years: not recommended; 30-90 kg + IgE >30-100 IU/ml 150 mg q 4 weeks; 90-150 kg + IgE >30-100 IU/ml or 30-90 kg + IgE >100-200 IU/ml or 30-60 kg + IgE >200-300 IU/ml 300 mg q 4 hours; >90-150 kg + IgE >100-200 IU/ml or >60-90 kg + IgE >200-300 IU/ml or 30-70 kg + IgE >300-400 IU/ml 225 mg q 2 weeks; >90-150 kg + IgE >200-300 IU/ml or >70-90 kg + IgE >300-400 IU/ml or 30-70 kg + IgE >400-500 IU/ml or 30-60 kg + IgE >500-600 IU/ml or 30-60 kg + IgE >600-700 IU/ml 375 mg q 2 weeks
Xolair *Vial:* 150 mg pwdr for SC injection after reconstitution (preservative-free)

 ATROPHIC VAGINITIS

Oral Estrogens *see* **Menopause** *page* 295

VAGINAL ESTROGEN PREPARATIONS

▷ *estradiol* (X)(G)
Vagifem Vaginal Tablet 1 tab intravaginally daily x 2 weeks; then 1 tab intravaginally twice weekly
Vag tab: 10 mcg (15 tabs w. applicators)
Yuvafem Vaginal Tablet 1 tab intravaginally daily x 2 weeks; then 1 tab intravaginally twice weekly
Vag tab: 10 mcg (15 tabs w. applicators)
▷ *estradiol* (X)
Estrace Vaginal Cream 2-4 gm daily x 1-2 weeks; then gradually reduce to 1/2 initial dose x 1-2 weeks; then maintenance dose of 1 gm 1-3 x/week
Vag crm: 0.01% (1 oz tube w. calib applicator)
▷ *estrogens, conjugated* (X)
Premarin Cream 2 gm/day intravaginally
Vag crm: 1.5 oz w. applicator marked in 1/2 gm increments to max 2 gm
▷ *estropipate* (X)
Ogen Cream 2-4 gm intravaginally daily x 3 weeks; discontinue 4th week; continue in this cyclical pattern
Vag crm: 1.5 mg/gm (42.5 gm w. calib applicator)

 ATTENTION DEFICIT HYPERACTIVITY DISORDER (ADHD)

SELECTIVE NOREPINEPHRINE REUPTAKE INHIBITORS (SNRIs)

▷ *atomoxetine* (C)(G) take one dose daily in the morning or in two divided doses in the morning and late afternoon or early evening; initially 40 mg/kg; increase after at least 3 days to 80 mg/kg; then after 2-4 weeks may increase to max 100 mg/day
Pediatric: <6 years: not recommended; ≥6 years, <70 kg: initially 0.5 mg/kg/day: increase after at least 3 days to 1.2 mg/kg/day; max 1.4 mg/kg/day or 100 mg/day (whichever is less); ≥6 years, >70 kg: same as adult
Strattera *Cap:* 10, 18, 25, 40, 60, 80, 100 mg
Comment: **Strattera** is not associated with stimulant or euphoric effects. May discontinue without tapering. Common adverse effects associated with *atomoxetine* in children and adolescents included upset stomach, decreased appetite, nausea or vomiting, dizziness, tiredness, and mood swings. For adult patients, the most common adverse side effects included constipation, dry mouth, nausea, decreased appetite, sexual side effects, problems passing urine, and dizziness. Other adverse

effects associated with *atomoxetine* included severe liver damage and potential for serious cardiovascular events. In addition, *atomoxetine* increases the risk of suicidal ideation in children and adolescents. Health Care providers should monitor patients taking this medication for clinical worsening, suicidality, and unusual changes in behavior, particularly within the first few months of initiation or during dose changes.

STIMULANTS

▷ *amphetamine, mixed salts of single entity amphetamine* (C)(II)

> **Adzenys ER** initially 12.5 mg (10 ml) once daily in the morning; take with or without food; individualize the dosage according to the therapeutic needs and response
>
> **Pediatric:** <6 years: not recommended; 6-17 years: take with or without food; individualize the dosage according to the therapeutic needs and response; 6-12 years: initially 6.3 mg (5 ml) once daily in the morning; max dose 18.8 mg (15 ml); 13-17 years:12.5 mg (10 ml) once daily in the morning; ≥17 years: same as adult
>
> *Oral susp:* 125 mg/ml ext-rel (450 ml) (orange)

Comment: Patients taking **Adderall XR** may be switched to **Adzenys ER** at the equivalent dose taken once daily; switching from any other amphetamine products (e.g., **Adderall** immediate-release), discontinue that treatment, and titrate with **Adzenys ER** using the titration schedule (see mfr pkg insert). To avoid substitution errors and overdosage, do not substitute for other amphetamine products on a mg-per-mg basis because of different amphetamine salt compositions and differing pharmacokinetic profiles. No dosage adjustments for renal or hepatic insufficiency are provided in the manufacturer's labeling.

> **Adzenys XR-ODT** take with or without food; individualize the dosage according to the therapeutic needs and response; initially 12.5 mg once daily; max recommended dose 18.8 mg once daily
>
> *Pediatric:* <6 years: not recommended; ≥6 years: take with or without food; individualize the dosage according to the therapeutic needs and response; 6-12 years: initially 6.3 mg once daily in the morning; increase in increments of 3.1 mg or 6.3 mg at weekly intervals; max recommended dose 18.8 mg once daily; ≥13 years: 12.5 mg (10 ml) once daily in the morning

Comment: Patients taking **Adderall XR** may be switched to **Adzenys XR-ODT** at the equivalent dose taken once daily; switching from any other amphetamine products (e.g., **Adderall** immediate-release), discontinue that treatment, and titrate with **Adzenys XR-ODT** using the titration schedule (see mfr pkg insert). To avoid substitution errors and overdosage, do not substitute for other amphetamine products on a mg-per-mg basis because of different amphetamine salt compositions and differing pharmacokinetic profiles. No dosage adjustments for renal or hepatic insufficiency are provided in the manufacturer's labeling.

> *ODT:* 3.1, 6.3, 9.4, 12.5, 15.7, 18.8 mg orally-disint ext-rel (orange) (fructose)
>
> **Dyanavel XR Oral Suspension** <6 years: not recommended; ≥6 years: initially 2.5 mg or 5 mg once daily in the morning; may increase in increments of 2.5 mg to 5 mg per day every 4-7 days; max 20 mg per day; shake bottle prior to administration
>
> *Oral susp:* 2.5 mg/ml (464 ml) ext-rel
>
> **Evekeo** <3 years: not recommended; ≥3-5 years: initially 2.5 mg once or twice daily at the same time(s) each day; may increase by 2.5 mg/day at weekly intervals; max 40 mg/day; >5 years: initially 5 mg once or twice daily at the same time(s) each day; may increase by 5 mg/day at weekly intervals; max 40 mg/day
>
> *Tab:* 5, 10 mg

Mydayis initially 12.5 mg once daily in the morning; may titrate at weekly intervals; max 50 mg/day

Pediatric: <13 years: not recommended; 13-17 years: initially 12.5 mg once daily in the morning; may titrate at weekly intervals; max 25 mg/day; >17 years: same as adult

Cap: 12.5, 25, 37.5, 50 mg ext-rel

▷ *dexmethylphenidate* (C)(II)(G) not indicated for adults

Focalin <6 years: not established; ≥6 years: initially 2.5 mg bid; allow at least 4 hours between doses; may increase at 1 week intervals; max 20 mg/day

Tab: 2.5, 5, 10*mg (dye-free)

Focalin ER <6 years: not established; ≥6 years: initially 5 mg weekly; usual dose 10-30 mg/day

Cap: 15, 30 mg ext-rel

Focalin XR <6 years: not established; ≥6 years: initially 5 mg weekly; usual dose 10-30 mg/day

Cap: 5, 10, 15, 20, 25, 30, 35, 40 mg ext-rel

▷ *dextroamphetamine sulfate* (C)(II)(G) initially start with 10 mg daily; increase by 10 mg at weekly intervals if needed; may switch to daily dose with sust-rel spansules when titrated

Pediatric: <3 years: not recommended; ≥3-5 years: 2.5 mg daily; may increase by 2.5 mg daily at weekly intervals if needed; 6-12 years: initially 5 mg daily or bid; may increase by 5 mg/day at weekly intervals; usual max 40 mg/day; >12 years: initially 10 mg daily; may increase by 10 mg/day at weekly intervals; max 40 mg/day

Dexedrine *Tab:* 5*mg (tartrazine)

Dexedrine Spansule *Cap:* 5, 10, 15 mg ext-rel

Dextrostat *Tab:* 5, 10 mg (tartrazine)

▷ *dextroamphetamine saccharate+dextroamphetamine sulfate+amphetamine aspartate+amphetamine sulfate* (C)(II)(G) not indicated for adults

Adderall initially 10 mg daily; may increase weekly by 10 mg/day; usual max 60 mg/day in 2-3 divided doses; first dose on awakening; then q 4-6 hours prn

Pediatric: <6 years: not indicated; ≥6-12 years: initially 5 mg daily; may increase by 5 mg/day at weekly intervals; >12 years: same as adult

Tab: 5**, 7.5**, 10**, 12.5**, 15**mg, 20**, 30**mg

Adderall XR 20 mg by mouth once daily in AM; may increase by 10 mg/day at weekly intervals; max: 60 mg/day

Pediatric: <6 years: not recommended; ≥6 years: initially 10 mg daily in the AM; may increase by 10 mg/day at weekly intervals; max 30 mg/day; 13-17 years: 10-20 mg by mouth daily in the AM; may increase by 10 mg/day at weekly intervals; max 40 mg/day; Do not chew; may sprinkle on apple sauce

Cap: 5, 10, 15, 20, 25, 30 mg ext-rel

▷ *lisdexamfetamine dimesylate* (C)(II) 30 mg once daily in the AM; may increase by 10-20 mg/day at weekly intervals; max 70 mg/day

Pediatric: <6 years: not recommended; ≥6 years: same as adult

Vyvanse *Cap:* 20, 30, 40, 50, 60, 70 mg

Comment: May dissolve **Vyvanse** capsule contents in water; take immediately.

▷ *methylphenidate (regular-acting)* (C)(II)(G)

Methylin, Methylin Chewable, Methylin Oral Solution usual dose 20-30 mg/day in 2-3 divided doses 30-45 minutes before a meal; max 60 mg/day

Pediatric: <6 years: not recommended; ≥6 years: initially 5 mg bid ac (breakfast and lunch); may increase 5-10 mg/day at weekly intervals; max 60 mg/day

Tab: 5, 10*, 20*mg; *Chew tab:* 2.5, 5, 10 mg; (grape) (phenylalanine); *Oral soln:* 5, 10 mg/5 ml (grape)

Ritalin 10-60 mg/day in 2-3 divided doses 30-45 minutes ac; max 60 mg/day

Pediatric: <6 years: not recommended; ≥6 years: initially 5 mg bid ac (breakfast and lunch); may increase by 5-10 mg at weekly intervals as needed; max 60 mg/day
>   *Tab:* 5, 10*, 20*mg

▷ *methylphenidate (long-acting)* (C)(II)

Concerta initially 18 mg q AM; may increase in 18 mg increments as needed; max 54 mg/day; do <u>not</u> crush <u>or</u> chew
Pediatric: <6 years: not recommended; ≥6-12 years: initially 18 mg daily; max 54 mg/day; ≥13-17 years: initially 18 mg daily; max 72 mg/day <u>or</u> 2 mg/kg, whichever is less
>   *Tab:* 18, 27, 36, 54 mg sust-rel

Cotempla XR-ODT take consistently with <u>or</u> without food in the morning
Pediatric: <6 years: not recommended; 6-17 years: initially 8.6 mg; may increase as needed and tolerated by 8.6 mg/day; Daily dosage >51.8 mg is not recommended.
>   *ODT:* 8.6, 17.3, 25.9 mg ext-rel orally-disint

Metadate CD (G) 1 cap daily in the AM; may sprinkle on food; do <u>not</u> crush <u>or</u> chew
Pediatric: <6 years: not recommended; ≥6 years: initially 20 mg daily; may gradually increase by 20 mg/day at weekly intervals as needed; max 60 mg/day
>   *Cap:* 10, 20, 30, 40, 50, 60 mg immed- and ext-rel beads

Metadate ER 1 tab daily in the AM; do <u>not</u> crush <u>or</u> chew
Pediatric: <6 years: not recommended; ≥6 years: use in place of regular-acting *methylphenidate* when the 8-hour dose of **Metadate-ER** corresponds to the titrated 8-hour dose of regular-acting *methylphenidate*
>   *Tab:* 10, 20 mg ext-rel (dye-free)

QuilliChew ER initially 1 x 10 mg chew tab once daily in the AM
Pediatric: <6 years: not recommended; initially 10 mg daily; may gradually increase by 20 mg/day at weekly intervals as needed; max 60 mg/day
>   *Chew tab:* 20*, 30*40 mg ext-rel

Quillivant XR initially 20 mg once daily in the AM, with <u>or</u> without food; may be titrated in increments of 10-20 mg/day at weekly intervals; daily doses above 60 mg have not been studied and are <u>not</u> recommended; shake the bottle vigorously for at least 10 seconds to ensure that the correct dose is administered
Pediatric: <6 years: not recommended; ≥6 years: same as adult
>   *Bottle:* 5 mg/ml, 25 mg/5 ml pwdr for reconstitution; 300 mg (60 ml), 600 mg (120 ml), 750 mg (150 ml), 900 mg (180 ml)

Comment: **Quillivant XR** must be reconstituted by a pharmacist, <u>not</u> by the patient <u>or</u> caregiver.

Ritalin LA (G) 1 cap daily in the AM
Pediatric: <6 years: not recommended; ≥6 years: use in place of regular-acting *methylphenidate* when the 8-hour dose of **Ritalin LA** corresponds to the titrated 8-hour dose of regular-acting *methylphenidate*; max 60 mg/day
>   *Cap:* 10, 20, 30, 40 mg ext-rel (immed- and ext-rel beads)

Ritalin SR 1 cap daily in the AM
Pediatric: <6 years: not recommended; ≥6 years: use in place of regular-acting *methylphenidate* when the 8-hour dose of **Ritalin SR** corresponds to the titrated 8-hour dose of regular-acting *methylphenidate*; max 60 mg/day
>   *Tab:* 20 mg sust-rel (dye-free)

▷ *methylphenidate* (transdermal patch) (C)(II)(G) not applicable >17 years
Pediatric: <6 years: not recommended; ≥6-17 years: initially 10 mg patch applied to hip 2 hours before desired effect daily in the AM; may increase by 5-10 mg at weekly intervals; max 60 mg/day
>   **Daytrana** *Transdermal patch:* 10, 15, 20, 30 mg

▷ *pemoline* (B)(IV) 18.75-112.5 mg/day; usually start with 37.5 mg in AM; may increase 18.75 mg/day at weekly intervals; max 112.5 gm/day
  Pediatric: <6 years: not recommended; ≥6 years: same as adult
    Cylert *Tab:* 18.75*, 37.5*, 75*mg
    Cylert Chewable *Chew tab:* 37.5*mg
Comment: Check baseline serum ALT and monitor every 2 weeks thereafter.

CENTRAL ALPHA-2 AGONIST

▷ *guanfacine* (B)(G) not applicable >17 years
  Pediatric: <6 years: not recommended; ≥6-17 years: initially 1 mg once daily; may increase by 1 mg/day at weekly intervals; usual max 4 mg/day
  Intuniv *Tab:* 1, 2, 3, 4 mg ext-rel
  Comment: Take **Intuniv** with water, milk, or other liquid. Do not take with a high-fat meal. Withdraw gradually by 1 mg every 3-7 days.

TRICYCLIC ANTIDEPRESSANTS (TCAs)

see Depression page 117

OTHER AGENTS

▷ *clonidine* (C)(G)
    Catapres 4-5 mcg/kg/day
    Pediatric: <12 years: not recommended; ≥12 years: same as adult
      Tab: 0.1*, 0.2*, 0.3*mg
    Catapres-TTS <12 years: not recommended; ≥12 years: initially 0.1 mg patch weekly; increase after 1-2 weeks if needed; max 0.6 mg/day
      Patch: 0.1, 0.2 mg/day (12/carton); 0.3 mg/day (4/carton)
    Kapvay not indicated for adults
    Pediatric: <6 years: not recommended; ≥6-12 years: initially 0.1 mg at bedtime x 1 week; then 0.1 mg bid x 1 week; then 0.1 mg AM and 0.2 mg PM x 1 week; then 0.2 mg bid; withdraw gradually by 0.1 mg/day at 3-7 day intervals
      Tab: 0.1, 0.2 mg ext-rel
    Nexiclon XR initially 0.18 mg (2 ml) suspension or 0.17 mg tab once daily; usual max 0.52 mg (6 ml suspension) once daily
    Pediatric: <12 years: not recommended; ≥12 years: same as adult
      Tab: 0.17, 0.26 mg ext-rel; *Oral susp:* 0.09 mg/ml ext-rel (4 oz)

AMINOKETONES (FOR THE TREATMENT OF ADHD)

▷ *bupropion HBr* (C)(G) initially 100 mg bid for at least 3 days; may increase to 375 or 400 mg/day after several weeks; then after at least 3 more days, 450 mg in 4 divided doses; max 450 mg/day, 174 mg/single dose
  Pediatric: <18 years: not recommended; ≥18 years: Safety and effectiveness in the pediatric population have not been established. When considering the use of **Aplenzin** in a child or adolescent, balance the potential risks with the clinical need
    Aplenzin *Tab:* 174, 348, 522 mg
▷ *bupropion HCl* (C)(G)
  Forfivo XL do not use for initial treatment; use immediate-release *bupropion* forms for initial titration; switch to **Forfivo XL** 450 mg once daily when total dose/day reaches 450 mg; may switch to **Forfivo XL** when total dose/day reaches 300 mg for 2 weeks and patient needs 450 mg/day to reach therapeutic target; swallow whole, do not crush or chew
    Pediatric: <18 years: not recommended; >18 years: same as adult; Safety and effectiveness of long-acting and extended-release *bupropion* in the pediatric

population have not been established. When considering the use of **Forfivo XL** in a child or adolescent, balance the potential risks with the clinical need
Tab: 450 mg ext-rel

Wellbutrin initially 100 mg bid for at least 3 days; may increase to 375 or 400 mg/ day after several weeks; then after at least 3 more days, 450 mg in 4 divided doses; max 450 mg/day, 150 mg/single dose
Pediatric: <12 years: not recommended; ≥12 years: same as adult
Tab: 75, 100 mg

Wellbutrin SR initially 150 mg in AM for at least 3 days; may increase to 150 mg bid if well tolerated; usual dose 300 mg/day; max 400 mg/day
Pediatric: <12 years: not recommended; ≥12 years: same as adult
Tab: 100, 150 mg sust-rel

Wellbutrin XL initially 150 mg in AM for at least 3 days; increase to 150 mg bid if well tolerated; usual dose 300 mg/day; max 400 mg/day
Pediatric: <12 years: not recommended; ≥12 years: same as adult
Tab: 150, 300 mg sust-rel

BACTERIAL ENDOCARDITIS: PROPHYLAXIS

Comment: Bacterial endocarditis prophylaxis is appropriate for persons with a history of previous infective endocarditis, persons with a prosthetic cardiac valve or prosthetic material used for valve repair, cardiac transplant patients who develop cardiac valvulopathy, congenital heart disease (CHD), unrepaired cyanotic CHD including palliative shunts and conduits, completely repaired congenital heart defect(s) with prosthetic material or device, whether placed by surgery or by catheter intervention, during the first 6 months after the procedure, repaired CHD with residual defects at the site or adjacent to the site of a prosthetic patch or prosthetic device (which may inhibit endothelialization), or any other condition deemed to place a patient at high risk.

DENTAL, ORAL, RESPIRATORY TRACT, ESOPHAGEAL PROCEDURES

➤ *amoxicillin* (B)(G) 2 gm PO 30-60 minutes before procedure as a single dose or 3 gm 1 hour before procedure and 1.5 gm 6 hours later
Pediatric: 50 mg/kg as a single dose or 50 mg/kg (max 3 gm) 1 hour before procedure and (max 1.5 gm) 25 mg/kg 6 hours later; ≥40 kg: same as adult; *see pages* 616- *for dose by weight*

    Amoxil *Cap:* 250, 500 mg; *Tab:* 875*mg; *Chew tab:* 125, 200, 250, 400 mg (cherry-banana-peppermint) (phenylalanine); *Oral susp:* 125, 250 mg/5 ml (80, 100, 150 ml) (strawberry); 200, 400 mg/5 ml (50, 75, 100 ml) (bubble gum); *Oral drops:* 50 mg/ml (30 ml) (bubble gum)

    Trimox *Tab:* 125, 250 mg; *Cap:* 250, 500 mg; *Oral susp:* 125, 250 mg/5 ml (80, 100, 150 ml) (raspberry-strawberry)

➤ *ampicillin* (B)(G) 2 gm PO/IM/IV 30-60 minutes before procedure
Pediatric: <12 years: 50 mg/kg PO/IM/IV 30-60 minutes before procedure; ≥12 years: same as adult

    Omnipen, Principen *Cap:* 250, 500 mg; *Oral susp:* 125, 250 mg/5 ml (100, 150, 200 ml) (fruit)

    Unasyn *Vial:* 1.5, 3 gm

➤ *azithromycin* (B)(G) 500 mg PO 30-60 minutes before procedure
Pediatric: <12 years: 15 mg/kg 30-60 minutes before procedure; max 500 mg; *see page* 621 *for dose by weight;* ≥12 years: same as adult

    Zithromax *Tab:* 250, 500, 600 mg; *Oral susp:* 100 mg/5 ml (15 ml); 200 mg/5 ml (15, 22.5, 30 ml) (cherry)

▷ *cefazolin* (B) 1 gm IM/IV 30-60 minutes before procedure
  Pediatric: <12 years: 25 mg/kg IM/IV 30-60 minutes before procedure; ≥12 years:
  same as adult
    Ancef *Vial:* 250, 500 mg; 1, 5 gm
    Kefzol *Vial:* 500 mg; 1 gm
▷ *ceftriaxone* (B)(G) 1 gm IM/IV as a single dose
  Pediatric: <12 years: 50 mg/kg IM/IV as a single dose; ≥12 years: same as adult
    Rocephin *Vial:* 250, 500 mg; 1, 2 gm
▷ *cephalexin* (B)(G) 2 gm as a single dose 30-60 minutes before procedure
  Pediatric: 50 mg/kg as a single dose 30-60 minutes before procedure; *see page 629 for
  dose by weight*
    Keflex *Cap:* 250, 333, 500, 750 mg; *Oral susp:* 125, 250 mg/5 ml (100, 200 ml)
    (strawberry)
▷ *clarithromycin* (C)(G) 500 mg or 500 mg ext-rel as a single dose 30-60 minutes before
  procedure
  Pediatric: 15 mg/kg as a single dose 30-60 minutes before procedure; *see page 630 for
  dose by weight*
    Biaxin *Tab:* 250, 500 mg
    Biaxin Oral Suspension *Oral susp:* 125, 250 mg/5 ml (50, 100 ml) (fruit-
    punch)
    Biaxin XL *Tab:* 500 mg ext-rel
▷ *clindamycin* (B)(G) 600 mg PO as a one-time single-dose or 300 mg 30-60 minutes
  before procedure and 150 mg 6 hours later; take with a full glass of water
  Pediatric: <12 years: 20 mg/kg (max 300 mg) 1 hour before procedure and 10 mg/
  kg (max 150 mg) 6 hours later; take with a full glass of water; *see page 631 for dose
  by weight*; ≥12 years: same as adult
    Cleocin (G) *Cap:* 75 (tartrazine), 150 (tartrazine), 300 mg; *Vial:* 150 mg/ml
    (2, 4 ml) (benzyl alcohol)
    Cleocin Pediatric Granules (G) *Oral susp:* 75 mg/ml (100 ml)(cherry)
▷ *erythromycin estolate* (B)(G) 1 gm 1 hour before procedure; then 500 mg 6 hours
  later
  Pediatric: <12 years: 20 mg/kg 1 hour before procedure; then 10 mg/kg 6 hours later;
  see page 634 for dose by weight; ≥12 years: same as adult
    Ilosone *Pulvule:* 250 mg; *Tab:* 500 mg; *Liq:* 125, 250 mg/5 ml (100 ml)
  Comment: *erythromycin* may increase INR with concomitant **warfarin**, as well as
  increase serum level of **digoxin**, benzodiazepines and statins.
▷ *penicillin v potassium* (B)(G) 2 gm 1 hour before procedure; then 1 gm 6 hours later
  or 2 gm 1 hour before procedure; then 1 gm q 6 hours x 8 doses
  Pediatric: <12 years, <60 lb: 1 gm 1 hour before procedure; then 500 mg 6 hours later
  or 1 gm 1 hour before procedure; then 500 mg q 6 hours x 8 doses; *see page 644 for
  dose by weight*; ≥12 years: same as adult
    Pen-Vee K *Tab:* 250, 500 mg; *Oral soln:* 125 mg/5 ml (100, 200 ml); 250 mg/5 ml
    (100, 150, 200 ml)

◯ BACTERIAL VAGINOSIS (BV) *GARDNERELLA VAGINALIS*

PROPHYLAXIS AND RESTORATION OF VAGINAL ACIDITY

▷ *acetic acid+oxyquinolone* (C) one full applicator intravaginally bid for up to 30 days
  Pediatric: <12 years: not recommended; ≥12 years: same as adult
    Relagard *Gel:* acet acid 0.9%+oxyq 0.025% (50 gm tube w. applicator)
Comment: The following treatment regimens for *bacterial vaginosis* are published in the
2015 CDC Sexually Transmitted Diseases Treatment Guidelines. Treatment regimens
are presented by generic drug name first, followed by information about brands and

dose forms. BV is associated with adverse pregnancy outcomes, including premature rupture of the membranes, preterm labor, preterm birth, intra-amniotic infection, and postpartum endometritis. Therefore, treatment is recommended for all pregnant women with symptoms <u>or</u> positive screen.

RECOMMENDED REGIMENS

Regimen 1
▷ *metronidazole* 500 mg bid x 7 days or *metronidazole er* 750 mg once daily x 7 days

Regimen 2
▷ *metronidazole* gel 0.75% one full applicatorful (5 gm) once daily x 5 days

Regimen 3
▷ *clindamycin* cream 2% one full applicatorful (5 gm) intravaginally once daily at bedtime x 5 days

ALTERNATE REGIMENS

Regimen 1
▷ *tinidazole* 2 gm once daily x 2 days

Regimen 2
▷ *tinidazole* 1 gm once daily x 5 days

Regimen 3
▷ *clindamycin* 300 mg bid x 7 days

Regimen 4
▷ *clindamycin* ovules 100 mg intravaginally once daily at bedtime x 3 days

Drug Brands and Dose Forms

▷ *clindamycin* (B)
    Cleocin (G) *Cap:* 75 (tartrazine), 150 (tartrazine), 300 mg
    Cleocin Pediatric Granules (G) *Oral susp:* 75 mg/5 ml (100 ml) (cherry)
    Cleocin Vaginal Cream *Vag crm:* 2% (21, 40 gm tubes w. applicator)
    Cleocin Vaginal Ovules *Vag supp:* 100 mg
▷ *metronidazole* (not for use in 1st; B in 2nd, 3rd)
    Flagyl *Tab:* 250*, 500*mg
    Flagyl 375 *Cap:* 375 mg
    Flagyl ER *Tab:* 750 mg ext-rel
    MetroGel-Vaginal, Vandazole *Vag gel:* 0.75% (70 gm w. applicator) (parabens)
▷ *tinidazole* (not for use in 1st; B in 2nd, 3rd)
    Tindamax *Tab:* 250*, 500*mg

BALDNESS: MALE PATTERN

TYPE II 5-ALPHA-REDUCTASE SPECIFIC INHIBITOR

▷ *finasteride* (X)(G) 1 mg daily
    Propecia *Tab:* 1 mg

    Comment: Pregnant women should <u>not</u> touch broken *finasteride* tabs. Use of **Propecia**, a 5-alpha reductase inhibitor, is associated with low but increased risk of high-grade prostate cancer.

PERIPHERAL VASODILATOR

▷ *minoxidil* topical soln (C)(G) 1 ml from dropper <u>or</u> 6 sprays bid
    Pediatric: <18 years: not recommended; ≥18 years: same as adult

Rogaine for Men (OTC) *Regular soln:* 2% (60 ml w. applicator) (alcohol 60%);
Extra strength soln: 5% (60 ml w. applicator) (alcohol 30%)
Rogaine for Women (OTC) *Regular soln:* 2% (60 ml w. applicator) (alcohol 60%);
Topical aerosol: 5%
Comment: Do not use *minoxidil* on abraded or inflamed scalp.

BELL'S PALSY

▷ *prednisone* (C)(G) 80 mg once daily x 3 days; then 60 mg daily x 3 days; then 40 mg
daily x 3 days; then 20 mg x 1 dose; then discontinue
Deltasone *Tab:* 2.5*, 5*, 10*, 20*, 50*mg

BENIGN ESSENTIAL TREMOR

ANTI-PARKINSON'S AGENT

▷ *amantadine* (C)(G) 200 mg daily or 100 mg bid; 4 tsp of syrup once daily or 2 tsp bid
Symmetrel *Tab:* 100 mg; *Syr:* 50 mg/5 ml (raspberry)

BETA-BLOCKER

▷ *propranolol* (C)(G)
Inderal initially 40 mg bid; usual range 160-240 mg/day
Tab: 10*, 20*, 40*, 60*, 80*mg
Inderal LA initially 80 mg once daily in a single dose; increase q 3-7 days; usual
range 120-160 mg/day; max 320 mg/day in a single dose
Cap: 60, 80, 120, 160 mg sust-rel
InnoPran XL initially 80 mg q HS; max 120 mg/day
Cap: 80, 120 mg ext-rel

BENIGN PROSTATIC HYPERPLASIA (BPH)

ALPHA-1 BLOCKERS

Comment: Educate patient regarding potential side effect of hypotension especially with
first dose. Usually start at lowest dose and titrate upward.
▷ *doxazosin* (C)
Cardura initially 1 mg daily; may double dose every 1-2 weeks; max 8 mg/day
Tab: 1*, 2*, 4*, 8*mg
Cardura XL initially 4 mg once daily with breakfast; may titrate after 3-4 weeks;
max 8 mg/day
Tab: 4, 8 mg ext-rel
▷ *silodosin* (B)(G) 8 mg once daily; *CrCl 30-50 mL/min:* 4 mg once daily
Rapaflo *Cap:* 4, 8 mg
▷ *terazosin* (C)(G) initially 1 mg q HS; titrate up to 10 mg once daily; max 20 mg/day
Hytrin *Cap:* 1, 2, 5, 10 mg

ALPHA-1A BLOCKERS

▷ *alfuzosin* (B)(G) 10 mg once daily taken immediately after the same meal each day
UroXatral *Tab:* 10 mg ext-rel
▷ *tamsulosin* (B)(G) initially 0.4 mg once daily; may increase to 0.8 mg daily after 2-4
weeks if needed
Flomax *Cap:* 0.4 mg
Comment: May take **Flomax** 0.4 mg plus **Imitrex** 0.5 mg once daily as
combination therapy.

TYPE II 5-ALPHA-REDUCTASE INHIBITOR

Comment: Pregnant women and women of childbearing age should not handle *finasteride*. Monitor for potential side effects of decreased libido and/or impotence. Low, but increased risk of being diagnosed with high-grade prostate cancer.

▷ *finasteride* (X) 5 mg once daily

   Proscar *Tab:* 5 mg

TYPES I AND II 5-ALPHA-REDUCTASE INHIBITOR

Comment: Pregnant women and women of childbearing age should not handle *dutasteride*. Monitor for potential side effects of decreased libido and/or impotence. Low, but increased risk of being diagnosed with high-grade prostate cancer.

▷ *dutasteride* (X)(G) 0.5 mg once daily

   Avodart *Cap:* 0.5 mg

   Comment: May take **Avodart** 0.5 mg with **Flomax** 0.4 mg once daily as combination therapy.

TYPE I AND II 5-ALPHA-REDUCTASE INHIBITOR+ALPHA-1A BLOCKER

▷ *dutasteride+tamsulosin* (X)(G) take 1 cap once daily after the same meal each day

   Jalyn *Cap:* duta 0.5 mg+tam 0.4 mg

PHOSPHODIESTERASE TYPE 5 (PDE5) INHIBITORS, CGMP-SPECIFIC

Comment: Oral PDE5 inhibitors are contraindicated in patients taking nitrates. Caution with history of recent MI, stroke, life-threatening arrhythmia, hypotension, hypertension, cardiac failure, unstable angina, retinitis pigmentosa, CYP3A4 inhibitors (e.g., *cimetidine*, the azoles, *erythromycin*, grapefruit juice), protease inhibitors (e.g., *ritonavir*), CYP3A4 inducers (e.g., *rifampin, carbamazepine, phenytoin, phenobarbital*), alcohol, antihypertensive agents. Side effects include headache, flushing, nasal congestion, rhinitis, dyspepsia, and diarrhea.

▷ *tadalafil* (B) 5 mg once daily at the same time each day; *CrCl 30-50 mL/min:* initially 2.5 mg; *CrCl <30 mL/min:* not recommended; *Concomitant alpha blockers:* not recommended

   Cialis *Tab:* 2.5, 5, 10, 20 mg

◯ BILE ACID DEFICIENCY

BILE ACID

▷ *ursodiol* (B)

   Dissolution of radiolucent non-calcified gallstones <20 mm diameter: 8-10 mg/kg/day in 2-3 divided doses; *Prevention:* 13-15 mg/kg/day in 4 divided doses
   Pediatric: <12 years: not recommended; ≥12 years: same as adult

   Actigall *Cap:* 300 mg

   Comment: *ursodiol* decreases the amount of cholesterol produced by the liver and absorbed by the intestines. It helps break down cholesterol that has formed into stones in the gallbladder. *ursodiol* increases bile flow in patients with primary biliary cirrhosis. It is used to treat small gallstones in people who cannot have cholecystectomy surgery and to prevent gallstones in overweight patients undergoing rapid weight loss. *ursodiol* is not for treating gallstones that are calcified.

◯ BINGE EATING DISORDER

CENTRAL NERVOUS SYSTEM (CNS) STIMULANT

▷ *lisdexamfetamine dimesylate* (C)(II) swallow whole or may open and mix/dissolve contents of cap in yogurt, water, orange juice and take immediately; 30 mg once daily in

the AM; may adjust in increments of 20 mg at weekly intervals; target dose 50-70 mg/day; max 70 mg/day; *GFR 15-<30 mL/min:* max 50 mg/day; *GFR <15 mL/min, ESRD:* max 30 mg/day
Pediatric: <18 years: not established; ≥18 years: same as adult
>   **Vyvanse** *Cap:* 10, 20, 30, 40, 50, 60 70 mg
>   Comment: **Vyvanse** is <u>not</u> approved <u>or</u> recommended for weight loss treatment of obesity.

 BIPOLAR DISORDER

Comment: Bipolar I Disorder is characterized by one or more manic episodes that last at least a week <u>or</u> require hospitalization. Severe mania may manifest symptoms of psychosis. Bipolar II Disorder is characterized by one or more depressive episodes accompanied by at least one hypomanic episode. When one parent has Bipolar Disorder, the risk to each child of developing the disorder is estimated to be 15-30%. When both parents have the disorder, the risk to each child increases to 50-75%. Symptoms of mood disorders may be difficult to diagnose in children and adolescents because they can be mistaken for age-appropriate emotions and behaviors <u>or</u> overlap with symptoms of other conditions such as ADHD. However, since anxiety and depression in children may be precursers to Bipolar Disorder, these behaviors should be carefully monitored and evaluated. The cornerstone of treatment for Bipolar Disorder is mood-stabilizers (*lithium* and *valproate*). Common adjunctive agents include antiepileptics, antipsychotics, and combination agents. Mounting evidence suggests that antidepressants aren't effective in the treatment of bipolar depression. A major study funded by the National Institute of Mental Health (NIMH) showed that adding an antidepressant to a mood stabilizer was no more effective in treating bipolar depression than using a mood stabilizer alone. Another NIMH study found that antidepressants work no better than placebo. If antidepressants are used at all, they should be combined with a mood stabilizer such as *lithium* <u>or</u> *valproic acid.* Antidepressants, without a concomitant mood stabilizer, can increase the frequency of mood cycling and trigger a manic episode. Many experts believe that over time, antidepressant use as monotherapy (i.e., without a mood stabilizer) in people with Bipolar Disorder has a mood destabilizing effect, increasing the frequency of manic and depressive episodes. Drugs and conditions that can mimic Bipolar Disorder include thyroid disorders, corticosteroids, antidepressants, adrenal disorders (e.g. Addison's disease, Cushing's syndrome), antianxiety drugs, drugs for Parkinson's disease, vitamin B12 deficiency, neurological disorders (e.g., epilepsy, multiple sclerosis).

MOOD STABILIZERS
Lithium Salts Mood Stabilizer
> *lithium carbonate* (D)(G) swallow whole; *Usual maintenance:* 900-1200 mg/day in 2-3 divided doses
Pediatric: <12 years: not recommended; ≥12 years: same as adult
>   **Lithobid** *Tab:* 300 mg slow-rel
>   Comment: Signs and symptoms of *lithium* toxicity can occur below 2 mEq/L and include blurred vision, tinnitus, weakness, dizziness, nausea, abdominal pains, vomiting, diarrhea to (severe) hand tremors, ataxia, muscle twitches, nystagmus, seizures, slurred speech, decreased level of consciousness, coma, death.

Valproate Mood Stabilizer
> *divalproex sodium* (D)(G) take once daily; swallow ext-rel form whole; initially 25 mg/kg/day in divided doses; max 60 mg/kg/day; *Elderly:* reduce initial dose and titrate slowly

Pediatric: <12 years: not recommended; ≥12 years: same as adult
Depakene *Cap:* 250 mg; *Syr:* 250 mg/5 ml (16 oz)
> **Depakote** *Tab:* 125, 250 mg
> **Depakote ER** *Tab:* 250, 500 mg ext-rel
> **Depakote Sprinkle** *Cap:* 125 mg

ANTIEPILEPTICS

▷ *carbamazepine* (D) ext-rel oral forms should be swallowed whole; may open caps and sprinkle on applesauce (do <u>not</u> crush <u>or</u> chew beads); initially 400 mg/day in 2 divided doses; adjust in increments of 200 mg/day; max 1.6 gm/day. *Elderly:* reduce initial dose and titrate slowly; oral doses are preferred; IV administration is recommended when the patient is unable to swallow an oral form (see **Carnexiv**)
Pediatric: <12 years: not recommended; ≥12 years: same as adult
> **Carbatrol** (G) *Cap:* 200, 300 mg ext-rel
> **Carnexiv** *Vial:* 10 mg/ml (20 ml)
> Comment: The total daily dose of **Carnexiv** is 70% of the total daily oral *carbamazepine* dose (see mfr pkg insert for dosage conversion table). The total daily dose should be equally divided into four 30-minute infusions, separated by 6 hours. Must be diluted prior to administration. Patients should be switched back to oral *carbamazepine* at their previous total daily oral dose and frequency of administration as soon as clinically appropriate. The use of **Carnexiv** for more than 7 consecutive days has not been studied.
> **Equetro** (G) *Cap:* 100, 200, 300 mg ext-rel
> **Tegretol** (G) *Tab:* 200*mg; *Chew tab:* 100*mg; *Oral susp:* 100 mg/5 ml (450 ml; citrus-vanilla)
> **Tegretol XR** (G) *Tab:* 100, 200, 400 mg ext-rel

Comment: *carbamazepine* is indicated in mixed episodes in bipolar I disorder.

▷ *lamotrigine* (C)(G) <u>Not taking an enzyme-inducing antiepileptic drug (EIAED) (e.g., *phenytoin, carbamazepine, phenobarbital, primidone, valproic acid*):</u> 25 mg once daily x 2 weeks; then 50 mg once daily x 2 weeks; then 100 mg once daily x 2 weeks; then target dose 200 mg once daily; *Concomitant valproic acid:* 25 mg every other day x 2 weeks; then 25 mg once daily x 2 weeks; then 50 mg once daily x 1 week; then target dose 100 mg once daily; *Concomitant EIAED, <u>not</u> valproic acid:* 50 mg once daily x 2 weeks; then 100 mg daily in divided doses; then increase weekly by 100 mg in divided doses to target dose 400 mg/day in divided doses daily
Pediatric: <12 years: not recommended; ≥12 years: same as adult
> **Lamictal** *Tab:* 25*, 100*, 150*, 200*mg
> **Lamictal Chewable Dispersible Tab** *Chew tab:* 2, 5, 25, 50 mg (black current)
> **Lamictal ODT** *ODT:* 25, 50, 100, 200 mg
> **Lamictal XR** *Tab:* 25, 50, 100, 200 mg ext-rel

Comment: *lamotrigine* is indicated for maintenance treatment of bipolar I disorder. See mfr pkg insert for drug interactions, interactions with contraceptives and hormone replacement therapy, and discontinuation protocol

ANTIPSYCHOTICS

Comment: Common side effects of antipsychotic drugs include drowsiness, weight gain, sexual dysfunction, dry mouth, constipation, blurred vision. *Neuroleptic Malignant Syndrome* (NMS) and *Tardive Dyskinesia* (TD) are adverse side effects (ASEs) most often associated with the older antipsychotic drugs. Risk is decreased with the newer "atypical" antipsychotic drugs. However, these syndromes can develop, although much less commonly, after relatively brief treatment periods at low doses. Given these considerations, antipsychotic drugs should be prescribed in a manner that is most likely to minimize the occurrence. NMS, a potentially fatal symptom complex, is characterized by hyperpyrexia, muscle rigidity, altered mental status and evidence of autonomic instability (irregular pulse or blood pressure, tachycardia, diaphoresis, and cardiac dysrhythmia). Additional signs may include elevated creatine phosphokinase (CPK), myoglobinuria (rhabdomyolysis), and acute renal failure (ARF). TD is a syndrome consisting of potentially irreversible, involuntary, dyskinetic movements that can develop in patients with antipsychotic drugs. Characteristics include repetitive involuntary movements, usually of the jaw, lips and tongue, such as grimacing, sticking out the tongue and smacking the lips. Some affected people also experience involuntary movement of the extremities difficulty breathing. The syndrome may remit, partially or completely, if antipsychotic treatment is withdrawn. If signs and symptoms of NMS and/or TD appear in a patient, management should include immediate discontinuation of antipsychotic drugs and other drugs not essential to concurrent therapy, intensive symptomatic treatment, medical monitoring, and treatment of any concomitant serious medical problems. The risk of developing NMS and/or TD, and the likelihood that either syndrome will become irreversible, is believed to increase as the duration of treatment and the total cumulative dose of antipsychotic drugs administered to the patient increase. The first and only FDA-approved treatment for TD is *valbenazine* (**Ingrezza**) (*see page 456*)

➢ *aripiprazole* (C)(G) initially 15 mg once daily; may increase to max 30 mg/day
  Pediatric: <10 years: not recommended; ≥10-17 years: initially 2 mg/day in a single dose for 2 days; then increase to 5 mg/day in a single dose for 2 days; then increase to target dose of 10 mg/day in a single dose; may increase by 5 mg/day at weekly intervals as needed to max 30 mg/day
    Abilify *Tab:* 2, 5, 10, 15, 20, 30 mg
    Abilify Discmelt *Tab:* 15 mg orally-disint (vanilla) (phenylalanine)
    Abilify Maintena *Vial:* 300, 400 mg ext-rel pwdr for IM injection after reconstitution; 300, 400 mg single dose prefilled dual-chamber syringes w. supplies
    Comment: **Abilify** is indicated for acute and maintenance treatment of mixed episodes in bipolar I disorder, as monotherapy or as adjunct to *lithium* or *valproic acid.*

➢ *asenapine* (C) allow SL tab to dissolve on tongue; do not split, crush, chew, or swallow; do not eat or drink for 10 minutes after administration; *Monotherapy:* 10 mg bid; *Adjunctive therapy:* 5 mg bid; may increase to max 10 mg bid
  Pediatric: <10 years: not established; 10-17 years: *Monotherapy:* initially 2.5 mg bid; may increase to 5 mg bid after 3 days; then to 10 mg bid after 3 more days; max 10 mg bid
    Saphris *SL tab:* 2, 5, 5, 10 mg (black cherry)
    Comment: **Saphris** is indicated for acute treatment of manic or mixed episodes in bipolar I disorder, as monotherapy or as adjunct to *lithium* or *valproic acid.*

➢ *cariprazine* initially 1.5 mg once daily; recommended therapeutic dose 3-6 mg/day
  Pediatric: <12 years: not established; ≥12 years: same as adult
    Vraylar *Cap:* 1.5, 3, 4.5, 6 mg; 7-count (1 x 1.5 mg, 6 x 3 mg) mixed blister pck
    Comment: **Vraylar** is an atypical antipsychotic with partial agonist activity at D2 and 5-HT1A receptors and antagonist activity at 5-HT2A receptors. It is indicated for acute treatment of mixed episodes in bipolar I disorder. There is a **Vraylar** pregnancy exposure registry that monitors pregnancy outcomes in women exposed to **Vraylar** during pregnancy. For more information, contact the National Pregnancy Registry for Atypical Antipsychotics at 1-866-961-2388 or visit https://womensmentalhealth.org/clinical-and-research-programs/pregnancyregistry. Safety and effectiveness in pediatric patients have not been established.

▷ *lurasidone* (B) initially 20 mg once daily; usual range 20 to max 120 mg/day; take with food; *CrCl <50 mL/min, moderate hepatic impairment (Child-Pugh 7-9):* max 80 mg/day; *Child-Pugh 10-15):* max 40 mg/day

Pediatric: <18 years: not established; ≥18 years: same as adult

  Latuda *Tab:* 20, 40, 60, 80, 120 mg

Comment: Latuda is indicated for major depressive episodes associated with bipolar I disorder as monotherapy and as adjunctive therapy with *lithium* or *valproic* acid. Contraindicated with concomitant strong CYP3A4 inhibitors (e.g., *ketoconazole, voriconazole, clarithromycin, ritonavir*) and inducers (e.g., *phenytoin, carbamazepine, rifampin, St. John's wort*); see mfr pkg insert if patient taking moderate CYP3A4 inhibitors (e.g., *diltiazem, atazanavir, erythromycin, fluconazole, verapamil*). The efficacy of **Latuda** in the treatment of mania associated with bipolar disorder has not been established.

▷ *quetiapine fumarate* (C)(G)

  SeroQUEL initially 25 mg bid, titrate q 2nd or 3rd day in increments of 25-50 mg bid-tid; usual maintenance 400-600 mg/day in 2-3 divided doses

  Pediatric: <10 years: not recommended; ≥10-17 years: initially 25 mg bid, titrate q 2nd or 3rd day in increments of 25-50 mg bid-tid; max 600 mg/day in 2-3 divided doses

   Tab: 25, 50, 100, 200, 300, 400 mg

  SeroQUEL XR swallow whole; administer once daily in the PM; *Day 1:* 50 mg; *Day 2:* 100 mg; *Day 3:* 200 mg; *Day 4:* 300 mg; usual range 400-600 mg/day

  Pediatric: <18 years: not recommended; ≥18 years: same as adult

   Tab: 50, 150, 200, 300, 400 mg ext-rel

▷ *risperidone* (C) *Tab:* initially 2-3 mg once daily; may adjust at 24 hour intervals by 1 mg/day; usual range 1-6 mg/day; max 6 mg/day; *Oral soln:* do not take with cola or tea; *M-tab:* dissolve on tongue with or without fluid; *Consta:* administer deep IM in the deltoid or gluteal; give with oral *risperidone* or other antipsychotic x 3 weeks; then stop oral form; 25 mg IM every 2 weeks; max 50 mg every 2 weeks

  Risperdal

  Pediatric: <5 years: not established; 5-10 years: initially 0.5 mg once daily at the same time each day adjust at 24 hour intervals by 0.5-1 mg to target dose 1-2.5 mg/day; usual range 1-6 mg/day; max 6 mg/day; >10 years: same as adult

   Tab: 0.25, 0.5, 1, 2, 3, 4 mg; *Oral soln:* 1 mg/ml (100 ml)

  Risperdal Consta

  Pediatric: <18 years: not established; ≥18 years: same as adult

   Vial: 12.5, 25, 37.5, 50 mg pwdr for long-acting IM inj after reconstitution, single-use, w. diluent and supplies

  Risperdal M-Tab

  Pediatric: <10 years: not established; ≥10 years: same as adult

   Tab: 0.5, 1, 2, 3, 4 mg orally-disint (phenylalanine)

Comment: **Risperdol** tabs, oral solution, and M-tabs are indicated for the short-term monotherapy of acute mania or mixed episodes associated with bipolar I disorder, or in combination with *lithium* or *valproic acid* in adults

  Risperdol Consta is indicated as monotherapy or adjunctive therapy to *lithium* or *valproic acid* for the maintenance treatment of mania and mixed episodes in bipolar I disorder.

▷ *ziprasidone* (C)(G) *Adult:* take with food; initially 40 mg bid; on day 2, may increase to 60-80 mg bid; *Elderly:* lower initial dose and titrate slowly

  Pediatric: <12 years: not recommended; ≥12 years: same as adult

  Geodon *Cap:* 20, 40, 60, 80 mg

Comment: **Geodon** is indicated for acute and maintenance treatment of mixed episodes in bipolar I disorder, as monotherapy or as adjunct to *lithium* or *valproic acid*.

COMBINATION AGENTS

Thienobenzodiazepine+Selective Serotonin Reuptake Inhibitor (SSRI) Combinations

▷ *olanzapine+fluoxetine* (C) initially 1 x 6/25 cap once daily in the PM; titrate; max 1 x 12/50 cap once daily in the PM
Pediatric: <10 years: not recommended; 10-17 years: initially 1 x 3/25 cap once daily in the PM; max 1 x 12/50 cap once daily in the PM
    Symbyax
      Cap: **Symbyax 3/25** olan 3 mg+fluo 25 mg
          Symbyax 6/25 olan 6 mg+fluo 25 mg
          Symbyax 6/50 olan 6 mg+fluo 50 mg
          Symbyax 12/25 olan 12 mg+fluo 25 mg
          Symbyax 12/50 olan 12 mg+fluo 50 mg

Comment: **Symbyax** is indicated for the treatment of depressive episode associated with bipolar I disorder and treatment-resistant depression (TRD).

 BITE: CAT

TETANUS PROPHYLAXIS

▷ *tetanus toxoid* vaccine (C) 0.5 ml IM x 1 dose if previously immunized
Vial: 5 Lf units/0.5 ml (0.5, 5 ml); *Prefilled syringe:* 5 Lf units/0.5 ml (0.5 ml)
see **Tetanus** *page 460 for patients not previously immunized*

ANTI-INFECTIVES

▷ *amoxicillin+clavulanate* (B)(G)
    Augmentin 500 mg tid or 875 mg bid x 10 days
    Pediatric: 40-45 mg/kg/day divided tid x 10 days or 90 mg/kg/day divided bid x 10 days *see pages 618-619 for dose by weight*
      Tab: 250, 500, 875 mg; *Chew tab:* 125, 250 mg (lemon-lime); 200, 400 mg (cherry-banana) (phenylalanine); *Oral susp:* 125 mg/5 ml (banana), 250 mg/5 ml (75, 100, 150 ml) (orange); 200, 400 mg/5 ml (50, 75, 100 ml) (orange) (phenylalanine)
    Augmentin ES-600 not recommended for adults
    Pediatric: <3 months: not recommended; ≥3 months, <40 kg: 90 mg/kg/day in 2 divided doses x 10 days; ≥40 kg: not recommended
      Oral susp: 42.9 mg/5 ml (50, 75, 100, 125, 150, 200 ml) (strawberry cream) (phenylalanine)
    Augmentin XR 2 tabs q 12 hours x 10 days
    Pediatric: <16 years: use other forms; ≥16 years: same as adult
      Tab: 1000*mg ext-rel
▷ *doxycycline* (D)(G) 100 mg bid day 1; then 100 mg daily x 10 days
Pediatric: <8 years: not recommended ≥8 years, <100 lb: 2 mg/lb on first day in 2 divided doses, followed by 1 mg/lb/day in 1-2 divided doses; *see page 633 for dose by weight;* ≥8 years, ≥100 lb: same as adult
    Acticlate *Tab:* 75, 150**mg
    Adoxa *Tab:* 50, 75, 100, 150 mg ent-coat
    Doryx *Tab:* 50, 75, 100, 150, 200 mg del-rel
    Doxteric *Tab:* 50 mg del-rel
    Monodox *Cap:* 50, 75, 100 mg
    Oracea *Cap:* 40 mg del-rel
    Vibramycin *Tab:* 100 mg; *Cap:* 50, 100 mg; *Syr:* 50 mg/5 ml (raspberry-apple) (sulfites); *Oral susp:* 25 mg/5 ml (raspberry)
    Vibra-Tab *Tab:* 100 mg film-coat

Comment: *doxycycline* is contraindicated <8 years-of-age, in pregnancy, and lactation (discolors developing tooth enamel). A side effect may be photosensitivity (photophobia). Do not take with antacids, calcium supplements, milk or other dairy, or within 2 hours of taking another drug.

▷ *penicillin v potassium* (B)(G) 500 mg PO qid x 3 days
Pediatric: <12 years: 15-50 mg/kg/day in 3-6 divided doses x 3 days; *see page 644 for dose by weight;* ≥12 years: same as adult
   Pen-Vee K *Tab:* 250, 500 mg; *Oral soln:* 125 mg/5 ml (100, 200 ml); 250 mg/5 ml (100, 150, 200 ml)

BITE: DOG

TETANUS PROPHYLAXIS

*see **Tetanus** page 460 for patients not previously immunized*

▷ *tetanus toxoid* vaccine (C) 0.5 ml IM x 1 dose if previously immunized
Vial: 5 Lf units/0.5 ml (0.5, 5 ml); *Prefilled syringe:* 5 Lf units/0.5 ml (0.5 ml)

ANTI-INFECTIVES

▷ *amoxicillin+clavulanate* (B)(G)
   Augmentin 500 mg tid <u>or</u> 875 mg bid x 10 days
   Pediatric: 40-45 mg/kg/day divided tid x 10 days <u>or</u> 90 mg/kg/day divided bid x 10 days *see pages 618-619 for dose by weight*
      Tab: 250, 500, 875 mg; *Chew tab:* 125, 250 mg (lemon-lime); 200, 400 mg (cherry-banana) (phenylalanine); *Oral susp:* 125 mg/5 ml (banana), 250 mg/5 ml (75, 100, 150 ml) (orange); 200, 400 mg/5 ml (50, 75, 100 ml) (orange) (phenylalanine)
   Augmentin ES-600 not recommended for adults
   Pediatric: <3 months: not recommended; ≥3 months, <40 kg: 90 mg/kg/day in 2 divided doses x 10 days; ≥40 kg: not recommended
      Oral susp: 42.9 mg/5 ml (50, 75, 100, 125, 150, 200 ml) (strawberry cream) (phenylalanine)
   Augmentin XR 2 tabs q 12 hours x 10 days
   Pediatric: <16 years: use other forms; ≥16 years: same as adult
      Tab: 1000*mg ext-rel
▷ *clindamycin* (B) (administer with fluoroquinolone in adult and TMP-SMX in children) 300 mg qid x 10 days
Pediatric: 8-16 mg/kg/day in 3-4 divided doses x 10 days; *see page 631 for dose by weight*
   Cleocin (G) *Cap:* 75 (tartrazine), 150 (tartrazine), 300 mg
   Cleocin Pediatric Granules (G) *Oral susp:* 75 mg/5 ml (100 ml) (cherry)
▷ *doxycycline* (D)(G) 100 mg bid
Pediatric: <8 years: not recommended ≥8 years, <100 lb: 2 mg/lb on first day in 2 divided doses, followed by 1 mg/lb/day in 1-2 divided doses; ≥8 years, ≥100 lb: same as adult; *see page 633 for dose by weight*
   Acticlate *Tab:* 75, 150**mg
   Adoxa *Tab:* 50, 75, 100, 150 mg ent-coat
   Doryx *Tab:* 50, 75, 100, 150, 200 mg del-rel
   Doxteric *Tab:* 50 mg del-rel
   Monodox *Cap:* 50, 75, 100 mg
   Oracea *Cap:* 40 mg del-rel
   Vibramycin *Tab:* 100 mg; *Cap:* 50, 100 mg; *Syr:* 50 mg/5 ml (raspberry-apple) (sulfites); *Oral susp:* 25 mg/5 ml (raspberry)
   Vibra-Tab *Tab:* 100 mg film-coat

Comment: *doxycycline* is contraindicated <8 years-of-age, in pregnancy, and lactation (discolors developing tooth enamel). A side effect may be photosensitivity (photophobia). Do not take with antacids, calcium supplements, milk or other dairy, or within 2 hours of taking another drug.

▷ *penicillin v potassium* (B)(G) 500 mg PO qid x 3 days
   Pediatric: 50 mg/kg/day in 4 divided doses x 3 days; ≥12 years: same as adult; *see page 644 for dose by weight*
   Pen-Vee K *Tab:* 250, 500 mg; *Oral soln:* 125 mg/5 ml (100, 200 ml); 250 mg/5 ml (100, 150, 200 ml)

 BITE: HUMAN

TETANUS PROPHYLAXIS

▷ *tetanus toxoid* vaccine (C) 0.5 ml IM x 1 dose if previously immunized
   Vial: 5 Lf units/0.5 ml (0.5, 5 ml)
   Prefilled syringe: 5 Lf units/0.5 ml (0.5 ml)

ANTI-INFECTIVES

▷ *amoxicillin+clavulanate* (B)(G)
   Augmentin 500 mg tid or 875 mg bid x 10 days
   Pediatric: 40-45 mg/kg/day divided tid x 10 days or 90 mg/kg/day divided bid x 10 days *see pages 618-619 for dose by weight*
      Tab: 250, 500, 875 mg; *Chew tab:* 125, 250 mg (lemon-lime); 200, 400 mg (cherry-banana) (phenylalanine); *Oral susp:* 125 mg/5 ml (banana), 250 mg/5 ml (75, 100, 150 ml) (orange); 200, 400 mg/5 ml (50, 75, 100 ml) (orange) (phenylalanine)
   Augmentin ES-600 not recommended for adults
   Pediatric: <3 months: not recommended; ≥3 months, <40 kg: 90 mg/kg/day in 2 divided doses x 10 days; ≥40 kg: not recommended
      Oral susp: 42.9 mg/5 ml (50, 75, 100, 125, 150, 200 ml) (strawberry cream) (phenylalanine)
   Augmentin XR 2 tabs q 12 hours x 10 days
   Pediatric: <16 years: use other forms; ≥16 years: same as adult
      Tab: 1000*mg ext-rel
▷ *cefoxitin* (B) 80-160 mg/kg/day IM in 3-4 divided doses x 10 days; max 12 gm/day
   Pediatric: <3 months: not recommended; ≥3 months: same as adult
   Mefoxin Injectable *Vial:* 1, 2 g
▷ *ciprofloxacin* (C) 500 mg bid x 10 days
   Pediatric: <18 years: not recommended; ≥18 years: same as adult
   Cipro (G) *Tab:* 250, 500, 750 mg; *Oral susp:* 250, 500 mg/5 ml (100 ml) (strawberry)
   Cipro XR *Tab:* 500, 1000 mg ext-rel
   ProQuin XR *Tab:* 500 mg ext-rel
▷ *erythromycin base* (B)(G) 250 mg qid x 10 days
   Pediatric: <45 kg: 30-40 mg/kg/day in 4 divided doses x 10 days; ≥45 kg: same as adult
   Ery-Tab *Tab:* 250, 333, 500 mg ent-coat
   PCE *Tab:* 333, 500 mg
Comment: *erythromycin* may increase INR with concomitant *warfarin*, as well as increase serum level of *digoxin, benzodiazepines*, and *statins*.
▷ *erythromycin ethylsuccinate* (B)(G) 400 mg qid x 10 days
   Pediatric: 30-50 mg/kg/day in 4 divided doses x 10 days; may double dose with severe infection; max 100 mg/kg/day; *see page 635 for dose by weight*

EryPed *Oral susp:* 200 mg/5 ml (100, 200 ml) (fruit); 400 mg/5 ml (60, 100, 200 ml) (banana); *Oral drops:* 200, 400 mg/5 ml (50 ml) (fruit); *Chew tab:* 200 mg wafer (fruit)

E.E.S. *Oral susp:* 200, 400 mg/5 ml (100 ml) (fruit)

E.E.S. Granules *Oral susp:* 200 mg/5 ml (100, 200 ml) (cherry)

E.E.S. 400 Tablets *Tab:* 400 mg

Comment: *erythromycin* may increase INR with concomitant *warfarin*, as well as increase serum level of *digoxin, benzodiazepines,* and *statins.*

➤ *trimethoprim+sulfamethoxazole (TMP-SMX)*(D)(G) bid x 10 days

Pediatric: <2 months: not recommended; ≥2 months: 40 mg/kg/day of *sulfamethoxazole* in 2 divided doses bid x 10 days; *see page 648 for dose by weight*

Bactrim, Septra 2 tabs bid x 10 days

Tab: trim 80 mg+*sulfa* 400 mg*

Bactrim DS, Septra DS 1 tab bid x 10 days

Tab: trim 160 mg+*sulfa* 800 mg*

Bactrim Pediatric Suspension, Septra Pediatric Suspension

Oral susp: trim 40 mg+*sulfa* 200 mg per 5 ml (100 ml) (cherry) (alcohol 0.3%)

BLEPHARITIS

OPHTHALMIC AGENTS

➤ *erythromycin* ophthalmic ointment **(B)** apply 1/2 inch bid-qid x 14 days; then q HS x 10 days

Pediatric: same as adult

Ilotycin *Oint:* 5 mg/gm (1/2 oz)

➤ *polymyxin b+bacitracin* ophthalmic ointment **(C)** apply 1/2 inch bid-qid x 14 days; then q HS

Pediatric: same as adult

Polysporin *Oint: poly b* 10,000 U+*baci* 500 U (3.75 gm)

➤ *polymyxin b+bacitracin+neomycin* ophthalmic ointment **(C)** apply 1/2 inch bid-qid x 14 days; then q HS

Pediatric: same as adult

Neosporin *Oint: poly b* 10,000 U+*baci* 400 U+*neo* 3.5 mg/gm (3.75 gm)

➤ *sodium sulfacetamide* **(C)**

Bleph-10 Ophthalmic Solution 2 drops q 4 hours x 7-14 days

Pediatric: <2 years: not recommended; ≥2 years: 1-2 drops q 2-3 hours during the day x 7-14 days

Ophth soln: 10% (2.5, 5, 15 ml) (benzalkonium chloride)

Bleph-10 Ophthalmic Ointment apply 1/2 inch qid and HS x 7-14 days

Pediatric: <2 years: not recommended; ≥2 years: same as adult

Ophth oint: 10% (3.5 gm) (phenylmercuric acetate)

SYSTEMIC AGENTS

➤ *tetracycline* **(D)(G)** 250 mg qid x 7 days

Pediatric: <8 years: not recommended; ≥8 years, <100 lb: 25-50 mg/kg/day in 2-4 divided doses x 7-10 days; ≥100 lb: same as adult; *see page 646 for dose by weight*

Achromycin V *Cap:* 250, 500 mg

Sumycin *Tab:* 250, 500 mg; *Cap:* 250, 500 mg; *Oral susp:* 125 mg/5 ml (100, 200 ml) (fruit) (sulfites)

Comment: *tetracycline* is contraindicated <8 years-of-age, in pregnancy, and lactation (discolors developing tooth enamel). A side effect may be photo-sensitivity (photophobia). Do not give with antacids, calcium supplements, milk or other dairy, or within two hours of taking another drug.

BREAST CANCER: PROPHYLAXIS

ANTI-ESTROGEN AGENTS

▷ *fulvestrant* (D) 250 mg IM once monthly; administer 2.5 ml IM in each buttock concurrently

Faslodex *Prefilled syringe:* 50 mg/ml (2 x 2.5 ml, 1 x 5 ml)

▷ *letrozole* (D)(G) 2.5 mg daily

Femara *Tab:* 2.5 mg film-coat

Comment: *letrozole* is indicated for the extended adjuvant treatment of early breast cancer in postmenopausal women, who have received 5 years of adjuvant *tamoxifen* therapy.

▷ *tamoxifen citrate* (D)(G) 20 mg once daily x 5 years

Tab: 10, 20 mg

Comment: Cautious use of *tamoxifen* with concomitant *coumarin*-type anticoagulation therapy, history of DVT, <u>or</u> history of pulmonary embolus.

 BRONCHIOLITIS

Inhaled Beta-2 Agonists (Bronchodilators) *see Asthma page* 30
Oral Beta-2 Agonists (Bronchodilators) *see Asthma page* 37
Inhaled Corticosteroids *see Asthma page* 32
Parenteral Corticosteroids *see page* 570
Oral Corticosteroids *see page* 569

 BRONCHITIS: ACUTE AND ACUTE EXACERBATION OF CHRONIC BRONCHITIS (AECB)

Comment: Antibiotics are seldom needed for treatment of acute bronchitis because the etiology is usually viral.

Inhaled Beta-2 Agonists (Bronchodilators) *see Asthma page* 30
Oral Beta-2 Agonists (Bronchodilators) *see Asthma page* 37
Decongestants *see page* 598
Expectorants *see page* 598
Antitussives *see page* 598

ANTI-INFECTIVES FOR SECONDARY BACTERIAL INFECTION

▷ *amoxicillin* (B)(G) 500-875 mg bid <u>or</u> 250-500 mg tid x 10 days

Pediatric: <40 kg (88 lb): 20-40 mg/kg/day in 3 divided doses x 10 days <u>or</u> 25-45 mg/kg/day in 2 divided doses x 10 days; ≥40 kg: same as adult; *see page* 616 *for dose by weight*

Amoxil *Cap:* 250, 500 mg; *Tab:* 875*mg; *Chew tab:* 125, 200, 250, 400 mg (cherry-banana-peppermint) (phenylalanine); *Oral susp:* 125, 250 mg/5 ml (80, 100, 150 ml) (strawberry); 200, 400 mg/5 ml (50, 75, 100 ml) (bubble gum); *Oral drops:* 50 mg/ml (30 ml) (bubble gum)

Moxatag *Tab:* 775 mg ext-rel

Trimox *Tab:* 125, 250 mg; *Cap:* 250, 500 mg; *Oral susp:* 125, 250 mg/5 ml (80, 100, 150 ml) (raspberry-strawberry)

▷ *amoxicillin+clavulanate* (B)(G)

Augmentin 500 mg tid <u>or</u> 875 mg bid x 7-10 days

Pediatric: 40-45 mg/kg/day divided tid x 10 days <u>or</u> 90 mg/kg/day divided bid x 10 days *see pages* 618-619 *for dose by weight*

Tab: 250, 500, 875 mg; *Chew tab*: 125, 250 mg (lemon-lime); 200, 400 mg (cherry-banana) (phenylalanine); *Oral susp*: 125 mg/5 ml (banana), 250 mg/5 ml (75, 100, 150 ml) (orange); 200, 400 mg/5 ml (50, 75, 100 ml) (orange) (phenylalanine)

Augmentin ES-600 not recommended for adults

Pediatric: <3 months: not recommended; ≥3 months, <40 kg: 90 mg/kg/day in 2 divided doses x 7-10 days; ≥40 kg: not recommended

Oral susp: 42.9 mg/5 ml (50, 75, 100, 125, 150, 200 ml) (strawberry cream) (phenylalanine)

Augmentin XR 2 tabs q 12 hours x 7-10 days

Pediatric: <16 years: use other forms; ≥16 years: same as adult

Tab: 1000*mg ext-rel

➤ *ampicillin* (B) 250-500 mg qid x 10 days

Pediatric: not recommended for bronchitis in children

Omnipen, Principen *Cap*: 250, 500 mg; *Oral susp*: 125, 250 mg/5 ml (100, 150, 200 ml) (fruit)

➤ *azithromycin* (B)(G) 500 mg x 1 dose on day 1, then 250 mg daily on days 2-5 <u>or</u> 500 mg once daily x 3 days <u>or</u> 2 gm in a single dose

Pediatric: not recommended for bronchitis in children

Zithromax *Tab*: 250, 500, 600 mg; *Oral susp*: 100 mg/5 ml (15 ml); 200 mg/5 ml (15, 22.5, 30 ml) (cherry); *Pkt*: 1 gm for reconstitution (cherry-banana)

Zithromax Tri-pak *Tab*: 3 x 500 mg tabs/pck

Zithromax Z-pak *Tab*: 6 x 250 mg tabs/pck

Zmax *Oral susp*: 2 gm ext-rel for reconstitution (cherry-banana) (148 mg Na$^+$)

➤ *cefaclor* (B)(G) 250-500 mg q 8 hours x 10 days; max 2 gm/day

Tab: 500 mg; *Cap*: 250, 500 mg; *Susp*: 125 mg/5 ml (75, 150 ml) (strawberry); 187 mg/5 ml (50, 100 ml) (strawberry); 250 mg/5 ml (75, 150 ml) (strawberry); 375 mg/5 ml (50, 100 ml) (strawberry)

Pediatric: <16 years: ext-rel not recommended; ≥16 years: same as adult

Cefaclor Extended Release *Tab*: 375, 500 mg ext-rel

➤ *cefadroxil* (B) 1-2 gm in 1-2 divided doses x 10 days

Pediatric: 30 mg/kg/day in 2 divided doses x 10 days; *see page 623 for dose by weight*

Duricef *Tab*: 1 gm; *Cap*: 500 mg; *Oral susp*: 250 mg/5 ml (100 ml); 500 mg/5 ml (75, 100 ml) (orange-pineapple)

➤ *cefdinir* (B) 300 mg bid x 5-10 days <u>or</u> 600 mg daily x 10 days

Pediatric: <6 months: not recommended; 6 months-12 years: 14 mg/kg/day in 1-2 divided doses x 10 days; ≥12 years: same as adult; *see page 624 for dose by weight*

Omnicef *Cap*: 300 mg; *Oral susp*: 125 mg/5 ml (60, 100 ml) (strawberry)

➤ *cefditoren pivoxil* (B) 400 mg bid x 10 days

Pediatric: <12 years: not recommended; ≥12 years: same as adult

Spectracef *Tab*: 200 mg

Comment: Spectracef is contraindicated with milk protein allergy <u>or</u> carnitine deficiency.

➤ *cefixime* (B)(G)

Pediatric: <6 months: not recommended; ≥6 months-12 years, <50 kg: 8 mg/kg/day in 1-2 divided doses x 10 days; ≥12 years, >50 kg: same as adult; *see page 625 for dose by weight*

Suprax *Tab*: 400 mg; *Cap*: 400 mg; *Oral susp*: 100, 200, 500 mg/5 ml (50, 75, 100 ml) (strawberry)

➤ *cefpodoxime proxetil* (B) 200 mg bid x 10 days

Pediatric: <2 months: not recommended; ≥2 months-12 years: 10 mg/kg/day (max 400 mg/dose) <u>or</u> 5 mg/kg/day bid (max 200 mg/dose) x 10 days; >12 years: same as adult; *see page 626 for dose by weight*

Vantin *Tab*: 100, 200 mg; *Oral susp*: 50, 100 mg/5 ml (50, 75, 100 mg) (lemon creme)

▷ *cefprozil* (B) 500 mg q 12 hours x 10 days
Pediatric: <2 years: not recommended; 2-12 years: 15 mg/kg q 12 hours x 10 days; see page 627 for dose by weight; >12 years: same as adult
    Cefzil *Tab:* 250, 500 mg; *Oral susp:* 125, 250 mg/5 ml (50, 75, 100 ml) (bubble gum) (phenylalanine)

▷ *ceftibuten* (B) 400 mg daily x 10 days
Pediatric: 9 mg/kg daily x 10 days; max 400 mg/day; see page 628 for dose by weight
    Cedax *Cap:* 400 mg; *Oral susp:* 90 mg/5 ml (30, 60, 90, 120 ml); 180 mg/5 ml (30, 60, 120 ml) (cherry)

▷ *ceftriaxone* (B)(G) 1-2 gm IM daily continued 2 days after signs of infection have disappeared; max 4 gm/day
Pediatric: 50 mg/kg IM daily and continued 2 days after clinical stability
    Rocephin *Vial:* 250, 500 mg; 1, 2 gm

▷ *cephalexin* (B)(G) 250-500 mg qid or 500 mg bid x 10 days
Pediatric: 25-50 mg/kg/day in 4 divided doses x 10 days; ≥12 years: same as adult; see page 629 for dose by weight
    Keflex *Cap:* 250, 333, 500, 750 mg; *Oral susp:* 125, 250 mg/5 ml (100, 200 ml) (strawberry)

▷ *clarithromycin* (C)(G) 500 mg or 500 mg ext-rel once daily x 7 days
Pediatric: <6 months: not recommended; ≥6 months: 7.5 mg/kg bid x 7 days; see page 630 for dose by weight; ≥12 years: same as adult
    Biaxin *Tab:* 250, 500 mg
    Biaxin Oral Suspension *Oral susp:* 125, 250 mg/5 ml (50, 100 ml) (fruit-punch)
    Biaxin XL *Tab:* 500 mg ext-rel

▷ *dirithromycin* (C)(G) 500 mg daily x 7 days
Pediatric: <12 years: not recommended; ≥12 years: same as adult
    Dynabac *Tab:* 250 mg

▷ *doxycycline* (D)(G) 100 mg bid x 10 days
Pediatric: <8 years: not recommended; ≥8 years, <100 lb: 2 mg/lb on first day in 2 divided doses, followed by 1 mg/lb/day in 1-2 divided doses; ≥8 years, ≥100 lb: same as adult; see page 633 for dose by weight
    Acticlate *Tab:* 75, 150**mg
    Adoxa *Tab:* 50, 75, 100, 150 mg ent-coat
    Doryx *Tab:* 50, 75, 100, 150, 200 mg del-rel
    Doxteric *Tab:* 50 mg del-rel
    Monodox *Cap:* 50, 75, 100 mg
    Oracea *Cap:* 40 mg del-rel
    Vibramycin *Tab:* 100 mg; *Cap:* 50, 100 mg; *Syr:* 50 mg/5 ml (raspberry-apple) (sulfites); *Oral susp:* 25 mg/5 ml (raspberry)
    Vibra-Tab *Tab:* 100 mg film-coat

Comment: *doxycycline* is contraindicated <8 years-of-age, in pregnancy, and lactation (discolors developing tooth enamel). A side effect may be photosensitivity (photophobia). Do not take with antacids, calcium supplements, milk or other dairy, or within 2 hours of taking another drug.

▷ *erythromycin ethylsuccinate* (B)(G) 400 mg qid x 7 days
Pediatric: 30-50 mg/kg/day in 4 divided doses x 7 days; may double dose with severe infection; max 100 mg/kg/day; see page 635 for dose by weight
    EryPed *Oral susp:* 200 mg/5 ml (100, 200 ml) (fruit); 400 mg/5 ml (60, 100, 200 ml) (banana); *Oral drops:* 200, 400 mg/5 ml (50 ml) (fruit); *Chew tab:* 200 mg wafer (fruit)
    E.E.S. *Oral susp:* 200, 400 mg/5 ml (100 ml) (fruit)
    E.E.S. Granules *Oral susp:* 200 mg/5 ml (100, 200 ml) (cherry)
    E.E.S. 400 Tablets *Tab:* 400 mg

Comment: *erythromycin* may increase INR with concomitant **warfarin**, as well as increase serum level of **digoxin**, benzodiazepines and statins.

➤ **gemifloxacin** (C) 320 mg daily x 5 days
  Pediatric: <18 years: not recommended; ≥18 years: same as adult
    Factive *Tab:* 320*mg

Comment: *gemifloxacin* is contraindicated <18 years-of-age and during pregnancy and lactation. Risk of tendonitis or tendon rupture.

➤ **levofloxacin** (C) *Uncomplicated:* 500 mg daily x 7 days; *Complicated:* 750 mg daily x 7 days
  Pediatric: <18 years: not recommended; ≥18 years: same as adult
    Levaquin *Tab:* 250, 500, 750 mg

Comment: *levofloxacin* is contraindicated <18 years-of-age and during pregnancy and lactation. Risk of tendonitis or tendon rupture.

➤ **loracarbef** (B) 200-400 mg bid x 7 days
  Pediatric: 30 mg/kg/day in 2 divided doses x 7 days; ≥12 years: same as adult; *see page 642 for dose by weight*
    Lorabid *Pulvule:* 200, 400 mg; *Oral susp:* 100 mg/5 ml (50, 100 ml); 200 mg/5 ml (50, 75, 100 ml) (strawberry bubble gum)

➤ **moxifloxacin** (C)(G) 400 mg daily x 5 days
  Pediatric: <18 years: not recommended; ≥18 years: same as adult
    Avelox *Tab:* 400 mg; *IV soln:* 400 mg/250 mg (latex-free, preservative-free)

Comment: *moxifloxacin* is contraindicated <18 years-of-age and during pregnancy and lactation. Risk of tendonitis or tendon rupture.

➤ **ofloxacin** (C)(G) 400 mg bid x 10 days
  Pediatric: <18 years: not recommended; ≥18 years: same as adult
    Floxin *Tab:* 200, 300, 400 mg

Comment: *ofloxacin* is contraindicated <18 years-of-age and during pregnancy and lactation. Risk of tendonitis or tendon rupture.

➤ **telithromycin** (C) 800 mg once daily x 7-10 days; *Severe renal impairment including dialysis:* 600 mg once daily; *Severe renal impairment with coexisting hepatic impairment:* 400 mg once daily.
  Pediatric: <18 years: not recommended; ≥18 years: same as adult
    Ketek *Tab:* 400, 500 mg

Comment: *telithromycin* is a ketolide indicated for the treatment of mild-to-moderate CAP). Fatal acute liver injury has been reported; discontinue immediately if signs and symptoms of hepatitis occur. There is increased risk for ventricular arrhythmias, including ventricular tachycardia and *torsades de pointes* with fatal outcomes; avoid use in patients with known QT prolongation, hypokalemia, and with class IA and III antiarrhythmics. Fatalities with **colchicine**, rhabdomyolysis with HMG-CoA reductase inhibitors (statins), and hypotension with calcium channel blockers (CCBs) have been reported; therefore, avoid concomitant use. Monitor for toxicity and consider dose reduction of the concomitant medication, if concomitant use is unavoidable. Evaluate for *C. difficile* if diarrhea occurs. Contraindications include: myasthenia gravis, concomtitant **cisapride** or **pimozide**, history of hepatitis or jaundice with any macrolide.

➤ **tetracycline** (D)(G) 250-500 mg qid x 7 days
  Pediatric: <8 years: not recommended; ≥8 years, <100 lb: 25-50 mg/kg/day in 2-4 divided doses x 7 days; ≥8 years, ≥100 lb: same as adult; *see page 646 for dose by weight*
    Achromycin V *Cap:* 250, 500 mg
    Sumycin *Tab:* 250, 500 mg; *Cap:* 250, 500 mg; *Oral susp:* 125 mg/5 ml (100, 200 ml) (fruit) (sulfites)

Comment: *tetracycline* is contraindicated <8 years-of-age, in pregnancy, and lactation (discolors developing tooth enamel). A side effect may be photo-sensitivity (photophobia). Do not give with antacids, calcium supplements, milk or other dairy, or within two hours of taking another drug.

▷ *trimethoprim/sulfamethoxazole (TMP-SMX)*(D)(G) bid x 10 days
Pediatric: <2 months: not recommended; ≥2 months: 40 mg/kg/day of *sulfamethoxazole* in 2 divided doses bid x 10 days; *see page* 648 *for dose by weight;* ≥12 years: same as adult
    Bactrim, Septra 2 tabs bid x 10 days
        Tab: trim 80 mg+sulfa 400 mg*
    Bactrim DS, Septra DS 1 tab bid x 10 days
        Tab: trim 160 mg+sulfa 800 mg*
    Bactrim Pediatric Suspension, Septra Pediatric Suspension
        Oral susp: trim 40 mg+sulfa 200 mg per 5 ml (100 ml) (cherry) (alcohol 0.3%)

BRONCHITIS: CHRONIC/CHRONIC OBSTRUCTIVE PULMONARY DISEASE (COPD)

Oral Beta-2 Agonists (Bronchodilators) *see Asthma page* 37
Inhaled Corticosteroids *see Asthma page* 32
Parenteral Corticosteroids *see page* 570
Oral Corticosteroids *see page* 569
Inhaled Beta-2 Agonists (Bronchodilators) *see Asthma page* 30

LONG-ACTING INHALED BETA-2 AGONIST (LABA)

▷ *indacaterol* (C) inhale contents of one 75 mcg cap daily
Pediatric: <12 years: not recommended; ≥12 years: same as adult
    Arcapta Neohaler *Neohaler Device/Cap:* 75 mcg pwdr for inhalation (5 blister cards, 6 caps/card)
Comment: Remove cap from blister cap immediately before use. For oral inhalation with **Neohaler** device only. *indacaterol* is indicated for the long-term maintenance treatment of bronchoconstriction in patients with COPD. Not indicated for treating asthma, for primary treatment of acute symptoms, or for acute deterioration of COPD.

▷ *indacaterol+glycopyrrolate* (C) inhale the contents of one cap twice daily
Pediatric: <18 years: not recommended; ≥18 years: same as adult
    Utibron Neohaler *Neohaler Device/Cap:* inda 27.5 mcg+glyco 15.6 mcg pwdr for inhalation (1, 10 blister cards, 6 caps/card)

▷ *olodaterol* (C)
Pediatric: <12 years: not recommended; ≥12 years: same as adult
    Striverdi Respimat 12 mcg q 12 hours
        Inhal soln: 2.5 mcg/cartridge (metered actuation) (40 gm, 60 metered actuations) (benzalkonium chloride)

▷ *salmeterol* (C)(G) 1 inhalation q 12 hours
Pediatric: <4 years: not recommended; ≥4 years: same as adult
    Serevent Diskus
Diskus (pwdr): 50 mcg/actuation (60 doses/disk)

INHALED ANTICHOLINERGICS

▷ *ipratropium bromide* (B)(G)
Pediatric: <12 years: not recommended; ≥12 years: same as adult
    Atrovent 2 inhalations qid; max 12 inhalations/day
        Inhaler: 14 gm (200 inh)
    Atrovent Inhalation Solution 500 mcg by nebulizer tid-qid
        Inhal soln: 0.02% (2.5 ml)

Comment: *ipratropium bromide* is contraindicated with severe hypersensitivity to milk proteins.

▷ *umeclidinium* (C) 1 inhalation once daily at the same time each day
   Pediatric: <12 years: not recommended; ≥12 years: same as adult
      Incruse Ellipta *Inhal pwdr:* 62.5 mcg/inhalation (30 doses) (lactose)
      Comment: **Incruse Ellipta** is contraindicated with allergy to *atropine* or its derivatives.

INHALED LONG-ACTING ANTI-CHOLINERGICS (LAA) (ANTIMUSCARINICS)

Comment: Inhaled LAAs are for prophylaxis and chronic treatment, only. Not for primary (rescue) treatment of acute attack. Avoid getting powder in eyes. Caution with narrow-angle glaucoma, BPH, bladder neck obstruction, and pregnancy. Contraindicated with allergy to atropine or its derivatives (e.g., *ipratropium*). Avoid other anticholinergic agents.

▷ *aclidinium bromide* (C) 1 inhalation twice daily using inhaler
   Pediatric: <12 years: not recommended; ≥12 years: same as adult
      Tudorza Pressair *Inhal device:* 400 mcg/actuation (60 doses per inhalation device)
▷ *tiotropium (as bromide monohydrate)* (C) 1 inhalation daily using inhaler; do not swallow caps
   Pediatric: <12 years: not recommended; ≥12 years: same as adult
      Spiriva HandiHaler *Inhal device:* 18 mcg/cap (5, 30, 90 caps w. inhalation device)

INHALED ANTI-CHOLINERGIC+LONG-ACTING BETA-2 AGONIST (LABA)

▷ *ipratropium/albuterol* (C) 1 inhalation qid; max 6 inhalations/day
   Pediatric: <12 years: not established; ≥12 years: same as adult
      Combivent Respimat *Inhal soln:* ipra 20 mcg+alb 100 mcg per inhalation (4 gm, 120 inhal)
Comment: **Combivent Respimat** is contraindicated with *atropine* allergy.
▷ *tiotropium+olodaterol* (C) 2 inhalations once daily at the same time each day; max 2 inhalations/day
   Pediatric: <12 years: not recommended; ≥12 years: same as adult
      Stiolto Respimat *Inhal soln:* tio 2.5 mcg+olo 2.5 mcg per actuation (4 gm, 60 inh) (benzalkonium chloride)
Comment: **Stiolto Respimat** is not for treating asthma, for relief of acute bronchospasm, or acutely deteriorating COPD.
▷ *umeclidinium+vilanterol* (C) 1 inhalation once daily at the same time each day
   Pediatric: <12 years: not recommended; ≥12 years: same as adult
      Anoro Ellipta *Inhal soln:* ume 62.5 mcg+vila 25 mcg per inhalation (30 doses)
Comment: **Anoro Ellipta** is contraindicated with severe hypersensitivity to milk proteins.

INHALED CORTICOSTEROID+LONG-ACTING BETA-2 AGONIST (LABA) COMBINATION

▷ *fluticasone furoate+vilanterol* (C) 1 inhalation 100/25 once daily at the same time each day
   Pediatric: <17 years: not recommended; ≥17 years: same as adult
      Breo Ellipta 100/25 *Inhal pwdr:* flu 100 mcg+vil 25 mcg dry pwdr per inhalation (30 doses)
      Breo Ellipta 200/25 *Inhal pwdr:* flu 200 mcg+vil 25 mcg dry pwdr per inhalation (30 doses)
      Comment: **Breo Ellipta** is contraindicated with severe hypersensitivity to milk proteins.

INHALED CORTICOSTEROID+ANTICHOLINERGIC+LONG-ACTING BETA-2 AGONIST (LABA) COMBINATION

▷ *fluticasone furoate+umeclidinium+vilanterol* one inhalation once daily

> Trelegy Ellipta flutic furo 100 mcg/umec 62.5 mcg/vilan 25 mcg dry pwdr

Comment: Trelegy Ellipta is maintenance therapy for patients with COPD, including chronic bronchitis and emphysema, who are receiving fixed-dose *furoate* and *vilanterol* for airflow obstruction and to reduce exacerbations, <u>or</u> receiving *umeclidinium* and a fixed-dose combination of *fluticasone furoate* and *vilanterol*. Trelegy Ellipta is the first FDA approved once-daily single-dose inhaler that combines *fluticasone furoate*, a corticosteroid, *umeclidinium*, a long-acting muscarinic antagonist, and *vilantero*, a long-acting beta-2 adrenergic agonist. Common adverse reactions reported with Trelegy Ellipta included headache, back pain, dysgeusia, diarrhea, cough, oropharyngeal pain, and gastroenteritis. Trelegy Ellipta has been found to increase the risk of pneumonia in patients with COPD, and increase the risk of asthma-related death in patients with asthma. Trelegy Ellipta is not indicated for the treatment of asthma <u>or</u> acute bronchospasm.

REFERENCE

Trelegy Ellipta approved as the first once-daily single inhaler triple therapy for the treatment of appropriate patients with COPD in the US [press release]. London, UK: GlaxoSmithKline plc, September 18, 2017. https://www.gsk.com/en-gb/media/press-releases/trelegy-ellipta-approved-as-the-first-once-daily-single-inhaler-triple-therapy-for-the-treatment-of-appropriate-patients-with-copd-in-the-us/

METHYLXANTHINES

Comment: Check serum theophylline level just before 5th dose is administered. Therapeutic theophylline level: 10-20 mcg/ml.

▷ *theophylline* (C)(G)

> **Theo-24** initially 300-400 mg once daily at HS; after 3 days, increase to 400-600 mg once daily at HS; max 600 mg/day
> *Pediatric:* <45 kg: initially 12-14 mg/kg/day; max 300 mg/day; increase after 3 days to 16 mg/kg/day to max 400 mg; after 3 more days increase to 30 mg/kg/day to max 600 mg/day; ≥45 kg: same as adult
> > *Cap:* 100, 200, 300, 400 mg ext-rel
>
> **Theo-Dur** initially 150 mg bid; increase to 200 mg bid after 3 days; then increase to 300 mg bid after 3 more days
> *Pediatric:* <6 years: not recommended; ≥6-15 years: initially 12-14 mg/kg/day in 2 divided doses; max 300 mg/day; then increase to 16 mg/kg in 2 divided doses; max 400 mg/day; then to 20 mg/kg/day in 2 divided doses; max 600 mg/day
> > *Tab:* 100, 200, 300 mg ext-rel
>
> **Theolair-SR**
> *Pediatric:* <12 years: not recommended; ≥12 years: same as adult
> > *Tab:* 200, 250, 300, 500 mg sust-rel
>
> **Uniphyl** 400-600 mg daily with meals
> *Pediatric:* <12 years: not recommended; ≥12 years: same as adult
> > *Tab:* 400*, 600*mg cont-rel

METHYLXANTHINE+EXPECTORANT COMBINATION

▷ *dyphylline+guaifenesin* (C)

> **Lufyllin GG** 1 tab qid <u>or</u> 15-30 ml qid
> > *Tab: dyphy* 200 mg+*guaif* 200 mg; *Elix: dyphy* 100 mg+*guaif* 100 mg per 15 ml

SELECTIVE PHOSPHODIESTERASE 4 (PDE4) INHIBITOR

▷ *roflumilast (C)* 500 mcg once daily
  Pediatric: <12 years: not recommended; ≥12 years: same as adult
    Daliresp *Tab:* 500 mcg
  Comment: *roflumilast* is indicated to reduce the risk of COPD exacerbations in severe COPD patients with chronic bronchitis and a history of exacerbations.

LONG-ACTING MUSCARINIC ANTAGONISTS (LAMA)

▷ *glycopyrrolate* (C)
Comment: There are no data on the safety of *glycopyrrolate* use in pregnancy or presence of *glycopyrrolate* or its metabolites in human milk or effects on the breastfed infant.
    Lonhala Magnair inhale the contents of 1 vial twice daily at the same times of day, AM and PM, via Magnair neb inhal device; do not swallow solution; do not use **Magnair** with any other medicine; length of treatment is 2-3 minutes; do not use 2 vials/treatment or more than 2 vials/day
    Pediatric: not indicated for use in children
      Neb soln: Vial: 25 mcg/1 ml single-dose for administration with Magnair neb inhal device; *Starter Kit:* 30 day supply (2 vials/pouch, 30 foil pouches/carton) and 1 complete MAGNAIR Nebulizer System; *Refill Kit:* (2 vials/pouch, 30 foil pouches/carton) and 1 complete MAGNAIR refill handset
Comment: **Lonhala Magnair** is the first nebulizing long-acting muscarinic antagonist (LAMA) approved for the treatment of COPD in the United States. Its approval was based on data from clinical trials in the Glycopyrrolate for Obstructive Lung Disease via Electronic Nebulizer (GOLDEN) program, including GOLDEN-3 and GOLDEN-4, 2 Phase 3, 12-week, randomized, double-blind, placebo-controlled, parallel-group, multicenter study.
    Seebri Neohaler inhale the contents of 1 capsule twice daily at the same time of day, AM and PM, using the neohaler; do not swallow caps
    Pediatric: not indicated for use in children
      Inhal cap: 15.6 mcg (60/blister pck) dry pwdr for inhalation w. 1 Neohaler device (lactose)

BULIMIA NERVOSA

SELECTIVE SEROTONIN REUPTAKE INHIBITOR (SSRI)

▷ *fluoxetine* (C)(G)
    Prozac initially 20 mg daily; may increase after 1 week; doses >20 mg/day may be divided into AM and noon doses; usual daily dose 60 mg; max 80 mg/day
    Pediatric: <8 years: not recommended; 8-17 years: initially 10-20 mg/day; start lower weight children at 10 mg/day; if starting at 10 mg daily, may increase after 1 week to 20 mg daily; >17 years: same as adult
      Cap: 10, 20, 40 mg; *Tab:* 30*, 60*mg; *Oral soln:* 20 mg/5 ml (4 oz) (mint)
    Prozac Weekly following daily *fluoxetine* therapy at 20 mg/day for 13 weeks, may initiate **Prozac Weekly** 7 days after the last 20 mg *fluoxetine* dose
    Pediatric: <12 years: not recommended; ≥12 years: same as adult
      Cap: 90 mg ent-coat del-rel pellets

BURN: MINOR

▷ *silver sulfadiazine* (C)(G) apply topically to burn 1-2 x daily
    Pediatric: <12 years: not recommended; ≥12 years: same as adult

Silvadene *Crm:* 1% (20, 50, 85, 400, 1000 gm jar; 20 gm tube)
Comment: *silver sulfadiazine* is contradicted in sulfa allergy.

TOPICAL & TRANSDERMAL ANESTHETICS

Comment: *lidocaine* should not be applied to non-intact skin.
▷ *lidocaine* burn gel (B)(G)
▷ *lidocaine* cream (B)
    LidaMantle *Crm:* 3% (1, 2 oz)
    Lidoderm *Crm:* 3% (85 gm)
▷ *lidocaine* lotion (B)
    LidaMantle *Lotn:* 3% (177 ml)
▷ *lidocaine* 5% patch (B)(G) apply up to 3 patches at one time for up to 12 hours/24-hour period (12 hours on/12 hours off); patches may be cut into smaller sizes before removal of the release liner; do not re-use
    Pediatric: <12 years: not recommended; ≥12 years: same as adult
    Lidoderm *Patch:* 5% (10x14 cm; 30/carton)
▷ *lidocaine* 2.5%+*prilocaine* 2.5% apply sparingly to the burn bid-tid prn
    Pediatric: <12 years: not recommended; ≥12 years: same as adult
    Emla Cream (B) 5, 30 gm/tube

BURSITIS

Acetaminophen for IV Infusion *see Pain page 344*
NSAIDs *see page 562*
Opioid Analgesics *see Pain page 345*
Topical and Transdermal NSAIDs *see Pain page 344*
Parenteral Corticosteroids *see page 570*
Oral Corticosteroids *see page 569*
Topical Analgesic and Anesthetic Agents *see page 560*

CANDIDIASIS: ABDOMEN, BLADDER, ESOPHAGUS, KIDNEY

▷ *voriconazole* (D)(G) *PO:* <40 kg: 100 mg q 12 hours; may increase to 150 mg q 12 hours if inadequate response; ≥40 kg: 200 mg q 12 hours; may increase to 300 mg q 12 hours if inadequate; *IV:* 6 mg/kg q 12 hours x 2 doses; then 4 mg/kg q 12 hour; max rate 3 mg/kg/hour over 1-2 hours; response
    Pediatric: <12 years: not recommended; ≥12 years: same as adult
    Vfend *Tab:* 50, 200 mg
    Vfend I.V. for Injection *Vial:* 200 mg pwdr for reconstitution (preservative-free)
    Vfend *Oral susp:* 40 mg/ml pwdr for reconstitution (75 ml) (orange)

CANDIDIASIS: ORAL (THRUSH)

ORAL ANTIFUNGALS

▷ *clotrimazole* (C) *Prophylaxis:* 1 troche dissolved in mouth tid; *Treatment:* 1 troche dissolved in mouth 5 x/day x 10-14 days
    Pediatric: <3 years: not recommended; ≥3 years: same as adult
    Mycelex Troches *Troche:* 10 mg
▷ *fluconazole* (C) 200 mg x 1 dose first day; then 100 mg once daily x 13 days
    Pediatric: >2 weeks: 6 mg/kg x 1 day; then 3 mg/kg/day for at least 3 weeks; *see page 638 for dose by weight*

> **Diflucan** *Tab:* 50, 100, 150, 200 mg; *Oral susp:* 10, 40 mg/ml (35 ml) (orange) (sucrose)

➤ *gentian violet* **(G)** apply to oral mucosa with a cotton swab tid x 3 days

➤ *itraconazole* **(C)(G)** 200 mg daily x 7-14 days
  Pediatric: 5 mg/kg daily x 7-14 days; max 200 mg/day; *see page* 631 *for dose by weight*
  > **Sporanox** *Oral soln:* 10 mg/ml (150 ml) (cherry-caramel)

➤ *miconazole* **(C)** One buccal tab once daily x 14 days; apply to upper gum region; hold in place 30 seconds; do not crush, chew, <u>or</u> swallow
  Pediatric: <16 years: not recommended; ≥16 years: same as adult
  > **Oravig** *Buccal tab:* 50 mg (14/pck)

➤ *nystatin* **(C)(G)**
  > **Mycostatin** 1-2 pastilles dissolved slowly in mouth 4-5 x/day x 10-14 days; max 14 days
  > *Pediatric:* same as adult
  > > *Pastille:* 200,000 units (30 pastilles/pck)
  > **Mycostatin Suspension** 4-6 ml qid swish and swallow
  > *Pediatric: Infants:* 1 ml in each cheek qid after feedings; *Older children:* same as adult
  > > *Oral susp:* 100,000 units/ml (60 ml w. dropper)

INVASIVE INFECTION

➤ *posaconazole* **(D)** take with food; 100 mg bid on day one; then 100 mg once daily x 13 days; refractory, 400 mg bid
  Pediatric: <13 years: not recommended; ≥13 years: same as adult
  > **Noxafil** *Oral susp:* 40 mg/ml (105 ml) (cherry)

  Comment: **Noxafil** is indicated as prophylaxis for invasive aspergillus and candida infections in patients >13-years-old who are at high risk due to being severely compromised.

CANDIDIASIS: SKIN

TOPICAL ANTIFUNGALS

➤ *butenafine* **(B)(G)** apply bid x 1 week <u>or</u> once daily x 4 weeks
  Pediatric: <12 years: not recommended; ≥12 years: same as adult
  > **Lotrimin Ultra** **(C)(OTC)** *Crm:* 1% (12, 24 gm)
  > **Mentax** *Crm:* 1% (15, 30 gm)

Comment: *butenafine* is a benzylamine, not an azole. Fungicidal activity continues for at least 5 weeks after the last application.

➤ *ciclopirox* **(B)**
  > **Loprox Cream** apply bid; max 4 weeks
  > *Pediatric:* <10 years: not recommended; ≥10 years: same as adult
  > > *Crm:* 0.77% (15, 30, 90 gm)
  > **Loprox Lotion** apply bid; max 4 weeks
  > *Pediatric:* <10 years: not recommended; ≥10 years: same as adult
  > > *Lotn:* 0.77% (30, 60 ml)
  > **Loprox Gel** apply bid; max 4 weeks
  > *Pediatric:* <16 years: not recommended; ≥16 years: same as adult
  > > *Gel:* 0.77% (30, 45 gm)

➤ *clotrimazole* **(B)** apply bid x 7 days
  Pediatric: <12 years: not recommended; ≥12 years: same as adult
  > **Lotrimin** *Crm:* 1% (15, 30, 45 gm)
  > **Lotrimin AF** **(OTC)** *Crm:* 1% (12 gm); *Lotn:* 1% (10 ml); *Soln:* 1% (10 ml)

▷ *econazole* (C) apply bid x 14 days
  Pediatric: <12 years: not recommended; ≥12 years: same as adult
    Spectazole *Crm:* 1% (15, 30, 85 gm)
▷ *ketoconazole* (C) apply once daily x 14 days
  Pediatric: <12 years: not recommended; ≥12 years: same as adult
    Nizoral Cream *Crm:* 2% (15, 30, 60 gm)
▷ *miconazole* 2% (C) apply once daily x 2 weeks
  Pediatric: <12 years: not recommended; ≥12 years: same as adult
    Lotrimin AF Spray Liquid (OTC) *Spray liq:* 2% (113 gm) (alcohol 17%)
    Lotrimin AF Spray Powder (OTC) *Spray pwdr:* 2% (90 gm) (alcohol 10%)
    Monistat-Derm *Crm:* 2% (1, 3 oz); *Spray liq:* 2% (3.5 oz); *Spray pwdr:* 2% (3 oz)
▷ *nystatin* (C) dust affected skin freely bid-tid
    Nystop Powder *Pwdr:* 100,000 U/gm (15 gm)

ORAL ANTIFUNGALS

▷ *amphotericin b* (B)
    Fungizone *Oral susp:* 100 mg/ml (24 ml w. dropper)
▷ *ketoconazole* (C) 400 mg once daily x 1-2 weeks
  Pediatric: <2 years: not recommended; ≥2 years: 3.3-6.6 mg/kg once daily
    Nizoral *Tab:* 200 mg

INVASIVE INFECTION

▷ *posaconazole* (D) take with food; 100 mg bid on day one; then 100 mg once daily x 13
  days; refractory, 400 mg bid x 13 days
  Pediatric: <13 years: not recommended; ≥13 years: same as adult
    Noxafil *Oral susp:* 40 mg/ml (105 ml) (cherry)
Comment: **Noxafil** is indicated as prophylaxis for invasive aspergillus and candida infections in patients >13 years old who are at high risk due to being severely compromised.

 CANDIDIASIS: VULVOVAGINAL (*MONILIASIS*)

PROPHYLAXIS

▷ *acetic acid+oxyquinolone* (C) one full applicator intravaginally bid for up to 30 days
  Pediatric: <12 years: not recommended; ≥12 years: same as adult
    Relagard *Gel:* acetic acid 0.9%+oxyquin 0.025% (50 gm tube w. applicator)

Comment: The following treatment regimens for vulvovaginal candidiasis (VVC) are published in the **2015 CDC Sexually Transmitted Diseases Treatment Guidelines**. Treatment regimens are presented by generic drug name first, followed by information about brands and dose forms. Complicated VVC (recurrent, severe, non-albicans, or women with uncontrolled diabetes, debilitation, or immunosuppression) may require more intensive treatment and/or longer duration of treatment. VVC frequently occurs during pregnancy. Only topical azole therapies, applied for 7 days, are recommended during pregnancy.

RX ORAL AGENT

▷ *fluconazole* 150 mg in a single dose; complicated VVC, 150 mg x 3 doses on days 1, 4,
  7 or weekly x 6 months

Rx INTRAVAGINAL AGENTS
Regimen 1

▷ *butoconazole* 2% cream (bioadhesive product) 5 gm intravaginally in a single dose

Regimen 2
▷ *nystatin* 100,000-unit vaginal tablet once daily x 14 days

Regimen 3
▷ *terconazole* 0.4% cream 5 gm intravaginally once daily x 7 days

Regimen 4
▷ *terconazole* 0.8% cream 5 gm intravaginally once daily x 3 days

Regimen 5
▷ *terconazole* 80 mg vaginal suppository intravaginally once daily x 3 days

OTC INTRAVAGINAL AGENTS
Regimen 1
▷ *butoconazole* 2% cream 5 gm intravaginally once daily x 3 days

Regimen 2
▷ *clotrimazole* 1% cream intravaginally once daily x 7-14 days

Regimen 3
▷ *clotrimazole* 2% cream intravaginally once daily x 3 days

Regimen 4
▷ *miconazole* 2% cream intravaginally once daily x 7 days

Regimen 5
▷ *miconazole* 4% cream intravaginally once daily x 3 days

Regimen 6
▷ *miconazole* 100 mg vaginal suppository intravaginally once daily x 7 days

Regimen 7
▷ *miconazole* 200 mg vaginal suppository intravaginally once daily x 3 days

Regimen 8
▷ *miconazole* 1,200 mg vaginal suppository intravaginally in a single application

Regimen 9
▷ *tioconazole* 6.5% ointment 5 gm intravaginally in a single application

DRUG BRANDS AND DOSE FORMS
▷ *butoconazole* cream 2% **(C)**
    Gynazole-12% Vaginal Cream *Prefilled vag applicator:* 5 g
    Femstat-3 Vaginal Cream (OTC) *Vag crm:* 2% (20 gm w. 3 applicators); *Prefilled vag applicator:* 5 gm (3/pck)
▷ *clotrimazole* **(B)(OTC)**
    Gyne-Lotrimin Vaginal Cream (OTC) *Vag crm:* 1% (45 gm w. applicator)
    Gyne-Lotrimin Vaginal Suppository (OTC) *Vag supp:* 100 mg (7/pck)

Gyne-Lotrimin 3 Vaginal Suppository (OTC) *Vag supp:* 200 mg (3/pck)
Gyne-Lotrimin Combination Pack (OTC) *Combination pck:* 7-100 mg supp <u>with</u> 7 gm 1% cream
Gyne-Lotrimin 3 Combination Pack (OTC) *Combination pck:* 200 mg supp (7/pck) <u>plus</u> 1% cream (7 gm)
Mycelex-G Vaginal Cream *Vag crm:* 1% (45, 90 gm w. applicator)
Mycelex-G Vaginal Tab 1 *Tab:* 500 mg (1/pck)
Mycelex Twin Pack *Twin pck:* 500 mg tab (7/pck) <u>with</u> 1% crm (7 gm)
Mycelex-7 Vaginal Cream (OTC) *Vag crm:* 1% (45 gm w. applicator)
Mycelex-7 Vaginal Inserts (OTC) *Vag insert:* 100 mg insert (7/pck)
Mycelex-7 Combination Pack (OTC) *Combination pck:* 100 mg inserts (7/pck) <u>plus</u> 1% crm (7 gm)
▷ *fluconazole* (C)
Diflucan *Tab:* 50, 100, 150, 200 mg; *Oral susp:* 10, 40 mg/ml (35 ml) (orange)
▷ *miconazole* (B)
Monistat-3 Combination Pack (OTC) *Combination pck:* 200 mg supp (3/pck) <u>plus</u> 2% crm (9 gm)
Monistat-7 Combination Pack (OTC) *Combination pck:* 100 mg supp (7/pck) <u>plus</u> 2% crm (9 gm)
Monistat-7 Vaginal Cream (OTC) *Vag crm:* 2% (45 gm w. applicator)
Monistat-7 Vaginal Suppositories (OTC) *Vag supp:* 100 mg (7/pck)
Monistat-3 Vaginal Suppositories (OTC) *Vag supp:* 200 mg (3/pck)
▷ *nystatin* (C)
Mycostatin *Vag tab:* 100,000 U (1/pck)
▷ *terconazole* (C)
Terazol-3 Vaginal Cream *Vag crm:* 0.8% (20 gm w. applicator)
Terazol-3 Vaginal Suppositories *Vag supp:* 80 mg supp (3/pck)
Terazol-7 Vaginal Cream *Vag crm:* 0.4% (45 gm w. applicator)
▷ *tioconazole* (C)
1-Day (OTC) *Vag oint:* 6.5% (prefilled applicator x 1)
Monistat 1 Vaginal Ointment (OTC) *Vag oint:* 6.5% (prefilled applicator x 1)
Vagistat-1 Vaginal Ointment (OTC) *Vag oint:* 6.5% (prefilled applicator x 1)

INVASIVE INFECTION

▷ *posaconazole* (D) take with food; 100 mg bid on day 1; then 100 mg once daily x 13 days; refractory, 400 mg bid
Pediatric: <13 years: not recommended; ≥13 years: same as adult
Noxafil *Oral susp:* 40 mg/ml (105 ml) (cherry)
Comment: **Noxafil** is indicated as prophylaxis for invasive aspergillus and candida infections in patients >13-years-old who are at high risk due to being severely compromised.

 CANNABINOID HYPEREMESIS SYNDROME (CHS)

Comment: cannabinoid hyperemesis syndrome (CHS) is indicated by recurrent episodes of refractory nausea and vomiting with vague diffuse abdominal pain (accompanied by compulsive, frequent, hot baths <u>or</u> showers for relief of abdominal pain; these behaviors are thought to be learned through their cyclical periods of emesis) in the setting of chronic cannabis use (at least weekly for >2 years. The nausea and vomiting typically do not respond to antiemetic medications. 5HT3 (e.g., ***ondansetron***), D2 (e.g., ***prochlorperazine***), H1 (e.g., ***promethazine***), <u>or</u> neurokinin-1 receptor antagonists (e.g., ***aprepitant***) can be tried, but these therapies often are ineffective. The recovery phase can last weeks to months despite continued cannabis use prior to returning to the hyperemetic phase. Symptoms that are worse in the morning, with normal bowel habits, and negative evaluation, including laboratory, radiography, and endoscopy. Resolution requires cannabis cessation from 1 to 3 months. Returning to cannabis use often results in the returning of CHS.

REFERENCE

Fleming, J. E., & Lockwood, S. (2017). Cannabinoid hyperemesis syndrome. *Fed Pract, 34*(10), 33–36.

PHENOTHIAZINES

▷ *chlorpromazine* (C)(G) 10-25 mg PO q 4 hours prn or 50-100 mg rectally q 6-8 hours prn
  Pediatric: <6 months: not recommended; ≥6 months: 0.25 mg/lb orally q 4-6 hours prn or 0.5 mg/lb rectally q 6-8 hours prn
    Thorazine *Tab:* 10, 25, 50, 100, 200 mg; *Spansule:* 30, 75, 150 mg sust-rel; *Syr:* 10 mg/5 ml (4 oz; orange custard); *Conc:* 30 mg/ml (4 oz); 100 mg/ml (2, 8 oz); *Supp:* 25, 100 mg

▷ *perphenazine* (C) 5 mg IM (may repeat in 6 hours) or 8-16 mg/day PO in divided doses; max 15 mg/day IM; max 24 mg/day PO
  Pediatric: <12 years: not recommended; ≥12 years: same as adult
    Trilafon *Tab:* 2, 4, 8, 16 mg; *Oral conc:* 16 mg/5 ml (118 ml); *Amp:* 5 mg/ml (1 ml)

▷ *prochlorperazine* (C)(G) 5-10 mg tid-qid prn; usual max 40 mg/day
    Compazine
    Pediatric: <2 years or <20 lb: not recommended; 20-29 lb: 2.5 mg daily bid prn; max 7.5 mg/day; 30-39 lb: 2.5 mg bid-tid prn; max 10 mg/day; 40-85 lb: 2.5 mg tid or 5 mg bid prn; max 15 mg/day
      Tab: 5, 10 mg; *Syr:* 5 mg/5 ml (4 oz) (fruit)
    Compazine Suppository 25 mg rectally bid prn; usual max 50 mg/day
    Pediatric: <2 years or <20 lb: not recommended; 20-29 lb: 2.5 mg daily-bid prn; max 7.5; mg/day; 30-39 lb: 2.5 mg bid-tid prn; max 10 mg/day; 40-85 lb: 2.5 mg tid or 5 mg bid prn; max 15 mg/day
      Rectal supp: 2.5, 5, 25 mg
    Compazine Injectable 5-10 mg tid or qid prn
    Pediatric: <2 years or <20 lb: not recommended; ≥2 years or ≥20 lb: 0.06 mg/kg x 1 dose
      Vial: 5 mg/ml (2, 10 ml)
    Compazine Spansule 15 mg q AM prn or 10 mg q 12 hours prn usual max 40 mg/day
    Pediatric: <12 years: not recommended; ≥12 years: same as adult
      Spansule: 10, 15 mg sust-rel

▷ *promethazine* (C)(G) 25 mg PO or rectally q 4-6 hours prn
  Pediatric: <2 years: not recommended; ≥2 years: 0.5 mg/lb or 6.25-25 mg q 4-6 hours prn
    Phenergan *Tab:* 12.5*, 25*, 50 mg; *Plain syr:* 6.25 mg/5 ml; *Fortis syr:* 25 mg/5 ml; *Rectal supp:* 12.5, 25, 50 mg

SUBSTANCE P/NEUROKININ 1 RECEPTOR ANTAGONIST

▷ *aprepitant* (B)(G) administer with 5HT-3 receptor antagonist; *Day 1:* 125 mg x 1 dose; *Starting Day 2:* 80 mg once daily in the morning
  Pediatric: <6 months: years: not recommended; ≥6 months: use oral suspension (see mfr pkg insert for dose by weight
    Emend *Cap:* 40, 80, 125 mg (2 x 80 mg bi-fold pck; 1 x 25 mg/2 x 80 mg tri-fold pck); *Oral susp:* 125 mg pwdr for oral suspension, single-dose pouch w. dispenser; *Vial:* 150 mg pwdr for reconstitution and IV infusion

SEROTONIN (5HT-3) RECEPTOR ANTAGONISTS

▷ **dolasetron (B)** administer 100 mg IV over 30 seconds; max 100 mg/dose
   Pediatric: <2 years: not recommended; 2-16 years: 1.8 mg/kg; >16 years: same as adult
       Anzemet *Tab:* 50, 100 mg; *Amp:* 12.5 mg/0.625 ml; *Prefilled carpuject syringe:* 12.5
       mg (0.625 ml); *Vial:* 100 mg/5 ml (single-use); *Vial:* 500 mg/25 ml (multi-dose)

▷ **granisetron**
       Kytril (B) administer IV over 30 seconds; max 1 dose/week
       Pediatric: <2 years: not recommended; ≥2 years: 10 mcg/kg
           Tab: 1 mg; *Oral soln:* 2 mg/10 ml (30 ml) (orange); *Vial:* 1 mg/ml (1 ml
           single-dose) (preservative-free); 1 mg/ml (4 ml multi-dose) (benzyl alcohol)
       Sancuso (B) apply 1 patch; remove 24 hours (minimum) to 7 days (maximum)
           Transdermal patch: 3.1 mg/day

▷ **Sustol** administer SC over 20-30 seconds (due to drug viscosity) and not more frequently than once every 7 days; *CrCl 30-59 mL/min:* repeat dose no more than every
   14th day; *CrCl <30 mL/min:* not recommended
   Pediatric: <18 years: not established; ≥18 years: same as adult
       Syringe: 10 mg/0.4 ml ext-rel; prefilled single-dose/kit

   Comment: At least 60 minutes prior to administration, remove the **Sustol** kit from
   refrigeration; activate a warming pouch and wrap the syringe in the warming pouch
   for 5-6 minutes to warm it to room temperature.

▷ **ondansetron (C)(G)** Oral Forms: 8 mg q 8 hours x 2 doses; then 8 mg q 12 hours
   Pediatric: <4 years: not recommended; 4-11 years: 4 mg q 4 hours x 3 doses; then 4
   mg q 8 hours
       Zofran *Tab:* 4, 8, 24 mg
       Zofran ODT *ODT:* 4, 8 mg (strawberry) (phenylalanine)
       Zofran Oral Solution *Oral soln:* 4 mg/5 ml (50 ml) (strawberry) (phenylalanine);
       Parenteral form: see mfr pkg insert
       Zofran Injection *Vial:* 2 mg/ml (2 ml single-dose); 2 mg/ml (20 ml muti-dose); 32
       mg/50 ml (50 ml multi-dose); *Prefilled syringe:* 4 mg/2 ml, single-use (24/ carton)
       Zuplenz Oral Soluble Film: 4, 8 mg oral-dis (10/carton) (peppermint)

▷ **palonosetron (B)(G)** administer 0.25 mg IV over 30 seconds; max 1 dose/week
   Pediatric: <1 month: not recommended; 1 month to 17 years: 20 mcg/kg; max 1.5 mg/
   single dose; infuse over 15 minutes
       Aloxi *Vial (single-use):* 0.075 mg/1.5 ml; 0.25 mg/5 ml (mannitol)

 CARCINOID SYNDROME DIARRHEA

TRYPTOPHAN HYDROXYLASE

▷ **telotristat** <18 years: not established; ≥18 years: take with food; 250 mg tid
       Xermelo *Tab:* 250 mg (4 x 7 daily dose pcks/carton)

Comment: Take **Xermelo** in combination with somatostatin analog (SSA) therapy to
treat patients inadequately controlled by SSA therapy. Breastfeeding females should
monitor the infant for constipation.

 CARPAL TUNNEL SYNDROME (CTS)

Acetaminophen for IV Infusion *see Pain page 344*
NSAIDs *see page 562*
Opioid Analgesics *see Pain page 345*
Topical and Transdermal NSAIDs *see Pain page 344*
Parenteral Corticosteroids *see page 570*

Oral Corticosteroids *see page* 569
Topical Analgesic and Anesthetic Agents *see page* 560

CAT SCRATCH FEVER (*BARTONELLA*)

Comment: Cat scratch fever is usually self-limited. Treatment should be limited to severe <u>or</u> debilitating cases.

ANTI-INFECTIVES

➤ *azithromycin* (B)(G) 500 mg x 1 dose on day 1, then 250 mg daily on days 2-5 <u>or</u> 500 mg daily x 3 days <u>or</u> **Zmax** 2 gm in a single dose
Pediatric: 12 mg/kg/day x 5 days; max 500 mg/day; *see page* 621 *for dose by weight*
Zithromax *Tab:* 250, 500, 600 mg; *Oral susp:* 100 mg/5 ml (15 ml); 200 mg/5 ml (15, 22.5, 30 ml) (cherry); *Pkt:* 1 gm for reconstitution (cherry-banana)
Zithromax Tri-pak *Tab:* 3 x 500 mg tabs/pck
Zithromax Z-pak *Tab:* 6 x 250 mg tabs/pck
Zmax *Oral susp:* 2 gm ext-rel for reconstitution (cherry-banana) (148 mg Na$^+$)
➤ *doxycycline* (D)(G) 100 mg daily bid
Pediatric: <8 years: not recommended ≥8 years, <100 lb: 2 mg/lb on first day in 2 divided doses, followed by 1 mg/lb/day in 1-2 divided doses; ≥8 years, ≥100 lb: same as adult; *see page* 633 *for dose by weight*
Acticlate *Tab:* 75, 150**mg
Adoxa *Tab:* 50, 75, 100, 150 mg ent-coat
Doryx *Tab:* 50, 75, 100, 150, 200 mg del-rel
Doxteric *Tab:* 50 mg del-rel
Monodox *Cap:* 50, 75, 100 mg
Oracea *Cap:* 40 mg del-rel
Vibramycin *Tab:* 100 mg; *Cap:* 50, 100 mg; *Syr:* 50 mg/5 ml (raspberry-apple) (sulfites); *Oral susp:* 25 mg/5 ml (raspberry)
Vibra-Tab *Tab:* 100 mg film-coat
➤ *erythromycin base* (B)(G) 500-1000 mg qid x 4 weeks
Pediatric: <45 kg: 30-50 mg in 2-4 divided doses x 4 weeks; ≥45 kg: same as adult
Ery-Tab *Tab:* 250, 333, 500 mg ent-coat
PCE *Tab:* 333, 500 mg

Comment: *erythromycin* may increase INR with concomitant *warfarin*, as well as increase serum level of *digoxin, benzodiazepines*, and *statins*.

➤ *erythromycin ethylsuccinate* (B)(G) 400 mg qid x 4 weeks
Pediatric: 30-50 mg/kg/day in 4 divided doses x 4 weeks; may double dose with severe infection; max 100 mg/kg/day; *see page* 635 *for dose by weight*
EryPed *Oral susp:* 200 mg/5 ml (100, 200 ml) (fruit); 400 mg/5 ml (60, 100, 200 ml) (banana); *Oral drops:* 200, 400 mg/5 ml (50 ml) (fruit); *Chew tab:* 200 mg wafer (fruit)
E.E.S. *Oral susp:* 200, 400 mg/5 ml (100 ml) (fruit)
E.E.S. Granules *Oral susp:* 200 mg/5 ml (100, 200 ml) (cherry)
E.E.S. 400 Tablets *Tab:* 400 mg

Comment: *erythromycin* may increase INR with concomitant *warfarin*, as well as increase serum level of *digoxin, benzodiazepines*, and *statins*.

➤ *trimethoprim+sulfamethoxazole (TMP-SMX)*(D)(G) bid x 10 days
Pediatric: <2 months: not recommended; ≥2 months: 40 mg/kg/day of *sulfamethoxazole* in 2 divided doses bid x 10 days; *see page* 648 *for dose by weight*
Bactrim, Septra 2 tabs bid x 10 days
Tab: trim 80 mg+sulfa 400 mg*

Bactrim DS, Septra DS 1 tab bid x 10 days
Tab: trim 160 mg+sulfa 800 mg*
Bactrim Pediatric Suspension, Septra Pediatric Suspension
Oral susp: trim 40 mg+sulfa 200 mg per 5 ml (100 ml) (cherry) (alcohol 0.3%)

 CELLULITIS

Comment: Duration of treatment should be 10-30 days. Obtain culture from site. Consider blood cultures.

ANTI-INFECTIVES

▷ *amoxicillin* (B)(G) 500-875 mg bid <u>or</u> 250-500 mg tid x 10 days
Pediatric: <40 kg (88 lb): 20-40 mg/kg/day in 3 divided doses x 10 days <u>or</u> 25-45 mg/kg/day in 2 divided doses x 10 days; ≥40 kg: same as adult; *see page* 616 *for dose by weight*
　　Amoxil *Cap:* 250, 500 mg; *Tab:* 875*mg; *Chew tab:* 125, 200, 250, 400 mg (cherry-banana-peppermint) (phenylalanine); *Oral susp:* 125, 250 mg/5 ml (80, 100, 150 ml) (strawberry); 200, 400 mg/5 ml (50, 75, 100 ml) (bubble gum); *Oral drops:* 50 mg/ml (30 ml) (bubble gum)
　　Moxatag *Tab:* 775 mg ext-rel
　　Trimox *Tab:* 125, 250 mg; *Cap:* 250, 500 mg; *Oral susp:* 125, 250 mg/5 ml (80, 100, 150 ml) (raspberry-strawberry)
▷ *amoxicillin+clavulanate* (B)(G)
　　Augmentin 500 mg tid <u>or</u> 875 mg bid x 7-10 days
　　Pediatric: 40-45 mg/kg/day divided tid x 10 days <u>or</u> 90 mg/kg/day divided bid x 10 days *see pages* 618-619 *for dose by weight*
　　　　Tab: 250, 500, 875 mg; *Chew tab:* 125, 250 mg (lemon-lime); 200, 400 mg (cherry-banana) (phenylalanine); *Oral susp:* 125 mg/5 ml (banana), 250 mg/5 ml (75, 100, 150 ml) (orange); 200, 400 mg/5 ml (50, 75, 100 ml) (orange) (phenylalanine)
　　Augmentin ES-600 not recommended for adults
　　Pediatric: <3 months: not recommended; ≥3 months, <40 kg: 90 mg/kg/day in 2 divided doses x 7-10 days; ≥40 kg: not recommended
　　　　Oral susp: 42.9 mg/5 ml (50, 75, 100, 125, 150, 200 ml) (strawberry cream) (phenylalanine)
　　Augmentin XR 2 tabs q 12 hours x 7-10 days
　　Pediatric: <16 years: use other forms; ≥16 years: same as adult
　　　　Tab: 1000*mg ext-rel
▷ *azithromycin* (B)(G) 500 mg x 1 dose on day 1, then 250 mg daily on days 2-5 <u>or</u> 500 mg daily x 3 days <u>or</u> **Zmax** 2 gm in a single dose
Pediatric: 12 mg/kg/day x 5 days; max 500 mg/day; *see page* 621 *for dose by weight*
　　Zithromax *Tab:* 250, 500, 600 mg; *Oral susp:* 100 mg/5 ml (15 ml); 200 mg/5 ml (15, 22.5, 30 ml) (cherry); *Pkt:* 1 gm for reconstitution (cherry-banana)
　　Zithromax Tri-pak *Tab:* 3 x 500 mg tabs/pck
　　Zithromax Z-pak *Tab:* 6 x 250 mg tabs/pck
　　Zmax *Oral susp:* 2 gm ext-rel for reconstitution (cherry-banana) (148 mg Na$^+$)
▷ *cefaclor* (B)(G) 250-500 mg q 8 hours x 10 days; max 2 gm/day
Pediatric: <1 month: not recommended; 20-40 mg/kg bid <u>or</u> q 12 hours x 10 days; max 1 gm/day; *see page* 622 *for dose by weight*
Tab: 500 mg; *Cap:* 250, 500 mg; *Susp:* 125 mg/5 ml (75, 150 ml) (strawberry); 187 mg/5 ml (50, 100 ml) (strawberry); 250 mg/5 ml (75, 150 ml) (strawberry); 375 mg/5 ml (50, 100 ml) (strawberry)

Cefaclor Extended Release
Pediatric: <16 years: ext-rel not recommended; ≥16 years: same as adult
> *Tab:* 375, 500 mg ext-rel

▷ *cefpodoxime proxetil* (B) 400 mg bid x 7-14 days
Pediatric: <2 months: not recommended; ≥2 months-12 years: 10 mg/kg/day (max 400 mg/dose) *or* 5 mg/kg/day bid (max 200 mg/dose) x 7-14 days; *see page 626 for dose by weight;* >12 years: same as adult
> **Vantin** *Tab:* 100, 200 mg; *Oral susp:* 50, 100 mg/5 ml (50, 75, 100 mg) (lemon creme)

▷ *cefprozil* (B) 500 mg q 12 hours x 10 days
Pediatric: <2 years: not recommended; 2-12 years: 15 mg/kg q 12 hours x 10 days; *see page 627 for dose by weight;* >12 years: same as adult
> **Cefzil** *Tab:* 250, 500 mg; *Oral susp:* 125, 250 mg/5 ml (50, 75, 100 ml) (bubble gum) (phenylalanine)

▷ *ceftaroline fosamil* (B) administer 600 mg once every 12 hours, by IV infusion over 5-60 minutes, x 5-14 days
Pediatric: <18 years: not established; ≥18 years: same as adult
> **Teflaro** *Vial:* 400, 600 mg pwdr for reconstitution, single-use (10/carton)
> Comment: **Teflaro** is indicated for the treatment of adults with acute bacterial skin and skin structures infection (ABSSSI).

▷ *ceftriaxone* (B)(G) 1-2 gm daily x 5-14 days IM; max 4 gm daily
Pediatric: 50-75 mg/kg IM in 1-2 divided doses x 5-14 days; max 2 gm/day
> **Rocephin** *Vial:* 250, 500 mg; 1, 2 gm

▷ *cephalexin* (B)(G) 500 mg bid x 10 days
Pediatric: 25-50 mg/kg/day in 4 divided doses x 10 days; *see page 629 for dose by weight*
> **Keflex** *Cap:* 250, 333, 500, 750 mg; *Oral susp:* 125, 250 mg/5 ml (100, 200 ml) (strawberry)

▷ *clarithromycin* (C)(G) 500 mg q 12 hours *or* 500 mg ext-rel once daily x 10 days
Pediatric: <6 months: not recommended; ≥6 months: 7.5 mg/kg bid x 10 days; *see page 630 for dose by weight*
> **Biaxin** *Tab:* 250, 500 mg
> **Biaxin Oral Suspension** *Oral susp:* 125, 250 mg/5 ml (50, 100 ml) (fruit-punch)
> **Biaxin XL** *Tab:* 500 mg ext-rel

▷ *dalbavancin* (C) 1000 mg administered once as a single dose via IV infusion over 30 minutes *or* initially 1,000 mg once, followed by 500 mg 1 week later; infuse over 30 minutes; *CrCl <30 mL/min:* not receiving dialysis: initially 750 mg, followed by 375 mg 1 week later
Pediatric: <18 years: not established; ≥18 years: same as adult
> **Dalvance** *Vial:* 500 mg pwdr for reconstitution, single-use (preservative-free)
> Comment: **Dalvance** is indicated for the treatment of adults with acute bacterial skin and skin structures infection (ABSSSI) caused by gram positive bacteria.

▷ *delafloxacin* IV infusion: administer 300 mg every 12 hours over 60 minutes x 5-14 days; *Tablet:* 450 mg every 12 hours x 5-14 days; dosage for patients with renal impairment is based on eGFR (see mfr pkg insert)
Pediatric: <18 years: not recommended; ≥18 years: same as adult
> **Baxdela** *Tab:* 450 mg; *Vial:* 300 mg pwdr for reconstitution and IV infusion
Comment: **Baxdela,** a fluoroquinolone, is indicated for the treatment of acute bacterial skin and skin structure infections (ABSSSI) caused by designated susceptible bacteria. Fluoroquinolones have been associated with disabling and potentially irreversible serious adverse reactions that have occurred together, including tendinitis and tendon rupture, peripheral neuropathy, and central nervous system effects. Discontinue **Baxdela** immediately and avoid the use of fluoroquinolones,

including **Baxdela,** in patients who experience any of these serious adverse reactions. Fluoroquinolones may exacerbate muscle weakness in patients with myasthenia gravis. Therefore, avoid **Baxdela** in patients with known history of myasthenia gravis. Most common adverse reactions are nausea, diarrhea, headache, transaminase elevations and vomiting. Closely monitor SCr in patients with severe renal impairment (eGFR 15-29 mL/min/1.73 m²) receiving intravenous *delafloxacin.* If SCr level increases occur, consider changing to oral *delafloxacin.* Discontinue **Baxdela** if eGFR decreases to <15 mL/min/1.73 m². The limited available data with **Baxdela** use in pregnant females are insufficient to inform a drug-associated risk of major birth defects and miscarriages. There are no data available on the presence of *delafloxacin* in human milk or the effects on the breast-fed infant. To report suspected adverse reactions, contact Melinta Therapeutics at (844) 635-4682 or FDA at 1-800FDA-1088 or www.fda.gov/medwatch

▷ *dicloxacillin* **(B)(G)** 500 mg q 6 hours x 10 days
   Pediatric: 12.5-25 mg/kg/day in 4 divided doses x 10 days; *see page 632 for dose by weight*
      Dynapen *Cap:* 125, 250, 500 mg; *Oral susp:* 62.5 mg/5 ml (80, 100, 200 ml)
▷ *dirithromycin* **(C)(G)** 500 mg once daily x 5-7 days
   Pediatric: <12 years: not recommended; ≥12 years: same as adult
      Dynabac *Tab:* 250 mg
▷ *erythromycin base* **(B)(G)** 250 mg qid or 333 mg tid or 500 mg bid x 7-10 days; then taper to lowest effective dose
   Pediatric: <45 kg: 30-50 mg in 2-4 divided doses x 7-10 days; ≥45 kg: same as adult
      Ery-Tab *Tab:* 250, 333, 500 mg ent-coat
      PCE *Tab:* 333, 500 mg

Comment: *erythromycin* may increase INR with concomitant *warfarin*, as well as increase serum level of *digoxin*, benzodiazepines and statins.

▷ *erythromycin ethylsuccinate* **(B)(G)** 400 mg qid x 7-10 days
   Pediatric: 30-50 mg/kg/day in 4 divided doses x 7-10 days; may double dose with severe infection; max 100 mg/kg/day; *see page 635 for dose by weight*
      EryPed *Oral susp:* 200 mg/5 ml (100, 200 ml) (fruit); 400 mg/5 ml (60, 100, 200 ml) (banana); *Oral drops:* 200, 400 mg/5 ml (50 ml) (fruit); *Chew tab:* 200 mg wafer (fruit)
      E.E.S. *Oral susp:* 200, 400 mg/5 ml (100 ml) (fruit)
      E.E.S. Granules *Oral susp:* 200 mg/5 ml (100, 200 ml) (cherry)
      E.E.S. 400 Tablets *Tab:* 400 mg

Comment: *erythromycin* may increase INR with concomitant *warfarin*, as well as increase serum level of *digoxin*, benzodiazepines and statins.

▷ *linezolid* **(C)(G)** 600 mg q 12 hours x 10-14 days
   Pediatric: <5 years: 10 mg/kg q 8 hours x 10-14 days; 5-11 years: 10 mg/kg q 12 hours x 10-14 days; >11 years: same as adult
      Zyvox *Tab:* 400, 600 mg; *Oral susp:* 100 mg/5 ml (150 ml) (orange) (phenylalanine)

Comment: *linezolid* is indicated to treat susceptible vancomycin-resistant *E. faecium* infections of skin and skin structures, including diabetic foot without osteomyelitis.

▷ *loracarbef* **(B)** 200 mg bid x 10 days
   Pediatric: 15 mg/kg/day in 2 divided doses x 10 days; *see page 642 for dose by weight*
      Lorabid *Pulvule:* 200, 400 mg; *Oral susp:* 100 mg/5 ml (50, 100 ml); 200 mg/5 ml (50, 75, 100 ml) (strawberry bubble gum)
▷ *moxifloxacin* **(C)(G)** 400 mg once daily x 5 days
   Pediatric: <18 years: recommended; ≥18 years: same as adult
      Avelox *Tab:* 400 mg; *IV soln:* 400 mg/250 mg (latex-free, preservative-free)

Comment: *moxifloxacin* is contraindicated <18 years-of-age and during pregnancy and lactation. Risk of tendonitis or tendon rupture.

▷ *oritavancin* (C) administer 1,200 mg as a single dose by IV infusion over 3 hours
  Pediatric: <18 years: not established; ≥18 years: same as adult
    Orbactiv *Vial:* 400 mg pwdr for reconstitution, single-use (10/carton) (mannitol; preservative-free)
Comment: Orbactiv is indicated for the treatment of adults with acute bacterial skin and skin structures infection (ABSSSI).

▷ *penicillin v potassium* (B) 250-500 mg q 6 hours x 5-7 days
  Pediatric: <12 years: see page 644 for dose by weight; >12 years: same as adult
    Pen-Vee K *Tab:* 250, 500 mg; *Oral soln:* 125 mg/5 ml (100, 200 ml); 250 mg/5 ml (100, 150, 200 ml)

▷ *tedizolid phosphate* (C) administer 200 mg once daily x 6 days, via PO or IV infusion over 1 hour
  Pediatric: <18 years: not established; ≥18 years: same as adult
    Sivextro *Tab:* 200 mg (6/blister pck)
    Comment: Sivextro is indicated for the treatment of adults with acute bacterial skin and skin structures infection (ABSSSI).

▷ *tigecycline* (D)(G) 100 mg as a single dose; then 50 mg q 12 hours x 5-14 days; with severe hepatic impairment (Child-Pugh Class C), 100 mg as a single dose; then 25 mg q 12 hours
  Pediatric: <18 years: not recommended; ≥18 years: same as adult
    Tygacil *Vial:* 50 mg pwdr for reconstitution and IV infusion (preservative-free)
Comment: Tygacil is contraindicated in pregnancy, and lactation (discolors developing tooth enamel). A side effect may be photo-sensitivity (photophobia). Do not give with antacids, calcium supplements, milk or other dairy, or within two hours of taking another drug.

CERUMEN IMPACTION

OTIC ANALGESIC

▷ *antipyrine+benzocaine+zinc acetate dihydrate* otic (C) fill ear canal with solution; then moisten cotton plug with solution and insert into meatus; may repeat every 1-2 hours prn
  Pediatric: same as adult
    Otozin *Otic soln:* antipyr 5.4%+benz 1%+zinc 1% per ml (10 ml w. dropper)

CERUMINOLYTICS

▷ *triethanolamine* (OTC)(G) fill ear canal and insert cotton plug for 15-30 minutes before irrigating with warm water
    Cerumenex *Soln:* 10% (6, 12 ml)

▷ *carbamide peroxide* (OTC)(G) instill 5-10 drops in ear canal; keep drops in ear several minutes; then irrigate with warm water; repeat bid for up to 4 days
    Debrox *Soln:* 15, 30 ml squeeze bottle w. applicator

CHAGAS DISEASE (AMERICAN TRYPANOSOMIASIS)

Comment: Chagas Disease is a protozoal parasite (*Trypanosoma cruzi*) infection with increasing prevalence in the US attributed to immigration from *T. cruzi*-endemic areas of South and Central Latin America. Approximately 300,000 persons in the US have chronic Chagas Disease and up to 30% of them will develop clinically evident cardiovascular and/or gastrointestinal disease. Chagas Disease is one of the five neglected parasitic infections (NPIs) targeted by CDC for public health action. Transmitted by the bite of the triatomine bug ("kissing bug") which feeds on human blood, maternal-fetus vertical transmission, blood transfusion, consumption of contaminated food, and organ donation. A clinical marker is Romaña sign (periorbital swelling), chagoma (skin nodule), Schizotrypanides (nonpruritic morbilliform rash). Only two antiparasitic drugs, *benznidazole* and *nifurtimox*, have demonstrated effectiveness altering the progression of this chronic disease. These drugs are not FDA approved and are available only from CDC under investigational protocols. Treatment is indicated for all cases of acute or reactivated Chagas Disease and for chronic *Trypanosoma cruzi* infection in children ≤18. Congenital infections are considered acute disease. Treatment is strongly recommended up to 50 years old with chronic infection who do not already have advanced Chagas cardiomyopathy. For adults older than 50 years with chronic *T. cruzi* infection, the decision to treat with antiparasitic drugs should be individualized, weighing the potential benefits and risks for the patient. Patients taking either of these drugs should have a CBC and CMP at the start of treatment and then bi-monthly for the duration of treatment to monitor for rare bone marrow suppression. Contraindications for treatment include severe hepatic and/or renal disease. As safety for infants exposed through breastfeeding has not been documented, withholding treatment while breastfeeding is also recommended. For emergencies (for example, acute Chagas Disease with severe manifestations, Chagas Disease in a newborn, or Chagas Disease in an immunocompromised person) outside of regular business hours, call the CDC Emergency Operations Center (770-488-7100) and ask for the person on call for Parasitic Diseases. For more detailed information about screening, assessment, and treatment of this public health threat, see McDonald, J, & Mattingly, J. (November, 2016). Chagas disease: Creeping into family practice in the United States, *Clinician Reviews*, pp. 38-45, or call 404-718-4745 or e-mail questions to chagas@cdc.gov.

ANTI-PARASITIC AGENTS

▷ *benznidazole* (NR)(G) take with a meal to avoid GI upset; <12 years: 5-7.5 mg/kg/day divided bid x 60 days; ≥12 years: 5-7 mg/kg/day divided bid x 60 days

Comment: Common side effects of *benznidazole* are allergic dermatitis, peripheral neuropathy, insomnia, anorexia with weight loss.

▷ *nifurtimox* (NR)(G) take with a meal to avoid GI upset; ≤10 years: 15-20 mg/kg/day divided tid-qid x 90 days; 11-16 years: 12.5-15 mg/kg/day divided tid-qid x 90 days; ≥17 years: 8-10 mg/kg/day divided tid-qid x 90 days

Comment: Common side effects of *nifurtimox* are anorexia and weight loss, nausea, vomiting, polyneuropathy, headache, dizziness or vertigo.

 CHANCROID

ANTI-INFECTIVES

▷ *azithromycin* (B)(G) 500 mg x 1 dose on day 1, then 250 mg daily on days 2-5 or 500 mg daily x 3 days or Zmax 2 gm in a single dose
  Pediatric: 12 mg/kg/day x 5 days; max 500 mg/day; *see page 621 for dose by weight*
    Zithromax *Tab:* 250, 500, 600 mg; *Oral susp:* 100 mg/5 ml (15 ml); 200 mg/5 ml (15, 22.5, 30 ml) (cherry); *Pkt:* 1 gm for reconstitution (cherry-banana)
    Zithromax Tri-pak *Tab:* 3 x 500 mg tabs/pck
    Zithromax Z-pak *Tab:* 6 x 250 mg tabs/pck
    Zmax *Oral susp:* 2 gm ext-rel for reconstitution (cherry-banana) (148 mg Na⁺)
▷ *ceftriaxone* (B)(G) 250 mg IM in a single dose
  Pediatric: <45 kg: 125 mg IM in a single dose; ≥45 kg: same as adult
    Rocephin *Vial:* 250, 500 mg; 1, 2 gm

▷ *ciprofloxacin* (C) 500 mg bid x 3 days
Pediatric: <18 years: not recommended; ≥18 years: same as adult
  Cipro *Tab:* 250, 500, 750 mg; *Oral susp:* 250, 500 mg/5 ml (100 ml) (strawberry)
  Cipro XR *Tab:* 500, 1000 mg ext-rel
  ProQuin XR *Tab:* 500 mg ext-rel
▷ *erythromycin base* (B)(G) 500 mg qid x 7 days
Pediatric: 30-50 mg/kg/day divided bid-qid; max 100 mg/kg/day
  Ery-Tab *Tab:* 250, 333, 500 mg ent-coat
  PCE *Tab:* 333, 500 mg

Comment: *erythromycin* may increase INR with concomitant *warfarin*, as well as increase serum level of *digoxin, benzodiazepines*, and *statins*.

▷ *erythromycin ethylsuccinate* (B)(G) 400 mg qid x 7 days
Pediatric: 30-50 mg/kg/day in 4 divided doses x 7 days; may double dose with severe infection; max 100 mg/kg/day; *see page 635 for dose by weight*
  EryPed *Oral susp:* 200 mg/5 ml (100, 200 ml) (fruit); 400 mg/5 ml (60, 100, 200 ml) (banana); *Oral drops:* 200, 400 mg/5 ml (50 ml) (fruit); *Chew tab:* 200 mg wafer (fruit)
  E.E.S. *Oral susp:* 200, 400 mg/5 ml (100 ml) (fruit)
  E.E.S. Granules *Oral susp:* 200 mg/5 ml (100, 200 ml) (cherry)
  E.E.S. 400 Tablets *Tab:* 400 mg

Comment: *erythromycin* may increase INR with concomitant *warfarin*, as well as increase serum level of *digoxin, benzodiazepines*, and *statins*.

CHEMOTHERAPY-RELATED NAUSEA/VOMITING

PHENOTHIAZINES

▷ *chlorpromazine* (C)(G) 10-25 mg PO q 4 hours prn <u>or</u> 50-100 mg rectally q 6-8 hours prn
Pediatric: <6 months: not recommended; ≥6 months: 0.25 mg/lb orally q 4-6 hours prn <u>or</u> 0.5 mg/lb rectally q 6-8 hours prn; >12 years: same as adult
  Thorazine *Tab:* 10, 25, 50, 100, 200 mg; *Spansule:* 30, 75, 150 mg sust-rel; *Syr:* 10 mg/5 ml (4 oz; orange custard); *Conc:* 30 mg/ml (4 oz); 100 mg/ml (2, 8 oz); *Supp:* 25, 100 mg
▷ *perphenazine* (C) 5 mg IM (may repeat in 6 hours) <u>or</u> 8-16 mg/day PO in divided doses; max 15 mg/day IM; max 24 mg/day PO
Pediatric: <12 years: not recommended; ≥12 years: same as adult
  Trilafon *Tab:* 2, 4, 8, 16 mg; *Oral conc:* 16 mg/5 ml (118 ml); *Amp:* 5 mg/ml (1 ml)
▷ *prochlorperazine* (C)(G) 5-10 mg tid-qid prn; usual max 40 mg/day
  Compazine
  Pediatric: <2 years <u>or</u> <20 lb: not recommended; 20-29 lb: 2.5 mg daily bid prn; max 7.5 mg/day; 30-39 lb: 2.5 mg bid-tid prn; max 10 mg/day; 40-85 lb: 2.5 mg tid <u>or</u> 5 mg bid prn; max 15 mg/day; >85 lb: same as adult
    Tab: 5, 10 mg; *Syr:* 5 mg/5 ml (4 oz) (fruit)
  Compazine Suppository 25 mg rectally bid prn; usual max 50 mg/day
  Pediatric: <2 years <u>or</u> <20 lb: not recommended; 20-29 lb: 2.5 mg daily-bid prn; max 7.5; mg/day; 30-39 lb: 2.5 mg bid-tid prn; max 10 mg/day; 40-85 lb: 2.5 mg tid <u>or</u> 5 mg bid prn; max 15 mg/day; >85 lb: same as adult
    Rectal supp: 2.5, 5, 25 mg
  Compazine Injectable 5-10 mg tid <u>or</u> qid prn
  Pediatric: <2 years <u>or</u> <20 lb: not recommended; ≥2 years <u>or</u> ≥20 lb: 0.06 mg/kg x 1 dose; >12 years: same as adult
    Vial: 5 mg/ml (2, 10 ml)

Compazine Spansule 15 mg q AM prn or 10 mg q 12 hours prn usual max 40 mg/day
Pediatric: <12 years: not recommended; ≥12 years: same as adult
  Spansule: 10, 15 mg sust-rel
▷ *promethazine* (C)(G) 25 mg PO or rectally q 4-6 hours prn
Pediatric: <2 years: not recommended; ≥2 years: 0.5 mg/lb or 6.25-25 mg q 4-6 hours prn; >12 years: same as adult
  Phenergan *Tab:* 12.5*, 25*, 50 mg; *Plain syr:* 6.25 mg/5 ml; *Fortis syr:* 25 mg/5 ml; *Rectal supp:* 12.5, 25, 50 mg

SUBSTANCE P/NEUROKININ 1 RECEPTOR ANTAGONIST

▷ *aprepitant* (B)(G) administer with corticosteroid and 5HT-3 receptor antagonist; *Day 1 of chemotherapy cycle:* 125 mg 1 hour prior to chemotherapy *Day 2 and 3:* 80 mg in the morning
Pediatric: <6 months: years: not recommended; ≥6 months-12 years: use oral suspension (see mfr pkg insert for dose by weight); >12 years: same as adult
  Emend *Cap:* 40, 80, 125 mg (2 x 80 mg bi-fold pck; 1 x 25 mg/2 x 80 mg tri-fold pck); *Oral susp:* 125 mg pwdr for oral suspension, single-dose pouch w. dispenser; *Vial:* 150 mg pwdr for reconstitution and IV infusion

5HT-3 RECEPTOR ANTAGONISTS

Comment: The selective 5HT-3 receptor antagonists indicated for prevention of nausea and vomiting associated with moderately to highly emetogenic chemotherapy.
▷ *dolasetron* (B) administer 100 mg IV over 30 seconds, 30 min prior to administration of chemotherapy or 2 hours before surgery; max 100 mg/dose
Pediatric: <2 years: not recommended; 2-16 years: 1.8 mg/kg; >16 years: same as adult
  Anzemet *Tab:* 50, 100 mg; *Amp:* 12.5 mg/0.625 ml; *Prefilled carpuject syringe:* 12.5 mg (0.625 ml); *Vial:* 100 mg/5 ml (single-use); *Vial:* 500 mg/25 ml (multi-dose)
▷ *granisetron*
  Kytril (B) 10 mcg/kg as a single dose; administer IV over 30 seconds, 30 min prior to administration of chemotherapy; max 1 dose/week
  Pediatric: <2 years: not recommended; ≥2 years: same as adult
    Tab: 1 mg; *Oral soln:* 2 mg/10 ml (30 ml; orange); *Vial:* 1 mg/ml (1 ml single-dose) (preservative-free); 1 mg/ml (4 ml multi-dose) (benzyl alcohol)
  Sancuso (B) apply 1 patch 24-48 hours before chemo; remove 24 hours (minimum) to 7 days (maximum) after completion of treatment
  Pediatric: <2 years: not recommended; ≥2 years: same as adult
    Transdermal patch: 3.1 mg/day
▷ **Sustol** administer SC over 20-30 seconds (due to drug viscosity) on Day 1 of chemotherapy and not more frequently than once every 7 days; *CrCl 30-59 mL/min:* repeat dose no more than every 14th day; *CrCl <30 mL/min:* not recommended; for patients receiving MEC, the recommended *dexamethasone* dosage is 8 mg IV on Day 1; for patients receiving AC combination chemotherapy regimens, the recommended *dexamethasone* dosage is 20 mg IV on Day 1, followed by 8 mg PO bid on Days 2, 3 and 4; if **Sustol** is administered with an NK₁ receptor antagonist, see that drug's mfr pkg insert for the recommended *dexamethasone* dosing
Pediatric: <18 years: not recommended; ≥18 years: same as adult
  Syringe: 10 mg/0.4 ml ext-rel; prefilled single-dose/kit
Comment: At least 60 minutes prior to administration, remove the **Sustol** kit from refrigeration; activate a warming pouch and wrap the syringe in the warming pouch for 5-6 minutes to warm it to room temperature.

▷ *ondansetron* (C)(G) Oral Forms: *Highly emetogenic chemotherapy:* 24 mg x 1 dose 30 min prior to start of single-day chemotherapy; *Moderately emetogenic chemotherapy:* 8 mg q 8 hours x 2 doses beginning 30 minutes prior to start of chemotherapy; then 8 mg q 12 hours x 1-2 days following
Pediatric: <4 years: not recommended; 4-11 years: *Moderately emetogenic chemotherapy:* 4 mg q 4 hours x 3 doses beginning 30 min prior to start; then 4 mg q 8 hours x 1-2 days following
Zofran *Tab:* 4, 8, 24 mg
Zofran ODT *ODT:* 4, 8 mg (strawberry) (phenylalanine)
Zofran Oral Solution *Oral soln:* 4 mg/5 ml (50 ml) (strawberry) (phenylalanine); *Parenteral form:* see mfr pkg insert
Zofran Injection *Vial:* 2 mg/ml (2 ml single-dose); 2 mg/ml (20 ml multi-dose); 32 mg/50 ml (50 ml multi-dose); *Prefilled syringe:* 4 mg/2 ml, single-use (24/carton)
Zuplenz Oral Soluble Film: 4, 8 mg oral-dis (10/carton) (peppermint)
▷ *palonosetron* (B)(G) *Chemotherapy:* administer 0.25 mg IV over 30 seconds, 30 min prior to administration of chemo; max 1 dose/week or 1 cap 1 hour before chemo; *Post-op:* administer 0.075 mg IV over 10 seconds immediately before induction of anesthesia
Pediatric: <1 month: not recommended; 1 month-17 years: 20 mcg/kg; max 1.5 mg single dose; infuse over 15 minutes beginning 30 minutes prior to administration of chemo
Aloxi *Vial (single-use):* 0.075 mg/1.5 ml; 0.25 mg/5 ml (mannitol)

CANNABINOID

▷ *dronabinol* (C)(III) initially 5 mg/m^2 1-3 hours before chemotherapy; then q 2-4 hours prn; max 4-6 doses/day, 15 mg/m^2
Pediatric: <18 years: not recommended; ≥18 years: same as adult
Marinol *Cap:* 2.5, 5, 10 mg (sesame seed oil)
▷ *nabilone* (C)(II) 1-2 mg bid; max 6 mg/day in 3 divided doses; initially 1-3 hours before chemotherapy; may give 1-2 mg the night before chemo; may continue 48 hours after each chemo cycle
Pediatric: <18 years: not recommended; ≥18 years: same as adult
Cesamet *Cap:* 1 mg (sesame seed oil)

CHICKENPOX (VARICELLA)

Antipyretics *see Fever page* 165

PROPHYLAXIS

▷ *Varicella virus* vaccine, live, attenuated (C)
Varivax 0.5 ml SC; repeat 4-8 weeks later
Pediatric: <12 months: not recommended; 12 months-12 years: 1 dose of 0.5 ml SC; repeat 4-6 weeks later
Vial: 1350 PFU/0.5 ml single-dose w. diluent (preservative-free)
Comment: Administer **Varivax** SC in the deltoid for adults and children.

ORAL ANTIPRURITICS

▷ *diphenhydramine* (B)(OTC)(G) 25-50 mg q 6-8 hours; max 100 mg/day
Pediatric: <2 years: not recommended; 2-6 years: 6.25 mg q 4-6 hours; max 37.5 mg/day; >6-12 years: 12.5-25 mg q 4-6 hours; max 150 mg/day; >12 years: same as adult

　　Benadryl (OTC) *Chew tab:* 12.5 mg (grape; phenylalanine); *Liq:* 12.5 mg/5 ml (4, 8 oz); *Cap:* 25 mg; *Tab:* 25 mg; *dye-free soft gel:* 25 mg; *Dye-free liq:* 12.5 mg/5 ml (4, 8 oz)

▷ *hydroxyzine* (C)(G) 50-100 mg qid; max 600 mg/day
　　Pediatric: <6 years: 50 mg/day divided qid; ≥6 years: 50-100 mg/day divided qid
　　　AtaraxR *Tab:* 10, 25, 50, 100 mg; *Syr:* 10 mg/5 ml (alcohol 0.5%)
　　　Vistaril *Cap:* 25, 50, 100 mg; *Oral susp:* 25 mg/5 ml (4 oz) (lemon)

ANTIVIRALS

▷ *acyclovir* (B)(G) 800 mg qid x 5 days
　　Pediatric: <2 years: not recommended; ≥2 years, <40 kg: 20 mg/kg qid x 5 days; ≥2 years, >40 kg: 800 mg qid x 5 days; *see page* 614 *for dose by weight*
　　　Zovirax *Cap:* 200 mg; *Tab:* 400, 800 mg
　　　Zovirax Oral Suspension *Oral susp:* 200 mg/5 ml (banana)

CHIKUNGUNYA VIRUS/CHIKUNGUNYA-RELATED ARTHRITIS

Comment: Chikungunya is a mosquito-borne viral disease first described during an outbreak in southern Tanzania in 1952. It is an RNA virus that belongs to the alphavirus genus of the family *Togaviridae.* The name "chikungunya" derives from a word in the Kimakonde language, meaning "to become contorted," and describes the stooped appearance of sufferers with joint pain (arthralgia). Acute infection with *chikungunya virus* is associated with fever, rash, headache, and muscle and joint pain, with outbreaks having been reported in Africa, Asia, the Indian and Pacific Ocean islands, and Europe. In 2013 for the first time the virus was first detected in the Caribbean region, and more than 1.2 million peoples in the Americas have now been infected. After transmission by an *Aedes aegypti* or *Aedes albopictus* mosquito bite, *chikungunya virus* undergoes local replication and then dissemination to lymphoid tissue," the researchers explained. Viremia is detectable for only 5 to 12 days, but animal studies have indicated that the virus can be found in lymphoid organs, joints, and muscles for several months and that viral RNA can be detected in muscle, liver, and spleen for long periods. But it is not known whether the remnants of the virus actually persist in humans and, if so, whether this can be causatively linked with chronic arthritis, which has implications for treatment. With no evidence of viral persistence, potential mechanisms for arthritis included epigenetic changes to host DNA, as has been observed with *Epstein Barr virus* infection, modification of macrophages, and molecular mimicry. There is currently no cure and no standard treatment for acute *chikungunya virus* infection or chikungunya-related arthritis, but various immunosuppressants such as **methotrexate** and **hydroxychloroquine** and biologics such as **adalimumab** (**Humira**) and **etanercept** (**Enbrel**) have been tried, despite concerns of renewed viral replication in the synovium and relapse of systemic viral infection. However, no relapses have been reported, and the lack of evidence of viral persistence in the joint seen in this analysis may provide some reassurance that treatment with immunosuppressant anti-rheumatic medications 2 years after infection is a viable option.

REFERENCES

Chang, A. Y., Martins, K. A. O., Encinales, L., Reid, S. P., Acuña, M., Encinales, C., . . . Firestein, G. S. (2017). A cross-sectional analysis of chikungunya arthritis patients 22-months post-infection demonstrate no detectable viral persistence in synovial fluid. *Arthritis & Rheumatology.* doi:10.1002/art.40383

Chang, A. Y., Encinales, L., Porras, A., Pachecho, N., Reid, S. P., Martins, K. A. O., . . . Simon, G. L. (2017). Frequency of Chronic Joint Pain following Chikungunya Infection: A Colombian Cohort Study. *Arthritis & Rheumatology.* doi:10.1002/art.40384

CHLAMYDIA TRACHOMATIS

Comment: The following treatment regimens for *C. trachomatis* are published in the **2015 CDC Sexually Transmitted Diseases Treatment Guidelines**. Treatment regimens are presented by generic drug name first, followed by information about brands and dose forms. Treat all sexual contacts. Patients who are HIV-positive should receive the same treatment as those who are HIV-negative. Sexual abuse must be considered a cause of chlamydial infection in preadolescent children, although perinatally transmitted *C. trachomatis* infections of the nasopharynx, urogenital tract, and rectum may persist for >1 year.

RECOMMENDED REGIMENS: ADOLESCENT AND ADULT, NON-PREGNANT
Regimen 1
▷ *azithromycin* 1 gm in a single dose

Regimen 2
▷ *doxycycline* 100 mg bid x 7 days

ALTERNATIVE REGIMENS: ADOLESCENT AND ADULT, NON-PREGNANT
Regimen 1
▷ *erythromycin base* 500 mg qid x 7 days

Regimen 2
▷ *erythromycin ethylsuccinate* 800 mg qid x 7 days

Regimen 3
▷ *levofloxacin* 500 mg once daily x 7 days

Regimen 4
▷ *ofloxacin* 300 mg bid x 7 days

RECOMMENDED REGIMENS: PREGNANCY
Regimen 1
▷ *azithromycin* 1 gm in a single dose

Regimen 2
▷ *amoxicillin* 500 mg tid x 7 days

ALTERNATE REGIMENS: PREGNANCY
Regimen 1
▷ *erythromycin base* 500 mg qid x 7 days

Regimen 2
▷ *erythromycin base* 250 mg qid x 14 days

Regimen 3
▷ *erythromycin ethylsuccinate* 800 mg qid x 7 days

Regimen 4

▷ *erythromycin ethylsuccinate* 400 mg qid x 14 days

ALTERNATE REGIMENS: CHILDREN (>8 YEARS)

Regimen 1

▷ *azithromycin* 1 gm in a single dose

Regimen 2

▷ *doxycycline* 100 mg bid x 7 days

ALTERNATE REGIMEN: CHILDREN (>45 KG; <8 YEARS)

Regimen 1

▷ *azithromycin* 1 gm in a single dose

ALTERNATE REGIMENS: INFANTS

Regimen 1

▷ *erythromycin base* 50 mg/kg/day in divided doses qid x 14 days

Regimen 2

▷ *erythromycin ethylsuccinate* 50 mg/kg/day divided qid x 14 days

DRUG BRANDS AND DOSE FORMS

▷ *azithromycin* (B)(G) 500 mg x 1 dose on day 1, then 250 mg daily on days 2-5 <u>or</u> 500 mg daily x 3 days <u>or</u> **Zmax** 2 gm in a single dose
  Pediatric: 12 mg/kg/day x 5 days; max 500 mg/day; *see page* 621 *for dose by weight*
    Zithromax *Tab:* 250, 500, 600 mg; *Oral susp:* 100 mg/5 ml (15 ml); 200 mg/5 ml (15, 22.5, 30 ml) (cherry); *Pkt:* 1 gm for reconstitution (cherry-banana)
    Zithromax Tri-pak *Tab:* 3 x 500 mg tabs/pck
    Zithromax Z-pak *Tab:* 6 x 250 mg tabs/pck
    Zmax *Oral susp:* 2 gm ext-rel for reconstitution (cherry-banana) (148 mg Na$^+$)
▷ *doxycycline* (D)(G)
    Acticlate *Tab:* 75, 150**mg
    Adoxa *Tab:* 50, 75, 100, 150 mg ent-coat
    Doryx *Tab:* 50, 75, 100, 150, 200 mg del-rel
    Doxteric *Tab:* 50 mg del-rel
    Monodox *Cap:* 50, 75, 100 mg
    Oracea *Cap:* 40 mg del-rel
    Vibramycin *Tab:* 100 mg; *Cap:* 50, 100 mg; *Syr:* 50 mg/5 ml (raspberry-apple) (sulfites); *Oral susp:* 25 mg/5 ml (raspberry)
    Vibra-Tab *Tab:* 100 mg film-coat
▷ *erythromycin base* (B)(G)
    Ery-Tab *Tab:* 250, 333, 500 mg ent-coat
    PCE *Tab:* 333, 500 mg
Comment: *erythromycin* may increase INR with concomitant **warfarin**, as well as increase serum level of **digoxin, benzodiazepines**, and **statins**.
▷ *erythromycin ethylsuccinate* (B)(G)
    EryPed *Oral susp:* 200 mg/5 ml (100, 200 ml) (fruit); 400 mg/5 ml (60, 100, 200 ml) (banana); *Oral drops:* 200, 400 mg/5 ml (50 ml) (fruit); *Chew tab:* 200 mg wafer (fruit)
    E.E.S. *Oral susp:* 200, 400 mg/5 ml (100 ml) (fruit)
    E.E.S. Granules *Oral susp:* 200 mg/5 ml (100, 200 ml) (cherry)
    E.E.S. 400 Tablets *Tab:* 400 mg

Comment: *erythromycin* may increase INR with concomitant *warfarin*, as well as increase serum level of *digoxin, benzodiazepines,* and *statins*.

▷ *levofloxacin* (C)

Levaquin *Tab:* 250, 500, 750 mg

Comment: *levofloxacin* is contraindicated; <18 years-of-age, and during pregnancy and lactation. Risk of tendonitis or tendon rupture.

▷ *ofloxacin* (C)(G)

Floxin *Tab:* 200, 300, 400 mg

Comment: *ofloxacin* is contraindicated <18 years-of-age, and during pregnancy and lactation. Risk of tendonitis or tendon rupture.

 CHOLANGITIS, PRIMARY BILIARY (PBC)

Comment: Monitor intensity of pruritis and administer antihistamines as appropriate for dermal pruritis. **Ocaliva** (*obeticholic acid*), a farnesoid X receptor (FXR) agonist, is indicated for the treatment of primary biliary cholangitis (PBC) in combination with *ursodeoxycholic acid* (UDCA), in adults with an inadequate response to UDCA, or as monotherapy in adults unable to tolerate UDCA. This indication is approved under accelerated approval based on a reduction in alkaline phosphatase (ALP). An improvement in survival or disease-related symptoms has not been established. Continued approval for this indication may be contingent upon verification and description of clinical benefit in confirmatory trials.

FARNESOID X RECEPTOR (FXR) AGONIST

▷ *obeticholic acid* initially 5 mg once daily (this lower starting dose is recommended to reduce pruritus); then after 3 months of treatment, if an adequate reduction in ALP and/or total bilirubin is not achieved, and if the patient is tolerating the drug, increase the dose to 10 mg once daily; take with or without food

Pediatric: <18 years: not recommended; ≥18 years: same as adult

Ocaliva *Tab:* 5, 10 mg

Comment: **Ocalvia** is contraindicated in patients with complete biliary obstruction. If this complication develops, discontinue **Ocaliva**. Because PBC management strategies include bile acid binding resin (e.g., *cholestyramine, colestipol,* or *colesevelam*), concurrent use with *obeticholic acid* should be separated by at least 4 hours. Concurrent use of *obeticholic acid* and *warfarin* may reduce the international normalized ratio (INR), monitor INR and adjust the *warfarin* dose as necessary. Monitor concentrations of CYP1A2 substrates with a narrow therapeutic index (e.g., *theophylline* and *tizanidine*) as *obeticholic acid* a CYP1A2 inhibitor). Reduce the dose of **Ocaliva** in patients with moderate or severe hepatic impairment, and monitor LFTs and lipid levels (especially reduction in HDL).

URSODEOXYCHOLIC ACID (UDCA)

▷ *ursodeoxycholic acid* (UDCA) (G) in the first 3 months of treatment, the total daily dose should be divided tid (morning, midday, evening); as liver function values improve, the total daily dose may be taken once a day at bedtime; (see mfr pkg insert for dose table based on kilograms weight); monitor hepatic function every 4 weeks for the first 3 months; then, monitor hepatic function once every 3 months

Pediatric: same as adult

Ursofalk *Tab:* 500 mg film-coat; *Cap:* 250 mg, *Oral susp:* 250 mg/5 ml

Comment: *ursodeoxycholic acid* (UDCA) is indicated for the dissolution of cholesterol gall stones that are radioluscent (not visible on plain x-ray), ≤15 mm, and the gall bladder must still be functioning despite the gall stones.

BILE ACID BINDING RESINS

Comment: This drug class may produce <u>or</u> severely worsen pre-existing constipation. The dosage should be increased gradually in patients to minimize the risk of developing fecal impaction. Increased fluid and fiber intake should be encouraged to alleviate constipation and a stool softener may occasionally be indicated. If the initial dose is well tolerated, the dose may be increased as needed by one dose/day (at monthly intervals) with periodic monitoring of serum lipoproteins. If constipation worsens <u>or</u> the desired therapeutic response is not achieved at one to six doses/day, combination therapy <u>or</u> alternate therapy should be considered. Bile acid sequestrants may decrease absorption of fat-soluble vitamins. Use caution in patients susceptible to fat-soluble vitamin deficiencies.

▷ *cholestyramine* (C)(G) starting dose: 1 packet <u>or</u> 1 scoopful of powder once daily for 5 to 7 days; then, increase to twice daily with monitoring of constipation and of serum lipoproteins, at least twice, 4 to 6 weeks apart; empty one packet into a glass <u>or</u> cup; add 1/2 to 1 cup (4 to 8 ounces) of water, fruit juice, <u>or</u> diet soft drink; stir well and drink immediately; do not swallow dry form; take with meals
Pediatric: 240 mg/kg/day of anhydrous cholestyramine resin in two to three divided doses, normally not to exceed 8 gm/day with dose titration based on response and tolerance.
   Prevalite *Pwdr:* 4 gm/pkt, 4 gm/scoopful (1 level tsp) for oral suspension

▷ *colestipol* (C)(G)
Starting dose tabs: 2 gm once <u>or</u> twice daily; then, increases should occur at one <u>or</u> two month intervals; usual dose is 2 to 16 gm/day given once daily <u>or</u> in divided doses
Starting dose granules: 1 packet <u>or</u> 1 scoopful (1 level tsp) of granules once daily for 5 to 7 days, increasing to twice daily with monitoring of constipation and of serum lipoproteins, at least twice, 4 to 6 weeks apart; empty one packet <u>or</u> one scoopful (1 level tsp) of granules into a glass <u>or</u> cup; add 1/2 to 1 cup (4 to 8 ounces) of water, fruit juice, <u>or</u> diet soft drink; stir well and drink immediately; do not swallow dry form; take with meals
Pediatric: <12 years: not established; ≥12 years: same as adult
   Colestid *Tab:* 1 gm; *Granules:* 5 gm/pkt, 5 gm/scoopful (1 level tsp) for oral suspension
   Flavored Colestid *Granules:* 5 gm/pkt, 5 gm/scoopful (1 level tsp) for oral suspension (orange)

▷ *colesevelam* (C)(G) <12 years: not recommended; >12 years:
Pediatric: <10 years: pre-menarchal; not recommended; ≥10 years, postmenarchal: same as adult
   Welchol recommended dose is 6 tablets once daily <u>or</u> 3 tablets twice daily; take with a meal and liquid
      Tab: 625 mg
   Welchol for Oral Suspension recommended dose is one 3.75 gm packet once daily <u>or</u> one 1.875 gm packet twice daily; empty one packet into a glass <u>or</u> cup; add 1/2 to 1 cup (4 to 8 ounces) of water, fruit juice, <u>or</u> diet soft drink; stir well and drink immediately; do not swallow dry form; take with meals
      Pwdr: 3.75 gm/pkt (30 pkt/carton), 1.875 gm/pkt (60 pkt/carton) for oral suspension

◯ CHOLELITHIASIS

▷ *ursodeoxycholic acid* (UDCA) (G) in the first 3 months of treatment, the total daily dose should be divided tid (morning, midday, evening); as liver function values improve, the total daily dose may be taken once a day at bedtime; (see mfr pkg insert for dose table based on kilograms weight); monitor hepatic function every 4 weeks for the

first 3 months; then, monitor hepatic function once every 3 months
Pediatric: same as adult
> **Ursofalk** *Tab:* 500 mg film-coat; *Cap:* 250 mg, *Oral susp:* 250 mg/5 ml

Comment: **ursodeoxycholic** (UDCA) is indicated for the dissolution of cholesterol gall
stones that are radioluscent (not visible on plain x-ray), ≤15 mm, and the gall bladder
must still be functioning despite the gall stones
➤ **ursodiol (B)** 8-10 mg/kg/day in 2-3 divided doses
Pediatric: <12 years: not recommended; ≥12 years: same as adult
> **Actigall** *Cap:* 300 mg

Comment: **Actigall** is indicated for the dissolution of radiolucent, noncalciferous,
gallstones <20 mm in diameter and for prevention of gallstones during rapid weight loss.

BILE ACID BINDING RESINS

Comment: This drug class may produce or severely worsen pre-existing constipation.
The dosage should be increased gradually in patients to minimize the risk of developing
fecal impaction. Increased fluid and fiber intake should be encouraged to alleviate
constipation and a stool softener may occasionally be indicated. If the initial dose is well
tolerated, the dose may be increased as needed by one dose/day (at monthly intervals)
with periodic monitoring of serum lipoproteins. If constipation worsens or the desired
therapeutic response is not achieved at one to six doses/day, combination therapy or
alternate therapy should be considered. Bile acid sequestrants may decrease absorption
of fat-soluble vitamins. Use caution in patients susceptible to fat-soluble vitamin
deficiencies.
➤ **cholestyramine (C)(G)** starting dose: 1 packet or 1 scoopful of powder once daily for 5
to 7 days; then, increase to twice daily with monitoring of constipation and of serum
lipoproteins, at least twice, 4 to 6 weeks apart; empty one packet into a glass or cup;
add 1/2 to 1 cup (4 to 8 ounces) of water, fruit juice, or diet soft drink; stir well and
drink immediately; do not swallow dry form; take with meals
Pediatric: <12 years: 240 mg/kg/day of anhydrous cholestyramine resin in 2 to 3
divided doses, normally not to exceed 8 gm/day with dose titration based on response
and tolerance.
> **Prevalite** *Pwdr:* 4 gm/pkt, 4 gm/scoopful (1 level tsp) for oral suspension
➤ **colestipol (C)(G)**
Starting dose tabs: 2 gm once or twice daily; then, increases should occur at one or
two month intervals; usual dose is 2 to 16 gm/day given once daily or in divided doses
Starting dose granules: 1 packet or 1 scoopful (1 level tsp) of granules once daily for
5 to 7 days, increasing to twice daily with monitoring of constipation and of serum
lipoproteins, at least twice, 4 to 6 weeks apart; empty one packet or one scoopful (1
level tsp) of granules into a glass or cup; add 1/2 to 1 cup (4 to 8 ounces) of water,
fruit juice, or diet soft drink; stir well and drink immediately; do not swallow dry
form; take with meals
Pediatric: <12 years: not established; ≥12 years: same as adult
> **Colestid** *Tab:* 1 gm; *Granules:* 5 gm/pkt, 5 gm/scoopful (1 level tsp) for oral
suspension
> **Flavored Colestid** *Granules:* 5 gm/pkt, 5 gm/scoopful (1 level tsp) for oral
suspension (orange)
➤ **colesevelam (C)(G)** <12 years: not recommended; >12 years:
> **Welchol** recommended dose is 6 tablets once daily or 3 tablets twice daily; take
with a meal and liquid
> *Tab:* 625 mg
> **Welchol for Oral Suspension** recommended dose is one 3.75 gm packet once
daily or one 1.875 gm packet twice daily; empty one packet into a glass or cup;

add 1/2 to 1 cup (4 to 8 ounces) of water, fruit juice, or diet soft drink; stir well and drink immediately; do not swallow dry form; take with meals

Pwdr: 3.75 gm/pkt (30 pkt/carton), 1.875 gm/pkt (60 pkt/carton) for oral suspension

 ## CHOLERA (*VIBRIO CHOLERAE*)

Comment: June 10, 2016, the FDA approved the first vaccine for the prevention of cholera caused by serogroup O1 (the most predominant cause of cholera globally [WHO]) in adults age 18-64 years traveling to cholera-affected areas. https://www.drugs.com/newdrugs/fda-approves-vaxchora-cholera-vaccine-live-oral-prevent-cholera-travelers-4396.html. **Vaxchora (R)** is the only FDA approved vaccine for the prevention of cholera. The bacterium *Vibrio cholerae* is acquired by ingesting contaminated water or food and causes nausea, vomiting, and watery diarrhea that may be mild to severe. Profuse fluid loss may cause life-threatening dehydration if antibiotics and fluid replacement are not initiated promptly.

VACCINE PROPHYLAXIS

▷ *Vibrio cholerae* vaccine

Vaxchora reconstitute the buffer component in 100 ml purified bottled water; then add the active component (lyophilized V. cholerae CVD 103-HgR); total dose after reconstitution is 100 ml; instruct the patient to avoid eating or drinking fluids for 60 minutes before and after ingestion of the dose

Comment: Vaxchora is a live, attenuated vaccine that is taken as a single oral dose at least 10 days before travel to a cholera-affected area and at least 10 days before starting antimalarial prophylaxis. Diminished immune response when taken concomitantly with *chloroquine*. Avoid concomitant administration with systemic antibiotics since these agents may be active against the vaccine strain. Do not administer to patients who have received an oral or parental antibiotic within 14 days prior to vaccination. **Vaxchora** may be shed in the stool of recipients for at least 7 days. There is potential for transmission of the vaccine strain to non-vaccinated and immunocompromised close contacts. The CDC and several health professional organizations state that vaccines given to a nursing mother do not affect the safety of breastfeeding for mothers or infants and that breastfeeding is not a contraindication to cholera vaccine. **Vaxchora** is not absorbed systemically, and maternal use is not expected to result in fetal exposure to the drug. The **Vaxchora** pregnancy exposure registry for reporting adverse events is 800-533-5899. There are 0 disease interactions, but at least 165 drug-drug interactions with **Vaxchora** (see mfr pkg insert).

TREATMENT

Comment: The first line treatment for *V. cholerae* is oral rehydration therapy (ORT) and intravenous fluid replacement as indicated. Antibiotic therapy may shorten the duration and severity of symptoms, but is optional in other than severe cases. Although *doxycycline* is contraindicated in pregnancy and in children under 7 years-of-age, the benefits may outweigh the risks (WHO, CDC, UNICEF). Although *ciprofloxacin* is contraindicated in children under 18 years-of-age, the benefits may outweigh the risks (WHO, CDC, UNICEF). Cholera is not transmitted from person to person, but rather the fecal-oral route. Therefore, chemoprophylaxis is not usually required with strict hand hygiene and sanitation measures, and avoidance of contaminated food and water. Drugs and dosages for chemoprophylaxis are the same as for treatment.

NON-PREGNANT FEMALES >15 YEARS
Regimen 1

▷ *doxycycline* (D)(G) 300 mg in a single dose
    Acticlate *Tab:* 75, 150**mg
    Adoxa *Tab:* 50, 75, 100, 150 mg ent-coat
    Doryx *Tab:* 50, 75, 100, 150, 200 mg del-rel
    Doxteric *Tab:* 50 mg del-rel
    Monodox *Cap:* 50, 75, 100 mg
    Oracea *Cap:* 40 mg del-rel
    Vibramycin *Tab:* 100 mg; *Cap:* 50, 100 mg; *Syr:* 50 mg/ml (raspberry-apple) (sulfites); *Oral susp:* 25 mg/5 ml (raspberry)
    Vibra-Tab *Tab:* 100 mg film-coat

Comment: *doxycycline* is contraindicated <8 years-of-age, in pregnancy, and lactation (discolors developing tooth enamel). A side effect may be photosensitivity (photophobia). Do not take with antacids, calcium supplements, milk or other dairy, or within 2 hours of taking another drug.

Regimen 2

▷ *azithromycin* (B)(G) 1000 mg in a single dose
    Zithromax *Tab:* 250, 500, 600 mg
    Zmax *Oral susp:* 2 gm ext-rel for reconstitution (cherry-banana) (148 mg Na^+)
    or
▷ *ciprofloxacin* (C)(G) 1000 mg in a single dose
    Cipro *Tab:* 250, 500, 750 mg;
    Cipro XR *Tab:* 500, 1000 mg ext-rel
    ProQuin XR *Tab:* 500 mg ext-rel

PREGNANT FEMALES >15 YEARS

▷ *azithromycin* (B)(G) 1000 mg in a single dose
    Zithromax *Tab:* 250, 500, 600 mg
    Zmax *Oral susp:* 2 gm ext-rel for reconstitution (cherry-banana) (148 mg Na^+)
    or
▷ *erythromycin* (B)(G) 500 mg q 6 hours x 3 days
    E.E.S. 400 Tablets *Tab:* 400 mg
    Ery-Tab *Tab:* 250, 333, 500 mg ent-coat
    PCE *Tab:* 333, 500 mg

CHILDREN 3-15 YEARS WHO CAN SWALLOW TABLETS
Regimen 1

▷ *erythromycin* (B)(G) 12.5 mg/kg q 6 hours x 3 days
    E.E.S. 400 Tablets *Tab:* 400 mg
    Ery-Tab *Tab:* 250, 333, 500 mg ent-coat
    PCE *Tab:* 333, 500 mg
    or
▷ *azithromycin* (B)(G) 20 mg/kg in a single dose; max 1 g
    Zithromax *Tab:* 250, 500, 600 mg
    Zmax *Oral susp:* 2 gm ext-rel for reconstitution (cherry-banana) (148 mg Na^+)

Regimen 2

▷ *ciprofloxacin* (D)(G) <18 years usually not recommended; *erythromycin* or *azithromycin* preferred; consider risk/benefit; 20 mg/kg in a single dose
    Cipro *Tab:* 250, 500, 750 mg;

> **Cipro XR** *Tab:* 500, 1000 mg ext-rel
> **ProQuin XR** *Tab:* 500 mg ext-rel
> or
▷ **doxycycline (D)(G)** <8 years usually not recommended; ***erythromycin*** or ***azithromycin*** preferred; consider risk benefit; >8 years: 2-4 mg/kg in a single dose
> **Acticlate** *Tab:* 75, 150**mg
>> **Adoxa** *Tab:* 50, 75, 100, 150 mg ent-coat
>> **Doryx** *Tab:* 50, 75, 100, 150, 200 mg del-rel
>> **Doxteric** *Tab:* 50 mg del-rel
>> **Monodox** *Cap:* 50, 75, 100 mg
>> **Oracea** *Cap:* 40 mg del-rel
>> **Vibramycin** *Tab:* 100 mg; *Cap:* 50, 100 mg; *Syr:* 50 mg/ml (raspberry-apple) (sulfites); *Oral susp:* 25 mg/5 ml (raspberry)
>> **Vibra-Tab** *Tab:* 100 mg film-coat

CHILDREN <3 YEARS
Regimen 1

▷ **erythromycin ethylsuccinate (B)(G)** 12.5 mg/kg q 6 hours x 3 days; use suspension
> **E.E.S.** *Oral susp:* 200, 400 mg/5 ml (100 ml) (fruit)
> **E.E.S. Granules** *Oral susp:* 200 mg/5 ml (100, 200 ml) (cherry, fruit); *Chew tab:* 200 mg wafer (fruit)
> **EryPed** *Oral susp:* 200 mg/5 ml (100, 200 ml) (fruit); 400 mg/5 ml (60, 100, 200 ml) (banana); *Oral drops:* 200, 400 mg/5 ml (50 ml) (fruit); *Chew tab:* 200 mg wafer (fruit)
> or
▷ **azithromycin (B)(G)** 20 mg/kg in a single dose; max 1 gm; use suspension
> **Zithromax** *Tab:* 250, 500, 600 mg; *Oral susp:* 100 mg/5 ml (15 ml); 200 mg/5 ml (15, 22.5, 30 ml) (cherry)
> **Zmax** *Oral susp:* 2 gm ext-rel for reconstitution (cherry-banana) (148 mg Na$^+$)

Regimen 2

▷ **ciprofloxacin (C)(G)** <18 years usually not recommended; ***erythromycin*** or ***azithromycin*** preferred; consider risk benefit; 20 mg/kg in a single dose; use suspension
> **Cipro** *Oral susp:* 250, 500 mg/5 ml (100 ml) (strawberry)
> or
▷ **doxycycline (D)(G)** <8 years usually not recommended; ***erythromycin*** or ***azithromycin*** preferred; consider risk benefit; 2-4 mg/kg in a single dose; use suspension or syrup
> **Vibramycin** *Syr:* 50 mg/5 ml (raspberry-apple) (sulfites); *Oral susp:* 25 mg/5 ml (raspberry)

 CLOSTRIDIUM DIFFICILE

Comment: Acid-suppressing drugs including proton pump inhibitors (PPIs), third- and fourth-generation cephalosporins, carbapenems, and ***piperacillin-tazobactam*** significantly increase the risk of hospital-onset Clostridium difficile infection (CDI), according to the results of a recent study. Patients who received tetracyclines, macrolides, or clindamycin had lower risk of developing hospital-onset CDI.

REFERENCE
Watson, T., Hickok, J., Fraker, S., Korwek, K., Poland, R. E., & Septimus, E. (2017). Evaluating the risk factors for hospital-onset Clostridium difficile infections in a large healthcare system. *Clinical Infectious Diseases*. doi:10.1093/cid/cix1112

HUMAN IGG1 MONOCLONAL ANTIBODY

Comment: *bezlotoxumab* is a human IgG1 monoclonal antibody that inhibits the binding of *Clostridium difficile* toxin B, preventing its effects on mammalian cells. *bezlotoxumab* does not bind to C. difficile toxin A. *bezlotoxumab* is indicated to reduce the recurrence of CDI in patients who are receiving antibacterial drug treatment of CDI and are at high risk for CDI recurrence. CDI recurrence is defined as a new episode of diarrhea associated with a positive stool test for toxigenic *C. difficile* following a clinical cure of the presenting CDI episode. It is not indicated for the primary treatment of CDI infection. It is to be used only in conjunction with appropriate primary drug treatment of CDI. Patients at high risk for CDI recurrence, studied in clinical trials establishing efficacy, include those ≥65 years-of-age, with a history of CDI in the previous 6 months, immunocompromised state, severe CDI at presentation, and *C. difficile* ribotype 027.

▷ *bezlotoxumab* (C) administer a single dose of 10 mg/kg via IV infusion over 60 minutes
   Pediatric: <18 years: not established; ≥18 years: same as adult
   Zinplava *Vial:* 40 ml single-use solution

COLIC: INFANTILE

▷ *hyoscyamine* (C)(G)
   Levsin Drops
      Pediatric: 3-4 kg: 4 drops q 4 hours prn; max 24 drops/day; 5 kg: 5 drops q 4 hours prn; max 30 drops/day; 7 kg: 6 drops q 4 hours prn; max 36 drops/day; 10 kg: 8 drops q 4 hours prn; max 40 drops/day; *Oral drops:* 0.125 mg/ml (15 ml) (orange) (alcohol 5%)
▷ *simethicone* (C) 0.3 ml qid pc and HS
   Mylicon Drops (OTC) *Oral drops:* 40 mg/0.6 ml (30 ml)

COLONOSCOPY PREP/COLON CLEANSE

▷ *sodium picosulfate+magnesium oxide+citric acid* reconstitute pwdr with cold water right before use; two dosing regimen options—each requires two separate dosing times; *Split Dose Method* (preferred): 1st dose during evening before the colonoscopy and 2nd dose the next day during the morning prior to the colonoscopy; *Day Before Method* (alternative, if split dose is not appropriate): 1st dose during afternoon or early evening before the colonoscopy and 2nd dose 6 hours later during evening before colonoscopy; additional clear liquids (no solid food or milk) must be consumed after every dose in both dosing regimens
   Pediatric: <18 years: not recommended; ≥18 years: same as adult
      Prepopik *Pwdr:* sod picos 10 mg+mag oxide 3.5 gm+anhy cit acid 12 gm/pkt pwdr for oral solution (2 pkts)
Comment: **Prepopik** is a combination of sodium picosulfate, a stimulant laxative, and magnesium oxide and anhydrous citric acid which form magnesium citrate, an osmotic laxative, indicated for cleansing of the colon as a preparation for colonoscopy in adults. Rule out diagnosis of suspected GI obstruction or perforation diagnosis before administration. **Prepopik** should be used during pregnancy only if clearly needed. **Prepopik** is contraindicated with severely reduced renal function (CrCl< 30 mL/min), GI obstruction or ileus, bowel perforation, toxic colitis or toxic megacolon, and gastric retention for any reason.

COMMON COLD (VIRAL UPPER RESPIRATORY INFECTION [URI])

Drugs for the Management of Allergy, Cough, and Cold Symptoms *see page* 598
Oral Decongestants *see page* 598
Oral Expectorants *see page* 598
Oral Antitussives *see page* 598
Oral Antipyretic-Analgesics *see Fever page* 165

NASAL SALINE DROPS AND SPRAYS

Comment: Homemade saline nose drops: 1/4 tsp salt added to 8 oz boiled water, then cool water.
▷ *saline* nasal spray (G)

> **Afrin Saline Mist w. Eucalyptol and Menthol (OTC)** 2-6 sprays in each nostril prn
> *Pediatric:* 1 month-2 years: 1-2 sprays in each nostril prn; >2-12 years: 1-4 sprays in each nostril prn; >12 years: same as adult
>> *Squeeze bottle:* 45 ml
> **Afrin Moisturizing Saline Mist (OTC)** 2-6 sprays in each nostril prn
> *Pediatric:* 1 month-2 years: 1-2 sprays in each nostril prn; 2-12 years: 1-4 sprays in each nostril prn; >12 years: same as adult
>> *Squeeze bottle:* 45 ml
> **Ocean Mist (OTC)** 2-6 sprays in each nostril prn
> *Pediatric:* 1 month-2 years: 1-2 sprays in each nostril prn; >2-12 years: 1-4 sprays in each nostril prn; >12 years: same as adult
>> *Squeeze bottle: saline* 0.65% (45 ml) (alcohol-free)
> **Pediamist (OTC)** 2-6 sprays in each nostril prn
> *Pediatric:* 1 month-2 years: 1-2 sprays in each nostril prn; >2-12 years: 1-4 sprays in each nostril prn; >12 years: same as adult
>> *Squeeze bottle: saline* 0.5% (15 ml) (alcohol-free)

NASAL SYMPATHOMIMETICS

▷ *oxymetazoline* (C)(OTC)
4-Hour Formulation: 2-3 drops <u>or</u> sprays in each nostril q 10-12 hours prn; max 2 doses/day; max duration 5 days
Pediatric: <6 years: not recommended; ≥6 years: same as adult
> **Afrin 4-Hour:**
12-hour Formulation: 2-3 drops <u>or</u> sprays q 4 hours prn; max duration 5 days
Pediatric: <12 years: not recommended; ≥12 years: same as adult
> **Afrin 12-Hour Extra Moisturizing Nasal Spray**
> **Afrin 12-Hour Nasal spray Pump Mist**
> **Afrin 12-Hour Original Nasal spray**
> **Afrin 12-Hour Original Nose Drops**
> **Afrin 12-Hour Severe Congestion Nasal Spray**
> **Afrin 12-Hour Sinus Nasal Spray**
>> *Nasal spray:* 0.05% (45 ml); *Nasal drops:* 0.05% (45 ml)
> **Afrin 4-Hour Nasal Spray**
> **Neo-Synephrine 12 Hour Nasal Spray**
> **Neo-Synephrine 12 Hour Extra Moisturizing Nasal Spray**
>> *Nasal spray:* 0.05% (15 ml)
▷ *phenylephrine* (C)
> **Afrin Allergy Nasal Spray (OTC)** 2-3 sprays in each nostril q 4 hours prn; max duration 5 days

Pediatric: <12 years: not recommended; ≥12 years: same as adult
    Nasal spray: 0.5% (15 ml)
Afrin Nasal Decongestant Childrens Pump Mist (OTC)
Pediatric: <6 years: not recommended; ≥6 years: 2-3 sprays in each nostril
q 4 hours prn; max duration 5 days
    Nasal spray: 0.25% (15 ml)
Neo-Synephrine Extra Strength (OTC) 2-3 sprays or drops in each nostril
q 4 hours prn; max duration 5 days
Pediatric: <12 years: not recommended; ≥12 years: same as adult
    Nasal spray: 0.1% (15 ml); *Nasal drops:* 0.1% (15 ml)
Neo-Synephrine Mild Formula (OTC) 2-3 sprays or drops in each nostril
q 4 hours prn; max duration 5 days
Pediatric: <6 years: not recommended; ≥6 years: same as adult
    Nasal spray: 0.25% (15 ml)
Neo-Synephrine Regular Strength (OTC) 2-3 sprays or drops in each nostril q 4
hours prn; max duration 5 days
Pediatric: <12 years: not recommended; ≥12 years: same as adult
    Nasal spray: 0.5% (15 ml); *Nasal drops:* 0.5% (15 ml)
➤ *tetrahydrozoline* (C)
Tyzine 2-4 drops or 3-4 sprays in each nostril q 3-8 hours prn; max duration
5 days
Pediatric: <6 years: not recommended; ≥6 years: same as adult
    Nasal spray: 0.1% (15 ml); *Nasal drops:* 0.1% (30 ml)
Tyzine Pediatric Nasal Drops 2-3 sprays or drops in each nostril q 3-6 hours prn
    Nasal drops: 0.05% (15 ml)

CONJUNCTIVITIS: ALLERGIC

Oral Antihistamines *see* **Drugs for the Management of Allergy, Cough, and Cold
Symptoms** *see page* 598

OPHTHALMIC CORTICOSTEROIDS

Comment: Concomitant contact lens wear is contraindicated during therapy.
Ophthalmic steroids are contraindicated with ocular, fungal, mycobacterial, viral
(except herpes zoster), and untreated bacterial infection. Ophthalmic steroids may mask
or exacerbate infection, and may increase intraocular pressure, optic nerve damage,
cataract formation, or corneal perforation. Limit ophthalmic steroid use to 2-3 days if
possible; usual max 2 weeks. With prolonged or frequent use, there is risk of corneal and
scleral thinning and cataract formation.
➤ *dexamethasone* (C) initially 1-2 drops hourly during the day and q 2 hours at night;
then prolong dosing interval to 4-6 hours as condition improves
Pediatric: <12 years: not recommended; ≥12 years: same as adult
    Maxidex *Ophth susp:* 0.1% (5, 15 ml) (benzalkonium chloride)
➤ *dexamethasone phosphate* (C) initially 1-2 drops hourly during the day and q 2 hours
at night; then 1 drop q 4-8 hours or more as condition improves
Pediatric: <12 years: not recommended; ≥12 years: same as adult
    Decadron *Ophth soln:* 0.1% (5 ml) (sulfites)
➤ *fluorometholone* (C) 1 drop bid-qid or 1/2 inch of ointment once daily-tid; may
increase dose frequency during initial 24-48 hours
Pediatric: <2 years: not recommended; ≥2 years: same as adult
    FML *Ophth susp:* 0.1% (5, 10, 15 ml) (benzalkonium chloride)
    FML Forte *Ophth susp:* 0.25% (5, 10, 15 ml) (benzalkonium chloride)
    FML S.O.P. Ointment *Ophth oint:* 0.1% (3.5 gm)

▷ *fluorometholone acetate* (C) initially 2 drops q 2 hours during the first 24-48 hours; then 1-2 drops qid as condition improves
   Pediatric: <12 years: not recommended; ≥12 years: same as adult
      Flarex *Ophth susp:* 0.1% (2.5, 5 10 ml) (benzalkonium chloride)
▷ *loteprednol etabonate* (C)
   Pediatric: <12 years: not recommended; ≥12 years: same as adult
      Alrex 1 drop qid
         Ophth susp: 0.2% (5, 10 ml) (benzalkonium chloride)
      Lotemax 1-2 drops qid
         Ophth susp: 0.5% (5, 10, 15 ml) (benzalkonium chloride)
▷ *medrysone* (C) 1 drop up to q 4 hours
   Pediatric: <12 years: not recommended; ≥12 years: same as adult
      HMS *Ophth susp:* 1% (10 ml) (benzalkonium chloride)
▷ *rimexolone* (C) initially 1-2 drops hourly while awake x 1 week; then 1 drop q 2 hours while awake x 1 week; then taper as condition improves
   Pediatric: <12 years: not recommended; ≥12 years: same as adult
      Vexol *Ophth susp:* 0.1% (5, 10 ml) (benzalkonium chloride)
▷ *prednisolone acetate* (C)(G)
   Pediatric: <12 years: not recommended; ≥12 years: same as adult
      Econopred 2 drops qid
         Ophth susp: 0.125% (5, 10 ml)
      Econopred Plus 2 drops qid
         Ophth susp: 1% (5, 10 ml)
      Pred Forte initially 2 drops hourly x 24-48 hours; then 1-2 drops bid-qid
         Ophth susp: 1% (1, 5, 10, 15 ml) (benzalkonium chloride, sulfites)
      Pred Mild initially 2 drops hourly x 24-48 hours; then 1-2 drops bid-qid
         Ophth susp: 0.12% (5, 10 ml) (benzalkonium chloride)
▷ *prednisolone sodium phosphate* (C) initially 1-2 drops hourly during the day and q 2 hours at night; then 1 drop q 4 hours; then 1 drop tid-qid as condition improves
   Pediatric: <12 years: not recommended; ≥12 years: same as adult
      Inflamase Forte *Ophth soln:* 1% (5, 10, 15 ml) (benzalkonium chloride)
      Inflamase Mild *Ophth soln:* 1/8% (5, 10 ml) (benzalkonium chloride)

OPHTHALMIC H1 ANTAGONISTS (ANTIHISTAMINES)

Comment: May insert contact lens 10 minutes after administration of ophthalmic antihistamine.
▷ *cetirizine* (C) 1 drop bid prn
   Pediatric: <2 years: not established; ≥2 years: same as adult
      Zerviate *Ophth soln:* 0.24%/ml (5 ml [7.5 ml bottle]; 7.5 ml [10 ml bottle])
▷ *emedastine* (C) 1 drop qid prn
   Pediatric: <3 years: not recommended; ≥3 years: same as adult
      Emadine *Ophth soln:* 0.05% (5 ml) (benzalkonium chloride)
▷ *levocabastine* (C) 1 drop qid prn
   Pediatric: <12 years: not recommended; ≥12 years: same as adult
      Livostin *Ophth susp:* 0.05% (2.5, 5, 10 ml) (benzalkonium chloride)

OPHTHALMIC MAST CELL STABILIZERS

Comment: Concomitant contact lens wear is contraindicated during treatment.
▷ *cromolyn sodium* (B) 1-2 drops 4-6 x/day at regular intervals
   Pediatric: <4 years: not recommended; ≥4 years: same as adult
      Crolom *Ophth soln:* 4% (10 ml) (benzalkonium chloride)
▷ *lodoxamide tromethamine* (B) 1-2 drops qid up to 3 months
   Pediatric: <2 years: not recommended; ≥2 years: same as adult
      Alomide *Ophth soln:* 1% (10 ml) (benzalkonium chloride)

▷ *nedocromil* (B) 1-2 drops bid
  Pediatric: <3 years: not recommended; ≥3 years: same as adult
    Alocril *Ophth soln:* 2% (5 ml) (benzalkonium chloride)
▷ *pemirolast potassium* (C) 1-2 drops qid
  Pediatric: <3 years: not recommended; ≥3 years: same as adult
    Alamast *Ophth soln:* 0.1% (10 ml) (lauralkonium chloride)

OPHTHALMIC ANTIHISTAMINE+MAST CELL STABILIZER COMBINATIONS

▷ *alcaftadine* (B) 1 drop each eye daily
  Pediatric: <2 years: not recommended; ≥2 years: same as adult
    Lastacaft *Ophth soln:* 0.25% (6 ml) (benzalkonium chloride)
Comment: May insert contact lens 10 minutes after ophthalmic administration.
▷ *azelastine* (C) 1 drop each eye bid
  Pediatric: <3 years: not recommended; ≥3 years: same as adult
    Optivar *Ophth soln:* 0.05% (6 ml) (benzalkonium chloride)
Comment: May insert contact lens 10 minutes after ophthalmic administration.
▷ *bepotastine besilate* (C) 1 drop each eye bid
  Pediatric: <2 years: not recommended; ≥2 years: same as adult
    Bepreve *Ophth soln:* 1.5% (10 ml) (benzalkonium chloride)
Comment: May insert contact lens 10 minutes after ophthalmic administration.
▷ *epinastine* (C)(G) 1 drop each eye bid
  Pediatric: <3 years: not recommended; ≥3 years: same as adult
    Elestat *Ophth soln:* 0.05% (5 ml) (benzalkonium chloride)
Comment: May insert contact lens 10 minutes after administration.
▷ *ketotifen fumarate* (C) 1 drop each eye q 8-12 hours
  Pediatric: <3 years: not recommended; ≥3 years: same as adult
    Alaway (OTC) *Ophth soln:* 0.025% (10 ml) (benzalkonium chloride)
    Claritin Eye (OTC) *Ophth soln:* 0.025% (5 ml) (benzalkonium chloride)
    Refresh Eye Itch Relief (OTC) *Ophth soln:* 0.025% (5 ml) (benzalkonium chloride)
    Zaditor (OTC) *Ophth soln:* 0.025% (5 ml) (benzalkonium chloride)
    Zyrtec Itchy Eye (OTC) *Ophth soln:* 0.025% (5 ml) (benzalkonium chloride)
Comment: May insert contact lens 10 minutes after administration.
▷ *olopatadine* (C) 1 drop each eye bid
  Pediatric: <3 years: not recommended; ≥3 years: same as adult
    Pataday (G) *Ophth soln:* 0.2% (2.5 ml) (benzalkonium chloride)
    Patanol (G) *Ophth soln:* 0.1% (5 ml) (benzalkonium chloride)
    Pazeo *Ophth soln:* 0.7% (2.5 ml) (benzalkonium chloride)
Comment: May insert contact lens 10 minutes after administration.

OPHTHALMIC VASOCONSTRICTORS

Comment: Concomitant contact lens wear is contraindicated during treatment.
▷ *naphazoline* (C) 1-2 drops each eye qid prn
  Pediatric: <12 years: not recommended; ≥12 years: same as adult
    Vasocon-A *Ophth soln:* 0.1% (15 ml) (benzalkonium chloride)
▷ *oxymetazoline* (OTC) 1-2 drops each eye qid prn
  Pediatric: <6 years: not recommended; ≥6 years: same as adult
    Visine L-R *Ophth soln:* 0.025% (15, 30 ml)
▷ *tetrahydrozoline* (OTC)(G) 1-2 drops each eye qid prn
  Pediatric: <6 years: not recommended; ≥6 years: same as adult
    Visine *Ophth soln:* 0.05% (15, 22.5, 30 ml)

OPHTHALMIC VASOCONSTRICTOR+MOISTURIZER COMBINATION

Comment: Concomitant contact lens wear is contraindicated during treatment.

▷ *tetrahydrozoline+polyethylene glycol 400+povidone+dextran 70* (OTC) 1-2 drops each eye qid prn
  Pediatric: <6 years: not recommended; ≥6 years: same as adult
    Advanced Relief Visine *Ophth soln: tetra* 0.025%+*poly* 1%+*pov* 1%+*dex* 0.1% (15, 30 ml)

OPHTHALMIC VASOCONSTRICTOR+ASTRINGENT COMBINATION

Comment: Concomitant contact lens wear is contraindicated during treatment.
▷ *tetrahydrozoline+zinc sulfate* (OTC) 1-2 drops each eye qid prn
  Pediatric: <6 years: not recommended; ≥6 years: same as adult
    Visine AC *Ophth soln: tetra* 0.025%+*zinc* 0.05% (15, 30 ml)

OPHTHALMIC VASOCONSTRICTOR+ANTI-HISTAMINE COMBINATIONS

Comment: Concomitant contact lens wear is contraindicated during treatment.
▷ *naphazoline+pheniramine* (C) 1-2 drops each eye qid
  Pediatric: <6 years: not recommended; ≥6 years: same as adult
    Naphcon-A (OTC) *Ophth soln: naph* 0.025%+*phen* 0.3% (15 ml)
    (benzalkonium chloride)

OPHTHALMIC NSAIDs

Comment: Concomitant contact lens wear is contraindicated during treatment.

▷ *bromfenac* (C)(G) 1 drop affected eye(s) bid
    Bromday Ophthalmic Solution *Ophth soln:* 0.09% (2.5 ml in 7.5 ml dropper bottle; 7.5 ml in 10 ml dropper bottle)
    Xibrom Ophthalmic Solution *Ophth soln:* 0.09% (2.5 ml in 7.5 ml dropper bottle; 7.5 ml in 10 ml dropper bottle)
▷ *diclofenac* (B) 1 drop affected eye(s) qid
  Pediatric: <12 years: not recommended; ≥12 years: same as adult
    Voltaren Ophthalmic Solution *Ophth soln:* 0.1% (2.5, 5 ml)
▷ *ketorolac tromethamine* (C) 1 drop affected eye(s) qid; max x 4 days
  Pediatric: <3 years: not recommended; ≥3 years: same as adult
    Acular *Ophth soln:* 0.5% (3, 5, 10 ml) (benzalkonium chloride)
    Acular LS *Ophth soln:* 0.4% (5 ml) (benzalkonium chloride)
    Acular PF *Ophth soln:* 0.5% (0.4 ml; 12 single-use vials/carton) (preservative-free)
▷ *nepafenac* (C) 1 drop affected eye(s) tid
  Pediatric: <10 years: not recommended; ≥10 years: same as adult
    Nevanac Ophthalmic Suspension *Ophth susp:* 0.1% (3 ml) (benzalkonium chloride)

 CONJUNCTIVITIS/BLEPHAROCONJUNCTIVITIS: BACTERIAL

OPHTHALMIC ANTI-INFECTIVES

▷ *azithromycin* (B)(G) ophthalmic solution (B)(G) 1 drop to affected eye(s) bid x 2 days; then 1 drop once daily for the next 5 days
  Pediatric: <1 year: not recommended; ≥1 year: same as adult
    AzaSite Ophthalmic Solution *Ophth susp:* 1% (2.5 ml) (benzalkonium chloride)
▷ *bacitracin* ophthalmic ointment (C)(G) apply 1/2 inch ribbon to the lower conjunctival sac of affected eye(s) 1-3 x daily x 7 days
  Pediatric: same as adult
    Bacitracin Ophthalmic Ointment *Ophth oint:* 500 units/gm (3.5 gm)

▷ *besifloxacin* ophthalmic solution (C) 1 drop to affected eye(s) tid x 7 days
Pediatric: <1 year: not recommended; ≥1 year: same as adult
 Besivance Ophthalmic Solution *Ophth susp:* 0.6% (5 ml) (benzalkonium chloride)
▷ *ciprofloxacin* ophthalmic ointment (C) apply 1/2 inch ribbon to the lower conjunctival sac of affected eye(s) tid x 2 days; then bid x 5 days
Pediatric: <2 years: not recommended; ≥2 years: same as adult
 Ciloxan Ophthalmic Ointment *Ophth oint:* 0.3% (3.5 gm)
▷ *ciprofloxacin* ophthalmic solution (C) 1-2 drops to affected eye(s) q 2 hours while awake x 2 days; then, q 4 hours while awake x 5 days
Pediatric: <1 year: not recommended; ≥1 year: same as adult
 Ciloxan Ophthalmic Solution *Ophth soln:* 0.3% (2.5, 5, 10 ml) (benzalkonium chloride)
▷ *erythromycin* ophthalmic ointment (B) apply 1/2 inch ribbon to the lower conjunctival sac of affected eye(s) up to 6 x/day
Pediatric: same as adult
 Ilotycin Ophthalmic Ointment *Ophth oint:* 5 mg/gm (1/8 oz)
▷ *gatifloxacin* ophthalmic solution (C)
Pediatric: <1 years: not recommended; ≥1 year: same as adult
 Zymar Ophthalmic Solution initially 1 drop to affected eye(s) q 2 hours while awake up to 8 x/day for 2 days; then 1 drop qid while awake x 5 more days
  Ophth soln: 0.3% (5 ml) (benzalkonium chloride)
 Zymaxid Ophthalmic Solution (G) initially 1 drop to affected eye(s) q 2 hours while awake up to 8 x/day on day 1; then 1 drop bid-qid while awake on days 2-7
  Ophth soln: 0.5% (2.5 ml) (benzalkonium chloride)
▷ *gentamicin sulfate* ophthalmic ointment (C)(G) apply 1/2 inch ribbon to the lower conjunctival sac of affected eye(s) bid-tid
Pediatric: same as adult
 Garamycin Ophthalmic Ointment *Ophth oint:* 3 mg/gm (3.5 gm) (preservative-free formulation available)
 Genoptic Ophthalmic Ointment *Ophth oint:* 3 mg/gm (3.5 gm)
 Gentacidin Ophthalmic Ointment *Ophth oint:* 3 mg/gm (3.5 gm)
▷ *gentamicin sulfate* ophthalmic solution (C)(G) 1-2 drops to affected eye(s) q 4 hours x 7-14 days; max 2 drops q 1 h
Pediatric: same as adult
 Garamycin Ophthalmic Solution *Ophth soln:* 0.3% (5 ml) (benzalkonium chloride)
 Genoptic Ophthalmic Solution *Ophth soln:* 0.3% (3, 5 ml)
▷ *levofloxacin* ophthalmic solution (C) 1-2 drops to affected eye(s) q 2 hours while awake on days 1 and 2 (max 8 x/day); then 1-2 drops q 4 hours while awake on days 3-7; max 4 x/day
Pediatric: <1 years: not recommended; ≥1 years: same as adult
 Quixin Ophthalmic Solution *Ophth soln:* 0.5% (2.5, 5 ml) (benzalkonium chloride)
▷ *moxifloxacin* ophthalmic solution (C)(G) 1 drop to affected eye(s) tid x 7 days
Pediatric: <1 years: not recommended; ≥1 year: same as adult
 Moxeza Ophthalmic Solution (G) *Ophth soln:* 0.5% (3 ml)
 Vigamox Ophthalmic Solution *Ophth soln:* 0.5% (3 ml)
▷ *ofloxacin* ophthalmic solution (C) 1-2 drops to affected eye(s) q 2-4 hours x 2 days; then qid x 5 days
Pediatric: <1 years: not recommended; ≥1 year: same as adult
 Ocuflox Ophthalmic Solution *Ophth soln:* 0.3% (5, 10 ml) (benzalkonium chloride)

▷ *sulfacetamide* ophthalmic solution and ointment **(C)**

    Bleph-10 Ophthalmic Solution 1-2 drops to affected eye(s) q 2-3 hours x 7-10 days

    Pediatric: <2 months: not recommended; ≥2 months: 1-2 drops q 2-3 hours during the day x 7-10 days

      Ophth soln: 10% (2.5, 5, 15 ml) (benzalkonium chloride)

    Bleph-10 Ophthalmic Ointment apply 1/2 inch ribbon to the lower conjunctival sac of affected eye(s) q 3-4 hours and HS x 7-10 days

    Pediatric: <2 years: not recommended; ≥2 years: same as adult

      Ophth oint: 10% (3.5 gm) (phenylmercuric acetate)

    Cetamide Ophthalmic Solution initially 1-2 drops to affected eye(s) q 2-3 hours; then increase dosing interval as condition improves

    Pediatric: <2 years: not recommended; ≥2 years: same as adult

      Ophth soln: 15% (5, 15 ml)

    Isopto Cetamide Ophthalmic Ointment initially 1/2 inch ribbon in lower conjunctival sac of affected eye(s) q 3-4 hours; then increase dosing interval as condition improves

    Pediatric: <2 years: not recommended; ≥2 years: same as adult

      Ophth oint: 10% (3.5 gm)

    Isopto Cetamide Ophthalmic Solution initially 1-2 drops to affected eye(s) q 2-3 hours; then increase dosing interval as condition improves

    Pediatric: <2 years: not recommended; ≥2 years: same as adult

      Ophth soln: 15% (5, 15 ml)

▷ *tobramycin* **(B)**

    Tobrex Ophthalmic Solution 1-2 drops to affected eye(s) q 4 hours

    Pediatric: same as adult

      Ophth soln: 0.3% (5 ml) (benzalkonium chloride)

    Tobrex Ophthalmic Ointment apply 1/2 inch ribbon to the lower conjunctival sac of affected eye(s) bid-tid

    Pediatric: same as adult

      Ophth oint: 0.3% (3.5 gm) (chlorobutanol)

OPHTHALMIC ANTI-INFECTIVE COMBINATIONS

▷ *polymyxin b sulfate+bacitracin* ophthalmic ointment **(C)** apply 1/2 inch ribbon to the lower conjunctival sac of affected eye(s) q 3-4 hours x 7-10 days

    Pediatric: same as adult

    Polysporin Ophthalmic Ointment *Ophth oint:* poly b 10,000 U+*bac* 500 U (3.75 gm)

▷ *polymyxin b sulfate+bacitracin zinc+neomycin sulfate* ophthalmic ointment **(C)** apply 1/2 inch ribbon to the lower conjunctival sac of affected eye(s) q 3-4 hours x 7-10 days

    Pediatric: same as adult

    Neosporin Ophthalmic Ointment *Ophth oint:* poly b 10,000 U+*bac* 400 U+*neo* 3.5 mg/gm (3.75 gm)

▷ *polymyxin b sulfate+gramicidin+neomycin* ophthalmic solution **(C)** 1-2 drops to affected eye(s) q 1 hour x 2-3 doses; then 1-2 drops bid-qid x 7-10 days

    Pediatric: <12 years: not recommended; ≥12 years: same as adult

    Neosporin Ophthalmic Solution *Ophth soln:* poly b 10,000 U+*grami* 0.025 mg+ neo 1.7 mg/gm (10 ml)

▷ *trimethoprim+polymyxin b sulfate* ophthalmic solution **(C)** 1 drop to affected eye(s) q 3 hours x 7-10 days; max 6 doses/day

    Pediatric: <2 years: not recommended; ≥2 years: same as adult

    Polytrim *Ophth soln:* trim 1 mg+*poly b* 10,000 U/ml (10 ml) (benzalkonium chloride)

OPHTHALMIC ANTI-INFECTIVE+STEROID COMBINATIONS

Comment: Ophthalmic corticosteroids are contraindicated after removal of a corneal foreign body, epithelial herpes simplex keratitis, *varicella*, other viral infections of the cornea or conjunctiva, fungal ocular infections, and mycobacterial ocular infections. Limit ophthalmic steroid use to 2-3 days if possible; usual max 2 weeks. With prolonged or frequent use, there is risk of corneal and scleral thinning and cataract formation.

▶ *gentamicin sulfate+prednisolone acetate* ophthalmic suspension (C)
    Pediatric: <12 years: not recommended; ≥12 years: same as adult
      Pred-G Ophthalmic Suspension 1 drop to affected eye(s) bid-qid; max 20 ml/therapeutic course
        Ophth susp: gent 0.3%+*pred* 1%/ml (2, 5, 10 ml) (benzalkonium chloride)
      Pred-G Ophthalmic Ointment apply 1/2 inch ribbon to the lower conjunctival sac of affected eye(s) once daily-tid; max 8 gm/therapeutic course
        Ophth oint: gent 0.3%+*pred* 0.6%/gm (3.5 gm)

▶ *neomycin sulfate+polymyxin b sulfate+dexamethasone* ophthalmic suspension (C)
    Pediatric: <12 years: not recommended; ≥12 years: same as adult
      Maxitrol Ophthalmic Suspension 1-2 drops to affected eye(s) q 1 hour (severe infection) or qid (mild to moderate infection)
        Ophth susp: neo 0.35%+*poly b* 10,000 U+*dexa* 1%/ml (5 ml) (benzalkonium chloride)
      Maxitrol Ophthalmic Ointment apply 1/2 inch ribbon to the lower conjunctival sac of affected eye(s) q 1 hour (severe infection) or qid (mild to moderate infection)
        Ophth oint: neo 0.35%+*poly b* 10,000 U+*dexa* 0.1%/gm (3.5 gm)

▶ *neomycin sulfate+polymyxin b sulfate+prednisolone acetate ophthalmic suspension* (C)
    Pediatric: <12 years: not recommended; ≥12 years: same as adult
      Poly-Pred Ophthalmic Suspension 1-2 drops to affected eye(s) q 3-4 hours; more often as necessary; max 20 ml/therapeutic course.
        Ophth susp: neo 0.35%+*poly b* 10,000 U+*pred* 0.5%/ml (10 ml)

▶ *polymyxin b sulfate+neomycin sulfate+hydrocortisone* ophthalmic suspension (C)
    Pediatric: <12 years: not recommended; ≥12 years: same as adult
      Cortisporin Ophthalmic Suspension 1-2 drops to affected eye(s) tid-qid; more often if necessary; max 20 ml/therapeutic course
        Ophth susp: poly b 10,000 U+*neo* 0.35%+*hydro* 1%/ml (7.5 ml) (thimerosal)

▶ *polymyxin b sulfate+neomycin sulfate+bacitracin zinc+hydrocortisone* ophthalmic ointment (C)
    Pediatric: <12 years: not recommended; ≥12 years: same as adult
      Cortisporin Ophthalmic Ointment apply 1/2 inch ribbon to the lower conjunctival sac of affected eye(s) tid-qid; more often if necessary; max 8 gm/therapeutic course
        Ophth oint: poly b 10,000 U+*neo* 0.35%+*bac* 400 U+*hydro* 1%/gm (3.5 gm)

▶ *sulfacetamide sodium+fluorometholone* suspension (C) 1 drop to affected eye(s) qid; max 20 ml/therapeutic course
    Pediatric: <12 years: not recommended; ≥12 years: same as adult
      FML-S *Ophth susp: sulfa* 10%+*fluoro* 0.1%+ml (5, 10, 15 ml) (benzalkonium chloride)

▶ *sulfacetamide sodium+prednisolone acetate* ophthalmic suspension and ointment (C)
    Pediatric: <6 years: not recommended; ≥6 years: same as adult
      Blephamide Liquifilm 2 drops to affected eye(s) qid and HS
        *Ophth susp: sulfa*10%+*pred* 0.2%/ml (5, 10 ml) (benzalkonium chloride)
      Blephamide S.O.P. Ophthalmic Ointment apply 1/2 inch ribbon to the lower conjunctival sac of affected eye(s) tid-qid
        Ophth oint: sulfa 10%+*pred* 0.2%/gm (3.5 gm) (benzalkonium chloride)

▷ **sulfacetamide sodium+prednisolone sodium phosphate** ophthalmic solution **(C)** 2 drops
to affected eye(s) q 4 hours
Pediatric: <6 years: not recommended; ≥6 years: same as adult
  Vasocidin Ophthalmic Solution *Ophth soln:* sulfa 10%+pred 0.25%/ml (5, 10 ml)
▷ **tobramycin+dexamethasone** ophthalmic solution and ointment **(C)**
  TobraDex Ophthalmic Solution 1-2 drops to affected eye(s) q 2-6 hours x 24-48
  hours; then 4-6 hours; reduce frequency of dose as condition improves; max 20
  ml per therapeutic course
  Pediatric: ≤2 years: not recommended; ≥2 years: 1-2 drops q 4-6 hours; may start
  with 1-2 drops q 2 hours first 1-2 days
    Ophth susp: tobra 0.3%+dexa 0.1%/ml (2.5, 5 ml) (benzalkonium chloride)
  TobraDex Ophthalmic Ointment apply 1/2 inch ribbon to the lower conjunctival
  sac of affected eye(s) tid-qid; may use at HS in conjunction with daytime drops;
  max 8 gm/therapeutic course
  Pediatric: <2 years: not recommended; ≥2 years: apply 1/2 inch ribbon to lower
  conjunctival sac tid-qid
    Ophth oint: tobra 0.3%/dexa 0.1%/gm (3.5 gm) (chlorobutanol chloride)
  TobraDex ST 1-2 drops to affected eye(s) q 2-6 hours x 24-48 hours; then 4-6 hours;
  reduce frequency of dose as condition improves; max 20 ml per therapeutic course
  Pediatric: <12 years: not recommended; ≥12 years: same as adult
    Ophth susp: tobra 0.3%/dexa 0.05%/ml (2.5, 5, 10 ml) (benzalkonium chloride)
▷ **tobramycin+loteprednol etabonate** ophthalmic suspension **(C)**
  Pediatric: <12 years: not recommended; ≥12 years: same as adult
    Zylet 1-2 drops to affected eye(s) q 1-2 hours first 24-48 hours; reduce frequency
    of dose to q 4-6 hours as condition improves; max 20 ml per therapeutic course
      Ophth susp: tobra 0.3%+lote etab 0.5%/ml (2.5, 5, 10 ml) (benzalkonium chloride)

CONJUNCTIVITIS: CHLAMYDIAL

Comment: A chlamydial etiology should be considered for all infants aged ≤30 days that
have conjunctivitis, especially if the mother has a history of chlamydia infection. Topical
antibiotic therapy alone is inadequate for treatment for *ophthalmia neonatorum* caused by
chlamydia and is unnecessary when systemic treatment is administered.

RECOMMENDED FIRST LINE REGIMEN

▷ **erythromycin base (B)(G)** 250 mg qid x 14 days <u>or</u> 500 mg qid x 7 days
  Pediatric: <45 kg: 50 mg/kg/day in 4 divided doses x 14 days; ≥45 kg: same as adult
    Ery-Tab *Tab:* 250, 333, 500 mg ent-coat
    PCE *Tab:* 333, 500 mg
Comment: *erythromycin* may increase INR with concomitant *warfarin*, as well as
increase serum level of *digoxin*, benzodiazepines and statins.
▷ **erythromycin ethylsuccinate (B)(G)** 400 mg qid x 14 days <u>or</u> 800 mg qid x 7 days
  Pediatric: 50 mg/kg/day in 4 divided doses x 7 days; max 100 mg/kg/day; *see page*
  635 *for dose by weight*
    EryPed *Oral susp:* 200 mg/5 ml (100, 200 ml) (fruit); 400 mg/5 ml (60, 100,
    200 ml) (banana); Oral drops: 200, 400 mg/5 ml (50 ml) (fruit); *Chew tab:*
    200 mg wafer (fruit)
    E.E.S. *Oral susp:* 200, 400 mg/5 ml (100 ml) (fruit)
    E.E.S. Granules *Oral susp:* 200 mg/5 ml (100, 200 ml) (cherry)
    E.E.S. 400 Tablets *Tab:* 400 mg
Comment: *erythromycin* may increase INR with concomitant *warfarin*, as well as
increase serum level of *digoxin*, benzodiazepines and statins.

ALTERNATE REGIMEN

➤ *azithromycin* (B)(G) 500 mg x 1 dose on day 1; then 250 mg once daily on days; 2-5 or 500 mg daily x 3 days or 2 gm in a single dose
Pediatric: 20 mg/kg in a single dose once daily x 3 days

Zithromax *Tab:* 250, 500, 600 mg; *Oral susp:* 100 mg/5 ml (15 ml); 200 mg/5 ml (15, 22.5, 30 ml) (cherry); *Pkt:* 1 gm for reconstitution (cherry-banana)
Zithromax Tri-pak *Tab:* 3 x 500 mg tabs/pck
Zithromax Z-pak *Tab:* 6 x 250 mg tabs/pck
Zmax *Oral susp:* 2 gm ext-rel for reconstitution (cherry-banana) (148 mg Na⁺)

CONJUNCTIVITIS: FUNGAL

➤ *natamycin* ophthalmic suspension (C) 1 drop q 1-2 hours x 3-4 days; then 1 drop every 6 hours; treat for 14-21 days; withdraw dose gradually at 4- to 7-day intervals
Pediatric: <1 year: not recommended; ≥1 year: same as adult
Natacyn Ophthalmic Suspension *Ophth susp:* 0.5% (15 ml) (benzalkonium chloride)

CONJUNCTIVITIS: GONOCOCCAL

RECOMMENDED REGIMENS

Regimen 1

➤ *ceftriaxone* (B)(G) 250 mg IM x 1 dose
Pediatric: <45 kg: 50 mg/kg IM x 1 dose; max 125 mg IM
Rocephin *Vial:* 250, 500 mg; 1, 2 gm

Regimen 2

➤ *erythromycin base* (B)(G) 250 mg qid x 10-14 days
Pediatric: <45 kg: 50 mg/kg/day in 4 divided doses x 10-14 days; ≥45 kg: same as adult
Ery-Tab *Tab:* 250, 333, 500 mg ent-coat
PCE *Tab:* 333, 500 mg
Comment: *erythromycin* may increase INR with concomitant *warfarin*, as well as increase serum level of *digoxin*, benzodiazepines and statins.

➤ *erythromycin ethylsuccinate* (B)(G) 400 mg qid x 14 days or 800 mg qid x 7 days
Pediatric: 50 mg/kg/day in 4 divided doses x 7 days; max 100 mg/kg/day; *see page 635 for dose by weight*
EryPed *Oral susp:* 200 mg/5 ml (100, 200 ml) (fruit); 400 mg/5 ml (60, 100, 200 ml) (banana); *Oral drops:* 200, 400 mg/5 ml (50 ml) (fruit); *Chew tab:* 200 mg wafer (fruit)
E.E.S. *Oral susp:* 200, 400 mg/5 ml (100 ml) (fruit)
E.E.S. Granules *Oral susp:* 200 mg/5 ml (100, 200 ml) (cherry)
E.E.S. 400 Tablets *Tab:* 400 mg
Comment: *erythromycin* may increase INR with concomitant *warfarin*, as well as increase serum level of *digoxin*, benzodiazepines and statins.

ALTERNATE REGIMEN

➤ *azithromycin* (B)(G) 500 mg x 1 dose on day 1; then 250 mg once daily on days; 2-5 or 500 mg daily x 3 days or 2 gm in a single dose
Pediatric: not recommended for bronchitis in children

Zithromax *Tab:* 250, 500, 600 mg; *Oral susp:* 100 mg/5 ml (15 ml); 200 mg/5 ml (15, 22.5, 30 ml) (cherry); Pkt: 1 gm for reconstitution (cherry-banana)
Zithromax Tri-pak *Tab:* 3 x 500 mg tabs/pck
Zithromax Z-pak *Tab:* 6 x 250 mg tabs/pck
Zmax *Oral susp:* 2 gm ext-rel for reconstitution (cherry-banana) (148 mg Na⁺)

CONJUNCTIVITIS: VIRAL

Comment: For prevention of secondary bacterial infection, see agents listed under bacterial conjunctivitis. Ophthalmic corticosteroids are contraindicated with herpes simplex, keratitis, *Varicella*, and other viral infections of the cornea.
▷ *trifluridine* ophthalmic suspension (C) 1 drop q 2 hours while awake; max 9 drops/day; after re-epithelialization, 1 drop q 4 h x 7 days (at least 5 drops/day); max 21 days of therapy
Pediatric: <6 years: not recommended; ≥6 years: same as adult
    Viroptic Ophthalmic Solution *Ophth soln:* 1% (7.5 ml) (thimerosal)

CONSTIPATION: OCCASIONAL, INTERMITTENT

BULK-FORMING AGENTS

▷ *calcium polycarbophil* (C) 2 tabs once daily to qid
Pediatric: <6 years: not recommended; 6-12 years: 1 tab daily to qid
    FiberCon (OTC) *Cplt:* 625 mg
    Konsyl Fiber Tablets (OTC) *Tab:* 625 mg
▷ *methylcellulose*
    Citrucel 1 heaping tbsp in 8 oz cold water tid
    Pediatric: <6 years: not recommended; 6-12 years: 1/2 adult dose
        Oral pwdr: 16, 24, 30 oz and single-dose pkts (orange)
    Citrucel Sugar-Free 1 heaping tbsp in 8 oz cold water tid
    Pediatric: <6 years: not recommended; 6-12 years: 1/2 adult dose
        Oral pwdr: 16, 24, 30 oz and single-dose pkts (orange) (sugar-free, phenylala-nine)
▷ *psyllium husk* (B)
    Pediatric: <6 years: not recommended; 6-12 years: 1/2 adult dose in 8 oz liquid tid
    Metamucil (OTC) wafer or cap or 1 pkt or 1 rounded tsp (1 rounded tbsp for sugar-containing form) in 8 oz liquid tid
        Cap: psyllium husk 5.2 gm (100, 150/carton); *Wafer: psyllium husk* 3.4 gm/rounded tsp (24/carton) (apple crisp, cinnamon spice); *Plain and flavored pwdr:* 3.4 gm/rounded tsp (15, 20, 24, 29, 30, 36, 44, 48 oz); *Efferv sugar-free flav pkts:* 3.4 gm/pkt (30/carton) (phenylalanine)
▷ *psyllium* hydrophilic mucilloid (B) 2 rounded tsp in 8 oz water qid
    Pediatric: <6 years: not recommended; 6-12 years: 1 rounded tsp in 8 oz liquid tid
    Konsyl (OTC) *Pwdr:* 6 gm/rounded tsp (10.6, 15.9 oz); *Pwdr pkt:* 6 gm/rounded tsp (30/carton)
    Konsyl-D (OTC) *Pwdr:* 3.4 gm/rounded tsp (11.5, 17.59 oz); *Pwdr pkt:* 3.4 gm/rounded tsp (30/carton)
    Konsyl Easy Mix Formula (OTC) *Pwdr:* 3.4 gm/rounded tsp (8 oz) (sugar-free, low sodium)
    Konsyl Orange (OTC) *Pwdr:* 3.4 gm/rounded tsp (19 oz); *Pwdr pkt:* 3.4 gm/rounded tsp (30/carton)
    Konsyl Orange SF (OTC) *Pwdr:* 3.5 gm/rounded tsp (15 oz) (phenylalanine); *Pwdr pkt:* 3.5 gm/rounded tsp (30/carton) (phenylalanine)

STOOL SOFTENERS

▷ *docusate sodium* (OTC) 50-200 mg/day
    Pediatric: <3 years: 10-40 mg/day; 3-6 years: 20-60 mg/day; >6 years: 40-120 mg/day
        Cap: 50, 100 mg; *Liq:* 10 mg/ml (30 ml w. dropper); *Syr:* 20 mg/5 ml (8 oz) (alcohol ≤1%)
    Dialose 1 tab q HS
    Pediatric: <6 years: not recommended; ≥6 years: same as adult
        Tab: 100 mg
    Surfak (OTC) 240 mg/day
    Pediatric: <12 years: not recommended; ≥12 years: same as adult
        Cap: 240 mg

OSMOTIC LAXATIVES

▷ *lactulose* (B)(G) take 10-20 gm dissolved in 4 oz water once daily prn; max 40 gm/day
    Pediatric: <12 years: not recommended; ≥12 years: same as adult
    Kristalose *Crystals for oral soln:* 10, 20 gm single-dose pkts (30/carton)
▷ *magnesium citrate* (B)(G) 1 full bottle (120-300 ml) once daily prn
    Pediatric: <2 years: not recommended; 2-6 years: 4-12 ml once daily prn; ≥6-12 years: 50-100 ml once daily prn
    Citrate of Magnesia (OTC) *Oral soln:* 300 ml
▷ *magnesium hydroxide* (B) 30-60 ml/day in a single or divided doses prn
    Pediatric: 2-5 years: 5-15 ml/day in a single or divided doses; 6-11 years: 15-30 ml/day in a single or divided doses; ≥12 years: same as adult
    Milk of Magnesia *Liq:* 390 mg/5 ml (10, 15, 20, 30, 100, 120, 180, 360, 720 ml)
▷ *polyethylene glycol (PEG)* (C)(OTC)(G) 1 tbsp (17 gm) dissolved in 4-8 oz water per day for up to max 7 days; may need 2-4 days for results
    Pediatric: ≤17: <12 years: not recommended; ≥12 years: same as adult
    GlycoLax Powder for Oral Solution *Oral pwdr:* 7, 14, 30, and 45 dose bottles w. 17 gm dosing cup (gluten-free, sugar-free); 17 gm single-dose pkts (20/ carton)
    MiraLAX Powder for Oral Solution *Oral pwdr:* 7, 14, 30, and 45 dose bottles w. 17 gm dosing cup (gluten-free, sugar-free)
    Polyethylene Glycol 3350 Powder for Oral Solution (G) *Oral pwdr:* 3350 gm w. dosing cup; 17 gm/scoop
Comment: *PEG* is an osmotic indicated for occasional constipation without affecting glucose and electrolyte levels. Contraindicated with suspected or known bowel obstruction.

STIMULANTS

▷ *bisacodyl* (B) 2-3 tabs or 1 suppository bid prn
    Dulcolax, Gentlax *Tab:* 5 mg; *Rectal supp:* 10 mg
    Pediatric: <12 years: 1/2 suppository once daily prn; 6-12 years: 1 tablet or 1/2 suppository once daily prn; >12 years: same as adult
    Senokot (OTC) initially 2-4 tabs or 1 level tsp at HS prn; max 4 tabs or 2 tsp bid
    Pediatric: <2 years: not recommended; 2-6 years: 1/4 tab or 1/2 tsp once daily prn; max 1 tab or 1/2 tsp bid; 6-12 years: 1 tab or 1/2 tsp once daily prn; max 2 tabs or 1 tsp once daily
        Tab: 8.6*mg; *Granules:* 15 mg/tsp (2, 6, 12 oz) (cocoa)
    Senokot Syrup (OTC) initially 10-15 ml at HS prn; max 15 ml bid
    Pediatric: use Childrens Syrup
        Syr: 8.8 mg/5 ml (2, 8 oz) (chocolate) (alcohol-free)
    Senokot Childrens Syrup (OTC)
    Pediatric: <2 years: not recommended; 2-6 years: 2.5-3.75 ml once daily prn; max 3.75 ml bid prn; ≥6-12 years: 5-7.5 ml once daily prn; max 7.5 ml bid
        Syr: 8.8 mg/5 ml (2.5 oz) (chocolate) (alcohol-free)

Senokot Xtra (OTC) 1 tab at HS prn; max 2 tabs bid
Pediatric: <2 years: not recommended; 2-6 years: use Childrens Syrup; 6-12 years: 1/2 tab once daily at HS; max 1 tab bid
Tab: 17*mg

BULK FORMING AGENT+STIMULANT COMBINATIONS

▷ *psyllium+senna* (B)
Perdiem (OTC) 1-2 rounded tsp swallowed with 8 oz cool liquid daily bid
Pediatric: <7 years: not recommended; 7-11 years: 1 rounded tsp swallowed with 8 oz cool liquid once daily-bid; ≥12 years: same as adult
Canister: 8.8, 14 oz; *Individual pkt:* 6 gm (6/pck)
SennaPrompt (OTC) initially 2-5 caps bid
Pediatric: <12 years: not recommended; ≥12 years: same as adult
Cap: psyl 500 mg+*senna* 9 mg

STOOL SOFTENER+STIMULANT COMBINATIONS

▷ *docusate+casanthranol* (C)
Doxidan (OTC) 1-3 caps/day; max 1 week
Pediatric: <2 years: not recommended; ≥2 years: 1 cap/day
Cap: doc 60 mg+cas 30 mg
Peri-Colace (OTC) 1-2 caps <u>or</u> 15-30 ml q HS; max 2 caps <u>or</u> 30 ml bid <u>or</u> 3 caps q HS
Pediatric: 5-15 ml q HS
Cap: doc 100 mg+cas 30 mg; *Syr:* doc 60 mg+cas 30 mg per 15 ml (8, 16 oz)
▷ *docusate+senna* concentrate (C)
Senokot S (OTC) 2 tabs q HS; max 4 tabs bid
Pediatric: <2 years: not recommended; 2-6 years: 1/2 tab daily; max 1 tab bid; >6-12 years: 1 tab daily; max 2 tabs bid
Tab: doc 50 mg+*senna* 8.6 mg

ENEMAS AND OTHER AGENTS

▷ *sodium biphosphate+sodium phosphate* enema (C)(OTC)
Fleets Adult 59-118 ml rectally
Pediatric: <2 years: not recommended; ≥2-12 years: 59 ml rectally
Enema: sod biphos 19 gm+sod phos 7 gm (59, 118 ml w. applicator)
Fleets Pediatric 59 ml
Pediatric: rectally
Enema: sod biphos 19 gm+sod phos 7 gm (59 ml w. applicator)
▷ *glycerin* suppositories (C)(OTC) 1 adult suppository
Pediatric: <6 years: 1 pediatric suppository; ≥6 years: 1 adult suppository

 CONSTIPATION: CHRONIC IDIOPATHIC (CIC)

GUANYLATE CYCLASE-C AGONISTS

Comment: Guanylate cyclase-c agonists increase intestinal fluid and intestinal transit time may induce diarrhea and bloating and therefore, are contraindicated with known <u>or</u> suspected mechanical GI obstruction.

▷ *linaclotide* (C) 145 mcg orally once daily <u>or</u> 72 mcg orally once daily based on individual presentation <u>or</u> tolerability; take on an empty stomach at least 30 minutes before the first meal of the day; swallow whole, do not crush <u>or</u> chew cap <u>or</u> cap contents; may open cap and administer with applesauce <u>or</u> water (e.g., NGT, PEG tube)

Pediatric: ≤18 years: not established (<6 years: contraindicated; 6-18 years: avoid); >18 years: same as adult

Linzess *Cap:* 72, 145, 290 mcg

Comment: *linaclotide* and its active metabolite are negligibly absorbed systemically following oral administration and maternal use is not expected to result in fetal exposure to the drug. There is no information regarding the presence of *plecanatide* in human milk <u>or</u> its effects on the breastfed infant.

▷ *plecanatide* take one tab once daily; if necessary, may crush and administer with apple-sauce <u>or</u> water (e.g., NGT, PEG tube)

Pediatric: ≤18 years: not established (<6 years: contraindicated; 6-18 years: avoid); >18 years: same as adult

Trulance *Tab:* 3 mg

Comment: Suspend *plecanatide* dosing and rehydrate if severe diarrhea occurs. Most common adverse reactions in CIC are sinusitis, URI, diarrhea, abdominal distension and tenderness, flatulence, increased liver enzymes. *plecanatide* and its active metabolite are negligibly absorbed systemically following oral administration and maternal use is not expected to result in fetal exposure to the drug. There is no information regarding the presence of *plecanatide* in human milk <u>or</u> its effects on the breastfed infant.

CHLORIDE CHANNEL ACTIVATOR

▷ *lubiprostone* (C) one 24 mcg cap bid with food and water; swallow whole, do not break apart <u>or</u> chew

Pediatric: <18 years: not recommended; ≥18 years: same as adult

Amitiza *Cap:* 8, 24 mcg

Comment: **Amitiza** increases intestinal fluid and intestinal transit time. Suspend dosing and rehydrate if severe diarrhea occurs. **Amitiza** is contraindicated with known <u>or</u> suspected mechanical GI obstruction. Most common adverse reactions in CIC are nausea, diarrhea, headache, abdominal pain, abdominal distension, and flatulence.

 CORNEAL EDEMA

▷ *sodium chloride* (G)

Pediatric: same as adult 1-2 drops or 1 inch ribbon q 3-4 hours prn; reduce frequency as edema subsides

Various (OTC)

Ophth soln: 2, 5% (15, 30 ml); *Ophth oint:* 5% (3.5 gm)

 CORNEAL ULCERATION

ANTIBACTERIAL OPHTHALMIC SOLUTION/OINTMENT

see Conjunctivitis/Blepharoconjunctivitis: Bacterial page 96

 COSTOCHONDRITIS (CHEST WALL SYNDROME)

Acetaminophen for IV Infusion *see Pain page 344*
NSAIDs *see page 562*
Opioid Analgesics *see Pain page 345*
Topical and Transdermal NSAIDs *see Pain page 344*
Parenteral Corticosteroids *see page 570*
Oral Corticosteroids *see page 569*
Topical Analgesic and Anesthetic Agents *see page 560*

COXSACKIEVIRUS (HAND, FOOT AND MOUTH DISEASE)

NSAIDs *see page* 553
Opioid Analgesics *see Pain page* 345
OTC Throat Lozenges
OTC Cough Drops and Cough Syrup

Comment: The hand, foot, and mouth disease occurs most commonly in children <10 years-of-age. Although adults are susceptible, most have built up natural immunity. The causative organism, *Coxsackievirus*, is transmitted via droplet spread (coughing and/ or sneezing) and contact with contaminated objects and surfaces (same as influenza). Clinical signs and symptoms are typically relatively mild and include fever, sore throat, feeling generally unwell, malaise, headache, and poor appetite. Red spots, some painful blister-like lesions, most often appear on the tongue and roof of the mouth, palms of the hands, and soles of the feet (but not necessarily all three), and are often faint or sparse. Lesions, which are not pruritic, may also be noted on the dorsal surfaces of the hands/ fingers and feet/ toes. Medical treatment, per se, is not required. Treatment in the home with age/ weight-dosed ibuprofen or acetaminophen for relief of sore throat, lesion pain, and fever. Other comfort measures include salt water gargles, throat lozenges, cough drops or cough syrup, and fluids. The disease typically resolves in 7 to 10 days.

CRAMPS: ABDOMINAL, INTESTINAL

ANTISPASMODIC-ANTICHOLINERGIC AGENTS

▷ *dicyclomine* **(B)(G)** initially 20 mg bid-qid; may increase to 40 mg qid PO; usual IM dose 80 mg/day divided qid; do not use IM route for more than 1-2 days
  Pediatric: <12 years: not recommended; ≥12 years: same as adult
    Bentyl *Tab:* 20 mg; *Cap:* 10 mg; *Syr:* 10 mg/5 ml (16 oz); *Vial:* 10 mg/ml (10 ml);
    Amp: 10 mg/ml (2 ml)
▷ *methscopolamine bromide* **(B)** 1 tab q 6 hours prn
  Pediatric: <12 years: not recommended; ≥12 years: same as adult
    Pamine *Tab:* 2.5 mg
    Pamine Forte *Tab:* 5 mg

ANTICHOLINERGICS

▷ *hyoscyamine* **(C)(G)**
    Anaspaz 1-2 tabs q 4 hours prn; max 12 tabs/day
    Pediatric: <2 years: not recommended; 2-12 years: 0.0625-0.125 mg q 4 hours prn;
    max 0.75 mg/day; ≥12 years: same as adult
      Tab: 0.125*mg
    Levbid 1-2 tabs q 12 hours prn; max 4 tabs/day
    Pediatric: <12 years: not recommended; ≥12 years: same as adult
      Tab: 0.375*mg ext-rel
    Levsin 1-2 tabs q 4 hours prn; max 12 tabs/day
    Pediatric: <6 years: not recommended; ≥6-12 years: 1 tab q 4 hours prn
      Tab: 0.125*mg
    Levsinex SL 1-2 tabs q 4 hours SL <u>or</u> PO; max 12 tabs/day
    Pediatric: 2-12 years: 1 tab SL <u>or</u> PO q 4 hours; max 6 tabs/day
      Tab: 0.125 mg sublingual
    Levsinex Timecaps 1-2 caps q 12 hours; may adjust to 1 cap q 8 hours
    Pediatric: 2-12 years: 1 cap q 12 hours; max 2 caps/day
      Cap: 0.375 mg time-rel

NuLev dissolve 1-2 tabs on tongue, with <u>or</u> without water, q 4 hours prn; max 12 tabs/day

Pediatric: <2 years: not recommended; 2-12 years: dissolve 1 tab on tongue, with <u>or</u> without water, q 4 hours prn; max 6 tabs/day; >12 years: same as adult

ODT: 0.125 mg (mint) (phenylalanine)

▷ *simethicone* (C)(G) 0.3 ml qid pc and HS

Mylicon Drops (OTC) *Oral drops:* 40 mg/0.6 ml (30 ml)

▷ *phenobarbital+hyoscyamine+atropine+scopolamine* (C)(IV)(G)

Donnatal 1-2 tabs ac and HS

Pediatric: <12 years: not recommended; ≥12 years: same as adult

Tab: pheno 16.2 mg+hyo 0.1037 mg+atro 0.0194 mg+scop 0.0065 mg

Donnatal Elixir 1-2 tsp ac and HS

Pediatric: 20 lb: 1 ml q 4 hours <u>or</u> 1.5 ml q 6 hours; 30 lb: 1.5 ml q 4 hours <u>or</u> 2 ml q 6 hours; 50 lb: 1/2 tsp q 4 hours <u>or</u> 3/4 tsp q 6 hours; 75 lb: 3/4 tsp q 4 hours <u>or</u> 1 tsp q 6 hours; 100 lb: 1 tsp q 4 hours <u>or</u> 1 tsp q 6 hours

Elix: pheno 16.2 mg+hyo 0.1037 mg+atro 0.0194 mg+scop 0.0065 mg per 5 ml (4, 16 oz)

Donnatal Extentabs 1 tab q 12 hours

Pediatric: <12 years: not recommended; ≥12 years: same as adult

Tab: pheno 48.6 mg+hyo 0.3111 mg+atro 0.0582 mg+scop 0.0195 mg ext-rel

ANTICHOLINERGIC+SEDATIVE COMBINATION

▷ *chlordiazepoxide+clidinium* (D)(IV) 1-2 caps ac and HS; max 8 caps/day

Pediatric: <12 years: not recommended; ≥12 years: same as adult

Librax *Cap:* chlor 5 mg+clid 2.5 mg

 CROHN'S DISEASE

Parenteral Corticosteroids *see page* 570
Oral Corticosteroids *see page* 569

Comment: Standard treatment regimen for active disease (flare) is: antibiotic, antispasmodic, and bowel rest; progress to clear liquids; then progress to high-fiber diet. Long term management of chronic disease includes salicylates, immune modulators, and tumor necrosis factor (TNF) blockers.

ORAL ANTI-INFECTIVES

▷ *metronidazole* (G) 500 mg tid <u>or</u> 750 mg bid; max 8 weeks

Pediatric: 35-50 mg/kg/day in 3 divided doses x 10 days

Flagyl *Tab:* 250*, 500*mg

Flagyl 375 *Cap:* 375 mg

Flagyl ER *Tab:* 750 mg ext-rel

Comment: Alcohol is contraindicated during treatment with oral *metronidazole* and for 72 hours after therapy due to a possible *disulfiram*-like reaction (nausea, vomiting, flushing, headache).

SALICYLATES

▷ *mesalamine* (B)(G)

Asacol 800 mg tid x 6 weeks; maintenance 1.6 gm/day in divided doses; swallow whole, do not crush <u>or</u> chew

Pediatric: <12 years: not recommended; ≥12 years: same as adult

Tab: 400 mg del-rel

Comment: 2 **Asacol** 400 mg tabs are not bioequivalent to 1 **Asacol HD** 800 mg tab.

Asacol HD 1600 mg tid x 6 weeks; swallow whole, do not crush <u>or</u> chew

Pediatric: <12 years: not recommended; ≥12 years: same as adult

Tab: 800 mg del-rel

Comment: 1 **Asacol HD** 800 mg tab is not bioequivalent to 2 **Asacol** 400 mg tabs

Canasa 1 gm qid for up to 8 weeks

Pediatric: <12 years: not recommended; ≥12 years: same as adult

Rectal supp: 1 gm del-rel (30, 42/pck)

Delzicol *Treatment:* 800 mg tid x 6 weeks; maintenance 1.6 gm/day in 2-4 divided doses daily; swallow whole; do not crush <u>or</u> chew

Pediatric: <5 years: not established; ≥5 years: same as adult

Cap: 400 mg del-rel

Comment: 2 **Delzicol** 400 mg caps are not bioequivalent to 1 *mesalamine* 800 mg del-rel tab

Lialda 2.4-4.8 gm daily in a single dose for up to 8 weeks; swallow whole, do not crush <u>or</u> chew

Pediatric: <18 years: not recommended; ≥18 years: same as adult

Tab: 1.2 gm del-rel

Pentasa 1 gm qid for up to 8 weeks; swallow whole, do not crush <u>or</u> chew

Pediatric: <12 years: not recommended; ≥12 years: same as adult

Cap: 250 mg cont-rel

Rowasa Enema 4 gm rectally by enema q HS; retain for 8 hours x 3-6 weeks

Pediatric: <12 years: not recommended; ≥12 years: same as adult

Enema: 4 gm/60 ml (7, 14, 28/pck; kit, 7, 14, 28/pck w. wipes)

Rowasa Suppository 1 suppository rectally bid x 3-6 weeks; retain for 1-3 hours <u>or</u> longer

Rectal supp: 500 mg

Sulfite-Free Rowasa Rectal Suspension 4 gm rectally by enema q HS; retain for 8 hours x 3-6 weeks

Enema: 4 gm/60 ml (7, 14, 28/pck; kit, 7, 14, 28/pck w. wipes)

▷ *olsalazine* (C)

Dipentum 1 gm/day in 2 divided doses; max 2 gm/day

Cap: 250 mg

Comment: Indicated in persons who cannot tolerate *sulfasalazine*.

▷ *sulfasalazine* (B)(G)

Azulfidine initially 1-2 gm/day; increase to 3-4 gm/day in divided doses pc until clinical symptoms controlled; maintenance 2 gm/day; max 4 gm/day

Tab: 500*mg

Pediatric: <2 years: not recommended; 2-16 years: initially 40-60 mg/kg/day in 3-6 divided doses; max 2 gm/day

Azulfidine EN initially 500 mg in the PM x 7 days; then 500 mg bid x 7 days; then 500 mg in the AM and 1 gm in the PM x 7 days; then 1 gm bid; max 4 gm/day

Pediatric: <12 years: not recommended; ≥12 years: same as adult

Tab: 500 mg ent-coat

▷ *budesonide micronized* (C) (G)

Pediatric: <12 years: not recommended; ≥12 years: same as adult

Entocort EC *Treatment* 9 mg once daily in the AM for up to 8 weeks; may repeat an 8-week course; *Maintenance of remission*: 6 mg once daily for up to 3 months

Cap: 3 mg ent-coat ext-rel granules

Comment: Taper other systemic steroids when transferring to **Entocort EC**. When corticosteroids are used chronically, systemic effects such as hypercorticism and adrenal suppression may occur. Corticosteroids can reduce the response of the hypothalamus-pituitary-adrenal (HPA) axis to stress. In situations where patients are subject to surgery <u>or</u>

other stress situations, supplementation with a systemic corticosteroid is recommended. General precautions concerning corticosteroids should be followed.

PURINE ANTIMETABOLITE IMMUNOSUPPRESSANT

➤ *azathioprine* (D)(G)

    Imuran *Tab:* 50*mg; *Injectable:* 100 mg

Comment: Imuran is usually administered on a daily basis. The initial dose should be approximately 1.0 mg/kg (50 to 100 mg) as a single dose or divided bid. Dose may be increased beginning at 6-8 weeks, and thereafter at 4-week intervals, if there are no serious toxicities and if initial response is unsatisfactory. Dose increments should be 0.5 mg/kg/day, up to max 2.5 mg/kg per day. Therapeutic response usually occurs after 6-8 weeks of treatment. An adequate trial should be a minimum of 12 weeks. Patients not improved after 12 weeks can be considered refractory. **Imuran** may be continued long-term in patients with clinical response, but patients should be monitored carefully, and gradual dosage reduction should be attempted to reduce risk of toxicities. Maintenance therapy should be at the lowest effective dose, and the dose given can be lowered decrementally with changes of 0.5 mg/kg or approximately 25 mg daily every 4 weeks while other therapy is kept constant. The optimum duration of maintenance **Imuran** has not been determined. **Imuran** can be discontinued abruptly, but delayed effects are possible.

TUMOR NECROSIS FACTOR (TNF) BLOCKERS

➤ *adalimumab* (B) 40 mg SC once every other week; may increase to once weekly without MTX; administer in abdomen or thigh; rotate sites

    Pediatric: <2 years, <10 kg: not recommended; 10-<15 kg: 10 mg every other week; 15-<30 kg: 20 mg every other week; ≥30 kg: 40 mg every other week; 2-17 years, supervise first dose

    Humira *Prefilled syringe:* 20 mg/0.4 ml; 40 mg/0.8 ml single-dose (2/pck; 2, 6/ starter pck) (preservative-free)

Comment: May use with *methotrexate* (MTX), DMARDS, corticosteroids, salicylates, NSAIDs, or analgesics.

➤ *adalimumab-adbm* (B) *First dose* (*Day 1*): 160 mg SC (4 x 40 mg injections in one day or 2 x 40 mg injections per day for two consecutive days); *Second dose two weeks later* (*Day 15*): 80 mg SC; *Two weeks later* (*Day 29*): begin a maintenance dose of 40 mg SC every other week

    Pediatric: <18 years: not recommended; ≥18 years: same as adult

    Cyltezo *Prefilled syringe:* 40 mg/0.8 ml single-dose (preservative-free)

Comment: Cyltezo is biosimilar to **Humira** (*adalimumab*).

➤ *certolizumab* (B) 400 mg SC (2 x 200 mg inj at two different sites on day 1); then, 400 mg SC at weeks 2 and 4; maintenance 400 mg SC every 4 weeks; administer in abdomen or thigh; rotate sites

    Pediatric: <12 years: not recommended; ≥12 years: same as adult

    Cimzia *Vial:* 200 mg (2/pck); *Prefilled syringe:* 200 mg/ml single-dose (2/pck; 2, 6/starter pck) (preservative-free)

➤ *infliximab* (*tumor necrosis factor-alpha blocker*) must be refrigerated at 2°C to 8°C (36°F to 46°F); administer dose intravenously over a period of not less than 2 hours; do not use beyond the expiration date as this product contains no preservative; 5 mg/ kg at 0, 2 and 6 weeks, then every 8 weeks.

    Pediatric: <6 years: not studied; ≥6-17 years: mg/kg at 0, 2 and 6 weeks, then every 8 weeks; ≥18 years: same as adult

    Remicade *Vial:* 100 mg for reconstitution to 10 ml administration volume, single-dose (preservative-free)

Comment: **Remicade** is indicated to reduce signs and symptoms, and induce and maintain clinical remission, in adults and children ≥6 years-of-age with moderately to severely active disease who have had an inadequate response to conventional therapy <u>and</u> reduce the number of draining enterocutaneous and rectovaginal fistulas, and maintain fistula closure, in adults with fistulizing disease. Common adverse effects associated with **Remicade** included abdominal pain, headache, pharyngitis, sinusitis, and upper respiratory infections. In addition, **Remicade** might increase the risk for serious infections, including tuberculosis, bacterial sepsis, and invasive fungal infections. Available data from published literature on the use of *infliximab* products during pregnancy have not reported a clear association with *infliximab* products and adverse pregnancy outcomes. *infliximab* products cross the placenta and infants exposed *in utero* should not be administered live vaccines for at least 6 months after birth. Otherwise, the infant may be at increased risk of infection, including disseminated infection which can become fatal. Available information is insufficient to inform the amount of *infliximab* products present in human milk <u>or</u> effects on the breast-fed infant. To report suspected adverse reactions, contact Merck Sharp & Dohme Corp., a subsidiary of Merck & Co. at 1-877-888-4231 <u>or</u> FDA at 1-800-FDA1088 <u>or</u> www.fda.gov/medwatch

▷ *infliximab-abda (tumor necrosis factor-alpha blocker)* **(B)**
    Renflexis: see *infliximab* (**Remicade**) above for full prescribing information
Comment: **Renflexis** is a biosimilar to **Remicade** for the treatment of immune disorders including Crohn's disease, ulcerative colitis, rheumatoid arthritis, ankylosing spondylitis, psoriatic arthritis and plaque psoriasis. **Renflexis** was approved under the FDA category for biosimilars and demonstrated no clinically meaningful differences for use, dosing regimens, strengths, dosage forms, and routes of administration from the FDA-approved biological product **Remicade**.

▷ *infliximab-qbtx (tumor necrosis factor-alpha blocker)* **(B)**
    Ifixi: see *infliximab* (**Remicade**) above for full prescribing information
Comment: **Ifixi** is a biosimilar to **Remicade** for the treatment of immune disorders including Crohn's disease, ulcerative colitis, rheumatoid arthritis, ankylosing spondylitis, psoriatic arthritis and plaque psoriasis. **Ifixi** was approved under the FDA category for biosimilars and demonstrated no clinically meaningful differences for use, dosing regimens, strengths, dosage forms, and routes of administration from the FDA-approved biological product **Remicade.**

▷ *infliximab-qbtx (tumor necrosis factor-alpha blocker)* **(B)**
    Ifixi: see *infliximab* (**Remicade**) above for full prescribing information
Comment: **Ifixi** is a biosimilar to **Remicade** for the treatment of immune disorders including Crohn's disease, ulcerative colitis, rheumatoid arthritis, ankylosing spondylitis, psoriatic arthritis and plaque psoriasis. **Ifixi** was approved under the FDA category for biosimilars and demonstrated no clinically meaningful differences for use, dosing regimens, strengths, dosage forms, and routes of administration from the FDA-approved biological product **Remicade.**

INTEGRIN RECEPTOR ANTAGONIST (IMMUNOMODULATOR)

▷ *natalizumab* **(C)** administer by IV infusion over 1 hour; monitor during and for 1 hour post-infusion; 300 mg every 4 weeks; discontinue after 12 weeks if no therapeutic response, or if unable to taper off chronic concomitant steroids within 6 months; may continue aminosalicylates
Pediatric: <18 years: not established; ≥18 years: same as adult
    Tysabri *Vial:* 300 mg single-dose, soln after dilution for IV infusion (preservative-free)

▷ *vedolizumab* **(B)** administer by IV infusion over 30 minutes; 300 mg at weeks 0, 2, 6; then once every 8 weeks
Pediatric: <18 years: not established; ≥18 years: same as adult

Entyvio *Vial:* 300 mg (20 ml) single-dose, pwdr for IV infusion after reconstitution (preservative-free)

Comment: To report suspected adverse reactions, contact Takeda Pharmaceuticals at 1-877-TAKEDA-7 (1-877-825-3327) or FDA at 1800-FDA-1088 or www.fda.gov/medwatch

CRIPTOSPORIDIOSIS (*CRYPTOSPORIDIUM PARVUM*)

➤ *nitazoxanide* (B) 500 mg by mouth q 12 hours x 3 days
Pediatric: 12-47 months: 5 ml q 12 hours x 3 days; 4-11 years: 10 ml q 12 hours x 3 days; ≥12 years: same as adult
Alinia *Oral susp:* 100 mg/5 ml (60 ml)

Comment: **Alinia** is an antiprotozoal for the treatment of diarrhea due to *G. lamblia* or *C. parvum.*

CYCLOSPORIASIS (*CYCLOSPORA CAVETANENSIS*)

Comment: The CDC, state and local health departments, and the US Food and Drug Administration have issued a Health Alert Network advisory after an increase in reported cases of cyclosporiasis, an intestinal illness caused by the parasite *Cyclospora cayetanensis.* Clinicians should consider a diagnosis of cyclosporiasis in patients who experience prolonged or remitting-relapsing diarrhea. Since May 1, 2017, 206 cases have been identified, more than twice the 88 cases reported from May 1 to August 3, 2016. Most laboratories in the United States do not routinely test for *Cyclospora,* even when a stool sample has been tested for parasites, so providers must specifically order the test. Several stool specimens may be required because *Cyclospora* oocysts may be shed intermittently and at low levels, even in persons with profuse diarrhea. Symptoms include watery diarrhea, which can be profuse, anorexia, fatigue, weight loss, nausea, flatulence, stomach cramps, myalgia, vomiting, and low-grade fever. Symptoms begin from 2 days to more than 2 weeks (average 7 days) after ingestion of the parasite. *Cyclospora* is food- and water-borne; it is not transmitted directly from person to person. The recommended treatment is *trimethoprim-sulfamethoxazole* (TMP/SMX). There are no effective alternatives for people who are allergic to or who cannot tolerate TMP/SMX; observation and symptomatic care is recommended for those patients. If untreated, illness may last for a few days to a month or longer.

➤ *trimethoprim+sulfamethoxazole (TMP-SMX)*(C)(G) bid x 10 days
Pediatric: <2 months: not recommended; ≥2 months: 40 mg/kg/day of *sulfamethoxazole* in 2 divided doses x 10 days; *see page 648 for dose by weight*
Bactrim, Septra 2 tabs bid x 10 days
Tab: trim 80 mg+sulfa 400 mg*
Bactrim DS, Septra DS 1 tab bid x 10 days
Tab: trim 160 mg+sulfa 800 mg*
Bactrim Pediatric Suspension, Septra Pediatric Suspension
Oral susp: trim 40 mg+sulfa 200 mg per 5 ml (100 ml) (cherry) (alcohol 0.3%)

CYSTIC FIBROSIS (CF)

➤ *acetylcysteine* (B)(G) administer via face mask, mouth piece, tracheostomy T-piece, mist tent, or croupette; routine tracheostomy care, 1 to 2 ml of a 10% to 20% solution may be administered by direct instillation into the tracheostomy every 1 to 4 hours
Pediatric: same as adult

Mucomyst *Vial:* 10, 20% (4, 10, 30 ml) soln for inhalation

Comment: **Mucomyst** is a mucolytic. For inhalation, the 10% concentration may be used undiluted; the 20% concentration should be diluted with sterile water or normal saline (either for injection or inhalation).

▷ **lumacaftor+ivacaftor (B)** 2 tabs q 12 hours; reduce dose with moderate to severe hepatic impairment
Pediatric: <12 years: not established; ≥12 years: same as adult

Orkambi *Tab: luma* 200 mg+*iva* 125 mg film-coat

CYSTIC FIBROSIS TRANSMEMBRANE CONDUCTANCE REGULATOR (CFTR) POTENTIATOR

▷ **ivacaftor (B)** 150 mg every 12 hours; administer with fat-containing food (e.g., eggs, butter, peanut butter, cheese pizza); avoid food and juices containing grapefruit or Seville oranges.
Pediatric: <2 years: not established; 2-6 years, <14 kg: one 50 mg packet mixed with 1 tsp (5 ml) soft food or liquid every 12 hours with fat-containing food; 2-6 years, ≥14 kg: one 75 mg packet mixed with 1 tsp (5 ml) soft food or liquid every 12 hours with fat-containing food; >6 years: same as adult

Kalydeco *Tab:* 150 mg film-coat; *Oral granules:* 50, 75 mg unit dose pkts (56 pkt/carton)

Comment: **ivacaftor** is indicated for the treatment of CF in patients who have a *G551D* co-mutation in the *CFTR* gene. If the patient's genotype is unknown, an FDA-cleared CF mutation test should be used to detect the presence of the *G551D* mutation. **Kalydeco** is not effective in patients with CF who are homozygous for the *F508del* mutation in the *CFTR* gene. Transaminases (ALT and AST) should be assessed prior to initiating **Kalydeco**, every 3 months during the first year of treatment, and annually thereafter. Patients who develop increased transaminase levels should be closely monitored until the abnormalities resolve. Dosing should be interrupted in patients with ALT or AST greater than 5 times the upper limit of normal (ULN). Following resolution of transaminase elevations, consider the benefits and risks of resuming **Kalydeco**. Concomitant use with strong CYP3A inducers (e.g., *rifampin*, St. John's wort) substantially decreases exposure of *Kalydeco* (which may diminish effectiveness); therefore, co-administration is not recommended. Reduce dose to 150 mg twice weekly when co-administered with strong CYP3A inhibitors (e.g., *ketoconazole*). Reduce dose to 150 mg once daily when co-administered with moderate CYP3A inhibitors. Caution is recommended in patients with severe renal impairment (CrCl ≤30 mL/min) or ESRD. No dose adjustment is necessary for patients with mild hepatic impairment (Child-Pugh Class A). A reduced dose of 150 mg once daily is recommended in patients with moderate hepatic impairment (Child-Pugh Class B). No studies have been conducted in patients with severe hepatic impairment (Child-Pugh Class C). The most commonly reported adverse reactions are headache, sore throat, nasopharyngitis, URI, nasal congestion, abdominal pain, nausea, diarrhea, dizziness, and rash. Excretion of **Kalydeco** into human milk is probable. To report suspected adverse reactions, contact Vertex Pharmaceuticals Incorporated at 1-877-752-5933 or FDA at 1-800-FDA-1088 or www.fda.gov/medwatch

URSODEOXYCHOLIC ACID (UDCA)

Comment: *ursodeoxycholic acid* (UDCA) is indicated for liver disease associated with cystic fibrosis in children 6-18 years-of-age.

▷ **ursodeoxycholic acid** (UDCA) **(G)** in the first 3 months of treatment, the total daily dose should be divided tid (morning, midday, evening); as liver function values

improve, the total daily dose may be taken once a day at bedtime; (see mfr pkg insert for dose table based on kilograms weight); monitor hepatic function every 4 weeks for the first 3 months; then, monitor hepatic function once every 3 months
Pediatric: 6-18 years: same as adult

Ursofalk *Tab:* 500 mg film-coat; *Cap:* 250 mg, *Oral susp:* 250 mg/5 ml
Comment: ursodeoxycholic (UDCA) is indicated for the dissolution of cholesterol gall stones that are radioluscent (not visible on plain x-ray), <15 mm, and the gall bladder must still be functioning despite the gall stones.

ANTI-INFECTIVE

▷ *ciprofloxacin* (C) <18 years: 20-40 mg/kg/day divided q 12 hours; ≥18 years: 500 mg bid x 7-10 days; max 1.5 gm/day
    Cipro (G) *Tab:* 250, 500, 750 mg; *Oral susp:* 250, 500 mg/5 ml (100 ml) (strawberry)
    Cipro XR *Tab:* 500, 1000 mg ext-rel
    ProQuin XR *Tab:* 500 mg ext-rel

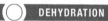

DEEP VEIN THROMBOSIS (DVT) PROPHYLAXIS

Anticoagulation Therapy *see page* 589

DEHYDRATION

ORAL REHYDRATION AND ELECTROLYTE REPLACEMENT THERAPY

▷ *oral electrolyte replacement* (OTC)(G)
    KaoLectrolyte 1 pkt dissolved in 8 oz water q 3-4 hours
    Pediatric: not indicated <2 years
      Pkt: sodium 12 mEq+*potassium* 5 mEq+*chloride* 10 mEq+*citrate* 7 mEq+*dextrose* 5 gm+calories 22 per 6.2 gm
    Pedialyte
    Pediatric: <2 years: as desired and as tolerated; ≥2 years: 1-2 liters/day
      Oral soln: dextrose 20 gm+*fructose* 5 gm+*sodium* 25 mEq+*potassium* 20 mEq+*chloride* 35 mEq+*citrate* 30 mEq+*calories* 100 per liter (8 oz, 1 L)
    Pedialyte Freezer Pops
    Pediatric: as desired and as tolerated
      Pops: dextrose 1.6 gm+sodium 2.8 mEq+potassium 1.25 mEq+chloride 2.2 mEq+citrate 1.88 mEq+calories 6.25 per 62.5 ml (2.1 fl oz) pop

DELIRIUM: END-OF-LIFE

Comment: "Ultimately ... it is essential for clinicians to focus on the humanness of medicine; to keep dying patients comfortable and as awake as they and their families would like them to be so they can make the last few hours or days of life meaningful; and to make reasonable efforts not to cloud their sensorium unless essential to alleviate patient pain or other severe symptoms" (Pandharipande, *et al*, 2017). In a preliminary randomized control study, Hui et al (2017) demonstrated that adding the benzodiazepine *lorazepam* to background *haloperidol* therapy significantly reduced agitated delirium at 8 hours compared with *haloperidol* alone in patients admitted to an acute palliative care unit with advanced cancer and a very short life-expectancy. Moreover, most of the effect the combination had on delirium was achieved in the first 30 minutes following administration (Hui, et al., 2017).

REFERENCES

Hui, D., Frisbee-Hume, S., Wilson, A., Dibaj, S. S., Nguyen, T., De La Cruz, M., … Bruera, E. (2017). Effect of Lorazepam With Haloperidol vs Haloperidol Alone on Agitated Delirium in Patients With Advanced Cancer Receiving Palliative Care. *JAMA, 318*(11), 1047. doi:10.1001/jama.2017.11468

Pandharipande, P. P., & Ely, E. W. (2017). Humanizing the Treatment of Hyperactive Delirium in the Last Days of Life. *JAMA, 318*(11), 1014. doi:10.1001/jama.2017.11466

BENZODIAZEPINE: INTERMEDIATE-ACTING

▷ *lorazepam* (D)(IV)(G) 1-10 mg/day in 2-3 divided doses
　　Pediatric: <12 years: not recommended; ≥12 years: same as adult
　　　　Ativan *Tab:* 0.5, 1*, 2*mg
　　　　Lorazepam Intensol *Oral conc:* 2 mg/ml (30 ml w. graduated dropper)

ANTIPSYCHOSIS AGENTS

▷ *haloperidol* (C)(G)
　　Oral route of administration: Moderate Symptomology: 0.5 to 2 mg orally 2 to 3 times a day; Severe symptomology: 3 to 5 mg orally 2 to 3 times a day; initial doses of up to 100 mg/day have been necessary in some severely resistant cases;
　　Maintenance: after achieving a satisfactory response, the dose should be adjusted as practical to achieve optimum control
　　Parenteral route of administration: Prompt control of acute agitation: 2 to 5 mg IM every 4 to 8 hours; *Maintenance:* frequency of IM administration should be determined by patient response and may be given as often as every hour; max: 20 mg/day
　　　　Haldol *Tab:* 0.5*, 1*, 2*, 5*, 10*, 20*mg
　　　　Haldol Lactate *Vial:* 5 mg for IM injection, single-dose
▷ *mesoridazine* (C) initially 25 mg tid; max 300 mg/day
　　　　Serentil *Tab:* 10, 25, 50, 100 mg; *Conc:* 25 mg/ml (118 ml)
▷ *olanzapine* (C) initially 2.5-10 mg daily; increase to 10 mg/day within a few days; then by 5 mg/day at weekly intervals; max 20 mg/day
　　　　Zyprexa *Tab:* 2.5, 5, 7.5, 10 mg
　　　　Zyprexa Zydis *ODT:* 5, 10, 15, 20 mg (phenylalanine)
▷ *quetiapine fumarate* (C)(G)
　　　　SeroQUEL initially 25 mg bid, titrate q 2nd <u>or</u> 3rd day in increments of 25-50 mg bid-tid; usual maintenance 400-600 mg/day in 2-3 divided doses
　　　　　　Tab: 25, 50, 100, 200, 300, 400 mg
　　　　SeroQUEL XR administer once daily in the PM; *Day 1:* 50 mg; *Day 2:* 100 mg; *Day 3:* 200 mg; *Day 4:* 300 mg; usual range 400-600 mg/day
　　　　　　Tab: 50, 150, 200, 300, 400 mg ext-rel
▷ *risperidone* (C) 0.5 mg bid x 1 day; adjust in increments of 0.5 mg bid; usual range 0.5-5 mg/day
　　　　Risperdal *Tab:* 1, 2, 3, 4 mg; *Oral soln:* 1 mg/ml (100 ml)
　　　　Risperdal M-Tab *Tab:* 0.5, 1, 2 mg
▷ *thioridazine* (C)(G) 10-25 mg bid
　　　　Mellaril *Tab:* 10, 15, 25, 50, 100, 150, 200 mg; *Oral susp:* 25 mg/5 ml, 100 mg/5 ml; *Oral conc:* 30 mg/ml, 100 mg/ml (4 oz)

 DEMENTIA

Alzheimer's Disease *see page* 12
Antidepressants *see Depression page* 117
Hypnotics/Sedatives *see Insomnia page* 231

ANTIPSYCHOTICS

Comment: Underlying cause should be explored, accurately diagnosed, and addressed. All antipsychotic agents are associated with increased risk of mortality in elderly patients with dementia-related psychosis (Black Box Warning.) APA recommends that non-emergency antipsychotic medication should only be used for the treatment of agitation or psychosis in patients with dementia when symptoms are severe, are dangerous and/or cause significant distress to the patient. APA recommends that before non-emergency treatment with an antipsychotic is initiated in patients with dementia, the potential risks and benefits are discussed with the patient and the patient's surrogate decision maker with input from family or others involved with the patient. *haloperidol injection* is not approved for the treatment of patients with dementia-related psychosis.

➤ *haloperidol* (C)(G) 0.5-1 mg q HS
   Haldol *Tab*: 0.5, 1, 2, 5, 10, 20 mg
➤ *mesoridazine* (C) initially 25 mg tid; max 300 mg/day
   Serentil *Tab*: 10, 25, 50, 100 mg; *Conc*: 25 mg/ml (118 ml)
➤ *olanzapine* (C) initially 2.5-10 mg daily; increase to 10 mg/day within a few days; then by 5 mg/day at weekly intervals; max 20 mg/day
   Zyprexa *Tab*: 2.5, 5, 7.5, 10 mg
   Zyprexa Zydis *ODT*: 5, 10, 15, 20 mg (phenylalanine)
➤ *quetiapine fumarate* (C)(G)
   SeroQUEL initially 25 mg bid, titrate q 2nd or 3rd day in increments of 25-50 mg bid-tid; usual maintenance 400-600 mg/day in 2-3 divided doses
      Tab: 25, 50, 100, 200, 300, 400 mg
   SeroQUEL XR administer once daily in the PM; *Day 1*: 50 mg; *Day 2*: 100 mg; *Day 3*: 200 mg; *Day 4*: 300 mg; usual range 400-600 mg/day
      Tab: 50, 150, 200, 300, 400 mg ext-rel
➤ *risperidone* (C) 0.5 mg bid x 1 day; adjust in increments of 0.5 mg bid; usual range 0.5-5 mg/day
   Risperdal *Tab*: 1, 2, 3, 4 mg; *Oral soln*: 1 mg/ml (100 ml)
   Risperdal M-Tab *Tab*: 0.5, 1, 2 mg
➤ *thioridazine* (C)(G) 10-25 mg bid
   Mellaril *Tab*: 10, 15, 25, 50, 100, 150, 200 mg; *Oral susp*: 25 mg/5 ml, 100 mg/5 ml; *Oral conc*: 30 mg/ml, 100 mg/ml (4 oz)

DENGUE FEVER (*DENGUE VIRUS*)

Dengue is the most common arthropod-borne viral (arboviral) illness in humans. The CDC reports that cases of dengue in returning US travelers have increased steadily during the past 20 years, and dengue has become the leading cause of acute febrile illness in US travelers returning from the Caribbean, South America, and Asia. Dengue is transmitted by mosquitoes of the genus *Aedes*, which are widely distributed in subtropical and tropical areas of the world. A small percentage of persons who have previously been infected by one dengue serotype develop bleeding and endothelial leak upon infection with another dengue serotype. This syndrome is termed "dengue hemorrhagic fever." Dengue fever is typically a self-limited disease, with a mortality rate of less than 1%. When treated, dengue hemorrhagic fever has a mortality rate of 2%-5%, but when left untreated, the mortality rate is as high as 50%. Dengue fever is usually a self-limited illness. Supportive care with analgesics, fluid replacement, and bed rest is usually sufficient. Acetaminophen may be used to treat fever and relieve other symptoms. *aspirin*, nonsteroidal anti-inflammatory drugs (NSAIDs), and corticosteroids should be avoided. Management of severe dengue requires careful attention to fluid management and proactive treatment of hemorrhage. Single dose methylprednisolone showed no mortality benefit in the treatment of dengue shock syndrome in a prospective, randomized, double-blind, placebo-controlled trial. **There is no specific antiviral treatment currently available for dengue fever. No vaccine is currently approved or in drug trials for the prevention of dengue infection.** Because lack of immunity to a single dengue strain is the major risk factor for dengue hemorrhagic fever and dengue shock syndrome, a vaccine must provide high levels of immunity to all 4 dengue strains to be clinically useful.

A live attenuated tetravalent vaccine against dengue was effective against all four serotypes of the virus and well-tolerated among children, according to researchers. Interim results from a phase II study showed that children at four study sites in dengue-endemic areas of Asia and Latin America who received the vaccine all had significantly higher levels of antibody titers 18 months later. The vaccine (TAK-003 or TDV) is comprised of a molecularly cloned attenuated strain of dengue serotype 2 (DENV-2), and engineered strains of dengue serotypes 1, 3 and 4 (DENV-1, DENV-3 and DENV-4). Prior phase I and phase II data found the vaccine was well-tolerated and immunogenic against all four dengue serotypes. The trial will take 48 months to complete. The trial is ongoing at three sites in the Dominican Republic (n=535), Panama (n=935), and the Philippines (n=330). Participants are "healthy" children, ages 2 to 17 years, randomized into three groups plus a placebo group. A phase III efficacy trial for the vaccine, entitled Tetravalent Immunization against Dengue Efficacy Study (TIDES) is currently being conducted in eight dengue-endemic countries, with data available in late 2018.

REFERENCES

Sáez-Llorens, X., Tricou, V., Yu, D., Rivera, L., Jimeno, J., Villarreal, A. C., . . . Wallace, D. (2017). Immunogenicity and safety of one versus two doses of tetravalent dengue vaccine in healthy children aged 2–17 years in Asia and Latin America: 18-month interim data from a phase 2, randomised, placebo-controlled study. *The Lancet Infectious Diseases.* doi:10.1016/s1473-3099(17)30632-1

Tricou, V., Sáez-Llorens, X., Yu, D., Rivera, L., Borkowski, A., & Wallace, D. *Progress in development of Takeda's tetravalent dengue vaccine candidate.* Paper presented at the 66th annual meeting of American Society of Tropical Medicine & Hygiene. Retrieved from http://www.abstractsonline.com/pp8/#!/4395/presentation/1438

Yoon, I.-K., & Thomas, S. J. (2017). Encouraging results but questions remain for dengue vaccine. *The Lancet Infectious Diseases.* doi:10.1016/s1473-3099(17)30634-5

DENTAL ABSCESS

ANTI-INFECTIVES

▷ *amoxicillin+clavulanate* (B)(G)

Augmentin 500 mg tid or 875 mg bid x 7-10 days
Pediatric: 40-45 mg/kg/day divided tid x 10 days or 90 mg/kg/day divided bid x 10 days *see pages 618-619 for dose by weight*
Tab: 250, 500, 875 mg; *Chew tab:* 125, 250 mg (lemon-lime); 200, 400 mg (cherry-banana) (phenylalanine); *Oral susp:* 125 mg/5 ml (banana), 250 mg/5 ml (75, 100, 150 ml) (orange); 200, 400 mg/5 ml (50, 75, 100 ml) (orange) (phenylalanine)

Augmentin ES-600 not recommended for adults
Pediatric: <3 months: not recommended; ≥3 months, <40 kg: 90 mg/kg/day in 2 divided doses x 7-10 days; ≥40 kg: not recommended
Oral susp: 42.9 mg/5 ml (50, 75, 100, 125, 150, 200 ml) (strawberry cream) (phenylalanine)

Augmentin XR 2 tabs q 12 hours x 7-10 days

> *Pediatric:* <16 years: use other forms; ≥16 years: same as adult
> > *Tab:* 1000*mg ext-rel

▷ *clindamycin* (B) (administer with fluoroquinolone in adults and TMP-SMX in children) 300 mg qid x 10 days
Pediatric: 8-16 mg/kg/day in 3-4 divided doses x 10 days
  Cleocin (G) *Cap:* 75 (tartrazine), 150 (tartrazine), 300 mg
  Cleocin Pediatric Granules (G) *Oral susp:* 75 mg/5 ml (100 ml) (cherry)

▷ *erythromycin base* (B)(G) 500 mg q 6 hours x 10 days
Pediatric: 30-40 mg/kg/day in 4 divided doses x 10 days
  Ery-Tab *Tab:* 250, 333, 500 mg ent-coat
  PCE *Tab:* 333, 500 mg
Comment: *erythromycin* may increase INR with concomitant *warfarin*, as well as increase serum level of *digoxin*, benzodiazepines and statins.

▷ *erythromycin ethylsuccinate* (B)(G) 400 mg qid x 7 days
Pediatric: 30-50 mg/kg/day in 4 divided doses x 7 days; may double dose with severe infection; max 100 mg/kg/day; *see page 635 for dose by weight*
  EryPed *Oral susp:* 200 mg/5 ml (100, 200 ml) (fruit); 400 mg/5 ml (60, 100, 200 ml) (banana); *Oral drops:* 200, 400 mg/5 ml (50 ml) (fruit); *Chew tab:* 200 mg wafer (fruit)
  E.E.S. *Oral susp:* 200, 400 mg/5 ml (100 ml) (fruit)
  E.E.S. Granules *Oral susp:* 200 mg/5 ml (100, 200 ml) (cherry)
  E.E.S. 400 Tablets *Tab:* 400 mg
Comment: *erythromycin* may increase INR with concomitant *warfarin*, as well as increase serum level of *digoxin*, benzodiazepines and statins.

▷ *penicillin v potassium* (B) 250-500 mg q 6 hours x 5-7 days
Pediatric: <12 years: 25-50 mg/kg/day divided q 6 hours x 5-7 days; *see page 644 for dose by weight*; ≥12 years: same as adult
  Pen-Vee K *Tab:* 250, 500 mg; *Oral soln:* 125 mg/5 ml (100, 200 ml); 250 mg/5 ml (100, 150, 200 ml)

 DENTURE IRRITATION

DEBRIDING AGENT/CLEANSER

▷ *carbamide peroxide 10%* (OTC) apply 10 drops to affected area; swish x 2-3 minutes, then spit; do not rinse; repeat treatment qid
Pediatric: with adult supervision only
  Gly-Oxide *Liq:* 10% (15, 60 ml, squeeze bottle w. applicator)

DEPRESSION, MAJOR DEPRESSIVE DISORDER (MDD)

Comment: Antidepressant monotherapy should be avoided until any presence of (hypo)mania or positive family history for bipolar spectrum disorder has been ruled out as antidepressant monotherapy can induce mania in the bilopar patient. Abrupt withdrawal or interruption of treatment with an antidepressant medication is sometimes associated with an antidepressant discontinuation syndrome which may be mediated by gradually tapering the drug over a period of two weeks or longer, depending on the dose strength and length of treatment. Common symptoms of antidepressant withdrawal include flu-like symptoms, insomnia, nausea, imbalance, sensory disturbances, and hyperarousal. These medications include SSRIs, TCAs, MAOIs, and atypical agents such as *venlafaxine* (Effexor), *mirtazapine* (Remeron), *trazodone* (Desyrel), and *duloxetine* (Cymbalta). Common symptoms of the serotonin discontinuation syndrome include flu-like symptoms (nausea, vomiting, diarrhea, headaches, sweating), sleep disturbances (insomnia, nightmares, constant sleepiness), mood disturbances (dysphoria, anxiety, agitation), cognitive disturbances (mental confusion, hyperarousal), sensory and movement disturbances (imbalance, tremors, vertigo, dizziness, electric-shock-like sensations in the brain, often described by sufferers as "brain zaps."

SELECTIVE SEROTONIN REUPTAKE INHIBITORS (SSRIs)

Comment: Co-administration of SSRIs with TCAs requires extreme caution. Concomitant use of MAOIs and SSRIs is absolutely contraindicated. Avoid St. John's wort and other serotonergic agents. A potentially fatal adverse event is *serotonin syndrome*, caused by serotonin excess. Milder symptoms require HCP intervention to avert severe symptoms which can be rapidly fatal without urgent/emergent medical care. Symptoms include restlessness, agitation, confusion, tachycardia, hypertension, dilated pupils, muscle twitching, muscle rigidity, loss of muscle coordination, diaphoresis, diarrhea, headache, shivering, piloerection, hyperpyrexia, cardiac arrhythmias, seizures, loss of consciousness, coma, death. Common symptoms of the *serotonin discontinuation syndrome* include flu-like symptoms (nausea, vomiting, diarrhea, headaches, sweating), sleep disturbances (insomnia, nightmares, constant sleepiness), mood disturbances (dysphoria, anxiety, agitation), cognitive disturbances (mental confusion, hyperarousal, hallucinations), sensory and movement disturbances (imbalance, tremors, vertigo, dizziness, electric-shock-like sensations in the brain, often described by sufferers as "brain zaps."

▷ *citalopram* (C)(G) initially 20 mg daily; may increase after one week to 40 mg; max 40 mg
   Pediatric: <12 years: not recommended; ≥12 years: same as adult
   Celexa *Tab:* 10, 20, 40 mg; *Oral soln:* 10 mg/5 ml (120 ml) (peppermint) (sugar-free, alcohol-free, parabens)

▷ *escitalopram* (C)(G) initially 10 mg daily; may increase to 20 mg daily after 1 week; elderly <u>or</u> hepatic impairment, 10 mg once daily
   Pediatric: <12 years: not recommended; 12-17 years: initially 10 mg daily; may increase to 20 mg daily after 3 weeks
   Lexapro *Tab:* 5, 10*, 20*mg
   Lexapro Oral Solution *Oral soln:* 1 mg/ml (240 ml) (peppermint) (parabens)

▷ *fluoxetine* (C)(G)
   Prozac initially 20 mg daily; may increase after 1 week; doses >20 mg/day should be divided into AM and noon doses; max 80 mg/day
   Pediatric: <8 years: not recommended; 8-17 years: initially 10 mg/day; may increase after 1 week to 20 mg/day; range 20-60 mg/day; range for lower weight children, 20-30 mg/day; >17 years: same as adult
      Cap: 10, 20, 40 mg; *Tab:* 30*, 60*mg; *Oral soln:* 20 mg/5 ml (4 oz) (mint)
   Prozac Weekly following daily fluoxetine therapy at 20 mg/day for 13 weeks, may initiate **Prozac Weekly** 7 days after the last 20 mg fluoxetine dose
   Pediatric: <12 years: not recommended; ≥12 years: same as adult
      Cap: 90 mg ent-coat del-rel pellets

▷ *levomilnacipran* (C) swallow whole; initially 20 mg once daily for 2 days; then increase to 40 mg once daily; may increase dose in 40 mg increments at intervals of ≥2 days; max 120 mg once daily; *CrCl 30-59 mL/min:* max 80 mg once daily; *CrCl 15-29 mL/min:* max 40 mg once daily
   Fetzima
   Pediatric: <12 years: not recommended; ≥12 years: same as adult
      Cap: 20, 40, 80, 120 mg ext-rel

▷ *paroxetine maleate* (D)(G)
   Pediatric: <12 years: not recommended; ≥12 years: same as adult

Paxil initially 20 mg daily in AM; may increase by 10 mg/day at weekly intervals as needed; max 60 mg/day

Tab: 10*, 20*, 30, 40 mg

Paxil CR initially 25 mg daily in AM; may increase by 12.5 mg at weekly intervals as needed; max 62.5 mg/day

Tab: 12.5, 25, 37.5 mg cont-rel ent-coat

Paxil Suspension initially 20 mg daily in AM; may increase by 10 mg/day at weekly intervals as needed; max 60 mg/day

Oral susp: 10 mg/5 ml (250 ml) (orange)

➤ *paroxetine mesylate* (D)(G) initially 7.5 mg daily in AM; may increase by 10 mg/day at weekly intervals as needed; max 60 mg/day

Pediatric: <12 years: not established; ≥12 years: same as adult

Brisdelle *Cap:* 7.5 mg

➤ *sertraline* (C)(G) initially 50 mg daily; increase at 1 week intervals if needed; max 200 mg daily; dilute oral concentrate immediately prior to administration in 4 oz water, ginger ale, lemon-lime soda, lemonade, <u>or</u> orange juice

Pediatric: <6 years: not recommended; 6-12 years: initially 25 mg daily; max 200 mg/day; 13-17 years: initially 50 mg daily; max 200 mg/day; ≥17 years: same as adult

Zoloft *Tab:* 25*, 50*, 100*mg; *Oral conc:* 20 mg per ml (60 ml) (alcohol 12%)

SEROTONIN-NOREPINEPHRINE REUPTAKE INHIBITORS (SNRIs)

➤ *desvenlafaxine* (C)(G) swallow whole; initially 50 mg once daily; max 120 mg/day

Pediatric: <12 years: not recommended; ≥12 years: same as adult

Pristiq *Tab:* 50, 100 mg ext-rel

➤ *duloxetine* (C)(G) swallow whole; initially 30 mg once daily x 1 week; then, increase to 60 mg once daily; max 120 mg/day

Pediatric: <12 years: not recommended; ≥12 years: same as adult

Cymbalta *Cap:* 20, 30, 40, 60 mg del-rel

➤ *levomilnacipran* (C) swallow whole; initially 20 mg once daily for 2 days; then increase to 40 mg once daily; may increase dose in 40 mg increments at intervals of ≥2 days; max 120 mg once daily; *CrCl 30-59 mL/min:* max 80 mg once daily; *CrCl 15-29 mL/min:* max 40 mg once daily

Pediatric: <12 years: not recommended; ≥12 years: same as adult

Fetzima *Cap:* 20, 40, 80, 120 mg ext-rel

➤ *venlafaxine* (C)(G)

Effexor initially 75 mg/day in 2-3 divided doses; may increase at 4 day intervals in 75 mg increments to 150 mg/day; max 225 mg/day

Pediatric: <18 years: not recommended; ≥18 years: same as adult

Tab: 37.5, 75, 150, 225 mg

Effexor XR initially 75 mg q AM; may start at 37.5 mg daily x 4-7 days, then increase by increments of up to 75 mg/day at intervals of at least 4 days; usual max 375 mg/day

Pediatric: <18 years: not recommended; ≥18 years: same as adult

Tab/Cap: 37.5, 75, 150 mg ext-rel

➤ *vortioxetine* (C) initially 10 mg once daily; max 30 mg/day

Pediatric: <18 years: not established; ≥18 years: same as adult

Brintellix *Tab:* 5, 10, 15, 20 mg

SELECTIVE SEROTONIN REUPTAKE INHIBITOR (SSRI)+5HT-14 RECEPTOR PARTIAL AGONIST COMBINATION

➤ *vilazodone* (C) take with food; initially 10 mg once daily x 7 days; then, 20 mg once daily x 7 days; then, 40 mg once daily

Pediatric: <18 years: not established; ≥18 years: same as adult
Viibryd *Tab:* 10, 20, 40 mg

THIENOBENZODIAZEPINE+SSRI COMBINATION

▷ *olanzapine+fluoxetine* (C) initially one 6/25 cap in the PM; titrate; max one 18/75 cap once daily in the PM
Pediatric: <10 years: not established; ≥10 years: same as adult
Symbyax
Cap: **Symbyax 3/25** olan 3 mg+fluo 25 mg
Symbyax 6/25 olan 6 mg+fluo 25 mg
Symbyax 6/50 olan 6 mg+fluo 50 mg
Symbyax 12/25 olan 12 mg+fluo 25 mg
Symbyax 12/50 olan 12 mg+fluo 50 mg
Comment: **Symbyax** is a thienobenzodiazepine-SSRI indicated for the treatment of depressive episodes associated with bipolar depression disorder and treatment resistant depression (TRD).

TRICYCLIC ANTIDEPRESSANTS (TCAs)

Comment: Co-administration of TCAs with SSRIs requires extreme caution.
▷ *amitriptyline* (C)(G) initially 75 mg/day in divided doses <u>or</u> 50-100 mg in a single dose at HS; max 300 mg/day
Pediatric: <12 years: not recommended; ≥12 years: same as adult
Tab: 10, 25, 50, 75, 100, 150 mg
▷ *amoxapine* (C) initially 50 mg bid-tid; after 1 week may increase to 100 mg bid-tid; usual effective dose 200-300 mg/day; if total dose exceeds 300 mg/day, give in divided doses (max 400 mg/day); may give as a single bedtime dose (max 300 mg q HS)
Pediatric: <12 years: not recommended; ≥12 years: same as adult
Tab: 25, 50, 100, 150 mg
▷ *desipramine* (C)(G) 100-200 mg/day in single <u>or</u> divided doses; max 300 mg/day
Pediatric: <12 years: not recommended; ≥12 years: same as adult
Norpramin *Tab:* 10, 25, 50, 75, 100, 150 mg
▷ *doxepin* (C)(G) 75 mg/day; max 150 mg/day
Pediatric: <12 years: not recommended; ≥12 years: same as adult
Cap: 10, 25, 50, 75, 100, 150 mg; *Oral conc:* 10 mg/ml (4 oz w. dropper)
▷ *imipramine* (C)(G)
Pediatric: <12 years: not recommended; ≥12 years: same as adult
Tofranil initially 75 mg daily (max 200 mg); adolescents initially 30-40 mg daily (max 100 mg/day); if maintenance dose exceeds 75 mg daily, may switch to **Tofranil PM** for divided <u>or</u> bedtime dose
Tab: 10, 25, 50 mg
Tofranil PM initially 75 mg daily 1 hour before HS; max 200 mg
Cap: 75, 100, 125, 150 mg
Tofranil Injection 50 mg IM; lower dose for adolescents; switch to oral form as soon as possible
Amp: 25 mg/2 ml (2 ml)
▷ *nortriptyline* (D)(G) initially 25 mg tid-qid; max 150 mg/day
Pediatric: <12 years: not recommended; ≥12 years: same as adult
Pamelor *Cap:* 10, 25, 50, 75 mg; *Oral soln:* 10 mg/5 ml (16 oz)
▷ *protriptyline* (C) initially 5 mg tid; usual dose 15-40 mg/day in 3-4 divided doses; max 60 mg/day
Pediatric: <12 years: not recommended; ≥12 years: same as adult
Vivactil *Tab:* 5, 10 mg

▷ *trimipramine* (C) initially 75 mg/day in divided doses; max 200 mg/day
　Pediatric: not recommended
　　Surmontil *Cap:* 25, 50, 100 mg

AMINOKETONES

▷ *bupropion HBr* (C)(G)
　Pediatric: Safety and effectiveness in the pediatric population have not been estab-
　lished; when considering the use of **bupropion** in a child <u>or</u> adolescent, balance the
　potential risks with the clinical need
　　Aplenzin initially 100 mg bid for at least 3 days; may increase to 375 <u>or</u> 400 mg/
　　day after several weeks; then after at least 3 more days, 450 mg in 4 divided doses;
　　max 450 mg/day, 174 mg/single dose
　　　Tab: 174, 348, 522 mg
▷ *bupropion HCl* (C)(G)
　Pediatric: Safety and effectiveness in the pediatric population have not been estab-
　lished; when considering the use of **bupropion** in a child or adolescent, balance the
　potential risks with the clinical need
　　Forfivo XL do not use for initial treatment; use immediate-release *bupropion*
　　forms for initial titration; switch to **Forfivo XL** 450 mg once daily when total
　　dose/day reaches 450 mg; may switch to **Forfivo XL** when total dose/day reaches
　　300 mg for 2 weeks and patient needs 450 mg/day to reach therapeutic target;
　　swallow whole, do not crush <u>or</u> chew
　　　Tab: 450 mg ext-rel
　　Wellbutrin initially 100 mg bid for at least 3 days; may increase to 375 <u>or</u> 400 mg/
　　day after several weeks; then after at least 3 more days, 450 mg in 4 divided doses;
　　max 450 mg/day, 150 mg/single dose
　　　Tab: 75, 100 mg
　　Wellbutrin SR initially 150 mg in AM for at least 3 days; increase to 150 mg bid if
　　well tolerated; usual dose 300 mg/day; max 400 mg/day
　　　Tab: 100, 150 mg sust-rel
　　Wellbutrin XL initially 150 mg in AM for at least 3 days; increase to 150 mg bid if
　　well tolerated; usual dose 300 mg/day; max 450 mg/day
　　　Tab: 150, 300 mg sust-rel

MONOAMINE OXIDASE INHIBITORS (MAOIs)

Comment: Many drug and food interactions with this class of drugs, use cautiously.
Should be reserved for refractory depression that has not responded to other classes of
antidepressants. Concomitant use of MAOIs and SSRIs is an absolute contraindication.
See mfr pkg insert for drug and food interactions.
▷ *isocarboxazid* (C)(G) initially 10 mg bid; increase by 10 mg every 2-4 days up to 40
　mg/day; may increase by 20 mg/week to max 60 mg/day divided bid-qid
　Pediatric: <16 years: not recommended; ≥16 years: same as adult
　　Marplan *Tab:* 10 mg
▷ *phenelzine* (C)(G) initially 15 mg tid; max 90 mg/day
　Pediatric: <16 years: not recommended; ≥16 years: same as adult
　　Nardil *Tab:* 15 mg
▷ *selegiline* (C) initially 10 mg tid; max 60 mg/day
　　Emsam *Transdermal patch:* 6 mg/24 Hr, 9 mg/24 Hr, 12 mg/24 Hr
Comment: With the **Emsam** transdermal patch 6 mg/24 h dose, the dietary restrictions
commonly required when using nonselective MAOIs are not necessary.
▷ *tranylcypromine* (C) initially 10 mg tid; may increase in 10 mg/day every 1-3 weeks;
　max 60 mg/day
　　Parnate *Tab:* 10 mg

TETRACYCLICS

▷ *maprotiline* (B)(G) initially 75 mg/day for 2 weeks then change gradually as needed in 25 mg increments; max 225 mg/day
Pediatric: <18 years: not recommended; ≥18 years: same as adult
Ludiomil *Tab:* 25, 50, 75 mg

▷ *mirtazapine* (C) initially 15 mg q HS; increase at intervals of 1-2 weeks; usual range 15-45 mg/day; max 45 mg/day
Pediatric: <12 years: not recommended; ≥12 years: same as adult
Remeron *Tab:* 15*, 30*, 45*mg
Remeron SolTab *ODT:* 15, 30, 45 mg (orange) (phenylalanine)

▷ *chlordiazepoxide+amitriptyline* (C)(IV)
Pediatric: <12 years: not recommended; ≥12 years: same as adult
Limbitrol 3-4 tabs in divided doses
Tab: chlor 5 mg+amit 12.5 mg
Limbitrol DS 3-4 tabs in divided doses; max 6 tabs/day
Tab: chlor 10 mg+amit 25 mg

▷ *trazodone* (C)(G) initially 150 mg/day in divided doses with food; increase by 50 mg/day q 3-4 days; max 400 mg/day in divided doses
Pediatric: <18 years: not recommended; ≥18 years: same as adult
Oleptro *Tab:* 50, 100*, 150*, 200, 250, 300 mg

ATYPICAL ANTIPSYCHOTICS

▷ *aripiprazole* (C)(G) initially 15 mg daily; may increase to max 30 mg/day
Pediatric: <10 years: not recommended; 10-17 years: initially 2 mg/day for 2 days; then, increase to 5 mg/day for 2 days; then, increase to target dose of 10 mg/day; may increase by 5 mg/day at 1 week intervals as needed to max 30 mg/day
Abilify *Tab:* 2, 5, 10, 15, 20, 30 mg
Abilify Discmelt *Tab:* 15 mg orally disintegrating (vanilla) (phenylalanine)
Abilify Maintena *Vial:* 300, 400 mg ext-rel pwdr for IM injection after reconstitution; 300, 400 mg single-dose prefilled dual-chamber syringes w. supplies

Comment: Abilify is indicated for acute and maintenance treatment of manic or mixed episodes in bipolar I disorder, as monotherapy or as an adjunct to *lithium* or *valproate*, as adjunct to antidepressants for major depressive disorder (MDD), and for irritability associated with autistic disorder.

▷ *brexpiprazole* (C) initially 0.5 or 1 mg once daily; titrate weekly up to target 2 mg/day; max 3 mg/day; *Moderate-severe hepatic impairment, renal impairment, or ESRD,* max 2 mg/day
Pediatric: <12 years: not established; ≥12 years: same as adult
Rexulti *Tab:* 0.25, 0.5, 1, 2, 3, 4 mg

 DERMATITIS: ATOPIC (ECZEMA)

Parenteral Corticosteroids *see page 570*
Oral Corticosteroids *see page 569*
Topical Corticosteroids *see page 566*

PHOSPHODIESTERASE 4 INHIBITOR

▷ *crisaborole 2%* (C) apply sparingly bid; max 4 weeks
Pediatric: <2 years: not recommended; ≥2 years: same as adult
Eucrisa *Oint:* 2% (60 gm)

MOISTURIZING AGENTS

Aquaphor Healing Ointment (OTC) *Oint:* 1.75, 3.5, 14 oz (alcohol)
Eucerin Daily Sun Defense (OTC) *Lotn:* 6 oz (fragrance-free)
Comment: Eucerin Daily Sun Defense is a moisturizer with SPF-15 sunscreen.
Eucerin Facial Lotion (OTC) *Lotn:* 4 oz
Eucerin Light Lotion (OTC) *Lotn:* 8 oz
Eucerin Lotion (OTC) *Lotn:* 8, 16 oz
Eucerin Original Creme (OTC) *Crm:* 2, 4, 16 oz (alcohol)
Eucerin Plus Creme (OTC) *Crm:* 4 oz
Eucerin Plus Lotion (OTC) *Lotn:* 6, 12 oz
Eucerin Protective Lotion (OTC) *Lotn:* 4 oz (alcohol)
Comment: Eucerin Protective Lotion is a moisturizer with SPF-25 sunscreen.
Lac-Hydrin Cream (OTC) *Crm:* 280, 385 gm
Lac-Hydrin Lotion (OTC) *Lotn:* 25, 400 gm
Lubriderm Dry Skin Scented (OTC) *Lotn:* 6, 10, 16, 32 oz
Lubriderm Dry Skin Unscented (OTC) *Lotn:* 3.3, 6, 10, 16 oz (fragrance-free)
Lubriderm Sensitive Skin Lotion (OTC) *Lotn:* 3.3, 6, 10, 16 oz (lanolin-free)
Lubriderm Dry Skin (OTC) *Lotn (scented):* 2.5, 6, 10, 16 oz;
    Lotn (fragrance-free): 1, 2.5, 6, 10, 16 oz
Lubriderm Bath 1-2 capfuls in bath or rub onto wet skin as needed, then rinse
    Oil: 8 oz
Moisturel (OTC) apply as needed
    Crm: 4, 16 oz; *Lotn:* 8, 12 oz; *Clnsr:* 8.75 oz

OATMEAL COLLOIDS

Aveeno (OTC) add to bath as needed
    Regular: 1.5 oz (8/pck); *Moisturizing:* 0.75 oz (8/pck)
Aveeno Oil (OTC) add to bath as needed
    Oil: 8 oz
Aveeno Moisturizing (OTC) apply as needed
    Lotn: 2.5, 8, 12 oz; *Crm:* 4 oz
Aveeno Cleansing Bar (OTC) *Bar:* 3 oz
Aveeno Gentle Skin Cleanser (OTC) *Liq clnsr:* 6 oz

TOPICAL OIL

▷ *fluocinolone acetonide* 0.01% topical oil (C)
Pediatric: <6 years: not recommended; ≥6 years: apply sparingly bid for up to 4 weeks
    Derma-Smoothe/FS Topical Oil apply sparingly tid
    Topical oil: 0.01% (4 oz) (peanut oil)

TOPICAL STEROIDS

Comment: Topical steroids should be applied sparingly and for the shortest time necessary. Do not use in the diaper area. Do not use an occlusive dressing. Systemic absorption of topical corticosteroids can induce reversible hypothalamic-pituitary-adrenal (HPA) axis suppression with the potential for clinical corticosteroid insufficiency.

▷ *desonide* 0.05% topical gel (C) apply sparingly bid-tid; max 4 weeks
Pediatric: <3 months: not recommended; ≥3 months: same as adult
    Desonate *Gel:* 0.05% (60 gm) (89% purified water; fragrance-free, surfactant-free, alcohol-free)

SECOND GENERATION ORAL ANTIHISTAMINES

Comment: The following drugs are second generation antihistamines. As such they minimally sedating, much less so than the first generation antihistamines. All antihistamines are excreted into breast milk.

▷ *cetirizine* (C)(OTC)(G) initially 5-10 mg once daily; 5 mg once daily; >65 years: use with caution

Pediatric: <6 years: not recommended; ≥6 years: same as adult

    Children's Zyrtec Chewable *Chew tab:* 5, 10 mg (grape)

    Children's Zyrtec Allergy Syrup *Syr:* 1 mg/ml (4 oz) (grape, bubble gum) (sugar-free, dye-free)

    Zyrtec *Tab:* 10 mg

    Zyrtec Hives Relief *Tab:* 10 mg

    Zyrtec Liquid Gels *Liq gel:* 10 mg

▷ *desloratadine* (C)

    Clarinex 1/2-1 tab once daily

    Pediatric: <6 years: not recommended; ≥6 years: same as adult

        Tab: 5 mg

    Clarinex RediTabs 5 mg once daily

    Pediatric: <6 years: not recommended; 6-12 years: 2.5 once daily; ≥12 years: same as adult

        ODT: 2.5, 5 mg (tutti-frutti) (phenylalanine)

    Clarinex Syrup 5 mg (10 ml) once daily

    Pediatric: <6 months: not recommended; 6-11 months: 1 mg (2 ml) once daily; 1-5 years: 1.25 mg (2.5 ml) once daily; 6-11 years: 2.5 (5 ml) once daily; ≥12 years: same as adult

        Syr: 0.5 mg per ml (4 oz) (tutti-frutti) (phenylalanine)

    Desloratadine ODT 1 tab once daily

    Pediatric: <6 years: not recommended; 6-11 years: 1/2 tab once daily; ≥12 years: same as adult

        ODT: 5 mg

▷ *fexofenadine* (C)(OTC)(G) 60 mg once daily-bid <u>or</u> 180 mg once daily; *CrCl <90 mL/min:* 60 mg once daily

Pediatric: <6 months: not recommended; 6 months-2 years: 15 mg bid; *CrCl ≤90 mL/min:* 15 mg once daily; 2-11 years: 30 mg bid; *CrCl ≤90 mL/min:* 30 mg once daily; ≥12 years: same as adult

    Allegra *Tab:* 30, 60, 180 mg film-coat

    Allegra Allergy *Tab:* 60, 180 mg film-coat

    Allegra ODT *ODT:* 30 mg (phenylalanine)

    Allegra Oral Suspension *Oral susp:* 30 mg/5 ml (6 mg/ml) (4 oz)

▷ *levocetirizine* (B)(OTC) administer dose in the PM; *Seasonal Allergic Rhinitis:* <2 years: not recommended; may start at ≥2 years; *Chronic Idiopathic Urticaria (CIU), Perennial Allergic Rhinitis:* <6 months: not recommended; may start at ≥ 6 months; *Dosing by Age:* 6 months-5 years: max 1.25 mg once daily; 6-11 years: max 2.5 mg once daily; ≥12 years: 2.5-5 mg once daily; *Renal Dysfunction <12 years:* contraindicated; *Renal Dysfunction ≥12 years:* CrCl 50-80 ml/min: 2.5 mg once daily; *CrCl 30-50 mL/min:* 2.5 mg every other day; CrCl: 10-30 mL/min: 2.5 mg twice weekly (every 3-4 days); CrCl <10 mL/min, ESRD <u>or</u> hemodialysis: contraindicated

    Children's Xyzal Allergy 24HR *Oral Soln:* 0.5 mg/ml (150 ml)

    Xyzal Allergy 24HR *Tab:* 5*mg

▷ *loratadine* (C)(OTC)(G) 5 mg bid <u>or</u> 10 mg once daily; *Hepatic <u>or</u> Renal Insufficiency:* see mfr pkg insert

Pediatric: <2 years: not recommended; 2-5 years: 5 mg once daily; ≥6 years: same as adult

    Children's Claritin Chewables *Chew tab:* 5 mg (grape) (phenylalanine)

Children's Claritin Syrup 1 mg/ml (4 oz) (fruit) (sugar-free, alcohol-free, dye-free; sodium 6 mg/5 ml)
Claritin *Tab:* 10 mg
Claritin Hives Relief *Tab:* 10 mg
Claritin Liqui-Gels *Liq gel:* 10 mg
Claritin RediTabs 12 Hours *ODT:* 5 mg (mint)
Claritin RediTabs 24 Hours *ODT:* 10 mg (mint)

FIRST GENERATION ANTIHISTAMINES

▷ *diphenhydramine* (B)(G) 25-50 mg q 6-8 hours; max 100 mg/day
Pediatric: <2 years: not recommended; 2-6 years: 6.25 mg q 4-6 hours; max 37.5 mg/day; >6-12 years: 12.5-25 mg q 4-6 hours; max 150 mg/day; >12 years: same as adult
Benadryl (OTC) *Chew tab:* 12.5 mg (grape) (phenylalanine); *Liq:* 12.5 mg/5 ml (4, 8 oz); *Cap:* 25 mg; *Tab:* 25 mg; *Dye-free soft gel:* 25 mg; *Dye-free liq:* 12.5 mg/5 ml (4, 8 oz)
▷ *diphenhydramine injectable* (B)(G) 25-50 mg IM immediately; then q 6 hours prn
Pediatric: <12 years: *See mfr pkg insert:* 1.25 mg/kg up to 25 mg IM x 1 dose; then q 6 hours prn; ≥12 years: same as adult
Benadryl Injectable *Vial:* 50 mg/ml (1 ml single-use); 50 mg/ml (10 ml multi-dose); *Amp:* 10 mg/ml (1 ml); *Prefilled syringe:* 50 mg/ml (1 ml)
▷ *hydroxyzine* (C)(G) 50 mg/day divided qid prn; 50-100 mg/day divided qid prn
Pediatric: <6 years: 50 mg/day divided qid prn; ≥6 years: same as adult
Atarax *Tab:* 10, 25, 50, 100 mg; *Syr:* 10 mg/5 ml (alcohol 0.5%)
Vistaril *Cap:* 25, 50, 100 mg; *Oral susp:* 25 mg/5 ml (4 oz) (lemon)
Comment: *hydroxyzine* is contraindicated in early pregnancy and in patients with a prolonged QT interval. It is not known whether this drug is excreted in human milk; therefore, *hydroxyzine* should not be given to nursing mothers.

TOPICAL ANALGESICS

▷ *capsaicin* cream (B)(G) apply tid-qid prn
Pediatric: <2 years: not recommended; ≥2 years: apply sparingly tid-qid prn
Axsain *Crm:* 0.075% (1, 2 oz)
Capsin (OTC) *Lotn:* 0.025, 0,075% (59 ml)
Capzasin-P (OTC) *Crm:* 0.025% (1.5 oz); *Lotn:* 0.025% (2 oz)
Capzasin-HP (OTC) *Crm:* 0.075% (1.5 oz); *Lotn:* 0.075% (2 oz)
Dolorac *Crm:* 0.025% (28 gm)
Double Cap (OTC) *Crm:* 0.05% (2 oz)
R-Gel *Gel:* 0.025% (15, 30 gm)
Zostrix (OTC) *Crm:* 0.025% (0.7, 1.5, 3 oz)
Zostrix HP (OTC) *Emol crm:* 0.075% (1, 2 oz)
Comment: Provides some relief by 1-2 weeks; optimal benefit may take 4-6 weeks. Avoid contact with mucous membranes.
▷ *doxepin* (B) cream apply to affected area qid at intervals of at least 3-4 hours; max 8 days
Pediatric: <12 years: not recommended; ≥12 years: same as adult
Prudoxin *Crm:* 5% (45 gm)
Zonalon *Crm:* 5% (30, 45 gm)
▷ *pimecrolimus* 1% cream (C) apply to affected area bid; do not occlude
Pediatric: <2 years: not recommended; ≥2 years: same as adult
Elidel *Crm:* 1% (30, 60, 100 gm)
Comment: *pimecrolimus* is indicated for short-term and intermittent long-term use. Discontinue use when resolution occurs. Contraindicated if the patient is immunosuppressed. Change to the 0.1% preparation or if secondary bacterial infection is present.

▷ *tacrolimus* (C) apply to affected area bid; do not occlude <u>or</u> apply to wet skin; continue for 1 week after clearing
Pediatric: <2 years: not recommended; 2-15 years: use 0.03% strength; apply to affected area bid; continue for 1 week after clearing; >15 years: same as adult
Protopic *Oint:* 0.03, 0.1% (30, 60, 100 gm)

TOPICAL ANESTHETIC

▷ *lidocaine* (B) apply to affected area bid-tid prn
Pediatric: reduce dosage commensurate with age, body weight, and physical condition
Lidoderm *Crm:* 3% (85 gm)

INTERLEUKIN-4 RECEPTOR ALPHA ANTAGONIST

dupilumab <18 years: not recommended; ≥18 years: administer SC into the upper arm, abdomen, <u>or</u> thigh; rotate sites; initially 600 mg (2 x 300 mg injections at different sites) followed by 300 mg SC once every other week; may use with <u>or</u> without topical corticosteroids; may use with calcineurin inhibitors, but reserve only for problem areas (e.g., face, neck, intertriginous, and genital areas); avoid live vaccines.
Dupixent *Prefill syr:* 300 mg/2 ml (2/pck without needle) (preservative-free)
Comment: *dupilumab* is a human monoclonal IgG4 antibody that inhibits interleukin-4 (IL-4) and interleukin-13 (IL-13) signaling by specifically binding to the IL4Rα subunit shared by the IL-4 and IL-13 receptor complexes, thereby inhibiting the release of pro-inflammatory cytokines, chemokines, and IgE. *dupilumab* is indicated for moderate-to-severe atopic dermatitis patients ≥18 years-of-age who are not adequately controlled with topical prescription therapies <u>or</u> when they are not advisable.

 DERMATITIS: CONTACT

Oral Prescription Drugs for the Management of Allergy, Cough, and Cold Symptoms
see page 598
Topical Corticosteroids *see page 566*
Parenteral Corticosteroids *see page 570*
Oral Corticosteroids *see page 569*

PROPHYLAXIS

▷ *bentoquatam* apply as a wet film to exposed skin at least 15 minutes prior to possible contact; reapply at least q 4 hours; remove with soap and water
Pediatric: <6 years: not recommended; ≥6 years: same as adult
IvyBlock (OTC) *Soln:* 120 ml
Comment: Provides protection against genus *Rhus* (poison ivy, oak, and sumac).

TREATMENT
Oatmeal Colloids

Aveeno (OTC) add to bath as needed
Regular: 1.5 oz (8/pck); *Moisturizing:* 0.75 oz (8/pck)
Aveeno Oil (OTC) add to bath as needed
Oil: 8 oz
Aveeno Moisturizing (OTC) apply as needed
Lotn: 2.5, 8, 12 oz; *Crm:* 4 oz
Aveeno Cleansing Bar (OTC) *Bar:* 3 oz
Aveeno Gentle Skin Cleanser (OTC) *Liq clnsr:* 6 oz

SECOND GENERATION ORAL ANTIHISTAMINES

Comment: The following drugs are second generation antihistamines. As such they minimally sedating, much less so than the first generation antihistamines. All antihistamines are excreted into breast milk.

▷ *cetirizine* (C)(OTC)(G) initially 5-10 mg once daily; 5 mg once daily; ≥65 years: use with caution

Pediatric: <6 years: not recommended; ≥6 years: same as adult

    Children's Zyrtec Chewable *Chew tab:* 5, 10 mg (grape)

    Children's Zyrtec Allergy Syrup *Syr:* 1 mg/ml (4 oz) (grape, bubble gum) (sugar-free, dye-free)

    Zyrtec *Tab:* 10 mg

    Zyrtec Hives Relief *Tab:* 10 mg

    Zyrtec Liquid Gels *Liq gel:* 10 mg

▷ *desloratadine* (C)

    Clarinex 1/2-1 tab once daily

    Pediatric: <6 years: not recommended; ≥6 years: same as adult

      Tab: 5 mg

    Clarinex RediTabs 5 mg once daily

    Pediatric: <6 years: not recommended; 6-12 years: 2.5 mg once daily; ≥12 years: same as adult

      ODT: 2.5, 5 mg (tutti-frutti) (phenylalanine)

    Clarinex Syrup 5 mg (10 ml) once daily

    Pediatric: <6 months: not recommended; 6-11 months: 1 mg (2 ml) once daily; 1-5 years: 1.25 mg (2.5 ml) once daily; 6-11 years: 2.5 mg (5 ml) once daily; ≥12 years: same as adult

      Syr: 0.5 mg per ml (4 oz) (tutti-frutti) (phenylalanine)

    Desloratadine ODT 1 tab once daily

    Pediatric: <6 years: not recommended; 6-11 years: 1/2 tab once daily; ≥12 years: same as adult

      ODT: 5 mg

▷ *fexofenadine* (C)(OTC)(G) 60 mg once daily-bid <u>or</u> 180 mg once daily; *CrCl <90 mL/ min:* 60 mg once daily

Pediatric: <6 months: not recommended; 6 months-2 years: 15 mg bid; *CrCl ≤90 mL/ min:* 15 mg once daily; 2-11 years: 30 mg bid; *CrCl ≤90 mL/min:* 30 mg once daily; ≥12 years: same as adult

    Allegra *Tab:* 30, 60, 180 mg film-coat

    Allegra Allergy *Tab:* 60, 180 mg film-coat

    Allegra ODT *ODT:* 30 mg (phenylalanine)

    Allegra Oral Suspension *Oral susp:* 30 mg/5 ml (6 mg/ml) (4 oz)

▷ *levocetirizine* (B)(OTC) administer dose in the PM; *Seasonal Allergic Rhinitis:* <2 years: not recommended; may start at ≥2 years; *Chronic Idiopathic Urticaria (CIU), Perennial Allergic Rhinitis:* <6 months: not recommended; may start at ≥ 6 months; *Dosing by Age:* 6 months-5 years: max 1.25 mg once daily; 6-11 years: max 2.5 mg once daily; ≥12 years: 2.5-5 mg once daily; *Renal Dysfunction <12 years:* contraindicated; *Renal Dysfunction ≥12 years:* CrCl 50-80 ml/min: 2.5 mg once daily; CrCl 30-50 mL/min: 2.5 mg every other day; CrCl: 10-30 mL/min: 2.5 mg twice weekly (every 3-4 days); CrCl <10 mL/min, ESRD <u>or</u> hemodialysis: contraindicated

    Children's Xyzal Allergy 24HR *Oral Soln:* 0.5 mg/ml (150 ml)

    Xyzal Allergy 24HR *Tab:* 5*mg

▷ *loratadine* (C)(OTC)(G) 5 mg bid <u>or</u> 10 mg once daily; *Hepatic <u>or</u> Renal Insufficiency:* see mfr pkg insert

Pediatric: <2 years: not recommended; 2-5 years: 5 mg once daily; ≥6 years: same as adult

    Children's Claritin Chewables *Chew tab:* 5 mg (grape) (phenylalanine)
    Children's Claritin Syrup 1 mg/ml (4 oz) (fruit) (sugar-free, alcohol-free,
    dye-free; sodium 6 mg/5 ml)
    Claritin *Tab:* 10 mg
    Claritin Hives Relief *Tab:* 10 mg
    Claritin Liqui-Gels *Lig gel:* 10 mg
    Claritin RediTabs 12 Hours *ODT:* 5 mg (mint)
    Claritin RediTabs 24 Hours *ODT:* 10 mg (mint)

FIRST GENERATION ORAL ANTIHISTAMINES

▷ *diphenhydramine* (B)(G) 25-50 mg q 6-8 hours; max 100 mg/day
  Pediatric: <2 years: not recommended; 2-6 years: 6.25 mg q 4-6 hours; max 37.5 mg/
  day; >6-12 years: 12.5-25 mg q 4-6 hours; max 150 mg/day; >12 years: same as adult
    Benadryl (OTC) *Chew tab:* 12.5 mg (grape) (phenylalanine); *Liq:* 12.5 mg/5 ml
    (4, 8 oz); *Cap:* 25 mg; *Tab:* 25 mg; *Dye-free soft gel:* 25 mg; *Dye-free liq:* 12.5 mg/5
    ml (4, 8 oz)
▷ *hydroxyzine* (C)(G) 50 mg/day divided qid prn; 50-100 mg/day divided qid prn
  Pediatric: <6 years: 50 mg/day divided qid prn; ≥6 years: same as adult
    Atarax *Tab:* 10, 25, 50, 100 mg; *Syr:* 10 mg/5 ml (alcohol 0.5%)
    Vistaril *Cap:* 25, 50, 100 mg; *Oral susp:* 25 mg/5 ml (4 oz) (lemon)
  Comment: *hydroxyzine* is contraindicated in early pregnancy and in patients with a
  prolonged QT interval. It is not known whether this drug is excreted in human milk;
  therefore, *hydroxyzine* should not be given to nursing mothers.

FIRST GENERATION PARENTERAL ANTIHISTAMINE

▷ *diphenhydramine* **injectable** (B)(G) 25-50 mg IM immediately; then q 6 hours prn
  Pediatric: <12 years: *See mfr pkg insert:* 1.25 mg/kg up to 25 mg IM x 1 dose; then q 6
  hours prn; ≥12 years: same as adult
    Benadryl Injectable *Vial:* 50 mg/ml (1 ml single-use); 50 mg/ml (10 ml multi-
    dose); *Amp:* 10 mg/ml (1 ml); *Prefilled syringe:* 50 mg/ml (1 ml)

 DERMATITIS: GENUS *RHUS* (POISON OAK, POISON IVY, POISON SUMAC)

Topical Corticosteroids *see page* 566
Parenteral Corticosteroids *see page* 570
Oral Corticosteroids *see page* 569
OTC Calamine Lotion
OTC Diphenhydramine Cream

PROPHYLAXIS

▷ *bentoquatam* <6 years: not recommended; ≥6 years: apply as a wet film to exposed
  skin at least 15 minutes prior to possible contact; reapply at least q 4 hours; remove
  with soap and water
    IvyBlock (OTC) *Soln:* 120 ml
  Comment: Provides protection against genus *Rhus* (poison oak, poison ivy, and
  poison sumac).

TREATMENT

Oatmeal Colloids
Aveeno (OTC) add to bath as needed
  Regular: 1.5 oz (8/pck); *Moisturizing:* 0.75 oz (8/pck)

Aveeno Oil (OTC) add to bath as needed
   Oil: 8 oz
Aveeno Moisturizing (OTC) apply as needed
   Lotn: 2.5, 8, 12 oz; *Crm:* 4 oz
Aveeno Cleansing Bar (OTC) *Bar:* 3 oz
Aveeno Gentle Skin Cleanser (OTC) *Liq clnsr:* 6 oz

SECOND GENERATION ORAL ANTIHISTAMINES

Comment: The following drugs are second generation antihistamines. As such they are minimally sedating, much less so than the first generation antihistamines. All antihistamines are excreted into breast milk.

➤ *cetirizine* (C)(OTC)(G) initially 5-10 mg once daily; 5 mg once daily; ≥65 years: use with caution
   Pediatric: <6 years: not recommended; ≥6 years: same as adult
      Children's Zyrtec Chewable *Chew tab:* 5, 10 mg (grape)
      Children's Zyrtec Allergy Syrup *Syr:* 1 mg/ml (4 oz) (grape, bubble gum) (sugar-free, dye-free)
      Zyrtec *Tab:* 10 mg
      Zyrtec Hives Relief *Tab:* 10 mg
      Zyrtec Liquid Gels *Liq gel:* 10 mg
➤ *desloratadine* (C)
      Clarinex 1/2-1 tab once daily
      Pediatric: <6 years: not recommended; ≥6 years: same as adult
         Tab: 5 mg
      Clarinex RediTabs 5 mg once daily
      Pediatric: <6 years: not recommended; 6-12 years: 2.5 mg once daily; ≥12 years: same as adult
         ODT: 2.5, 5 mg (tutti-frutti) (phenylalanine)
      Clarinex Syrup 5 mg (10 ml) once daily
      Pediatric: <6 months: not recommended; 6-11 months: 1 mg (2 ml) once daily; 1-5 years: 1.25 mg (2.5 ml) once daily; 6-11 years: 2.5 mg (5 ml) once daily; ≥12 years: same as adult
         Syr: 0.5 mg per ml (4 oz) (tutti-frutti) (phenylalanine)
      Desloratadine ODT 1 tab once daily
      Pediatric: <6 years: not recommended; 6-11 years: 1/2 tab once daily; ≥12 years: same as adult
         ODT: 5 mg
➤ *fexofenadine* (C)(OTC)(G) 60 mg once daily-bid <u>or</u> 180 mg once daily; *CrCl <90 mL/min:* 60 mg once daily
   Pediatric: <6 months: not recommended; 6 months-2 years: 15 mg bid; *CrCl ≤90 mL/min:* 15 mg once daily; 2-11 years: 30 mg bid; *CrCl ≤90 mL/min:* 30 mg once daily; ≥12 years: same as adult
      Allegra *Tab:* 30, 60, 180 mg film-coat
      Allegra Allergy *Tab:* 60, 180 mg film-coat
      Allegra ODT *ODT:* 30 mg (phenylalanine)
      Allegra Oral Suspension *Oral susp:* 30 mg/5 ml (6 mg/ml) (4 oz)
➤ *levocetirizine* (B)(OTC) administer dose in the PM; *Seasonal Allergic Rhinitis:* <2 years: not recommended; may start at ≥2 years; *Chronic Idiopathic Urticaria (CIU), Perennial Allergic Rhinitis:* <6 months: not recommended; may start at ≥ 6 months; *Dosing by Age:* 6 months-5 years: max 1.25 mg once daily; 6-11 years: max 2.5 mg once daily; ≥12 years: 2.5-5 mg once daily; *Renal Dysfunction <12 years:* contraindicated; *Renal Dysfunction ≥12 years:* CrCl 50-80 ml/min: 2.5 mg

once daily; CrCl 30-50 mL/min: 2.5 mg every other day; CrCl: 10-30 mL/min: 2.5 mg twice weekly (every 3-4 days); CrCl <10 mL/min, ESRD <u>or</u> hemodialysis: contraindicated

   Children's Xyzal Allergy 24HR *Oral Soln:* 0.5 mg/ml (150 ml)
   Xyzal Allergy 24HR *Tab:* 5*mg

▷ *loratadine* (C)(OTC)(G) 5 mg bid <u>or</u> 10 mg once daily; *Hepatic <u>or</u> Renal Insufficiency:* see mfr pkg insert
   Pediatric: <2 years: not recommended; 2-5 years: 5 mg once daily; ≥6 years: same as adult
   Children's Claritin Chewables *Chew tab:* 5 mg (grape) (phenylalanine)
   Children's Claritin Syrup 1 mg/ml (4 oz) (fruit) (sugar-free, alcohol-free, dye-free, sodium 6 mg/5 ml)
   Claritin *Tab:* 10 mg
   Claritin Hives Relief *Tab:* 10 mg
   Claritin Liqui-Gels *Liq gel:* 10 mg
   Claritin RediTabs 12 Hours *ODT:* 5 mg (mint)
   Claritin RediTabs 24 Hours *ODT:* 10 mg (mint)

FIRST GENERATION ANTIHISTAMINES

▷ *diphenhydramine* (B)(G) 25-50 mg q 6-8 hours; max 100 mg/day
   Pediatric: <2 years: not recommended; 2-6 years: 6.25 mg q 4-6 hours; max 37.5 mg/day; >6-12 years: 12.5-25 mg q 4-6 hours; max 150 mg/day; >12 years: same as adult
   Benadryl (OTC) *Chew tab:* 12.5 mg (grape) (phenylalanine); *Liq:* 12.5 mg/5 ml (4, 8 oz); *Cap:* 25 mg; *Tab:* 25 mg; *Dye-free soft gel:* 25 mg; *Dye-free liq:* 12.5 mg/5 ml (4, 8 oz)

▷ *diphenhydramine* injectable (B)(G) 25-50 mg IM immediately; then q 6 hours prn
   Pediatric: <12 years: *See mfr pkg insert:* 1.25 mg/kg up to 25 mg IM x 1 dose; then q 6 hours prn; ≥12 years: same as adult
   Benadryl Injectable *Vial:* 50 mg/ml (1 ml single-use); 50 mg/ml (10 ml multi-dose); *Amp:* 10 mg/ml (1 ml); *Prefilled syringe:* 50 mg/ml (1 ml)

▷ *hydroxyzine* (C)(G) 50 mg/day divided qid prn; 50-100 mg/day divided qid prn
   Pediatric: <6 years: 50 mg/day divided qid prn; ≥6 years: same as adult
   Atarax *Tab:* 10, 25, 50, 100 mg; *Syr:* 10 mg/5 ml (alcohol 0.5%)
   Vistaril *Cap:* 25, 50, 100 mg; *Oral susp:* 25 mg/5 ml (4 oz) (lemon)

Comment: *hydroxyzine* is contraindicated in early pregnancy and in patients with a prolonged QT interval. It is not known whether this drug is excreted in human milk; therefore, *hydroxyzine* should not be given to nursing mothers.

 DERMATITIS: SEBORRHEIC

ANTIFUNGAL SHAMPOOS AND TOPICAL AGENTS

▷ *chloroxine* shampoo (C) massage onto wet scalp; wait 3 minutes, rinse, repeat, and rinse thoroughly; use twice weekly
   Pediatric: <12 years: not recommended; ≥12 years: same as adult
   Capitrol Shampoo *Shampoo:* 2% (4 oz)

▷ *ciclopirox* (B) apply gel once daily <u>or</u> apply cream <u>or</u> lotion twice daily, x 4 weeks <u>or</u> shampoo twice weekly; massage shampoo onto wet scalp; wait 3 minutes, rinse, repeat, and rinse thoroughly; shampoo twice weekly
   Loprox Cream
      Pediatric: <10 years: not recommended; ≥10 years: same as adult
      Crm: 0.77% (15, 30, 90 gm)
   Loprox Gel
      Pediatric: <16 years: not recommended; ≥16 years: same as adult

> *Gel:* 0.77% (30, 45 gm)

Loprox Lotion
> *Pediatric:* <10 years: not recommended; ≥10 years: same as adult
> *Lotn:* 0.77% (30, 60 ml)

Loprox Shampoo *Shampoo:* 1% (120 ml)

▷ *coal tar* (C)(G)
Pediatric: same as adult

Scytera (OTC) apply once daily-qid; use lowest effective dose
> *Foam:* 2%

T/Gel Shampoo Extra Strength (OTC) use every other day; max 4 x/week; massage into wet scalp for 5 minutes; rinse; repeat *Shampoo:* 1%

T/Gel Shampoo Original Formula (OTC) use every other day; max 7 x/week; massage into wet scalp for 5 minutes; rinse; repeat
> *Shampoo:* 0.5%

T/Gel Shampoo Stubborn Itch Control (OTC) use every other day; max 7 x/week; massage into wet scalp for 5 minutes; rinse; repeat
> *Shampoo:* 0.5%

▷ *fluocinolone acetonide* (C)

Derma-Smoothe/FS Shampoo apply up to 1 oz to scalp daily, lather, and leave on x 5 minutes, then rinse twice
Pediatric: <12 years: not recommended; ≥12 years: same as adult
> *Shampoo:* 0.01% (4 oz)

Derma-Smoothe/FS Topical Oil *fluocinolone acetonide* 0.01% topical oil (C) apply sparingly tid; for scalp psoriasis wet <u>or</u> dampen hair <u>or</u> scalp, then apply a thin film, massage well, cover with a shower cap and leave on for at least 4 hours <u>or</u> overnight, then wash hair with regular shampoo and rinse
Pediatric: <6 years: not recommended; ≥6 years: apply sparingly bid for up to 4 weeks
> *Topical oil:* 0.01% (4 oz) (peanut oil)

▷ *ketoconazole* (C) apply cream <u>or</u> gel once daily x 4 week <u>or</u> apply up to 1 oz shampoo to scalp daily, lather, leave on x 5 minutes, then rinse twice
Pediatric: <12 years: not recommended; ≥12 years: same as adult

Nizoral Cream *Crm:* 2% (15, 30, 60 gm)
Nizoral Shampoo *Shampoo:* 2% (4 oz)
Xolegel *Gel:* 2% (45 gm)
Xolegel Duo *Kit:* **Xolegel** *Gel:* 2% (45 gm) + **Xolex** *Shampoo:* 2% (4 oz)

▷ *selenium sulfide* (C) massage cream into scalp twice weekly x 2 weeks <u>or</u> massage into wet scalp, wait 2-3 minutes, rinse; repeat twice weekly x 2 weeks; may continue treatment with lotion of shampoo 1-2 x weekly as needed
Pediatric: <12 years: not recommended; ≥12 years: same as adult

Exsel Shampoo *Shampoo:* 2.5% (4 oz)
Selsun Rx *Lotn:* 2.5% (4 oz)
Selsun Shampoo *Shampoo:* 1% (120, 210, 240, 330 ml); 2.5% (120 ml)

▷ *sodium sulfacetamide+sulfur* (C)

Clenia Emollient Cream apply daily tid
> *Emol crm: sod sulfa* 10%+*sulfur* 5% (10 oz)

Clenia Foaming Wash wash 1-2 x/day
> *Wash: sod sulfa* 10%+*sulfur* 5% (6, 12 oz)

Rosula Gel apply daily tid
> *Gel: sod sulfa* 10%+*sulfur* 5% (45 ml)

Rosula Lotion apply daily tid
> *Lotn: sod sulfa* 10%+*sulfur* 5% (45 ml) (alcohol-free)

Rosula Wash wash bid
> *Clnsr: sod sulfa* 10%+*sulfur* 5% (335 ml)

TOPICAL STEROID

▷ **betamethasone valerate** 0.12% foam (C)(G) apply twice daily in AM and PM; invert can and dispense a small amount of foam onto a clean saucer <u>or</u> other cool surface (do not apply directly to hand) and massage a small amount into affected area until foam disappears
Pediatric: <12 years: not recommended; ≥12 years: same as adult
   Luxiq *Foam:* 100 g

 DIABETIC PERIPHERAL NEUROPATHY (DPN)

Other Oral Analgesics *see Pain page* 344

NUTRITIONAL SUPPLEMENT

▷ **L-methylfolate calcium (as metafolin)+pyridoxyl 5-phosphate+methylcobalamin** 1 cap twice daily <u>or</u> 2 caps once daily
Pediatric: <12 years: not recommended; ≥12 years: same as adult
   Metanx *Cap: meta* 3 mg+*pyr* 35 mg+*methyl* 2 mg
Comment: Metanx is indicated as adjunct treatment for patients with endothelial cell dysfunction, who have loss of protective sensation and neuropathic pain associated with diabetic peripheral neuropathy.

ORAL ANALGESICS

▷ **acetaminophen** (B)(G) *see Fever page* 165
▷ **aspirin** (D)(G) *see Fever page* 165
   Comment: *aspirin*-containing medications are contraindicated with history of allergic-type reaction to **aspirin**, children and adolescents with *Varicella* <u>or</u> other viral illness, and 3rd trimester of pregnancy.
▷ **tramadol** (C)(IV)(G)
Comment: *tramadol* is known to be excreted in breast milk. The FDA and the European Medicines Agency (EMA) are investigating the safety of using **tramadol**-containing medications to treat pain in children 12-18 years because of the potential for serious side effects, including slowed or difficult breathing.
   Rybix ODT initially 100 mg once daily; may increase by 100 mg every 5 days; max 300 mg/day; *CrCl <30 mL/min* <u>or</u> *severe hepatic impairment*: not recommended; *Cirrhosis:* max 50 mg q 12 hours
   Pediatric: <18 years: not recommended; ≥18 years: same as adult
      ODT: 50 mg (mint) (phenylalanine)
   Ryzolt initially 100 mg once daily; may increase by 100 mg every 5 days; max 300 mg/day; *CrCl <30 mL/min* <u>or</u> *severe hepatic impairment*: not recommended
   Pediatric: <18 years: not recommended; ≥18 years: same as adult
      Tab: 100, 200, 300 mg ext-rel
   Ultram 50-100 mg q 4-6 hours prn; max 400 mg/day; *CrCl <30 mL/min*, max 100 mg q 12 hours; cirrhosis, max 50 mg q 12 hours
   Pediatric: <18 years: not recommended; ≥18 years: same as adult
      Tab: 50*mg
   Ultram ER initially 100 mg once daily; may increase by 100 mg every 5 days; max 300 mg/day; *CrCl <30 mL/min* <u>or</u> *severe hepatic impairment*: not recommended
      Pediatric: <18 years: not recommended; ≥18 years: same as adult
      Tab: 100, 200, 300 mg ext-rel
▷ **tramadol+acetaminophen** (C)(IV)(G) 2 tabs q 4-6 hours; max 8 tabs/day x 5 days; *CrCl <30 mL/min:* max 2 tabs q 12 hours; max 4 tabs/day x 5 days
Pediatric: <18 years: not recommended; ≥18 years: same as adult

Ultracet *Tab: tram* 37.5+*acet* 325 mg
Comment: *Tramadol* is known to be excreted in breast milk. The FDA and the European Medicines Agency (EMA) are investigating the safety of using *tramadol*-containing medications to treat pain in children 12-18 years because of the potential for serious side effects, including slowed or difficult breathing.

TOPICAL ANALGESICS

▷ *capsaicin* cream (B)(G) apply tid-qid after lesions have healed
Pediatric: <2 years: not recommended; ≥2 years: same as adult
Axsain *Crm:* 0.075% (1, 2 oz)
Capsin *Lotn:* 0.025, 0.075% (59 ml)
Capsaicin-P (OTC) *Crm:* 0.025% (1.5 oz); *Lotn:* 0.025% (2 oz)
Capsaicin-HP (OTC) *Crm:* 0.075% (1.5 oz); *Lotn:* 0.075% (2 oz); *Crm:* 0.025% (45, 90 gm)
Dolorac *Crm:* 0.025% (28 gm)
Double Cap (OTC) *Crm:* 0.05% (2 oz)
R-Gel *Gel:* 0.025% (15, 30 gm)
Zostrix (OTC) *Crm:* 0.025% (0.7, 1.5, 3 oz)
Zostrix HP *Emol crm:* 0.075% (1, 2 oz)
▷ *capsaicin* 8% patch (B) apply up to 4 patches for one 60-minute application to clean dry skin; may prep area with topical anesthetic; wear nonlatex gloves; patches may be cut to size/shape; treatment may be repeated every 3 months
Pediatric: <18 years: not recommended; ≥18 years: same as adult
Qutenza *Patch:* 8% 1640 mcg/cm (179 mg) (1 or 2 patches w. 1-50 gm tube cleansing gel/carton)
▷ *lidocaine* 5% patch (B)(G) apply up to 3 patches at one time for up to 12 hours/24-hour period (12 hours on/12 hours off); patches may be cut into smaller sizes before removal of the release liner; do not re-use
Pediatric: <12 years: not recommended; ≥12 years: same as adult
Lidoderm *Patch:* 5% 10x14 cm (30 patches/carton)

ANTICONVULSANTS

Gamma Aminobutyric Acid Analog

▷ *gabapentin* (C)
Pediatric: <3 years: not recommended; 3-12 years: initially 10-15 mg/kg/day in 3 divided doses; max 12 hours between doses; titrate over 3 days; 3-4 years: titrate to 40 mg/kg/day; 5-12 years: titrate to 25-35 mg/kg/day; max 50 mg/kg/day
Gralise (C) initially 300 mg on Day 1; then 600 mg on Day 2; then 900 mg on Days 3-6; then 1200 mg on Days 7-10; then 1500 mg on Days 11-14; titrate up to 1800 mg on Day 15; take entire dose once daily with the evening meal; do not crush, split, or chew
Tab: 300, 600 mg
Neurontin (G) *Tab:* 600*, 800*mg; *Cap:* 100, 300, 400 mg; *Oral soln:* 250 mg/5 ml (480 ml) (strawberry-anise)
▷ *gabapentin enacarbil* (C) 600 mg once daily at about 5:00 PM; if dose not taken at recommended time, next dose should be taken the following day; swallow whole; take with food; CrCl 30-59 mL/min: 600 mg on Day 1, Day 3, and every day thereafter; CrCl <30 mL/min: or on hemodialysis: not recommended
Pediatric: <12 years: not recommended; ≥12 years: same as adult
Horizant *Tab:* 300, 600 mg ext-rel
Comment: Avoid abrupt cessation of *gabapentin* and *gabapentin enacarbil*. To discontinue, withdraw gradually over 1 week or longer.

▷ *pregabalin (GABA analog)* **(C)(V)**
Pediatric: <12 years: not recommended; ≥12 years: same as adult
 Lyrica initially 50 mg tid; may titrate to 100 mg tid within one week; max 600 mg divided tid; discontinue over 1 week
  Cap: 25, 50, 75, 100, 150, 200, 225, 300 mg; *Oral soln:* 20 mg/ml
 Lyrica CR *Tab:* usual dose: 165 mg once daily; may increase to 330 mg/day within 1 week; max 660 mg/day
  Tab: 82.5, 165, 330 mg ext-rel

TRICYCLIC ANTIDEPRESSANTS (TCAs)

Comment: Co-administration of TCAs with SSRIs requires extreme caution.
▷ *amitriptyline* **(C)(G)** titrate to achieve pain relief; max 300 mg/day
Pediatric: <12 years: not recommended; ≥12 years: same as adult
 Tab: 10, 25, 50, 75, 100, 150 mg
▷ *amoxapine* **(C)** titrate to achieve pain relief; if total dose exceeds 300 mg/day, give in divided doses; max 400 mg/day
Pediatric: <12 years: not recommended; ≥12 years: same as adult
 Tab: 25, 50, 100, 150 mg
▷ *desipramine* **(C)(G)** titrate to achieve pain relief; max 300 mg/day
Pediatric: <12 years: not recommended; ≥12 years: same as adult
 Norpramin *Tab:* 10, 25, 50, 75, 100, 150 mg
▷ *doxepin* **(C)(G)** titrate to achieve pain relief; max 150 mg/day
Pediatric: <12 years: not recommended; ≥12 years: same as adult
 Cap: 10, 25, 50, 75, 100, 150 mg; *Oral conc:* 10 mg/ml (4 oz w. dropper)
▷ *imipramine* **(C)(G)**
Pediatric: <12 years: not recommended; ≥12 years: same as adult
 Tofranil titrate to achieve pain relief; max 200 mg/day; adolescents max 100 mg/day; if maintenance dose exceeds 75 mg/day, may switch to **Tofranil PM** at bedtime
  Tab: 10, 25, 50 mg
 Tofranil PM titrate to achieve pain relief; initially 75 mg at HS; max 200 mg at HS
  Cap: 75, 100, 125, 150 mg
 Tofranil Injection 50 mg IM; lower dose for adolescents; switch to oral form as soon as possible
  Amp: 25 mg/2 ml (2 ml)
▷ *nortriptyline* **(D)(G)** titrate to achieve pain relief; initially 10-25 mg tid-qid; max 150 mg/day; lower doses for elderly and adolescents
Pediatric: <12 years: not recommended; ≥12 years: same as adult
 Pamelor titrate to achieve pain relief; max 150 mg/day
  Cap: 10, 25, 50, 75 mg; *Oral soln:* 10 mg/5 ml (16 oz)
▷ *protriptyline* **(C)** titrate to achieve pain relief; initially 5 mg tid; max 60 mg/day
Pediatric: <12 years: not recommended; ≥12 years: same as adult
 Vivactil *Tab:* 5, 10 mg
▷ *trimipramine* **(C)** titrate to achieve pain relief; max 200 mg/day
Pediatric: <12 years: not recommended; ≥12 years: same as adult
 Surmontil *Cap:* 25, 50, 100 mg

 DIABETIC RETINOPATHY

VASCULAR ENDOTHELIAL GROWTH FACTOR (VEGF) INHIBITOR

Comment: Diabetic retinopathy is the leading cause of blindness among working-age adults in the US. **Lucentis** *(ranibizumab)* is only one FDA-approved drug for the treatment of diabetic retinopathy. Additional labeled indications include treatment of diabetic macular edema (DME), treatment of neovascular (wet) age-related macular degeneration (AMD), treatment of macular edema following retinal vein occlusion (RVO), and treatment of myopic choroidal neovascularization (mCNV).

▷ *ranibizumab* (D)

Pediatric: <18 years: not established; ≥18 years: same as adult

DR: *Diabetic retinopathy:* Intravitreal: 0.3 mg once a month (approximately every 28 days)

DME: *Diabetic macular edema:* Intravitreal: 0.3 mg once a month (approximately every 28 days); in clinical trials, monthly doses of 0.5 mg were also studied

AMD: *Neovascular (wet) Age-related Macular Degeneration:* Intravitreal: 0.5 mg once a month (approximately every 28 days). Frequency may be reduced (e.g., 4 to 5 injections over 9 months) after the first 3 injections or may be reduced after the first 4 injections to once every 3 months if monthly injections are not feasible. *Note:* A regimen averaging 4 to 5 doses over 9 months is expected to maintain visual acuity and an every 3-month dosing regimen has reportedly resulted in a ~5 letter (1 line) loss of visual acuity over 9 months, as compared to monthly dosing which may result in an additional ~1 to 2 letter gain

RVO: *macular edema following retinal vein occlusion:* Intravitreal: 0.5 mg once a month (approximately every 28 days)

mCNV: *myopic choroidal neovascularization:* Intravitreal: 0.5 mg once a month (approximately every 28 days) for up to 3 months; may re-treat if necessary

   Lucentis *Prefilled Syringe:* 0.3 mg/0.05 mL (0.05 ml); 0.5 mg/0.05 ml (0.05 ml); for intravitreal injection (preservative free); *Vial:* 10 mg/ml (**Lucentis** 0.5 mg); 6 mg/ml solution (**Lucentis** 0.3 mg); single-use; a 5-micron sterile filter needle (19 gauge x 1½ inch) is required for preparation, but not included; keep refrigerated; do not freeze; protect vial from light; see mfr pkg insert for other precautions

Comment: *ranibizumab* is a recombinant humanized monoclonal antibody fragment which binds to and inhibits human vascular endothelial growth factor A (VEGF-A). **Lucentis** inhibits VEGF from binding to its receptors and thereby suppressing neovascularization and slowing vision loss. Contraindications include ocular or periocular infection, and active intraocular inflammation. For ophthalmic intravitreal injection only. Each vial or prefilled syringe should only be used for the treatment of a single eye. If the contralateral eye requires treatment, a new vial or prefilled syringe should be used and the sterile field, syringe, gloves, drapes, eyelid speculum, filter, and injection needles should be changed before **Lucentis** is administered to the other eye. Adequate anesthesia and a topical broad-spectrum antimicrobial agent should be administered prior to the procedure. Refer to manufacturer labeling for additional detailed information. Based on its mechanism of action, adverse effects on pregnancy would be expected. Information related to use in pregnancy is limited. The intravitreal injection procedure should be carried out under controlled aseptic conditions, which include the use of sterile gloves, a sterile drape, and a sterile eyelid speculum (or equivalent). Adequate anesthesia and a broad-spectrum microbicide should be given prior to the injection. Prior to and 30 minutes following the intravitreal injection, patients should be monitored for elevation in intraocular pressure using tonometry. Each prefilled syringe or vial should only be used for the treatment of a single eye. If the contralateral eye requires treatment, a new prefilled syringe or vial should be used and the sterile field, syringe, gloves, drapes, eyelid speculum, filter needle (vial only), and injection needles should be changed.

REFERENCE

Solomon, SD, Chew, E, Duh, EJ, et al. Diabetic retinopathy: A position statement by the American Diabetes Association [published online February 21, 2017]. ADA.

DIAPER RASH

Topical Corticosteroids *see page* 566
Comment: Low to intermediate potency topical corticosteroids are indicated if inflammation is present.

BARRIER AGENTS

▷ *aloe+vitamin E+zinc oxide* ointment apply at each diaper change after thoroughly cleansing skin
    Balmex *Oint:* 2, 4 oz tube; 16 oz jar
▷ *vitamin A and D* (G) ointment apply at each diaper change after thoroughly cleansing skin
    A&D Ointment *Oint:* 1.5, 4 oz
▷ *zinc oxide* (G) cream and ointment apply at each diaper change after thoroughly cleansing the skin
    A&D Ointment with Zinc Oxide *Oint:* 10% (1.5, 4 oz)
    Desitin *Oint:* 40% (1, 2, 4, 9 oz)
    Desitin Cream *Crm:* 10% (2, 4 oz)

TOPICAL ANTIFUNGALS

Comment: Use if caused by *Candida albicans*.
▷ *butenafine* (B)(G) apply bid x 1 week <u>or</u> once daily x 4 weeks
Pediatric: <12 years: not recommended; ≥12 years: same as adult
    Lotrimin Ultra (C)(OTC) *Crm:* 1% (12, 24 gm)
    Mentax *Crm:* 1% (15, 30 gm)
Comment: *butenafine* is a benzylamine, not an azole. Fungicidal activity continues for at least 5 weeks after last application.
▷ *clotrimazole* (B) apply to affected area bid x 7 days
Pediatric: same as adult
    Lotrimin (OTC) *Crm:* 1% (15, 30, 45 gm)
    Lotrimin AF (OTC) *Crm:* 1% (12 gm); *Lotn:* 1% (10 ml); *Soln:* 1% (10 ml)
▷ *econazole* (C) apply bid x 7 days
    Spectazole *Crm:* 1% (15, 30, 85 gm)
▷ *ketoconazole* (C)(G)
    Nizoral Cream *Crm:* 2% (15, 30, 60 gm)
▷ *miconazole* 2% (C)(G) apply bid x 7 days
Pediatric: same as adult
    Lotrimin AF Spray Liquid (OTC) *Spray liq:* 2% (113 gm) (alcohol 17%)
    Lotrimin AF Spray Powder (OTC) *Spray pwdr:* 2% (90 gm) (alcohol 10%)
    Monistat-Derm *Crm:* 2% (1, 3 oz); *Spray liq:* 2% (3.5 oz); *Spray pwdr:* 2% (3 oz)
▷ *nystatin* (C)(G) apply bid x 7 days
    Mycostatin *Crm:* 100,000 U/gm (15, 30 gm)

COMBINATION AGENT

▷ *clotrimazole+betamethasone* (C)(G) cream apply bid x 7 days
    Lotrisone *Crm:* 15, 45 g

 DIARRHEA: ACUTE

▷ *attapulgite* (C)
    Donnagel (OTC) 30 ml after each loose stool; max 7 doses/day x 2 days
    Pediatric: <3 years: not recommended; 3-6 years: 7.5 ml; >6-12 years: 15 ml; >12 years: same as adult

Liq: 600 mg/15 ml (120, 240 ml)

Donnagel Chewable Tab (OTC) 2 tabs after each loose stool; max 14 tabs/day
Pediatric: <3 years: not recommended; 3-6 years: 1/2 tab after each loose stool; max 7 doses/day; >6-12 years: 1 tab after each loose stool; max 7 tabs/day
   Chew tab: 600 mg

Kaopectate (OTC) 30 ml after each loose stool; max 7 doses/day x 2 days
Pediatric: <3 years: not recommended; 3-6 years: 7.5 ml after each loose stool; >6-12 years: 15 ml after each loose stool; >12 years: same as adult
   Liq: 600 mg/15 ml (120, 240 ml)

▷ *bismuth subsalicylate* (C; D in 3rd)(G)

Pepto-Bismol (OTC) 2 tabs or 30 ml q 30-60 minutes as needed; max 8 doses/day
Pediatric: <3 years (14-18 lb): 2.5 ml q 4 hours; max 6 doses/day; <3 years (18-28 lb): 5 ml q 4 hours; max 6 doses/day; 3-6 years: 1/3 tab or 5 ml 30-60 minutes; max 8 doses/day; >6-9 years: 2/3 tab or 10 ml q 30-60 minutes; max 8 doses/day; >9-12 years: 1 tab or 15 ml q 30-60 minutes; max 8 doses/day
   Chew tab: 262 mg; *Liq:* 262 mg/15 ml (4, 8, 12, 16 oz)

Pepto-Bismol Maximum Strength (OTC) 30 ml q 60 minutes; max 4 doses/day
Pediatric: <3 years: not recommended; 3-6 years: 5 ml q 60 minutes; max 4 doses/day; >6-9 years: 10 ml q 60 minutes; max 4 doses/day; >9-12 years: 15 ml q 60 minutes; max 4 doses/day
   Liq: 525 mg/15 ml (4, 8, 12, 16 oz)

Comment: *aspirin*-containing medications are contraindicated with history of allergic-type reaction to *aspirin*, children and adolescents with *Varicella* or other viral illness, and 3rd trimester of pregnancy.

▷ *calcium polycarbophil* (C)
Pediatric: <6 years: not recommended; 6-12 years: 1 tab daily qid; >12 years: same as adult

Fibercon (OTC) 2 tabs daily qid
   Cplt: 625 mg

▷ *crofelemer* (C) 2 tabs once daily; swallow whole with or without food; do not crush or chew
Pediatric: <12 years: not established; ≥12 years: same as adult

Mytesi *Tab:* 125 mg del-rel

Comment: *crofelemer* is indicated for the symptomatic relief of non-infectious diarrhea in adult patients with HIV/AIDS on antiretroviral therapy.

▷ *difenoxin+atropine* (C)
Pediatric: <2 years: not recommended; ≥2 years: same as adult

Motofen 2 tabs, then 1 tab after each loose stool or 1 tab q 3-4 hours as needed; max 8 tab/day x 2 days
   Tab: dif 1 mg+atro 0.025 mg

▷ *diphenoxylate+atropine* (C)(V)(G)
Pediatric: <2 years: not recommended; 2-12 years: initially 0.3-0.4 mg/kg/day in 4 divided doses; >12 years: same as adult

Lomotil 2 tabs or 10 ml qid until diarrhea is controlled
   Tab: diphen 2.5 mg+atrop 0.025 mg; *Liq:* diphen 2.5 mg+atrop 0.025 mg per 5 ml (2 oz)

▷ *loperamide* (B)(OTC)(G)

Imodium 4 mg initially, then 2 mg after each loose stool; max 16 mg/day x 2 days
Pediatric: <5 years: not recommended; ≥5 years: same as adult
   Cap: 2 mg

Imodium A-D 4 mg initially, then 2 mg after each loose stool; usual max 8 mg/day x 2 days
Pediatric: <2 years: not recommended; 2-5 years (24-47 lb): 1 mg up to tid x 2 days; 6-8 years (48-59 lb): 2 mg initially, then 1 mg after each loose stool; max 4

mg/day x 2 days; 9-11 years (60-95 lb): 2 mg initially, then 1 mg after each loose stool; max 6 mg/day x 2 days

Cplt: 2 mg; *Liq:* 1 mg/5 ml (2, 4 oz) (cherry-mint) (alcohol 0.5%)

▷ *loperamide+simethicone* (B)(OTC)(G)

Imodium Advanced 2 tabs chewed after loose stool, then 1 after the next loose stool; max 4 tabs/day

Pediatric: 6-8 years: chew 1 tab after loose stool, then chew 1/2 tab after next loose stool; 9-11 years: chew 1 tab after loose stool, then chew 1/2 tab after next loose stool; max 3 tabs/day; ≥12 years: same as adult

Chew tab: loper 2 mg+*simeth* 125 mg (vanilla-mint)

ORAL REHYDRATION AND ELECTROLYTE REPLACEMENT THERAPY

▷ *oral electrolyte replacement* (OTC)

CeraLyte 50 dissolve in 8 oz water

Pediatric: <4 years: not indicated; ≥4 years, same as adult

Pkt: sodium 50 mEq+*potassium* 20 mEq+*chloride* 40 mEq+*citrate* 30 mEq+*rice syrup solids* 40 gm+*calories* 190 per liter (mixed berry) (gluten-free)

CeraLyte 70 dissolved in 8 oz water

Pediatric: <4 years: not indicated; ≥4 years: same as adult

Pkt: sodium 70 mEq+*potassium* 20 mEq+*chloride* 60 mEq+*citrate* 30 mEq+*rice syrup solids* 40 gm+*calories* 165 per liter (natural, lemon) (gluten-free)

KaoLectrolyte 1 pkt dissolved in 8 oz water q 3-4 hours

Pediatric: <2 years: not indicated; ≥2 years: same as adult

Pkt: sodium 12 mEq+*potassium* 5 mEq+*chloride* 10 mEq+*citrate* 7 mEq+ *dextrose* 5 gm+*calories* 22 per 6.2 gm

Pedialyte

Pediatric: <2 years: as desired and as tolerated; ≥2 years: 1-2 L/day

Oral soln: dextrose 20 gm+*fructose* 5 gm+*sodium* 25 mEq+*potassium* 20 mEq+*chloride* 35 mEq+*citrate* 30 mEq+*calories* 100 per liter (8 oz, 1 L)

Pedialyte Freezer Pops

Pediatric: as desired and as tolerated

Pops: dextrose 1.6 gm+*sodium* 2.8 mEq+*potassium* 1.25 mEq+*chloride* 2.2 mEq+*citrate* 1.88 mEq+*calories* 6.25 per 6.25 ml pop (8 oz, 1 L)

 DIARRHEA: CARCINOID SYNDROME

TRIPTOPHAN HYDROXYLASE

▷ *telotristat* take with food; 250 mg tid

Pediatric: <18 years: not established; ≥18 years: same as adult

Xermelo *Tab:* 250 mg (4 x 7 daily dose pcks/carton)

Comment: Take **Xermelo** in combination with somatostatin analog (SSA) therapy to treat patients inadequately controlled by SSA therapy. Breastfeeding females should monitor the infant for constipation. ESRD requiring dialysis not studied.

 DIARRHEA: CHRONIC

▷ *cholestyramine* (C)

Questran Powder for Oral Suspension initially 1 pkt or scoop daily; usual maintenance 2-4 pkts or scoops daily in 2 doses; max 6 pkts or scoops daily

Oral pwdr: 9 gm pkts; 9 gm equal 4 gm *anhydrous cholestyramine resin* (60/pck); *Bulk can:* 378 gm w. scoop

Questran Light initially 1 pkt <u>or</u> scoop daily; usual maintenance 2-4 pkts <u>or</u> scoops daily in 2 doses

Light: 5 gm pkts; 5 gm equals 4 gm *anhydrous cholestyramine resin* (60/pck); *Bulk can:* 210 gm w. scoop

Comment: Use *cholestyramine* only if diarrhea is due to bile salt malabsorption.

▷ *crofelemer* **(C)** 2 tabs once daily; swallow whole with <u>or</u> without food; do not crush <u>or</u> chew

Pediatric: <12 years: not established; ≥12 years: same as adult

Mytesi *Tab:* 125 mg del-rel

Comment: *crofelemer* is indicated for the symptomatic relief of non-infectious diarrhea in adult patients with HIV/AIDS on antiretroviral therapy.

▷ *difenoxin+atropine* **(C)** 2 tabs, then 1 tab after each loose stool <u>or</u> 1 tab q 3-4 hours prn; max 8 tab/day x 2 days

Pediatric: <2 years: not recommended; ≥2 years: same as adult

Motofen *Tab:* dif 1 mg+atrop 0.025 mg

▷ *diphenoxylate+atropine* **(B)(V)(G)**

Pediatric: <2 years: not recommended; 2-12 years: initially 0.3-0.4 mg/kg/day in 4 divided doses; >12 years: same as adult

Lomotil 5-20 mg/day in divided doses

Tab: diphen 2.5 mg+atrop 0.025 mg; *Liq:* diphen 2.5 mg+atrop 0.025 mg per 5 ml (2 oz w. dropper)

▷ *attapulgite* **(C)(G)**

Donnagel (OTC) 30 ml after each loose stool; max 7 doses/day

Pediatric: <2 years: not recommended; 2-6 years: 7.5 ml after each loose stool; >6 years: same as adult

Liq: 600 mg/15 ml (120, 240 ml)

Donnagel Chewable Tab 2 tabs after each loose stool; max 14 tabs/day

Pediatric: <3 years: not recommended; 3-6 years: 1/2 tab after each stool; max 7 doses/day; >6-12 years: 1 tab after each loose stool; max 7 tabs/day; >12 years: same as adult

▷ *loperamide* **(B)(OTC)(G)**

Imodium (OTC) 4-16 mg/day in divided doses

Pediatric: <5 years: not recommended; ≥5 years: same as adult

Cap: 2 mg

Imodium A-D (OTC) 4-16 mg/day in divided doses

Pediatric: <2 years: not recommended; 2-5 years (24-47 lb): 1 mg up to tid x 2 days; 6-8 years (48-59 lb): 2 mg initially, then 1 mg after each loose stool; max 4 mg/day x 2 days; 9-11 years (60-95 lb): 2 mg initially, then 1 mg after each loose stool; max 6 mg/day x 2 days; ≥12 years: same as adult

Cplt: 2 mg; *Liq:* 1 mg/5 ml (2, 4 oz)

▷ *loperamide+simethicone* **(B)(OTC)(G)**

Imodium Advanced 2 tabs chewed after loose stool, then 1 after the next loose stool; max 4 tabs/day

Pediatric: 6-8 years: chew 1 tab after loose stool, then chew 1/2 tab after next loose stool; 9-11 years: chew 1 tab after loose stool, then chew 1/2 tab after next loose stool; max 3 tabs/day

Chew tab: loper 2 mg+simeth 125 mg

◯ DIARRHEA: TRAVELER'S

ANTI-INFECTIVES

▷ *ciprofloxacin* **(C)** 500 mg bid x 3 days

Pediatric: <18 years: not recommended; ≥18 years: same as adult

Cipro (G) *Tab:* 250, 500, 750 mg; *Oral susp:* 250, 500 mg/5 ml (100 ml) (strawberry)
Cipro XR *Tab:* 500, 1000 mg ext-rel
ProQuin XR *Tab:* 500 mg ext-rel

▷ *rifaximin* (C) 200 mg tid x 3 days; discontinue if diarrhea worsens <u>or</u> persists more than 24 hours; not for use if diarrhea is accompanied by fever <u>or</u> blood in the stool <u>or</u> if causative organism other than *E. coli* is suspected.
Pediatric: <12 years: not recommended; ≥12 years: same as adult
Xifaxan *Tab:* 200 mg

▷ *trimethoprim+sulfamethoxazole (TMP-SMX)* (C)(G) bid x 10 days
Pediatric: <2 months: not recommended; ≥2 months: 40 mg/kg/day of *sulfamethoxazole* in 2 divided doses x 10 days; *see page 648* for dose by weight
Bactrim, Septra 2 tabs bid x 10 days
Tab: trim 80 mg+*sulfa* 400 mg*
Bactrim DS, Septra DS 1 tab bid x 10 days
Tab: trim 160 mg+*sulfa* 800 mg*
Bactrim Pediatric Suspension, Septra Pediatric Suspension
Oral susp: trim 40 mg+*sulfa* 200 mg per 5 ml (100 ml) (cherry) (alcohol 0.3%)

 DIGITALIS TOXICITY

Comment: The digitalis therapeutic index is narrow, 0.8-1.2 ng/mL. Whether acute <u>or</u> chronic toxicity, the patient should be treated in the emergency department <u>and/or</u> admitted to in-patient service for continued monitoring and care. Signs and symptoms of digitalis toxicity include: loss of appetite, nausea, vomiting, abdominal pain, diarrhea, visual disturbances (diplopia, blurred, <u>or</u> yellow vision, yellow-green halos around lights and other visual images, spots, blind spots), decreased urine output, generalized edema, orthopnea, confusion, delirium, decreased consciousness, potentially lethal cardiac arrhythmias (ranging from ventricular tachycardia (VT) and ventricular fibrillation (VF) to sino-atrial heart block AVB). Treatment measures include repeated doses of charcoal via NG tube administered after gastric lavage for acute ingestion (methods to induce vomiting are usually discouraged because vomiting can worsen bradyarrhythmias), digitalis binders. Monitoring includes: serial ECGs, serum digitalis level, chemistries, potassium (hyperkalemia), magnesium (hypomagnesemia), BUN and creatinine.

DIGOXIN BINDER

▷ *digoxin (immune fab [ovine])* (B)
Digibind contents of one vial of **Digibind** neutralizes 0.5 mg digoxin; dose based on amount of *digoxin* <u>or</u> *digitoxin* to be neutralized; see mfr pkg insert
Pediatric: see mfr pkg insert
Vial: 38 mg
Digifab dose is based on amount of digoxin <u>or</u> digitoxin to be neutralized (see mfr pkg insert for dosage; contents of 1 vial neutralizes 0.5 mg digoxin.
Pediatric: see mfr pkg insert
Vial: 40 mg for IV injection after reconstitution (preservative-free)

DIPHTHERIA

Prophylaxis *see Childhood Immunizations page 546*

POST-EXPOSURE PROPHYLAXIS FOR NON-IMMUNIZED PERSONS

▷ *erythromycin base* **(B)(G)** 500 mg qid x 14 days
    Pediatric: <45 kg: 50 mg/kg/day in 4 divided doses x 14 days; ≥45 kg: same as adult
        Ery-Tab *Tab:* 250, 333, 500 mg ent-coat
        PCE *Tab:* 333, 500 mg
Comment: *erythromycin* may increase INR with concomitant *warfarin*, as well as increase serum level of *digoxin*, benzodiazepines and statins.
▷ *erythromycin ethylsuccinate* **(B)(G)** 400 mg qid x 14 days
    Pediatric: 30-50 mg/kg/day in 4 divided doses x 14 days; may double dose with severe infection; max 100 mg/kg/day; *see page 635 for dose by weight*
        EryPed *Oral susp:* 200 mg/5 ml (100, 200 ml) (fruit); 400 mg/5 ml (60, 100, 200 ml) (banana); *Oral drops:* 200, 400 mg/5 ml (50 ml) (fruit); *Chew tab:* 200 mg wafer (fruit)
        E.E.S. *Oral susp:* 200, 400 mg/5 ml (100 ml) (fruit)
        E.E.S. Granules *Oral susp:* 200 mg/5 ml (100, 200 ml) (cherry)
        E.E.S. 400 Tablets *Tab:* 400 mg
Comment: *erythromycin* may increase INR with concomitant *warfarin*, as well as increase serum level of *digoxin*, benzodiazepines and statins.
▷ *Immunization Series*
    See Childhood Immunizations page 546

POST-EXPOSURE PROPHYLAXIS FOR IMMUNIZED PERSONS

▷ *Diphtheria* immunization booster

 DIVERTICULITIS

ANTI-INFECTIVES

▷ *amoxicillin* **(B)(G)** 500 mg q 8 hours or 875 mg q 12 hours x 7 days
    Amoxil *Cap:* 250, 500 mg; *Tab:* 875*mg; *Chew tab:* 125, 200, 250, 400 mg (cherry-banana-peppermint) (phenylalanine); *Oral susp:* 125, 250 mg/5 ml (80, 100, 150 ml) (strawberry); 200, 400 mg/5 ml (50, 75, 100 ml) (bubble gum); *Oral drops:* 50 mg/ml (30 ml) (bubble gum)
    Moxatag *Tab:* 775 mg ext-rel
    Trimox *Tab:* 125, 250 mg; *Cap:* 250, 500 mg; *Oral susp:* 125, 250 mg/5 ml (80, 100, 150 ml) (raspberry-strawberry)
▷ *amoxicillin+clavulanate* **(B)(G)**
    Augmentin 500 mg tid or 875 mg bid x 7-10 days
    Pediatric: 40-45 mg/kg/day divided tid x 10 days or 90 mg/kg/day divided bid x 10 days *see pages 618-619 for dose by weight*
        Tab: 250, 500, 875 mg; *Chew tab:* 125, 250 mg (lemon-lime); 200, 400 mg (cherry-banana) (phenylalanine); *Oral susp:* 125 mg/5 ml (banana), 250 mg/5 ml (75, 100, 150 ml) (orange); 200, 400 mg/5 ml (50, 75, 100 ml) (orange) (phenylalanine)
    Augmentin ES-600 not recommended for adults
    Pediatric: <3 months: not recommended; ≥3 months, <40 kg: 90 mg/kg/day in 2 divided doses x 7-10 days; ≥40 kg: not recommended
        Oral susp: 42.9 mg/5 ml (50, 75, 100, 125, 150, 200 ml) (strawberry cream) (phenylalanine)
    Augmentin XR 2 tabs q 12 hours x 7-10 days
    Pediatric: <16 years: use other forms; ≥16 years: same as adult
        Tab: 1000*mg ext-rel

▷ **ciprofloxacin (C)** 500 mg bid x 7 days
    Cipro (G) *Tab:* 250, 500, 750 mg; *Oral susp:* 250, 500 mg/5 ml (100 ml)
    (strawberry)
    Cipro XR *Tab:* 500, 1000 mg ext-rel
    ProQuin XR *Tab:* 500 mg ext-rel
▷ **metronidazole (not for use in 1st; B in 2nd, 3rd)(G)** 250-500 mg q 8 hours or 750 mg
  q 12 hours x 7 days
    Flagyl *Tab:* 250*, 500*mg
    Flagyl 375 *Cap:* 375 mg
    Flagyl ER *Tab:* 750 mg ext-rel
▷ **trimethoprim+sulfamethoxazole (TMP-SMX) (D)(G)** bid x 7 days
    Bactrim, Septra 2 tabs bid x 7 days
      Tab: trim 80 mg+*sulfa* 400 mg*
    Bactrim DS, Septra DS 1 tab bid x 7 days
      Tab: trim 160 mg+*sulfa* 800 mg*
    Bactrim Pediatric Suspension, Septra Pediatric Suspension 20 ml bid x 7 days
      Oral susp: trim 40 mg+sulfa 200 mg per 5 ml (100 ml) (cherry) (alcohol 0.3%)

 DIVERTICULOSIS

BULK-PRODUCING AGENTS
*see **Constipation** page* 102

 DRY EYE SYNDROME

OPHTHALMIC IMMUNOMODULATOR/ANTI-INFLAMMATORY

▷ **cyclosporine (C)** 1 drop q 12 hours
  Pediatric: <16 years: not recommended; ≥16 years: same as adult
    Restasis *Ophth emul:* 0.05% (0.4 ml) (preservative-free)
Comment: Ophthalmic Immunomodulators are contraindicated with active ocular
infection. Allow at least 15 minutes between doses of artificial tears. May re-insert
contact lenses 15 minutes after treatment.

OCULAR LUBRICANTS
Comment: Remove contact lens prior to using an ocular lubricant.
▷ **dextran 70+hypromellose** 1-2 drops prn
  Pediatric: same as adult
    Bion Tears (OTC) *Ophth soln:* single-use containers (28/pck) (preservative-free)
▷ **hydroxypropyl cellulose apply** 1/2 inch ribbon or 1 insert in each inferior cul-de-sac
  1-2 x/day prn
  Pediatric: same as adult
    Lacrisert *Ophth inserts:* 5 mg (60/pck) (preservative-free)
    Hypotears Ophthalmic Ointment (OTC) *Ophth oint:* 1% (3.5 gm)
    (preservative-free)
Comment: Place insert in the inferior cul-de-sac of the eye, beneath the base of the tarsus,
not in apposition to the cornea nor beneath the eyelid at the level of the tarsal plate.
▷ **hydroxypropyl methylcellulose** 1-2 drops prn
  Pediatric: same as adult
    GenTeal Mild, GenTeal Moderate (OTC) *Ophth soln:* (15 ml) (perborate)
    GenTeal Severe (OTC) *Ophth soln:* (15 ml) (carbopol 980, perborate)

➢ *petrolatum+mineral oil* apply 1/2 inch ribbon prn
　Pediatric: same as adult
　　Hypotears Ophthalmic Ointment (OTC) *Ophth oint:* 1% (3.5 gm) (benzalkonium chloride, alcohol 1%)
　　Hypotears PF Ophthalmic Ointment (OTC) *Ophth oint:* 1% (3.5 gm) (preservative-free, alcohol 1%)
　　Lacri-Lube (OTC) *Ophth oint:* 1% (3.5, 7 gm)
　　Lacri-Lube NP (OTC) *Ophth oint:* 1% (0.7 gm, 24/pck) (preservative-free)
➢ *petrolatum+lanolin+mineral oil* apply 1/4 inch ribbon prn
　Pediatric: same as adult
　　Duratears Naturale (OTC) *Ophth oint:* 3.5 gm (preservative-free)
➢ *polyethylene glycol+glycerin+hydroxypropyl methylcellulose* 1-2 drops prn
　Pediatric: same as adult
　　Visine Tears (OTC) *Ophth soln:* 1% (15, 30 ml)
➢ *polyethylene glycol* 400 0.4%*+propylene glycol* 0.3% 1-2 drops prn
　Pediatric: same as adult
　　Systane (OTC) *Ophth soln:* (15, 30, 40 ml) (polyquaternium-1, zinc chloride); *Vial:* 0.01 oz (28) (preservative-free)
　　Systane Ultra (OTC) *Ophth soln:* (10, 20 ml) (aminomethylpropanol, polyquaternium-1, sorbitol (zinc chloride); *Vial:* 0.01 oz (24) (preservative-free)
➢ *polyvinyl alcohol* 1-2 drops prn
　Pediatric: same as adult
　　Hypotears (OTC) *Ophth soln:* 1% (15, 30 ml)
　　Hypotears PF (OTC) 1-2 drops q 3-4 hours prn
　　　Ophth soln: 1% (0.02 oz single-use containers, 30/pck) (preservative-free)
➢ *propylene glycol* 0.6% 1-2 drops prn
　Pediatric: same as adult
　　Systane Balance (OTC) *Ophth soln:* (10 ml) (polyquaternium-1)

DUCHENNE MUSCULAR DYSTROPHY (DMD)

➢ *deflazacort* (B) 0.9 mg/kg/day administered once daily; take with <u>or</u> without food; may crush and mix with applesauce (then take immediately)
　Pediatric: <5 years: not established; ≥ 5 years: same as adult
　　Emflaza *Tab:* 6, 18, 30, 36 mg; *Oral susp:* 22.75 mg/ml (13 ml)
Comment: (**Emflaza**) is the first and only FDA-approved indicated for DMD to decrease inflammation and reduce the activity of the immune system. The side effects caused by **Emflaza** are similar to those experienced with other corticosteroids. The most common side effects include facial puffiness (cushingoid appearance), weight gain, increased appetite, upper respiratory tract infection, cough, extraordinary daytime urinary frequency (pollakiuria), hirsutism, and central obesity. Other side effects that are less common include problems with endocrine function, increased susceptibility to infection, elevation in blood pressure, risk of gastrointestinal perforation, serious skin rashes, behavioral and mood changes, decrease in the density of the bones and vision problems such as cataracts. Patients receiving immunosuppressive doses of corticosteroids should not be given live <u>or</u> live attenuated vaccines (LAVs). Moderate <u>or</u> strong CYP3A4 inhibitors, give one third of the recommended dosage of **Emflaza**. Avoid use of moderate <u>or</u> strong CYP3A4 inducers with **Emflaza**, as they may reduce efficacy. Dosage must be decreased gradually if the drug has been administered for more than a few days. Use only the oral dispenser provided with the product. After withdrawing the appropriate dose into the oral dispenser, slowly add the oral suspension into 3 to 4 ounces of juice <u>or</u> milk and mix well and then the dose should then be administered immediately. Do not administer

with grapefruit. Discard any unused **Emflaza** oral suspension remaining after 1 month of first opening the bottle.

REFERENCE
FDA News Release: FDA approves drug to treat Duchenne muscular dystrophy (2/9/17) https://www.fda.gov/
NewsEvents/Newsroom/PressAnnouncements/ucm540945.htm

 eteplirsen 30 mg/kg via IV infusion over 35-60 minutes once weekly
> *Pediatric:* same as adult
> **Exondys** *Vial:* 100 mg/2 ml (50 mg/ml), 500 mg/10 ml

Comment: Exondys is indicated for patients who have a confirmed mutation of the dystrophin gene amenable to exon 51 skipping (which affects about 13% of patients with DMD.

DYSHIDROSIS (DYSHIDROTIC ECZEMA) POMPHYLOX

Topical Corticosteroids *see page* 566
Comment: Intermediate to high potency ophthalmic steroid treatment is indicated for dyshidrosis.

DYSFUNCTIONAL UTERINE BLEEDING (DUB)

NSAIDs *see page* 562
Opioid Analgesics *see **Pain** page* 345
Oral and Injectable Progesterone-only Contraceptives *page* 558
Combined Oral Contraceptives *page* 538

 medroxyprogesterone acetate (X) 10 mg daily x 10-13 days
> **Provera** *Tab:* 2.5, 5, 10 mg
> *combined oral contraceptive* (X) with 35 mcg estrogen equivalent

DYSLIPIDEMIA (HYPERCHOLESTEROLEMIA, HYPERLIPIDEMIA, MIXED DYSLIPIDEMIA)

Comment: As recommended by the American Heart, Lung, and Blood Institute, children and adolescents should be screened for dyslipidemia once between 9 and 11 years and once between 17 and 21 years.

OMEGA 3-FATTY ACID ETHYL ESTERS

Comment: *Vascepa, Lovaza,* and *Epanova* are indicated for the treatment of TG ≥500 mg/dL.

 icosapent ethyl (omega 3-fatty acid ethyl ester of EPA) (C) 2 caps bid with food; max 4 gm/day; swallow whole, do not crush or chew
> *Pediatric:* <18 years: not recommended; ≥18 years: same as adult
> **Vascepa** *sgc:* 0.5, 1 gm (α-tocopherol 4 mg/cap)
> *omega 3-acid ethyl esters* (C)(G) 2 gm bid or 4 gm once daily; swallow whole, do not crush or chew
> *Pediatric:* <18 years: not recommended; ≥18 years: same as adult
> **Lovaza** *Soft gel cap:* 1 gm (α-tocopherol 4 mg/cap)
> **Epanova** *Gelcap:* 1 gm

MICROSOMAL TRIGLYCERIDE-TRANSFER PROTEIN (MTP) INHIBITOR

➤ *lomitapide mesylate* (X) 10 mg daily
  Pediatric: <12 years: not established; ≥12 years: same as adult
    Juxtapid *Cap:* 5, 10, 20 mg
Comment: **Juxtapid** is an adjunct to low-fat diet and other lipid-lowering treatments, including LDL apheresis where available, to reduce LDL-C, total cholesterol, apoB, and non-HDL-C in patients with homozygous familial hypercholesterolemia (HoFH); not for patients with hypercholesterolemia who do not have HoFH.

OLIGONUCLEOTIDE INHIBITOR OF APO B-100 SYNTHESIS

➤ *mipomersen* (B) administer 200 mg SC once weekly, on the same day, in the upper arm, abdomen, or thigh; administer 1st injection under appropriate professional supervision
  Pediatric: <12 years: not established; ≥12 years: same as adult
    Kynamro *Vial/Prefilled syringe:* 200 mg mg/ml soln for SC inj single-use vial (preservative-free)
Comment: **Kynamro** is an adjunct to low-fat diet and other lipid-lowering treatments, to reduce LDL-C, apo-B, total cholesterol (TC), non-HDL-C in patients with homozygous familial hypercholesterolemia (HoFH).

CHOLESTEROL ABSORPTION INHIBITOR

➤ *ezetimibe* (C)(G) 10 mg daily
  Pediatric: <10 years: not recommended; ≥10 years: same as adult
    Zetia *Tab:* 10 mg
Comment: *ezetimibe* is contraindicated with concomitant statins in liver disease, persistent elevations in serum transaminase, pregnancy, and nursing mothers. Concomitant fibrates are not recommended. Potentiated by *fenofibrate*, *gemfibrozil*, and possibly *cyclosporine*. Separate dosing of bile acid sequestrants is required; take *ezetimibe* at least 2 hours before or 4 hours after.

PROPROTEIN CONVERTASE SUBTILISIN KEXIN TYPE 9 (PCSK9) INHIBITOR

Comment: PCSK9 inhibitors are an adjunct to maximally tolerated statin therapy in persons who require additional lowering of LDL-C. There is currently no information regarding the use of PCSK9 inhibitors in pregnancy or the presence of PCSK9 inhibitors in human milk.

➤ *alirocumab* administer SC in the upper outer arm, abdomen, or thigh; initially 75 mg SC once every 2 weeks; measure LDL 4-8 weeks after initiation or titration; if inadequate response, may increase to 150 mg SC every 2 weeks or 300 mg SC once monthly
  Pediatric: <18 years: not established; ≥18 years: same as adult
    Praluent *Soln for SC inj:* 75, 150 mg/ml single-use prefilled syringe (preservative-free)
Comment: The FDA has approved a new once-monthly 300 mg dosing option for **Praluent** injection, for the treatment of patients with high low-density lipoprotein (LDL) cholesterol. The drug is indicated as an adjunct to diet and statin therapy for patients with heterozygous familial hypercholesterolemia (HeFH) or clinical atherosclerotic cardiovascular disease (ASCVD) who require additional LDL lowering. The most common side effects of **Praluent** include injection site reactions, symptoms of the common cold, and flu-like symptoms. Each 150 mg pen delivers the dose over 20 seconds. A 300 mg once monthly dose = administration of 2 x 150 mg pens. **Praluent** is contraindicated in the 2nd and 3rd trimester of pregnancy.

➤ *evolocumab* administer SC in the upper outer arm, elbow, or thigh; measure LDL 4-8 weeks after initiation; *HeFH or primary hyperlipidemia:* 140 mg SC once every 2 weeks or 420 mg once monthly; *HoFH:* 420 mg once monthly

Pediatric: HeFH, primary hyperlipidemia: not established; HoFH: <13 years: not established; ≥13 years: same as adult

Repatha *Soln for SC inj:* single-use prefilled syringe; 140 mg/syringe; single-use prefilled SureClick autoinjector (140 mg/syringe preservative-free)

Comment: To administer 420 mg of **Repatha**, administer 150 mg SC x 3 within 30 minutes. Although **Repatha**, does not have an assigned pregnancy category, it is contraindicated in pregnancy.

HMG-COA REDUCTASE INHIBITORS (STATINS)

Comment: The statins decrease total cholesterol, LDL-C, TG, and apo-B, and increase HDL-C. Before initiating and at 4-6 weeks, 3 months, and 6 months of therapy, check fasting lipid profile and LFTs. Side effects include myopathy and increased liver enzymes. Relative contraindications include concomitant use of cyclosporine, a macrolide antibiotic, various oral antifungal agents, and CYP-450 inhibitors. An absolute contraindication is active or chronic liver disease.

▷ *atorvastatin* **(X)(G)** initially 10 mg daily; usual range 10-80 mg/day
Pediatric: <10 years: not recommended; ≥10 years (female post-menarche): same as adult
    Lipitor *Tab:* 10, 20, 40, 80 mg

▷ *fluvastatin* **(X)(G)** initially 20-40 mg q HS; usual range 20-80 mg/day
Pediatric: <18 years: not recommended; ≥18 years: same as adult
    Lescol *Cap:* 20, 40 mg
    Lescol XL *Tab:* 80 mg ext-rel

▷ *lovastatin* **(X)**
    Mevacor initially 20 mg daily at evening meal; may increase at 4-week intervals; max 80 mg/day in single or divided doses; if concomitant fibrates, *niacin*, or *CrCl <30 mL/min*, usual max 20 mg/day
    Pediatric: <10 years: not recommended; 10-17 years: initially 10-20 mg daily at evening meal; may increase at 4-week intervals; max 40 mg daily
        Tab: 10, 20, 40 mg
    Altoprev initially 20 mg daily at evening meal; may increase at 4-week intervals; max 60 mg/day; if concomitant fibrates, or *niacin*; >1 gm/day, usual max 40 mg/day; if concomitant *cyclosporine, amiodarone*, or *verapamil*, or *CrCl <30 mL/min*, usual max 20 mg/day
    Pediatric: <20 years: not recommended
        Tab: 10, 20, 40, 60 mg ext-rel

▷ *pitavastatin* **(X)(G)** initially 2 mg q HS; may increase to 4 mg after 4 weeks; max 4 mg/day; if concomitant *erythromycin* or *CrCl <60 ml/min;* 1 mg/day with usual max 2 mg/day; if concomitant rifampin, max 2 mg once daily
Pediatric: <12 years: not established; ≥12 years: same as adult
    Livalo *Tab:* 1, 2, 4 mg
    Nikita *Tab:* 1, 2, 4 mg

▷ *pravastatin* **(X)** initially 10-20 mg q HS; usual range 10-40 mg/day; may start at 40 mg/day
Pediatric: <8 years: not recommended; 8-13 years: 20 mg daily; 14-18 years: 40 mg daily
    Pravachol *Tab:* 10, 20, 40, 80 mg

▷ *rosuvastatin* **(X)(G)** initially 10-20 mg q HS; usual range 5-40 mg/day; adjust at 4-week intervals
Pediatric: <10 years: not recommended; 10-17 years: 5-20 mg/day; max 20 mg/day
    Crestor *Tab:* 5, 10, 20, 40 mg

▷ *simvastatin* **(X)** initially 20 mg q PM; usual range 5-80 mg/day; adjust at 4-week intervals
Pediatric: <10 years: not recommended; ≥10 years (female post-menarche): same as adult
    Zocor *Tab:* 5, 10, 20, 40, 80 mg

CHOLESTEROL ABSORPTION INHIBITOR+HMG-COA REDUCTASE INHIBITOR COMBINATION

➤ *ezetimibe+atorvastatin* (X)(G) Take once daily in the PM; may start at 10/40; swallow whole, do not cut, crush, or chew
  Pediatric: <17 years: not recommended; ≥17 years: same as adult
      Tab: **Liptruzet 10/10** ezet 10 mg+atorva 10 mg
           Liptruzet 10/20 ezet 10 mg+atorva 20 mg
           Liptruzet 10/40 ezet 10 mg+atorva 40 mg
           Liptruzet 10/80 ezet 10 mg+atorva 80 mg
➤ *ezetimibe+simvastatin* (X)(G) Take once daily in the PM; may start at 10/40; swallow whole, do not cut, crush, or chew
  Pediatric: <17 years: not recommended; ≥17 years: same as adult
      Tab: **Vytorin 10/10** *ezet* 10 mg+*simva* 10 mg
           Vytorin 10/20 *ezet* 10 mg+*simva* 20 mg
           Vytorin 10/40 *ezet* 10 mg+*simva* 40 mg
           Vytorin 10/80 *ezet* 10 mg+*simva* 80 mg

Comment: These agents decrease total cholesterol, LDL-C, and TG; increase HDL-C. They are indicated when the primary problem is very high TG level. Side effects include epigastric discomfort, dyspepsia, abdominal pain, cholelithiasis, myopathy, and neutropenia. Before initiating, and at 4-6 weeks, 3 months, and 6 months of therapy, check fasting CBC, lipid profile, LFT, and serum creatinine. Absolute contraindications include severe renal disease and severe hepatic disease.

ISOBUTYRIC ACID DERIVATIVES

➤ *gemfibrozil* (C)(G) 600 mg bid 30 minutes before AM and PM meal
  Pediatric: <12 years: not recommended; ≥12 years: same as adult
      Lopid *Tab:* 600*mg

FIBRATES (FIBRIC ACID DERIVATIVES)

➤ *fenofibrate* (C)(G) take with meals; adjust at 4- to 8-week intervals; discontinue if inadequate response after 2 months; lowest dose or contraindicated with renal impairment and the elderly
  Pediatric: <12 years: not recommended; ≥12 years: same as adult
      Antara 43-130 mg daily; max 130 mg/day
          Cap: 43, 87, 130 mg
      Fenoglide 40-120 mg daily; max 120 mg/day
          Tab: 40, 120 mg
      FibriCor 30-105 mg daily; max 105 mg/day
          Tab: 30, 105 mg
      TriCor 48-145 mg daily; max 145 mg/day
          Tab: 48, 145 mg
      TriLipix 45-135 mg daily; max 135 mg/day
          Cap: 45, 135 mg del-rel
      Lipofen 50-150 mg daily; max 150 mg/day
          Cap: 50, 150 mg
      Lofibra 67-200 mg daily; max 200 mg/day
          Tab: 67, 134, 200 mg

NICOTINIC ACID DERIVATIVES

Comment: Nicotinic acid derivatives decrease total cholesterol, LDL-C, and TG; increase HDL-C. Before initiating and at 4-6 weeks, 3 months, and 6 months of therapy, check fasting lipid profile, LFT, glucose, and uric acid. Side effects include hyperglycemia, upper GI distress, hyperuricemia, hepatotoxicity, and significant transient skin flushing.

Take with food and take **aspirin** 325 mg 30 minutes before **niacin** dose to decrease flushing. *Relative contraindications:* diabetes, hyperuricemia (gout), and PUD Absolute contraindications severe gout and chronic liver disease.

▷ *niacin* (C)

> **Niaspan** (G) 375 mg daily for 1st week, then 500 mg daily for 2nd week, then 750 mg daily for 3rd week, then 1 gm daily for weeks 4-7; may increase by 500 mg q 4 weeks; usual range 1-2 gm/day; max 2 gm/day
>
> *Pediatric:* <21 years: not recommended; ≥21 years: same as adult
>
>> *Tab:* 500, 750, 1000 mg ext-rel
>
> **Slo-Niacin** one 250 or 500 mg tab q AM or HS or one-half 750 mg tab q AM or HS
>
> *Pediatric:* <12 years: not recommended; ≥12 years: same as adult
>
>> *Tab:* 250, 500, 750 mg cont-rel

BILE ACID SEQUESTRANTS

Comment: Bile acid sequestrants decrease total cholesterol, LDL-C, and increase HDL-C, but have no effect on triglycerides. A relative contraindication is TG ≥200 mg/dL and an absolute contraindication is TG ≥400 mg/dL. Before initiating and at 4-6 weeks, 3 months, and 6 months of therapy, check fasting lipid profile. Side effects include sandy taste in mouth, abdominal gas, abdominal cramping, and constipation. These agents decrease the absorption of many other drugs.

▷ *cholestyramine* (C)

Pediatric: see mfr pkg insert

> **Questran Powder for Oral Suspension** initially 1 pkt or scoop daily; usual maintenance 2-4 pkts or scoops daily in 2 divided doses; max 6 pkts or scoops daily
>
>> *Pwdr:* 9 gm pkts; 9 gm equals 4 gm anhydrous *cholestyramine* resin for reconstitution (60/pck); *Bulk can:* 378 gm w. scoop
>
> **Questran Light** initially 1 pkt or scoop daily; usual maintenance 2-4 pkts or scoops daily in 2 doses
>
>> *Light:* 5 gm pkts; 5 gm equals 4 gm anhydrous *cholestyramine* resin (60/pck): *Bulk can:* 210 gm w. scoop

▷ *colesevelam* (B)

> **Monotherapy:** 3 tabs bid or 6 tabs once daily or one 1.875 gm pkt bid or one 3.75 gm pkt once daily
>
> *Pediatric:* <12 years: not recommended; ≥12 years: same as adult
>
> **WelChol** *Tab:* 625 mg; *Pwdr for oral susp:* 1.875 gm pwdr pkts (60/carton); 3.75 gm pwdr pkts (30/carton) (citrus) (phenylalanine)
>
> **Comment:** **WelChol** is indicated as adjunctive therapy to improve glycemic control in adults with type 2 diabetes. It can be added to *metformin*, sulfonylureas, or insulin alone or in combination with other antidiabetic agents

▷ *colestipol* (C)

Comment: *colestipol* lowers LDL and total cholesterol.

Pediatric: <12 years: not recommended; ≥12 years: same as adult

> **Colestid** tabs: 2-16 gm daily in a single or divided doses; granules: 5-30 gm daily in a single or divided dose
>
>> *Tabs:* 1 gm (120); *Granules:* unflavored: 5 gm pkt (30, 90/carton); unflavored bulk: 300, 500 gm w. scoop; orange-flavored: 7.5 gm pkt (60/carton) (aspartame); orange-flavored bulk: 450 gm w. scoop (aspartame) flavored: 7.5 gm pkt; flavored bulk: 450 gm w. scoop
>
> **Colestid Tab** initially 2 gm bid; increase by 2 gm bid at 1-2-month intervals; usual maintenance 2-16 gm/day
>
>> *Tab:* 1 gm

ANTILIPID COMBINATIONS

Nicotinic Acid Derivative+HMG-CoA Reductase Inhibitors Combinations

Comment: Nicotinic acid derivatives decrease total cholesterol, LDL-C, and TG; increase HDL-C. Before initiating and at 4-6 weeks, 3 months, and 6 months of therapy, check fasting lipid profile, LFT, glucose, and uric acid. Side effects include hyperglycemia, upper GI distress, hyperuricemia, hepatotoxicity, and significant transient skin flushing. Take with food and take *aspirin* 325 mg 30 minutes before *niacin* dose to decrease flushing. Relative contraindications: diabetes, hyperuricemia (gout), and PUD. *Absolute contraindications:* severe gout and chronic liver disease.

▷ *niacin+lovastatin* (X)

Pediatric: <18 years: not recommended; ≥18 years: same as adult

Advicor swallow whole at bedtime with a low-fat snack; may pretreat with aspirin; start at lowest niacin dose; may titrate niacin by no more than 500 mg/day every 4 weeks; max 2000/40 daily

Tab: **Advicor 500/20** *nia* 500 mg ext-rel+*lova* 20 mg
Advicor 750/20 *nia* 750 mg ext-rel+*lova* 20 mg
Advicor 1000/20 *nia* 1000 mg ext-rel+*lova* 20 mg
Advicor 1000/40 *nia* 1000 mg ext-rel+*lova* 40 mg

▷ *niacin+simvastatin* (X)

Pediatric: <18 years: not recommended; ≥18 years: same as adult

Simcor swallow whole at bedtime with a low-fat snack; may pretreat with *aspirin*; to reduce niacin reaction. Start at lowest *niacin* dose; may titrate *niacin* by no more than 500 mg/day every 4 weeks; max 2000/40 daily

Tab: **Simcor 500/20** *nia* 500 mg ext-rel+*simva* 20 mg
Simcor 750/20 *nia* 750 mg ext-rel+*simva* 20 mg
Simcor 1000/20 *nia* 1000 mg ext-rel+*simva* 20 mg
Simcor 500/40 *nia* 500 mg ext-rel+*simva* 40 mg
Simcor 1000/40 *nia* 1000 mg ext-rel+*simva* 40 mg

ANTIHYPERTENSIVE+ANTILIPID COMBINATIONS

Calcium Channel Blocker+HMG-CoA Reductase Inhibitor (Statin) Combinations

▷ *amlodipine+atorvastatin* (X)(G)

Caduet select according to blood pressure and lipid values; titrate amlodipine over 7-14 days; titrate atorvastatin according to monitored lipid values; max amlodipine 10 mg/day and max atorvastatin 80 mg/day; refer to contraindications and precautions for CCB and statin therapy

Pediatric: <10 years: not recommended; ≥10 years (female, post-menarche): same as adult

Tab: **Caduet 5/10** amlo 5 mg+ator 10 mg
Caduet 5/20 *amlo* 5 mg+*ator* 20 mg
Caduet 5/40 *amlo* 5 mg+*ator* 40 mg
Caduet 5/80 *amlo* 5 mg+*ator* 80 mg
Caduet 10/10 *amlo* 10 mg+*ator* 10 mg
Caduet 10/20 *amlo* 10 mg+*ator* 20 mg
Caduet 10/40 *amlo* 10 mg+*ator* 40 mg
Caduet 10/80 *amlo* 10 mg+*ator* 80 mg

 DYSMENORRHEA: PRIMARY

NSAIDs *see page 562*
Opioid Analgesics *see Pain page 345*
Combined Oral Contraceptives *see page 548*

BENZENEACETIC ACID DERIVATIVE

▷ *diclofenac* (C) 50-100 mg once; then 50 tid
  Pediatric: <14 years: not recommended; ≥14 years: same as adult
    Cataflam *Tab:* 50 mg
    Voltaren *Tab:* 25, 50, 75 mg ent-coat
    Voltaren-XR *Tab:* 100 mg ext-rel
  Comment: *diclofenac* is contraindicated with *aspirin* allergy and late (≥30 weeks) pregnancy.

FENAMATE

Comment: Avoid *aspirin* with a fenamate.
▷ *mefenamic acid* (C) 500 mg once; then 250 mg q 6 hours for up to 2-3 days; take with food
  Pediatric: <14 years: not recommended; ≥14 years: same as adult
    Ponstel *Cap:* 250 mg

COX-2 INHIBITORS

Comment: Cox-2 inhibitors are contraindicated with history of asthma, urticaria, and allergic-type reactions to *aspirin*, other NSAIDs, and sulfonamides, 3rd trimester of pregnancy, and coronary artery bypass graft (CABG) surgery.
▷ *celecoxib* (C)(G) 400 mg x 1 dose; then 200 mg more on 1st day if needed; then 400 mg daily-bid; max 800 mg/day
  Pediatric: <18 years: not recommended; ≥18 years: same as adult
    Celebrex *Cap:* 50, 100, 200, 400 mg
▷ *meloxicam* (C)(G)
    Mobic <2 years, <60 kg: not recommended; ≥2, >60 kg: 0.125 mg/kg; max 7.5 mg once daily; ≥18 years: initially 7.5 mg once daily; max 15 mg once daily; *Hemodialysis:* max 7.5 mg/day
      Tab: 7.5, 15 mg; *Oral susp:* 7.5 mg/5 ml (100 ml) (raspberry)
    Vivlodex <18 years: not established; ≥18 years: initially 5 mg qd; may increase to max 10 mg/day; *Hemodialysis:* max 5 mg/day
      Cap: 5, 10 mg

 DYSPAREUNIA, POSTMENOPAUSAL PAINFUL INTERCOURSE

Oral and Transdermal Hormonal Therapy *see Menopause page 295*

NON-HORMONAL THERAPY

▷ *prasterone (dehydroepiandrosterone [DHEA])* (X) insert 1 tab intravaginally daily at bedtime
    Intrarosa *Vaginal inserts:* 6.5 mg (20 tabs+28 applicators/carton)
Comment: Intrarosa is the first local (intravaginal) non-estrogen drug approved for moderate-to-severe dyspareunia. **prosterone** is an active endogenous steroid converted into active androgens <u>and/or</u> estrogens.

HORMONAL THERAPY

Comment: Estrogen-alone therapy should not be used for the prevention of cardiovascular Disease <u>or</u> dementia. The Women's Health Initiative (WHI) estrogen-alone sub-study reported increased risks of stroke and deep vein thrombosis (DVT). The WHI Memory Study (WHIMS) estrogen-alone ansillary study of WHI reported an increased risk of probable dementia in postmenopausal women 65 years-of-age and older. *Contraindications:* undiagnosed abnormal genital bleeding, known <u>or</u> suspected estrogen-dependent neoplasia (e.g., breast cancer), active DVT, pulmonary embolism

(PE), or history of these conditions; active arterial thromoembolic disease (e.g., stroke, myocardial infarction [AMI]), or history of these conditions; known or suspected pregnancy; severe hepatic impairment (Child-Pugh Class C).

➢ *estradiol* (X)(G)
   Yuvafem Vaginal Tablet insert one 10 mcg or 25 mcg vaginal tablet once daily x 2 weeks; then twice weekly x 2 weeks (e.g., tues/fri); consider the addition of a progestin with intact uterus
      Vag tab: 10, 25 mcg (8, 18/blister pck with applicator)

ESTROGEN AGONIST-ANTAGONIST

➢ *ospemifene* take 1 tab daily
   Osphena *Tab:* 60 mg
Comment: *ospemifene* is an estrogen agonist-antagonist with tissue selective effects. In the endometrium, OSPHENA has estrogen agonistic effects. There is an increased risk of endometrial cancer in a woman with a uterus who uses unopposed estrogens. Adding a progestin to estrogen therapy reduces the risk of endometrial hyperplasia, which may be a precursor to endometrial cancer. Estrogen-alone therapy has an increased risk of stroke and deep vein thrombosis (DVT). **Osphena** 60 mg had cerebral thromboembolic and hemorrhagic stroke incidence rates of 0.72 and 1.45 per thousand women, respectively vs. 1.04 and 0 per thousand women, respectively in placebo. For DVT, the incidence rate for **Osphena** 60 mg is 1.45 per thousand women vs. 1.04 per thousand women in placebo. Do not use estrogen or estrogen agonist/antagonist concomitantly with **Osphena**. *fluconazole* increases serum concentration of **Osphena**. *rifampin* decreases serum concentration of **Osphena**).

EDEMA

THIAZIDE DIURETICS

➢ *chlorthalidone* (B)(G) initially 30-60 mg daily or 60 mg on alternate days; max 90-120 mg/day
   Thalitone *Tab:* 15 mg
➢ *chlorothiazide* (B)(G) 0.5-1 gm/day in a single or divided doses; max 2 gm/day
   Pediatric: <6 months: up to 15 mg/lb/day in 2 divided doses; ≥6 months: 10 mg/lb/day in 2 divided doses; max 375 mg/day
      Diuril *Tab:* 250*, 500*mg; *Oral susp:* 250 mg/5 ml (237 ml)
➢ *hydrochlorothiazide* (B)(G)
   Pediatric: <12 years: not recommended; ≥12 years: same as adult
      Esidrix 25-200 mg daily
         Tab: 25, 50, 100 mg
      Microzide 12.5 mg daily; usual max 50 mg/day
         Cap: 12.5 mg
➢ *hydroflumethiazide* (B) 50-200 mg/day in a single or 2 divided doses
   Pediatric: <12 years: not recommended; ≥12 years: same as adult
      Saluron *Tab:* 50 mg
➢ *methyclothiazide+deserpidine* (B) initially 2.5 mg daily; max 5 mg daily
   Pediatric: <12 years: not recommended; ≥12 years: same as adult
      Enduronyl *Tab: methy* 5 mg+*deser* 0.25 mg*
      Enduronyl Forte *Tab: methy* 5 mg+*deser* 0.5 mg*
➢ *polythiazide* (C) 1-4 mg daily
   Pediatric: <12 years: not recommended; ≥12 years: same as adult
      Renese *Tab:* 1, 2, 4 mg

POTASSIUM-SPARING DIURETICS

▷ **amiloride** (B)(G) initially 5 mg; may increase to 10 mg; max 20 mg
  Pediatric: <12 years: not recommended; ≥12 years: same as adult
      Tab: 5 mg

▷ **spironolactone** (D) initially 25-200 mg in a single or divided doses; titrate at 2-week intervals
  Pediatric: <12 years: not recommended; ≥12 years: same as adult
      Aldactone (G) *Tab:* 25, 50*, 100*mg
      CaroSpir *Oral susp:* 25 mg/5 ml (118, 473 ml) (banana)

▷ **triamterene** (B) 100 mg bid; max 300 mg
  Pediatric: <12 years: not recommended; ≥12 years: same as adult
      Dyrenium *Cap:* 50, 100 mg

LOOP DIURETICS

▷ **bumetanide** (C)(G) 0.5-2 mg daily; *Tab:* 5 mg; may repeat at 4-5 hour intervals; max 10 mg/day
  Pediatric: <18 years: not recommended; ≥18 years: same as adult
      Tab: 1*mg
  Comment: *bumetanide* is contraindicated with sulfa drug allergy.

▷ **ethacrynic acid** (B)(G) initially 50-100 mg once daily-bid; max 400 mg/day
  Pediatric: Infants: not recommended; ≥1 month: initially 25 mg/day; then adjust dose in 25 mg increments
      Edecrin *Tab:* 25, 50 mg

▷ **ethacrynate sodium** for IV injection (B)(G) administer smallest dose required to produce gradual weight loss (about 1-2 pounds per day); onset of diuresis usually occurs at 50-100 mg in children ≥12 years; after diuresis has been achieved, the minimally effective dose (usually 50-200 mg/day) may be administered on a continuous or intermittent dosage schedule; dose titrations are usually in 25-50 mg increments to avoid derangement electrolyte and water excretion; the patient should be weighed under standard conditions before and during administration of *ethacrynate sodium;* the following schedule may be helpful in determining the lowest effective dose: *Day 1:* 50 mg once daily after a meal; *Day 2:* 50 mg bid after meals, if necessary; *Day 3:* 100 mg in the morning and 50-100 mg following the afternoon or evening meal, depending upon response to the morning dose; a few patients may require initial and maintenance doses as high as 200 mg bid; these higher doses, which should be achieved gradually, are most often required in patients with severe, refractory edema
  Pediatric: <1 month: not recommended; ≥1 month-12 years: use the smallest effective dose; initially 25 mg; then careful stepwise increments in dosage of 25 mg to achieve effective maintenance
      Sodium Edecrin *Vial:* 50 mg single-dose
  Comment: *ethacrynate sodium* in is more potent than more commonly used loop and thiazide diuretics. Treatment of the edema associated with congestive heart failure, cirrhosis of the liver, and renal disease, including the nephrotic syndrome, short-term management of ascites due to malignancy, idiopathic edema, and lymphedema, short-term management of hospitalized pediatric patients, other than infants, with congenital heart disease or the nephrotic syndrome. IV **Sodium Edecrin** is indicated when a rapid onset of diuresis is desired, e.g., in acute pulmonary edema or when gastrointestinal absorption is impaired or oral medication is not practical.

▷ **furosemide** (C)(G) initially 20-80 mg as a single dose
  Pediatric: <12 years: not recommended; ≥12 years: same as adult
      Lasix *Tab:* 20, 40*, 80 mg; *Oral soln:* 10 mg/ml (2, 4 oz w. dropper)

Comment: *furosemide* is contraindicated with sulfa drug allergy.

▷ *torsemide* (B) 5 mg daily; may increase to 10 mg daily
  Pediatric: <12 years: not recommended; ≥12 years: same as adult
    Demadex *Tab:* 5*, 10*, 20*, 100*mg

OTHER DIURETICS

▷ *indapamide* (B) initially 1.25 mg daily; may titrate every 4 weeks if needed; max
  5 mg/day
  Pediatric: <12 years: not recommended; ≥12 years: same as adult
    Lozol *Tab:* 1.25, 2.5 mg
  Comment: *indapamide* is contraindicated with sulfa drug allergy.

▷ *metolazone* (B)
  Pediatric: <12 years: not recommended; ≥12 years: same as adult
    Mykrox initially 0.5 mg q AM; max 1 mg/day
      Tab: 0.5 mg
    Zaroxolyn 2.5-5 mg once daily
      Tab: 2.5, 5, 10 mg
  Comment: *metolazone* is contraindicated with sulfa drug allergy.

DIURETIC COMBINATIONS

▷ *amiloride+hydrochlorothiazide* (B)(G) initially 1 tab daily; may increase to 2 tabs/day
  in a single <u>or</u> divided doses
  Pediatric: <12 years: not recommended; ≥12 years: same as adult
    Moduretic *Tab: amil* 5 mg+*hctz* 50 mg*

▷ *spironolactone+hydrochlorothiazide* (D)(G) usual maintenance is 100 mg each of
  spironolactone and *hydrochlorothiazide* daily, in a single-dose <u>or</u> in divided doses;
  range 25-200 mg of each component daily depending on the response to the initial
  titration
  Pediatric: <12 years: not recommended; ≥12 years: same as adult
    Aldactazide
      Tab: **Aldactazide 25** *spiro* 25 mg+*hctz* 25 mg
        Aldactazide 50 *Tab: spiro* 50 mg+*hctz* 50 mg

▷ *triamterene+hydrochlorothiazide* (C)(G)
  Pediatric: <12 years: not recommended; ≥12 years: same as adult
    Dyazide 1-2 caps once daily
      Cap: triam 37.5 mg+*hctz* 25 mg
    Maxzide 1 tab once daily
      Tab: triam 75 mg+*hctz* 50 mg*
    Maxzide-25 1-2 tabs once daily
      Tab: triam 37.5 mg+*hctz* 25 mg*

 EMPHYSEMA

Inhaled Corticosteroids *see Asthma page 32*
Parenteral Corticosteroids *see page 570*
Oral Corticosteroids *see page 569*
Inhaled Beta Agonists (Bronchodilators) *see Asthma page 30*
Oral Beta-Agonists (Bronchodilators) *see Asthma page 37*

METHYLXANTHINES

see Asthma page 30

LONG-ACTING INHALED BETA-2 AGONIST (LABA)

▷ *indacaterol* (C)

Arcapta Neohaler inhale contents of one 75 mcg cap once daily

Neohaler Device/Cap: 75 mcg (5 blister cards, 6 caps/card)

Comment: Remove cap from blister cap immediately before use. For oral inhalation with neohaler device only. **Arcapta Neohaler** is indicated for the long-term maintenance treatment of bronchoconstriction in persons with COPD. It is not indicated for treating asthma, for primary treatment of acute symptoms, or for acute deterioration of COPD.

▷ *olodaterol* (C)

Striverdi Respimat 12 mcg q 12 hours

Inhal soln: 2.5 mcg/cartridge (metered actuation) (40 gm, 60 metered actuations) (benzalkonium chloride)

CORTICOSTEROID+INHALED LONG-ACTING BETA-2 AGONIST (LABA)

▷ *fluticasone furoate/vilanterol* (C) 1 inhalation 100/25 or 200/25 once daily at the same time each day

Breo Ellipta 100/25 *Inhal pwdr: flu* 100 mcg+*vil* 25 mcg dry pwdr per inhal (30 doses)

Breo Ellipta 200/25 *Inhal pwdr: flu* 200 mcg+*vil* 25 mcg dry pwdr per inhal (30 doses)

Comment: **Breo Ellipta** is contraindicated with severe hypersensitivity to milk proteins.

INHALED ANTICHOLINERGICS (ANTIMUSCARINICS)

▷ *ipratropium* (B)(G)

Atrovent 2 inhalations qid; max 12 inhalations/day

Inhaler: 14 gm (200 inh)

Atrovent Inhaled Solution 500 mcg by nebulizer tid to qid

Inhal soln: 0.02%; 500 mcg (2.5 ml)

LONG-ACTING MUSCARINIC ANTAGONISTS (LAMA)

Comment: Inhaled LAMA's are indicated for prophylaxis and chronic treatment, only. Not for primary (rescue) treatment of acute attack. Avoid getting powder/nebulizer solution in the eyes. Caution with narrow-angle glaucoma, BPH, bladder neck obstruction, and pregnancy. Contraindicated with allergy to atropine or its derivatives (e.g., *ipratropium*). Avoid other anticholinergic agents.

▷ *aclidinium bromide* (C) 1 inhalation twice daily using inhaler

Tudorza Pressair *Inhal device:* 400 mcg/actuation (60 doses per inhalation device)

INHALED LONG-ACTING MUSCARENIC-ANTAGONISTS (LAMAS)

▷ *glycopyrrolate* (C)

Comment: There are no data on the safety of *glycopyrrolate* use in pregnancy or presence of *glycopyrrolate* or its metabolites in human milk or effects on the breastfed infant.

Lonhala Magnair inhale the contents of 1 vial twice daily at the same times of day, AM and PM, via Magnair neb inhal device; do not swallow solution; do not use **Magnair** with any other medicine; length of treatment is 2-3 minutes; do not use 2 vials/treatment or more than 2 vials/day

Neb soln: Vial: 25 mcg/1 ml single-dose for administration with Magnair neb inhal device; *Starter Kit:* 30 day supply (2 vials/pouch, 30 foil pouches/carton) and 1 complete MAGNAIR Nebulizer System; *Refill Kit:* (2 vials/pouch, 30 foil pouches/carton) and 1 complete MAGNAIR refill handset

Comment: **Lonhala Magnair** is the first nebulizing long-acting muscarinic antagonist (LAMA) approved for the treatment of COPD in the United States. Its approval was based on data from clinical trials in the Glycopyrrolate for Obstructive Lung Disease via Electronic Nebulizer (GOLDEN) program, including GOLDEN-3 and GOLDEN-4, 2 Phase 3, 12-week, randomized, double-blind, placebo-controlled, parallel-group, multicenter study.

>> **Seebri Neohaler** inhale the contents of 1 capsule twice daily at the same time of day, AM and PM, using the neohaler; do not swallow caps
>> *Inhal cap:* 15.6 mcg (60/blister pck) dry pwdr for inhalation w. 1 Neohaler device (lactose)

▷ *tiotropium (as bromide monohydrate)* (C) 2 inhalations once daily using inhalation device; do not swallow caps
>> **Spiriva HandiHaler** *Inhal device:* 18 mcg/cap pwdr for inhalation (5, 30, 90 caps w. inhalation device)
>> **Spiriva Respimat** *Inhal device:* 1.25, 2.5 mcg/actuation cartridge w. inhalation device (4 gm, 60 metered actuations) (benzylkonian chloride)

Comment: *tiotropium* is for prophylaxis and chronic treatment, only. Not for primary (rescue) treatment of acute attack. Avoid getting powder in eyes. Caution with narrow-angle glaucoma, BPH, bladder neck obstruction, and pregnancy. Contraindicated with allergy to *atropine* or its derivatives (e.g., *ipratropium*).

▷ *umeclidinium* (C) one inhalation once daily at the same time each day
>> **Incruse Ellipta** *Inhal pwdr:* 62.5 mcg/inhalation (30 doses) (lactose)
>> Comment: **Incruse Ellipta** is contraindicated with allergy to atropine or its derivatives.

INHALED BRONCHODILATOR+ANTICHOLINERGIC COMBINATION

▷ *ipratropium/albuterol* (C) 2 inhalations qid; max 12 inhalations/day
>> **Combivent MDI** *Inhaler:* 14.7 gm (200 inh)

INHALED ANTICHOLINERGIC+LONG-ACTING BETA-2 AGONIST (LABA) COMBINATIONS

▷ *indacaterol+glycopyrrolate* (C)
>> **Utibron Neohaler** inhale the contents of 1 capsule 2 x/day at the same times of day, AM and PM, using the neohaler; do not swallow caps
>> *Inhal cap:* indac 27.5 mcg+*glycop* 15.6 mcg per cap (60/blister pck) dry pwdr for inhalation w. 1 Neohaler device (lactose)

▷ *ipratropium+albuterol* (C) 1 inhalation qid; max 6 inhalations/day
>> **Combivent Respimat** *Inhal soln:* ipra 20 mcg+*alb* 100 mcg per inhal (4 gm, 120 inhal)
>> Comment: When the labeled number of metered actuations (120) has been dispensed from the **Combivent Respimat** inhaler, the locking mechanism engages and no more actuations can be dispensed. **Combivent Respimat** is contraindicated with atropine allergy.

▷ *tiotropium+olodaterol* (C) 2 inhalations once daily at the same time each day; max 2 inhalations/day
>> **Stiolto Respimat** *Inhal soln:* tio 2.5 mcg+*olo* 2.5 mcg per actuation (4 gm, 60 inh) (benzalkonium chloride)
>> Comment: **Stiolto Respimat** is not for treating asthma, for relief of acute bronchospasm, or acutely deteriorating COPD.

▷ *umeclidinium+vilanterol* (C) 1 inhalation once daily at the same time each day
>> **Anoro Ellipta** *Inhal soln:* ume 62.5 mcg+*vila* 25 mcg per inhal (30 doses)
>> Comment: **Anoro Ellipta** is contraindicated with severe hypersensitivity to milk proteins.

INHALED CORTICOSTEROID+ANTICHOLINERGIC+ LONG-ACTING BETA AGONIST (LABA) COMBINATION

▷ *fluticasone furoate+umeclidinium+vilanterol* one inhalation once daily
     Trelegy Ellipta *flutic furo* 100 mcg/*umec* 62.5 mcg/*vilan* 25 mcg dry pwdr
Comment: **Trelegy Ellipta** is maintenance therapy for patients with COPD, including chronic bronchitis and emphysema, who are receiving fixed-dose *furoate* and *vilanterol* for airflow obstruction and to reduce exacerbations, or receiving *umeclidinium* and a fixed-dose combination of *fluticasone furoate* and *vilanterol*. **Trelegy Ellipta** is the first FDA approved once-daily single-dose inhaler that combines *fluticasone furoate*, a corticosteroid, *umeclidinium*, a long-acting muscarinic antagonist, and *vilantero*, a long-acting beta2-adrenergic agonist. Common adverse reactions reported with **Trelegy Ellipta** included headache, back pain, dysgeusia, diarrhea, cough, oropharyngeal pain, and gastroenteritis. **Trelegy Ellipta** has been found to increase the risk of pneumonia in patients with COPD, and increase the risk of asthma-related death in patients with asthma. **Trelegy Ellipta** is not indicated for the treatment of asthma or acute bronchospasm.

REFERENCE

Trelegy Ellipta approved as the first once-daily single inhaler triple therapy for the treatment of appropriate patients with COPD in the US [press release]. London, UK: GlaxoSmithKline plc, September 18, 2017 https://www.gsk.com/en-gb/media/press-releases/trelegy-ellipta-approved-as-the-first-once-daily-single-inhaler-triple-therapy-for-the-treatment-of-appropriate-patients-with-copd-in-the-us/

METHYLXANTHINE+EXPECTORANT COMBINATION

▷ *dyphylline+guaifenesin* (C)
    Pediatric: <12 years: not recommended; ≥12 years: same as adult
        Lufyllin GG 1 tab qid
            Tab: dyph 200 mg+*guaif* 200 mg
        Lufyllin GG Elixir 30 ml qid
            Elix: dyph 100 mg+*guaif* 100 mg per 15 ml (16 oz)

OTHER METHYLXANTHINE COMBINATION

▷ *theophylline+potassium iodide+ephedrine+phenobarbital* (X)(II) 1 tab tid-qid prn; add an additional dose q HS as needed
    Pediatric: <6 years: not recommended; ≥6-12 years: 1/2 tab tid
        Quadrinal *Tab: theo* 130 mg+*pot iod* 320 mg+*ephed* 24 mg+*phenol 24 mg*

 ENCOPRESIS

INITIAL BOWEL EVACUATION

▷ *mineral oil* (C) 1 oz x 1 day
Comment: Mineral oil can inhibit absorption of the fat-soluble vitamins (A, D, E, and K).
▷ *bisacodyl* (B) 1 suppository daily prn
    Pediatric: <12 years: 1/2 suppository daily prn
        Dulcolax *Rectal supp:* 10 mg
▷ *glycerin* suppository (A) 1 adult suppository
    Pediatric: <6 years: 1 pediatric suppository; ≥6 years: same as adult

MAINTENANCE

▷ *mineral oil* (C) 5-15 ml once daily
    Comment: Mineral oil can inhibit absorption of the fat-soluble vitamins (A, D, E, and K).

ENDOMETRIOSIS

Acetaminophen for IV Infusion *see Pain page* 344
NSAIDs *see page* 562
Opioid Analgesics *see Pain page* 345
Other Contraceptives *see page* 548
➤ *medroxyprogesterone* **(X)** 30 mg daily
 Provera *Tab:* 2.5, 5, 10 mg
➤ *medroxyprogesterone acetate* injectable **(X)** 100-400 mg IM monthly
 Depo-Provera Injectable: 300 mg/ml (2.5, 10 ml)
➤ *norethindrone acetate* **(X)** initially 5 mg daily x 2 weeks; then increase by 2.5 mg/day
 every 2 weeks up to 15 mg/day maintenance dose; then continue for 6 to 9 months
 unless breakthrough bleeding is intolerable
 Aygestin *Tab:* 5*mg

GONADOTROPIN-RELEASING HORMONE ANALOGS

➤ *goserelin (GnRH analog)* implant **(X)** implant SC into upper abdominal wall; 1 SC
 implant q 28 days for up to 6 months; re-treatment not recommended
 Pediatric: <18 years: not recommended; ≥18 years: same as adult
 Zoladex SC implant in syringe: 3.6 mg
➤ *leuprolide acetate (GnRH analog)* **(X)**
 Pediatric: <18 years: not recommended; ≥18 years: same as adult
  Lupron Depot 3.75 mg 3.75 mg SC monthly for up to 6 months; may repeat one
  6-month cycle
   Syringe: 3.75 mg (single-dose depo susp for SC injection)
  Lupron Depot-3 Month 22.5 mg SC q 3 months (84 days); max 2 injections
   Syringe: 22.5 mg (single-dose depo susp for IM injection)
Comment: Do not split doses.
➤ *nafarelin acetate* **(X)** 1 spray (200 mcg) into one nostril q AM, then 1 spray (200 mcg)
 into the other nostril q PM x 6 months; if no response after 2 months, may increase to
 2 sprays (400 mcg) bid
 Pediatric: <18 years: not recommended; ≥18 years: same as adult
 Synarel *Nasal spray:* 2 mg/ml (10 ml)
Comment: Start *nafarelin acetate* **(Synarel)** on the 3rd or 4th day of the menstrual period
or after a negative pregnancy test.

OTHER AGENTS

➤ *danazol* **(X)** start on 3rd or 4th day of menstrual period or after a negative pregnancy
 test; initially 400 mg bid; gradual downward titration of dosage may be considered
 dependent upon patient response; mild cases may respond to 100-200 mg bid
 Pediatric: <18 years: not recommended; ≥18 years: same as adult
 Danocrine *Cap:* 50, 100, 200 mg
Comment: *danazol* is a synthetic steroid derived from ethisterone. It suppresses
the pituitary-ovarian axis. This suppression is probably a combination of depressed
hypothalamic-pituitary response to lowered *estrogen* production, the alteration of
sex steroid metabolism, and interaction of *danazol* with sex hormone receptors.
The only other demonstrable hormonal effects are weak androgenic activity and
depression of both follicle-stimulating hormone (FSH) and luteinizing hormone
(LH) output. Recent evidence suggests a direct inhibitory effect at gonadal sites and
a binding of **Danocrine** to receptors of gonadal steroids at target organs. In addition,
Danocrine has been shown to significantly decrease IgG, IgM and IgA levels, as well
as phospholipid and IgG isotope autoantibodies in patients with endometriosis and
associated elevations of autoantibodies, suggesting this could be another mechanism

by which it facilitates regression of endometrial lesions. **Danocrine** alters the normal and ectopic endometrial tissue so that it becomes inactive and atrophic. Complete resolution of endometrial lesions occurs in the majority of cases. Changes in the menstrual pattern may occur. Generally, the pituitary-suppressive action of **Danocrine** is reversible. Ovulation and cyclic bleeding usually return within 60 to 90 days when therapy with **Danocrine** is discontinued. **Danocrine** is also used to treat fibrocystic breast disease (reduces breast tissue nodularity and breast pain) and hereditary angioedema (to prevent attacks). Contraindications include pregnancy, breastfeeding, active or history of thromboembolic disease/event, porphyria, undiagnosed abnormal genital bleeding, androgen-dependent tumor, and markedly impaired hepatic, renal, or cardiac function.

 ENURESIS: PRIMARY, NOCTURNAL

VASOPRESSIN

▷ *desmopressin acetate* (B)
> DDAVP usual dosage 0.2 mg before bedtime
> *Pediatric:* <6 years: not recommended; ≥6 years: same as adult
> *Tab:* 0.1*, 0.2*mg
> DDAVP Rhinal Tube 10 mcg or 0.1 ml of soln each nostril (20 mcg total dose) before bedtime
> *Pediatric:* <6 years: not recommended; ≥6 years: same as adult
> *Nasal spray:* 10 mcg/actuation (5 ml, 50 sprays); *Rhinal tube:* 0.1 mg/ml (2.5 ml)

TRICYCLIC ANTIDEPRESSANTS (TCAs)

Comment: Co-administration of SSRIs and TCAs requires extreme caution.
▷ *amitriptyline* (C)(G) initially 10 mg before bedtime; use lowest effective dose
Pediatric: <12 years: not recommended; ≥12 years: same as adult
> *Tab:* 10, 25, 50, 75, 100, 150 mg
Pediatric: <12 years: not recommended; ≥12 years: same as adult
▷ *amoxapine* (C) initially 25 mg before bedtime; use lowest effective dose
> *Tab:* 25, 50, 100, 150 mg
▷ *clomipramine* (C)(G) initially 25 mg before bedtime; use lowest effective dose
Pediatric: <10 years: not recommended; ≥10 years: same as adult
> **Anafranil** *Cap:* 25, 50, 75 mg
▷ *desipramine* (C)(G) initially 25 mg before bedtime; use lowest effective dose
Pediatric: <12 years: not recommended; ≥12 years: same as adult
> **Norpramin** *Tab:* 10, 25, 50, 75, 100, 150 mg
▷ *doxepin* (C)(G) initially 10 mg before bedtime; use lowest effective dose
Pediatric: <12 years: not recommended; ≥12 years: same as adult
> *Cap:* 10, 25, 50, 75, 100, 150 mg; Oral conc: 10 mg/ml (4 oz w. dropper)
▷ *imipramine* (C)(G) initially 10 mg before bedtime; use lowest effective dose
Pediatric: <12 years: not recommended; ≥12 years: same as adult
> **Tofranil** initially 10 at bedtime; use lowest effective dose; if bedtime dose exceeds 75 mg daily, may switch to **Tofranil PM**
> *Tab:* 10, 25, 50 mg
> **Tofranil PM** initially 75 mg before bedtime; use lowest effective dose
> *Cap:* 75, 100, 125, 150 mg
▷ *nortriptyline* (D)(G)
Pediatric: <12 years: not recommended; ≥12 years: initially 10 mg before bedtime; use lowest effective dose
> **Pamelor** *Cap:* 10, 25, 50, 75 mg; *Oral soln:* 10 mg/5 ml (16 oz)

▷ *protriptyline* (C) initially 5 mg before bedtime; use lowest effective dose
  Pediatric: <12 years: not recommended; ≥12 years: same as adult
    Vivactil *Tab:* 5, 10 mg
▷ *trimipramine* (C) initially 25 mg before bedtime; use lowest effective dose
  Pediatric: <12 years: not recommended; ≥12 years: same ad adult
    Surmontil *Cap:* 25, 50, 100 mg

 ## EOSINOPHILIC GRANULOMATOSIS WITH POLYANGITIS (FORMERLY, CHURG-STRAUSS SYNDROME)

Comment: Eosinophilic granulomatosis with polyangiitis (EGPA) is a rare autoimmune disease that causes vasculitis, an inflammation in the wall of blood vessels of the body. EGPA is a characterized by asthma, high levels of eosinophils, and inflammation of small- to medium-sized blood vessels affecting organ systems including the lungs, GI tract, skin, heart, and nervous system. **Nucala** *(mepolizumab)* is the first FDA-approved therapy specifically to treat EGPA. This expanded indication of **Nucala** meets a critical, unmet need for EGPA patients. It's notable that patients taking **Nucala** in clinical trials reported a significant improvement in their symptoms. The FDA granted this application Priority Review and Orphan Drug designations. Orphan Drug designation provides incentives to assist and encourage the development of drugs for rare diseases.

REFERENCE
https://www.fda.gov/NewsEvents/Newsroom/PressAnnouncements/ucm588594.htm

HUMANIZED INTERLEUKIN-5 ANTAGONIST MONOCLONAL ANTIBODY

▷ *mepolizumab* 100 mg SC once every 4 weeks in upper arm, abdomen, <u>or</u> thigh
  Pediatric: <12 years: not recommended; ≥12 years: same as adult
    Nucala *Vial:* 100 mg pwdr for reconstitution, single-use (preservative-free)
Comment: Nucala is an add-on maintenance treatment for severe asthma. There is a pregnancy exposure registry that monitors pregnancy outcomes in women exposed to **Nucala** during pregnancy. Healthcare providers can enroll patients <u>or</u> encourage patients to enroll themselves by calling 1-877-311-8972 <u>or</u> visiting www.mothertobaby.org/asthma.

 ## EPICONDYLITIS

Acetaminophen for IV Infusion *see Pain page* 344
NSAIDs *see page* 562
Opioid Analgesics *see Pain page* 345
Topical and Transdermal NSAIDs *see Pain page* 344
Parenteral Corticosteroids *see page* 570
Oral Corticosteroids *see page* 569
Topical Analgesic and Anesthetic Agents *see page* 560

 ## EPIDIDYMITIS

Comment: The following treatment regimens for epididymitis are published in the **2015 CDC Transmitted Diseases Treatment Guidelines.** Treatment regimens are presented by generic drug name first, followed by information about brands and dose forms. Empiric treatment requires concomitant treatment of chlamydia. Treat all sexual contacts. Patients who are HIV-positive should receive the same treatment as those who are HIV-negative.

RECOMMENDED REGIMEN

Regimen 1

▷ *ceftriaxone* (B)(G) 250 mg IM in a single dose
    plus
▷ *doxycycline* (D)(G) 100 mg bid x 10 days

RECOMMENDED REGIMENS: LIKELY CAUSED BY ENTERIC ORGANISMS

Regimen 1

▷ *levofloxacin* (C) 500 mg daily x 10 days

Regimen 2

▷ *ofloxacin* (C)(G) 300 mg bid x 10 day

DRUG BRANDS AND DOSE FORMS

▷ *ceftriaxone* (B)(G)
    Rocephin *Vial:* 250, 500 mg; 1, 2 gm
▷ *doxycycline* (D)(G)
    Acticlate *Tab:* 75, 150**mg
    Adoxa *Tab:* 50, 75, 100, 150 mg ent-coat
    Doryx *Tab:* 50, 75, 100, 150, 200 mg del-rel
    Doxteric *Tab:* 50 mg del-rel
    Monodox *Cap:* 50, 75, 100 mg
    Oracea *Cap:* 40 mg del-rel
    Vibramycin *Tab:* 100 mg; *Cap:* 50, 100 mg; *Syr:* 50 mg/5 ml (raspberry-apple)
    (sulfites); *Oral susp:* 25 mg/5 ml (raspberry)
    Vibra-Tab *Tab:* 100 mg film-coat
Comment: *doxycycline* is contraindicated <8 years-of-age, in pregnancy, and
lactation (discolors developing tooth enamel). A side effect may be photo-sensitivity
(photophobia). Do not take with antacids, calcium supplements, milk or other dairy, or
within 2 hours of taking another drug.
▷ *levofloxacin* (C)
    Levaquin *Tab:* 250, 500, 750 mg; *Oral soln:* 25 mg/ml (480 ml) (benzyl alcohol)
Comment: *levofloxacin* is contraindicated <18 years-of-age, and during pregnancy, and
lactation. Risk of tendonitis or tendon rupture.
▷ *ofloxacin* (C)(G)
    Floxin *Tab:* 200, 300, 400 mg
Comment: *ofloxacin* is contraindicated <18 years-of-age, and during pregnancy and
lactation. Risk of tendonitis or tendon rupture.

 ERECTILE DYSFUNCTION (ED)

Comment: Due to a degree of cardiac risk with sexual activity, consider cardiovascular
status of patient before instituting therapeutic measures for erectile dysfunction.

PHOSPHODIESTERASE TYPE 5 (PDE5) INHIBITORS, CGMP-SPECIFIC

Comment: Oral PDE5 inhibitors (**Cialis, Levitra, Staxyn, Viagra**) are contraindicated
in patients taking nitrates. Caution with history of recent MI, stroke, life-threatening
arrhythmia, hypotension, hypertension, cardiac failure, unstable angina, retinitis
pigmentosa, CYP3A4 inhibitors (e.g., *cimetidine*, the azoles, *erythromycin*,
grapefruit juice), protease inhibitors (e.g., *ritonavir*), CYP3A4 inducers (e.g.,
rifampin, *carbamazepine*, *phenytoin*, *phenobarbital*), alcohol, antihypertensive

agents. Side effects include headache, flushing, nasal congestion, rhinitis, dyspepsia, and diarrhea. Use with caution in patients with anatomical deformation of the penis (e.g., angulation, cavernosal fibrosis, or Peyronie's disease) or in patients who have conditions, which may predispose them to priapism (e.g., sickle cell anemia, multiple myeloma, or leukemia). In the event of an erection that persists longer than 4 hours, the patient should seek immediate medical assistance. If priapism (painful erection greater than 6 hours in duration) is not treated immediately, penile tissue damage and permanent loss of potency could result.

➤ *avanafil* (B) initially 100 mg taken 30 min prior to sexual activity; may decrease to 50 mg or increase to 200 mg based on response; max one administration/day
   Stendra *Tab:* 50, 100, 200 mg

➤ *sildenafil citrate* (B)(G) one dose about 1 hour (range 30 min-4 hrs) before sexual activity; usual initial dose 50 mg; may decrease to 25 mg or increase to max 100 mg/dose based on response; max one administration/day
   Viagra *Tab:* 25, 50, 100 mg

➤ *tadalafil* (B) initially 10 mg prior to sexual activity up to once daily; may decrease to 5 mg or increase to 20 mg based on response; max one administration/day; effect may last 36 hours
   Cialis *Tab:* 2.5, 5, 10, 20 mg

➤ *vardenafil* (B) initially 10 mg taken 60 min prior to sexual activity; may decrease to 5 mg or increase to 20 mg based on response; max one administration/day
   Levitra *Tab:* 2.5, 5, 10, 20 mg film-coat
Comment: **Levitra** is not interchangeable with **Staxyn**.

➤ *vardenafil (as HCl)* (B)(G) dissolve 1 tab on tongue 60 min prior to sexual activity, max once daily
   Staxyn *Tab:* 10 mg orally disintegrating (peppermint) (phenylalanine)
Comment: **Staxyn** is not interchangeable with **Levitra**.

➤ *alprostadil* (X) *urethral suppository* initially 125 or 250 mcg inserted in the urethra after urination; adjust dose in stepwise manner on separate occasions; max two administrations/day
   Muse *Urethral supp:* 125, 250, 500, 1000 mcg
Comment: Contraindicated with urethral stricture, balanitis, severe hypospadias and curvature, urethritis, predisposition to venous thrombosis, hyperviscosity syndrome. Extreme caution with anticoagulant therapy (e.g., warfarin, heparin). Potential for hypotension and/or syncope.

➤ *alprostadil* (X) *injection* inject over 5-10 seconds into the dorsal lateral aspect of the proximal third of the penis; avoid visible veins; rotate injection sites and sides; if no initial response, may give next higher dose within 1 hour; if partial response, give next higher dose after 24 hours; max 60 mcg and 3 self-injections/week; allow at least 24 hours between doses; reduce dose if erection lasts >1 hour.
   Caverject *Vial:* 5, 10, 20, 40 mcg/vial (pwdr for reconstitution w. diluent)
   Caverject Impulse *Cartridge:* 10, 20 mcg (2 cartridge starter and refill pcks)
   Edex *Vial:* 5, 10, 20, 40 mcg (6/pck); *Syringe:* 5, 10, 20, 40 mcg (4/pck); *Cartridge:* 10, 20, 40 mcg (2 cartridge starter and refill pcks)
Comment: Determine dose of injectable prostaglandins in the office. Contraindicated with predisposition to priapism, penile angulation, cavernosal fibrosis, Peyronies disease, penile implant. Extreme caution with anticoagulant therapy (e.g., *warfarin, heparin*).

◯ ERYSIPELAS

Comment: Erysipelas is most commonly due to GABHS (Group A beta-hemolytic *Streptococcus*).

TREATMENT OF CHOICE

▷ *penicillin v potassium* (B) 250-500 mg q 6 hours x 10 days
   Pediatric: 25-50 mg/kg/day divided q 6 hours x 10 days; *see page 644 for dose by weight*
      Pen-Vee K *Tab:* 250, 500 mg; *Oral soln:* 125 mg/5 ml (100, 200 ml); 250 mg/5 ml (100, 150, 200 ml)

TREATMENT IF PENICILLIN ALLERGIC

▷ *erythromycin base* (B)(G) 250 mg q 6 hours x 10 days
   Pediatric: 30-40 mg/kg/day divided q 6 hours x 10 days; >40 kg: same as adult
      Ery-Tab *Tab:* 250, 333, 500 mg ent-coat
      PCE *Tab:* 333, 500 mg
Comment: *erythromycin* may increase INR with concomitant *warfarin*, as well as increase serum level of *digoxin*, benzodiazepines and statins.
▷ *erythromycin ethylsuccinate* (B)(G) 400 mg qid x 7 days
   Pediatric: 30-50 mg/kg/day in 4 divided doses x 7 days; may double dose with severe infection; max 100 mg/kg/day; *see page 635 for dose by weight*
      EryPed *Oral susp:* 200 mg/5 ml (100, 200 ml) (fruit); 400 mg/5 ml (60, 100, 200 ml) (banana); *Oral drops:* 200, 400 mg/5 ml (50 ml) (fruit); *Chew tab:* 200 mg wafer (fruit)
      E.E.S. *Oral susp:* 200, 400 mg/5 ml (100 ml) (fruit)
      E.E.S. Granules *Oral susp:* 200 mg/5 ml (100, 200 ml) (cherry)
      E.E.S. 400 Tablets *Tab:* 400 mg
Comment: *erythromycin* may increase INR with concomitant *warfarin*, as well as increase serum level of *digoxin*, benzodiazepines and statins.

ESOPHAGITIS, EROSIVE

Antacids *see GERD page* 173
H2 Antagonists *see GERD page* 173
Proton Pump Inhibitors *see GERD page* 173
▷ *sucralfate* (B)(G) *Active ulcer:* 1 gm qid; *Maintenance:* 1 gm bid
      Carafate *Tab:* 1*g; *Oral susp:* 1 gm/10 ml (14 oz)

EXOCRINE PANCREAS INSUFFICIENCY (EPI)/PANCREATIC ENZYME DEFICIENCY

Comment: Seen in chronic pancreatitis, post-pancreatectomy, cystic fibrosis, post-GI tract bypass surgery (Whipple procedure), and ductal obstruction from neoplasia. May sprinkle cap; however, do not crush <u>or</u> chew cap <u>or</u> tab. May mix with applesauce <u>or</u> other acidic food; follow with water <u>or</u> juice. Do not let any drug remain in mouth. Take dose with (not before <u>or</u> after) each meal <u>and</u> snack (half dose with snacks). Base dose on lipase units; adjust per diet and clinical response (i.e., steatorrhea). Pancrelipase products are interchangeable. Contraindicated with pork protein hypersensitivity.

PANCRELIPASE PRODUCTS

▷ *pancreatic enzymes* (C)
      Creon 500 units/kg per meal; max 2,500 units/kg per meal <u>or</u> <10,000 units/kg per day <u>or</u> <4,000 units/gm fat ingested per day
      Pediatric: <12 months: 2,000-4,000 units per 120 ml formula <u>or</u> per breast-feeding (do not mix directly into formula <u>or</u> breast milk; 12 months to 4 years: 1,000 units/kg per meal; max 2,500 units/kg per meal <10,000 units/kg per day; >4 years: same as adult

    Cap: **Creon 3000** lip 3,000 units+pro 9,500 units+amyl 15,000 units del-rel
        Creon 6000 lip 6,000 units+pro 19,000 units+amyl 30,000 units del-rel
        Creon 12000 lip 12,000 units+pro 38,000 units+amyl 60,000 units del-rel
        Creon 24000 lip 24,000 units+pro 76,000 units+amyl 120,000 units del-rel
        Creon 36000 lip 36,000 units+pro 114,000 units+amyl 180,000 units del-rel
Cotazym 1-3 tabs just prior to each meal <u>or</u> snack
Pediatric: <12 years: not recommended; ≥12 years: same as adult
    Tab: **Cotazym** lip 1,000 units+pro 12,500 units+amyl 12,500 units del-rel
        Cotazym-S lip 5,000 units+pro 20,000 units+amyl 20,000 units del-rel
Donnazyme 1-3 caps just prior to each meal <u>or</u> snack
Pediatric: <12 years: not recommended; ≥12 years: same as adult
    Cap: **Donnazyme** lip 5,000 units+pro 20,000 units+amyl 20,000 units del-rel
Ku-Zyme 1-2 caps just prior to each meal <u>or</u> snack
Pediatric: <12 years: not recommended; ≥12 years: same as adult
    Cap: **Ku-Zyme:** lip 12,000 units+pro 15,000 units+amyl 15,000 units del-rel
Kutrase 1-2 caps just prior to each meal <u>or</u> snack
Pediatric: <12 years: not recommended; ≥12 years: same as adult
    Cap: **Kutrase:** lip 12,000 units+pro 30,000 units+amyl 30,000 units del-rel
Pancreaze 2,500 lipase units/kg per meal <u>or</u> <10,000 lipase units/kg per day <u>or</u> <4,000 lipase units/gm fat ingested per day
Pediatric: <12 months: 2,000-4,000 lipase units per 120 ml formula <u>or</u> per breast-feeding; >12 months to <4 years 1,000 lipase units/kg per meal; ≥4 years: 500 lipase units/kg per meal; max: adult dose
    Cap: **Pancreaze 4200** *lip* 4,200 units+*pro* 10,000 units+*amyl* 17,500 units ec-microtabs
        Pancreaze 10500 lip 10,500 units+pro 25,000 units+amyl 43,750 units ec microtabs
        Pancreaze 16800 lip 16,800 units+pro 40,000 units+amyl 70,000 units ec-microtabs
        Pancreaze 21000 lip 21,000 units+pro 37,000 units+amyl 61,000 units ec-microtabs
Pertyze *12 months to 4 years and ≥8 kg:* initially 1,000 lipase units/kg per meal; *≥4 years and ≥16 kg:* initially 500 lipase units/kg per meal; *Both:* 2,500 lipase units/kg per meal <u>or</u> <10,000 units/kg per day <u>or</u> <4,000 lipase units/gm fat ingested per day
    Cap: **Pertyze 8000** lip 8,000 units+pro 28,750 units+amyl 30,250 units del-rel
        Pertyze 16000 lip 16,000 units+pro 57,500 units+amyl 65,000 units del-rel
Ultrase 1-3 tabs just prior to each meal <u>or</u> snack
Pediatric: same as adult
    Cap: **Ultrase** *lip* 4,500 units+*pro* 20,000 units+*amyl* 25,000 units del-rel
        Ultrase MT lip 12,000 units+pro 39,000 units+amyl 39,000 units del-rel
        Ultrase MT 18 lip 18,000 units+pro 58,500 units+amyl 58,500 units del-rel
        Ultrase MT 20 lip 20,000 units+pro 65,000 units+amyl 65,000 units del-rel
Viokace initially 500 lip units/kg per meal; max 2,500 lipase units/kg per meal, <u>or</u> <10,000 lipase units/kg per meal, <u>or</u> <4,000 units/gm fat ingested per day
Pediatric: same as adult
    Tab: **Viokace 8** lip 8,000 units+pro 30,000 units+amyl 30,000 units
        Viokace 16 lip 16,000 units+pro 60,000 units amyl 60,000 units
        Viokace 0440 lip 10,440 units+pro 39,150 units amyl 39,150 units
        Viokace 20880 lip 20,880 units+pro 78,300 units amyl 78,300 units
Comment: **Viokace 10440** and **Viokase 20880** should be taken with a daily proton pump inhibitor.
Viokace Powder 1/4 tsp (0.7 gm) with meals
Viokace Powder lip 16,800 units+pro 70,000 units+amyl 70,000 units per 1/4 tsp (8 oz)

Zenpep 500 units/kg per meal; max 2,500 units/kg per meal <u>or</u> <10,000 units/kg per day <u>or</u> <4,000 units/gm fat ingested per day
> *Pediatric:* <12 months: 2,000-4,000 units per 120 ml formula <u>or</u> per breast feeding (do not mix directly into formula <u>or</u> breast milk); 12 months-4 years: 1,000 units/kg per meal; max 2,500 units/kg per meal <10,000 units/kg per day; >4 years: same as adult
> *Cap:* **Zenpep 5000** lip 5,000 units+pro 17,000 units+amyl 27,000 units del-rel
> **Zenpep 10000** lip 10,000 units+pro 34,000 units+amyl 55,000 units del-rel
> **Zenpep 15000** lip 15,000 units+pro 51,000 units+amyl 82,000 units del-rel
> **Zenpep 20000** lip 20,000 units+pro 68,000 units+amyl 109,000 units del-rel

Zymase 1-3 caps just prior to each meal <u>or</u> snack
Pediatric: <12 years: not recommended; ≥12 years: same as adult
> *Cap:* **Zymase** lip 12,000 units+prot 24,000 units+amyl 24,000 units del-rel

 EYE PAIN

Acetaminophen for IV Infusion *see Pain page* 344
Ibuprofen for IV Infusion *see Pain page* 344

OPHTHALMIC NSAIDs
Comment: Concomitant contact lens wear is contraindicated during therapy. Etiology of eye pain must be known prior to use of these agents
➤ *diclofenac* (B) 1 drop affected eye qid
Pediatric: <12 years: not recommended; ≥12 years: same as adult
> **Voltaren Ophthalmic Solution** *Ophth soln:* 0.1% (2.5, 5 ml)
➤ *ketorolac tromethamine* (C) 1 drop affected eye qid for up to 4 days
Pediatric: <3 years: not recommended; ≥3 years: same as adult
> **Acular** *Ophth soln:* 0.5% (3, 5, 10 ml; benzalkonium chloride)
> **Acular LS** *Ophth soln:* 0.4% (5 ml; benzalkonium chloride)
> **Acular PF** *Ophth soln:* 0.5% (0.4 ml; 12 single-use vials/carton) (preservative-free)
➤ *nepafenac* (C) 1 drop affected eye tid
Pediatric: <10 years: not recommended; ≥10 years: same as adult
> **Nevanac Ophthalmic Suspension** *Ophth susp:* 0.1% (3 ml) (benzalkonium chloride)

OPHTHALMIC STEROIDS
Comment: Contraindications: ocular fungal, viral, <u>or</u> mycobacterial infections. Effectiveness of treatment should be assessed after 2 days. The corticosteroid should be tapered and treatment concluded within 14 days if possible due to risk of corneal <u>and/or</u> scleral thinning with prolonged use.
➤ *difluprednate* (C) 1 drop affected eye qid; *Post-op Pain:* beginning 24 hours after surgery, 1 drop affected eye qid; continue for 2 weeks post-op; then bid x 1 week; then taper until resolved
Pediatric: <12 years: not recommended; ≥12 years: same as adult
> **Durezol Ophthalmic Solution** *Ophth emul:* 0.05% (5 ml)
➤ *etabonate* (C) 1 drop affected eye qid
Pediatric: <12 years: not recommended; ≥12 years: same as adult
> **Alrex Ophthalmic Solution** *Ophth emul:* 0.2% (5 ml) (benzylkonium chloride)

 FACIAL HAIR, EXCESSIVE/UNWANTED

TOPICAL HAIR GROWTH RETARDANT
➤ *eflornithine* 13.9% cream (C) apply a thin layer to affected areas of face and under the chin bid at least 8 hours apart; rub in thoroughly; do not wash treated area for at least 4 hours following application

Pediatric: <12 years: not recommended; ≥12 years: same as adult
Vaniqa *Crm:* 13.9% (30, 60 gm)
Comment: After **Vaniqa** dries, may apply cosmetics or sunscreen. Hair removal techniques may be continued as needed.

FECAL ODOR

▷ *bismuth subgallate powder* (B)(OTC) 1-2 tabs tid with meals
Devron *Chew tab:* 200 mg; *Cap:* 200 mg
Comment: **Devron** is an internal (oral) deodorant for control of odors from ileostomy or colostomy drainage or fecal incontinence.

FEVER (PYREXIA)

ACETAMINOPHEN FOR IV INFUSION

▷ *acetaminophen* injectable (B)(G) administer by IV infusion over 15 minutes; 1000 mg q 6 hours prn or 650 mg q 4 hours prn; max 4,000 mg/day
Pediatric: <2 years: not recommended; 2-13 years <50 kg: 15 mg/kg q 6 hours prn or 12.5 mg/kg q 4 hours prn; max 750 mg/single dose; max 75 mg/kg per day
Ofirmev *Vial:* 10 mg/ml (100 ml) (preservative-free)
Comment: The **Ofirmev** vial is intended for single-use. If any portion is withdrawn from the vial, use within 6 hours. Discard the unused portion. For pediatric patients, withdraw the intended dose and administer via syringe pump. Do not ad-mix **Ofirmev** with any other drugs. **Ofirmev** is physically incompatable with diazepam and chlorpromazine hydrochloride.

▷ *acetaminophen* (B)(G)
Children's Tylenol (OTC) 10-20 mg/kg q 4-6 hours prn
Oral susp: 80 mg/tsp
4-11 months (12-17 lb): 1/2 tsp q 4 hours prn; 12-23 months (18-23 lb): 3/4 tsp q 4 hours prn; 2-3 years (24-35 lb): 1 tsp q 4 hours prn; 4-5 years (36-47 lb): 1 tsp q 4 hours prn; 6-8 years (48-59 lb): 2 tsp q 4 hours prn; 9-10 years (60-71 lb): 2 tsp q 4 hours prn; 11 years (72-95 lb): 3 tsp q 4 hours prn; All: max 5 doses/day
Elix: 160 mg/5 ml (2, 4 oz)
Chew tab: 80 mg
2-3 years (24-35 lb): 2 tabs q 4 hours prn; 4-5 years (36-47 lb): 3 tabs q 4 hours prn; 6-8 years (48-59 lb): 4 tabs q 4 hours prn; 9-10 years (60-71 lb): 5 tabs q 4 hours prn; 11 years (72-95 lb): 6 tabs q 4 hours prn; All: max 5 doses/day
Junior Strength:
6-8 years: 2 tabs q 4 hours prn; 9-10 years: 2 tabs q 4 hours prn; 11 years: 3 tabs q 4 hours prn; 12 years: 4 tabs q 4 hours prn; All: max 5 doses/day
Chew tab: 160 mg
Junior cplt: 160 mg
Infant's Drops and Suspension: 80 mg/0.8 ml (1/2, 1 oz)
<3 months: 0.4 ml q 4 hours prn; 4-11 months: 0.8 ml q 4 hours prn; 12-23 months: 1.2 ml q 4 hours prn; 2-3 years (24-35 lb): 1.6 ml q 4 hours prn; 4-5 years (36-47 lb): 2.4 ml q 4 hours prn; All: max 5 doses/day
Extra Strength Tylenol (OTC) 1 gm q 4-6 hours prn; max 4 gm/day
Pediatric: <12 years: not recommended; ≥12 years: same as adult
Tab/Cplt/Gel tab/Gel cap: 500 mg; *Liq:* 500 mg/15 ml (8 oz)

FeverAll Extra Strength Tylenol (OTC)
Pediatric: <3 months: not recommended; 3-36 months: 80 mg q 4 hours prn; 3-6 years: 120 mg q 4 hours prn; ≥6 years: 325 mg q 4 hours prn; *Rectal supp:* 80, 120, 325 mg (6/carton)

Maximum Strength Tylenol Sore Throat (OTC) 500-1000 mg q 4-6 hours prn
Pediatric: <12 years: not recommended; ≥12 years: same as adult
   Liq: 1000 mg/30 ml (8 oz)

Tylenol (OTC) 650 mg q 4-6 hours; max 4 gm/day
Pediatric: <6 years: not recommended; 6-11 years: 325 mg q 4-6 hours prn; max 1.625 gm/day; ≥12 years: same as adult

▷ *aspirin* (D)(G)
Bayer (OTC) 325-650 mg q 4 hours prn; max: 5 doses/day
Pediatric: <12 years: not recommended; ≥12 years: same as adult
   Tab/Cplt: 325 mg ext-rel

Extra Strength Bayer (OTC) 500 mg-1 gm q 4-6 hours prn; max 4 gm/day
Pediatric: <12 years: not recommended; ≥12 years: same as adult
   Cplt: 500 mg

Extended-Release Bayer 8 Hour (OTC) 650-1300 mg q 8 hours prn
Pediatric: <12 years: not recommended; ≥12 years: same as adult
   Cplt: 650 mg ext-rel

Comment: *aspirin*-containing medications are contraindicated with history of allergic-type reaction to *aspirin*, children and adolescents with *Varicella* or other viral illness, and 3rd trimester pregnancy.

▷ *aspirin+caffeine* (D)(G)
Anacin (OTC) 800 mg q 4 hours prn; max 4 gm/day
Pediatric: <6 years: not recommended; 6-12 years: 400 mg q 4 hours prn; max 2 gm/day; ≥12 years: same as adult
   Tab/Cplt: 400 mg

Anacin Maximum Strength (OTC) 1 gm tid-qid
Pediatric: <12 years: not recommended; ≥12 years: same as adult
   Tab: 500 mg

Comment: *aspirin*-containing medications are contraindicated with history of allergic-type reaction to *aspirin*, children and adolescents with *Varicella* or other viral illness, and 3rd trimester pregnancy.

▷ *aspirin+antacid* (D)(G)
Extra Strength Bayer Plus (OTC) 500 mg-1 gm q 4-6 hours prn; usual max 4 gm/day
Pediatric: <12 years: not recommended; ≥12 years: same as adult
   Cplt: 500 mg aspirin+calcium carbonate

Bufferin (OTC) 650 mg q 4 hours; max 3.9 mg/day
Pediatric: <12 years: not recommended; ≥12 years: same as adult
   Tab: 325 mg aspirin+calcium carbonate+magnesium carbonate+magnesium oxide

Comment: *aspirin*-containing medications are contraindicated with history of allergic-type reaction to *aspirin*, children and adolescents with *Varicella* or other viral illness, and 3rd trimester of pregnancy.

▷ *ibuprofen* (B; not for use in 3rd)(G)
Comment: *ibuprofen* is contraindicated in children <6 months-of-age.
Children's Advil (OTC), ElixSure IB (OTC), Motrin (OTC), PediaCare (OTC), PediaProfen (OTC)
Pediatric: 5-10 mg/kg q 6-8 hours; max 40 mg/kg/day; <24 lb (<2 years): individualize; 24-35 lb (2-3 years): 5 ml q 6-8 hours prn; 36-47 lb (4-5 years): 7.5 ml q 6-8 hours prn; 48-59 lb (6-8 years): 10 ml or 2 tabs q 6-8 hours prn; 60-71 lb

(9-10 years): 12.5 ml <u>or</u> 2 tabs q 6-8 hours prn; 72-95 lb (11 years): 15 ml <u>or</u> 3 tabs q 6-8 hours prn

Oral susp: 100 mg/5 ml (2, 4 oz) (berry); *Junior tabs:* 100 mg

Children's Motrin Drops (OTC), PediaCare Drops (OTC)

Pediatric: <24 lb (<2 years): individualize; 24-35 lb (2-3 years): 2.5 ml q 6-8 hours prn

Oral drops: 50 mg/1.25 ml (15 ml; berry)

Children's Motrin Chewables and Caplets (OTC)

Pediatric: 48-59 lb (6-8 years): 200 mg q 6-8 hours prn; 60-71 lb (9-10 years): 250 mg q 6-8 hours prn; 72-95 lb (11 years): 300 mg q 6-8 hours prn; ≥12 years: same as adult

Chew tab: 100*mg (citrus; phenylalanine); *Cplt:* 100 mg

Motrin (OTC) 400 mg q 6 hours prn

Pediatric: <6 months: not recommended; ≥6 months, fever <102.5: 5 mg/kg q 6-8 hours prn; >6 months, fever >102.5: 10 mg/kg q 6-8 hours prn

All: max 40 mg/kg/day

Tab: 400 mg; *Cplt:* 100*mg; *Chew tab:* 50*, 100*mg (citrus; phenylalanine); *Oral susp:* 100 mg/5 ml (4, 16 oz) (berry); *Oral drops:* 40 mg/ml (15 ml) (berry)

Advil (OTC), Motrin IB (OTC), Nuprin (OTC) 200-400 mg q 4-6 hours; max 1.2 gm/day

Pediatric: <12 years: not recommended; ≥12 years: same as adult

Tab/Cplt/Gel cap: 200 mg

▷ *naproxen* (B)(G)

Pediatric: <2 years: not recommended; ≥2 years: 2.5-5 mg/kg bid-tid; max: 15 mg/kg/day

Aleve (OTC) 400 mg x 1 dose; then 200 mg q 8-12 hours prn; max 10 days

Tab/Cplt/Gel cap: 200 mg

Anaprox 550 mg x 1 dose; then 550 mg q 12 hours <u>or</u> 275 mg q 6-8 hours prn; max 1.375 gm first day and 1.1 gm/day thereafter

Tab: 275 mg

Anaprox DS 1 tab bid

Tab: 550 mg

EC-Naprosyn 375 <u>or</u> 500 mg bid prn; may increase dose up to max 1500 mg/day as tolerated

Tab: 375, 500 mg del-rel

Naprelan 1 gm daily <u>or</u> 1.5 gm daily for limited time; max 1 gm/day thereafter

Tab: 375, 500 mg

Naprosyn initially 500 mg, then 500 mg q 12 hours <u>or</u> 250 mg q 6-8 hours prn; max 1.25 gm first day and 1 gm/day thereafter

Tab: 250, 375, 500 mg; *Oral susp:* 125 mg/5 ml (473 ml) (pineapple-orange)

FIBROCYSTIC BREAST DISEASE

Contraceptives *see page* 548

▷ *spironolactone* (D) 10 mg bid premenstrually

Aldactone (G) *Tab:* 25, 50*, 100*mg

CaroSpir *Oral susp:* 25 mg/5 ml (118, 473 ml) (banana)

▷ *vitamin E* (A) 400-600 IU daily

▷ *vitamin B6* (A) 50-100 mg daily

▷ *danazol* (X) start on 3rd or 4th day of menstrual period or after a negative pregnancy test; 50-200 mg bid x 2-6 months

Pediatric: <18 years: not recommended; ≥18 years: same as adult

Danocrine *Cap:* 50, 100, 200 mg

Comment: *danazol* is a synthetic steroid derived from ethisterone. It suppresses the pituitary-ovarian axis. This suppression is probably a combination of depressed hypothalamic-pituitary response to lowered *estrogen* production, the alteration of sex steroid metabolism, and interaction of *danazol* with sex hormone receptors. The only other demonstrable hormonal effects are weak androgenic activity and depression of both follicle-stimulating hormone (FSH) and luteinizing hormone (LH) output. Recent evidence suggests a direct inhibitory effect at gonadal sites and a binding of **Danocrine** to receptors of gonadal steroids at target organs. In addition, **Danocrine** has been shown to significantly decrease IgG, IgM and IgA levels, as well as phospholipid and IgG isotope autoantibodies in patients with endometriosis and associated elevations of autoantibodies, suggesting this could be another mechanism by which it facilitates regression of fibrocystic breast disease. **Danocrine** usually produces partial to complete disappearance of breast tissue nodularity and complete relief of pain and tenderness. Changes in the menstrual pattern may occur. Generally, the pituitary-suppressive action of **Danocrine** is reversible. Ovulation and cyclic bleeding usually return within 60 to 90 days when therapy with **Danocrine** is discontinued. **Danocrine** is also used to treat endometriosis (to relieve associated abdominal pain) and hereditary angioedema (to prevent attacks). Contraindications include pregnancy, breastfeeding, active o̲r history of thromboembolic disease/event, porphyria, undiagnosed abnormal genital bleeding, androgen-dependent tumor, and markedly impaired hepatic, renal, o̲r cardiac function.

 FIBROMYALGIA

Acetaminophen for IV Infusion *see Pain page 344*
NSAIDs *see page 562*
Opioid Analgesics *see Pain page 345*
Topical and Transdermal NSAIDs *see Pain page 344*
Parenteral Corticosteroids *see page 570*
Oral Corticosteroids *see page 569*
Topical Analgesic and Anesthetic Agents *see page 560*

SEROTONIN-NOREPINEPHRINE REUPTAKE INHIBITORS (SNRIs)

▷ *duloxetine* (C)(G) swallow whole; initially 30 mg once daily x 1 week; then increase to 60 mg once daily; max 120 mg/day
  Pediatric: <12 years: not recommended; ≥12 years: same as adult
  Cymbalta *Cap:* 20, 30, 60 mg ent-coat pellets
▷ *milnacipran* (C)(G) *Day 1:* 12.5 mg once; *Days 2-3:* 12.5 mg bid; *Days 4-7:* 25 mg bid; max 100 mg bid
  Pediatric: <17 years: not recommended; ≥17 years: same as adult
  Savella *Tab:* 12.5, 25, 50, 100 mg

GAMMA-AMINOBUTYRIC ACID ANALOG

▷ *gabapentin* (C) initially 300 mg on Day 1; then 600 mg on Day 2; then 900 mg on Days 3-6; then 1200 mg on Days 7-10; then 1500 mg on Days 11-14; titrate up to 1800 mg on Day 15; take entire dose once daily with the evening meal; do not crush, split, o̲r chew
  Pediatric: <3 years: not recommended; 3-12 years: initially 10-15 mg/kg/day in 3 divided doses; max 12 hours between doses; titrate over 3 days; 3-4 years: titrate to 40 mg/kg/day; 5-12 years: titrate to 25-35 mg/kg/day; max 50 mg/kg/day; >12 years: same as adult
  Gralise *Tab:* 300, 600 mg

Neurontin (G) 100 mg daily x 1 day; then 100 mg bid x 1 day; then 100 mg tid continuously <u>or</u> 300 mg bid; max 900 mg tid
> *Tab:* 600*, 800*mg; *Cap:* 100, 300, 400 mg; *Oral soln:* 250 mg/5 ml (480 ml) (strawberry-anise)

▷ *gabapentin enacarbil* (C) 600 mg once daily at about 5:00 PM; if dose not taken at recommended time, next dose should be taken the following day; swallow whole; take with food; *CrCl 30-59 mL/min:* 600 mg on Day 1, Day 3, and every day thereafter; *CrCl <30 mL/min:* <u>or</u> on hemodialysis: not recommended
> *Pediatric:* <12 years: not recommended; ≥12 years: same as adult
> **Horizant** *Tab:* 300, 600 mg ext-rel

Comment: Avoid abrupt cessation of *gabapentin* and *gabapentin enacarbil*. To discontinue, withdraw gradually over 1 week <u>or</u> longer.

ALPHA-2 DELTA LIGAND

▷ *pregabalin (GABA analog)* (C)(V)
> *Pediatric:* <18 years: not recommended; ≥18 years: same as adult
> **Lyrica** initially 50 mg tid; may titrate to 100 mg tid within one week; max 600 mg divided tid; discontinue over 1 week
> > *Cap:* 25, 50, 75, 100, 150, 200, 225, 300 mg; *Oral soln:* 20 mg/ml
>
> **Lyrica CR** *Tab:* usual dose: 165 mg once daily; may increase to 330 mg/day within 1 week; max 660 mg/day
> > *Tab:* 82.5, 165, 330 mg ext-rel

OTHER AGENTS

▷ *amitriptyline* (C)(G) 20 mg q HS; may increase gradually to max 50 mg q HS
> *Pediatric:* <12 years: not recommended; ≥12 years: same as adult
> *Tab:* 10, 25, 50, 75, 100, 150 mg

▷ *cyclobenzaprine* (B)(G) 10 mg tid; usual range 20-40 mg/day in divided doses; max 60 mg/day x 2-3 weeks <u>or</u> 15 mg ext-rel once daily; max 30 mg ext-rel/day x 2-3 weeks
> *Pediatric:* <15 years: not recommended; ≥15 years: same as adult
> **Amrix** *Cap:* 15, 30 mg ext-rel
> **Fexmid** *Tab:* 7.5 mg
> **Flexeril** *Tab:* 5, 10 mg

▷ *eszopiclone* (C)(IV)(G) (pyrrolopyrazine) 1-3 mg; max 3 mg/day x 1 month; do not take if unable to sleep for at least 8 hours before required to be active again; delayed effect if taken with a meal
> *Pediatric:* <18 years: not recommended; ≥18 years: same as adult
> **Lunesta** *Tab:* 1, 2, 3 mg

▷ *flurazepam* (X)(IV)(G) 15 mg q HS; may increase to 30 mg q HS
> *Pediatric:* <18 years: not recommended; ≥18 years: same as adult
> **Dalmane** *Cap:* 15, 30 mg

▷ *trazodone* (C)(G) 50 mg q HS
> *Pediatric:* <18 years: not recommended; ≥18 years: same as adult
> **Desyrel** *Tab:* 50, 100, 150, 300 mg

▷ *triazolam* (X)(IV)(G) 0.125 mg q HS, may increase gradually to 0.5 mg
> **Halcion** *Tab:* 0.125, 0.25*mg

▷ *zaleplon* (C)(IV) (imidazopyridine) 5-10 mg at HS <u>or</u> after going to bed if unable to sleep; do not take if unable to sleep for at least 4 hours before required to be active again; max 20 mg/day x 1 month; delayed effect if taken with a meal
> *Pediatric:* <12 years: not recommended; ≥12 years: same as adult
> **Sonata** *Cap:* 5, 10 mg (tartrazine)

Comment: **Sonata** is indicated for the treatment of insomnia when a middle-of the-night awakening is followed by difficulty returning to sleep.

▷ *zolpidem* oral solution spray **(C)(IV)(G)** (imidazopyridine hypnotic) 2 actuations (10 mg) immediately before bedtime; *Elderly, debilitated,* or *hepatic impairment:* 2 actuations (5 mg); max 2 actuations (10 mg)
   Pediatric: <18 years: not recommended; ≥18 years: same as adult
   ZolpiMist *Oral soln spray:* 5 mg/actuation (60 metered actuations) (cherry)
Comment: The lowest dose of *zolpidem* in all forms is recommended for persons >50 years-of-age and women as drug elimination is slower than in men.
▷ *zolpidem* tabs **(B)(IV)(G)** (pyrazolopyrimidine hypnotic) 5-10 mg or 6.25-12.5 extrel q HS prn; max 12.5 mg/day x 1 month; do not take if unable to sleep for at least 8 hours before required to be active again; delayed effect if taken with a meal
   Pediatric: <18 years: not recommended; ≥18 years: same as adult
   Ambien *Tab:* 5, 10 mg
   Ambien CR *Tab:* 6.25, 12.5 mg ext-rel
Comment: The lowest dose of *zolpidem* in all forms is recommended for persons >50 years-of-age and women as drug elimination is slower than in men.
▷ *zolpidem* sublingual tabs (imidazopyridine hypnotic) **(C)(IV)** dissolve 1 tab under the tongue; allow to disintegrate completely before swallowing; take only once per night and only if at least 4 hours of bedtime remain before planned time for awakening
   Pediatric: <18 years: not recommended; ≥18 years: same as adult
   Edluar *SL Tab:* 5, 10 mg
   Intermezzo *SL Tab:* 1.75, 3.5 mg
Comment: **Intermezzo** is indicated for the treatment of insomnia when a middle-of-the-night awakening is followed by difficulty returning to sleep. The lowest dose of *zolpidem* in all forms is recommended for persons >50 years-of-age and women as drug elimination is slower than in men.

◯ FIFTH DISEASE (*ERYTHEMA INFECTIOSUM*)

Antipyretics *see Fever page 165*

◯ FLATULENCE

▷ *simethicone* **(C)(G)**
   Gas-X (OTC) 2-4 tabs pc and HS prn
      Tab: 40, 80, 125 mg; *Cap:* 125 mg
   Mylicon (OTC) 2-4 tabs pc and HS prn
      Tab: 40, 80, 125 mg; *Cap:* 125 mg
   Phazyme-95 1-2 tabs with each meal and HS prn
      Tab: 95 mg
   Phazyme Infant Oral Drops
   Pediatric: <2 years: 0.3 ml qid pc and HS prn; 2-12 years: 0.6 ml qid pc and HS prn; >12 years: 1.2 ml qid pc and HS prn
      Oral drops: 40 mg/0.6 ml (15, 30 ml w. calibrated dropper) (orange) (alcohol-free)
   Maximum Strength Phazyme 1-2 caps with each meal and HS prn
      Cap: 125 mg

◯ FLUORIDATION, WATER, <0.6 PPM

▷ *fluoride* **(G)**
   Luride
   Pediatric: Water fluoridation 0.3-0.6 ppm: <3 years: use drops; 3-6 years: 0.25 mg daily; 7-16 years: 0.5 mg daily; *Water fluoridation <0.3 ppm:* <3 years: use drops; 6 months-3 years: 0.25 mg daily; 4-6 years: 0.5 mg daily; 7-16 years: 1 mg daily

Chew tab: 0.25, 0.5, 1 mg (sugar-free)

Luride Drops

Pediatric: Water fluoridation 0.3-0.6 ppm: 6 months-3 years: 0.25 ml once daily; 4-6 years: 0.5 ml once daily; 7-16 years: 1 ml once daily; *Water fluoridation <0.3 ppm:* 6 months-3 years: 0.5 ml once daily; 4-6 years: 1 ml once daily; 7-16 years: 2 ml daily

Oral drops: 0.5 mg/ml (50 ml) (sugar-free)

COMBINATION AGENTS

▷ *fluoride+vitamin A+vitamin D+vitamin C* (G)

Pediatric: Water fluoridation 0.3-0.6 ppm: <3 years: not recommended; 3-6 years: 0.25 mg fluoride/day; 7-16 years: 0.5 mg fluoride/day; *Water fluoridation <0.3 ppm:* <6 months: not recommended; 6 months-3 years: 0.25 mg fluoride/day; 4-6 years: 0.5 mg fluoride/day; 7-16 years: 1 mg fluoride/day

Tri-Vi-Flor Drops

Oral drops: fluoride 0.25 mg+*vit a* 1500 u+*vit d* 400 u+*vit c* 35 mg per ml (50 ml)

Oral drops: fluoride 0.5 mg+*vit a* 1500 u+*vit d* 400 u+*vit c* 35 mg per ml (50 ml)

▷ *fluoride+vitamin A+vitamin D+vitamin C+iron*

Pediatric: Water fluoridation 0.3-0.6 ppm: <3 years: not recommended; 3-6 years: 0.25 mg fluoride/day; 7-16 years: 0.5 mg fluoride/day; *Water fluoridation <0.3 ppm:* <6 months: not recommended; 6 months-3 years: 0.25 mg fluoride/day; 4-6 years: 0.5 mg fluoride/day; 7-16 years: 1 mg fluoride/day

Tri-Vi-Flor w. Iron Drops

Oral drops: fluoride 0.25 mg+vit a 1500 u+vit d 400 u+vit c 35 mg+iron 10 mg per ml (50 ml)

◯ FOLLICULITIS BARBAE

Topical Corticosteroids *page* 558

TOPICAL AGENTS

▷ *benzoyl peroxide* (B) apply after shaving; may discolor clothing and linens.

Benzac-W initially apply to affected area once daily; increase to bid-tid as tolerated

Gel: 2.5, 5, 10% (60 gm)

Benzac-W Wash wash affected area bid

Wash: 5% (4, 8 oz); 10% (8 oz)

Benzagel apply to affected area one or more x/day

Gel: 5, 10% (1.5, 3 oz) (alcohol 14%)

Benzagel Wash wash affected area bid

Gel: 10% (6 oz)

Desquam X₅ wash affected area bid

Wash: 5% (5 oz)

Desquam X₁₀ wash affected area bid

Wash: 10% (5 oz)

Triaz apply to affected area daily bid

Lotn: 3, 6, 9% (bottle), 3% (tube); *Pads:* 3, 6, 9% (jar)

ZoDerm apply once or twice daily

Gel: 4.5, 6.5, 8.5% (125 ml); *Crm:* 4.5, 6.5, 8.5% (125 ml); *Clnsr:* 4.5, 6.5, 8.5% (400 ml)

▷ *clindamycin* topical (B) apply bid
  Pediatric: same as adult
    Cleocin T *Pad:* 1% (60/pck; alcohol 50%); *Lotn:* 1% (60 ml); *Gel:* 1% (30, 60 gm);
    Soln w. applicator: 1% (30, 60 ml) (alcohol 50%)
    Clindagel *Gel:* 1% (42, 77 gm)
    Clindets *Pad:* 1% (60/pck)
    Evoclin *Foam:* 1% (50, 100 gm) (alcohol)
▷ *clindamycin+benzoyl peroxide* topical (C)
  Pediatric: <12 years: not recommended; ≥12 years: same as adult
    Acanya (G) apply once daily-bid
      Gel: clin 1.2%+*benz* 2.5% (50 gm)
    BenzaClin apply bid
      Gel: clin 1%+*benz* 5% (25, 50 gm)
    Duac apply daily in the evening
      Gel: clin 1%+*benz* 5% (45 gm)
    Onexton Gel apply once daily
      Gel: clin 1.2%+*benz* 3.75% (50 gm pump) (alcohol-free) (preservative-free)
▷ *dapsone* topical (C)(G) apply bid
  Pediatric: <12 years: not recommended; ≥12 years: same as adult
    Aczone *Gel:* 5% (30 gm)
▷ *tazarotene* (X)(G) apply daily at HS
  Pediatric: <12 years: not recommended; ≥12 years: same as adult
    Avage Cream *Crm:* 0.1% (30 gm)
    Tazorac Cream *Crm:* 0.05, 0.1% (15, 30, 60 gm)
    Tazorac Gel *Gel:* 0.05, 0.1% (30, 100 gm)
▷ *tretinoin* (C) apply q HS
  Pediatric: <12 years: not recommended; ≥12 years: same as adult
    Atralin Gel *Gel:* 0.05% (45 gm)
    Avita *Crm:* 0.025% (20, 45 gm); *Gel:* 0.025% (20, 45 gm)
    Renova *Crm:* 0.02% (40 gm); 0.05% (40, 60 gm)
    Retin-A Cream *Crm:* 0.025, 0.05, 0.1% (20, 45 gm)
    Retin-A Gel *Gel:* 0.01, 0.025% (15, 45 gm; alcohol 90%)
    Retin-A Liquid *Soln:* 0.05% (alcohol 55%)
    Retin-A Micro Gel *Gel:* 0.04, 0.08, 0.1% (20, 45 gm)
    Tretin-X Cream *Crm:* 0.075% (35 gm) (parabens-free, alcohol-free, propylene glycol-free)
    Retin-A Micro *Microspheres:* 0.04, 0.1% (20, 45 gm)

◯ FOREIGN BODY: ESOPHAGUS

▷ *glucagon* (B) 0.02 mg/kg IV or IM with serial x-rays; max 1 mg
    Glucagon (rDNA origin or beef/pork derived)
      Vial: 1 mg/ml w. diluent
  Comment: *glucagon* facilitates passage of foreign body from esophagus into stomach.

◯ FOREIGN BODY: EYE

▷ *proparacaine* 1-2 drops to anesthetize surface of eye; then flush with normal saline
    Ophthaine *Ophth soln:* 0.5% (15 ml)
  Comment: *proparacaine* facilitates the search, location, and removal of foreign body and examination of the cornea.

GASTRITIS

Antacids *see GERD page* 173
H2 Antagonists *see GERD page* 175

 GASTRITIS-RELATED NAUSEA/VOMITING

OTC ANTI-EMETIC

▷ *phosphorylated carbohydrate* solution (C)(G) 1-2 tbsp q 15 minutes until nausea subsides; max 5 doses/day
  Pediatric: 1-2 tsp q 15 minutes until nausea subsides; max 5 doses/day
    Emetrol (OTC) *Soln:* dextrose 1.87 gm+fructose 1.87 gm+phosphoric acid 21.5 mg per 5 ml (4, 8, 16 oz)

Rx ANTI-EMETICS

▷ *ondansetron* (C)(G) 8 mg q 8 hours x 2 doses; then 8 mg q 12 hours
  Pediatric: <4 years: not recommended; 4-11 years: 4 mg q 4 hours x 3 doses; then 4 mg q 8 hours
    Zofran *Tab:* 4, 8, 24 mg
    Zofran ODT *ODT:* 4, 8 mg (strawberry) (phenylalanine)
    Zofran Oral Solution *Oral soln:* 4 mg/5 ml (50 ml) (strawberry) (phenylalanine); *Parenteral form:* see mfr pkg insert
    Zofran Injection *Vial:* 2 mg/ml (2 ml single-dose); 2 mg/ml (20 ml multi-dose); 32 mg/50 ml (50 ml multi-dose); *Prefilled syringe:* 4 mg/2 ml, single-use (24/carton)
    Zuplenz Oral Soluble Film: 4, 8 mg oral-dis (10/carton) (peppermint)
▷ *promethazine* (C)(G) 25 mg PO or rectally q 4-6 hours prn
  Pediatric: <2 years: not recommended; ≥2 years: 0.5 mg/lb or 6.25-25 mg q 4-6 hours prn
    Phenergan *Tab:* 12.5*, 25*, 50 mg; *Plain syr:* 6.25 mg/5 ml; *Fortis syr:* 25 mg/5 ml; *Rectal supp:* 12.5, 25, 50 mg

 GASTROESOPHAGEAL REFLUX (GER), IDIOPATHIC GASTRIC ACID HYPERSECRETION (IGAH), GASTROESOPHAGEAL REFLUX DISEASE (GERD)

Comment: Precipitators of gastric reflux include narcotics, benzodiazepines, calcium antagonists, alcohol, nicotine, chocolate, and peppermint. Issues associated with H2 secretion and gastrointestinal health (e.g., chronic remitting gastritis, Barrett's esophagitis, peptic ulcer disease [PUD]), other organ system impairments (e.g., CVD, metabolic syndrome, hepatitis, autoimmune and immune-deficiency disorders, renal insufficiency, iatrogenic consequences of treatments (e.g., steroids, NSAIDs, immune modulators), (advanced age,) and lifestyle (dietary habits and general nutritional health). Risk/benefit discussions with patients can be challenging, but are necessary for informed decision-making and prudent prescribing.

ANTACIDS

Comment: Antacids with *aluminum hydroxide* may potentiate constipation. Antacids with *magnesium hydroxide* may potentiate diarrhea.
▷ *aluminum hydroxide* (C)
    ALTernaGEL (OTC) 5-10 ml between meals and HS prn; max 90 ml/day

Pediatric: <12 years: not recommended; ≥12 years: same as adult
  Liq: 500 mg/5 ml (5, 12 oz)
Amphojel (OTC) 10 ml 5-6 x/day between meals and HS prn; max 60 ml/day
Pediatric: <12 years: not recommended; ≥12 years: same as adult
  Oral susp: 320 mg/5 ml (12 oz)
Amphojel Tab (OTC) 600 mg 5-6 x/day between meals and HS prn; max 3.6 gm/day
Pediatric: <12 years: not recommended; ≥12 years: same as adult
  Tab: 300, 600 mg

▷ *aluminum hydroxide+magnesium hydroxide* (C)(OTC)(G)
  Maalox 10-20 ml qid and HS prn
  Pediatric: <12 years: not recommended; ≥12 years: same as adult
    Oral susp: alum 225 mg+mag 200 mg per 5 ml (5, 12, 26 oz) (mint, lemon, cherry)
  Maalox Therapeutic Concentrate 10-20 ml qid pc and HS prn
  Pediatric: <12 years: not recommended; ≥12 years: same as adult
    Oral susp: alum 600 mg+mag 300 mg per 5 ml (12 oz) (mint)

▷ *aluminum hydroxide+magnesium hydroxide+simethicone* (C)(OTC)(G)
  Maalox Plus 10-20 ml qid pc and HS prn
  Pediatric: <12 years: not recommended; ≥12 years: same as adult
    Tab: alum 200 mg+mag 200 mg+sim 25 mg
  Extra Strength Maalox Plus 10-20 ml qid pc and HS prn
  Pediatric: <12 years: not recommended; ≥12 years: same as adult
    Tab: alum 350 mg+mag 350 mg+sim 30 mg
    Oral susp: alum 500 mg+mag 450 mg+sim 40 mg per 5 ml (5, 12, 26 oz)
  Extra Strength Maalox Plus Tab 1-3 tabs qid pc and HS prn
  Pediatric: <12 years: not recommended; ≥12 years: same as adult
    Tab: alum 350 mg+mag 350 mg+sim 30 mg
  Mylanta 10-20 ml between meals and HS prn
  Pediatric: <12 years: not recommended; ≥12 years: same as adult
    Liq: alum 200 mg+mag 200 mg+sim 20 mg per 5 ml (5, 12, 24 oz)
  Mylanta Double Strength 10-20 ml between meals and HS prn
  Pediatric: <12 years: not recommended; ≥12 years: same as adult
    Liq: alum 700 mg+mag 400 mg+sim 40 mg per 5 ml (5, 12, 24 oz)

▷ *aluminum hydroxide+magnesium carbonate* (C)(OTC)(G)
  Maalox HRF 10-20 ml qid pc and HS prn
  Pediatric: <12 years: not recommended; ≥12 years: same as adultss
    Oral susp: alum 280 mg+mag 350 mg per 10 ml (10 oz)

▷ *aluminum hydroxide+magnesium trisilicate* (C)(OTC)(G)
  Gaviscon chew 2-4 tabs qid pc and HS prn
  Pediatric: <12 years: not recommended; ≥12 years: same as adult
    Tab: alum 80 mg+mag 20 mg
  Gaviscon Liquid 15-30 ml qid pc and HS prn
  Pediatric: <12 years: not recommended; ≥12 years: same as adult
    Liq: alum 95 mg+mag 359 mg per 15 ml (6, 12 oz)
  Gaviscon Extra Strength 2-4 tabs qid pc and HS prn
  Pediatric: <12 years: not recommended; ≥12 years: same as adult
    Tab: alum 160 mg+mag 105 mg
  Gaviscon Extra Strength Liquid 10-20 ml qid prn
  Pediatric: <12 years: not recommended; ≥12 years: same as adult
    Liq: alum 508 mg+mag 475 mg per 10 ml (12 oz)

▷ *aluminum hydroxide+magnesium hydroxide+simethicone* (C)(OTC)(G)
  Maalox Maximum Strength 10-20 ml qid prn; max 60 ml/day
  Pediatric: <12 years: not recommended; ≥12 years: same as adult

>> *Oral susp:* alum 500 mg+*mag* 450 mg+*sim* 40 mg per 5 ml (5, 12, 26 oz) (mint, cherry)

▷ *calcium carbonate* (C)(OTC)(G)

Children's Mylanta Tab
Pediatric: <2 years: not recommended; 2-5 years (24-47 lb): 1 tab as needed up to tid; 6-11 years (48-95 lb): 2 tabs as needed up to tid
Tab: 400 mg

Children's Mylanta
Pediatric: <2 years: not recommended; 2-5 years (24-47 lb): 1 tab as needed up to tid; 6-11 years (48-95 lb): 2 tabs as needed up to tid
Liq: 400 mg/5 ml (4 oz)

Maalox Tab chew 2-4 tabs prn; max 12 tabs/day
Pediatric: <12 years: not recommended; ≥12 years: same as adult
Chew tab: 600 mg (wild berry, lemon, wintergreen) (phenylalanine)

Maalox Maximum Strength Tab 1-2 tabs prn; max 8 tabs/day
Pediatric: <12 years: not recommended; ≥12 years: same as adult
Tab: 1 gm (wild berry, lemon, wintergreen; phenylalanine)

Rolaids Extra Strength 1-2 tabs dissolved in mouth or chewed q 1 hour prn; max 8 tabs/day
Tab: 1000 mg

Tums 1-2 tabs dissolved in mouth or chewed q 1 hour prn; max 16 tabs/day
Tab: 500 mg

Tums E-X 1-2 tabs dissolved in mouth or chewed q 1 hour prn; max 16 tabs/day
Tab: 750 mg

▷ *calcium carbonate+magnesium hydroxide* (C)

Mylanta Tab 2-4 tabs between meals and HS prn
Pediatric: <12 years: not recommended; ≥12 years: same as adult
Tab: calib 350 mg+*mag* 150 mg

Mylanta DS Tab 2-4 tabs between meals and HS prn
Pediatric: <12 years: not recommended; ≥12 years: same as adult
Tab: calib 700 mg+*mag* 300 mg

Rolaids Sodium-Free 1-2 tabs dissolved in mouth or chewed q 1 hour as needed
Tab: calib 317 mg+*mag* 64 mg

▷ *calcium carbonate+magnesium carbonate* (C)

Mylanta Gel Caps (OTC) 2-4 caps prn
Gel cap: calib 550 mg+*mag* 125 mg

▷ *dihydroxyaluminum*

Rolaids (OTC) 1-2 tabs dissolved in mouth or chewed q 1 hour prn; max 24 tabs/day
Tab: 334 mg

H2 ANTAGONISTS

▷ *cimetidine* (B)(OTC)(G) 800 mg bid or 400 mg qid; max 12 weeks
Pediatric: <16 years: not recommended; ≥16 years: same as adult

Tagamet 800 mg bid or 400 mg qid; max 12 weeks
Tab: 200, 300, 400*, 800*mg

Tagamet HB *Prophylaxis:* 1 tab ac; *Treatment:* 1 tab bid
Tab: 200 mg

Tagamet HB Oral Suspension *Prophylaxis:* 1-3 tsp ac; *Treatment:* 1 tsp bid
Oral susp: 200 mg/20 ml (12 oz)

Tagamet Liquid *Liq:* 300 mg/5 ml (mint-peach) (alcohol 2.8%)

▷ *famotidine* (B)(OTC)(G)
Pediatric: 0.5 mg/kg/day q HS prn or in 2 divided doses; max 40 mg/day

Maximum Strength Pepcid AC 1 tab ac
Tab: 20 mg

Pepcid 20-40 mg bid; max 6 weeks
Tab: 20 mg; *Tab:* 40 mg; *Oral susp:* 40 mg/5 ml (50 ml)
Pepcid AC 1 tab ac; max 2 doses/day
Tab/Rapid dissolving tab: 10 mg
Pepcid Complete (OTC) 1 tab ac; max 2 doses/day
Tab: fam 10 mg+$CaCO_2$ 800 mg+*mag hydroxide* 165 mg
Pepcid RPD *Tab:* 20, 40 mg rapid dissolv

▷ *nizatidine* **(B)(OTC)(G)** 150 mg bid or 300 mg once daily
Pediatric: <12 years: not recommended; ≥12 years: same as adult
Axid *Cap:* 150, 300 mg; *Oral soln:* 15 mg/ml (480 ml) (bubble gum)

▷ *ranitidine* **(B)(OTC)(G)**
Pediatric: <1 month: not recommended; 1 month to 16 years: 2-4 mg/kg/day in 2 divided doses; max 300 mg/day; *Duodenal/Gastric Ulcer:* 2-4 mg/kg/day divided bid; max 300 mg/day; *Erosive Esophagitis:* 5-10 mg/kg/day divided bid; max 300 mg/day; 20 lb, 9 kg: 0.6 ml; 30 lb, 13.6 kg: 0.9 ml; 40 lb, 18.2 kg: 1.2 ml; 50 lb, 22.7 kg: 1.5 ml; 60 lb, 27.3 kg: 1.8 ml; 70 lb, 31.8 kg: 2.1 ml
Zantac 150 mg bid or 300 mg q HS
Tab: 150, 300 mg
Zantac 75 1 tab ac
Tab: 75 mg
Zantac EFFERdose dissolve 25 mg tab in 5 ml water and dissolve 150 mg tab in 6-8 oz water
Efferdose: 25, 150 mg effervescent
Zantac Syrup *Syr:* 15 mg/ml (peppermint) (alcohol 7.5%)

▷ *ranitidine bismuth citrate* **(C)** 400 mg bid
Pediatric: <12 years: not recommended; ≥12 years: same as adult
Tritec *Tab:* 400 mg

PROTON PUMP INHIBITORS (PPIs)

Comment: A recent study of 144,032 incident users of acid suppression therapy, including 125,596 PPI users and 18,436 histamine H2 receptor antagonist users were followed over 5 years. The researchers reported PPI users had an increased risk of having an eGFR <60 mL/min/1.73m², incident CKD, eGFR decline over 30%, and ESRD or eGFR decline over 50%, as compared to those taking H2 blockers. They concluded, "reliance on antecedent acute kidney injury (AKI) as a warning sign to guard against the risk of chronic kidney disease (CKD) among PPI users is not sufficient as a sole mitigation strategy." Further, timely PPI discontinuation is warranted if there is a first AKI to avoid progression to CKD.

REFERENCE
Xie, Y., Bowe, B., Li, T., Xian, H., Yan, Y., & Al-Aly, Z. (2017). Long-term kidney outcomes among users of proton pump inhibitors without intervening acute kidney injury. *Kidney International, 91*(6), 1482–1494. doi:10.1016/j.kint.2016.12.021

Comment: Practice guidelines from the American Gastroenterological Association (AGA) address risks and recommendations for prescribing PPI therapy based on an extensive review of the literature. PPI use may increase the risk for fracture, vitamin B12 deficiency, hypomagnesemia, iron-deficiency anemia, small intestinal bacterial overgrowth (SIBO), *C. difficile* infection, kidney disease, cardiovascular disease (CVD), pneumonias, and dementia. Health care providers are advised to discuss the risks/benefits of PPI therapy with respect to each individual patient's situation.

REFERENCE

Freedberg, D. E., Kim, L. S., & Yang, Y.-X. (2017). The risks and benefits of long-term use of proton pump inhibitors: Expert review and best practice advice from the American Gastroenterological Association. *Gastroenterology, 152*(4), 706–715. doi:10.1053/j.gastro.2017.01.031

▷ *dexlansoprazole* (B)(G) 30-60 mg daily for up to 4 weeks
  Pediatric: <18 years: not recommended; ≥18 years: same as adult
    Dexilant *Cap:* 30, 60 mg ent-coat del-rel granules; may open and sprinkle on applesauce; do not crush <u>or</u> chew granules
    Dexilant SoluTab *Tab:* 30 mg del-rel orally disint

▷ *esomeprazole* (B)(OTC)(G) 20-40 mg once daily; max 8 weeks; take 1 hour before food; swallow whole <u>or</u> mix granules with food <u>or</u> juice and take immediately; do not crush <u>or</u> chew granules
  Pediatric: <1 month: not established; 1 month-<1 year, 3-5 kg: 2.5 mg; 5-7.5 kg: 5 mg; 7.5-12 kg: 10 mg; 1-11 years, <20 kg: 10 mg; ≥20 kg: 10-20 mg; 12-17 years: 20 mg; max 8 weeks; >17 years: same as adult
    Nexium *Cap:* 20, 40 mg ent-coat del-rel pellets
    Nexium for Oral Suspension *Oral susp:* 10, 20, 40 mg ent-coat del-rel granules/pkt; mix in 2 tbsp water and drink immediately; 30 pkt/carton

▷ *lansoprazole* (B)(OTC)(G) 15-30 mg daily for up to 8 weeks; may repeat course; take before eating
  Pediatric: <1 year: not recommended; 1-11 years, <30 kg: 15 mg once daily; >11 years: same as adult
    Prevacid *Cap:* 15, 30 mg ent-coat del-rel granules; swallow whole <u>or</u> mix granules with food <u>or</u> juice and take immediately; do not crush <u>or</u> chew granules; follow with water
    Prevacid for Oral Suspension *Oral susp:* 15, 30 mg ent-coat del-rel granules/pkt; mix in 2 tbsp water and drink immediately; 30 pkt/carton (strawberry)
    Prevacid SoluTab *ODT:* 15, 30 mg (strawberry) (phenylalanine)
    Prevacid 24HR 15 mg ent-coat del-rel granules; swallow whole <u>or</u> mix granules with food <u>or</u> juice and take immediately; do not crush <u>or</u> chew granules; follow with water

▷ *omeprazole* (C)(OTC)(G) 20-40 mg daily for 14 days; may repeat course in 4 months; take before eating; swallow whole <u>or</u> mix granules with applesauce and take immediately; do not crush <u>or</u> chew granules; follow with water
    Prilosec *Cap:* 10, 20, 40 mg ent-coat del-rel granules
    Pediatric: <1 year: not recommended; ≥1 year: 5-<10 kg: 5 mg daily; 10-<20 kg: 10 mg daily; ≥20 kg: same as adult
    Prilosec OTC *Tab:* 20 mg del-rel (regular, wildberry)
    Pediatric: <18 years: not recommended; ≥18 years: same as adult

▷ *pantoprazole* (B)(G) 40 mg daily
  Pediatric: <12 years: not recommended; ≥12 years: same as adult
    Protonix
    Tab: 40 mg ent-coat del-rel
    Protonix for Oral Suspension *Oral susp:* 40 mg ent-coat del-rel granules/pkt; mix in 1 tsp apple juice for 5 seconds <u>or</u> sprinkle on 1 tsp apple sauce, and swallow immediately; do not mix in water <u>or</u> any other liquid <u>or</u> food; take approximately 30 minutes prior to a meal; 30 pkt/carton

▷ *rabeprazole* (B)(OTC)(G) *Tab:* 20 mg daily after breakfast; do not crush <u>or</u> chew; *Cap:* open cap and sprinkle contents on a small amount of soft food <u>or</u> liquid
  Pediatric: <1 year: not recommended; 1-11 years, <15 kg: 5 mg once daily for up to 12 weeks; ≥12 years, ≥15 kg: same as adult
    AcipHex *Tab:* 20 mg ent-coat del-rel
    AcipHex Sprinkle *Cap:* 5, 10 mg del-rel

PROTON PUMP INHIBITORS+SODIUM BICARBONATE COMBINATION

▷ *omeprazole+sodium bicarbonate* (B)(G) 20 mg daily; do not crush or chew; max 8 weeks
  Pediatric: <18 years: not recommended; ≥18 years: same as adult
    Zegerid *Cap:* omep 20 mg+*sod bicarb* 1100 mg; *omep* 40 mg+*sod bicarb* 1100 mg
    Zegerid OTC (OTC) *Cap:* omep 20 mg+*sod bicarb* 1100 mg
    Zegerid for Oral Suspension *Pwdr for oral susp:* omep 20 mg+*sod bicarb* 1680 mg; *omep* 40 mg+*sod bicarb* 1680 mg (30 pkt/carton)

PROMOTILITY AGENT

▷ *metoclopramide* (B)(G) 10-15 mg qid 30 minutes ac and HS prn; up to 20 mg prior to provoking situation; max 12 weeks per therapeutic course
  Pediatric: <18 years: not recommended; ≥18 years: same as adult
    Metozolv ODT *ODT:* 5, 10 mg (mint)
    Reglan *Tab:* 5*, 10 mg; *Syr:* 5 mg/5 ml
    Reglan ODT *ODT:* 5, 10 mg (orange)
Comment: *metoclopramide* is contraindicated when stimulation of GI motility may be dangerous. Observe for tardive dyskinesia and Parkinsonism. Avoid concomitant drugs which may cause an extrapyramidal reaction (e.g., phenothiazines, *haloperidol*).

 GIANT CELL ARTERITIS (GCA), TEMPORAL ARTERITIS

  Acetaminophen for IV Infusion *see Pain page 344*
  NSAIDs *see page 562*
  Opioid Analgesics *see Pain page 345*
  Topical and Transdermal NSAIDs *see Pain page 344*
  Parenteral Corticosteroids *see page 570*
  Oral Corticosteroids *see page 569*

Comment: Giant cell arteritis (GCA), or temporal arteritis, is a systemic inflammatory vasculitis of unknown etiology that occurs in persons ≥50 years-of-age (median age of onset is 75 years) and can result in a wide variety of systemic, neurologic, and ophthalmologic complications. GCA is the most common form of systemic vasculitis in adults. Other names for GCA include arteritis cranialis, Horton disease, granulomatous arteritis, and arteritis of the aged. GCA typically affects the superficial temporal arteries—hence the term temporal arteritis. In addition, GCA most commonly affects the ophthalmic, occipital, vertebral, posterior ciliary, and proximal vertebral arteries. It has also been shown to involve medium- and large-sized vessels, including the aorta and the carotid, subclavian, and iliac arteries. Common early symptoms include headache and visual difficulties. Potential consequences include blindness and aortic aneurysms. Newly recognized GCA should be considered a true neuro-ophthalmic emergency. Prompt initiation of treatment may prevent blindness and other potentially irreversible ischemic sequelae. Corticosteroids are the mainstay of therapy. In steroid-resistant cases, drugs such as *cyclosporine*, *azathioprine*, or *methotrexate* may be used as steroid-sparing agents. GCA is the most common systemic vasculitis affecting elderly patients. (http://emedicine.medscape.com/article/332483-overview)

INTERLEUKIN-6 RECEPTOR ANTAGONIST

▷ *tocilizumab* (B) <100 kg: 162 mg SC every other week on the same day followed by an increase according to clinical response; ≥100 kg: 162 mg SC once weekly on the same day; SC injections may be self-administered

Actemra *Vial:* 80 mg/4 ml, 200 mg/10 ml, 400 mg/20 ml, single-use, for IV infusion after dilution; *Prefilled syringe:* 162 mg (0.9 ml, single-dose)

Comment: **Actemra** received FDA approval in May, 2017 to treat GCA. This is the first FDA-approved drug specifically for the treatment of this form of vasculitis. *tocilizumab* is an interleukin-6 receptor-α inhibitor also indicated for use in moderate-to-severe rheumatoid arthritis (RA) that has not responded to conventional therapy, and some subtypes of juvenile idiopathic arthritis (JIA). **Actemra** may be used alone or in combination with *methotrexate* and in RA, other DMARDs may be used. Monitor patient for dose-related laboratory changes including elevated LFTs, neutropenia, and thrombocytopenia. **Actemra** should not be initiated in patients with an absolute neutrophil count (ANC) <2000/mm³, platelet count <100,000/mm³, or who have ALT or AST above 1.5 times the upper limit of normal (ULN). Registration in the Pregnancy Exposure Registry (1-877-311-8972) is encouraged for monitoring pregnancy outcomes in women exposed to **Atemra** during pregnancy. The limited available data with **Actemra** in pregnant women are not sufficient to determine whether there is a drug-associated risk for major birth defects and miscarriage. Monoclonal antibodies, such as *tocilizumab*, are actively transported across the placenta during the third trimester of pregnancy and may affect immune response in the infant exposed *in utero*. It is not known whether *tocilizumab* passes into breast milk; therefore, breastfeeding is not recommended while using **Actemra**.

GIARDIASIS (*GIARDIA LAMBLIA*)

 metronidazole (not for use in 1st; B in 2nd, 3rd)(G) 250 mg tid x 5-10 days
Pediatric: 35-50 mg/kg/day in 3 divided doses x 10 days
Flagyl *Tab:* 250*, 500*mg
Flagyl 375 *Cap:* 375 mg
Flagyl ER *Tab:* 750 mg ext-rel

 tinidazole (not for use in 1st; B in 2nd, 3rd) 2 gm in a single dose; take with food
Pediatric: <3 years: not recommended; ≥3 years: 50 mg/kg daily in a single dose; take with food; max 2 gm
Tindamax *Tab:* 250*, 500*mg

▷ *nitazoxanide* (B) 500 mg q 12 hours x 3 days; take with food
Pediatric: <1 year: not recommended; 1-3 years: 100 mg q 12 hours x 3 days; 4-11 years: 200 mg q 12 hours x 3 days; ≥12 years: same as adult
Alinia *Tab:* 500 mg; *Oral susp:* 100 mg/5 ml (60 ml)
Comment: **Alinia** is an antiprotozoal for the treatment of diarrhea due to *G. lamblia* or *C. parvum*.

GINGIVITIS/PERIODONTITIS

ANTI-INFECTIVE ORAL RINSES

Comment: Oral treatments should be preceded by brushing and flossing the teeth. Avoid foods and liquids for 2-3 hours after a treatment.

▷ *chlorhexidine gluconate* (B)(G) swish 15 ml undiluted for 30 seconds bid; do not swallow; do not rinse mouth after treatment.
Peridex, PerioGard *Oral soln:* 0.12% (480 ml)

GLAUCOMA: OPEN ANGLE

Comment: Other ophthalmic medications should not be administered within 5-10 minutes of administering an ophthalmic antiglaucoma medication. Contact lenses should be removed prior to instillation of antiglaucoma medications and may be replaced 15 minutes later. Interactions with ophthalmic anti-glaucoma agents include MAOIs, CNS depressants, beta-blockers, tricyclic antidepressants, and hypoglycemics. Choices for medical treatment in progressive cases include *betaxolol* eye drops which have a beneficial effect on optic nerve blood flow in addition to intraocular pressure IOP reduction. Other beta blockers and adrenergic drugs (such as **dipivefrine**) should better be avoided because of the probability of nocturnal systemic hypotension and optic nerve hypoperfusion (e.g., in patients with untreated obstructive sleep apnea). Prostaglandin derivatives tend to have greater IOP-lowering effect which may be of overriding consideration. *dorzolamide-timolol* fixed combination is a safe and effective IOP-lowering agent in patients with normal tension glaucoma (NTG). *brimonidine* significantly improved retinal vascular autoregulation in NTG patients.

REFERENCE

Mallick, J., Devi, L., Malik, P., & Mallick, J. (2016). Update on normal tension glaucoma. *Journal of Ophthalmic and Vision Research, 11*(2), 204. doi:10.4103/2008-322x.183914

OPHTHALMIC ALPHA-2 AGONISTS

Comment: Ophthalmic alpha-2 agonists are contraindicated with concomitant MAOI use. Cautious use with CNS depressants, beta-blockers (ocular and systemic), antihypertensives, cardiac glycosides, and tricyclic antidepressants.
▷ *apraclonidine* ophthalmic solution (**C**) 1-2 drops affected eye tid
   Pediatric: <12 years: not recommended; ≥12 years: same as adult
     Iopidine *Ophth soln:* 0.5% (5 ml) (benzalkonium chloride)
▷ *brimonidine tartrate* ophthalmic solution (**B**) 1 drop affected eye q 8 hours
   Pediatric: <2 years: not recommended; ≥2 years: 1 drop affected eye q 8 hours
     Alphagan P *Ophth soln:* 0.1, 0.15% (5, 10, 15 ml) (purite)

OPHTHALMIC CARBONIC ANHYDRASE INHIBITORS

Comment: Ophthalmic carbonic anhydrase inhibitors are contraindicated in patients with sulfa allergy.
▷ *brinzolamide* ophthalmic suspension (**C**) 1 drop affected eye tid
   Pediatric: <12 years: not recommended; ≥12 years: same as adult
     Azopt *Ophth susp:* 1% (2.5, 5, 10, 15 ml) (benzalkonium chloride)
▷ *dorzolamide* ophthalmic solution (**C**)(**G**) 1 drop affected eye tid
   Pediatric: same as adult
     Trusopt *Ophth soln:* 2% (10 ml) (benzalkonium chloride)

OPHTHALMIC ALPHA-2 ADRENERGIC RECEPTOR AGONIST+CARBONIC ANHYDRASE INHIBITOR

▷ *brimonidine+brinzolamide* (**C**) 1 drop affected eye tid
   Pediatric: <12 years: not recommended; ≥12 years: same as adult
     Simbrinza *Ophth soln:* brim 1% mg+brinz 0.2% per ml (10 ml)

OPHTHALMIC CHOLINERGICS (MIOTICS)

▷ *carbachol+hydroxypropyl methylcellulose* ophthalmic solution (**C**) 2 drops affected eye tid
   Pediatric: <12 years: not recommended; ≥12 years: same as adult
     Isopto Carbachol *Ophth soln:* carb 0.75% <u>or</u> 2.25%+hydroxy 1% (15 ml); carb 1.5% <u>or</u> 3%+hydroxy 1% (15, 30 ml) (benzalkonium chloride)

▷ *pilocarpine* (C)(G)
  Pediatric: <12 years: not recommended; ≥12 years: same as adult
    Isopto Carpine 2 drops affected eye tid-qid
      Ophth soln: 1, 2, 4% (15 ml) (benzalkonium chloride)
    Ocusert Pilo change ophthalmic insert once weekly
      Ophth inserts: 20 mcg/Hr (8/pck)
    Pilocar Ophthalmic Solution 1-2 drops affected eye 1-6 x/day
      Ophth soln: 0.5, 1, 2, 3, 4, 6, 8% (15 ml)
    Pilopine HS apply 1/2 inch ribbon in lower conjunctival sac q HS
      Opth gel: 4% (4 gm)

OPHTHALMIC CHOLINESTERASE INHIBITORS

▷ *demecarium bromide* ophthalmic solution (X) 1-2 drops affected eye q 12-48 hours
  Pediatric: <12 years: not recommended; ≥12 years: same as adult
    Humorsol Ocumeter *Ophth soln:* 0.125, 0.25% (5 ml)
▷ *echothiophate iodide* ophthalmic solution (C) initially 1 drop of 0.03% affected eye
  bid; then increase strength as needed
  Pediatric: <12 years: not recommended; ≥12 years: same as adult
    Phospholine Iodide *Ophth soln:* 0.03, 0.06, 0.125, 0.25% (5 ml)

OPHTHALMIC CARDIOSELECTIVE BETA-BLOCKERS

Comment: Ophthalmic beta-blockers are generally contraindicated in severe COPD,
history of <u>or</u> current bronchial asthma, sinus bradycardia, 2nd <u>or</u> 3rd degree AV
block.
▷ *betaxolol* ophthalmic solution (C)(G) 1-2 drops affected eye bid
  Pediatric: <12 years: not recommended; ≥12 years: same as adult
    Betoptic *Ophth soln:* 0.5% (5, 10, 15 ml) (benzalkonium chloride)
    Betoptic S *Ophth soln:* 0.25% (2.5, 5, 10, 15 ml) (benzalkonium chloride)

OPHTHALMIC BETA-BLOCKERS (NONCARDIOSELECTIVE)

Comment: Ophthalmic beta-blockers are generally contraindicated in severe COPD,
history of <u>or</u> current bronchial asthma, sinus bradycardia, 2nd <u>or</u> 3rd degree AV block.
▷ *carteolol* ophthalmic solution (C)(G) 1 drop affected eye bid
  Pediatric: <12 years: not recommended; ≥12 years: same as adult
    Ocupress *Ophth soln:* 1% (5, 10, 15 ml) (benzalkonium chloride)
▷ *levobunolol* ophthalmic solution (C) 1-2 drops affected eye bid
  Pediatric: <12 years: not recommended; ≥12 years: same as adult
    Betagan *Ophth soln:* 0.5% (5, 10, 15 ml) (benzalkonium chloride)
▷ *metipranolol* ophthalmic solution (C)(G) 1 drop affected eye bid
  Pediatric: <12 years: not recommended; ≥12 years: same as adult
    OptiPranolol *Ophth soln:* 0.3% (5, 10 ml) (benzalkonium chloride)
▷ *timolol* ophthalmic solution and gel (C)(G)
  Pediatric: <12 years: not recommended; ≥12 years: same as adult
    Betimol 1 drop affected eye bid
      Ophth soln: 0.25, 0.5% (5, 10, 15 ml) (benzalkonium chloride)
    Istalol 1 drop affected eye daily
      Ophth soln: 0.5% (2.5, 5 ml) (preservative-free)
    Timoptic 1 drop affected eye bid
      Ophth soln: 0.25, 0.5% (5, 10, 15 ml) (benzalkonium chloride)
    Timoptic Ocudose 1 drop bid
      Ophth soln: 0.25, 0.5% (0.2 ml/dose, 60 dose) (preservative-free)
    Timoptic-XE 1 drop affected eye bid
      Ophth gel: 0.25, 0.5% (2.5, 5 ml) (preservative-free)

OPHTHALMIC ALPHA-2 AGONIST+ NON-CARDIOSELECTIVE BETA-BLOCKER COMBINATION

Comment: Generally contraindicated in severe COPD, history of <u>or</u> current bronchial asthma, sinus bradycardia, 2nd <u>or</u> 3rd degree AV block.

▷ *brimonidine tartrate+timolol* ophthalmic solution (C) 1 drop affected eye bid
Pediatric: <2 years: not recommended; ≥2 years: same as adult
Combigan *Ophth soln: brimo 0.2%+timo 0.5%* (5, 10, 15 ml) (benzalkonium chloride)

OPHTHALMIC PROSTAMIDE ANALOGS

▷ *bimatoprost* ophthalmic solution (C)(G) 1 drop q affected eye HS
Pediatric: <16 years: not recommended; ≥16 years: same as adult
Lumigan *Ophth soln: 0.01, 0.03%* (2.5, 5, 7.5 ml) (benzalkonium chloride)
▷ *latanoprost* ophthalmic solution (C) 1 drop affected eye q HS
Pediatric: <12 years: not recommended; ≥12 years: same as adult
Xalatan *Ophth soln: 0.005%* (2.5 ml) (benzalkonium chloride)
▷ *tafluprost* ophthalmic solution (C) 1 drop affected eye q HS
Pediatric: <12 years: not recommended; ≥12 years: same as adult
Zioptan *Ophth soln: 0.0015%* (0.3 ml single-use, 30-60/carton) (preservative-free)
▷ *travoprost* ophthalmic solution (C)(G) 1 drop affected eye q HS
Pediatric: <16 years: not recommended; ≥16 years: same as adult
Travatan *Ophth soln: 0.004%* (2.5, 5 ml) (benzalkonium chloride)
Travatan Z *Ophth soln: 0.004%* (2.5, 5 ml) (boric acid, propylene glycol, sorbitol, zinc chloride)

OPHTHALMIC SYMPATHOMIMETICS

Comment: Contraindicated in narrow-angle glaucoma. Use with caution in cardiovascular disease, hypertension, hyperthyroidism, diabetes, and asthma.

▷ *dipivefrin* ophthalmic solution (B) 1 drop affected eye q 12 hours
Propine *Ophth soln: 0.1%* (5, 10, 15 ml) (benzalkonium chloride)

OPHTHALMIC CARBONIC ANHYDRASE INHIBITOR+NON-CARDIOSELECTIVE BETA-BLOCKER

▷ *dorzolamide+timolol* ophthalmic solution (C) 1 drop affected eye bid
Pediatric: <12 years: not recommended; ≥12 years: same as adult
Cosopt *Ophth soln: dorz 2%+tim 0.5%* (10 ml) (benzalkonium chloride)
Cosopt PF *Ophth soln: dorz 2%+tim 0.5%* (10 ml) (preservative-free)

OPHTHALMIC SYNTHETIC DOCOSANOID

▷ *unoprostone isopropyl* ophthalmic solution (C) 1 drop affected eye bid
Pediatric: <12 years: not recommended; ≥12 years: same as adult
Rescula *Ophth soln: 0.15%* (5 ml) (benzalkonium chloride)

OPHTHALMIC RHO KINASE INHIBITOR

▷ *netarsudil* ophthalmic solution (C) 1 drop affected eye once daily in the PM
Pediatric: <18 years: not established; ≥18 years: same as adult
Rhopressa *Ophth soln: 0.02%* (0.2 mg/ml, 2.5 ml) (benzalkonium chloride)

OPHTHALMIC ORAL CARBONIC ANHYDRASE INHIBITORS

▷ *acetazolamide* (C) 250-1000 mg/day in divided doses <u>or</u> 500 mg bid sust-rel tabs; max 1 gm/day

Pediatric: <12 years: not recommended; ≥12 years: same as adult
> **Diamox** *Tab:* 125*, 250*mg
> **Diamox Sequels** *Tab:* 500 mg sust-rel
▷ *methazolamide* (C)(G) 50-100 mg bid-tid times daily
  Pediatric: <12 years: not recommended; ≥12 years: same as adult
    Neptazane *Tab:* 25, 50 mg
Comment: Administer ophthalmic osmotic and miotic agents concomitantly.

GONORRHEA (*NEISSERIA GONORRHOEAE*)

Comment: The following treatment regimens for *N. gonorrhoeae* are published in the **2015 CDC Transmitted Diseases Treatment Guidelines**. Treatment regimens are presented by generic drug name first, followed by information about brands and dose forms. Empiric treatment requires concomitant treatment of chlamydia. Treat all sexual contacts. Patients who are HIV-positive should receive the same treatment as those who are HIV-negative. Sexual abuse must be considered a cause of gonococcal infection in preadolescent children.

RECOMMENDED REGIMENS, >12 YEARS: UNCOMPLICATED INFECTIONS OF THE CERVIX, URETHRA, AND RECTUM
Regimen 1
▷ *ceftriaxone* 250 mg IM in a single dose
    plus
▷ *azithromycin* 1 gm in a single dose

Regimen 2
▷ *ceftriaxone* 250 mg IM in a single dose
    plus
▷ *doxycycline* 100 mg bid x 7 days

RECOMMENDED REGIMENS, >12 YEARS: UNCOMPLICATED INFECTIONS OF THE PHARYNX
Regimen 1
▷ *ceftriaxone* 250 mg IM in a single dose
    plus
▷ *azithromycin* 1 gm in a single dose

Regimen 2
▷ *ceftriaxone* 250 mg IM in a single dose
    plus
▷ *doxycycline* 100 mg bid x 7 days

RECOMMENDED REGIMENS, CHILDREN ≥45 KG, ≥8 YEARS; UNCOMPLICATED INFECTIONS OF THE CERVIX, URETHRA, AND RECTUM
Regimen 1
▷ *ceftriaxone* 250 mg IM in a single dose
    plus
▷ *azithromycin* 1 gm in a single dose

RECOMMENDED REGIMEN: CHILDREN >45 KG

Regimen 1

▷ *ceftriaxone* 250 mg IM in a single dose

RECOMMENDED REGIMEN: CHILDREN >45 KG WHO HAVE GONOCOCCAL BACTEREMIA <u>OR</u> GONOCOCCAL ARTHRITIS

Regimen 1

▷ *ceftriaxone* 50 mg/kg IM <u>or</u> IV in a single dose daily x 7 days

RECOMMENDED REGIMENS, CHILDREN <45 KG, <8 YEARS: UNCOMPLICATED GONOCOCCAL VULVOVAGINITIS, CERVICITIS, URETHRITIS, PHARYNGITIS, <u>OR</u> PROCTITIS

Regimen 1

▷ *ceftriaxone* 250 mg IM in a single dose

RECOMMENDED REGIMEN, CHILDREN <45 KG, <8 YEARS: GONOCOCCAL BACTEREMIA <u>OR</u> ARTHRITIS

Regimen 1

▷ *ceftriaxone* 50 mg/kg (max dose 1 gm) IM <u>or</u> IV in a single dose daily x 7 days

DRUG BRANDS AND DOSE FORMS

▷ *azithromycin* (B)(G)
   Zithromax *Tab:* 250, 500, 600 mg; *Oral susp:* 100 mg/5 ml (15 ml); 200 mg/5 ml (15, 22.5, 30 ml) (cherry); *Pkt:* 1 gm for reconstitution (cherry-banana)
   Zithromax Tri-pak *Tab:* 3 x 500 mg tabs/pck
   Zithromax Z-pak *Tab:* 6 x 250 mg tabs/pck
   Zmax *Oral susp:* 2 gm ext-rel for reconstitution (cherry-banana) (148 mg Na$^+$)
▷ *ceftriaxone* (B)(G)
   Rocephin *Vial:* 250, 500 mg; 1, 2 gm
▷ *doxycycline* (D)(G)
   Acticlate *Tab:* 75, 150**mg
   Adoxa *Tab:* 50, 75, 100, 150 mg ent-coat
   Doryx *Tab:* 50, 75, 100, 150, 200 mg del-rel
   Doxteric *Tab:* 50 mg del-rel
   Monodox *Cap:* 50, 75, 100 mg
   Oracea *Cap:* 40 mg del-rel
   Vibramycin *Tab:* 100 mg; *Cap:* 50, 100 mg; *Syr:* 50 mg/5 ml (raspberry-apple) (sulfites); *Oral susp:* 25 mg/5 ml (raspberry)
   Vibra-Tab *Tab:* 100 mg film-coat

ALTERNATIVE THERAPY

▷ *azithromycin* (B)(G) 2 gm x 1 dose
   Pediatric: not recommended for treatment of gonorrhea in children
   Zithromax *Tab:* 250, 500, 600 mg; *Oral susp:* 100 mg/5 ml (15 ml); 200 mg/5 ml (15, 22.5, 30 ml) (cherry); *Pkt:* 1 gm for reconstitution (cherry-banana)
   Zithromax Tri-pak *Tab:* 3 x 500 mg tabs/pck
   Zithromax Z-pak *Tab:* 6 x 250 mg tabs/pck
   Zmax *Oral susp:* 2 gm ext-rel for reconstitution (cherry-banana) (148 mg Na$^+$)
▷ *cefotaxime* 500 mg IM x 1 dose
   Claforan *Vial:* 500 mg; 1, 2 gm

▷ *cefotetan* 1 gm IM x 1 dose
  Pediatric: <12 years: not recommended; ≥12 years: same as adult
    Cefotan *Vial:* 1, 2 gm
▷ *cefoxitin* (B) 2 gm IM x 1 dose
  Pediatric: <3 months: not recommended; ≥3 months: same as adult
    Mefoxin *Vial:* 1, 2 gm
      plus
▷ *probenecid* (B)(G)
    Benemid 1 gm 30 minutes before *cefoxitin*
      Pediatric: <2 years: not recommended; 2-14 years: 25 mg/kg 30 minutes before
      cefoxitin; ≥14 years: same as adult
      Tab: 500*mg; *Cap:* 500 mg
▷ *cefpodoxime proxetil* (B) 200 mg x 1 dose
  Pediatric: <2 months: not recommended; 2 months-12 years: 10 mg/kg/day (max 400
  mg/dose) or 5 mg/kg/day bid (max 200 mg/dose)
    Vantin *Tab:* 100, 200 mg; *Oral susp:* 50, 100 mg/5 ml (50, 75, 100 mg) (lemon creme)
▷ *ceftizoxime* (B) 1 gm IM x 1 dose
  Pediatric: <6 months: not recommended; ≥6 months: same as adult
    Cefizox *Vial:* 500 mg; 1, 2, 10 g
▷ *demeclocycline* (X) 600 mg initially, followed by 300 mg q 12 hours x 4 days (total 3 gm)
  Pediatric: <8 years: not recommended; ≥8 years: same as adult
    Declomycin *Tab:* 300 mg
Comment: *demeclocycline* is contraindicated <8 years-of-age, in pregnancy, and
lactation (discolors developing tooth enamel). A side effect may be photo-sensitivity
(photophobia). Do not give with antacids, calcium supplements, milk or other dairy, or
within two hours of taking another drug.
▷ *enoxacin* (C) 400 mg x 1 dose
  Pediatric: <18 years: not recommended; ≥18 years: same as adult
    Penetrex *Tab:* 200, 400 mg
▷ *imipramine* (C) 400 mg x 1 dose
  Pediatric: <18 years: not recommended; ≥18 years: same as adult
    Maxaquin *Tab:* 400 mg
▷ *norfloxacin* (C) 800 mg x 1 dose
  Pediatric: <18 years: not recommended; ≥18 years: same as adult
    Noroxin *Tab:* 400 mg
▷ *spectinomycin* (B) 2 gm IM x 1 dose
  Pediatric: 40 mg/kg IM x 1 dose
    Trobicin *Vial:* 2 g

 GOUT (HYPERURICEMIA)

Pseudogout *see page* 400
Acetaminophen for IV Infusion *see page* 344
NSAIDs *see page* 562
Opioid Analgesics *see Pain page* 345
Topical and Transdermal NSAIDs *see Pain page* 344
Parenteral Corticosteroids *see page* 570
Oral Corticosteroids *see page* 569

XANTHINE OXIDASE INHIBITORS (PROPHYLAXIS)

▷ *allopurinol* (C)(G) initially 100 mg daily; increase by 100 mg weekly; max 800 mg/
  day and 300 mg/dose; usual range for mild symptoms 200-300 mg/day; for severe
  symptoms 400-600 mg/day; take with food

Pediatric: <6 years: max 150 mg/day; 6-10 years: max 400 mg/day; max single dose
300 mg; >10 years: same as adult
  Zyloprim *Tab:* 100*, 300*mg
  Zyloprim *Tab:* 100*, 300*mg
Comment: Do not take concurrent with *colchicine.* Gout flares may occur after
initiation of urate lowering therapy, such as allopurinol, due to changing serum uric
acid concentrations resulting in mobilization of urate from tissue deposits. If a gout flare
occurs during treatment, allopurinol does not need to be discontinued. Manage the flare
concurrently, as appropriate for the individual patient. The correct dose and frequency
of dosage for maintaining the serum uric acid concentration within the normal range
are best determined by using the serum uric acid concentration as an index. Allopurinol
is not recommended for the treatment of asymptomatic hyperuricemia. Discontinue
allopurinol when the potential for overproduction of uric acid is no longer present.

ACUTE ATTACK

▷ *colchicine* (C)(G) 0.6-1.2 mg at first sign of attack; then 0.6 mg every hour <u>or</u> 1.2 mg
   every 2 hours until pain relief; then consider 0.6 mg/day <u>or</u> every other day for maintenance
   Pediatric: <12 years: not recommended; ≥12 years: same as adult
     Colcrys *Tab:* 0.6 mg
     Mitigare *Cap:* 0.6 mg
Comment: Do not take *colchicine* concurrently with *allopurinol.*
▷ *febuxostat* (C)(G) initially 40 mg daily; after 2 weeks, may increase to 80 mg daily.
   Pediatric: <18 years: not recommended; ≥18 years: same as adult
     Uloric *Tab:* 40, 80 mg
Comment: Gout flare prophylaxis with *colchicine* <u>or</u> NSAID is recommended on
initiation of *febuxostat* and up to 6 months.

PEGYLATED URIC ACID SPECIFIC ENZYME

▷ *pegloticase* (C) premedicate with antihistamine and corticosteroid; 8 mg once every
   2 weeks; administer IV infusion after dilution over at least 2 hours; observe at least 1
   hour post-infusion
   Pediatric: <18 years: not recommended; ≥18 years: same as adult
     Krystexxa *Vial:* 8 mg/ml (1 ml) single-use pwdr for IV infusion after dilution
Comment: Slow rate, <u>or</u> stop and restart at lower rate, if infusion reaction occurs
(e.g., **Krystexxa** is contraindicated with G6PD deficiency; screen patients of African
<u>or</u> Mediterranean descent). **Krystexxa** is not for the treatment of asymptomatic
hyperuricemia.

URICOSURIC AGENT

▷ *probenecid* (C)(G) 250 mg bid x 1 week; maintenance 500 mg bid
   Pediatric: <18 years: not recommended; ≥18 years: same as adult
     Tab: 500*mg; *Cap:* 500 mg
   Comment: Avoid concomitant use of *probenecid* and salicylates.

URICOSURIC+ANTI-INFLAMMATORY COMBINATIONS

▷ *probenecid+colchicine* (G) 1 tab once daily x 1 week; then, 1 tab bid thereafter
   Pediatric: <18 years: not recommended; ≥18 years: same as adult
     Tab: prob 500 mg+colch 0.5 mg
Comment: *probenecid+colchicine* is contraindicated in the treatment of acute gout
attack, patients with blood dyscrasias, and patients with uric acid kidney stones.
Concomitant salicylates antagonize the uricosuric effects.

➤ *sulfinpyrazone* (C) initially 200-400 mg bid; may gradually increase to 800 mg bid
  Pediatric: <18 years: not recommended; ≥18 years: same as adult
     Anturane *Cap:* 100, 200 mg
Comment: Goal is serum uric acid <6.5 mg/dL.

XANTHINE OXIDASE INHIBITOR

➤ *febuxostat* (C) 40 mg once daily x 2 weeks; if serum uric acid is not <6 mg/dL, may
  increase to 80 mg once daily
  Pediatric: <18 years: not established; ≥18 years: same as adult
     Uloric *Tab:* 40, 80 mg

XANTHINE OXIDASE INHIBITOR+URATI INHIBITOR COMBINATION

➤ *allopurinol+lesinurad* take 1 tab once daily
  Pediatric: <18 years: not established; ≥18 years: same as adult
     Duzallo *Tab:* 200/200, 300/200 mg
Comment: The US Food and Drug Administration recently approved **Duzallo** for the
treatment of hyperuricemia associated with gout in patients who have not achieved
target serum uric acid (sUA) levels with *allopurinol* alone. **Duzallo** is the first drug to
combine *allopurinol*, the current standard of care for hyperuricemia associated with
gout, and *lesinurad*, the most recent FDA-approved treatment for this condition. The
fixed-dose combination addresses the overproduction and underexcretion of serum
uric acid. Patients with asymptomatic hyperuricemia are not recommended to receive
Duzallo. Common adverse reactions associated with **Duzallo** include headache,
influenza, higher levels of blood creatinine, and heart burn. In addition, **Duzallo** has
a boxed warning for the risk of acute renal failure associated with *lesinurad*. There
are no available human data on use of **Duzallo** or *lesinurad* in pregnancy to inform a
drug-associated risk of adverse developmental outcomes. Limited published data on
allopurinol use in pregnancy do not demonstrate a clear pattern or increase in frequency
of adverse development outcomes. There is no information regarding the presence of
Duzallo or *lesinurad* in human milk or the effects on the breastfed infant. Based on
information from a single case report, *allopurinol* and its active metabolite, *oxypurinol*,
were detected in the milk of a mother at five weeks postpartum. The effect of *allopurinol*
on the breastfed infant is unknown. CrCl 45-< 60 mL/min: adjust the allopurinol to a
medically appropriate dose (200 mg). CrCl <45, *allopurinol* not recommended. Max
lesinurad 200 mg/day. In clinical trials evaluating the safety and efficacy of this
combined therapy among adult patients with gout who failed to achieve target sUA
levels on *allopurinol* alone, **Duzallo** was found to nearly double the number of patients
who achieved target sUA at 6 months, mean sUA was reduced to less than 6 mg/dL by 1
month, and this level was maintained through 12 months.

◯ GOUTY ARTHRITIS

Acetaminophen for IV Infusion see *Pain page* 344
NSAIDs see *page* 562
Opioid Analgesics see *Pain page* 345
Topical and Transdermal NSAIDs see *Pain page* 344
Parenteral Corticosteroids see *page* 570
Oral Corticosteroids see *page* 569
Topical Analgesic and Anesthetic Agents see *page* 560

TOPICAL ANALGESICS

➤ *capsaicin* (B)(G) apply tid-qid prn to intact skin
  Pediatric: <2 years: not recommended; ≥2 years: same as adult

Axsain *Crm:* 0.075% (1, 2 oz)
Capsin *Lotn:* 0.025, 0.075% (59 ml)
Capzasin-P (OTC) *Crm:* 0.025% (1.5 oz); *Lotn:* 0.025% (2 oz)
Dolorac *Crm:* 0.025% (28 gm)
Double Cap (OTC) *Crm:* 0.05% (2 oz)
R-Gel *Gel:* 0.025% (15, 30 gm)
Zostrix (OTC) *Crm:* 0.025% (0.7, 1.5, 3 oz)
Zostrix HP (OTC) *Emol crm:* 0.075% (1, 2 oz)
Comment: Provides some relief by 1-2 weeks; optimal benefit may take 4-6 weeks.

ORAL SALICYLATE

▷ *indomethacin* (C) initially 25 mg bid-tid; increase as needed at weekly intervals by
25-50 mg/day; max 200 mg/day
Pediatric: <14 years: usually not recommended; ≤2-14 years, if risk warranted: 1-2
mg/kg/day in divided doses; max 3-4 mg/kg/day (or 150-200 mg/day, whichever is
less); ≤14 years: ER cap not recommended; >14 years: same as adult
Cap: 25, 50 mg; *Susp:* 25 mg/5 ml (pineapple-coconut, mint; alcohol 1%); *Supp:*
50 mg; *ER Cap:* 75 mg ext-rel
Comment: *indomethacin* is indicated only for acute painful flares. Administer with food
and/or antacids. Use lowest effective dose for shortest duration.

NSAID PLUS PPI

▷ *esomeprazole+naproxen* (C; not for use in 3rd)(G) 1 tab bid; use lowest effective
dose for the shortest duration; swallow whole; take at least 30 minutes before a meal
Pediatric: <18 years: not recommended; ≥18 years: same as adult
Vimovo *Tab:* nap 375 mg+eso 20 mg ext-rel; nap 500 mg+eso 20 mg ext-rel

COX-2 INHIBITORS

Comment: Cox-2 inhibitors are contraindicated with history of asthma, urticaria, and
allergic-type reactions to *aspirin*, other NSAIDs, and sulfonamides, 3rd trimester of
pregnancy, and coronary artery bypass graft (CABG) surgery.
▷ *celecoxib* (C)(G) 100-400 mg bid; max 800 mg/day
Pediatric: <18 years: not recommended; ≥18 years: same as adult
Celebrex *Cap:* 50, 100, 200, 400 mg
▷ *meloxicam* (C)(G)
Mobic initially 7.5 mg once daily; max 15 mg once daily; Hemodialysis: max 7.5
mg/day
Pediatric: <2 years, <60 kg: not recommended; ≥2 years, >60 kg-12 years: 0.125
mg/kg; max 7.5 mg once daily; ≥12 years: same as adult
Tab: 7.5, 15 mg; *Oral susp:* 7.5 mg/5 ml (100 ml) (raspberry)
Vivlodex initially 5 mg qd; may increase to max 10 mg/day; Hemodialysis: max 5
mg/day
Cap: 5, 10 mg

GRANULOMA INGUINALE (DONOVANOSIS)

Comment: The following treatment regimens are published in the **2015 CDC Sexually
Transmitted Diseases Treatment Guidelines**. Treatment regimens are for adults only;
consult a specialist for treatment of patients less than 18 years-of-age. Treatment
regimens are presented by generic drug name first, followed by information about
brands and dose forms. Persons who have sexual contact with a patient who has had
granuloma inguinale within the past 60 days before onset of the patient's symptoms

should be examined and offered therapy. Patients who are HIV-positive should receive the same treatment as those who are HIV-negative; however, the addition of a parenteral aminoglycoside (e.g., *gentamicin*) can also be considered.

RECOMMENDED REGIMEN

➤ *doxycycline* 100 mg bid x at least 3 weeks and until all lesions have completely healed

ALTERNATE REGIMENS

➤ *azithromycin* 1 gm once weekly for at least 3 weeks and until all lesions have completely healed

➤ *ciprofloxacin* 750 mg bid x at least 3 weeks and until all lesions have completely healed

➤ *erythromycin base* 500 mg qid x 14 days or *erythromycin ethylsuccinate* 400 mg qid x 14 days

➤ *trimethoprim+sulfamethoxazole* take 1 double-strength (160/800) dose bid x at least 3 weeks and until all lesions have completely healed

DRUG BRANDS AND DOSE FORMS

➤ *azithromycin* (B)(G)
  Zithromax *Tab:* 250, 500, 600 mg; *Oral susp:* 100 mg/5 ml (15 ml); 200 mg/5 ml (15, 22.5, 30 ml) (cherry); *Pkt:* 1 gm for reconstitution (cherry-banana)
  Zithromax Tri-pak *Tab:* 3 x 500 mg tabs/pck
  Zithromax Z-pak *Tab:* 6 x 250 mg tabs/pck
  Zmax *Oral susp:* 2 gm ext-rel for reconstitution (cherry-banana) (148 mg Na⁺)
➤ *ciprofloxacin* (C)
  Cipro (G) *Tab:* 250, 500, 750 mg; *Oral susp:* 250, 500 mg/5 ml (100 ml) (strawberry)
  Cipro XR *Tab:* 500, 1000 mg ext-rel
  ProQuin XR *Tab:* 500 mg ext-rel
➤ *doxycycline* (D)(G)
  Acticlate *Tab:* 75, 150**mg
  Adoxa *Tab:* 50, 75, 100, 150 mg ent-coat
  Doryx *Tab:* 50, 75, 100, 150, 200 mg del-rel
  Doxteric *Tab:* 50 mg del-rel
  Monodox *Cap:* 50, 75, 100 mg
  Oracea *Cap:* 40 mg del-rel
  Vibramycin *Tab:* 100 mg; *Cap:* 50, 100 mg; *Syr:* 50 mg/5 ml (raspberry-apple) (sulfites); *Oral susp:* 25 mg/5 ml (raspberry)
  Vibra-Tab *Tab:* 100 mg film-coat
➤ *erythromycin base* (B)(G)
  Ery-Tab *Tab:* 250, 333, 500 mg ent-coat
  PCE *Tab:* 333, 500 mg
➤ *erythromycin ethylsuccinate* (B)(G)
  EryPed *Oral susp:* 200 mg/5 ml (100, 200 ml) (fruit); 400 mg/5 ml (60, 100, 200 ml) (banana); *Oral drops:* 200, 400 mg/5 ml (50 ml) (fruit); *Chew tab:* 200 mg wafer (fruit)
  E.E.S. *Oral susp:* 200, 400 mg/5 ml (100 ml) (fruit)
  E.E.S. Granules *Oral susp:* 200 mg/5 ml (100, 200 ml) (cherry)
  E.E.S. 400 Tablets *Tab:* 400 mg
➤ *trimethoprim+sulfamethoxazole* (TMP-SMX)(C)(G)
  Bactrim, Septra
    Tab: trim 80 mg+*sulfa* 400 mg*

Bactrim DS, Septra DS
Tab: trim 160 mg+*sulfa* 800 mg*
Bactrim Pediatric Suspension, Septra Pediatric Suspension
Oral susp: trim 40 mg+*sulfa* 200 mg per 5 ml (100 ml) (cherry)
(alcohol 0.3%)

 GROWTH FAILURE

Comment: Administer growth hormones by SC injection into thigh, buttocks, or abdomen. Rotate sites with each dose. Contraindicated in children with fused epiphyses or evidence of neoplasia.

▷ *mecasermin* (recombinant human insulin-like growth factor-1 [rhIGF-1])
Increlex (B) see mfr pkg insert
Vial: 10 mg/ml (benzyl alcohol)
Comment: **Increlex** is indicated for growth failure in children with severe primary IGF-1 deficiency (primary IGFD) or in those with growth hormone (GH) gene deletion who have developed neutralizing antibodies to GH.

▷ *somatropin* (rDNA origin)
Genotropin (B) initially not more than 0.04 mg/kg/week divided into 6-7 doses; may increase at 4-8 week intervals; max 0.08 mg/kg/week divided into 6-7 doses
Pediatric: usually 0.16-0.024 mg/kg/week divided into 6-7 doses
Intra-Mix Device: 1.5 mg (1.3 mg/ml after reconstitution), 5.8 mg (5 mg/ml after reconstitution) (two-chamber cartridge w. diluent); *Pen or Intra-Mix Device:* 5.8 mg (5 mg/ml after reconstitution), 13.8 mg (512 mg/ml after reconstitution) (2-chamber cartridge w. diluent)
Genotropin Miniquick (B) initially not more than 0.04 mg/kg/week divided into 6-7 doses; may increase at 4-8-week intervals; max 0.08 mg/kg/week divided into 6-7 doses
Pediatric: usually 0.16-0.024 mg/kg/week divided into 6-7 doses
MiniQuick: 0.2, 0.4, 0.6, 0.8, 1, 1.2, 1.4, 1.6, 1.8, 2 mg/0.25 ml (pwdr for SC injection after reconstitution) (2-chamber cartridge w. diluent)
Humatrope (C)
Pediatric: initially 0.18 mg/kg/week IM or SC divided into equal doses given either on 3 alternate days or 6 x/week; max 0.3 mg/kg/week
Vial: 5 mg w. 5 ml diluent
Norditropin (C)
Pediatric: 0.024-0.034 mg/kg 6-7 x/week SC
Vial: 4 mg (12 IU), 8 mg (24 IU); *Cartridge for inj:* 5, 10, 15 mg/1.5 ml; *FlexPro prefilled pen:* 5, 10, 15 mg/1.5 ml
NordiFlex prefilled pen: 5, 10, 15 mg/1.5 ml; 30 mg/3 ml
Nutropin (C)
Pediatric: 0.7 mg/kg/week SC in divided daily doses
Vial: 5, 10 mg/vial w. diluent
Nutropin AQ (C)
<35 years: initially not more than 0.006 mg/kg SC daily; may increase to max 0.025 mg/kg SC daily; ≥35 years: initially not more than 0.006 mg/kg SC daily; may increase to max 0.0125 mg/kg SC daily
Pediatric: Prepubertal: up to 0.043 mg/kg SC daily; *Pubertal:* up to 0.1 mg/kg SC daily; *Turner Syndrome:* up to 0.0375 mg/kg/week divided into equal doses 3-7 x/week
Vial: 5 mg/ml (2 ml)
Nutropin Depot (C) 1.5 mg/kg SC monthly on same day each month; max 22.5 mg/inj; divide injection if >22.5 mg

Pediatric: same as adult
   Vial: 13.5, 18, 22.5 mg/vial (pwdr for injection after reconstitution; single-use w. diluent and needle)
Omnitrope (B) 0.16-0.24 mg/kg/week SC divided 3-7 x/week
   Vial: 5.8 mg
Omnitrope Pen 5 (B) 0.16-0.24 mg/kg/week SC divided 3-7 x/week
   Cartridge for inj: 5 mg/1.5 ml
Omnitrope Pen 10 (B) 0.16-0.24 mg/kg/week SC divided 3-7 x/week
   Cartridge for inj: 10 mg/1.5 ml
Saizen (B)(G) 0.18 mg/kg/week IM <u>or</u> SC divided 3-7 x/week
   Vial: 5 mg (pwdr for SC injection w. diluent)
Serostim (B) 0.1 mg/kg SC once daily at HS; max 6 mg
   Vial: 5, 4, 6, 8.8 mg (pwdr for SC injection w. diluent) (benzyl alcohol)

HEADACHE: MIGRAINE, CLUSTER, VASCULAR

ERGOTAMINE AGENTS

Comment: Do not use an ergotamine-type drug within 24 hours of any triptan <u>or</u> other 5-HT agonist.
▶ *dihydroergotamine mesylate* **(X)**
   DHE 45 1 mg SC, IM, <u>or</u> IV; may repeat at 1 hour intervals; max 3 mg/day SC <u>or</u> IM/day; max 2 mg IV/day; max 6 mg/week
   Pediatric: <12 years: not recommended; ≥12 years: same as adult
     Amp: 1 mg/ml (1 ml)
   Migranal 1 spray in each nostril; may repeat 15 minutes later; max 6 sprays/day and 8 sprays/week
   Pediatric: <12 years: not recommended; ≥12 years: same as adult
     Nasal spray: 4 mg/ml; 0.5 mg/spray (caffeine)
▶ *ergotamine* **(X)(G)** 1 tab SL at onset of attack; then q 30 minutes as needed; max 3 tabs/day and 5 tabs/week
   Tab: 2 mg
▶ *ergotamine+caffeine* **(X)(G)**
   Pediatric: <12 years: not recommended; ≥12 years: same as adult
   Cafergot 2 tabs at onset of attack; then 1 tab every 1/2 hour if needed; max 6 tabs/attack and 10 tabs/week
   Tab: ergot 1 mg+*caf* 100 mg
   Cafergot Suppository 1 suppository rectally at onset of headache; may repeat x 1 after 1 hour; max 2/attack, 5/week
   Rectal supp: ergot 2 mg+*caf* 100 mg

5-HT RECEPTOR AGONISTS

Comment: Contraindications to 5-HT receptor agonists include cardiovascular disease, ischemic heart disease, cerebral vascular syndromes, peripheral vascular disease, uncontrolled hypertension, hemiplegic <u>or</u> basilar migraine. Do not use any triptan within 24 hours of ergot-type drugs <u>or</u> other 5-HT1A agonists, <u>or</u> within 2 weeks of taking an MAOI.
▶ *almotriptan* **(C)(G)** 6.25 <u>or</u> 12.5 mg; may repeat once after 2 hours; max 2 doses/day
   Pediatric: <12 years: not recommended; ≥12 years: same as adult
   Axert *Tab:* 6.25 mg (6/card), 12.5 mg (12/card)
   Comment: *almotriptan* is indicated for patients 12-17 years-of-age with PMHx migraine headache lasting ≥4 hours untreated.

▷ *eletriptan* (C)(G) 20 <u>or</u> 40 mg; may repeat once after 2 hours; max 80 mg/day
  Pediatric: <18 years: not recommended; ≥18 years: same as adult
    Relpax *Tab:* 20, 40 mg
▷ *frovatriptan* (C)(G) 2.5 mg with fluids; may repeat once after 2 hours; max 7.5 mg/day
  Pediatric: <18 years: not recommended; ≥18 years: same as adult
    Frova *Tab:* 2.5 mg
▷ *naratriptan* (C) 1 <u>or</u> 2.5 mg with fluids; may repeat once after 4 hours; max 5 mg/day
  Pediatric: <18 years: not recommended; ≥18 years: same as adult
    Amerge *Tab:* 1, 2.5 mg
▷ *rizatriptan* (C) initially 5 <u>or</u> 10 mg; may repeat in 2 hours if needed; max 30 mg/day
  Pediatric: <18 years: not recommended; ≥18 years: same as adult
    Maxalt *Tab:* 5, 10 mg
    Maxalt-MLT *ODT:* 5, 10 mg (peppermint) (phenylalanine)
▷ *sumatriptan* (C)(G)
  Pediatric: <18 years: not recommended; ≥18 years: same as adult
    Alsuma 6 mg SC to the upper arm <u>or</u> lateral thigh only; may repeat after 1 hour if
    needed; max 2 doses/day
      Prefilled syringe: 6 mg/0.5 ml (2/pck with auto injector)
    Imitrex Injectable 4-6 mg SC; may repeat after 1 hour if needed; max 2 doses/day
      Prefilled syringe: 4, 6 mg/0.5 ml (2/pck with <u>or</u> without autoinjector)
    Imitrex Nasal Spray (G) 5-20 mg intranasally; may repeat once after 2 hours if
    needed; max 40 mg/day
      Nasal spray: 5, 20 mg/spray (single-dose)
    Imitrex Tab 25-200 mg x 1 dose; may be repeated at intervals of at least 2 hours if
    needed; max 200 mg/day
      Tab: 25, 50, 100 mg rapid-rel
    Imitrex STATdose Pen 6 mg/0.5 mg SC; may repeat once after 2 hours if needed;
    max 2 doses/day
      Prefilled needle-free autoinjector delivery system: 6 mg/0.5 ml (6/pck)
    Onzetra Xsail each disposable white nosepiece contains half a dose of medication
    (11 mg of sumatriptan). A full dose is 22 mg. Do not use more than 2 nosepieces
    per dose; attach the mouthpiece and one nasal piece; then press the white button
    on the delivery device to pierce the capsule in the nasal piece, then insert the nasal
    piece into one nostril and blow into the mouth piece to deliver the nasal powder
    in the contents of one capsule (11 mg); repeat in the opposite nostril for a total
    single 22 mg dose
      Cap: 11 mg nasal pwdr; *Kit:* nosepieces (2), capsules (2), reusable breath pow-
      ered delivery device (1)
    Sumavel DosePro 6 mg SC to the upper arm <u>or</u> lateral thigh only; may repeat after
    1 hour if needed; max 2 doses/day
      Prefilled needle-free delivery system: 6 mg/0.5 ml (6/pck)
    Zembrace SymTouch administer 3 mg SC at onset of headache; may repeat hour-
    ly; max 12 mg/24 hours
    Pediatric: <18 years: not recommended; ≥18 years: same as adult
      Autoinjector: 3 mg/0.5 ml (prefilled single-dose disposable autoinjector)
▷ *zolmitriptan* (C)(G) initially 2.5 mg; may repeat after 2 hours if needed; max
  10 mg/day
  Pediatric: <18 years: not recommended; ≥18 years: same as adult
    Zomig *Tab:* 2.5*, 5 mg
    Zomig Nasal Spray *Nasal spray:* 5 mg/spray single-dose (6/carton)
    Zomig-ZMT *ODT:* 2.5 mg (6 tabs), 5*mg (3 tabs) (orange) (phenylalanine)
Comment: Do not use any ***triptan*** within 24 hours of ergotamine-type drugs <u>or</u> other
5-HT agonists, <u>or</u> within 2 weeks of taking an MAOI.

5-HT IB+ID RECEPTOR AGONIST+NSAID COMBINATION

▷ *sumatriptan+naproxen* (C; D in 3rd)
Pediatric: <18 years: not recommended; ≥18 years: same as adult
Treximet initially 1 tab; may repeat after 2 hours; max 2 doses/day
Tab: suma 85 mg+*naprox* 500 mg (9/blister card)
Comment: Do not use **sumatriptan** within 24 hours of ergot-type drugs or other 5-HT agonists, or within 2 weeks of taking an MAOI.

OTHER ANALGESICS

▷ *acetaminophen+aspirin+caffeine* (D)(G)
Comment: *aspirin*-containing medications are contraindicated with history of allergic-type reaction to **aspirin**, children and adolescents with *Varicella* or other viral illness, and 3rd trimester of pregnancy.
Excedrin Migraine (OTC) 2 tabs q 6 hours prn; max 8 tabs/day x 2 days
Pediatric: <18 years: not recommended; ≥18 years: same as adult
Tab: acet 250 mg+*asp* 250 mg+*caf* 65 mg
▷ *diclofenac potassium powder for oral solution* (C; D ≥30 weeks)(G) empty the contents of one pkt into a cup containing 1-2 oz or 2-4 tbsp (30-60 ml) of water, mix well, and drink immediately; water only, no other liquids; take on an empty stomach; use the closest effective dose for the shortest duration of time; safety and effectiveness of a 2nd dose has not been established
Pediatric: <18 years: not established; ≥18 years: same as adult
Cambia *Pwdr for oral soln:* 50 mg/pkt (3 pkts/set, conjoined with a perforated border
Comment: **Cambia** is not indicated for migraine prophylaxis. May not be bioequivalent with other *diclofenac* forms (e.g., *diclofenac sodium* ent-coat tabs, *diclofenac sodium* ext-rel tabs, *diclofenac potassium* immed-rel tabs) even of the mg strength is the same, therefore, it is not possible to convert dosing from any other diclofenac formulation to **Cambia**. **Cambia** is contraindicated in the setting of coronary artery bypass graft. Use of **Cambia** should not be considered with hepatic impairment, gastric/duodenal ulcer, starting at 30 weeks gestation (risk of premature closure of the ductus arteriosus in the fetus), concomitant NSAIDs, SSRIs, anticoagulants/antiplatelets, any risk factor for potential bleeding.
▷ *isometheptene mucate+dichloralphenazone+acetaminophen* (C)(IV)
Midrin 2 caps initially; then 1 cap q 1 hour until relieved; max 5 caps/12 hours
Pediatric: <12 years: not recommended; ≥12 years: same as adult
Cap: iso 65 mg+*dichlor* 100 mg+*acet* 325 mg

PROPHYLAXIS

▷ *topiramate* (D)(G) initially 25 mg daily in the PM and titrate up daily as tolerated; then 25 mg bid; then, 25 mg in the AM and 50 mg in the PM; then, 50 mg bid
Pediatric: <12 years: not recommended; ≥12 years: same as adult
Topamax *Tab:* 25, 50, 100, 200 mg
Topamax Sprinkle Caps *Cap:* 15, 25 mg
Trokendi XR *Cap:* 25, 50, 100, 200 mg ext-rel
Quedexy XR *Cap:* 25, 50, 100, 150, 200 mg ext-rel

BETA-BLOCKERS

▷ *atenolol* (D)(G) initially 25 mg bid; max 150 mg/day in divided doses
Pediatric: <12 years: not recommended; ≥12 years: same as adult
Tenormin *Tab:* 25, 50, 100 mg

▷ *metoprolol succinate* (C)
  Pediatric: <12 years: not recommended; ≥12 years: same as adult
    ToprolR-XL initially 25-100 mg in a single dose daily; increase weekly if needed;
    max 400 mg/day
      Tab: 25*, 50*, 100*, 200*mg ext-rel
▷ *metoprolol tartrate* (C)
  Pediatric: <12 years: not recommended; ≥12 years: same as adult
    Lopressor (G) initially 25-50 mg bid; increase weekly if needed; max 400 mg/day
      Tab: 25, 37.5, 50, 75, 100 mg
▷ *nadolol* (C)(G) initially 20 mg daily; max 240 mg/day in divided doses
  Pediatric: <12 years: not recommended; ≥12 years: same as adult
    Corgard *Tab:* 20*, 40*, 80*, 120*, 160*mg
▷ *propranolol* (C)(G)
  Pediatric: <12 years: not recommended; ≥12 years: same as adult
    Inderal initially 10 mg bid; usual range 160-320 mg/day in divided doses
      Tab: 10*, 20*, 40*, 60*, 80*mg
    Inderal LA initially 80 mg daily in a single dose; increase q 3-7 days; usual range
    120-160 mg/day; max 320 mg/day in a single dose
      Cap: 60, 80, 120, 160 mg sust-rel
    InnoPran XL initially 80 mg q HS; max 120 mg/day
      Cap: 80, 120 mg ext-rel
▷ *timolol* (C)(G) initially 5 mg bid; max 60 mg/day in divided doses
  Pediatric: <12 years: not recommended; ≥12 years: same as adult
    Blocadren *Tab:* 5, 10*, 20*mg

CALCIUM ANTAGONISTS

▷ *diltiazem* (C)(G)
  Pediatric: <12 years: not recommended; ≥12 years: same as adult
    Cardizem initially 30 mg qid; may increase gradually every 1-2 days; max
    360 mg/day in divided doses
      Tab: 30, 60, 90, 120 mg
    Cardizem CD initially 120-180 mg once daily; adjust at 1- to 2-week intervals;
    max 480 mg/day
      Cap: 120, 180, 240, 300, 360 mg ext-rel
    Cardizem LA initially 180-240 mg once daily; titrate at 2-week intervals; max 540
    mg/day
      Tab: 120, 180, 240, 300, 360, 420 mg ext-rel
    Cardizem SR initially 60-120 mg bid; adjust at 2-week intervals; max 360 mg/day
      Cap: 60, 90, 120 mg sust-rel
▷ *nifedipine* (C)(G)
  Pediatric: <12 years: not recommended; ≥12 years: same as adult
    Adalat initially 10 mg tid; usual range 10-20 mg tid; max 180 mg/day
      Cap: 10, 20 mg
    Procardia initially 10 mg tid; titrate over 7-14 days: max 30 mg/dose and 180 mg/
    day in divided doses
      Cap: 10, 20 mg
    Procardia XL initially 30-60 mg daily; titrate over 7-14 days; max 90 mg/day in
    divided doses
▷ *verapamil* (C)(G)
  Pediatric: <12 years: not recommended; ≥12 years: same as adult
    Calan 80-120 mg tid; increase daily <u>or</u> weekly if needed
      Tab: 40, 80*, 120*mg
    Covera HS initially 180 mg q HS; titrate in steps to 240 mg; then to 360 mg; then
    to 480 mg if needed

Tab: 180, 240 mg ext-rel

Isoptin initially 80-120 mg tid
Tab: 40, 80, 120 mg

Isoptin SR initially 120-180 mg in the AM; may increase to 240 mg in the AM; then, 180 mg q 12 hours <u>or</u> 240 mg in the AM and 120 mg in the PM; then, 240 mg q 12 hours
Tab: 120, 180*, 240*mg sust-rel

TRICYCLIC ANTIDEPRESSANTS (TCAs)

Comment: Co-administration of TCAs with SSRIs requires extreme caution.

▷ *amitriptyline* (C)(G) 10-20 mg q HS
Pediatric: <12 years: not recommended; ≥12 years: same as adult
Tab: 10, 25, 50, 75, 100, 150 mg

▷ *doxepin* (C)(G) 10-200 mg q HS
Pediatric: <12 years: not recommended; ≥12 years: same as adult
Cap: 10, 25, 50, 75, 100, 150 mg; *Oral conc:* 10 mg/ml (4 oz w. dropper)

▷ *imipramine* (C)(G) 10-200 mg q HS
Tofranil 25-50 mg; max 200 mg/day; if maintenance dose exceeds 75 mg daily, may switch to **Tofranil PM**
Pediatric: <6 years: not recommended; 6-12 years: initially 25 mg; >12 years: 50 mg max 2.5 mg/kg/day
Tab: 10, 25, 50 mg
Tofranil PM initially 75 mg once daily 1 hour before HS; max 200 mg
Cap: 75, 100, 125, 150 mg

▷ *nortriptyline* (D)(G) 10-150 mg q HS
Pediatric: <12 years: not recommended; ≥12 years: same as adult
Pamelor *Cap:* 10, 25, 50, 75 mg; *Oral soln:* 10 mg/5 ml (16 oz)

SELECTIVE SEROTONIN REUPTAKE INHIBITORS (SSRIs)

Comment: Co-administration of SSRIs with TCAs requires extreme caution. Concomitant use of MAOIs and SSRIs is absolutely contraindicated. Avoid other serotonergic drugs. A potentially fatal adverse event is Serotonin Syndrome, caused by serotonin excess. Milder symptoms require HCP intervention to avert severe symptoms which can be rapidly fatal without urgent/emergent medical care. Symptoms include restlessness, agitation, confusion, hallucinations, tachycardia, hypertension, dilated pupils, muscle twitching, muscle rigidity, loss of muscle coordination, diaphoresis, diarrhea, headache, shivering, piloerection, hyperpyrexia, cardiac arrhythmias, seizures, loss of consciousness, coma, death. Abrupt withdrawal <u>or</u> interruption of treatment with an antidepressant medication is sometimes associated with an Antidepressant Discontinuation Syndrome which may be mediated by gradually tapering the drug over a period of two weeks <u>or</u> longer, depending on the dose strength and length of treatment. Common symptoms of the Serotonin Discontinuation Syndrome include flu-like symptoms (nausea, vomiting, diarrhea, headaches, sweating), sleep disturbances (insomnia, nightmares, constant sleepiness), mood disturbances (dysphoria, anxiety, agitation), cognitive disturbances (mental confusion, hyperarousal), sensory and movement disturbances (imbalance, tremors, vertigo, dizziness, electric-shock-like sensations in the brain, often described by sufferers as "brain zaps."

▷ *fluoxetine* (C)(G)
Prozac initially 20 mg daily; may increase after 1 week; doses >20 mg/day may be divided into AM and noon doses; max 80 mg/day
Pediatric: <8 years: not recommended; 8-17 years: initially 10-20 mg/day; start lower weight children at 10 mg/day; if starting at 10 mg daily, may increase after 1 week to 20 mg once daily
Cap: 10, 20, 40 mg; *Tab:* 30*, 60*mg; *Oral soln:* 20 mg/5 ml (4 oz) (mint)

Prozac Weekly following daily fluoxetine therapy at 20 mg/day for 13 weeks, may initiate **Prozac Weekly** 7 days after the last 20 mg fluoxetine dose
Pediatric: <12 years: not recommended; ≥12 years: same as adult
Cap: 90 mg ent-coat del-rel pellets

ANTICONVULSANT

▷ **divalproex sodium** (D) *Delayed-release:* initially 250 mg bid; titrate weekly to usual max 500 mg bid; *Extended-release:* initially 500 mg once daily; may increase after one week to 1 gm once daily
Pediatric: <10 years: not recommended; ≥10 years: same as adult
Depakene *Cap:* 250 mg del-rel; syr: 250 mg/5 ml (16 oz)
Depakote *Tab:* 125, 250, 500 mg del-rel
Depakote ER *Tab:* 250, 500 mg ext-rel
Depakote Sprinkle *Cap:* 125 mg del-rel

OTHER AGENT

▷ **methysergide maleate** (X) 4-8 mg daily in divided doses with food; max 8 mg/day; max 6 month treatment course; wean off over last 2-3 weeks of treatment course; separate treatment courses by 3-4 week drug-free interval
Pediatric: <18 years: not recommended; ≥18 years: same as adult
Sansert *Tab:* 2 mg
Comment: *methysergide maleate* is indicated for the prevention or reduction of intensity and frequency of vascular headaches. It is contraindicated in pregnancy due to its oxytocic actions. *methysergide maleate* is a semi-synthetic compound structurally related to ergotamine, and thus it may appear in breast milk. Ergot alkaloids have been reported to cause nausea, vomiting, diarrhea and weakness in the nursing infant and suppression of prolactin secretion and lactation in the mother.

MAGNESIUM SUPPLEMENTS

▷ **magnesium** (B)
Slow-Mag 2 tabs daily
Tab: 64 mg (as chloride)+110 mg (as carbonate)
▷ **magnesium oxide** (B)
Mag-Ox 400 1-2 tabs daily
Tab: 400 mg

HEADACHE: TENSION (MUSCLE CONTRACTION)

Acetaminophen for IV Infusion *see Pain page* 344
NSAIDs *see page* 562
Opioid Analgesics *see Pain page* 345
Topical and Transdermal NSAIDs *see Pain page* 344
Parenteral Corticosteroids *see page* 570
Oral Corticosteroids *see page* 569
Topical Analgesic and Anesthetic Agents *see page* 560

ORAL ANALGESICS COMBINATIONS

Other Oral Analgesics *see Pain page* 338
▷ **butalbital+acetaminophen** (C)(G)
Pediatric: <12 years: not recommended; ≥12 years: same as adult
Phrenilin 1-2 tabs q 4 hours prn; max 6 tabs/day

   Tab: but 50 mg+*acet* 325 mg

  Phrenilin Forte 1 tab <u>or</u> cap q 4 hours prn; max 6 caps/day

   Cap/Tab: but 50 mg+*acet* 650 mg

▷ *butalbital+acetaminophen+caffeine* (C)(G)

 Pediatric: <12 years: not recommended; ≥12 years: same as adult

  Fioricet 1-2 tabs q 4 hours prn; max 6/day

   Tab: but 50 mg+*acet* 325 mg+*caf* 40 mg

  Zebutal 1 cap q 4 hours prn; max 5/day

   Cap: but 50 mg+*acet* 500 mg+*caf* 40 mg

▷ *butalbital+acetaminophen+codeine+caffeine* (C)(III)(G)

 Pediatric: <18 years: not recommended; ≥18 years: same as adult

  Fioricet with Codeine 1-2 tabs at onset q 4 hours prn; max 6 tabs/day

   Tab: but 50 mg+*acet* 325 mg+*cod* 30 mg+*caf* 40 mg

Comment: *Codeine* is known to be excreted in breast milk. <12 years: not recommended; 12-<18: use extreme caution; not recommended for children and adolescents with asthma <u>or</u> other chronic breathing problem. The FDA and the European Medicines Agency (EMA) are investigating the safety of using *codeine* containing medications to treat pain, cough and colds, in children 12-<18 years because of the potential for serious side effects, including slowed <u>or</u> difficult breathing.

▷ *butalbital+aspirin+caffeine* (C)(III)(G)

 Pediatric: <12 years: not recommended; ≥12 years: same as adult

  Fiorinal 1-2 tabs <u>or</u> caps q 4 hours prn; max 6 caps/tabs/day

   Tab/Cap: but 50 mg+*asa* 325 mg+*caf* 40 mg

Comment: *aspirin*-containing medications are contraindicated with history of allergic-type reaction to *aspirin*, children and adolescents with *Varicella* or other viral illness, and 3rd trimester of pregnancy.

▷ *butalbital+aspirin+codeine+caffeine* (C)(III)(G)

 Pediatric: 18 years: not recommended; ≥18 years: same as adult

  Fiorinal with Codeine 1-2 caps q 4 hours prn; max 6 caps/day

   Cap: but 50 mg+*asp* 325 mg+*cod* 30 mg+*caf* 40 mg

Comment: *Codeine* is known to be excreted in breast milk. <12 years: not recommended; 12-<18: use extreme caution; not recommended for children and adolescents with asthma <u>or</u> other chronic breathing problem. The FDA and the European Medicines Agency (EMA) are investigating the safety of using *codeine* containing medications to treat pain, cough and colds, in children 12-<18 years because of the potential for serious side effects, including slowed <u>or</u> difficult breathing. *aspirin*-containing medications are contraindicated with history of allergic-type reaction to *aspirin*, children and adolescents with *Varicella* or other viral illness, and 3rd trimester of pregnancy.

▷ *butorphanol tartrate* (C)(IV)(G) initially 1 spray (1 mg) in one nostril and may repeat after 60-90 minutes (*Elderly* 90-120 minutes) in opposite nostril if needed <u>or</u> 1 spray in each nostril and may repeat q 3-4 hours prn

 Pediatric: <18 years: not recommended; ≥18 years: same as adult

  Butorphanol Nasal Spray *Nasal spray:* 1 mg/actuation (10 mg/ml, 2.5 ml)

  Stadol Nasal Spray *Nasal spray:* 10 mg/ml, 1 mg/actuation (10 mg/ml, 2.5 ml)

▷ *tramadol* (C)(IV)(G) initially 100 mg once daily; may increase by 100 mg every 5 days; max 300 mg/day; *CrCl <30 mL/min* <u>or</u> *severe hepatic impairment*: not recommended; *Cirrhosis:* max 50 mg q 12 hours

  Rybix ODT *ODT:* 50 mg (mint) (phenylalanine)

  Ryzolt *Tab:* 100, 200, 300 mg ext-rel

  Ultram *Tab:* 50*mg

  Ultram ER *Tab:* 100, 200, 300 mg ext-rel

Comment: *tramadol* is known to be excreted in breast milk. The FDA and the European Medicines Agency (EMA) are investigating the safety of using *tramadol*-containing medications to treat pain in children 12-18 years because of the potential for serious side effects, including slowed or difficult breathing.

▷ *tramadol+acetaminophen* (C)(IV)(G) 2 tabs q 4-6 hours prn; max 8 tabs/day; 5 days; *CrCl <30 mL/min:* max 2 tabs q 12 hours; max 4 tabs/day x 5 days; *Cirrhosis or other liver disease:* contraindicated

Pediatric: <18 years: not recommended; ≥18 years: same as adult

Ultracet *Tab:* tram 37.5+acet 325 mg

Comment: *tramadol* is known to be excreted in breast milk. The FDA and the European Medicines Agency (EMA) are investigating the safety of using *tramadol*-containing medications to treat pain in children 12-18 years because of the potential for serious side effects, including slowed or difficult breathing.

TRICYCLIC ANTIDEPRESSANTS (TCAs)

Comment: Co-administration of TCAs with SSRIs requires extreme caution.

▷ *amitriptyline* (C)(G) 50-100 mg/day
Pediatric: <12 years: not recommended; ≥12 years: same as adult
Tab: 10, 25, 50, 75, 100, 150 mg

▷ *desipramine* (C)(G) 50-100 mg bid
Pediatric: <12 years: not recommended; ≥12 years: same as adult
Norpramin *Tab:* 10, 25, 50, 75, 100, 150 mg

▷ *imipramine* (C)(G)
Pediatric: <12 years: not recommended; ≥12 years: same as adult
Tofranil initially 75 mg daily (max 200 mg); adolescents initially 30-40 mg daily (max 100 mg/day); if maintenance dose exceeds 75 mg daily, may switch to Tofranil PM for divided or bedtime dosing
Tab: 10, 25, 50 mg
Tofranil PM initially 75 mg once daily 1 hour before HS; max 200 mg
Cap: 75, 100, 125, 150 mg
Tofranil Injection 50 mg IM; lower dose for adolescents; switch to oral form as soon as possible
Amp: 25 mg/2 ml (2 ml)

▷ *nortriptyline* (D)(G) 25-50 mg/day
Pediatric: <12 years: not recommended; ≥12 years: same as adult
Pamelor *Cap:* 10, 25, 50, 75 mg; *Oral soln:* 10 mg/5 ml (16 oz)

MAGNESIUM SUPPLEMENTS

▷ *magnesium* (B)
Slow-Mag 2 tabs daily
Tab: 64 mg (as chloride)/110 mg (as carbonate)

▷ *magnesium oxide* (B)
Mag-Ox 400 1-2 tabs daily
Tab: 400 mg

 HEART FAILURE (HF)

HEART FAILURE AND DIABETES

Comment: Heart failure (HF) in the presence of type 2 diabetes (T2DM) has a 5-year survival rate on par with some of the worst diseases, such as lung cancer, because diabetes makes the pathophysiology of heart failure worse. Diabetes amplifies the neurohormonal response to heart failure, so it drives progressive heart failure and increases the risk for sudden death. **As left ventricular function decreases, patients with diabetes have heightened activation of the renin angiotensin system (RAS). They have** increased left ventricular hypertrophy, and they have increased sympathetic nervous system activation. A "four Ds" framework that clinicians can use to improve prognosis in these patients: (1) *Loop diuretics* to get the patient out of congestive cardiac syndrome as quickly as possible; (2) *Disease modification* with beta-blockers (β and ACE inhibitors, to the maximal dose tolerated, the mainstays of treatment for patients with heart failure (ACEI's protect these patients against cardiac myocyte cell death and vasoconstriction and beta-blockers protect against the activation of the sympathetic nervous system [SNS]); (3) Consider *device therapy* (including defibrillators and resynchronization therapy); and (4) *Optimize diabetes management*.

REFERENCE

Reported by Mark Kearney, MD, Director of the Leeds Institute of Cardiovascular & Metabolic Medicine at Leeds (England) University, the World Congress on Insulin Resistance, Diabetes & Cardiovascular Disease [published online January 28, 2018]. https://www.mdedge.com/clinicalendocrinologynews/article/157198/diabetes/learn-four-ds-approach-heart-failure-diabetes

ACE INHIBITORS (ACEIs)

▷ *captopril* **(C; D in 2nd, 3rd)(G)** initially 25 mg tid; after 1-2 weeks may increase to 50 mg tid; max 450 mg/day
 Pediatric: <12 years: not recommended; ≥12 years: same as adult
  Capoten *Tab:* 12.5*, 25*, 50*, 100*mg

▷ *enalapril* **(D)** initially 5 mg daily; usual dosage range 10-40 mg/day; max 40 mg/day
 Pediatric: <12 years: not recommended; ≥12 years: same as adult
  Epaned Oral Solution *Oral soln:* 1 mg/ml (150 ml) (mixed berry)
  Vasotec (G) *Tab:* 2.5*, 5*, 10, 20 mg

▷ *fosinopril* **(C; D in 2nd, 3rd)** initially 10 mg daily, usual maintenance 20-40 mg/day in a single or divided doses
 Pediatric: <6 years, <50 kg: not recommended; 6-12 years, ≥50 kg: 5-10 mg daily; ≥12 years: same as adult
  Monopril *Tab:* 10*, 20, 40 mg

▷ *lisinopril* **(D)** initially 5 mg daily
  Prinivil initially 10 mg daily; usual range 20-40 mg/day
  Pediatric: <12 years: not recommended; ≥12 years: same as adult
   Tab: 5*, 10*, 20*, 40 mg
  Qbrelis Oral Solution administer as a single dose once daily
  Pediatric: <6 years, GFR <30 mL/min: not recommended; ≥6 years, GFR >30 mL/min: initially 0.07 mg/kg, max 5 mg; adjust according to BP up to a max 0.61 mg/kg (40 mg) once daily
   Oral soln: 1 mg/ml (150 ml)
  Zestril initially 10 mg daily; usual range 20-40 mg/day
  Pediatric: <12 years: not recommended; ≥12 years: same as adult
   Tab: 2.5, 5*, 10, 20, 30, 40 mg

▷ *quinapril* **(C; D in 2nd, 3rd)** initially 5 mg bid; increase weekly to 10-20 mg bid
 Pediatric: <12 years: not recommended; ≥12 years: same as adult
  Accupril *Tab:* 5*, 10, 20, 40 mg

▷ *ramipril* **(C; D in 2nd, 3rd)** initially 2.5 mg bid; usual maintenance 5 mg bid
 Pediatric: <12 years: not recommended; ≥12 years: same as adult
  Altace *Tab/Cap:* 1.25, 2.5, 5, 10 mg

▷ *trandolapril* **(C; D in 2nd, 3rd)** initially 1 mg daily; titrate to dose of 4 mg daily as tolerated
 Pediatric: <12 years: not recommended; ≥12 years: same as adult
  Mavik *Tab:* 1*, 2, 4 mg

BETA-BLOCKERS (CARDIOSELECTIVE)

▷ *carvedilol* (C)(G)

Coreg initially 3.125 mg bid; may increase at 1-2 week intervals to 12.5 mg bid; usual max 50 mg bid

Pediatric: <18 years: not recommended; ≥18 years: same as adult

Tab: 3.125, 6.25, 12.5, 25 mg

Coreg CR initially 10 mg once daily x 2 weeks; may double dose at 2 week intervals; max 80 mg once daily; may open caps and sprinkle on food

Pediatric: <18 years: not recommended; ≥18 years: same as adult

Cap: 10, 20, 40, 80 mg cont-rel

▷ *metoprolol succinate* (C)

Pediatric: <12 years: not recommended; ≥12 years: same as adult

Toprol-XL initially 12.5-25 mg in a single dose daily; increase weekly if needed; reduce if symptomatic bradycardia occurs; max 400 mg/day

Tab: 25*, 50*, 100*, 200*mg ext-rel

▷ *metoprolol tartrate* (C)

Pediatric: <12 years: not recommended; ≥12 years: same as adult

Lopressor (G) initially 25-50 mg bid; increase weekly if needed; max 400 mg/day

Tab: 25, 37.5, 50, 75, 100 mg

ANGIOTENSIN II RECEPTOR BLOCKERS (ARBs)

▷ *valsartan* (C; D in 2nd, 3rd) initially 40 mg bid; increase to 160 mg bid as tolerated or 320 mg daily after 2-4 weeks; usual range 80-320 mg/day

Pediatric: <12 years: not recommended; ≥12 years: same as adult

Diovan *Tab:* 40*, 80, 160, 320 mg

NEPRILYSIN INHIBITOR+ARB COMBINATION

▷ *sacubitril+valsartan* (D) initially 49/51 bid; double dose after 2-4 weeks; maintenance 97/103 bid; *GFR <30 mL/min or moderate hepatic impairment:* initially 24/26 bid; double dose every 2-4 weeks to target maintenance 97/103 bid

Pediatric: <12 years: not established; ≥12 years: same as adult

Entresto

Tab: **Entresto 24/26:** *sacu* 24 mg+*val* 26 mg

Entresto 49/51: *sacu* 49 mg+*val* 51 mg

Entresto 97/103: *sacu* 97 mg+*val* 103 mg

ALDOSTERONE RECEPTOR BLOCKER

▷ *eplerenone* (B) initially 25 mg once daily; titrate within 4 weeks to 50 mg once daily; adjust dose based on serum K⁺

Pediatric: <12 years: not recommended; ≥12 years: same as adult

Inspra *Tab:* 25, 50 mg

Comment: Inspra is contraindicated with concomitant potent CYP3A4 inhibitors. Risk of hyperkalemia with concomitant ACEI or ARB. Monitor serum potassium at baseline, 1 week, and 1 month. Caution with serum *Cr >2 mg/dL* (male) or >1.8 mg/dL (female) and/or *CrCl <50 mL/min*, and DM with proteinuria.

THIAZIDE DIURETICS

Comment: Monitor hydration status, blood pressure, urine output, serum K⁺.

▷ *chlorothiazide* (C)(G) 0.5-1 gm/day in single or divided doses; max 2 gm/day

Pediatric: <6 months: up to 15 mg/lb/day in 2 divided doses; ≥6 months: 10 mg/lb/day in 2 divided doses

Diuril *Tab:* 250*, 500*mg; *Oral susp:* 250 mg/5 ml (237 ml)

▷ *hydrochlorothiazide* (B)(G)
  Pediatric: <12 years: not recommended; ≥12 years: same as adult
    Esidrix 25-100 mg once daily
      Tab: 25, 50, 100 mg
    Microzide 12.5 mg daily; usual max 50 mg/day
      Cap: 12.5 mg
▷ *methyclothiazide+deserpidine* (B) initially 2.5 mg once daily; max 5 mg once daily
  Pediatric: <12 years: not recommended; ≥12 years: same as adult
    Enduronyl *Tab: methy* 5 mg+*deser* 0.25 mg*
    Enduronyl Forte *Tab: methy* 5 mg+*deser* 0.5 mg*
▷ *polythiazide* (C) 2-4 mg once daily
  Pediatric: <12 years: not recommended; ≥12 years: same as adult
    Renese *Tab:* 1, 2, 4 mg

POTASSIUM-SPARING DIURETICS

Comment: Monitor hydration status, blood pressure, urine output, serum K⁺.
▷ *amiloride* (B) initially 5 mg once daily; may increase to 10 mg; max 20 mg
  Pediatric: <12 years: not recommended; ≥12 years: same as adult
    Midamor *Tab:* 5 mg
▷ *spironolactone* (D) initially 50-100 mg in a single or divided doses; titrate at 2 week intervals
  Pediatric: <12 years: not established; ≥12 years: same as adult
    Aldactone (G) *Tab:* 25, 50*, 100*mg
    CaroSpir *Oral susp:* 25 mg/5 ml (118, 473 ml) (banana)

LOOP DIURETICS

Comment: Monitor hydration status, blood pressure, urine output, serum K⁺.
▷ *bumetanide* (C)(G) 0.5-2 mg as a single dose; may repeat at 4-5 hour intervals; max 10 mg/day
  Pediatric: <18 years: not recommended; ≥18 years: same as adult
    Bumex *Tab:* 0.5*, 1*, 2*mg
Comment: **bumetanide** is contraindicated with sulfa drug allergy.
▷ *ethacrynic acid* (B)(G) initially 50-200 mg once daily
  Pediatric: infants: not recommended; >1 month: initially 25 mg/day; then adjust dose in 25 mg increments
    Edecrin *Tab:* 25, 50 mg
▷ *ethacrynate sodium* (B)(G) for IV injection
    Sodium Edecrin *Vial:* 50 mg single-dose
Comment: **Sodium Edecrin** is more potent than more commonly used loop and thiazide diuretics.
▷ *furosemide* (C)(G) initially 40 mg bid
  Pediatric: <12 years: not recommended; ≥12 years: same as adult
    Lasix *Tab:* 20, 40*, 80 mg; *Oral soln:* 10 mg/ml (2, 4 oz w. dropper)
Comment: **furosemide** is contraindicated with sulfa drug allergy.
▷ *torsemide* (B) 5 mg once daily; may increase to 10 mg daily
  Pediatric: <12 years: not recommended; ≥12 years: same as adult
    Demadex *Tab:* 5*, 10*, 20*, 100*mg

OTHER DIURETICS

Comment: Monitor hydration status, blood pressure, urine output, serum K⁺.
▷ *indapamide* (B) initially 1.25 mg once daily; may titrate dosage upward every 4 weeks if needed; max 5 mg/day
    Lozol *Tab:* 1.25, 2.5 mg

Comment: *indapamide* is contraindicated with sulfa drug allergy.
▷ *metolazone* (B) 2.5-5 mg once daily
  Pediatric: <12 years: not recommended; ≥12 years: same as adult
    Zaroxolyn *Tab:* 2.5, 5, 10 mg
Comment: *metolazone* is contraindicated with sulfa drug allergy.

DIURETIC COMBINATIONS

Comment: Monitor hydration status, blood pressure, urine output, serum K⁺.
▷ *amiloride+hydrochlorothiazide* (B)(G) initially 1 tab once daily; may increase to
  2 tabs/day in a single or divided doses
  Pediatric: <12 years: not recommended; ≥12 years: same as adult
    Moduretic *Tab:* amil 5 mg+hctz 50 mg*
▷ *spironolactone+hydrochlorothiazide* (D)(G)
  Pediatric: <12 years: not recommended; ≥12 years: same as adult
    Aldactazide 25 usual maintenance 50-100 mg in a single or divided doses
      Tab: spiro 25 mg+hctz 25 mg
    Aldactazide 50 usual maintenance 50-100 mg in a single or divided doses
      Tab: spiro 50 mg+hctz 50 mg
▷ *triamterene+hydrochlorothiazide* (C)(G)
  Pediatric: <12 years: not recommended; ≥12 years: same as adult
    Dyazide 1-2 caps daily
      Cap: triam 37.5 mg+hctz 25 mg
    Maxzide 1 tab once daily
      Tab: triam 75 mg+hctz 50 mg*
    Maxzide-25 1-2 tabs once daily
      Tab: triam 37.5 mg+hctz 25 mg*

NITRATE+PERIPHERAL VASODILATOR COMBINATION

▷ *isosorbide dinitrate+hydralazine* (C) initially 1 tab tid; may reduce to 1/2 tab tid if
  not tolerated; titrate as tolerated after 3-5 days; max 2 tabs tid
  Pediatric: <12 years: not recommended; ≥12 years: same as adult
    BiDil *Tab:* isosor 20 mg+hydral 37.5 mg
    Comment: BiDil is an adjunct to standard therapy in self-identified black persons
    to improve survival, to prolong time to hospitalization for heart failure, and to
    improve patient-reported functional status.

CARDIAC GLYCOSIDES

Comment: Therapeutic serum level of is 0.8-2 mcg/ml.
▷ *digoxin* (C)(G) 1-1.5 mg IM, IV, or PO in divided doses over 1-3 days as a loading
  dose; usual maintenance 0.125-0.5 mg/day
  Pediatric: Total oral pediatric digitalizing dose (in 24 hours): <2 years: 40-50 mcg/kg; 2-10
  years: 30-40 mcg/kg; >10 years: 0.75-1.5 mg; *Daily oral pediatric maintenance dose (single
  dose):* <2 years: 10-12 mcg/kg; 2-10 years: 8-10 mcg/kg; >10 years: 0.125–0.5 mg
  Comment: For more information on the use of digoxin in pediatric heart failure, see
  Jain, S. & Vaidyanathan, B. Ann Pediatr Cardiol. Jul-Dec 2009: 2(2): 149-152.
    Lanoxicaps
    Pediatric: <10 years: use elixir or parenteral form
      Cap: 0.05, 0.1, 0.2 mg soln-filled (alcohol)
    Lanoxin
    Pediatric: <10 years: use elixir or parenteral form
      Tab: 0.0625, 0.125*, 0.1875, 0.25*mg; *Elix:* 0.05 mg/ml (2 oz w. dropper) (lime)
      (alcohol 10%)
    Lanoxin Injection *Amp:* 0.25 mg/ml (2 ml)
    Lanoxin Injection Pediatric *Amp:* 0.1 mg/ml (1 ml)

HYPERPOLARIZATION-ACTIVATED CYCLIC NUCLEOTIDE-GATED CHANNEL BLOCKER

➤ *ivabradine* (D) initially 5 mg bid with food; assess after 2 weeks and adjust dose to achieve a resting heart rate 50-60 bpm; thereafter, adjust dose as needed based on resting heart rate and tolerability; max 7.5 mg bid; in patients with a history of conduction defects, <u>or</u> for whom bradycardia could lead to hemodynamic compromise, initiate at 2.5 mg bid before increasing the dose based on heart rate
Pediatric: <18 years: not established; ≥18 years: same as adult
   Corlanor *Tab:* 5, 7.5 mg

Comment: **Corlanor** is indicated to reduce the risk of hospitalization for worsening heart failure in patients with stable, symptomatic, chronic heart failure with left ventricular ejection fraction (LVEF) ≤35%, who are in sinus rhythm with resting heart rate ≤70 bpm and either are on maximally tolerated doses of beta-blockers <u>or</u> have a contraindication to beta-blocker use. **Corlanor** is contraindicated with acute decompensated heart failure, BP <90/50, sick sinus syndrome (SSS), sinoatrial block, and 3rd degree AV block (unless patient has a functioning demand pacemaker). **Corlanor** may cause fetal toxicity when administered pregnant women based on embryo-fetal toxicity and cardiac teratogenic to effects observed in animal studies. Therefore, females should be advised to use effective contraception when taking this drug.

 HELICOBACTER PYLORI (H. PYLORI)

ERADICATION REGIMENS

Comment: There are many H2 receptor blocker-based and PPI-based treatment regimens suggested in the professional literature for the eradication of the *H. pylori* organism and subsequent ulcer healing. Generally, regimens range from 10-14 days for eradication and 2-6 more weeks of continued gastric acid suppression. A three- <u>or</u> four-antibiotic combination may increase treatment effectiveness and decrease the likelihood of resistant strain emergence. Empirical treatment is not recommended. Diagnosis should be confirmed before treatment is started. Antibiotic choices include *doxycycline, tetracycline, amoxicillin, amoxicillin+clavulanate, clarithromycin, clindamycin,* and *metronidazole.* Follow-up visits are recommended at 2 and 6 weeks to evaluate treatment outcomes.

➤ **Regimen 1: Helidac Therapy (D)** *bismuth subsalicylate* 525 mg qid + *tetracycline* 500 mg qid + *metronidazole* 250 mg qid x 14 days
Pediatric: <12 years: not recommended; ≥12 years: same as adult
Pack: bismuth subsalicylate chew tab: 262.4 mg (112/pck); *tetracycline cap:* 500 mg (56/pck); *metronidazole Tab:* 250 mg (56/pck)
➤ **Regimen 2: PrevPac (D)(G)** *amoxicillin* 500 mg 2 caps bid + *lansoprazole* 30 mg bid + *clarithromycin* 500 mg bid x 14 days (one card per day)
Pediatric: <12 years: not recommended; ≥12 years: same as adult
Kit: lansoprazole cap: 30 mg (2/card); *amoxicillin cap:* 500 mg (4/card); *clarithromycin tab:* 500 mg (2/card) (14 daily cards/carton)
➤ **Regimen 3: Pylera (D)** take 3 caps qid after meals and at bedtime x 10 days; take with 8 oz water <u>plus</u> *omeprazole* 20 mg bid, with breakfast and dinner, for 10 days
Pediatric: <12 years: not recommended; ≥12 years: same as adult
Cap: bismuth subsalicylate 140 mg+*tetracycline* 125 mg+*metronidazole* 125 mg (120 caps)
Comment: *omeprazole* not included with **Pylera**.
➤ **Regimen 4: Omeclamox-Pak (C)** *omeprazole* 20 mg bid + *amoxicillin* 1000 mg bid + *clarithromycin* 500 mg bid x 10 days
Kit: omeprazole cap: 20 mg (2/pck); *amoxicillin cap:* 500 mg (4/pck); *clarithromycin tab:* 500 mg (2/pck) (10 pcks/carton)

▷ **Regimen 5:** (C) *omeprazole* 40 mg daily + *clarithromycin* 500 mg tid x 2 weeks; then continue *omeprazole* 10-40 mg daily x 6 more weeks
▷ **Regimen 6:** (B) *lansoprazole* 30 mg tid + *amoxicillin* 1 gm tid x 10 days; then continue *lansoprazole* 15-30 mg daily x 6 more weeks
▷ **Regimen 7:** (C) *omeprazole* 40 mg daily + *amoxicillin* 1 gm bid + *clarithromycin* 500 mg bid x 10 days; then continue *omeprazole* 10-40 mg daily x 6 more weeks
▷ **Regimen 8:** (D) *bismuth subsalicylate* 525 mg qid + *metronidazole* 250 mg qid + *tetracycline* 500 mg qid + H2 receptor agonist x 2 weeks; then continue H2 receptor agonist x 6 more weeks
▷ **Regimen 9:** (not for use in 1st; B in 2nd, 3rd) *bismuth subsalicylate* 525 mg qid + *metronidazole* 250 mg qid + *amoxicillin 500 mg qid + H2 receptor agonist x 2 weeks; then continue H2 receptor agonist x 6 more weeks* receptor agonist x 2 weeks; then continue H2 receptor agonist x 6 more weeks
▷ **Regimen 10:** (C) *ranitidine bismuth citrate* 400 mg bid + *clarithromycin* 500 mg bid x 2 weeks; then continue *ranitidine bismuth citrate* 400 mg bid x 2 more weeks
▷ **Regimen 11:** (D) *omeprazole* 20 mg or *lansoprazole* 30 mg q AM + *bismuth subsalicylate* 524 mg qid + *metronidazole* 500 mg tid + *tetracycline* 500 mg qid x 2 weeks; then continue *omeprazole* 20 mg or *lansoprazole* 30 mg q AM for 6 more weeks

HEMOPHILIA A (CONGENITAL FACTOR VIII DEFICIENCY) WITH FACTOR VIII INHIBITORS

▷ *emicizumab-kxwh* initially 3 mg/kg by SC injection once weekly for the first 4 weeks; followed by 1.5 mg/kg once weekly
  Pediatric: same as adult
    Hemlibra *Vial:* 30 mg/ml (single-dose); 60 mg/0.4 ml (single-dose); 105 mg 0.7 ml (single-dose); 150 mg/ml (single-dose)
Comment: Hemlibra is a bispecific factor IXa- and factor X-directed antibody indicated for routine prophylaxis to prevent or reduce the frequency of bleeding episodes in adult and pediatric patients with hemophilia A (congenital factor VIII deficiency) with factor VIII inhibitors. Laboratory *Coagulation Test Interference*: **Hemlibra** interferes with activated clotting time (ACT), activated partial thrombo-plastin time (aPTT), and coagulation laboratory tests based on aPTT, including one stage aPTT-based single-factor assays, aPTT-based Activated Protein C Resistance (APC-R), and Bethesda assays (clotting-based) for factor VIII (FVIII) inhibitor titers. Intrinsic pathway clotting-based laboratory tests should not be used. Black Box Warning (BBW): Cases of thrombotic microangiopathy and thrombotic events were reported when on average a cumulative amount of >100 U/kg/24 hours of activated prothrombin complex concentrate (aPCC) was administered for 24 hours or more to patients receiving Hemlibra prophylaxis. Monitor for the development of thrombotic microangiopathy and thrombotic events if aPCC is administered. Discontinue aPCC and suspend dosing of Hemlibra if symptoms occur. Most common adverse reactions (incidence are injection site reactions, headache, and arthralgia. There are no available data on **Hemlibra** use in pregnant women to inform a drug-associated risk of major birth defects and miscarriage. Women of childbearing potential should use contraception while receiving **Hemlibra** and **Hemlibra** should be used during pregnancy only if the potential benefit for the mother outweighs the risk to the fetus. There is no information regarding the presence of *emicizumab-kxwh* in human milk or effects on the breastfed child. To report suspected adverse reactions, contact Genentech at 1-888-835-2555 or FDA at 1-800-FDA-1088 or www.fda.gov/medwatch

HEMORRHOIDS

▷ *dibucaine* (C)(OTC)(G) 1 applicatorful <u>or</u> suppository bid and after each stool; max 6/day

Pediatric: <12 years: not recommended; ≥12 years: same as adult

 Nupercainal (OTC) *Rectal oint:* 1% (30, 60 gm); *Rectal supp:* 1% (12, 14/pck)

▷ *hydrocortisone* (C)(OTC)(G)

Pediatric: <12 years: not recommended; ≥12 years: same as adult

 Anusol-HC 1 suppository rectally bid-tid <u>or</u> 2 suppositories bid x 2 weeks

 Rectal supp: 25 mg (12, 24/pck)

 Anusol-HC Cream 2.5% apply bid-qid prn

 Rectal crm: 2.5% (30 gm)

 Anusol HC-1 apply tid-qid prn; max 7 days

 Rectal crm: 1% (0.7 oz)

 Hydrocortisone Rectal Cream

 Rectal crm: 1, 2.5% (30 gm)

 Nupercainal apply tid-qid prn

 Rectal crm: 1% (30 gm)

 Proctocort 1 suppository rectally bid-tid prn <u>or</u> 2 suppositories bid
 x 2 weeks

 Rectal supp: 30 mg (12/pck)

 Proctocream HC 2.5% apply rectally bid-qid prn

 Rectal crm: 2.5% (30 gm)

 Proctofoam HC 1% apply rectally tid-qid prn

 Rectal foam: 1% (14 applications/10 gm)

▷ *hydrocortisone+pramoxine* (C) 1 applicatorful tid-qid and after each stool; max 2 weeks

Pediatric: <12 years: not recommended; ≥12 years: same as adult

 Procort *Rectal crm:* hydrocort 1.85%+pramox 1.15% (30 gm)

▷ *hydrocortisone+lidocaine* (B) apply bid-tid prn

Pediatric: <12 years: not recommended; ≥12 years: same as adult

 AnaMantle HC, LidaMantle HC *Crm/Lotn:* hydrocort 5%+lido 3% (1 oz)

▷ *petrolatum+mineral oil+shark liver oil+phenylephrine* (C)(OTC)(G)

 Preparation H Ointment apply up to qid prn

 Rectal oint: 1, 2 oz

▷ *petrolatum+glycerin+shark liver oil+phenylephrine* (C)(OTC)(G)

 Preparation H Cream apply up to qid prn

 Rectal crm: 0.9, 1.8 oz

▷ *phenylephrine+cocoa butter+shark liver oil* (C)(OTC)(G)

 Preparation H Suppositories 1 suppository <u>or</u> 1 application of rectal ointment <u>or</u>
 cream, up to qid

 Rectal supp: phenyle 0.25%+cocoa 85.5%+shark 3% (12, 24, 45/pck); *Rectal
 oint:* phenyle 0.25%+petro 1.9%+mineral oil 14%+shark liv 3% (1, 2 oz); *Rectal
 crm:* phenyle 0.25%+petro 18%+gly 12%+shark liv 3% (0.9, 1.8 oz)

▷ *witch hazel* topical soln/gel (OTC)

 Tucks apply up to 6 x/day; leave on x 5-15 minutes

 Pad: 12, 40, 100/pck; *Gel:* 19.8 g

▷ *lidocaine* 3% cream (B) apply bid-tid prn

Pediatric: reduce dosage commensurate with age, body weight, and physical condition

 LidaMantle *Crm:* 3% (1 oz)

Bulk-Forming Agents, Stool Softeners, and Stimulant Laxatives *see Constipation*
page 104

HEPATITIS A (HAV)

Comment: Administer a 2-dose series. Schedule first immunization at least 2 weeks before expected exposure. Booster dose recommended 6-12 months later. Under 1 year-of-age administer in the vastus lateralis; over 1 year-of-age administer in deltoid.

PROPHYLAXIS (HEPATITIS A)

▷ *hepatitis A vaccine, inactivated* (C)

> **Havrix** 1,440 El.U IM; repeat in 6-12 months
> *Pediatric:* <2 years: not recommended; 2-18 years: 720 El.U IM; repeat in 6-12 months or 360 El.U IM; repeat in 1 month
> **Vaqta** 25 U (1 ml) IM; repeat in 6 months
> *Pediatric:* <2 years: not recommended; 2-18 years: 0.5 ml IM; repeat in 6-18 months
>> *Vial:* 25 U/ml single-dose (preservative-free); *Prefilled syringe:* 25 U/ml, (0.5, 1 ml, single-dose)

PROPHYLAXIS VACCINE (HAV+HBV COMBINATION)

▷ *hepatitis A inactivated+hepatitis b surface antigen (recombinant vaccine)* (C)

> *Pediatric:* <18 years: not recommended; ≥18 years: same as adult
> **Twinrix** 1 ml IM in deltoid; repeat in 1 month and 6 months
>> *Vial (soln):* hepatitis a inactivated 720 IU+*hepatitis b* surface antigen (recombinant) 20 mcg/ml (1, 10 ml); *Prefilled syringe:* hepatitis a inactivated 720 IU+*hepatitis b* surface antigen (recombinant) 20 mcg/ml

 HEPATITIS B (HBV)

PROPHYLAXIS VACCINE (HBV)

Comment: Administer IM; under 1 year-of-age, administer in vastus lateralis. Over 1 year-of-age, administer in the deltoid. Administer a 3-dose series; *First dose:* newborn (or now); *Second dose:* 1-2 months after first dose; *Third dose:* 6 months after first dose.

▷ *hepatitis B recombinant vaccine* (C)

> **Engerix-B Adult** 20 mcg (1 ml) IM; repeat in 1 and 6 months
> *Pediatric:* infant-19 years: 10 mcg (1/2 ml) IM; repeat in 1 and 6 months
>> *Vial:* 20 mcg/ml single-dose (preservative-free, thimerosal); *Prefilled syringe:* 20 mcg/ml
> **Engerix-B Pediatric/Adolescent**
> *Pediatric:* infant-19 years: 10 mcg IM; repeat in 1 and 6 months; *Vial:* 10 mcg/0.5 ml single-dose (preservative-free, thimerosal)
>> *Prefilled syringe:* 10 mcg/0.5 ml
> **Recombivax HB Adult** 10 mcg (1 ml) IM in deltoid; repeat in 1 and 6 months
>> *Vial:* 10 mcg/ml single-dose; *Vial:* 10 mcg/3 ml multi-dose
> **Recombivax HB Pediatric/Adolescent** 5 mcg (0.5 ml) IM; repeat in 1 and 6 months
> *Pediatric:* birth-19 years: 5 mcg (0.5 ml) IM; repeat in 1 and 6 months; >19 years: use adult formulation or 10 mcg (1 ml) pediatric/adolescent formulation
>> *Vial:* 5 mcg/0.5 ml single-dose

PROPHYLAXIS VACCINE (HAV+HBV COMBINATION)

Comment: Administer IM; under 1 year-of-age, administer in vastus lateralis. Over 1 year-of-age, administer in the deltoid. Administer a 3-dose series; *First dose:* newborn (or now); *Second dose:* 1-2 months after first dose; *Third dose:* 6 months after first dose.

▷ *hepatitis A inactivated+hepatitis b surface antigen (recombinant) vaccine* (C)
  Pediatric: <18 years: not recommended; ≥18 years: same as adult
    Twinrix 1 ml IM in deltoid; repeat in 1 months and 6 months
      Vial (soln): hepatitis A inactivated 720 IU+*hepatitis b* surface antigen (recombinant) 20 mcg/ml (1, 10 ml); *Prefilled syringe: hepatitis A* inactivated 720 IU+*hepatitis b* surface antigen (recombinant) 20 mcg/ml

TREATMENT CHRONIC HBV INFECTION

Nucleoside Analogs (Reverse Transcriptase Inhibitors and HBV Polymerase Inhibitors)

Comment: Nucleoside analogs are indicated for chronic hepatitis infection with viral replication and either elevated ALT/AST or histologically active disease.

▷ *adefovir dipivoxil* (C)(G) 10 mg daily; *CrCl 20-49 mL/min:* 10 mg q 48 hours; *CrCl 10-19 mL/min:* 10 mg q 72 hours
  Pediatric: <12 years: not recommended; ≥12 years: same as adult
    Hepsera *Tab:* 10 mg
▷ *entecavir* (C)(G) take on an empty stomach;
  Nucleoside naïve: 0.5 mg daily; *Nucleoside naïve, CrCl 30-49 mL/min:* 0.25 mg daily; *Nucleoside naïve, CrCl 10-29 mL/min:* 0.15 mg daily; *Nucleoside naïve, CrCl <10 mL/min:* 0.05 mg daily; *lamivudine-refractory:* 1 mg daily; *lamivudine-refractory, renal impairment:* see mfr pkg insert
  Pediatric: <18 years: not recommended; ≥18 years: same as adult
    Baraclude *Tab:* 0.5, 1 mg; *Oral Soln:* 0.05 mg/ml (orange; parabens)
▷ *lamivudine* (C)(G) 100 mg daily; *CrCl <5 mL/min:* 35 mg for 1st dose, then 10 mg once daily; *CrCl 5-14 mL/min:* 35 mg for 1st dose, then 15 mg once daily; *CrCl 15-29 mL/min:* 100 mg for 1st dose, then 25 mg once daily; *CrCl 30-49 mL/min:* 100 mg for 1st dose, then 50 mg once daily
  Pediatric: <2 years: not recommended; 2-17 years: 3 mg/kg (max 100 mg) once daily
    Epivir-HBV *Tab:* 100 mg
    Epivir-HBV Oral Solution *Oral Soln:* 5 mg/ml (240 ml) (strawberry-banana)
▷ *telbivudine* (C) 600 mg daily; *CrCl <40 mL/min:* 600 mg q 72 hours; *CrCl 30-49 mL/min:* 600 mg q 48 hours
  Pediatric: <16 years: not recommended; ≥16 years: same as adult
    Tyzeka *Tab:* 600 mg
▷ *tenofovir alafenamide (TAF)* (C) take with food; take 1 tab once daily with concomitant carbamazepine 2 tablets
  Pediatric: <18 years: not established; ≥18 years: same as adult
    Vemlidy *Tab:* 25 mg
    Comment: No dosage adjustment of **Vemlidy** is required in patients with mild hepatic impairment (Child-Pugh Class A). The safety and efficacy of **Vemlidy** in patients with decompensated cirrhosis (Child-Pugh Class B or C) have not been established; therefore **Vemlidy** is not recommended in patients with decompensated (Child-Pugh Class B or C) hepatic impairment, Healthcare providers are encouraged to register patients by calling the Antiretroviral Pregnancy Registry (APR) at 1-800-258-4263.

Interferon Alpha

▷ *interferon alfa-2b* (C) 5 million IU SC or IM daily or 10 million IU SC or IM 3 x/week x 16 weeks; reduce dose by half or interrupt dose if WBCs, granulocyte count, or platelet count decreases
  Pediatric: <1 year: not recommended; ≥1 year: 3 million IU/m², 3 x/week x 1 week; then increase to 6 million IU/m², 3 x/week to 16-24 weeks; max 10 million IU/dose; reduce dose by half or interrupt dose if WBCs, granulocyte count, or platelet count decreases

Intron A *Vial (pwdr):* 5, 10, 18, 25, 50 million IU/vial (pwdr+diluent; single-dose) (benzoyl alcohol); *Vial (soln):* 3, 5, 10 million IU/vial (single-dose); *Multi-dose vials (soln):* 18, 25 million IU/vial soln; *Multi-dose pens (soln):* 3, 5, 10 million IU/0.2 ml (6 doses/pen)

 ## HEPATITIS C (HCV)

CHRONIC HCV INFECTION TREATMENT
Nucleoside Analogs (Reverse Transcriptase Inhibitors)
Comment: Nucleoside analogs are indicated for patients with compensated liver disease previously untreated with *alpha interferon* <u>or</u> who have relapsed after *alpha interferon* therapy. Primary toxicity is hemolytic anemia. Contraindicated in male partners of pregnant women; use 2 forms of contraception during therapy and for 6 months after discontinuation.

▷ *ribavirin* **(X)(G)** take with food in 2 divided doses; *Genotype 2, 3:* 800 mg/day x 24 weeks; *Genotype 1, 4, <75 kg:* 1 gm/day x 48 weeks; ≥75 km 1.2 gm/day x 48 weeks; *HIV co-infection:* 800 mg/day x 48 weeks; *CrCl 30-50 mL/min:* alternate 200 mg and 400 mg every other day; *CrCl <30 mL/min <u>or</u> hemodialysis:* reduce dose <u>or</u> discontinue if hematologic abnormalities occur
Pediatric: <5 years: not established; ≥5-<18 years: 23-33 kg: 400 mg/day; 34-46 kg: 600 mg/day; 47-59 kg: 800 mg/day; 60-75 kg: 1 gm/day; 1.2 gm/day; ≥75 kg: *Genotype 2, 3:* treat for 24 weeks; *Genotype 1, 4:* treat for 48 weeks; reduce dose <u>or</u> discontinue if hematologic abnormalities occur; ≥18 years: same as adult
    Copegus *Tab:* 200 mg
    Rebetol *Cap:* 200 mg
    Rebetol Oral Solution *Oral soln:* 40 mg/ml (120 ml) (bubble gum)
    Ribasphere RibaPak 600 mg *Tab:* 600 mg (14/pck)
    Virazole *Vial:* 6 gm for inhalation

Interferon Alpha
▷ *interferon alfacon-1* **(C)**
  Pediatric: <18 years: not recommended; ≥18 years: same as adult
    Infergen 9 mcg SC 3 x/week x 24 weeks, then 15 mcg SC 3 x/week x 6 months; allow at least 48 hours between doses
      Vial (soln): 9, 15 mcg/vial soln (6 single-dose/pck) (preservative-free)
▷ *interferon alfa-2b* **(C)**
    Intron A *Vial (pwdr):* 5, 10, 18, 25, 50 million IU/vial (pwdr w. diluent; single-dose) (benzoyl alcohol); *Vial (soln):* 3, 5, 10 million IU/vial (single-dose); *Multi-dose vials (soln):* 18, 25 million IU/vial; *Multi-dose pens (soln):* 3, 5, 10 million IU/0.2 ml (6 doses/pen)
▷ *peginterferon alfa-2a* **(C)** administer 180 mcg SC once weekly (on the same day of the week); treat for 48 weeks; consider discontinuing if adequate response after 12-24 weeks
  Pediatric: <18 years: not recommended; ≥18 years: same as adult
    PEGasys *Vial:* 180 mcg/ml (single-dose); *Monthly pck (vials):* 180 mcg/ml (1 ml, 4/pck)
▷ *peginterferon alfa-2b* **(C)** administer SC once weekly (on the same day of the week); treat for 1 year; consider discontinuing if inadequate response after 24 weeks; 37-45 kg: 40 mcg (100 mg/ml, 0.4 ml); 46-56 kg: 50 mcg (100 mg/ml, 0.5 ml); 57-72 kg: 64 mcg (160 mg/ml, 0.4 ml); 73-88 kg: 80 mcg (160 mg/ml, 0.5 ml); 89-106 kg: 96 mcg (240 mg/ml, 0.4 ml); 107-136 kg: 120 mcg (240 mg/ml, 0.5 ml); 137-160 kg: 150 mcg (300 mg/ml, 0.5 ml)

Pediatric: <18 years: not recommended; ≥18 years: same as adult
  PEG-Intron *Vial:* 50, 80, 120, 150 mcg/ml (single-dose)
  PEG-Intron Redipen *Pen:* 50, 80, 120, 150 mcg/ml (disposable pens)

HCV NS5A Inhibitor

▷ *daclatasvir* **(X)** 60 mg once daily for 12 weeks (with *sofosbuvir*); if *sofosbuvir* is discontinued, daclatasvir should also be discontinued; with concomitant CY3P inhibitors, reduce dose to 30 mg once daily; with concomitant CY3P inducers, increase dose to 90 mg once daily
  Daklinza *Tab:* 30, 60 mg

Comment: **Daklinza** is indicated in combination with *sofosbuvir* with or without *ribavirin*, for the treatment of HCV genotypes 1 and 3, and in patients with co-morbid HIV-1 infection, advanced cirrhosis, or post-liver transplant recurrence of HCV.

HCV NS5A Inhibitor+HCV NS3+4A Protease Inhibitor Combinations

▷ *elbasvir+grazoprevir* 1 tab as a single dose once daily; see mfr pkg insert for length of treatment
  Pediatric: <18 years: not recommended; ≥18 years: same as adult
  Zepatier *Tab:* elba 50 mg+grazo 100 mg

Comment: **Zepatier** is contraindicated with moderate or severe hepatic impairment, concomitant *atazanavir, carbamazepine, cyclosporine, darunavir, efavirenz, lopinavir, phenytoin, rifampin, saquinavir,* St. John's wort, *tipranavir*. When co-administered with *ribavirin,* pregnancy category **(X)**

▷ *glecaprevir+pibrentasvir* take 3 tablets (total daily dose: *glecaprevir* 300 mg and *pibrentasvir* 120 mg) once daily with food
  Pediatric: <18 years: not recommended; ≥18 years: same as adult
  Mavyret *Tab:* gleca 100 mg+pibre 40 mg

Comment: **Mavyret** is a drug for the treatment of adults who have chronic Hepatitis C virus genotypes 1, 2, 3, 4, 5 or 6 infection and who do not have cirrhosis or who have early stage cirrhosis. **Mavyret** may cause serious liver problems including liver failure and death in patients who had hepatitis B virus infection. This is because the hepatitis B virus could become active again (i.e., reactivated) during or after treatment with **Mavyret**. Test all patients for HBV infection by measuring HBsAg and anti-HBc prior to initiating therapy with **Mavyret**. The most common side effects of **Mavyret** are headache and tiredness. See mfr insert for table of recommended duration of treatment based on patient characteristics. No adequate human data are available to establish whether or not **Mavyret** poses a risk to pregnancy outcomes. It is not known whether the components of **Mavyret** are excreted in human breast milk or have effects on the breastfed infant.

HCV NS5A Inhibitor+HCV NS3/4A Protease Inhibitor+ CYP3A Inhibitor Combinations

▷ *ombitasvir+paritaprevir+ritonavir* **(B)** take 2 tabs once daily in the AM x 12 weeks
  Pediatric: <18 years: not established; ≥18 years: same as adult
  Technivie *Tab:* omvi 25 mg+pari 75 mg+rito 50 mg (4 x 7 daily dose pcks/carton)

Comment: **Technivie** is indicated for use in chronic HCV genotype 4 without cirrhosis. **Technivie** is not for use with moderate hepatic impairment.

HCV NS3/4A Protease Inhibitor

▷ *simeprevir* **(C)** 150 mg once daily; swallow whole; take with food, not for monotherapy; do not reduce dose or interrupt therapy; if discontinued, do not reinitiate; discontinue if HCV-RNA levels indicate futility; discontinue if *peginterferon, ribavirin,* or *sofosbuvir* is permanently discontinued; *Treatment naïve, treatment relapses, with or without cirrhosis:* treat x 12 weeks (*simeprevir* + *peginterferon* + *ribavirin*) followed by additional 12 weeks *peginterferon + ribavirin* (total = 24 weeks). *Partial and non-responders, with or without cirrhosis:* treat x 12 weeks (*simeprevir + peginterferon + ribavirin*) followed by additional 36 weeks *peginterferon + ribavirin* (total = 48 weeks); *Treatment naïve or treatment experienced without cirrhosis:* treat x 12 weeks (*simeprevir + sofosbuvir*); *Treatment naïve or treatment experienced with cirrhosis:* treat x 24 weeks (*simeprevir + sofosbuvir*)

 Olysio *Cap:* 150 mg

HCV NS5A Inhibitor+HCV NS5B Polymerase Inhibitor Combinations

▷ *ledipasvir+sofosbuvir Treatment naïve, without cirrhosis, with pretreatment HCV RNA <6 million IU/ml:* 1 tab daily x 8 weeks; *Treatment naïve with or without cirrhosis or treatment-experienced without cirrhosis:* 1 tab daily x 12 weeks; *Treatment-experienced with cirrhosis:* 1 tab daily x 24 weeks; *In combination with ribavirin:* 1 tab daily x 12 weeks
 Pediatric: <18 years: not established; ≥18 years: same as adult
 Harvoni *Tab:* ledi 90 mg+*sofo* 400 mg

Comment: Harvoni is indicated for patients with advanced liver disease, genotype 1, 4, 5, or 6 infection: chronic HCV genotype 1- or 4-infected liver transplant recipients with or without cirrhosis or with compensated cirrhosis (Child-Pugh Class A), and for HCV genotype 1-infected patients with decompensated cirrhosis (Child-Pugh Class B or C), including those who have undergone liver transplantation. No adequate human data are available to establish whether or not Harvoni poses a risk to pregnancy outcomes; the background risk of major birth defects and miscarriage for the indicated population is unknown. If Harvoni is administered with *ribavirin*, the combination regimen is contraindicated (X) in pregnant women and in men whose female partners are pregnant. It is not known whether Harvoni and its metabolites are present in human breast milk, affect human milk production or have effects on the breastfed infant. If Harvoni is administered with *ribavirin*, the nursing mother's information for *ribavirin* also applies to this combination regimen.

▷ *sofosbuvir+velpatasvir Without cirrhosis or compensated cirrhosis (Child-Pug A):* 1 tablet daily x 12 weeks; *Decompensated cirrhosis (Child Pugh Class B or C):* 1 tablet daily plus *ribavirin* (RBV)
 Pediatric: <18 years: not established; ≥18 years: same as adult
 Epclusa *Tab:* sofo 400 mg+velpa 100 mg

Comment: Epclusa is indicated for patients with chronic HCV with genotype 1, 2, 3, 4, 5, or 6 infection.

HCV NS5A Inhibitor+HCV NS3/4A Protease Inhibitor+CYP3A Inhibitor Combination

▷ *sofosbuvir+velpatasvir* (B) 1 tab daily
 Pediatric: <12 years: not established; ≥12 years: same as adult
 Viekira XR *Tab:* dasa 200 mg+omvi 8.33 mg+pari 50 mg+rito 33.33 mg ext-rel (4 weekly cartons, each containing 7 daily dose pcks/carton)

Comment: Viekira XR is indicated for HCV genotype 1 with mild liver dysfunction (Child-Pugh Class A). Viekira XR is contraindicated for moderate (Child-Pugh Class B) to severe (Child-Pugh Class C) liver dysfunction. No adjustment is recommended with mild, moderate, or severe renal dysfunction.

HCV NS5A Inhibitor+HCV NS3/4A Protease Inhibitor+CYP3A Inhibitor PLUS HCV NS5B Polymerase Inhibitor Combination

▷ *ombitasvir+paritaprevir+ritonavir* plus *dasabuvir* (B)
 Pediatric: <12 years: not established; ≥12 years: same as adult
 Viekira Pak *ombitasvir+paritaprevir+ritonavir* fixed-dose combination tablet: 2 tablets orally once a day (in the morning); *dasabuvir:* 250 mg orally twice a day (morning and evening)

Tab: omvi 12.5 mg+*pari* 75 mg+*rito* 50 mg plus *Tab:* dasa 250 mg (28 day supply/pck)

Comment: **Viekira Pak** is indicated for mild liver dysfunction (Child-Pugh Class A). **Viekira Pak** is contraindicated for moderate (Child-Pugh Class B) to severe (Child-Pugh Class C) liver dysfunction. No adjustment is recommended with mild, moderate, or severe renal dysfunction.

HCV NS5B Polymerase Inhibitor+HCV NS5A Inhibitor+HCV NS3/4A Protease Inhibitor Combination

▷ *sofosbuvir+velpatasvir+voxilaprevir* 1 tablet once daily with food x 12 weeks; pre-test for HBV infection by measuring HBsAg and anti-HBc prior to the initiation of therapy

Pediatric: <12 years: not established; ≥12 years: same as adult

Vosevi *Tab:* sofo 400 mg+velpa 100 mg+voxil 100 mg fixed-dose combination

Comment: **Vosevi** is not recommended in patients with moderate or severe hepatic impairment (Child-Pugh Class B or C). A dosage recommendation cannot be made for patients with severe renal impairment or end stage renal disease. **Vosevi** is contraindicated while taking any medicines containing *rifampin* (Rifater, Rifamate, Rimactane, Rifadin). **Vosevi** is indicated for the treatment of adult patients with chronic HCV infection without cirrhosis or with compensated cirrhosis (Child-Pugh Class A) who have: (1) genotype 1, 2, 3, 4, 5, or 6 infection and have previously been treated with an HCV regimen containing an NS5A inhibitor or (2) genotype 1a or 3 infection and have previously been treated with an HCV regimen containing *sofosbuvir* without an NS5A inhibitor. Duration of treatment is 12 weeks. Additional benefit of **Vosevi** over *sofosbuvir+velpatasvir* has not been demonstrated with genotype 1b, 2, 4, 5, or 6 infection previously treated with *sofosbuvir* without an NS5A inhibitor. Because there is risk of Hepatitis B virus reactivation, test all patients for evidence of current or prior HBV infection before initiation of HCV treatment. Monitor HCV/HBV co-infected patients for HBV reactivation and hepatitis flare during HCV treatment and post-treatment follow-up. Initiate appropriate patient management for HBV infection as clinically indicated. The most common adverse reactions are headache, fatigue, diarrhea, and nausea. To report a suspected adverse reaction, contact Gilead Sciences at 1-800-GILEAD-5 or FDA at 1-800-FDA-1088 or www.fda.gov/medwatch

DUAL TREATMENT REGIMEN
Harvoni+Sovaldi

Comment: Patients who are co-infected with hepatitis B are at risk for HBV reactivation during or after treatment with HCV direct-acting retrovirals. Therefore, patients should be screened for current or past HBV infection before starting this treatment protocol.

TRIPLE TREATMENT REGIMEN
Sovaldi+Harvoni+Ribavirin

Comment: For this FDA-approved triple therapy regimen, follow the recommended regimen for each individual drug. Patients who are co-infected with hepatitis B are at risk for HBV reactivation during or after treatment with HCV direct-acting retrovirals. Therefore, patients should be screened for current or past HBV infection before starting this triple therapy regimen.

HEREDITARY ANGIOEDEMA (HAE)/
C1 ESTERASE INHIBITOR DEFICIENCY

Comment: Agents administered for the treatment of hereditary angioedema carry a risk of hypersensitivity reactions, which are similar to HAE attacks, and the patient should be monitored closely for signs and symptoms accordingly (e.g., hives, urticaria, tightness of the chest, wheezing, hypotension and/or anaphylaxis).

HAE PROPHYLAXIS

▷ *danazol* (X) *Females:* start on 3rd or 4th day of menstrual period or after a negative pregnancy test; *Males/Females:* dosage requirements for continuous treatment of hereditary angioedema should be adjusted based on individual clinical response; initially 200 mg bid-tid; after a favorable initial response is achieved (prevention of episodes of edematous attacks), continuing dosage should be determined by decreasing the dosage by 50% or less at intervals of 1 to 3 months or longer if frequency of attacks prior to treatment dictates; if an attack occurs, daily dosage may be increased by up to 200 mg. During the dose adjusting phase, close monitoring of the patient's response is indicated, particularly if the patient has a history of airway involvement.
Pediatric: <18 years: not recommended; ≥18 years: same as adult
    Danocrine *Cap:* 50, 100, 200 mg
Comment: *danazol* is a synthetic steroid derived from ethisterone. It suppresses the pituitary-ovarian axis. This suppression is probably a combination of epressed hypothalamic-pituitary response to lowered *estrogen* production, the alteration of sex steroid metabolism, and interaction of *danazol* with sex hormone receptors. The only other demonstrable hormonal effects are weak androgenic activity and depression of both follicle-stimulating hormone (FSH) and luteinizing hormone (LH) output. Recent evidence suggests a direct inhibitory effect at gonadal sites and a binding of **Danocrine** to receptors of gonadal steroids at target organs. In addition, **Danocrine** has been shown to significantly decrease IgG, IgM and IgA levels, as well as phospholipid and IgG isotope autoantibodies in patients with endometriosis and associated elevations of autoantibodies, suggesting this could be another mechanism by which it facilitates regression of fibrocystic breast disease. Changes in the menstrual pattern may occur. Generally, the pituitary-suppressive action of **Danocrine** is reversible. Ovulation and cyclic bleeding usually return within 60 to 90 days when therapy with **Danocrine** is discontinued. In the treatment of hereditary angioedema, **Danocrine** at effective doses prevents attacks of the disease characterized by episodic edema of the abdominal viscera, extremities, face, and airway which may be disabling and, if the airway is involved, fatal. In addition, **Danocrine** corrects partially or completely the primary biochemical abnormality of hereditary angioedema by increasing the levels of the deficient C1 esterase inhibitor (C1EI). As a result of this action the serum levels of the C4 component of the complement system are also increased. **Danocrine** is also used to treat endometriosis (to relieve associated abdominal pain) and fibrocystic breast disease (to reduce breast tissue nodularity and breast pain/tenderness. Contraindications include pregnancy, breastfeeding, active or history of thromboembolic disease/event, porphyria, undiagnosed abnormal genital bleeding, androgen-dependent tumor, and markedly impaired hepatic, renal, or cardiac function.

C1 ESTERASE INHIBITOR [HUMAN]

▷ *C1 esterase inhibitor (human)* administer 60 International Units per kg body weight SC in the abdomen twice weekly (every 3 or 4 days); administer at room temperature within 8 hours after reconstitution; use a silicone-free syringe for reconstitution and administration; use either the Mix2Vial transfer set provided with **Haegarda** or a commercially available 566 double-ended needle and vented filter spike
Pediatric: <12 years: not recommended; ≥12 years: same as adult
    Haegarda *Vial:* 2000, 3000 IU C1 INH pwdr for reconstitution, single-use
Comment: **Haegarda is** a plasma-derived concentrate of C1 esterase inhibitor [human], a serine proteinase inhibitor. Indicated for routine prophylaxis to prevent HAE attacks in adults and adolescents. It is <u>not</u> indicated for treating acute attacks of

HAE. **Haegarda** is the first C1 esterase inhibitor (human) SC injection approved for self-administration by the patient or caregiver after healthcare provider instruction. An international consensus panel states that human plasma-derived C1 esterase inhibitor is considered to be the therapy of choice for both treatment and prophylaxis of maternal hereditary angioedema during lactation. There are no prospective clinical data from **Haegarda** use in pregnant women. C1-INH is a normal component of human plasma. There is no information regarding the excretion of **Haegarda** in human milk or effect the breastfed infant. The developmental and health benefits of breastfeeding should be considered along with the mother's clinical need for **Haegarda** and any potential adverse effects on the breastfed infant from **Haegarda** or from the underlying maternal condition.

HAE ACUTE ATTACK
C1 ESTERASE INHIBITORS [HUMAN]

▷ *C1 esterase inhibitor [human]* (C) reconstitute pwdr using the sterile water provided; administer 20 IU/kg body weight via IVP injection at approximately 4 ml/min, at room temperature within 8 hours of reconstitution; store the vial at room temperature in the original carton to protect from light; appropriately trained patients may self-administer upon recognition of an HAE attack; hypersensitivity reactions may occur, therefore, have epinephrine immediately available for treatment of acute severe hypersensitivity reaction

Pediatric: <12 years: not established; ≥12 years: same as adult

> **Berinert** *Vial:* 500 Units/10 ml vial, single-use, pwdr for reconstitution with the 10 ml sterile water diluent (provided)

Comment: To report suspected adverse reactions, contact the CSL Behring Pharmacovigilance Department at 1-866-915-6958 or to the FDA at 1-800-FDA-1088 or www.fda.gov/medwatch

▷ *C1 esterase inhibitor [human]* (C) administer 1,000 Units (2 x 500 U vials) via IVP injection, after reconstitution with 5 ml sterile H2O/vial; reconstitute 1,000 U pwdr in a 10 ml syringe with 10 ml sterile water; administer over 10 minutes (1 ml/min) at room temperature within 3 hours of reconstitution; each 1,000 Unit treatment is administered every 3-4 days; hypersensitivity reactions may occur, therefore, have epinephrine immediately available for treatment of acute severe hypersensitivity reaction

Pediatric: <16 years: not established; ≥16 years: same as adult

> **Cinryze** *Vial:* 500 Units/8 ml vial pwdr for reconstitution (sterile water diluent not provided)

Comment: No adequate and well-controlled studies have been conducted in pregnant women. It is not known whether **Cinryze** can cause fetal harm when administered to a pregnant woman or can affect reproduction capacity. **Cinryze** should be administered to a pregnant woman only if clearly needed. It is not known whether **Cinryze** is excreted in human milk. **Cinryze** is made from human plasma and may contain infectious agents (e.g viruses and, theoretically, the Creutzfeldt-Jakob disease agent). To report suspected adverse reactions, contact ViroPharma Medical Information at (866) 331-5637 or FDA at 1-800-FDA-1088 or www.fda.gov/medwatch

HAE ACUTE ATTACK
C1 Esterase Inhibitor [HUMAN]

▷ *C1 esterase inhibitor [human]* (C) reconstitute pwdr using the sterile water provided; administer 20 IU/kg body weight via IVP injection at approximately 4 ml/min, at room temperature within 8 hours of reconstitution; store the vial at room temperature in the original carton to protect from light; appropriately trained patients may self-administer upon recognition of an HAE attack; hypersensitivity reactions may occur, therefore, have epinephrine immediately available for treatment of acute severe hypersensitivity reaction

Pediatric: <12 years: not established; ≥12 years: same as adult

> Berinert *Vial:* 500 Units/10 ml vial, single-use, pwdr for reconstitution with the 10 ml sterile water diluent (provided)

Comment: To report suspected adverse reactions, contact the CSL Behring Pharmacovigilance Department at 1-866-915-6958 or to the FDA at 1-800-FDA-1088 or www.fda.gov/medwatch

C1 Esterase Inhibitor [Recombinant]

▷ *C1 esterase inhibitor [recombinant]* (B) reconstitute 2.100 IU pwdr (1 vial) with 14 ml sterile H2O; administer reconstituted solution at room temperature, slow IVP injection over approximately 5 minutes; appropriately trained patients may self-administer upon recognition of HAE attack; Weight-based dose: <84 kg: 50 IU /kg [wt in kg ÷ 3 = vol (ml) reconst soln for administration]; ≥84 kg: 4,200 IU (28 ml, 2 vials); if the attack symptoms persist, an additional (second) dose can be administered at the recommended dose level; do not exceed 4200 IU per dose; max two doses within a 24 hour period; hypersensitivity reactions may occur, therefore, have epinephrine immediately available for treatment of acute severe hypersensitivity reaction

Pediatric: <13 years: not established; ≥13 years: same as adult

> Ruconest *Vial:* 2,100 IU, pwdr, single-use for IVP injection after reconstitution (sterile water diluent not provided)

Comment: To report **Ruconest** suspected adverse reactions, contact Salix Pharmaceuticals, Inc. at 1-800-508-0024 or FDA at 1-800-FDA-1088 or www.fda.gov/medwatch

Bradykinen B2 Receptor Antagonist

▷ *icatibant* (C) administer 30 mg SC injection in the abdominal area; if response is inadequate or symptoms recur, additional injections of 30 mg may be administered at intervals of at least 6 hours; max 3 injections/24 hours; patients may self-administer upon recognition of an HAE attack

Pediatric: <18 years: not established; ≥18 years: same as adult

> Firazyr *Prefilled syringe:* 10 mg/ml (3 ml) single-dose w. 25 gauge luer lock needle (1/carton, 3 cartons/pck)

Comment: **Firazyr**, as a bradykinin B2 receptor antagonist, may attenuate the antihypertensive effect of ACE inhibitors. The most commonly reported adverse reaction is injection site reaction (97% in clinical trials). To report suspected adverse reactions, contact Shire Human Genetic Therapies OnePath at 1-800-828-2088 or FDA at 1-800-FDA-1088 or www.fda.gov/medwatch

Plasma Kallikrein Inhibitor

▷ *ecallantide* (C) administer 30 mg (3 ml) SC in three 10 mg (I ml) injections; if an attack persists, an additional dose of 30 mg may be administered within a 24 hour period; should only be administered by a healthcare professional with appropriate medical support to manage anaphylaxis and hereditary angioedema

Pediatric: <12 years: not established; ≥12 years: same as adult

> Kalbitor *Vial:* 10 mg/ml (1/carton, 3 vials/pkg) single-use

Comment: Anaphylaxis has occurred in 3.9% of patients treated with **Kalbitor**. Therefore, **Kakbitor** should only be administered in a setting equipped to manage anaphylaxis and hereditary angioedema. Given the similarity in hyper sensitivity symptoms and acute HAE symptoms, monitor patients closely for hypersensitivity reactions. To report suspected adverse reactions, contact Dyax Corp at 1-888-452-5248 or FDA at 1-800-FDA-1088 or ww.fda.gov/medwatch

 HERPANGINA

Other Oral Analgesics *see Pain page* 338

ORAL ANALGESICS

▷ *acetaminophen* (B) *see Fever page* 165

▷ *tramadol* (C)(IV)(G)

Comment: *tramadol* is known to be excreted in breast milk. The FDA and the European Medicines Agency (EMA) are investigating the safety of using *tramadol*-containing medications to treat pain in children 12-18 years because of the potential for serious side effects, including slowed or difficult breathing.

Rybix ODT initially 100 mg once daily; may increase by 100 mg every 5 days; max 300 mg/day; *CrCl <30 mL/min or severe hepatic impairment:* not recommended; *Cirrhosis:* max 50 mg q 12 hours
Pediatric: <18 years: not recommended; ≥18 years: same as adult
ODT: 50 mg (mint) (phenylalanine)

Ryzolt initially 100 mg once daily; may increase by 100 mg every 5 days; max 300 mg/day; *CrCl <40 mL/min or severe hepatic impairment:* not recommended
Pediatric: <18 years: not recommended; ≥18 years: same as adult
Tab: 100, 200, 300 mg ext-rel

Ultram 50-100 mg q 4-6 hours prn; max 400 mg/day; *CrCl <40 mL/min:* max 100 mg q 12 hours; *Cirrhosis:* max 50 mg q 12 hours
Pediatric: <18 years: not recommended; ≥18 years: same as adult
Tab: 50*mg

Ultram ER initially 100 mg once daily; may increase by 100 mg every 5 days; max 300 mg/day; *CrCl <40 mL/min or severe hepatic impairment:* not recommended
Pediatric: <18 years: not recommended; ≥18 years: same as adult
Tab: 100, 200, 300 mg ext-rel

Comment: *tramadol* is known to be excreted in breast milk. The FDA and the European Medicines Agency (EMA) are investigating the safety of using *tramadol*-containing medications to treat pain in children 12-18 years because of the potential for serious side effects, including slowed or difficult breathing.

▷ *tramadol+acetaminophen* (C)(IV)(G) 2 tabs q 4-6 hours; max 8 tabs/day; 5 days; *CrCl <40 mL/min:* max 2 tabs q 12 hours; max 4 tabs/day x 5 days
Pediatric: <18 years: not recommended; ≥18 years: same as adult
Ultracet *Tab:* tram 37.5+acet 325 mg

Comment: *tramadol* is known to be excreted in breast milk. The FDA and the European Medicines Agency (EMA) are investigating the safety of using *tramadol*-containing medications to treat pain in children 12-18 years because of the potential for serious side effects, including slowed or difficult breathing.

TOPICAL ANESTHETICS

▷ *lidocaine* viscous soln (B) 15 ml gargle or mouthwash; repeat after 3 hours; max 8 doses/day
Pediatric: <4 years: apply 1.25 ml to affected area with cotton-tipped applicator; may repeat after 3 hours; max 8 doses/day
Xylocaine 2% Viscous Solution *Viscous soln:* 2% (20, 100, 450 ml)
Antipyretics *see Fever page* 165

HERPES GENITALIS (HSV TYPE II)

Comment: The following treatment regimens are published in the **2015 CDC Sexually Transmitted Diseases Treatment Guidelines**. Treatment regimens are for adults only; consult a specialist for treatment of patients less than 18 years-of-age. Treatment regimens are presented in alphabetical order by generic drug name, followed by brands and dose forms.

RECOMMENDED REGIMENS: FIRST CLINICAL EPISODE
Regimen 1
▷ *acyclovir* 400 mg tid x 7-10 days <u>or</u> 200 mg 5 x/day x 10 days <u>or</u> until clinically resolved

Regimen 2
▷ *acyclovir* cream apply q 3 hours 6 x/day x 7 days

Regimen 3
▷ *famciclovir* 250 mg tid x 7-10 days <u>or</u> until clinically resolved

Regimen 4
▷ *valacyclovir* 1 gm bid x 10 days <u>or</u> until clinically resolved

RECOMMENDED RECURRENT/EPISODIC REGIMENS
Comment: Initiate treatment of recurrent episodes within 1 day of onset of lesions.

Regimen 1
▷ *acyclovir* 200 mg 5 x/day x 5 days

Regimen 2
▷ *famciclovir* 125 mg bid x 5 days

Regimen 3
▷ *valacyclovir* 500 mg bid x 3-5 days <u>or</u> until clinically resolved

SUPPRESSION THERAPY REGIMENS
Regimen 1
▷ *acyclovir* 400 mg bid x 1 year

Regimen 2
▷ *famciclovir* 250 mg bid x 1 year

Regimen 3
▷ *valacyclovir* 500 mg daily x 1 year (for ≤9 recurrences/year) <u>or</u> 1 gm daily x 1 year (for ≥10 recurrences/year)

DAILY SUPPRESSIVE REGIMENS FOR PERSONS WITH HIV
Regimen 1
▷ *acyclovir* 400-800 mg bid-tid

Regimen 2
▷ *famciclovir* 500 mg bid

Regimen 3
▷ *valacyclovir* 500 mg bid

RECURRENT/EPISODIC REGIMENS FOR PERSONS WITH HIV
Regimen 1
▷ *acyclovir* 400 mg tid x 5-10 days

Regimen 2
▷ *famciclovir* 500 mg bid x 5-10 days

Regimen 3
▷ *valacyclovir* 1 gm bid x 5-10 days

DRUG BRANDS AND DOSE FORMS
▷ *acyclovir* (B)(G)
    Zovirax *Cap:* 200 mg; *Tab:* 400, 800 mg
    Zovirax Oral Suspension *Oral susp:* 200 mg/5 ml (banana)
    Zovirax Cream *Crm:* 5% (3, 15 gm); *Oint:* 5% (3, 15 gm)
▷ *famciclovir* (B)
    Famvir *Tab:* 125, 250, 500 mg
▷ *valacyclovir* (B)
    Valtrex *Cplt:* 500, 1 gm

 HERPES LABIALIS/HERPES FACIALIS (HERPES SIMPLEX VIRUS TYPE I, COLD SORE, FEVER BLISTER)

PRIMARY INFECTION
▷ *acyclovir* (B)(G) do not chew, crush, <u>or</u> swallow the buccal tab; apply within 1 hour of symptom onset and before appearance of lesion; apply a single buccal tab to the upper gum region on the affected side and hold in place for 30 seconds
    Sitavig *Buccal tab:* 50 mg
    Pediatric: see page 614 *for dose by weight*
    Comment: **Sitavig** is contraindicated with allergy to milk protein concentrate.
▷ *valacyclovir* (B) 2 gm q 12 hours x 1 day
Pediatric: <12 years: not recommended; ≥12 years: same as adult
    Valtrex *Cplt:* 500, 1,000 mg

SUPPRESSION THERAPY (≥6 OUTBREAKS/YEAR)
▷ *acyclovir* (B)(G) 200 mg 2-5 x/day x 1 year
Pediatric: <2 years: not recommended; ≥2 years, <40 kg: 20 mg/kg 2-5 x/day x 1 year; ≥2 years, >40 kg: 200 mg 2-5 x/day x 1 year; *see page* 614 *for dose by weight*
    Zovirax *Cap:* 200 mg; *Tab:* 400, 800 mg
    Zovirax Oral Suspension *Oral susp:* 200 mg/5 ml (banana)

TOPICAL ANTIVIRAL THERAPY
▷ *acyclovir* (B)(G) apply q 3 hours 6 x/day x 7 days
Pediatric: <2 years: not recommended; ≥2 years: same as adult
    Zovirax Cream *Crm:* 5% (3, 15 gm); *Oint:* 5% (3, 15 gm)
▷ *docosanol* (B) apply and gently rub in 5 x daily until healed
Pediatric: <12 years: not recommended; ≥12 years: same as adult
    Abreva (OTC) *Crm:* 10% (2 gm)

▷ *penciclovir* (B) apply q 2 hours while awake x 4 days
  Pediatric: <12 years: not recommended; ≥12 years: same as adult
    Denavir *Crm:* 1% (2 gm)

TOPICAL ANTIVIRAL+CORTICOSTEROID THERAPY

▷ *acyclovir+hydrocortisone* (B)(G) cream apply to affected area 5 x/day x 5 days
  Pediatric: <12 years: not recommended; ≥12 years: same as adult
    Crm: 1% (2, 5 gm)

 HERPES ZOSTER (HZ, SHINGLES)

Other Oral Analgesics *see Pain page 314*
Postherpetic Neuralgia *see page 387*

PROPHYLAXIS VACCINE

Comment: Herpes zoster (shingles) vaccine is indicated for adults ≥50 years-of-age
(<50 years: not recommended). The vaccine is not for preventing primary infection
(chickenpox).
▷ *zoster vaccine recombinant, adjuvanted* administer one 0.5 mL dose at month 0
  followed by second dose anytime between 2–6 months later; administer immediately
  upon reconstitution or store refrigerated and use within 6 hours.
  Pediatric: <18 years: not established
    Shingrix *Vial:* 0.5 ml single-dose susp for IM injection after reconstitution with
    diluent (10/carton) (preservative-free)

ORAL ANTIVIRALS

▷ *acyclovir* (B)(G) 800 mg 5 x/day x 7-10 or 14 days
  Pediatric: <2 years: not recommended; ≥2 years, <40 kg: 20 mg/kg 5 x/day x 7-10
  days; *see page 614 for dose by weight;* >2 years, >40 kg: 800 mg 5 x/day x 7-10 days;
    Zovirax *Cap:* 200 mg; *Tab:* 400, 800 mg
    Zovirax Oral Suspension *Oral susp:* 200 mg/5 ml (banana)
▷ *famciclovir* (B) 500 mg tid x 7-10 days
  Pediatric: <18 years: not recommended; ≥18 years: same as adult
    Famvir *Tab:* 125, 250, 500 mg
▷ *valacyclovir* (B) 1 gm tid x 7-10 days
  Pediatric: <12 years: not recommended; ≥12 years: same as adult
    Valtrex *Cplt:* 500, 1,000 mg

PROPHYLAXIS AGAINST SECONDARY INFECTION

▷ *silver sulfadiazine* (B) apply qid
  Pediatric: <12 years: not recommended; ≥12 years: same as adult
    Silvadene *Crm:* 1% (20, 50, 85, 400, 1,000 gm jar; 20 gm tube)

ORAL ANALGESICS

Other Oral Analgesics *see Pain page 338*

▷ *acetaminophen* (B) *see Fever page 165*
▷ *aspirin* (D)(G) *see Fever page 166*
Comment: *aspirin*-containing medications are contraindicated with history of
allergic-type reaction to *aspirin*, children and adolescents with *varicella* or other viral
illness, and 3rd trimester pregnancy.

▷ *tramadol* (C)(IV)(G)

Comment: *tramadol* is known to be excreted in breast milk. The FDA and the European Medicines Agency (EMA) are investigating the safety of using *tramadol*-containing medications to treat pain in children 12-18 years because of the potential for serious side effects, including slowed or difficult breathing.

Rybix ODT initially 100 mg once daily; may increase by 100 mg every 5 days; max 300 mg/day; *CrCl <30 mL/min or severe hepatic impairment:* not recommended; *Cirrhosis:* max 50 mg q 12 hours
Pediatric: <18 years: not recommended; ≥18 years: same as adult
ODT: 50 mg (mint) (phenylalanine)

Ryzolt initially 100 mg once daily; may increase by 100 mg every 5 days; max 300 mg/day; *CrCl <30 mL/min or severe hepatic impairment,* not recommended
Pediatric: <18 years: not recommended; ≥18 years: same as adult
Tab: 100, 200, 300 mg ext-rel

Ultram 50-100 mg q 4-6 hours prn; max 400 mg/day; *CrCl <40 mL/min:* max 100 mg q 12 hours; *Cirrhosis:* max 50 mg q 12 hours
Pediatric: <18 years: not recommended; ≥18 years: same as adult
Tab: 50*mg

Ultram ER initially 100 mg once daily; may increase by 100 mg every 5 days; max 300 mg/day; *CrCl <30 mL/min or severe hepatic impairment:* not recommended
Pediatric: <18 years: not recommended; ≥18 years: same as adult
Tab: 100, 200, 300 mg ext-rel

▷ *tramadol+acetaminophen* (C)(IV)(G) 2 tabs q 4-6 hours; max 8 tabs/day x 5 days; *CrCl <40 mL/min:* max 2 tabs q 12 hours; max 4 tabs/day x 5 days
Pediatric: <18 years: not recommended; ≥18 years: same as adult
Ultracet Tab: tram 37.5+acet 325 mg

Comment: *tramadol* is known to be excreted in breast milk. The FDA and the European Medicines Agency (EMA) are investigating the safety of using *tramadol*-containing medications to treat pain in children 12-18 years because of the potential for serious side effects, including slowed or difficult breathing.

SECONDARY INFECTION PROPHYLAXIS

▷ *silver sulfadiazine* (B) apply qid
Pediatric: <12 years: not recommended; ≥12 years: same as adult
Silvadene Crm: 1% (20, 50, 85, 400, 1,000 gm/jar; 20 gm tube)

 HERPES ZOSTER OPHTHMICUS (HZO)

Parenteral Corticosteroids *see page* 563
Oral Corticosteroids *see page* 561

Comment: Herpes Zoster ophthalmicus (HZO) is an ophthalmologic emergency. Standard therapy involves initiating systemic (oral or intravenous) antiviral therapy as soon as possible. Pharmacotherapy options include *acyclovir*, *valacyclovir*, and *famciclovir*. IV acyclovir is recommended for immunocompromised persons. Duration of treatment is 7-10 or 14 days, depending on severity. Ocular complications include conjunctivitis with or without superimposed bacterial infections, episcleritis, scleritis, keratitis, and uveitis, involvement of the 3rd, 4th, and 5th cranial nerves, acute optic neuritis, and necrotizing retinopathy (that often leads to permanent vision loss). Corticosteroids reduce the duration of pain during the acute phase, however, they have not been shown to decrease the incidence of postherpetic neuralgia and can exacerbate some ocular complications. Ophthalmology consultation is mandatory before initiating corticosteroid therapy.

REFERENCES

Anderson, E., Fantus, R. J., & Haddadin, R. I. (2017). Diagnosis and management of herpes zoster ophthalmicus. *Disease-a-Month, 63*(2), 38–44.

Vrcek, I., Choudhury, E., & Durairaj, V. (2017). Herpes Zoster Ophthalmicus: A Review for the Internist. *The American Journal of Medicine, 130*(1), 21–26.

ORAL ANTIVIRALS

▷ *acyclovir* (B)(G) 800 mg 5 x/day x 7-10 days
  Pediatric: <2 years: not recommended; 2 years, ≤40 kg: 20 mg/kg 5 x/day x 7-10 days; 2 years, >40 kg: 800 mg 5 x/day x 7-10 days; *see page 614 for dose by weight*
    Zovirax *Cap:* 200 mg; *Tab:* 400, 800 mg; *IVF bag:* 500 mg, 1 gm pre-mixed in 0.9% NS
    Zovirax Oral Suspension *Oral susp:* 200 mg/5 ml (banana)
▷ *famciclovir* (B) 500 mg tid x 7-10 days
  Pediatric: <18 years: not recommended; ≥18 years: same as adult
    Famvir *Tab:* 125, 250, 500 mg
▷ *valacyclovir* (B) 1 gm tid x 7-10 days
  Pediatric: <12 years: not recommended; ≥12 years: same as adult
    Valtrex *Cplt:* 500, 1 gm

◯ HICCUPS: INTRACTABLE

▷ *chlorpromazine* (C) 25-50 mg tid-qid
  Pediatric: <6 months: not recommended; ≥6 months: 0.25 mg/lb orally q 4-6 hours prn <u>or</u> 0.5 mg/lb rectally q 6-8 hours prn
    Thorazine *Tab:* 10, 25, 50, 100, 200 mg; *Spansule:* 30, 75, 150 mg sust-rel; *Syr:* 10 mg/5 ml (4 oz; orange custard); *Oral conc:* 30 mg/ml (4 oz); 100 mg/ml (2, 8 oz); *Supp:* 25, 100 mg

◯ HIDRADENITIS SUPPURATIVA

ORAL ANTI-INFECTIVES

▷ *doxycycline* (D)(G) 100 mg bid x 7-14 days
  Pediatric: <8 years: not recommended; ≥8 years, <100 lb: 2 mg/lb on first day in 2 divided doses, followed by 1 mg/lb/day in 1-2 divided doses; ≥8 years, ≥100 lb: same as adult; *see page 633 for dose by weight*
    Acticlate *Tab:* 75, 150**mg
    Adoxa *Tab:* 50, 75, 100, 150 mg ent-coat
    Doryx *Tab:* 50, 75, 100, 150, 200 mg del-rel
    Doxteric *Tab:* 50 mg del-rel
    Monodox *Cap:* 50, 75, 100 mg
    Oracea *Cap:* 40 mg del-rel
    Vibramycin *Tab:* 100 mg; *Cap:* 50, 100 mg; *Syr:* 50 mg/5 ml (raspberry-apple); (sulfites); *Oral susp:* 25 mg/5 ml (raspberry)
    Vibra-Tab *Tab:* 100 mg film-coat
▷ *erythromycin base* (B)(G) 1-1.5 gm divided qid x 7-14 days
  Pediatric: <45 kg: 30-50 mg in 2-4 divided doses x 7-14 days; ≥45 kg: same as adult
    Ery-Tab *Tab:* 250, 333, 500 mg ent-coat
    PCE *Tab:* 333, 500 mg

Comment: *erythromycin* may increase INR with concomitant *warfarin*, as well as increase serum level of *digoxin, benzodiazepines*, and *statins*.

➤ *erythromycin ethylsuccinate* (B)(G) 1200-1600 mg divided qid x 7-14 days
Pediatric: 30-50 mg/kg/day in 4 divided doses x 7 days; may double dose with severe infection; max 100 mg/kg/day; *see page 635 for dose by weight*

    EryPed *Oral susp:* 200 mg/5 ml (100, 200 ml) (fruit); 400 mg/5 ml (60, 100, 200 ml) (banana); *Oral drops:* 200, 400 mg/5 ml (50 ml) (fruit); *Chew tab:* 200 mg wafer (fruit)

    E.E.S. *Oral susp:* 200, 400 mg/5 ml (100 ml) (fruit)

    E.E.S. Granules *Oral susp:* 200 mg/5 ml (100, 200 ml) (cherry)

    E.E.S. 400 Tablets *Tab:* 400 mg

Comment: *erythromycin* may increase INR with concomitant *warfarin*, as well as increase serum level of *digoxin*, benzodiazepines and statins.

➤ *minocycline* (D)(G) 100 mg bid x 7-14 days
Pediatric: <8 years: not recommended, ≥8 years: same as adult

    Dynacin *Cap:* 50, 100 mg

    Minocin *Cap:* 50, 75, 100 mg; *Oral susp:* 50 mg/5 ml (60 ml) (custard) (sulfites, alcohol 5%)

Comment: *minocycline* is contraindicated <8 years-of-age, in pregnancy, and lactation (discolors developing tooth enamel). A side effect may be photo-sensitivity (photophobia). Do not give with antacids, calcium supplements, milk or other dairy, or within two hours of taking another drug.

➤ *tetracycline* (D)(G) 250 mg qid or 500 mg tid x 7-14 days
Pediatric: <8 years: not recommended; ≥8 years, <100 lb: 25-50 mg/kg/day in 2-4 divided doses x 7-14 days; ≥8 years, ≥100 lb: same as adult; *see page 646 for dose by weight*

    Achromycin V *Cap:* 250, 500 mg

    Sumycin *Tab:* 250, 500 mg; *Cap:* 250, 500 mg; *Oral susp:* 125 mg/5 ml (100, 200 ml) (fruit, sulfites)

TOPICAL ANTI-INFECTIVES

➤ *clindamycin* (B) topical apply bid x 7-14 days

    Cleocin T *Pad:* 1% (60/pck; alcohol 50%); *Lotn:* 1% (60 ml); *Gel:* 1% (30, 60 gm); *Soln w. applicator:* 1% (30, 60 ml; alcohol 50%)

HOOKWORM (UNCINARIASIS, CUTANEOUS LARVAE MIGRANS)

ANTHELMINTICS

➤ *albendazole* (C) 400 mg as a single dose; may repeat in 3 weeks
Pediatric: <2 years: 200 mg daily x 3 days; may repeat in 3 weeks; ≥2-12 years: 400 mg daily x 3 days; may repeat in 3 weeks

    Albenza *Tab:* 200 mg

➤ *ivermectin* (C) take with water; chew or crush and mix with food; may repeat in 3 months if needed; <15 kg: not recommended; ≥15 kg: 200 mcg/kg as a single dose
Pediatric: <15 kg: not recommended; ≥15 kg: same as adult

    Stromectol *Tab:* 3, 6*mg

➤ *mebendazole* (C)(G) chew, swallow, or mix with food; 100 mg bid x 3 days; may repeat in 3 weeks if needed; take with a meal
Pediatric: <2 years: not recommended; ≥2 years: same as adult

    Emverm *Chew tab:* 100 mg

    Vermox *Chew tab:* 100 mg

▷ *pyrantel pamoate* (C) 11 mg/kg x 1 dose; max 1 gm/dose
  Pediatric: 25-37 lb: 1/2 tsp x 1 dose; 38-62 lb: 1 tsp x 1 dose; 63-87 lb: 1 tsp x 1 dose;
  88-112 lb: 2 tsp x 1 dose; 113-137 lb: 2 tsp x 1 dose; 138-162 lb: 3 tsp x 1 dose; 163-
  187 lb: 3 tsp x 1 dose; >187 lb: 4 tsp x 1 dose
    Antiminth *Cap:* 180 mg; *Liq:* 50 mg/ml (30 ml); 144 mg/ml (30 ml); *Oral susp:* 50
    mg/ml (60 ml)
      Pin-X (OTC) *Cap:* 180 mg; *Liq:* 50 mg/ml (30 ml); 144 mg/ml (30 ml); *Oral susp:*
      50 mg/ml (30 ml)
▷ *thiabendazole* (C) take with a meal; may crush and mix with food; treat x 7 days; <30
  lb: consult mfr pkg insert; ≥30 lb: 25 mg/kg/dose bid with meals; 30-50 lb: 250 mg bid
  with meals; >50 lb: 10 mg/lb/dose bid with meals; max 1.5 gm/dose; max 3 gm/day
  Pediatric: same as adult
    Mintezol *Chew tab:* 500*mg (orange); *Oral susp:* 500 mg/5 ml (120 ml) (orange)
Comment: *thiabendazole* is not for prophylaxis. May impair mental alertness. May not
be available in the US.

**HUMAN IMMUNODEFICIENCY VIRUS (HIV) INFECTION; HIV
PRE-EXPOSURE PROPHYLAXIS (PrEP); HIV OCCUPATIONAL
POST-EXPOSURE PROPHYLAXIS (oPEP); HIV NON-OCCUPATIONAL
POST-EXPOSURE PROPHYLAXIS (nPEP)**

ANTIRETROVIRAL HIV POST-EXPOSURE PROPHYLAXIS (oPEP and nPEP)

Comment: Antiretroviral prophylactic treatment regimens for occupational HIV
post-exposure prophylaxis (oPEP) and non-occupational HIV post-exposure
prophylaxis (nPEP) are referenced from the **2015 CDC Sexually Transmitted Diseases
Treatment Guidelines, MMWR, and NIH** available at: https://www.cdc.gov/hiv/pdf/
programresources/cdc-hiv-npep-guidelines.pdf

In this section, the 2015 CDC-recommended highly active antiretroviral treatment
(HAART) regimens are followed by a listing of the single and combination drugs with
dosing regimens and dose forms. Appendix S is an alphabetical listing of the HIV
drugs and dose forms. For more information on the management of HIV infection in
adults and adolescents, see *Guidelines for the Use of Antiretroviral Agents in HIV-1-
Infected Adults and Adolescents:* https://aidsinfo.nih.gov/contentfiles/lvguidelines/
adultandadolescentgl.pdf.

For specific dosing information in the management of HIV infection in children, see
Guidelines for Use of Antiretroviral Agents in Pediatric HIV Infection: https://www.
aidsinfo.nih.gov/contentfiles/lvguidelines/pediatricguidelines.pdf. Providers should
consult, and/or refer HIV-infected patients to, a specialist and/or specialty community
services for age-appropriate dosing regimens and other patient-specific needs.

Initiation of oPEP/nPEP with ART as soon as possible increases the likelihood of
prophylactic benefit. Treatment regimens must be initiated ≥72 hours following
exposure. A 28-day course of ART is recommended for persons with *substantial
risk for HIV exposure* (i.e., exposure of vagina, rectum, eye, mouth, or other mucous
membrane, non-intact skin, or percutaneous contact with blood, semen, vaginal
secretions, breast milk, or any body fluid that is visibly contaminated with blood,
when the source is known to be infected with HIV). ART is not recommended for
persons with *negligible risk for HIV exposure* (i.e., exposure of vagina, rectum,
eye, mouth, or other mucus membrane, intact or non-intact skin, or percutaneous
contact with urine, nasal secretions, saliva, sweat, or tears, if not visibly contaminated

with blood, regardless of the known or suspected HIV status of the source). There is no evidence indicating any specific antiretroviral medication, or combination of medications is optimal for suppressing local viral replication. There is no evidence to indicate that a 3-drug ART regimen is any more beneficial than a 2-drug regimen. When the source person is available for interview and testing, his or her history of retroviral medication use and most recent/current viral load measurement should be considered when selecting an ART treatment regimen (e.g., to help avoid prescribing an antiretroviral medication to which the source virus is likely to be resistant). Register pregnant patients exposed to antiretroviral agents to the Antiretroviral Pregnancy Registry (APR) at 800-258-4263. The CDC recommends that HIV-infected mothers not breastfeed their infants to avoid risking postnatal transmission of HIV infection.

ANTIRETROVIRAL HIV POST-EXPOSURE PROPHYLAXIS (PEP)

Comment: **Truvada** is indicated for treatment of HIV-1 infection and pre-exposure prophylaxis (PrEP) to reduce the risk of sexually acquired HIV-1 in persons at high risk for exposure, ≥18 years-of-age, in combination with safe sex practices.

➤ Truvada (B)(G) *emtricitabine+tenofovir disoproxil fumarate*
   Pediatric: <17 kg: not established; 17-<22 kg: 100/150 once daily; 22-<28 kg: 133/200 once daily; 28-35 kg: 167/250 once daily; ≥35 kg: 200/300 once daily
      Tab: **Truvada 100/150** emt 100 mg+teno 150 mg
            Truvada 133/200 emt 133 mg+teno 200 mg
            Truvada 167/250 emt 167 mg+teno 250 mg
            Truvada 200/300 emt 200 mg+teno 300 mg

HIV INFECTION ANTIRETROVIRAL TREATMENT REGIMENS
Nonnucleoside Reverse Transcriptase Inhibitor (NNRTI)-Based Regimen

➤ *efavirenz* plus (*lamivudine* or *emtricitabine*) plus (*zidovudine* or *tenofovir*)

Protease Inhibitor (PI)-Based Regimens

➤ *lopinavir+ritonavir* (co-formulated as **Kaletra**) plus (*lamivudine* or *emtricitabine*) plus *zidovudine*
➤ *darunavir+cobicistat* (co-formulated as **Prezcobix**) plus *other retroviral agents*

ALTERNATIVE REGIMENS
NNRTI-Based Regimen

➤ *efavirenz* plus (*lamivudine* or *emtricitabine*) plus (*abacavir* or *didanosine* or *stavudine*)
   Comment: *efavirenz* should be avoided in pregnant women and women of child-bearing potential.

Protease Inhibitor-Based Regimens
Regimen 1

➤ *atazanavir* plus (*lamivudine* or *emtricitabine*) plus (*zidovudine* or *stavudine* or *abacavir* or *didanosine*) or (*tenofovir* plus *ritonavir* (100 mg/day)

Regimen 2

➤ *fosamprenavir* plus (*lamivudine* or *emtricitabine*) plus (*zidovudine* or *stavudine*) or (*abacavir* or *tenofovir* or *didanosine*)

Regimen 3

▷ *fosamprenavir+ritonavir* plus (*lamivudine* or *emtricitabine*) plus (*zidovudine* or *stavudine* or *abacavir* or *tenofovir* or *didanosine*)

Regimen 4

▷ *indinavir+ritonavir* plus (*lamivudine* or *emtricitabine*) plus (*zidovudine* or *stavudine* or *abacavir* or *tenofovir* or *didanosine*)

Comment: Using *ritonavir* with *indinavir* may increase risk for renal adverse events.

Regimen 5

▷ *lopinavir+ritonavir* (co-formulated as **Kaletra**) plus (*lamivudine* or *emtricitabine*) plus (*stavudine* or *abacavir* or *tenofovir* or *didanosine*)

Regimen 6

▷ *nelfinavir* plus (*lamivudine* or *emtricitabine*) plus (*zidovudine* or *stavudine* or *abacavir* or *tenofovir* or *didanosine*)

Regimen 7

▷ *saquinavir+ritonavir* plus (*lamivudine* or *emtricitabine*) plus (*zidovudine* or *stavudine* or *abacavir* or *tenofovir* or *didanosine*)

Triple Nucleoside Reverse Transcriptase Inhibitor (NRTI)-Based Regimen

abacavir plus *lamivudine* plus *zidovudine*

Comment: Triple NRTI therapy should be used only when an NNRTI- or PI-based regimen cannot or should not be used.

BRAND NAMES, DOSING AND DOSE FORMS: SINGLE AGENTS

Integrase Strand Transfer Inhibitors (INSTIs)

▷ *dolutegravir* (C) *Treatment naïve or treatment experienced but INSTI naïve:* 50 mg once daily; *Treatment experienced or naïve and co-administered with efavirenz, FPV/r, TPV/r, or rifampin:* 50 mg bid; *INSTI experienced with certain INSTI-associated resistance substitutions:* 50 mg bid
Pediatric: <12 years, <40 kg: not established; ≥12 years, ≥40 kg: same as adult
    Tivicay *Tab:* 10, 25, 50 mg

▷ *raltegravir (as potassium)* (C) 400 mg (one film-coat tab) bid; take with concomitant **rifampin** 800 mg bid; swallow whole; do not crush or chew
Pediatric: ≥4 weeks, 3-11 kg [oral susp] 3-<4 kg: 20 mg bid; 4-<6 kg: 30 mg bid; 6-<8 kg: 40 mg bid; 8-<11 kg: 60 mg bid; ≥11-<25 kg [oral susp/chew tab]; 6 mg/kg/dose bid; see mfr pkg insert for dose by weight; ≥25 kg and unable to swallow tablet **use** chewable tab; 25-<28 kg: 150 mg bid; 28-<40 kg: 200 mg bid; ≥40 kg: 300 mg bid; 6 years, ≥**25** kg, and able to swallow tablets use film-coat tab; 400 mg bid
    Isentress *Tab:* 400 mg film-coat; *Chew tab:* 25, 100*mg (orange banana) (phenylalanine)
    Isentress HD *Tab:* 600 mg film-coat
    Isentress Oral Suspension *Oral susp:* 100 mg/pkt pwdr for oral susp (banana)
Comment: Oral suspension, chewable tablets and film-coat *raltegravir* tablets are not bioequivalent. Maximum dose for chewable tablets is 300 mg twice daily. Previously, the maximum dose for film-coat tablets was 400 mg twice daily. However, the US Food and Drug Administration has recently approved a new 1200 mg daily dosage of **Isentress HD** (*raltegravir*) for the treatment of HIV-1 infection in adults, and pediatric patients who weigh ≥ 40 kg and are treatment-naïve or

whose virus has been suppressed on an initial regimen of 400 mg twice-daily dose of **Isentress HD**. **Isentress HD** is administered as two 600 mg film-coat oral tablets in combination with other antiretroviral agents, and can be taken with o̲r without food. Co-administration of **Isentress HD** can include a wide range of antiretroviral agents and non-antiretroviral agents, however aluminum an̲d̲/o̲r̲ magnesium-containing antacids, calcium carbonate antacids, *rifampin, tipranavir+ritonavir, etravirine*, and other strong inducers of drug metabolizing enzymes are not recommended to be combined with **Isentress HD**. Health care providers should consider the potential for drug-drug interactions prior to and during treatment with **Isentress HD** and any other recommended agents. Adverse effects associated with treatment included abdominal pain, diarrhea, vomiting and decreased appetite. In addition, severe, potentially life-threatening and fatal skin reactions can occur, including Stevens-Johnson syndrome, hypersensitivity reaction, and toxic epidermal necrolysis. Treatment should be immediately discontinued if severe hypersensitivity, severe rash, o̲r rash with systemic symptoms o̲r liver aminotransferase elevations develop.

Nucleoside Reverse Transcriptase Inhibitors (NRTIs)

▷ *abacavir sulfate* (C)(G) 600 mg once daily o̲r 300 mg bid; *Mild hepatic impairment:* use oral solution for titration
Pediatric: 3 months-16 years: [tab/oral soln] 16 mg/kg qd o̲r 8 mg/kg bid; max 300 mg bid; >14 kg: see mfr pkg insert for tablet dosing by weight band
    Ziagen (as sulfate) *Tab:* 300*mg
    Ziagen Oral Solution *Oral soln:* 20 mg/ml (240 ml) (strawberry-banana) (parabens, propylene glycol)

▷ *didanosine* (C)
    Videx EC take once daily on an empty stomach; swallow whole; <20 kg: use oral solution; 20-<25 kg: 200 mg; 25-<60 kg: 250 mg; ≥60 kg: 400 mg; *CrCl 30-59 mL/min:* <60 kg: 125 mg; ≥60 kg: 200 mg; *CrCl 10-29 mL/min:* 125 mg; *CrCl<10 mL/min o̲r dialysis:*<60 kg: use oral solution ≥60 kg: 125 mg
    Pediatric: same as adult
        Cap: 125, 200, 250, 400 mg ent-coat del-rel; *Chew tab:* 25, 50, 100, 150, 200 mg (mandarin orange) (buffered with calcium carbonate and magnesium hydroxide, phenylalanine)
    Videx Pediatric Pwdr for Solution <60 kg: 125 mg bid; ≥60 kg: 200 mg bid; *If once daily dosing required:* <60 kg: 250 mg once daily; ≥60 kg: 400 mg once daily; *CrCl 30-59 mL/min:* <60 kg: 150 mg once daily o̲r 75 mg bid; ≥60 kg: 200 mg once daily o̲r 100 mg bid; *CrCl 10-29 mL/min:* <60 kg: 100 mg once daily; ≥60 kg: 150 mg once daily; *CrCl <10 mL/min o̲r dialysis:* <60 kg: 75 mg once daily; ≥60 kg: 100 mg once daily; take on an empty stomach
    Pediatric: <2 weeks: not recommended; 2 weeks-8 months: 100 mg/m² bid; >8 months: 120 mg/m² bid; *Renal impairment:* consider reducing dose o̲r increasing dosing interval; take on an empty stomach
        Pwdr for oral soln: 2, 4 gm (120, 240 ml)
    Comment: *didanosine* is contraindicated with concomitant *allopurinal* o̲r *ribavirin*.

▷ *emtricitabine* (B) 200 mg once daily; *CrCl 30-49 mL/min:* 200 mg q 48 hours; *CrCl 15-29 mL/min:* 200 mg q 72 hours; *CrCl <15 mL/min o̲r dialysis:* 200 mg q 96 hours
Pediatric: <3 months: 3 mg/kg oral soln once daily; 3 months-17 years, 6 mg/kg once daily; ≤33 kg: use oral soln, max 240 mg (24 ml); >33 kg: 200 mg cap once daily; max 240 mg/day; ≥18 years: same as adult
    Emtriva *Cap:* 200 mg
    Emtriva Oral Solution *Oral soln:* 10 mg/ml (170 ml) (cotton candy)

▷ *lamivudine* (C)(G) *CrCl* ≥50 mL/min: 300 mg qd or 150 mg bid; *CrCl* >30-50 mL/min: 150 mg qd; *CrCl 15-29*: first dose 150 mg, then 100 mg once daily; *CrCl 5-14 mL/min*: first dose 150 mg, then 50 mg qd; *CrCl <5/min*: first dose 50 mg, the 25 mg once daily; max 8 mg/kg once daily or 150 mg bid
Pediatric: <3 months: not established; 3 months-16 years: 4 mg/kg oral soln or tab bid; [tab] 14-<20 kg: 150 mg once daily or 75 mg bid; ≥20-<25 kg: 225 mg once daily or 75 mg in the AM and 150 mg in the PM; ≥25 kg: 300 mg once daily or 150 mg bid; max 8 mg/kg once daily or 150 mg bid or 300 mg once daily

    Epivir *Tab*: 150*, 300 mg
    Epivir Oral Solution *Oral soln*: 10 mg/ml (240 ml) (strawberry-banana)
    (sucrose 3 gm/15 ml)

Comment: With renal impairment reduce *lamivudine* dose or extend dosing interval.

▷ *stavudine* (C)(G) ≥60 kg: 40 mg q 12 hours; ≤60 kg: 30 mg q 12 hours; *If peripheral neuropathy develops*: discontinue; *After resolution, ≥60 kg*: may re-start at 20 mg q 12 hours; *After resolution, ≤60 kg*: may restart at 15 mg q 12 hours; *if neuropathy returns*: consider permanent discontinuation; *CrCl 10-50 mL/min, ≥60 kg*: 20 mg q 12 hours; *CrCl 10-50 mL/min, ≥60 kg*: 15 mg q 12 hours; *Hemodialysis, ≥60 kg*: 20 mg q 24 hours; *Hemodialysis, ≤60 kg*: 15 mg q 24 hours; administer at the same time of day; *Hemodialysis*: administer at the end of dialysis
Pediatric: birth-13 days: [tab/oral soln] 0.5 mg/kg q 12 hours; >14 days, <30 kg: [tab/oral soln] 1 mg/kg q 12 hours; ≥30-<60 kg: 30 mg q 12 hours; ≥60 kg: 40 mg q 12 hours

    Zerit *Cap*: 15, 20, 30, 40 mg
    Zerit for Oral Solution *Oral soln*: 1 mg/ml pwdr for reconstitution (fruit) (dye-free)

Comment: Withdraw *stavudine* if peripheral neuropathy occurs. After complete resolution, may restart at half the recommended dose. If peripheral neuropathy recurs consider permanent discontinuation.

▷ *tenofovir disoproxil fumarate* (C)(G) 300 mg once daily; *CrCl 30-49 mL/min*: 300 mg q 48 hours; *CrCl 10-29*: 300 mg q 72-96 hours; *Hemodialysis*: 300 mg once every 7 days or after a total of 12 hours of dialysis; *CrCl <10 mL/min*: not recommended
Pediatric: <2 years: not established; 2-12 years: 8 mg/kg once daily; >12 years, 35 kg: 300 mg once daily; mix oral pwdr with 2-4 oz soft food

    Viread *Tab*: 150, 200, 250, 300 mg; *Oral pwdr*: 40 mg/gm (60 gm w. dosing scoop)

▷ *zidovudine* (C)(G) 600 mg daily divided bid-tid; *ESRD/dialysis*: 100 mg q 6-8 hours; *Vertical transmission, severe anemia, or neutropenia*: see mfr pkg insert
Pediatric: Treatment of HIV-1 infection: 4-<9 kg: 24 mg/kg/day divided bid or tid; ≥9-<30 kg: 18 mg/kg/day divided bid or tid; ≥30 kg: 600 mg/day divided bid or tid; *Prevention of maternal-fetal neonatal transmission*: <12 hours after birth until 6 weeks of age: [Soln] 2 mg/kg q 6 hours until 6 weeks-of-age; [IV] 1.5 mg/kg infused over 30 minutes q 6 hours until 6 weeks-of-age; max 200 mg q 8 hours

    Retrovir Tablets *Tab*: 300 mg
    Retrovir Capsules *Cap*: 100 mg
    Retrovir Syrup *Syrup*: 50 mg/5 ml (strawberry)
    Retrovir IV *Vial*: 10 mg/ml after dilution (20 ml) (preservative-free)

Nonnucleoside Reverse Transcriptase Inhibitors (NNRTIs)

▷ *delavirdine mesylate* (C) 400 mg (4 x 100-mg or 2 x 200 mg) tablets tid in combination with other antiretroviral agents
Pediatric: <16 years: not established; ≥16 years: same as adult

    Rescriptor *Tab*: 100, 200 mg

Comment: The 100 mg **Rescriptor** tablets may be dispersed in water prior to consumption. To prepare a dispersion, add four 100 mg Rescriptor tablets to at least 3 ounces of water, allow to stand for a few minutes, and then stir until a uniform dispersion occurs. The dispersion should be consumed promptly. The glass should be rinsed with water and the rinse swallowed to insure the entire dose is consumed. The 200 mg tablets should be taken as intact tablets, because they are not readily dispersed in water.

▷ *efavirenz* (D)(G) 600 mg once daily
Pediatric: >3 months, 3.5 kg: [tab/cap] 3.5-< 5 kg: 100 mg once daily 5-<7.5 kg: 150 mg once daily; 7.5-<15 kg: 200 mg once daily; 15-<20 kg: 250 mg once daily; 20-<25 kg: 300 mg once daily; 25-<32.5 kg: 350 mg once daily; 32.5-<40 kg: 400 mg once daily; >40 kg: 600 mg once daily; max 600 mg once daily

Comment: For children who cannot swallow capsules, the capsule contents can be administered with a small amount of food or infant formula using the capsule sprinkle method of administration. See mfr pkg insert for instructions. Tablets should not be crushed or chewed. Administer at bedtime to limit CNS effects.
    Sustiva *Tab:* 75, 150, 600, 800 mg; *Cap:* 50, 200 mg

▷ *etravirine* (B) 200 mg (1 x 200 mg tablet or 2 x 100 mg tablets) bid following a meal
Pediatric: <3 year: not recommended; ≥3 years, >16 kg: 16-< 20 kg: 100 mg bid; 20-<25 kg: 125 mg bid; 25-<30 kg: 150 mg bid; ≥30 kg: 200 mg bid; max 200 mg bid; take following a mail
    Intelence *Tab:* 25*, 100, 200 mg

▷ *nevirapine* (B)(G) initially one 200 mg tablet of immediate-release **Viramune** once daily for the first 14 days in combination with other antiretroviral agents; then, one 400 mg tablet of **Viramune XR** once daily

Comment: The 14-day lead-in period has been found to lessen the frequency of rash.
Pediatric: <6 years: not recommended; 6-<18 years: BSA 0.58-0.83 kg/m²: 200 mg once daily; BSA 0.84-1.16 kg/m²: 300 mg once daily; BSA ≥1.17 kg/m²: 400 mg; once daily; max 400 mg once daily

Comment: Children must initiate therapy with immediate-release **Viramune** for the first 14 days; ≥15 days: [oral susp/tab]: 150 mg/m² once daily for 14 days, then 150 mg/m² bid
    Viramune *Tab:* 200*mg
    Viramune Oral Suspension *Oral susp:* 50 mg/5 ml (240 ml)
    Viramune XR *Tab:* 100, 400 mg ext-rel

▷ *rilpivirine* (D) 25 mg once daily; *If concomitant* **rifabutin**: 50 mg once daily; *If concomitant* **rifabutin** *stopped:* 25 mg once daily
Pediatric: <12 years: not recommended; ≥12 years, >35 kg: same adult
    Edurant *Tab:* 25 mg

Nucleoside and Nonnucleoside Reverse Transcriptase Inhibitor (NRTI/NNRTI) Combinations

▷ Atripla (B) *efavirenz+emtricitabine+tenofovir disoproxil fumarate* 1 tab once daily preferably at HS; take on an empty stomach; *Concomitant* **rifabutin**: >50 kg: take additional *efavirenz* 200 mg/day
Pediatric: <12 years: not recommended; ≥12 years, 40 kg: same as adult
    Tab: efa 600 mg+emtri 200 mg+teno dis fum 300 mg

▷ Complera (B) *emtricitabine+tenofovir disoproxil fumarate+rilpivirine* 1 tab once daily; CrCl <50 mL/min: not recommended; *Concomitant* **rifabutin**: take additional **ribavirin** 25 mg qd
Pediatric: <12 years, <35 kg: not established; ≥12 years, ≥35 kg: same as adult
    Tab: emtri 200 mg+teno dis 300 mg+rilpiv 25 mg

Protease Inhibitors (PIs)

▷ *atazanavir* (B)(G) *Treatment naive: Recommended regimen:* 300 mg plus **ritonavir** 100 mg once daily; *Unable to tolerate* **ritonavir**: 400 mg once daily; *In combination with* **efavirenz**: 400 mg plus **ritonavir** 100 mg once daily; *Treatment experienced:*

Recommended regimen: 300 mg plus *ritonavir* 100 mg once daily; *In combination with both an H2-blocker or PPI and tenofovir:* 400 mg plus *ritonavir* 100 mg once daily; take with food

Pediatric: <3 months: not recommended; ≥3 months, 5 kg: [oral pwdr] 5-<15 kg: 200 mg (4 packets) plus *ritonavir* 80 mg once daily; 15-<25 kg: 250 mg (5 packets) plus *ritonavir* 80 mg once daily; ≥25 kg, unable to swallow capsules: 300 mg (6 packets) plus *ritonavir* once daily; 6 years, <15 kg: [cap] 15-<20 kg: 150 mg plus *ritonavir* 100 mg once daily; 20-<40 kg: 200 mg plus *ritonavir* 100 mg once daily; ≥40 kg: 300 mg plus *ritonavir* 100 mg once daily; [capsule]15-<20 kg: 150 mg plus *ritonavir* 100 mg once daily; 20-<40 kg: 200 mg plus *ritonavir* 100 mg once daily; ≥40 kg: 300 mg plus *ritonavir* 100 mg once daily; max dose 400 mg once daily; take with food

> **Reyataz** *Cap:* 100, 150, 200, 300 mg; *Oral pwdr:* 50 mg/pkt (30/carton) (phenylalanine)

Comment: Administration of *atazanavir* with *ritonavir* is preferred. Dose for treatment-naïve children ≥13 years of age and ≥40 kg unable to tolerate *ritonavir*, administer 400 mg once daily. See mfr pkg insert for special dosing considerations when combining *atazanavir* with other retrovirals.

▷ *darunavir* (C)(G) *Treatment naïve and treatment experienced with no darunavir resistance associated substitutions:* 800 mg once daily with *ritonavir* 100 mg once daily; *Treatment-experienced with at least one darunavir resistance associated substitution:* 600 mg bid with ritonavir 100 mg bid; *Severe hepatic impairment:* not recommended

Pediatric: ≥3 years, 10 kg [oral soln/tab/cap] *Treatment naïve or experienced without darunavir-associated substitutions:* 10-<15 kg: 35 mg/kg once daily plus *ritonavir* 7 mg/kg once daily; 15-<30 kg: 600 mg plus *ritonavir* 100 mg once daily; 30-<40 kg: 675 mg plus *ritonavir* 100 mg once daily; >40 kg: 800 mg plus *ritonavir* 100 mg once daily; *Treatment experienced with ≥1 darunavir-associated substitution(s):* 10-15 kg: 20 mg/kg bid plus *ritonavir* 3 mg/kg bid; 15-<30 kg: 375 mg plus *ritonavir* 48 mg bid; 30-<40 kg: 450 mg plus *ritonavir* 60 mg bid; >40 kg: 600 mg plus *ritonavir* 100 mg bid

> **Prezista** *Tab:* 75, 150, 600, 800 mg film-coat
> **Prezista Oral Suspension** *Susp:* 100 mg/ml (strawberry cream)

Comment: **Prezista** is FDA approved for treatment of HIV-1-infected pregnant women and for the treatment of children >3 years-of-age in combination with *ritonavir* and other antiretrovirals.

▷ *fosamprenavir* (C)(G) *Treatment-naïve:* 1,400 mg bid or 1,400 mg once daily plus *ritonavir* 200 mg once daily or 1,400 mg once daily plus *ritonavir* 100 mg once daily or 700 mg bid plus *ritonavir* 100 mg bid; *Protease inhibitor-experienced:* 700 mg bid plus *ritonavir* 100 mg bid

Pediatric: <4 weeks: not recommended; *Protease inhibitor-naïve, ≥4 weeks or protease inhibitor-experienced:* ≥6 Months, <11 kg: 45 mg/kg plus *ritonavir* 7 mg/kg bid; 11-<15 kg: 30 mg/kg plus *ritonavir* 3 mg/kg bid; 15 kg-<20 kg: 23 mg/kg plus *ritonavir* 3 mg/kg bid; ≥20 kg: 18 mg/kg plus *ritonavir* 3 mg/kg bid; *Protease-inhibitor naïve, ≥2 years:* 30 mg/kg bid without *ritonavir*: max dose 700 mg plus *ritonavir* 100 mg bid

> **Lexiva** *Tab: 700 mg film-coat*
> **Lexiva Oral Suspension** *Oral susp:* 50 mg/ml (225 ml) (grape-bubble gum-peppermint)

Comment: *fosamprenavir* 1 ml is equivalent to approximately 43 mg of *amprenavir* 1 ml.

▷ *indinavir sulfate* (C) 800 mg q 8 hours; *Concomitant rifabutin:* 1 gm q 8 hours and reduce *rifabutin* dose by half; *Hepatic insufficiency or concomitant ketoconazole, itraconazole, or delavirdine:* 600 mg q 8 hours; take with water on an empty stomach or with a light meal

Pediatric: <3 years: not established ≥3-18 years, doses of 500 mg/m² every 8 hours have been used; see mfr pkg insert

Crixivan *Cap:* 100, 200, 333, 400 mg

➤ *nelfinavir mesylate* **(B)** 1250 mg (5 x 250 mg tablets or 2 x 625 mg tablets) bid or 750 mg (3 x 250 mg tablets) tid; take with a meal; may dissolve tablets in a small amount of water; max 2500 mg/day

Pediatric: <2 years: not established; 2-13 years: 45-55 mg/kg bid or 25-35 mg/kg tid; take with a meal; max 2500 mg/day; ≥13 years: same as adult

Viracept *Tab:* 250, 625 mg

Viracept Oral Powder *Oral pwdr:* 50 mg/gm (144 gm) (phenylalanine)

Comment: The 250 mg **Viracept** tabs are interchangeable with oral powder, the 625 mg tabs are not.

➤ *raltegravir (as potassium)* **(C)** 400 mg bid

Pediatric: ≥4 weeks, 3-11 kg: [oral susp] 3-<4 kg: 20 mg bid; 4-<6 kg: 30 mg bid; 6-<8 kg: 40 mg bid; 8-<11 kg: 60 mg bid; ≥11-<25 kg: [oral susp/chew tab] 6 mg/kg/dose bid; see mfr pkg insert for dosage by weight; ≥25 kg and unable to swallow tablet: [chew tab] 25-<28 kg: 150 mg bid; 28-<40 kg: 200 mg bid; ≥40 kg: 300 mg bid; ≥6 years, ≥25 kg, able to swallow tablets: 400 mg film-coat tablet bid

Comment: Oral suspension, chewable tablets, and film-coat tablets are not bioequivalent. Chewable tablet max dose 300 mg bid. Film-coat tablets max dose 400 mg bid. Oral suspension max dose 100 mg bid

Isentress *Tab:* 400 mg film-coat; *Chew tab:* 25, 100*mg (orange-banana) (phenylalanine)

Isentress Oral Suspension *Oral susp:* 100 mg/pkt pwdr for oral susp (banana)

➤ *ritonavir* **(B)(G)** initially 300 mg bid; increase at 2-3 day intervals by 100 mg bid; max 600 mg bid

Pediatric: <1 month: not recommended; ≥1 month: 350-400 mg/m² bid; initiate at 250 mg/m² bid and titrate upward every 2-3 days by 50 mg/m² bid; max dose 600 mg bid

Comment: Lower doses of *ritonavir* have been used to boost other protease inhibitors but the *ritonavir* doses used for boosting have not been specifically approved in children.

Norvir *Tab:* 100 mg film-coat; *Gel cap:* 100 mg (alcohol)

Norvir Oral Solution *Oral soln:* 80 mg/ml, 600 mg/7.5 ml (8 oz) (peppermint-caramel) (alcohol)

Comment: **Norvir** tablets should be swallowed whole. Take **Norvir** with meals. Patients may improve the taste of **Norvir Oral Solution** by mixing with chocolate milk, **Ensure,** or **Advera** within one hour of dosing. Dose reduction of **Norvir** is necessary when used with other protease inhibitors (*atazanavir, darunavir, fosamprenavir, saquinavir,* and *tipranavir*. Patients who take the 600 mg gel cap bid may experience more gastrointestinal side effects such as nausea, vomiting, abdominal pain or diarrhea when switching from the gel cap to the tablet because of greater maximum plasma concentration (Cmax) achieved with the tablet. These adverse events (gastrointestinal or paresthesias) may diminish as treatment is continued.

➤ *saquinavir mesylate* **(B)**

Pediatric: <16 years: not established; ≥16 years: same as adult

Fortovase *Tab/Cap:* 200 mg

Invirase *Tab:* 500 mg; *Cap:* 200 mg

➤ *tipranavir* **(C)** 500 mg bid plus ritonavir 200 mg bid

Pediatric: <2 years: not recommended; 2-18 years: [cap/oral soln] 14 mg/kg plus *ritonavir* 6 mg/kg bid or 375 mg/m² plus *ritonavir* 150 mg/m² bid; max 500 mg plus *ritonavir* 200 mg bid

Aptivus *Gel cap:* 250 mg (alcohol)

Aptivus Oral Solution *Oral soln:* 100 mg/ml (buttermint-butter toffee) (Vit E 116 IU/ml)

FUSION INHIBITORS—CCR5 CO-RECEPTOR ANTAGONISTS

▷ *enfuvirtide* (B) 90 mg (1 ml) SC bid; administer in upper arm, abdomen, or anterior thigh; rotate injection sites
Pediatric: <6 years: not established; 6-16 years: administer 2 mg/kg SC bid; max 90 mg SC bid; >16 years: same as adult; rotate injection sites
  Fuzeon *Vial:* 90 mg/ml pwdr for SC inj after reconstitution (1 ml, 60 vials/kit) (preservative-free)

▷ *maraviroc* (B) must be administered concomitant with other retrovirals; *Concomitant potent CYP3A inhibitors (with or without a potent CYP3A inducer) including protease inhibitors (except tipranavir+ritonavir), delavirdine, ketoconazole, itraconazole, clarithromycin, other potent CYP3A inhibitors (e.g., nefazodone, telithromycin): CrCl ≥30 mL/min:* 150 mg bid; *<30 mL/min, dialysis:* not recommended; *Potent CYP3A inducers (without a potent CYP3A inhibitor) including efavirenz, rifampin, etravirine, carbamazepine, phenobarbital, and phenytoin: CrCl ≥30 mL/min:* 600 mg bid; *<30 mL/min:* not recommended; *Other concomitant agents, including tipranavir+ritonavir, nevirapine, raltegravir, all NRTIs, and enfuvirtide:* 300 mg bid
Pediatric: <16 years: not established; ≥16 years: same as adult
  Selzentry *Tab:* 150, 300 mg film-coat

BRAND NAMES, DOSING, AND DOSE FORMS: COMBINATION AGENTS

▷ **Atripla** (B) *efavirenz+emtricitabine+tenofovir disoproxil fumarate* 1 tablet once daily on an empty stomach; bedtime dosing may improve the tolerability of nervous system symptoms; *CrCl <50 mL/min:* not recommended
Pediatric: <12 years, <40 kg: not established; ≥12 years, ≥40 kg: same as adult
  Tab: efa 600 mg+emtri 200 mg+teno dis fum 300 mg film-coat

▷ **Combivir** (C)(G) *lamivudine+zidovudine*
Pediatric: <12 years: not recommended; ≥12 years, ≥30 kg: 1 tablet bid with food
  Tab: lami 150 mg+zido 300 mg

▷ **Complera** (B) *emtricitabine+tenofovir disoproxil fumarate+rilpivirine* 1 tablet once daily; *CrCl <50 mL/min:* not recommended
Pediatric: <12 years, <40 kg: not recommended; ≥12 years, ≥40 kg: same as adult
  Tab: emtri 200 mg+teno dis 300 mg+**rilpiv** 25 mg

▷ **Descovy** (D) *emtricitabine+tenofovir alafenamide* 1 tablet once daily with or without food; *CrCl <30 mL/min:* not recommended
Pediatric: <12 years, <35 kg: not recommended; ≥12 years, ≥35 kg: same as adult
  Tab: emtri 200 mg+teno ala 25 mg

Comment: Patients with HIV-1 should be tested for the presence of chronic hepatitis B virus (HBV) before initiating antiretroviral therapy. **Descovy** is not approved for the treatment of chronic HBV infection, and the safety and efficacy of **Descovy** have not been established in patients co-infected with HIV-1 and HBV.

▷ **Epzicom** (B) *abacavir sulfate+lamivudine* 1 tab daily; *Mild hepatic impairment or CrCl<50 mL/min:* not recommended
Pediatric: <25 kg: use individual components; ≥25 kg: one tablet once daily; *Mild hepatic impairment or CrCl<50 mL/min:* not recommended
  Tab: aba 600 mg/lami 300 mg

▷ **Evotaz** (B) *atazanavir+cobicistat* 1 tab once daily
Pediatric: <12 years, <35 kg: not established; ≥12 years, ≥35 kg: same as adult
  Tab: ataz 600 mg+cobi 300 mg

▷ **Genvoya** (B) *elvitegravir+cobicistat+emtricitabine+tenofovir alafenamide* 1 tab once daily; *Severe hepatic impairment or CrCl <30 mL/min:* not recommended; take with food
Pediatric: <12 years, <35 kg: not established; ≥12 years, ≥35 kg: same as adult
  Tab: elvi 150 mg+cobi 150 mg+emtri 200 mg+teno 10 mg

▷ **Kaletra, Kaletra Oral Solution (C)(G)** *lopinavir+ritonavir* 800+200 mg (4 tablets or 10 ml) once daily or 400/100 (2 tablets or 5 ml) bid; *May administer once daily or bid:* patients with <3 *lopinavir* resistance-associated substitutions; *May dose bid only:* patients with ≥3 resistance-associated substitutions; *Dose must be increased:* when administered in combination with *efavirenz, nevirapine,* or *nelfinavir* (500 mg/125 mg (2 x 200/50 tab plus 1 x 100/25 tab) bid or 520/130 (6.5 ml) bid; *Once daily dosing regimen not recommended:* in combination with ≥3 *lopinavir* resistance-associated substitutions or in combination with: *carbamazepine, phenobarbital,* or *phenytoin;* Patients receiving *nevirapine* or *efavirenz* with **Kaletra** should have their **Kaletra** dose increased; swallow whole with or without food
Pediatric: dose calculation is based on the *lopinavir* component; 14 days-6 months: 16 mg/kg bid; 6 months-12 years: [tab/cap/soln] 7-<15 kg: 12 mg/kg bid (13 mg/kg plus *nevirapine*); 15-40 kg: 10 mg/kg bid (11 mg/kg plus *nevirapine*), ≥40 kg, >12 years: *lopinavir* 400 mg bid (533 mg plus *nevirapine*); max *lopinavir* 400 mg bid for patients who are not receiving *nevirapine* or *efavirenz;* **Kaletra** should not be used in combination with NNRTIs in children <6 months-of-age; see mfr pkg insert for BSA-based dosing
  Tab: **Kaletra 100/25** *lopin* 100 mg+*riton* 25 mg
         Kaletra 200/50 *lopin* 200 mg+*riton* 50 mg
  Oral Soln: *lopin* 80 mg+*riton* 20 mg per ml, *lopin* 400 mg+*riton* 500 mg per 5 ml (160 ml) (cotton candy) (alcohol 42.4%)
▷ **Odefsey (D)** *emtricitabine+rilpivirine+tenofovir alafenamide* 1 tab once daily with food; *CrCl <30 mL/min:* not recommended
Pediatric: <12 years, <35 kg: not established; ≥12 years, >35 kg: same as adult
  Tab: *emtri* 200 mg+*rilpi* 25 mg+*teno alafen* 25 mg
▷ **Prezcobix (C)** *darunavir+cobicistat* 1 tab once daily; *Treatment naïve and treatment experienced with no darunavir resistance-associated substitution:* 800 mg once daily plus *ritonavir* 100 mg once daily; *Treatment experienced with at least one darunavir resistance associated substitution:* 600 mg bid plus *ritonavir* 100 mg bid; take with food; *CrCl <70 mL/min:* not recommended
Pediatric: not recommended
  Tab: *darun* 800 mg+*cobi* 150 mg
▷ **Stribild (B)(G)** *elvitegravir+cobicistat+emtricitabine+tenofovir disoproxil fumarate* 1 tab once daily; *CrCl <70 mL/min:* not recommended; *if CrCl declines to <50 mL/min during treatment:* discontinue; *Severe hepatic impairment:* not recommended
Pediatric: <12 years: not recommended; ≥12 years: same as adult
  Tab: *elvi* 150 mg+*cobi* 150 mg+*emtri* 200 mg+*teno dis fum* 300 mg
▷ **Triumeq (C)(G)** *abacavir sulfate+dolutegravir+lamivudine* 1 tab once daily
Pediatric: <12 years: not recommended; ≥12 years: same as adult
  Tab: *aba* 600 mg+*dolu* 50 mg+*lami* 300 mg
▷ **Trizivir (C)(G)** *abacavir sulfate+lamivudine+zidovudine* 1 tab bid
Pediatric: <40 kg: not recommended; ≥40 kg: same as adult
  Tab: *aba* 300 mg+*lami* 150 mg+*zido* 300 mg

 HUMAN PAPILLOMAVIRUS (HPV, VENEREAL WART)

TREATMENT
see Wart: Venereal page 521

PROPHYLAXIS
Comment: Administer IM in deltoid. Administer a 3-dose series; *First dose* females (10-25 years-of-age) and males (9-15 years-of-age); *Second dose:* 1-2 months after first dose;

Third dose: 6 months after first dose. HPV vaccination is indicated for the prevention of cervical, vulvar, vaginal, and anal cancers. Register pregnant patients exposed to **Gardasil** by calling 800-986-8999.

▷ **bivalent human papillomavirus types 16 and 18 vaccine, aluminum adsorbed** (B)
   Pediatric: <10 years: not recommended
      Cervarix administer in the deltoid; 1st dose 0.5 ml IM on elected date; then, 2nd dose 0.5 ml IM 1 month later; then, 3rd dose 0.5 ml IM 6 months after the first dose
         Vial: susp for IM inj (single-dose); *Prefilled syringe* (single-dose) (preservative-free)

▷ **quadrivalent human papillomavirus types 6, 11, 16, and 18 vaccine, recombinant, aluminum adsorbed** (B)
   Pediatric: >9 years: not recommended
      Gardasil administer in the deltoid or upper thigh; 1st dose 0.5 ml IM on elected date; then, 2nd dose 0.5 ml IM 2 months later; then, 3rd dose 0.5 ml IM 6 months after the first dose
         Vial: susp for IM inj (single-dose); *Prefilled syringe* w. needles or tip caps (single-dose) (preservative-free)

▷ **quadrivalent human papillomavirus types 6, 11, 16, 18, 31, 33, 45, 52, and 58 vaccine, recombinant, aluminum adsorbed** (B)
      Gardasil 9 *Adults and Children: 9-26 Years-of-Age:* administer IM in the deltoid or thigh; administer the 1st dose; administer the 2nd dose 2 months after the 1st dose; administer the 3rd dose 6 months after the 1st dose (4 months after the 2nd dose).
         Vial: susp for IM inj 0.5 ml (single-dose); *Prefilled syringe* w. needles or tip caps (single-dose) (preservative-free)

⬤ HUNTINGTON DISEASE-ASSOCIATED CHOREA

VESICULAR MONOAMINE TRANSPORTER 2 (VMAT2) INHIBITOR

▷ **deutetrabenazine** take with food; initially 6 mg once daily; titrate up at weekly intervals by 6 mg per day to a tolerated dose that reduces chorea; administer total daily dosages ≥12 mg in two divided doses; max recommended daily dose 36 mg/day divided bid (18 mg twice daily); swallow whole; do not chew, crush, or break; if switching from *tetrabenazine,* discontinue *tetrabenazine* and initiate *Austedo* the following day; see mfr pkg insert for full prescribing information and for a recommended conversion table
   Pediatric: <12 years: not established; ≥12 years: same as adult
      Austedo *Tab:* 6, 9, 12 mg

Comment: The most common adverse effects of *deutetrabenazine* are somnolence, diarrhea, dry mouth, fatigue, and sedation, as well as an increased risk of depression and suicidal thoughts and behaviors. **Austedo** is contraindicated for patients with untreated or inadequately treated depression, who are suicidal, have hepatic impairment, are taking MAOIs, *reserpine,* or *tetrabenazine.* **Austedo** may increase the risk of akathisia, agitation and restlessness, and may cause parkinsonism in patients with Huntington disease. There are no adequate data on the developmental risk associated with the use of **Austedo** in pregnant women or lactation.

▷ **trabenazine** individualization of dose with careful weekly titration is required. *Week 1:* starting dose is 12.5 mg daily; *Week 2:* 25 mg (12.5 mg twice daily); then slowly titrate dose by 12.5 mg/day at weekly intervals as tolerated to a dose that reduces chorea; doses of 37.5 mg and up to 50 mg per day should be administered in three divided doses per day with a maximum recommended single dose not to exceed 25 mg; patients requiring doses above 50 mg per day should be genotyped for the drug metabolizing enzyme CYP2D6 to determine if the patient is a poor metabolizer (PM) or an extensive metabolizer (EM); max daily dose in PMs is 50 mg with a max single dose of 25 mg

Pediatric: <12 years: not established; ≥12 years: same as adult

Xenazine *Tab:* 12.5, 25*mg

Comment: Most common adverse reactions are sedation/somnolence, fatigue, insomnia, depression, akathisia, anxiety/anxiety aggravated, nausea. BBW:

Xenazine increases the risk of depression and suicidal thoughts and behavior (suicidality) in patients with Huntington's disease. Balance risks of depression and suicidality with the clinical need for control of chorea when considering the use of **Xenazine**. Monitor patients for the emergence or worsening of depression, suicidality, or unusual changes in behavior. Inform patients, caregivers and families of the risk of depression and suicidality and instruct to report behaviors of concern promptly to the treating health care provider. Exercise caution when treating patients with a history of depression or prior suicide attempts or ideation.

Xenazine is contraindicated in patients who are actively suicidal, and in patients with untreated or inadequately treated depression, hepatic impairment, concomitant an MAOI or reserpine, taking *deutetrabenazine* or *valbenazine*.

▷ *valbenazine* initially 40 mg once daily; after one week, increase to the recommended 80 mg once daily; take with or without food; recommended dose for patients with moderate or severe hepatic impairment is 40 mg once daily; consider dose reduction based on tolerability in known CYP2D6 poor metabolizers; concomitant use of strong CYP3A4 inducers is not recommended; avoid concomitant use of MAOIs

Pediatric: <18 years: not established; ≥18 years: same as adult

Ingrezza *Cap:* 40 mg

Comment: Safety and effectiveness of **Ingrezza** have not been established in pediatric patients. No dose adjustment is required for elderly patients. The limited available data on **Ingrezza** use in pregnant women are insufficient to inform a drug-associated risk. There is no information regarding the presence of **Ingrezza** or its metabolites in human milk, the effects on the breastfed infant, or the effects on milk production. However, women are advised not to breastfeed during treatment and for 5 days after the final dose. To report suspected adverse reactions, contact Neurocrine Biosciences, Inc. at 877-641-3461 or FDA at 1-800-FDA-1088 or www.fda.gov/medwatch

HYPEREMESIS GRAVIDARUM NAUSEA AND VOMITING OF PREGNANCY

ANTIHISTAMINE+VITAMIN B ANALOG

▷ *doxylamine* *succinate+pyridoxine* **hydrochloride** one tab at HS prn; if symptoms are not adequately controlled, the dose can be increased to max one tablet in the AM and one tab at HS

Pediatric: <18 years: not established; ≥18 years: same as adult

Bonjesta *Tab:* doxy 20 mg+pyri 20 mg ext-rel

Comment: **Bonjesta** is indicated for nausea/vomiting of pregnancy in women who do not respond to conservative management. Somnolence (severe drowsiness) can occur when used in combination with alcohol or other sedating medications. Use with caution in patients with asthma, increased intraocular pressure, narrow angle glaucoma, stenosing peptic ulcer, pyloroduodenal obstruction and urinary bladder-neck obstruction.

HYPERHIDROSIS (PERSPIRATION, EXCESSIVE)

Comment: Hyperhidrosis is a common, self-limiting problem that affects 2% to3% of the US population. Patients may complain of localized sweating of the hands, feet, face, or underarms, or more systemic, generalized sweating in multiple locations and report a significant impact on their quality of life.

REFERENCE

Varella, A. Y., Fukuda, J. M., Telvelis, M. P., Campos, J. R., Kauffman, P., Cucato, G. G., . . . Wolosker, N. (2016). Translation and validation of hyperhidrosis disease severity scale. *Revista da Associação Médica Brasileira, 62*(9), 843–847.

▷ *aluminum chloride* 20% solution apply q HS; wash treated area the following morning; after 1-2 treatments, may reduce frequency to 1-2 x/week
    Drysol *Soln:* 35, 60 ml (alcohol 93%) cont-rel
Comment: Apply to clean dry skin (e.g., underarms). Do not apply to broken, irritated, or recently shaved skin.

ANTICHOLINERGIC

Comment: *oxybutynin*, a cholinergic antagonist commonly prescribed for overactive bladder, is the first oral agent to emerge as a treatment option for hyperhidrosis.

REFERENCES

Scholhammer, M., Brenaut, E., Menard-Andivot, N., Pillette-Delarue, M., Zagnoli, A., Chassain-Le Lay, M., . . . Le Gal, G. (2015). Oxybutynin as a treatment for generalized hyperhidrosis: A randomized, placebo-controlled trial. *British Journal of Dermatology, 173*(5), 1163–1168.

Wolosker, N., de Campos, J. R., Kauffman, P., & Puech-Leão, P. (2012). A randomized placebo-controlled trial of oxybutynin for the initial treatment of palmer and axillary hyperhidrosis. *Journal of Vascular Surgery, 55*(6), 1696–1700.

▷ *oxybutynin chloride* (B)
    Ditropan 5 mg bid-tid; max 20 mg/day
    Pediatric: <5 years: not recommended; 5-12 years: 5 mg bid; max 15 mg/day; ≥16 years: same as adult
        Tab: 5*mg; *Syr:* 5 mg/5 ml
    Ditropan XL initially 5 mg daily; may increase weekly in 5-mg increments as needed; max 30 mg/day
    Pediatric: <6 years: not recommended; ≥6 years: initially 5 mg once daily; may increase weekly in 5-mg increments as needed; max 20 mg/day
        Tab: 5, 10, 15 mg ext-rel
    GelniQUE 3 mg Pump: apply 3 pumps (84 mg) once daily to clean dry intact skin on the abdomen, upper arm, shoulders, or thighs; rotate sites; wash hands; avoid washing application site for 1 hour after application
    Pediatric: <12 years: not recommended; ≥12 years: same as adult
        Gel: 3% (92 gm, metered pump dispenser) (alcohol)
    GelniQUE 1 gm Sachet: apply 1 gm gel (1 sachet) once daily to dry intact skin on abdomen, upper arms/shoulders, or thighs; rotate sites; wash hands; avoid washing application site for 1 hour after application
    Pediatric: <12 years: not recommended; ≥12 years: same as adult
        Gel: 10%, 1 gm/sachet (30/carton) (alcohol)
    Oxytrol Transdermal Patch (OTC): apply patch to clean dry area of the abdomen, hip, or buttock; one patch twice weekly; rotate sites
    Pediatric: <12 years: not recommended; ≥12 years: same as adult
        Transdermal patch: 3.9 mg/day

 HYPERHOMOCYSTEINEMIA

Comment: Elevated homocysteine is associated with cognitive impairment, vascular dementia, and dementia of the Alzheimer's type.

HOMOCYSTEINE-LOWERING NUTRITIONAL SUPPLEMENTS

▷ *L-methylfolate calcium (as metafolin)+pyridoxyl 5-phosphate+methylcobalamin* take 1 cap daily

Pediatric: <12 years: not recommended; ≥12 years: same as adult

Metanx *Cap:* metafo 3 mg+pyrid 35 mg+methyl 2 mg (gluten-free, yeast-free, lactose-free)

Comment: **Metanx** is indicated as adjunct treatment of endothelial dysfunction and/or hyperhomocysteinemia in patients who have lower extremity ulceration.

▷ *L-methylfolate calcium (as metafolin)+methylcobalamin+n-acetylcysteine* take 1 cap daily

Pediatric: <12 years: not recommended; ≥12 years: same as adult

Cerefolin *Cap:* metafo 5.6 mg+methyl 2 mg+N-ace 600 mg (gluten-free, yeast-free, lactose-free)

Comment: **Cerefolin** is indicated in the dietary management of patients treated for early memory loss, with emphasis on those at risk for neurovascular oxidative stress, hyperhomocysteinemia, mild to moderate cognitive impairment with or without vitamin B12 deficiency, vascular dementia, or Alzheimer's disease.

 HYPERKALEMIA

HYPERKALEMIA CATION EXCHANGE RESINS

Comment: Normal serum K^+ range is approximately 3.5-5.5 mEq/L. Hyperkalemia is associated with cardiac dysrhythmias and metabolic acidosis. Risk factors include kidney disease, heart failure, and drugs that inhibit the renin-angiotensin-aldosterone system (RAAS) including ACEIs, ARBs, direct renin inhibitors, and aldosterone antagonists. Cation exchange resins are not for emergency treatment of life-threatening hyperkalemia, severe constipation, bowel obstruction or impaction. May cause GI irritability, ulceration, necrosis, sodium retention, hypocalcemia, hypomagnesemia, fecal impaction, ischemic colitis. Avoid non-absorbable cation-donating antacids and laxatives (e.g., *magnesium hydroxide, aluminum hydroxide*). Concomitant sorbitol should be avoided because it may cause intestinal necrosis.

▷ *patiromer sorbitex calcium* (B) initially 8.4 gm once daily; adjust dosage as prescribed based on potassium concentration and target range; may increase dosage at 1-week (or longer) intervals in increments of 8.4 gm; max dose 25.2 gm once daily; prepare immediately prior to administration; do not take in dry form; administer with food; measure 1/3 cup of water and pour half into a glass; then add **Veltassa** and stir; add the remaining water and stir well; the powder will not dissolve and the mixture will look cloudy; add more water as needed for desired consistency; do not heat or mix with heated food or fluids

Veltassa *Pkt:* 8, 4, 16.8, 25.2 gm pwdr for oral susp, 30 single-use pkts/carton

Comment: Take **Veltassa** at least 3 hours before or 3 hours after any other medicine taken by mouth. Store packets in the refrigerator. It stored at room temperature, product must be used within 3 months.

▷ *sodium polystyrene sulfonate* (C)(G)

Pediatrics: Use 1 gm/1 mEq of K^+ as basis of calculation; see mfr literature

Kayexalate *Susp:* 15 gm 1-4 times daily; *Rectal Enema:* 30-50 gm in 100 ml every 6 hours

 HYPERPARATHYROIDISM

▷ *calcifediol* (C)(G) 1 cap daily

Pediatric: <18 years: not established; ≥18 years: same as adult

Rayaldee *Cap:* 30 mcg ext-rel

Comment: **Rayaldee** is indicated for the prevention and treatment of secondary hyperparathyroidism associated with chronic kidney disease (CKD), stage 3 or 4 and serum total 25-hydroxyvitamin D levels <30 mg/mL.

▷ *paricalcitol* (C)(G) administer 0.04-1 mcg/kg (2.8-7 mcg) IV bolus, during dialysis, no more than every other day; may be increased by 2-4 mcg every 2-4 weeks; monitor serum calcium and phosphorus during dose adjustment periods; if Ca x P ≥75, immediately reduce dose or discontinue until these levels normalize; discard unused portion of single-use vials immediately
Pediatric: <18 years: not established; ≥18 years: same as adult

Zemplar *Vial:* 2, 5 mcg/ml soln for inj

Comment: **Zemplar** is indicated for the prevention and treatment of secondary hyperparathyroidism associated with chronic kidney disease (CKD), stage 5.

 HYPERPHOSPHATEMIA

PHOSPHATE BINDERS

Comment: Monitor for development of hypercalcemia. Normal serum PO_4^- is 2.5-4.5 mg/dL and normal serum calcium is 8.5-10.5 mg/dL.

▷ *calcium acetate* (C)(G) initially 2 tabs or caps with each meal; then titrate gradually to keep serum phosphate at <6 mg/dL; usual maintenance is 3-4 tabs or caps with each meal
Pediatric: <12 years: not recommended; ≥12 years: same as adult

PhosLo *Tab:* 667 mg; *Cap:* 667 mg

▷ *lanthanum carbonate* (C)(G) initially 750 mg to 1.5 gm per day in divided doses; take with meals; titrate at 2-3-week intervals in increments of 750 mg/day based on serum phosphate; usual range 1.5-3 gm/day; usual max 3,750 mg/day
Pediatric: <12 years: not recommended; ≥12 years: same as adult

Fosrenol *Chew tab:* 250, 500, 750 mg; 1 gm

▷ *sevelamer* (C)(G) for patients not taking a phosphate binder, take tid with meals; swallow whole; titrate by 1 tab per meal at 1-week intervals to keep serum phosphorus 3.5-5.5 mg/dL; switching from calcium acetate to *sevelamer*, see mfr pkg insert. *Serum phosphorus* ≥5.5 to ≤7.5 mg/dL: 800 mg tid; *Serum phosphorus 7.5-9:* 1.2-1.6 gm tid
Pediatric: <12 years: not recommended; ≥12 years: same as adult

Renagel *Tab:* 400, 800 mg
Renvela *Tab:* 800 mg

 HYPERPIGMENTATION

Comment: Depigmenting agents may be used for hyperpigmented skin conditions including chloasma, melasma, freckles, senile lentigines. Limit treatments to small areas at one time. Sunscreen ≥30 SPF recommended.

▷ *hydroquinone* (C)(G) apply sparingly to affected area and rub in bid
Lustra *Crm:* 4% (1, 2 oz) (sulfites)
Lustra AF *Crm:* 4% (1, 2 oz) (sunscreen, sulfites)

▷ *monobenzone* (C) apply sparingly to affected area and rub in bid-tid; depigmentation occurs in 1-4 months
Benoquin *Crm:* 20% (1.25 oz)

▷ *tazarotene* (X)(G) apply daily at HS
Pediatric: <12 years: not recommended; ≥12 years: same as adult
Avage Cream *Crm:* 0.1% (30 gm)
Tazorac Cream *Crm:* 0.05, 0.1% (15, 30, 60 gm)
Tazorac Gel *Gel:* 0.05, 0.1% (30, 100 gm)

▷ *tretinoin* (C) apply daily at HS
Pediatric: <12 years: not recommended; ≥12 years: same as adult
 Avita *Crm/Gel:* 0.025% (20, 45 gm)
 Renova *Crm:* 0.02% (40 gm); 0.05% (40, 60 gm)
 Retin-A Cream *Crm:* 0.025, 0.05, 0.1% (20, 45 gm)
 Retin-A Gel *Gel:* 0.01, 0.025% (15, 45 gm) (alcohol 90%)
 Retin-A Liquid *Liq:* 0.05% (28 ml) (alcohol 55%)
 Retin-A Micro *Microspheres:* 0.04, 0.1% (20, 45 gm)

COMBINATION AGENTS

▷ *hydroquinone+fluocinolone+tretinoin* (C) apply sparingly to affected area and rub in daily at HS
Pediatric: <12 years: not recommended; ≥12 years: same as adult
 Tri-Luma *Crm:* hydroquin 4%+*fluo* 0.01%+*tretin* 0.05% (30 gm) (parabens, sulfites)
▷ *hydroquinone+padimate o+oxybenzone+octyl methoxycinnamate* (C) apply sparingly to affected area and rub in bid
Pediatric: <12 years: not recommended; ≥16 years: same as adult
 Glyquin *Crm:* 4% (1 oz jar)
▷ *hydroquinone+ethyl dihydroxypropyl PABA+dioxybenzone+oxybenzone* (C) apply sparingly to affected area and rub in bid; max 2 months
Pediatric: <12 years: not recommended; ≥12 years: same as adult
 Solaquin *Crm:* hydroquin 2%+*PABA* 5%+*dioxy* 3%+*oxy* 2% (1 oz) (sulfites)
▷ *hydroquinone+padimate+dioxybenzone+oxybenzone* (C) apply sparingly to affected area and rub in bid; max 2 months
Pediatric: <12 years: not recommended; ≥12 years: same as adult
 Solaquin Forte *Crm:* hydroquin 4%+*pad* 0.5%+*dioxy* 3%+*oxy* 2% (1oz) (sunscreen, sulfites)
▷ *hydroquinone+padimate+dioxybenzone* (C) apply sparingly to affected area and rub in bid; max 2 months
Pediatric: <12 years: not recommended; ≥12 years: same as adult
 Solaquin Forte Gel: hydroquin 4%+*pad* 0.5%+*dioxy* 3% (1 oz) (alcohol, sulfites)

 HYPERPROLACTINEMIA

DOPAMINE RECEPTOR AGONIST

▷ *dostinex* (B)(G) initial therapy is 0.25 mg twice a week; may increase by 0.25 mg twice weekly up to 1 mg twice a week according to the patient's serum prolactin level; dose increases should not occur more than every 4 weeks; after a normal serum prolactin level has been maintained for 6 months, may be discontinued, with periodic monitoring of serum prolactin level to determine if/when treatment should be reinstituted
Pediatric: <12 years: not established; ≥12 years: same as adult
 Cabergoline *Tab:* 0.5 mg

Comment: **Cabergoline** is indicated to treat hyperprolactinemia disorders due to idiopathic <u>or</u> pituitary adenoma.

 HYPERTENSION: PRIMARY, ESSENTIAL

see JNC-8 Recommendations page 535

BETA-BLOCKERS (CARDIOSELECTIVE)

Comment: Cardioselective beta-blockers are less likely to cause bronchospasm, peripheral vasoconstriction, <u>or</u> hypoglycemia than non-cardioselective beta-blockers.

▷ *acebutolol* (B)(G) initially 400 mg in 1-2 divided doses; usual range 200-800 mg/day; max 1.2 gm/day in 2 divided doses
Pediatric: <12 years: not recommended; ≥12 years: same as adult
   Sectral *Cap:* 200, 400 mg

▷ *atenolol* (D)(G) initially 50 mg daily; may increase after 1-2 weeks to 100 mg daily; max 100 mg/day
Pediatric: <12 years: not recommended; ≥12 years: same as adult
   Tenormin *Tab:* 25, 50, 100 mg

▷ *betaxolol* (C) initially 10 mg daily; may increase to 20 mg/day after 7-14 days; usual max 20 mg/day
Pediatric: <12 years: not recommended; ≥12 years: same as adult
   Kerlone *Tab:* 10*, 20 mg

▷ *bisoprolol* (C) 5 mg daily; max 20 mg daily
Pediatric: <12 years: not recommended; ≥12 years: same as adult
   Zebeta *Tab:* 5*, 10 mg

▷ *metoprolol succinate* (C)
Pediatric: <12 years: not recommended; ≥12 years: same as adult
   Toprol-XL initially 25-100 mg in a single dose once daily; increase weekly if needed; max 400 mg/day; as monotherapy <u>or</u> with a diuretic
      Tab: 25*, 50*, 100*, 200*mg ext-rel

▷ *metoprolol tartrate* (C) initially 25-50 mg bid; increase weekly if needed; max 400 mg/day; as monotherapy or with a diuretic
Pediatric: <12 years: not recommended; ≥12 years: same as adult
   Lopressor (G) *Tab:* 25, 37.5, 50, 75, 100 mg

▷ *nebivolol* (C)(G) initially 5 mg daily; may increase at 2 week intervals; max 40 mg/day
Pediatric: <12 years: not recommended; ≥12 years: same as adult
   Bystolic *Tab:* 2.5, 5, 10, 20 mg

BETA-BLOCKERS (NON-CARDIOSELECTIVE)

Comment: Non-cardioselective beta-blockers are more likely to cause bronchospasm, peripheral vasoconstriction, <u>and/or</u> hypoglycemia than cardioselective beta-blockers.

▷ *nadolol* (C)(G) initially 40 mg daily; usual maintenance 40-80 mg daily; max 320 mg/day
Pediatric: <12 years: not recommended; ≥12 years: same as adult
   Corgard *Tab:* 20*, 40*, 80*, 120*, 160*mg

▷ *penbutolol* (C) 10-20 mg once daily
Pediatric: <12 years: not recommended; ≥12 years: same as adult
   Levatol *Tab:* 20*mg

▷ *pindolol* (B)(G) initially 5 mg bid; may increase after 3-4 weeks in 10 mg increments; max 60 mg/day
Pediatric: <12 years: not recommended; ≥12 years: same as adult
   Pindolol *Tab:* 5, 10 mg
   Visken *Tab:* 5, 10 mg

▷ *propranolol* (C)(G)
   Inderal initially 40 mg bid; usual maintenance 120-240 mg/day; max 640 mg/day
   Pediatric: initially 1 mg/kg/day; usual range 2-4 mg/kg/day in 2 divided doses; max 16 mg/kg/day
      Tab: 10*, 20*, 40*, 60*, 80*mg
   Inderal LA initially 80 mg daily in a single dose; increase q 3-7 days; usual range 120-160 mg/day; max 320 mg/day in a single dose

Pediatric: <12 years: not recommended; ≥12 years: same as adult
  Cap: 60, 80, 120, 160 mg sust-rel
InnoPran XL initially 80 mg q HS; max 120 mg/day
Pediatric: <12 years: not recommended; ≥12 years: same as adult
  Cap: 80, 120 mg ext-rel

▷ *timolol* (C)(G) initially 10 mg bid, increase weekly if needed; usual maintenance 20-40 mg/day; max 60 mg/day in 2 divided doses
Pediatric: <12 years: not recommended; ≥12 years: same as adult
  Blocadren *Tab:* 5, 10*, 20*mg

BETA-BLOCKER (NON-CARDIOSELECTIVE)+ALPHA-1 BLOCKER COMBINATIONS

▷ *carvedilol* (C)(G)
Pediatric: <18 years: <12 years: not recommended; ≥12 years: same as adult
  Coreg initially 6.25 mg bid; may increase at 1-2-week intervals to 12.5 mg bid; max 25 mg bid
    Tab: 3.125, 6.25, 12.5, 25 mg
  Coreg CR initially 20 mg once daily for 2 weeks; may increase at 1-2-week intervals; max 80 mg once daily
    Tab: 10, 20, 40, 80 mg cont-rel

▷ *carteolol* (C) initially 2.5 mg daily, gradually increase to 5 or 10 mg daily; usual maintenance 2.5-5 mg daily
Pediatric: <12 years: not recommended; ≥12 years: same as adult
  Cartrol *Tab:* 2.5, 5 mg

▷ *labetalol* (C)(G) initially 100 mg bid; increase after 2-3 days if needed; usual maintenance 200-400 mg bid; max 2.4 gm/day
Pediatric: <12 years: not recommended; ≥12 years: same as adult
  Normodyne *Tab:* 100*, 200*, 300 mg
  Trandate *Tab:* 100*, 200*, 300*mg

DIURETICS

Thiazide Diuretics

▷ *chlorthalidone* (B)(G) initially 15 mg daily; may increase to 30 mg once daily based on clinical response; max 45-60 mg/day
Pediatric: <12 years: not established; ≥12 years: same as adult
  Chlorthalidone *Tab:* 25, 50 mg
  Thalitone *Tab:* 15 mg

▷ *chlorothiazide* (B)(G) 0.5-1 gm/day in a single or divided doses; max 2 gm/day
Pediatric: <6 months: up to 15 mg/lb/day in 2 divided doses; ≥6 months: 10 mg/lb/day in 2 divided doses
  Diuril *Tab:* 250*, 500*mg; *Oral susp:* 250 mg/5 ml (237 ml)

▷ *hydrochlorothiazide* (B)(G)
Pediatric: <12 years: not recommended; ≥12 years: same as adult
  Esidrix 25-100 mg once daily
    Tab: 25, 50, 100 mg
  Hydrochlorothiazide 12.5 mg once daily; usual max 50 mg/day
    Tab: 25*, 50*mg
  Microzide 12.5 mg once daily; usual max 50 mg/day
    Cap: 12.5 mg

▷ *methyclothiazide+deserpidine* (B) initially 5/0.25 mg once daily; titrate individual components
Pediatric: <12 years: not recommended; ≥12 years: same as adult
  Enduronyl *Tab: methy* 5 mg+*deser* 0.25 mg*
  Enduronyl Forte *Tab: methy* 5 mg+*deser* 0.5 mg*

▷ *polythiazide* (C) 2-4 mg once daily
  Pediatric: <12 years: not recommended; ≥12 years: same as adult
    Renese *Tab:* 1, 2, 4 mg

Potassium-Sparing Diuretics

▷ *amiloride* (B)(C) initially 5 mg; may increase to 10 mg; max 20 mg
  Pediatric: <12 years: not recommended; ≥12 years: same as adult
    Midamor *Tab:* 5 mg
▷ *spironolactone* (D)(G) initially 50-100 mg in a single <u>or</u> divided doses; titrate at 2-week intervals
  Pediatric: <12 years: not established; ≥12 years: same as adult
    Aldactone *Tab:* 25, 50*, 100*mg
    CaroSpir *Oral susp:* 25 mg/5 ml (118, 473 ml) (banana)
▷ *triamterene* (B) 100 mg bid; max 300 mg
  Pediatric: <12 years: not recommended; ≥12 years: same as adult
    Dyrenium *Cap:* 50, 100 mg

Loop Diuretics

▷ *bumetanide* (C)(G) 0.5-2 mg daily; may repeat at 4-5-hour intervals; max 10 mg/day
  Pediatric: <18 years: not recommended; ≥18 years: same as adult
    Tab: 1*mg
  Comment: *bumetanide* is contraindicated with sulfa drug allergy.
▷ *ethacrynic acid* (B)(G) initially 50-200 mg/day
  Pediatric: <1 month: not recommended; ≥1 month: initially 25 mg/day; then adjust dose in 25-mg increments
    Edecrin *Tab:* 25, 50 mg
▷ *ethacrynate sodium* (B)(G) for IV injection; see mfr pkg insert
  Pediatric: <12 years: not recommended; ≥12 years: same as adult
    Sodium Edecrin *Vial:* 50 mg single-dose
Comment: *ethacrynate sodium* is more potent than more commonly used loop and thiazide diuretics.
▷ *furosemide* (C)(G) initially 40 mg bid
  Pediatric: <12 years: not recommended; ≥12 years: same as adult
    Lasix *Tab:* 20, 40*, 80 mg; *Oral Soln:* 10 mg/ml (2, 4 oz w. dropper)
Comment: *furosemide* is contraindicated with sulfa drug allergy.
▷ *torsemide* (B) 5 mg once daily; may increase to 10 mg once daily
  Pediatric: <12 years: not recommended; ≥12 years: same as adult
    Demadex *Tab:* 5*, 10*, 20*, 100*mg

Indoline Diuretic

▷ *indapamide* (B) initially 1.25 mg daily; may titrate dosage upward q 4 weeks if needed; max 5 mg/day
  Pediatric: <12 years: not recommended; ≥12 years: same as adult
    Lozol *Tab:* 1.25, 2.5 mg
Comment: *indapamide* is contraindicated with sulfa drug allergy.

Quinazoline Diuretic

▷ *metolazone* (B) 2.5-5 mg daily
  Pediatric: <12 years: not recommended; ≥12 years: same as adult
    Zaroxolyn 2.5-5 mg daily
    Tab: 2.5, 5, 10 mg
Comment: *metolazone* is contraindicated with sulfa drug allergy.

DIURETIC COMBINATIONS

▷ *amiloride+hydrochlorothiazide* (B)(G) initially 1 tab daily; may increase to 2 tabs/day in a single <u>or</u> divided doses
Pediatric: <12 years: not recommended; ≥12 years: same as adult
  Moduretic *Tab:* amil 5 mg+*hydrochlor* 50 mg*

▷ *deserpidine+methylclothiazide* (C)
Pediatric: <12 years: not recommended; ≥12 years: same as adult
  Enduronyl
    Tab: **Enduronyl 0.25/5** *deser* 0.25 mg+*methy* 5 mg*
    Enduronyl 0.5/5 *deser* 0.5 mg+*methy* 5 mg*

▷ *spironolactone+hydrochlorothiazide* (D)(G)
Pediatric: <12 years: not recommended; ≥12 years: same as adult
  Aldactazide 25 usual maintenance 1-4 tabs in a single <u>or</u> divided doses
    Tab: spiro 25 mg+*hctz* 25 mg
  Aldactazide 50 usual maintenance 1-2 tabs in a single <u>or</u> divided doses
    Tab: spiro 50 mg+*hctz* 50 mg

▷ *triamterene+hydrochlorothiazide* (C)(G)
Pediatric: <12 years: not recommended; ≥12 years: same as adult
  Dyazide 1-2 caps once daily
    Cap: triam 37.5 mg/*hctz* 25 mg
  Maxzide 1 tab once daily
    Tab: triam 75 mg/*hctz* 50 mg*
  Maxzide-25 1-2 tabs once daily
    Tab: triam 37.5 mg/*hctz* 25 mg*

ANGIOTENSIN CONVERTING ENZYME INHIBITORS (ACEIs)

Comment: Black patients receiving ACEI monotherapy have been reported to have a higher incidence of angioedema compared to non-Blacks. Non-Blacks have a greater decrease in BP when ACEIs are used compared to Black patients.

▷ *benazepril* (D)(G) initially 10 mg daily; usual maintenance 20-40 mg/day in 1-2 divided doses; usual max 80 mg/day
Pediatric: <12 years: not recommended; ≥12 years: same as adult
  Lotensin *Tab:* 5, 10, 20, 40 mg

▷ *captopril* (D)(G) initially 25 mg bid-tid; after 1-2 weeks increase to 50 mg bid-tid
Pediatric: <12 years: not recommended; ≥12 years: same as adult
  Capoten *Tab:* 12.5*, 25*, 50*, 100*mg

▷ *enalapril* (D) initially 5 mg daily; usual dosage range 10-40 mg/day; max 40 mg/day
Pediatric: <12 years: not recommended; ≥12 years: same as adult
  Epaned Oral Solution *Oral soln:* 1 mg/ml (150 ml) (mixed berry)
  Vasotec (G) *Tab:* 2.5*, 5*, 10, 20 mg

▷ *fosinopril* (D) initially 10 mg daily; usual maintenance 20-40 mg/day in a single <u>or</u> divided doses; max 80 mg/day
Pediatric: <6 years, <50 kg: not recommended; ≥6-12 years, ≥50 kg: 5-10 mg once daily
  Monopril *Tab:* 10*, 20, 40 mg

▷ *lisinopril* (D)
  Prinivil initially 10 mg daily; usual range 20-40 mg/day
  Pediatric: <12 years: not recommended; ≥12 years: same as adult
    Tab: 5*, 10*, 20*, 40 mg
  Qbrelis Oral Solution administer as a single dose once daily
  Pediatric: <6 years, GFR <30 mL/min: not recommended; ≥6 years, GFR >30 mL/min: initially 0.07 mg/kg, max 5 mg; adjust according to BP up to a max 0.61 mg/kg (40 mg) once daily
    Oral soln: 1 mg/ml (150 ml)

Zestril initially 10 mg daily; usual range 20-40 mg/day
> *Pediatric:* <12 years: not recommended; ≥12 years: same as adult
>> *Tab:* 2.5, 5*, 10, 20, 30, 40 mg

▷ *moexipril* (D) initially 7.5 mg daily; usual range 15-30 mg/day in 1-2 divided doses; max 30 mg/day
> *Pediatric:* <12 years: not recommended; ≥12 years: same as adult
>> Univasc *Tab:* 7.5*, 15*mg

▷ *perindopril* (D) initially 2-8 mg daily-bid; max 16 mg/day
> *Pediatric:* <12 years: not recommended; ≥12 years: same as adult
>> Aceon *Tab:* 2*, 4*, 8*mg

▷ *quinapril* (D) initially 10 mg once daily; usual maintenance 20-80 mg daily in 1-2 divided doses
> *Pediatric:* <12 years: not recommended; ≥12 years: same as adult
>> Accupril *Tab:* 5*, 10, 20, 40 mg

▷ *ramipril* (C; D in 2nd, 3rd) initially 2.5 mg bid; usual maintenance 2.5-20 mg in 1-2 divided doses
> *Pediatric:* <12 years: not established; ≥12 years: same as adult
>> Altace *Tab/Cap:* 1.25, 2.5, 5, 10 mg

▷ *trandolapril* (D) initially 1-2 mg once daily; adjust at 1-week intervals; usual range 2-4 mg in 1-2 divided doses; max 8 mg/day
> *Pediatric:* <12 years: not recommended; ≥12 years: same as adult
>> Mavik *Tab:* 1*, 2, 4 mg

ANGIOTENSIN II RECEPTOR BLOCKERS (ARBs)

▷ *azilsartan medoxomil* (D) *Monotherapy, not volume depleted:* 80 mg once daily; *Volume-depleted (concomitant high-dose diuretic):* initially 40 mg once daily
> *Pediatric:* <12 years: not recommended; ≥12 years: same as adult
>> Edarbi *Tab:* 40, 80 mg

▷ *candesartan* (D)(G) initially 16 mg daily; range 8-32 mg in 1-2 divided doses
> *Pediatric:* <12 years: not recommended; ≥12 years: same as adult
>> Atacand *Tab:* 4, 8, 16, 32 mg

▷ *eprosartan* (D)(G) initially 400 mg bid <u>or</u> 600 mg once daily; max 800 mg/day
> *Pediatric:* <12 years: not established; ≥12 years: same as adult
>> Teveten *Tab:* 400, 600 mg

▷ *irbesartan* (D)(G) initially 150 mg daily; titrate up to 300 mg
> *Pediatric:* <12 years: not recommended; ≥12 years: same as adult
>> Avapro *Tab:* 75, 150, 300 mg

▷ *losartan* (D)(G) initially 50 mg daily; max 100 mg/day
> *Pediatric:* <12 years: not recommended; ≥12 years: same as adult
>> Cozaar *Tab:* 25, 50, 100 mg

▷ *olmesartan medoxomil* (D)(G) initially 20 mg once daily; after 2 weeks, may increase to 40 mg daily
> *Pediatric:* <6 years: not recommended; ≥6-16 years: 20-35 kg: initially 10 mg once daily; after 2 weeks, may increase to max 20 mg once daily; ≥6-16 years: >35 kg: initially 20 mg once daily; after 2 weeks, may increase to max 40 mg once daily
>> Benicar *Tab:* 5, 20, 40 mg

▷ *telmisartan* (D)(G) initially 40 mg once daily; usual dose 20-80 mg
> *Pediatric:* <12 years: not recommended; ≥12 years: same as adult
>> Micardis *Tab:* 20, 40, 80 mg

▷ *valsartan* (D)(G) initially 80 mg once daily; may increase to 160 <u>or</u> 320 mg once daily after 2-4 weeks; usual range 80-320 mg/day
> *Pediatric:* <12 years: not recommended; ≥12 years: same as adult
>> Diovan *Tab:* 40*, 80, 160, 320 mg

CALCIUM CHANNEL BLOCKERS (CCBs)

Benzothiazepines

▷ *diltiazem* (C)(G)

  Pediatric: <12 years: not established; ≥12 years: same as adult

  Cardizem initially 30 mg qid; may increase gradually every 1-2 days; max 360 mg/day in divided doses

  Tab: 30, 60, 90, 120 mg

  Cardizem CD initially 120-180 mg daily; adjust at 1-2-week intervals; max 480 mg/day

  Cap: 120, 180, 240, 300, 360 mg ext-rel

  Cardizem LA initially 180-240 mg daily; titrate at 2-week intervals; max 540 mg/day

  Tab: 120, 180, 240, 300, 360, 420 mg ext-rel

  Cardizem SR initially 60-120 mg bid; adjust at 2-week intervals; max 360 mg/day

  Cap: 60, 90, 120 mg sust-rel

  Cartia XT initially 180 or 240 mg once daily; max 540 mg once daily

  Cap: 120, 180, 240, 300 mg ext-rel

  Dilacor XR initially 180 or 240 mg in AM; usual range 180-480 mg/day; max 540 mg/day

  Cap: 120, 180, 240 mg ext-rel

  Tiazac (G) initially 120-240 mg daily; adjust at 2-week intervals; usual max 540 mg/day

  Cap: 120, 180, 240, 300, 360, 420 mg ext-rel

▷ *diltiazem maleate* (C) initially 120-180 mg daily; adjust at 2-week intervals; usual range 120-480 mg daily

  Pediatric: <12 years: not recommended; ≥12 years: same as adult

  Tiamate *Cap:* 120, 180, 240 mg ext-rel

Dihydropyridines

▷ *amlodipine* (C) initially 5 mg once daily; max 10 mg/day

  Pediatric: <12 years: not recommended; ≥12 years: same as adult

  Norvasc *Tab:* 2.5, 5, 10 mg

▷ *clevidipine butyrate* (C) administer by IV infusion; initially 1-2 mg/hour; double dose at 90-second intervals until BP approaches goal; then titrate slower; adjust at 5-10-minute intervals; maintenance 4-6 mg/hour; usual max, 16-32 mg/hour; do not exceed 1,000 ml (21 mg/hour for 24 hours) due to lipid load

  Pediatric: <18 years: not recommended; ≥18 years: same as adult

  Cleviprex *Vial:* 0.5 mg/ml soln for IV infusion (single-use, 50, 100 ml) (lipids)

Comment: **Cleviprex** is indicated to reduce blood pressure when oral therapy is not feasible or desirable. **Cleviprex** is contraindicated with egg or soy allergy.

▷ *felodipine* (C)(G) initially 5 mg daily; usual range 2.5-10 mg daily; adjust at 2-week intervals; max 10 mg/day

  Pediatric: <12 years: not recommended; ≥12 years: same as adult

  Plendil *Tab:* 2.5, 5, 10 mg ext-rel

▷ *isradipine* (C)

  Pediatric: <12 years: not recommended; ≥12 years: same as adult

  DynaCirc initially 2.5 mg bid; adjust in increments of 5 mg/day at 2-4-week intervals; max 20 mg/day

  Cap: 2.5, 5 mg

  DynaCirc CR initially 5 mg daily; adjust in increments of 5 mg/day at 2-4-week intervals; max 20 mg/day

  Tab: 5, 10 mg cont-rel

▷ *nicardipine* (C)(G)
   Pediatric: <18 years: not recommended; ≥18 years: same as adult
      Cardene initially 10-20 mg tid; adjust at intervals of at least 3 days; max 120 mg/day
         Cap: 20, 30 mg
      Cardene SR 30-60 mg bid
         Cap: 30, 45, 60 mg sust-rel
▷ *nifedipine* (C)(G)
   Pediatric: <12 years: not recommended; ≥12 years: same as adult
      Adalat initially 10 mg tid; usual range 10-20 mg tid; max 180 mg/day
         Cap: 10, 20 mg
      Adalat CC initially 10 mg tid; usual range 10-20 mg tid; max 180 mg/day
         Cap: 30, 60, 90 mg ext-rel
      Afeditab CR initially 30 mg once daily; titrate over 7-14 days; max 90 mg/day
         Cap: 30, 60 mg ext-rel
      Procardia initially 10 mg tid; titrate over 7-14 days; max 30 mg/dose and 180 mg/day in divided doses
         Cap: 10, 20 mg
      Procardia XL initially 30-60 mg daily; titrate over 7-14 days; max dose 90 mg/day
         Tab: 30, 60, 90 mg ext-rel
▷ *nisoldipine* (C) initially 20 mg daily; may increase by 10 mg weekly; usual maintenance 20-40 mg/day; max 60 mg/day
   Pediatric: <12 years: not recommended; ≥12 years: same as adult
      Sular *Tab:* 10, 20, 30, 40 mg ext-rel

Diphenylalkylamines

▷ *verapamil* (C)(G)
   Pediatric: <12 years: not recommended; ≥12 years: same as adult
      Calan 80-120 mg tid; may titrate up; usual max 360 mg in divided doses
         Tab: 40, 80*, 120*mg
      Calan SR initially 120 mg in the AM; may titrate up; max 480 mg/day in divided doses
         Cplt: 120, 180*, 240*mg sust-rel
      Covera HS initially 180 mg q HS; titrate to 240 mg; then to 360 mg; then to 480 mg if needed
         Tab: 180, 240 mg ext-rel
      Isoptin initially 80-120 mg tid
         Tab: 40, 80, 120 mg
      Isoptin SR initially 120-180 mg in the AM; may increase to 240 mg in the AM; then 180 mg q 12 hours or 240 mg in the AM and 120 mg in the PM; then 240 mg q 12 hours
         Tab: 120, 180*, 240*mg sust-rel
      Verelan initially 240 mg once daily; adjust in 120 mg increments; max 480 mg/day
         Cap: 120, 180, 240, 360 mg sust-rel
      Verelan PM initially 200 mg q HS; may titrate upward to 300 mg; then 400 mg if needed
         Cap: 100, 200, 300 mg ext-rel

ALPHA-1 ANTAGONISTS

Comment: Educate the patient regarding potential side effects of hypotension when taking an alpha-1 antagonist, especially with first dose ("first dose effect"). Start at lowest dose and titrate upward.

▷ *doxazosin* (C)(G) initially 1 mg once daily at HS; increase dose slowly every 2 weeks if needed; max 16 mg/day

Pediatric: <12 years: not recommended; ≥12 years: same as adult

    Cardura *Tab:* 1*, 2*, 4*, 8*mg

    Cardura XL *Tab:* 4, 8 mg

▷ *prazosin* (C)(G) first dose at HS, 1 mg bid-tid; increase dose slowly; usual range 6-15 mg/day in divided doses; max 20-40 mg/day

Pediatric: <12 years: not recommended; ≥12 years: same as adult

    Minipress *Cap:* 1, 2, 5 mg

▷ *terazosin* (C) 1 mg q HS, then increase dose slowly; usual range 1-5 mg q HS; max 20 mg/day

Pediatric: <12 years: not recommended; ≥12 years: same as adult

    Hytrin *Cap:* 1, 2, 5, 10 mg

CENTRAL ALPHA-AGONISTS

▷ *clonidine* (C)

Pediatric: <12 years: not recommended; ≥12 years: same as adult

    Catapres initially 0.1 mg bid; usual range 0.2-0.6 mg/day in divided doses; max 2.4 mg/day

        Tab: 0.1*, 0.2*, 0.3*mg

    Catapres-TTS initially 0.1 mg patch weekly; increase after 1-2 weeks if needed; max 0.6 mg/day

        Patch: 0.1, 0.2 mg/day (12/carton); 0.3 mg/day (4/carton)

    Kapvay (G) initially 0.1 mg bid; usual range 0.2-0.6 mg/day in divided doses; max 2.4 mg/day

        Tab: 0.1, 0.2 mg

    Nexiclon XR initially 0.18 mg (2 ml) suspension <u>or</u> 0.17 mg tab once daily; usual max 0.52 mg (6 ml suspension) once daily

        Tab: 0.17, 0.26 mg ext-rel; *Oral susp:* 0.09 mg/ml ext-rel (4 oz)

▷ *guanabenz* (C)(G) initially 4 mg bid; may increase by 4-8 mg/day every 1-2 weeks; max 32 mg/day

Pediatric: <12 years: not recommended; ≥12 years: same as adult

    Tab: 4, 8 mg

▷ *guanfacine* (B)(G) initially 1 mg/day q HS; may increase to 2 mg/day q HS; usual max 3 mg/day

Pediatric: <12 years: not recommended; ≥12 years: same as adult

    Tenex *Tab:* 1, 2 mg

▷ *methyldopa* (B)(G) initially 250 mg bid-tid; titrate at 2-day intervals; usual maintenance 500 mg/day to 2 gm/day; max 3 gm/day

Pediatric: initially 10 mg/kg/day in 2-4 divided doses; max 65 mg/kg/day <u>or</u> 3 gm/day, whichever is less

    Aldomet *Tab:* 125, 250, 500 mg; *Oral susp:* 250 mg/5 ml (473 ml)

ALDOSTERONE RECEPTOR BLOCKER

▷ *eplerenone* (B) initially 25-50 mg daily; may increase to 50 mg bid; max 100 mg/day

Pediatric: <12 years: not recommended; ≥12 years: same as adult

    Inspra *Tab:* 25, 50 mg

Comment: Contraindicated with concomitant potent CYP3A4 inhibitors. Risk of hyperkalemia with concomitant ACE-I <u>or</u> ARB. Monitor serum potassium at baseline, 1 week, and 1 month. Caution with serum Cr >2 mg/dL (male) <u>or</u> >1.8 mg/dL (female) <u>and/or</u> CrCl <50 mL/min, and DM with proteinuria.

PERIPHERAL ADRENERGIC BLOCKER

▷ *guanethidine* (C) initially 10 mg daily; may adjust dose at 5-7 day intervals; usual range 25-50 mg/day
   Pediatric: <12 years: not recommended; ≥12 years: same as adult
      Ismelin *Tab:* 10, 25 mg

DIRECT RENIN INHIBITOR

▷ *aliskiren* (D) initially 150 mg once daily; max 300 mg/day
   Pediatric: <18 years: not recommended; ≥18 years: same as adult
      Tekturna *Tab:* 150, 300 mg

PERIPHERAL VASODILATORS

▷ *hydralazine* (C)(G) initially 10 mg qid x 2-4 days; then increase to 25 mg qid for remainder of 1st week; then increase to 50 mg qid; max 300 mg/day
   Pediatric: initially 0.75 mg/kg/day in 4 divided doses; increase gradually over 3-4 weeks; max 7.5 mg/kg/day or 2,000 mg/day
      Tab: 10, 25, 50, 100 mg
▷ *minoxidil* (C) initially 5 mg daily; may increase at 3-day intervals to 10 mg/day, then 20 mg/day, then 40 mg/day; usual range 10-40 mg/day; max 100 mg/day
   Pediatric: initially 0.2 mg/kg daily; may increase in 50%-100% increments every 3 days; usual range 0.25-1 gm/kg/day; max 50 mg/day
      Loniten *Tab:* 2.5*, 10*mg

ACEI+DIURETIC COMBINATIONS

▷ *benazepril+hydrochlorothiazide* (D)
   Pediatric: <12 years: not recommended; ≥12 years: same as adult
      Lotensin HCT
         Tab: Lotensin HCT 5/6.25 *benaz* 5 mg+*hctz* 6.25 mg*
               Lotensin HCT 10/12.5 *benaz* 10 mg+*hctz* 12.5 mg*
               Lotensin HCT 20/12.5 *benaz* 20 mg+*hctz* 12.5 mg*
               Lotensin HCT 20/25 *benaz* 20 mg+*hctz* 25 mg*
▷ *captopril+hydrochlorothiazide* (D)(G)
   Pediatric: <12 years: not recommended; ≥12 years: same as adult
      Capozide 1 tab once daily; titrate individual components
         Tab: Capozide 25/15 *capt* 25 mg+*hctz* 15 mg*
               Capozide 25/25 *capt* 25 mg+*hctz* 25 mg*
               Capozide 50/15 *capt* 50 mg+*hctz* 15 mg*
               Capozide 50/25 *capt* 50 mg+*hctz* 25 mg*
▷ *enalapril+hydrochlorothiazide* (D)
   Pediatric: <12 years: not recommended; ≥12 years: same as adult
      Vaseretic 1 tab once daily; titrate individual components
         Tab: Vaseretic 5/12.5 *enal* 5 mg+*hctz* 12.5 mg
               Vaseretic 10/25 *enal* 10 mg+*hctz* 25 mg
▷ *lisinopril+hydrochlorothiazide* (D)
   Pediatric: <12 years: not recommended; ≥12 years: same as adult
      Prinzide 1 tab once daily; titrate individual components
         Tab: Prinzide 10/12.5 *lis* 10 mg+*hctz* 12.5 mg
               Prinzide 20/12.5 *lis* 20 mg+*hctz* 12.5 mg
               Prinzide 20/25 *lis* 20 mg+*hctz* 25 mg
      Zestoretic 1 tab once daily; titrate individual components; *CrCl <40 mL/min:* not recommended

        Tab: **Zestoretic 10/12.5** *lis* 10 mg+*hctz* 12.5 mg
           Zestoretic 20/12.5 *lis* 20 mg+*hctz* 12.5 mg*
           Zestoretic 20/25 *lis* 20 mg+*hctz* 25 mg

▷ *moexipril+hydrochlorothiazide* (D)
    Pediatric: <12 years: not recommended; ≥12 years: same as adult
      Uniretic 1 tab once daily; titrate individual components
      Tab: **Uniretic 7.5/12.5** *moex* 7.5 mg+*hctz* 12.5 mg*
         Uniretic 15/12.5 *moex* 15 mg+*hctz* 12.5 mg*
         Uniretic 15/25 *moex* 15 mg+*hctz* 25 mg*

▷ *quinapril+hydrochlorothiazide* (D)
    Pediatric: <12 years: not recommended; ≥12 years: same as adult
      Accuretic 1 tab once daily; titrate individual components
      Tab: **Accuretic 10/12.5** *quin* 10 mg+*hctz* 12.5 mg*
         Accuretic 20/12.5 *quin* 20 mg+*hctz* 12.5 mg*
         Accuretic 20/25 *quin* 20 mg+*hctz* 25 mg*

ARB+DIURETIC COMBINATIONS

▷ *azilsartan+chlorthalidone* (D)
    Pediatric: <18 years: not recommended; ≥18 years: same as adult
      Edarbyclor 1 tab once daily; titrate individual components
      Tab: **Edarbyclor 40/12.5** *azil* 40 mg+*chlor* 12.5 mg
         Edarbyclor 40/25 *azil* 40 mg+*chlor* 25 mg

▷ *candesartan+hydrochlorothiazide* (D)
    Pediatric: <12 years: not recommended; ≥12 years: same as adult
      Atacand HCT
      Tab: **Atacand HCT 16/12.5** *cande* 16 mg+*hctz* 12.5 mg
         Atacand HCT 32/12.5 *cande* 32 mg+*hctz* 12.5 mg

▷ *eprosartan+hydrochlorothiazide* (D)
    Pediatric: <12 years: not recommended; ≥12 years: same as adult
      Teveten HCT 1 tab once daily; titrate individual components
      Tab: **Teveten HCT 600/12.5** *epro* 600 mg+*hctz* 12.5 mg
         Teveten HCT 600/25 *epro* 600 mg+*hctz* 25 mg

▷ *irbesartan+hydrochlorothiazide* (D)
    Pediatric: <12 years: not recommended; ≥12 years: same as adult
      Avalide 1 tab once daily; titrate individual components
      Tab: **Avalide 150/12.5** *irbes* 150 mg+*hctz* 12.5 mg
         Avalide 300/12.5 *irbes* 300 mg+*hctz* 12.5 mg

▷ *losartan+hydrochlorothiazide* (D)(G)
    Pediatric: <12 years: not recommended; ≥12 years: same as adult
      Hyzaar 1 tab once daily; titrate individual components
      Tab: **Hyzaar 50/12.5** *losar* 50 mg+*hctz* 12.5 mg
         Hyzaar 100/12.5 *losar* 100 mg+*hctz* 12.5 mg
         Hyzaar 100/25 *losar* 100 mg+*hctz* 25 mg

▷ *olmesartan medoxomil+hydrochlorothiazide* (D)(G)
    Pediatric: <12 years: not recommended; ≥12 years: same as adult
      Benicar HCT 1 tab once daily; titrate individual components
      Tab: **Benicar HCT 20/12.5** *olmi* 20 mg+*hctz* 12.5 mg
         Benicar HCT 40/12.5 *olmi* 40 mg+*hctz* 12.5 mg
         Benicar HCT 40/25 *olmi* 40 mg+*hctz* 25 mg

▷ *telmisartan+hydrochlorothiazide* (D)(G)
    Pediatric: <12 years: not recommended; ≥12 years: same as adult

    Micardis HCT 1 tab once daily; titrate individual components

      Tab: **Micardis HCT 40/12.5** *telmi* 40 mg+*hctz* 12.5 mg

        Micardis HCT 80/12.5 *telmi* 80 mg+*hctz* 12.5 mg

        Micardis HCT 80/25 *telmi* 80 mg+*hctz* 25 mg

▷ *valsartan+hydrochlorothiazide* (D)

  Pediatric: <12 years: not recommended; ≥12 years: same as adult

    Diovan HCT 1 tab once daily; titrate individual components

      Tab: **Diovan HCT 80/12.5** *vals* 80 mg+*hctz* 12.5 mg

        Diovan HCT 160/12.5 *vals* 160 mg+*hctz* 12.5 mg

        Diovan HCT 160/25 *vals* 160 mg+*hctz* 25 mg

        Diovan HCT 320/12.5 *vals* 320 mg+*hctz* 12.5 mg

        Diovan HCT 320/25 *vals* 320 mg+*hctz* 25 mg

CENTRAL ALPHA-AGONIST+DIURETIC COMBINATIONS

▷ *clonidine+chlorthalidone* (C)

  Pediatric: <12 years: not recommended; ≥12 years: same as adult

    Combipres 1 tab daily-bid

      Tab: **Combipres 0.1** *clon* 0.1 mg+*chlor* 15 mg*

        Combipres 0.2 *clon* 0.2 mg+*chlor* 15 mg*

        Combipres 0.3 *clon* 0.3 mg+*chlor* 15 mg*

▷ *methyldopa+hydrochlorothiazide* (C)(G)

  Pediatric: <12 years: not recommended; ≥12 years: same as adult

    Aldoril initially **Aldoril 15** bid-tid or **Aldoril 25** bid; titrate individual components

      Tab: **Aldoril 15** *meth* 250 mg+*hctz* 15 mg

        Aldoril 25 *meth* 250 mg+*hctz* 25 mg

        Aldoril D30 *meth* 500 mg+*hctz* 30 mg

        Aldoril D50 *meth* 500 mg+*hctz* 50 mg

BETA-BLOCKER (CARDIOSELECTIVE)+DIURETIC COMBINATIONS

▷ *atenolol+chlorthalidone* (D)(G)

  Pediatric: <12 years: not recommended; ≥12 years: same as adult

    Tenoretic initially *tenoretic* 50 mg once daily; may increase to *tenoretic* 100 mg once daily

      Tab: **Tenoretic 50/25** *aten* 50 mg+*chlor* 25 mg*

        Tenoretic 100/25 *aten* 100 mg+*chlor* 25 mg

▷ *bisoprolol+hydrochlorothiazide* (C)

  Pediatric: <12 years: not recommended; ≥12 years: same as adult

    Ziac initially one 2.5/6.25 mg tab daily; adjust at 2 week intervals; max two 10/6.25 mg tabs daily

      Tab: **Ziac 2.5** *biso* 2.5 mg+*hctz* 6.25 mg

        Ziac 5 *biso* 5 mg+*hctz* 6.25 mg

        Ziac 10 *biso* 10 mg+*hctz* 6.25 mg

▷ *metoprolol succinate+hydrochlorothiazide* (C)

  Pediatric: <12 years: not recommended; ≥12 years: same as adult

    Lopressor HCT titrate individual components

      Tab: **Lopressor HCT 50/25** *meto succ* 50 mg+*hctz* 25 mg*

        Lopressor HCT 100/25 *meto succ* 100 mg+*hctz* 25 mg*

        Lopressor HCT 100/50 *meto succ* 100 mg+*hctz* 50 mg*

▷ *metoprolol succinate+ext-rel hydrochlorothiazide* (C)

  Pediatric: <12 years: not established; ≥12 years: same as adult

    Dutoprol titrate individual components; may titrate to max 200/25 mg once daily

      Tab: **Dutoprol 25/12.5** *meto succ* 25 mg+*hctz* 12.5 mg *ext-rel*

> Dutoprol 50/12.5 *meto succ* 50 mg+*hctz* 12.5 mg *ext-rel*
> Dutoprol 100/12.5 *meto succ* 100 mg+*hctz* 12.5 mg *ext-rel*

BETA-BLOCKER (NON-CARDIOSELECTIVE)+DIURETIC COMBINATIONS

▷ *nadolol+bendroflumethiazide* (C)
  Pediatric: <12 years: not recommended; ≥12 years: same as adult
    Corzide titrate individual components
      Tab: Corzide 40/5 *nado* 40 mg+*bend* 5 mg*
        Corzide 80/5 *nado* 80 mg+*bend* 5 mg*
▷ *propranolol+hydrochlorothiazide* (C)(G)
  Pediatric: <12 years: not recommended; ≥12 years: same as adult
    Inderide titrate individual components
      Tab: Inderide 40/25 *prop* 40 mg+*hctz* 25 mg*
        Inderide 80/25 *prop* 80 mg+*hctz* 25 mg*
    Inderide LA titrate individual components
      Cap: Inderide LA 80/50 *prop* 80 mg+*hctz* 50 mg sust-rel
        Inderide LA 120/50 *prop* 120 mg+*hctz* 50 mg sust-rel
        Inderide LA 160/50 *prop* 160 mg+*hctz* 50 mg sust-rel
▷ *timolol+hydrochlorothiazide* (C)
  Pediatric: <12 years: not recommended; ≥12 years: same as adult
    Timolide usual maintenance 2 tabs/day in a single or 2 divided doses
      Tab: *timo* 10 mg+*hctz* 25 mg

BETA-BLOCKER (CARDIOSELECTIVE)+ARB COMBINATION

▷ *nebivolol+valsartan* (X) 1 tab daily; may initiate when inadequately controlled on
  nebivolol 10 mg or *valsartan* 80 mg
  Pediatric: <12 years: not established; ≥12 years: same as adult
    Byvalson *Tab:* nebi 5 mg+val 80 mg

ALPHA-1 ANTAGONIST+DIURETIC COMBINATIONS

▷ *prazosin+polythiazide* (C)
  Pediatric: <12 years: not recommended; ≥12 years: same as adult
    Minizide titrate individual components
      Cap: Minizide 1 *praz* 1 mg+*poly* 0.5 mg
        Minizide 2 *praz* 2 mg+*poly* 0.5 mg
        Minizide 5 *praz* 5 mg+*poly* 0.5 mg

PERIPHERAL ADRENERGIC BLOCKER+HCTZ COMBINATIONS

▷ *guanethidine+hydrochlorothiazide* (C)
  Pediatric: <12 years: not recommended; ≥12 years: same as adult
    Esimil titrate individual components
      Tab: Esimil 10/25 *guan* 1 mg+*hctz* 25 mg

ACEI+CCB COMBINATIONS

▷ *amlodipine+benazepril* (D)
  Pediatric: <12 years: not recommended; ≥12 years: same as adult
    Lotrel titrate individual components
      Cap: Lotrel 2.5/10 *amlo* 2.5 mg+*benaz* 10 mg
        Lotrel 5/10 *amlo* 5 mg+*benaz* 10 mg
        Lotrel 5/20 *amlo* 5 mg+*benaz* 20 mg
        Lotrel 10/20 *amlo* 10 mg+*benaz* 20 mg
        Lotrel 5/40 *amlo* 5 mg+*benaz* 40 mg
        Lotrel 10/40 *amlo* 10 mg+*benaz* 40 mg

▷ **amlodipine+perindopril** (D)
  Pediatric: <12 years: not recommended; ≥12 years: same as adult
    Prolastin titrate individual components
      Cap: **Prolastin 2.5/3.5** *amlo* 2.5 mg+*peri* 3.5 mg
        Prolastin 5/7 *amlo* 5 mg+*peri* 7 mg
        Prolastin 5/14 *amlo* 5 mg+*peri* 14 mg
▷ **enalapril+diltiazem** (D)
  Pediatric: <12 years: not recommended; ≥12 years: same as adult
    Teczem titrate individual components
      Tab: **enal** 5 mg+*dil* 180 mg ext-rel
▷ **enalapril+felodipine** (D)
  Pediatric: <18 years: not recommended; ≥18 years: same as adult
    Lexxel titrate individual components
      Tab: **Lexxel 5/2.5** *enal* 5 mg+*felo* 2.5 mg ext-rel
        Lexxel 5/5 *enal* 5 mg+*felo* 5 mg ext-rel
▷ **perindopril+amlodipine** (D)
  Pediatric: <12 years: not established; ≥12 years: same as adult
    Prestalia titrate individual components; max 14/10 once daily
      Tab: **Prestalia 3.5/2.5** *peri* 3.5 mg+*amlo* 2.5 mg
        Prestalia 7/5 *peri* 7 mg+*amlo* 5 mg
        Prestalia 14/10 *peri* 14 mg+*amlo* 10 mg
▷ **trandolapril+verapamil** (D)
  Pediatric: <12 years: not established; ≥12 years: same as adult
    Tarka titrate individual components
      Tab: **Tarka 1/240** *tran* 1 mg+*ver* 240 mg ext-rel
        Tarka 2/180 *tran* 2 mg+*ver* 180 mg ext-rel
        Tarka 2/240 *tran* 2 mg+*ver* 240 mg ext-rel
        Tarka 4/240 *tran* 4 mg+*ver* 240 mg ext-rel

DRI+HCTZ COMBINATIONS

▷ **aliskiren+hydrochlorothiazide** (D) initially *aliskiren* 150 mg once daily; max *aliskiren*
300 mg/day
  Pediatric: <18 years: not recommended; ≥18 years: same as adult
    Tekturna HCT
      Tab: **Tekturna HCT 150/12.5** *alisk* 150 mg+*hctz* 12.5 mg
        Tekturna HCT 150/25 *alisk* 150 mg+*hctz* 25 mg
        Tekturna HCT 300/12.5 *alisk* 300 mg+*hctz* 12.5 mg
        Tekturna HCT 300/25 *alisk* 300 mg+*hctz* 25 mg

DRI+ARB COMBINATION

▷ **aliskiren+valsartan** (D)
  Pediatric: <12 years: not recommended; ≥12 years: same as adult
    Valturna initially 150/160 once daily; may increase to max 300/320 once daily
      Tab: **Valturna 150/160** *alisk* 150 mg+*vals* 160 mg
        Valturna 300/320 *alisk* 300 mg+*vals* 320 mg

DRI+CCB COMBINATIONS

▷ **aliskiren+amlodipine** (D)
  Pediatric: <12 years: not recommended; ≥12 years: same as adult
    Tekamlo initially 150/5 once daily; may increase to max 300/10 once daily
      Tab: **Tekamlo 150/5** *alisk* 150 mg+*amlo* 5 mg
        Tekamlo 150/10 *alisk* 150 mg+*amlo* 10 mg

Tekamlo 300/5 *alisk* 300 mg+*amlo* 5 mg
Tekamlo 300/10 *alisk* 300 mg+*amlo* 10 mg

DRI+CCB+HCTZ COMBINATIONS

▷ *aliskiren+amlodipine+hydrochlorothiazide* (D)
Pediatric: <12 years: not established; ≥12 years: same as adult
Amturnide initially 150/5/12.5 once daily; may increase to max 300/10/25 once daily
Tab: **Amturnide 150/5/12.5** *alisk* 150 mg+*amlo* 5 mg+*hctz* 12.5 mg
Amturnide 300/5/12.5 *alisk* 300 mg+*amlo* 5 mg+*hctz* 12.5 mg
Amturnide 300/5/25 *alisk* 300 mg+*amlo* 5 mg+*hctz* 25 mg

ARB+CCB COMBINATIONS

▷ *amlodipine+valsartan medoxomil* (D)(G)
Pediatric: <12 years: not recommended; ≥12 years: same as adult
Exforge 1 tab daily; titrate individual components at 1-week intervals; max 10/320 daily
Tab: **Exforge 5/160** *amlo* 5 mg+*vals* 160 mg
Exforge 5/320 *amlo* 5 mg+*vals* 320 mg
Exforge 10/160 *amlo* 10 mg+*vals* 160 mg
Exforge 10/320 *amlo* 10 mg+*vals* 320 mg
▷ *amlodipine+olmesartan* (D)(G)
Pediatric: <12 years: not established; ≥12 years: same as adult
Azor titrate individual components
Tab: **Azor 5/20** *amlo* 5 mg+*olme* 20 mg
Azor 10/20 *amlo* 10 mg+*olme* 20 mg
Azor 5/40 *amlo* 5 mg+*olme* 40 mg
Azor 10/40 *amlo* 10 mg+*olme* 40 mg
▷ *telmisartan+amlodipine* (D)
Pediatric: <12 years: not established; ≥12 years: same as adult
Twynsta initially 40/5 once daily; titrate at 1 week intervals; max 80/10 once daily
Tab: **Twynsta 40/5** *telmi* 40 mg+*amlo* 5 mg
Twynsta 40/10 *telmi* 40 mg+*amlo* 10 mg
Twynsta 80/5 *telmi* 80 mg+*amlo* 5 mg
Twynsta 80/10 *telmi* 80 mg+*amlo* 10 mg

ARB+CCB+HCTZ COMBINATIONS

▷ *amlodipine+valsartan medoxomil+hydrochlorothiazide* (D)(G)
Pediatric: <12 years: not recommended; ≥12 years: same as adult
Exforge HCT: initially 5/160/12.5 once daily; may titrate at 1-week intervals to max 10/320/25 once daily
Tab: **Exforge HCT 5/160/12.5** *amlo* 5 mg+*vals* 160 mg+*hctz* 12.5 mg
Exforge HCT 5/160/25 *amlo* 5 mg+*vals* 160 mg+*hctz* 25 mg
Exforge HCT 10/160/12.5 *amlo* 10 mg+*vals* 160 mg+*hctz* 12.5 mg
Exforge HCT 10/160/25 *amlo* 10 mg+*vals* 160 mg+*hctz* 25 mg
Exforge HCT 10/320/25 *amlo* 10 mg+*vals* 320 mg+*hctz* 25 mg
▷ *olmesartan medoxomil+amlodipine+hydrochlorothiazide* (D)(G)
Pediatric: <12 years: not recommended; ≥12 years: same as adult
Tribenzor: initially 40/5/12.5 once daily; may titrate at 1-week intervals to max 40/10/25 daily
Tab: **Tribenzor 40/5/12.5** *olme* 40 mg+*amlo* 5 mg+*hctz* 12.5 mg
Tribenzor 40/5/25 *olme* 40 mg+*amlo* 5 mg+*hctz* 25 mg

Tribenzor 40/10/12.5 *olme* 40 mg+*amlo* 10 mg+*hctz* 12.5 mg
Tribenzor 40/10/25 *olme* 40 mg+*amlo* 10 mg+*hctz* 25 mg

OTHER COMBINATION AGENTS

▷ *clonidine+chlorthalidone* (C)
  Pediatric: <12 years: not recommended; ≥12 years: same as adult
    Clorpres initially 0.1/15 once daily; may titrate to max 0.3/15 bid
      Tab: Clorpres 0.1/15 *clon* 0.1 mg+*chlor* 15 mg
        Clorpres 0.2/15 *clon* 0.2 mg+*chlor* 15 mg
        Clorpres 0.3/15 *clon* 0.3 mg+*chlor* 15 mg
▷ *reserpine+hydroflumethiazide* (C)
  Pediatric: <12 years: not recommended; ≥12 years: same as adult
    Salutensin initially 1.25/25 once daily; may titrate to 1.25/25 bid or 1.25/50 once
    daily
      Tab: Salutensin 1.25/25 *enal* 1.25 mg+*hydro* 25 mg
        Salutensin 1.25/50: *enal* 1.25 mg+*hydro* 50 mg

ANTIHYPERTENSION+ANTILIPID COMBINATIONS
CCB+Statin Combinations

▷ *amlodipine/atorvastatin* (X)
  Pediatric: <10 years: not established; ≥10 years (female postmenarche): same as adult
    Caduet select according to blood pressure and lipid values; titrate *amlodipine* over
    7-14 days; titrate *atorvastatin* according to monitored lipid values; max *amlodipine*
    10 mg/day and max *atorvastatin* 80 mg/day; refer to contraindications and precau-
    tions for CCB and statin therapy
      Tab: Caduet 2.5/10 *amlo* 2.5 mg+*ator* 10 mg
        Caduet 2.5/20 *amlo* 2.5 mg+*ator* 20 mg
        Caduet 5/10 *amlo* 5 mg+*ator* 10 mg
        Caduet 5/20 *amlo* 5 mg+*ator* 20 mg
        Caduet 5/40 *amlo* 5 mg+*ator* 40 mg
        Caduet 5/80 *amlo* 5 mg+*ator* 80 mg
        Caduet 10/10 *amlo* 10 mg+*ator* 10 mg
        Caduet 10/20 *amlo* 10 mg+*ator* 20 mg
        Caduet 10/40 *amlo* 10 mg+*ator* 40 mg
        Caduet 10/80 *amlo* 10 mg+*ator* 80 mg

◯ HYPERTHYROIDISM

▷ *methimazole* (D) initially 15-60 mg/day in 3 divided doses; maintenance 5-15 mg/day
  Pediatric: initially 0.4 mg/kg/day in 3 divided doses; maintenance 0.2 mg/kg/day or
  1/2 initial dose
    Tapazole *Tab:* 5*, 10*mg
Comment: *methimazole* potentiates anticoagulants. Contraindicated in nursing
mothers.
▷ *propylthiouracil (ptu)* (D)(G)
    Propyl-Thyracil initially 100-900 mg/day in 3 divided doses; maintenance usually
    50-600 mg/day in 2 divided doses
      Pediatric: <6 years: not recommended; ≥6-10 years: initially 50-150 mg/day or
      5-7 mg/kg/day in 3 divided doses; ≥10 years: initially 150-300 mg/day or 5-7
      mg/kg/day in 3 divided doses; *maintenance:* 0.2 mg/kg/day or 1/2-2/3 of initial
      dose
        Tab: 50*mg

Comment: Preferred agent in pregnancy. Side effects include dermatitis, nausea, agranulocytosis, and hypothyroidism. Should be taken regularly for 2 years. Do not discontinue abruptly.

BETA-ADRENERGIC BLOCKER

▷ *propranolol* (C)(G) 40-240 mg daily
 Pediatric: <12 years: not recommended; ≥12 years: same as adult
  Inderal *Tab:* 10*, 20*, 40*, 60*, 80*mg
  Inderal LA initially 80 mg daily in a single dose; increase q 3-7 days; usual range 120-160 mg/day; max 320 mg/day in a single dose
   Cap: 60, 80, 120, 160 mg sust-rel
  InnoPran XL initially 80 mg q HS; max 120 mg/day
   Cap: 80, 120 mg ext-rel

HYPERTRIGLYCERIDEMIA

OMEGA 3-FATTY ACID ETHYL ESTERS

Comment: **Vascepa, Lovaza,** and **Epanova** are indicated for the treatment of TG ≥500 mg/dL.
▷ *icosapent ethyl (omega 3-fatty acid ethyl ester of EPA)* (C) 2 caps bid with food; max 4 gm/day; swallow whole, do not crush <u>or</u> chew
 Pediatric: <18 years: not recommended; ≥18 years: same as adult
  Vascepa *sgc:* 0.5, 1 gm (α-tocopherol 4 mg/cap)
▷ *omega 3-fatty acid ethyl esters* (C)(G) 2 gm bid <u>or</u> 4 gm daily; swallow whole, do not crush <u>or</u> chew
 Pediatric: <18 years: not recommended; ≥18 years: same as adult
  Lovaza *Gelcap:* 1 gm (α-tocopherol 4 mg/cap) *omega 3-carcartonyl acids* (C) take 2-4 gel aps (2-4 gm) daily without regard to meals
  Epanova *Gelcap:* 1 gm

ISOBUTYRIC ACID DERIVATIVE

▷ *gemfibrozil* (C)(G)
 Pediatric: <12 years: not recommended; ≥12 years: same as adult
  Lopid 600 mg bid 30 minutes before AM and PM meals
   Tab: 600*mg

FIBRATES (FIBRIC ACID DERIVATIVES)

▷ *fenofibrate* (C) take with meals; adjust at 4-8-week intervals; discontinue if inadequate response after 2 months; lowest dose <u>or</u> contraindicated with renal impairment and the elderly
 Pediatric: <12 years: not recommended; ≥12 years: same as adult
  Antara 43-130 mg once daily; max 130 mg/day
   Cap: 43, 87, 130 mg
  FibriCor 30-105 mg once daily; max 105 mg/day
   Tab: 30, 105 mg
  TriCor (G) 48-145 mg once daily; max 145 mg/day
   Tab: 48, 145 mg
  TriLipix (G) 45-135 mg once daily; max 135 mg/day
   Cap: 45, 135 mg del-rel
  Lipofen (G) 50-150 mg once daily; max 150 mg/day
   Cap: 50, 150 mg
  Lofibra 67-200 mg daily; max 200 mg/day
   Tab: 67, 134, 200 mg

NICOTINIC ACID DERIVATIVES

Comment: Contraindicated in liver disease. Decrease total cholesterol, LDL-C, and TG; increase HDL-C. Before initiating and at 4-6 weeks, 3 months, and 6 months of therapy, check fasting lipid profile *or* as indicated by manufacturer, LFT, glucose, and uric acid. Significant side effect of transient skin flushing. Take with food and take *aspirin* 325 mg 30 minutes before *niacin* dose to decrease flushing.

▷ *niacin* (C)

Niaspan 375 mg daily for 1st week, then 500 mg daily for 2nd week, then 750 mg daily for 3rd week, then 1 gm daily for weeks 4-7; may increase by 500 mg q 4 weeks; usual range 1-3 gm/day
Pediatric: <12 years: not recommended; ≥12 years: same as adult
 Tab: 500, 750, 1,000 mg ext-rel
Slo-Niacin 250 mg *or* 500 mg *or* 750 mg q AM *or* HS
Pediatric: <12 years: not recommended; ≥12 years: same as adult
 Tab: 250, 500, 750 mg cont-rel

HMG-COA REDUCTASE INHIBITORS (STATINS)

▷ *atorvastatin* (X)(G) initially 10 mg daily; usual range 10-80 mg daily
Pediatric: <10 years: not recommended; ≥10 years (female post-menarche): same as adult
Lipitor *Tab:* 10, 20, 40, 80 mg
▷ *fluvastatin* (X)(G) initially 20-40 mg q HS; usual range 20-80 mg/day
Pediatric: <18 years: not established; ≥18 years: same as adult
Lescol *Cap:* 20, 40 mg
Lescol XL *Tab:* 80 mg ext-rel
▷ *lovastatin* (X) initially 20 mg daily at evening meal; may increase at 4 week intervals; max 80 mg/day in a single *or* divided doses; *Concomitant fibrates, niacin, or CrCl <40 mL/min:* usual max 20 mg/day
Pediatric: <10 years: not recommended; 10-17 years: initially 10-20 mg daily at evening meal; may increase at 4 week intervals; max 40 mg daily; *Concomitant fibrates, niacin, or CrCl <40 mL/min:* usual max 20 mg/day
Mevacor *Tab:* 10, 20, 40 mg
▷ *pravastatin* (X)(G) initially 10-20 mg q HS; usual range 10-80 mg/day; may start at 40 mg/day
Pediatric: <8 years: not recommended; 8-13 years: 20 mg q HS; 14-17 years: 40 mg q HS; >17 years: same as adult
Pravachol *Tab:* 10, 20, 40, 80 mg
▷ *rosuvastatin* (X) initially 20 mg q HS; usual range 5-40 mg/day; adjust at 4 week intervals
Pediatric: <10 years: not recommended; 10-17 years: 5-20 mg q HS; max 20 mg q HS; >17 years: same as adult
Crestor *Tab:* 5, 10, 20, 40 mg
▷ *simvastatin* (X)(G) initially 20 mg q HS; usual range 5-80 mg/day; adjust at 4 week intervals
Pediatric: <10 years: not recommended; 10-17 years: initially 10 mg q HS; may increase at 4 week intervals; max 40 mg q HS; >17 years: same as adult
Zocor *Tab:* 5, 10, 20, 40, 80 mg

NICOTINIC ACID DERIVATIVE+HMG-COA REDUCTASE INHIBITOR COMBINATION

Comment: Nicotinic acid derivatives decrease total cholesterol, LDL-C, and TG; increase HDL-C. Before initiating and at 4-6 weeks, 3 months, and 6 months of therapy, check fasting lipid profile, LFT, glucose, and uric acid. Side effects include hyperglycemia, upper GI distress, hyperuricemia, hepatotoxicity, and significant transient skin flushing. Take with food and take *aspirin* 325 mg 30 minutes before *niacin* dose to decrease flushing. *Relative contraindications:* diabetes, hyperuricemia (gout), and PUD. *Absolute contraindications:* severe gout and chronic liver disease.

▷ *niacin+lovastatin* (X)
    Pediatric: <18 years: not recommended; ≥18 years: same as adult
        Advicor monitor lab values; may titrate up to max 1,000/20 once daily
            Tab: **Advicor 500/20** *niac* 500 mg ext-rel+*lova* 20 mg
                  Advicor 750/20 *niac* 750 mg ext-rel+*lova* 20 mg
                  Advicor 1,000/20 *niac* 1,000 mg ext-rel+*lova* 20 mg

HYPOCALCEMIA

Comment: Hypocalcemia resulting in metabolic bone disease may be secondary to hyperparathyroidism, pseudoparathyroidism, and chronic renal disease. Normal serum Ca^{++} range is approximately 8.5-12 mg/dL. Signs and symptoms of hypocalcemia include confusion, increased neuromuscular excitability, muscle spasms, paresthesias, hyperphosphatemia, positive Chvostek's sign, and positive Trousseau's sign. Signs and symptoms of hypercalcemia include fatigue, lethargy, decreased concentration and attention span, frank psychosis, anorexia, nausea, vomiting, constipation, bradycardia, heart block, shortened QT interval. Foods high in calcium include almonds, broccoli, baked beans, salmon, sardines, buttermilk, turnip greens, collard greens, spinach, pumpkin, rhubarb, and bran. Recommended daily calcium intake: 1-3 years: 700 mg; 4-8 years: 1,000 mg; 9-18 years: 1,300 mg; 19-50 years: 1,000 mg: 51-70 years (males): 1,000 mg; ≥51 years (females): 1,200 mg; pregnancy <u>or</u> nursing: 1,000-1,300 mg. Recommended daily vitamin D intake: >1 year: 600 IU; 50+ years: 800-1,000 IU. The American Academy of Rheumatology (AAR) recommends the following daily doses for anyone on a chronic oral corticosteroid regimen: Calcium 1,200-1,500 mg/day and vitamin D 800-1,000 IU/day.

CALCIUM SUPPLEMENTS

Comment: Take *calcium* supplements after meals to avoid gastric upset. Dosages of *calcium* over 2,000 mg/day have not been shown to have any additional benefit. *Calcium* decreases *tetracycline* absorption. *Calcium* absorption is decreased by corticosteroids.
▷ *calcitonin-salmon* (C)
        Miacalcin 200 units (1 spray intranasally) once daily; alternate nostrils each day
            Nasal spray: 14 dose (2 ml)
        Miacalcin injection 100 units/day SC <u>or</u> IM
            Vial: 2 ml
▷ *calcium carbonate* (C)(OTC)(G)
        Rolaids chew 2 tabs bid; max 14 tabs/day
            Tab: calcium carbonate: 550 mg
        Rolaids Extra Strength chew 2 tabs bid; max 8 tabs/day
            Tab: 1,000 mg
        Tums chew 2 tabs bid; max 16 tabs/day
            Tab: 500 mg
        Tums Extra Strength chew 2 tabs bid; max 10 tabs/day
            Tab: 750 mg
        Tums Ultra chew 2 tabs bid; max 8 tabs/day
            Tab: 1,000 mg
        Os-Cal 500 (OTC) 1-2 tab bid-tid
            Tab: elemental calcium carbonate 500 mg
▷ *calcium carbonate+vitamin D* (C)(G)
        Os-Cal 250+D (OTC) 1-2 tabs tid
            Tab: elemental calcium carbonate 250 mg+*vit d* 125 IU

Os-Cal 500+D (OTC) 1-2 tabs bid-tid
Tab: elemental calcium carbonate 500 mg+*vit d* 125 IU
Viactiv (OTC) 1 tab tid
Chew tab: elemental calcium 500 mg+*vit d and vit a*100 IU+*Vit k* 40 mEq
▷ *calcium citrate*
Citracal (OTC) 1-2 tabs bid
Tab: elemental calcium citrate 200 mg
▷ *calcium citrate+vitamin D* (C)(G)
Citracal+D (OTC) 1-2 cplts bid
Cplt: elemental calcium citrate 315 mg+*vit d* 200 IU
Citracal 250+D (OTC) 1-2 tabs bid
Tab: elemental calcium citrate 250 mg+*vit d* 62.3 IU

VITAMIN D ANALOGS

Comment: Concurrent *vitamin D* supplementation is contraindicated for patients taking *calcitriol* or *doxercalciferol* due to the risk of *vitamin D* toxicity. Symptoms of hypervitaminosis D: hypercalcemia, hypercalciuria, elevated creatinine, erythema multiforme, hyperphosphatemia. Maintain adequate daily calcium and fluid intake. Keep serum calcium times phosphate (Ca x P) product below 70. Monitor serum calcium (esp. during dose titration), phosphorus, other lab values (see literature for frequency).

▷ *calcitriol* (C)(G) *Predialysis:* initially 0.25 mcg daily; may increase to 0.5 mcg daily; *Dialysis:* initially 0.25 mcg daily; may increase by 0.25 mcg/day at 4-8-week intervals; usual maintenance 0.5-1 mcg/day; *Hypoparathyroidism:* initially 0.25 mcg q AM; may increase by 0.25 mcg/day at 4-8 week intervals; usual maintenance 0.5-2 mcg/day *Pediatric:* <12 years: *Predialysis:* <3 years: 10-15 ng/kg per day; ≥3 years: initially 0.25 mcg daily; may increase to 0.5 mcg daily; *Dialysis:* not recommended; *Hypoparathyroidism:* initially 0.25 mcg daily in the AM; may increase by 0.25 mcg/day at 2-4 week intervals; usual maintenance: (1-5 years): 0.25-0.75 mcg daily; (≥6 years): 0.5-2 mcg daily; *Pseudohypoparathyroidism:* (<6 years): insufficient data, see mfr pkg insert; ≥12 years: *Predialysis:* initially 0.25 mcg daily; may increase to 0.5 mcg daily *Dialysis:* initially 0.25 mcg daily; may increase by 0.25 mcg daily at 4-8 week intervals; usual maintenance: 0.5-1 mcg daily.
Rocaltrol *Cap:* 0.25, 0.5 mcg
Rocaltrol Solution *Soln:* 1 mcg/ml (15 ml, single-use dispensers)
Comment: *calcitriol* is indicated for the treatment of secondary hyperparathyroidism and resultant metabolic bone disease in predialysis patients (CrCl 15-55 mL/min), hypocalcemia and resultant metabolic bone disease in patients on chronic renal dialysis, hypocalcemia in hypoparathyroidism, and pseudohypoparathyroidism.
▷ *doxercalciferol* (C)(G) *Dialysis:* initially 10 mcg 3 x/week at dialysis; adjust to maintain intact parathyroid hormone (iPTH) between 150-300 pg/mL; if iPTH is not lowered by 50% and fails to reach target range, may increase by 2.5 mcg at 8-week intervals; max 20 mcg 3 x/week; if iPTH <100 pg/mL, suspend for 1 week, then resume at a dose that is at least 2.5 mcg lower; *Predialysis:* initially 1 mcg once daily; may increase by 0.5 mcg at 2 week intervals to target iPTH levels; max 3.5 mcg/day *Pediatric:* <12 years: not established; ≥12 years: same as adult
Hectorol *Cap:* 0.25, 0.5, 1, 2.5 mcg
Comment: Oral **Hectorol** is indicated for the treatment of secondary hyperparathyroidism in patients with chronic kidney disease (CKD) on dialysis; Predialysis stage 3 or 4 CKD: use oral form only.
Hectoral Injection <12 years: not recommended; ≥12 years: 4 mcg 3 x weekly after dialysis; adjust dose to maintain intact parathyroid hormone (iPTH) between 150-300 pg/mL; if iPTH is not lowered by 50% and fails to reach target range, may

increase by 1-2 mcg at 8 week intervals; max 18 mcg/week; if iPTH <100 pg/mL, suspend for 1 week, then resume at a dose that is at least 1 mcg lower
> *Vial:* 2 mcg/ml (1, 2 ml single-dose; 2 ml multi-dose)

Comment: **Hectorol Injection** is indicated for the treatment of secondary hyperparathyroidism in patients with chronic kidney disease (CKD) on dialysis.

➤ *paricalcitol* **(C)(G)** administer 0.04-1 mcg/kg (2.8-7 mcg) IV bolus, during dialysis, no more than every other day; may be increased by 2-4 mcg/dose every 2-4 weeks; monitor serum calcium and phosphorus during dose adjustment periods; if Ca x P >75, immediately reduce dose or discontinue until these levels normalize; discard unused portion of single-use vials immediately
Pediatric: <18 years: not established; ≥18 years: same as adult
Zemplar *Vial:* 2, 5 mcg/ml soln for inj

Comment: *paricalcitol* is indicated for the prevention and treatment of secondary hyperparathyroidism associated with chronic kidney disease (CKD) stage 5.

BIOENGINEERED REPLICA OF HUMAN PARATHYROID HORMONE

➤ *bioengineered replica of human parathyroid hormone* **(C)** before starting, confirm 25-hydroxyvitamin D stores are sufficient; if insufficient, replace to sufficient levels per standard of care; confirm serum calcium is above 7.5 mg/dL; the goal of treatment is to achieve serum calcium within the lower half of the normal range; administer SC into the thigh once daily; alternate thighs; initially, 50 mcg/day; when initiating, decrease dose of active vitamin D by 50%, if serum calcium is above 7.5 mg/dL; monitor serum calcium levels every 3 to 7 days after starting or adjusting dose and when adjusting either active vitamin D or calcium supplements dose. Abrupt interruption or discontinuation of **Natpara** can result in severe hypocalcemia. Resume treatment with, or increase the dose of, an active form of vitamin D and calcium supplements. Monitor for signs and symptoms of hypocalcemia and monitor serum calcium levels, In the case of a missed dose, the next **Natpara** dose should be administered as soon as reasonably feasible and additional exogenous calcium should be taken in the event of hypocalcemia.
Natpara *Soln for inj:* 25, 50, 75, 100 mcg (2/pkg) multiple dose, dual-chamber glass cartridge containing a sterile powder and diluent

Comment: **Natpara** is indicated as an adjunct to calcium and vitamin D in patients with hypoparathyroidism. Because of a potential risk of osteosarcoma, use **Natpara** only in patients who cannot be well-controlled on calcium and active forms of vitamin D alone and for whom the potential benefits are considered to outweigh the potential risk. Avoid use of **Natpara** in patients who are at increased baseline risk for osteosarcoma, such as patients with Paget's disease of bone or unexplained elevations of alkaline phosphatase, pediatric and young adult patients with open epiphyses, patients with hereditary disorders predisposing to osteosarcoma or patients with a prior history of external beam or implant radiation therapy involving the skeleton. Because of the risk of osteosarcoma, **Natpara** is available only through a restricted program under a Risk Evaluation and Mitigation Strategy (REMS) (www.natparaREMS.com).

HYPOKALEMIA

Comment: Normal serum K+ range is approximately 3.5-5.5 mEq/L. Signs and symptoms of hypokalemia include neuromuscular weakness, muscle twitching and cramping, hyporeflexia, postural hypotension, anorexia, nausea and vomiting, depressed ST segments, flattened T waves, and cardiac tachyarrhythmias. Signs and symptoms of hyperkalemia include peaked T waves, elevated ST segment, and widened QRS complexes.

PROPHYLAXIS

Comment: Usual dose range is 8-10 mEq/day.

TREATMENT OF HYPOKALEMIA: NONEMERGENCY (K⁺ <3.5 mEq/L)

Comment: Usual dose range 40-120 mEq/day in divided doses. Solutions are preferred; potentially serious GI side effects may occur with tablet formulations <u>or</u> when taken on an empty stomach.

POTASSIUM SUPPLEMENTS

Comment: Potassium supplements should be taken with food. Solutions are the preferred form. Extended-release and sustained-release forms should be swallowed whole; do not crush <u>or</u> chew. Potassium supplementation is indicated for hypokalemia including that caused by diuretic use, and digitalis intoxication without atrioventricular (AV) block.

▷ *potassium* (C)(G)
   Pediatric: <12 years: not established; ≥12 years: same as adult
      KCL Solution Oral soln: 10% (30 ml unit dose, 50/case)
      K-Dur (as chloride) *Tab:* 10, 20* mEq sust-rel
      K-Lor for Oral Solution (as chloride) *Pkts* for reconstitution: 20 mEq/pkt (fruit)
      Klor-Con/25 (as chloride) *Pkts* for reconstitution: 25 mEq/pkt
      Klor-Con/EF 25 (as bicarbonate) *Pkts* for reconstitution: 25 mEq/pkt (effervescent) (fruit)
      Klor-Con Extended-Release (as chloride) *Tab:* 8, 10 mEq ext-rel
      Klor-Con M (as chloride) *Tab:* 10, 15*, 20* mEq ext-rel
      Klor-Con Powder (as chloride) 20, 25 mEq *Pkts* for reconstitution: (30/carton) (fruit)
      Klorvess (as bicarbonate and citrate) *Tab:* 20 mEq effervescent for solution; *Granules:* 20 mEq/pkt effervescent for solution; *Oral liq:* 20 mEq/15 ml (16 oz)
      Klotrix (as chloride) *Tab:* 10 mEq sust-rel
      K-Lyte (as bicarbonate and citrate) *Tab:* 25 mEq effervescent for solution (lime, orange)
      K-Lyte/CL (as chloride) *Tab:* 25 mEq effervescent for solution (citrus, fruit)
      K-Lyte/CL 50 (as chloride) *Tab:* 50 mEq effervescent for solution (citrus, fruit)
      K-Lyte/DS (as bicarbonate and citrate) *Tab:* 50 mEq effervescent for solution (lime, orange)
      K-Tab (as chloride) *Tab:* 10 mEq sust-rel
      Micro-K (as chloride) *Cap:* 8, 10 mEq sust-rel
      Potassium Chloride Extended Release Caps *Cap:* 8, 10 mEq ext-rel
      Potassium Chloride Sust-Rel Tabs *Tab/Cap:* 10 mEq sust-rel
      Potassium Chloride ER *Tab:* 8 mEq (600 mg), 10 mEq (750 mg)

 HYPOMAGNESEMIA

Comment: Normal serum Mg⁺⁺ range is approximately 1.2-2.6 mEq/L. Signs and symptoms of hypomagnesemia include confusion, disorientation, hallucinations, hyperreflexia, tetany, convulsions, tachyarrhythmia, positive Chvostek's sign, and positive Trousseau's sign. Signs and symptoms of hypermagnesemia include drowsiness, lethargy, muscle weakness, hypoactive reflexes, slurred speech, bradycardia, hypotension, convulsions, and cardiac arrhythmias.

MAGNESIUM SUPPLEMENTS

▷ *magnesium* (B) 2 tabs daily
   Slow-Mag
      Tab: 64 mg (as chloride)+110 mg (as carbonate)

➤ *magnesium oxide* (B) 1-2 tabs daily
    Mag-Ox 400
      Tab: 400 mg

 HYPOPARATHYROIDISM

VITAMIN D ANALOGS

Comment: Concurrent vitamin D supplementation is contraindicated for patients taking *calcitriol* or *doxecalciferol* owing to the risk of vitamin D toxicity.
➤ *calcitriol* (C) initially 0.25 mcg q AM; may increase by 0.25 mcg/day at 4-8-week intervals; usual maintenance 0.5-2 mcg/day
    Pediatric: initially 0.25 mcg daily; may increase by 0.25 mcg/day at 2-4-week intervals; usual maintenance (1-5 years) 0.25-0.75 mcg/day, (≥6 years) 0.5-2 mcg/day
      Rocaltrol *Cap:* 0.25, 0.5 mcg
      Rocaltrol Solution *Soln:* 1 mcg/ml (15 ml, single-use dispensers)
➤ *doxecalciferol* (C) initially 0.25 mcg q AM; may increase by 0.25 mcg/day at 4-8-week intervals; usual maintenance 0.5-2 mcg/day
    Pediatric: initially 0.25 mcg daily; may increase by 0.25 mcg/day at 2-4-week intervals; usual maintenance (1-5 years) 0.25-0.75 mcg/day, (≥6 years) 0.5-2 mcg/day
      Hectorol *Cap:* 0.25, 0.5 mcg

HUMAN PARATHYROID HORMONE

➤ *teriparatide* (C) 20 mcg SC daily in the thigh or abdomen; may treat for up to 2 years
    Forteo *Multi-dose pen:* 250 mcg/ml (3 ml)
Comment: **Forteo** is indicated for the treatment of postmenopausal osteoporosis in women who are at high risk for fracture and to increase bone mass in men with primary or hypogonadal osteoporosis who are at high risk for fracture.

HUMAN PARATHYROID HORMONE RELATED PEPTIDE (PTHrP) ANALOG

➤ *abaloparatide* (C) Administer 80 mcg SC once daily into the periumbilical region of the abdomen; sit or lie down in case of orthostatic hypotension, especially for first dose; patients should receive supplemental calcium and vitamin D if dietary intake is inadequate
    Tymlos *Multi-dose pen:* 3120 mcg/1.56 *ml* (2000 mcg/ml, 30 daily doses) disposable
Comment: **Tymlos** is indicated for the treatment of postmenopausal osteoporosis in women who are at high risk for fracture (defined as a history of osteoporotic fracture, or multiple risk factors for fracture, or patients who have failed or are intolerant to other available osteoporosis therapy. **Tymlos** is not recommended in patients who are at risk for osteosarcoma (boxed warning). Cumulative use of **Tymlos** or other parathyroid analogs (e.g., *teriparatide*) for >2 years during a patient's lifetime is not recommended (boxed warning). Avoid use in patients with pre-existing hypercalcemia and those known to have an underlying hypercalcemic disorder, such as primary hyperparathyroidism. Monitor urine calcium if preexisting hypercalciuria or active urolithiasis are suspected.

BIOENGINEERED REPLICA OF HUMAN PARATHYROID HORMONE

➤ *bioengineered replica of human parathyroid hormone* (C) initially inject mg IM into the thigh once daily; when initiating, decrease dose of active vitamin D by 50% if serum calcium is above 7.5 mg/dL; monitor serum calcium levels every 3-7 days after starting or adjusting dose and when adjusting either active vitamin D or calcium supplements dose

Natpara *Soln for inj:* 25, 50, 75, 100 mcg (2/pkg) multiple dose, dual-chamber glass cartridge containing a sterile powder and diluent

Comment: Natpara is indicated as an adjunct to calcium and vitamin D in patients with parathyroidism.

 HYPOPHOSPHATASIA (OSTEOMALACIA, RICKETS)

Comment: Hypophosphatasia (HPP) is an inborn error of metabolism marked by abnormally low serum alkaline phosphatase activity and phosphoethanolamine in the urine. It is manifested by osteomalacia in adults and rickets in infants and children. It is most severe in infants under 6 months-of-age. With congenital absence of alkaline phosphatase, an enzyme essential to the calcification of bone tissue, complications include vomiting, growth retardation, and often death in infancy. Surviving children have numerous skeletal abnormalities and dwarfism.

▷ *asfotase alfa* 6 mg/kg/week SC, administered as 2 mg/kg or 1 mg/kg 6 x/week; max 9 mg/kg/week SC administered as 3 mg/kg 3 x/week
Pediatric: same as adult
　　Strensiq *Vial:* 18 mg/0.45 ml, 28 mg/0.7 ml, 40 mg/ml, 80 mg/0.8 ml for SC inj, single-use (1, 12/carton) (preservative-free)

Comment: Strensiq is the first FDA-approved (2015) treatment for perinatal, infantile, and juvenile onset HPP. Prior to the availability of **Strensiq**, there was no effective treatment and patient prognosis was very poor.

 HYPOTENSION: NEUROGENIC, ORTHOSTATIC

ALPHA-1 AGONIST

▷ *midodrine* (C)(G) 10 mg tid at 3-4-hour intervals; take while upright; take last dose at least 4 hours before bedtime
Pediatric: <12 years: not recommended; ≥12 years: same as adult
　　ProAmatine *Tab:* 2.5*, 5*, 10*mg

SYNTHETIC AMINO ACID PRECURSOR OF NOREPINEPHRINE

▷ *droxidopa* (C) initially 100 mg, taken 3 x/day (upon arising in the morning, at mid-day, and in the late afternoon at least 3 hours prior to bedtime (to reduce the potential for supine hypertension during sleep); administer with or without; swallow whole; titrate to symptomatic response, in increments of 100 mg tid every 24-48 hours; max 600 mg tid (max total 1,800 mg/day)
Pediatric: <12 years: not recommended; ≥12 years: same as adult
　　Northera *Cap:* 100, 200, 300 mg

Comment: Northera is indicated for the treatment of orthostatic dizziness, lightheadedness, or feeling about to black out in adult patients with symptomatic neurogenic orthostatic hypotension (NOH) caused by primary autonomic failure [Parkinson's disease (PD), multiple system atrophy (MSA) and pure autonomic failure], dopamine beta-hydroxylase deficiency, and nondiabetic autonomic neuropathy. Effectiveness beyond 2 weeks of treatment has not been established. The continued effectiveness of **Northera** should be assessed. Administering **Northera** in combination with other agents that increase blood pressure (e.g., norepinephrine, ephedrine, midodrine, triptans) would be expected to increase the risk for supine hypertension.

HYPOTHYROIDISM

Comment: Take thyroid replacement hormone in the morning on an empty stomach. For the elderly, start thyroid hormone replacement at 25 mcg/day. Target TSH is 0.4-5.5 mIU/L; target T4 is 4.5-12.5 ng/L. Signs and symptoms of thyroid toxicity include tachycardia, palpitations, nervousness, chest pain, heat intolerance, and weight loss.

ORAL THYROID HORMONE SUPPLEMENTS
T3

▷ *liothyronine* (A) initially 25 mcg daily; may increase by 25 mcg every 1-2 weeks as needed; usual maintenance 25-75 mcg/day
Pediatric: initially 5 mcg/day; may increase by 5 mcg/day every 3-4 days; *Cretinism:* maintenance dose: <1 year: 20 mcg/day; 1-3 years: 50 mcg/day; >3 years: same as adult

   Cytomel *Tab:* 5, 25, 50 mcg

T4

▷ *levothyroxine* (A)(G)
   Levoxyl initially 25-100 mcg/day; increase by 25 mcg/day q 2-3 weeks as needed; maintenance 100-200 mcg/day
   Pediatric: <6 months: 8-10 mcg/kg/day; 6-12 months: 6-8 mcg/kg/day; >1-5 years: 5-6 mcg/kg/day; 6-12 years: 4-5 mcg/kg/day; >12 years: same as adult
      Tab: 25*, 50* (dye-free), 75*, 88*, 100*, 112*, 125*, 137*, 150*, 175*, 200*, 300*mcg
   Synthroid initially 50 mcg/day; increase by 25 mcg/day q 2-3 weeks as needed; max 300 mcg/day
   Pediatric: <6 months: 8-10 mcg/kg/day; 6-12 months: 6-8 mcg/kg/day; >1-5 years: 5-6 mcg/kg/day; 6-12 years: 4-5 mcg/kg/day; >12 years: same as adult
      Tab: 25*, 50* (dye-free), 75*, 88*, 100*, 112*, 125*, 137*, 150*, 175*, 200*, 300*mcg
   Unithroid initially 50 mcg/day; increase by 25 mcg/day q 2-3 weeks as needed; max 300 mcg/day
   Pediatric: 0-3 months: 10-15 mcg/kg/day; 3-6 months: 8-10 mcg/kg/day; 6-12 months: 6-8 mcg/kg/day; 1-5 years: 5-6 mcg/kg/day; 6-12 years: 4-5 mcg/kg/day; >12 years: 2-3 mcg/kg/day; *Growth and puberty complete:* same as adult
      Tab: 25*, 50* (dye-free), 75*, 88*, 100*, 112*, 125*, 150*, 175*, 200*, 300*mcg

T3+T4 Combination

▷ *liothyronine+levothyroxine* (A) initially 15-30 mg/day; increase by 15 mg/day q 2-3 weeks to target goal; usual maintenance 60-120 mg/day
   Pediatric: <6 months: 4.6-6 mcg/kg/day; 6-12 months: 3.6-4.8 mcg/kg/day; >1-5 years: 3-3.6 mcg/kg/day; 6-12 years: 2.4-3 mcg/kg/day; >12 years: 1.2-1.8 mcg/kg/day; *Growth and puberty complete:* same as adult
      Armour Thyroid Tab *Tab:* per grain: T3 9 mcg+T4 38 mcg: 1/4, 1/2, 1, 1, 2, 3*, 4*, 5* gr; 15, 30, 60, 90, 120, 180*, 240*, 300*mg
      Thyrolar *Tab:* per grain: T3 12.5 mcg+T4 50 mcg: 1/4, 1/5, 1, 2, 3 gr

PARENTERAL THYROID HORMONE SUPPLEMENT

▷ *levothyroxine sodium* (A)(G) 1/2 oral dose by IV or IM and titrate; *Myxedema Coma:* 200-500 mcg IV x 1 dose; may administer 100-300 mcg (or more) IV on second day if needed; then 50-100 mcg IV daily; switch to oral form as soon as possible
   Pediatric: <12 years: not recommended; ≥12 years: same as adult
      T4 *Vial:* 100, 200, 500 mcg (pwdr for IM or IV administration after reconstitution)

HYPOTRICHOSIS (THIN/SPARSE EYELASHES)

PROSTAGLANDIN ANALOG

▷ *bimatoprost* ophthalmic solution **(C)(G)** apply one drop nightly directly to the skin of the upper eyelid margin at the base of the eyelashes using the accompanying applicators; blot any excess solution beyond the eyelid margin; dispose of the applicator after one use; repeat for the opposite eyelid margin using a new sterile applicator. Repeat treatment of the opposite eye using a new applicator

Pediatric: <16 years: not recommended; ≥16 years: same as adult

Latisse *Ophth soln:* 0.03% (3 ml in 5 ml bottle w. 70 disposable sterile applicators; 5 ml in 5 ml bottle w. 140 disposable sterile applicators)

Comment: **Latisse** is indicated to treat hypotrichosis of the eyelashes by increasing their growth including length, thickness and darkness. Ensure the face is clean, all makeup is removed, and contact lenses removed. Place one drop of **Latisse** on the disposable sterile applicator and brush cautiously along the skin of the upper eyelid margin at the base of the eyelashes. Do not to apply to the lower eyelash line. If eyelid skin darkening occurs, it may be reversible after discontinuation of **Latisse**. If any **Latisse** solution gets into the eye proper, it will not cause harm; the eye should not be rinsed. Any excess solution outside the upper eyelid margin should be blotted with a tissue or other absorbent material. Onset of effect is gradual but is not significant in the majority of patients until 2 months. The effect is not permanent and can be expected to gradually return to previous. Additional applications of **Latisse** will not increase the growth of eyelashes.

 IDIOPATHIC PULMONARY FIBROSIS (IPF)

Parenteral Corticosteroids *see page* 570
Oral Corticosteroids *see page* 569

Comment: Idiopathic pulmonary fibrosis (IPF) is a chronic, progressive, interstitial lung disease of unknown etiology. There are few effective therapies and the mortality rate is high. New treatments for IPF are urgently needed. Antiinflammatory therapy with corticosteroids or immunosuppressants fails to significantly improve the survival time of patients with IPF. Other pharmacological interventions, which include *nintedanib, etanercept, warfarin, gleevec,* and *bosentan,* remain controversial. *pirfenidone* was approved by the European Medicines Agency in 2011. In a 2016 study, *N-Acetylcysteine* was found to have a significant effect only on decreases in percentage of predicted vital capacity and 6 minutes walking test distance. *N*-acetylcysteine showed no beneficial effect on changes in forced vital capacity, changes in predicted carbon monoxide diffusing capacity, rates of adverse events, or death rates.

REFERENCES

Canestaro, W. J., Forrester, S. H., Raghu, G., Ho, L., & Devine, B. E. (2016). Drug treatment of idiopathic pulmonary fibrosis: Systematic review and network meta-analysis. *Chest, 149*(3), 756–766.

Sun, T., Liu, J., & Zhao, D. W. (2016). Efficacy of *N*-Acetylcysteine in idiopathic pulmonary fibrosis: A systematic review and meta-analysis. *Medicine, 95*(19), e3629. doi:10.1097/md.0000000000003629

▷ *azathioprine* **(D)** 1 mg/kg/day in a single or divided doses; may increase by 0.5 mg/kg/day q 4 weeks; max 2.5 mg/kg/day; minimum trial to ascertain effectiveness is 12 weeks

Pediatric: <12 years: not recommended; ≥12 years: same as adult

Azasan *Tab* 75*, 100*mg
Imuran *Tab* 50*mg

➤ *nintedanib* (D) take with food at the same time each day; take 150 mg bid, 12 hours apart; max 300 mg/day
Pediatric: <12 years: not established; ≥12 years: same as adult
   Ofev *Cap:* 100, 150 mg
Comment: Monitor liver enzymes. If elevated LFTs (3 < AST/ALT <5 XULN) without severe liver damage, interrupt therapy or reduce dose to 100 mg bid. When liver enzymes return to baseline, restart at 100 mg bid and titrate up.
➤ *pirfenidone* (C) take with food at the same time each day; *Days 1-7:* 1 cap tid; *Days 8-14:* 2 caps tid; *Days 15 and ongoing:* 3 caps tid; max 9 caps/day
Pediatric: <12 years: not established; ≥12 years: same as adult
   Esbriet *Gelcap:* 267 mg

IMPETIGO CONTAGIOSA (INDIAN FIRE)

Comment: The most common infectious organisms are *Staphylococcus aureus* and *Streptococcus pyogenes*.

TOPICAL ANTI-INFECTIVES

➤ *mupirocin* (B)(G) apply to lesions bid; apply to walls of nares bid
Pediatric: same as adult
   Bactroban *Oint:* 2% (22 gm); *Crm:* 2% (15, 30 gm)
   Centany *Oint:* 2% (15, 30 gm)

ORAL ANTI-INFECTIVES

➤ *amoxicillin* (B)(G) 500-875 mg bid or 250-500 mg tid x 10 days
Pediatric: <40 kg (88 lb): 20-40 mg/kg/day in 3 divided doses x 10 days or 25-45 mg/kg/day in 2 divided doses x 10 days; ≥40 kg: same as adult; *see page 616 for dose by weight*
   Amoxil *Cap:* 250, 500 mg; *Tab:* 875*mg; *Chew tab:* 125, 200, 250, 400 mg (cherry-banana-peppermint) (phenylalanine); *Oral susp:* 125, 250 mg/5 ml (80, 100, 150 ml) (strawberry); 200, 400 mg/5 ml (50, 75, 100 ml) (bubble gum); Oral drops: 50 mg/ml (30 ml) (bubble gum)
   Moxatag *Tab:* 775 mg ext-rel
   Trimox *Tab:* 125, 250 mg; *Cap:* 250, 500 mg; *Oral susp:* 125, 250 mg/5 ml (80, 100, 150 ml) (raspberry-strawberry)
➤ *amoxicillin+clavulanate* (B)(G)
   Augmentin 500 mg tid or 875 mg bid x 7-10 days
   Pediatric: 40-45 mg/kg/day divided tid x 10 days or 90 mg/kg/day divided bid x 10 days *see pages 618-619 for dose by weight*
     Tab: 250, 500, 875 mg; *Chew tab:* 125, 250 mg (lemon-lime); 200, 400 mg (cherry-banana) (phenylalanine); *Oral susp:* 125 mg/5 ml (banana), 250 mg/5 ml (75, 100, 150 ml) (orange); 200, 400 mg/5 ml (50, 75, 100 ml) (orange) (phenylalanine)
   Augmentin ES-600 not recommended for adults
   Pediatric: <3 months: not recommended; ≥3 months, <40 kg: 90 mg/kg/day in 2 divided doses x 7-10 days; ≥40 kg: not recommended
     Oral susp: 42.9 mg/5 ml (50, 75, 100, 125, 150, 200 ml) (strawberry cream) (phenylalanine)
   Augmentin XR 2 tabs q 12 hours x 7-10 days
   Pediatric: <16 years: use other forms; ≥16 years: same as adult
     Tab: 1000*mg ext-rel
➤ *azithromycin* (B)(G) 500 mg x 1 dose on day 1, then 250 mg daily on days 2-5 or 500 mg daily x 3 days or 2 gm in a single dose

Zithromax *Tab:* 250, 500, 600 mg; *Oral susp:* 100 mg/5 ml (15 ml); 200 mg/5 ml (15, 22.5, 30 ml) (cherry); *Pkt:* 1 gm for reconstitution (cherry-banana)

Zithromax Tri-pak *Tab:* 3 x 500 mg tabs/pck

Zithromax Z-pak *Tab:* 6 x 250 mg tabs/pck

Zmax *Oral susp:* 2 gm ext-rel for reconstitution (cherry-banana) (148 mg Na$^+$)

▷ *cefaclor* (B)(G) 250-500 mg q 8 hours x 10 days; max 2 gm/day
Pediatric: <1 month: not recommended; 20-40 mg/kg bid or q 12 hours x 10 days; max 1 gm/day; *see page 622 for dose by weight*
    Tab: 500 mg; *Cap:* 250, 500 mg; *Susp:* 125 mg/5 ml (75, 150 ml) (strawberry); 187 mg/5 ml (50, 100 ml) (strawberry); 250 mg/5 ml (75, 150 ml) (strawberry); 375 mg/5 ml (50, 100 ml) (strawberry)
    Cefaclor Extended Release *Tab:* 375, 500 mg ext-rel
    Pediatric: <16 years: ext-rel not recommended; ≥16 years: same as adult

▷ *cefadroxil* (B) 1-2 gm in 1-2 divided doses x 10 days
Pediatric: 30 mg/kg/day in 2 divided doses x 10 days; *see page 623 for dose by weight*
    Duricef *Cap:* 500 mg; *Tab:* 1 gm; *Oral susp:* 250 mg/5 ml (100 ml); 500 mg/5 ml (75, 100 ml) (orange-pineapple)

▷ *cefpodoxime proxetil* (B) 200 mg bid x 10 days
Pediatric: <2 months: not recommended; 2 months-12 years: 10 mg/kg/day (max 400 mg/dose) or 5 mg/kg/day bid (max 200 mg/dose) x 10 days; *see page 626 for dose by weight*
    Vantin *Tab:* 100, 200 mg; *Oral susp:* 50, 100 mg/5 ml (50, 75, 100 mg) (lemon creme)

▷ *cefprozil* (B) 500 mg bid x 10 days
Pediatric: ≤6 months: not recommended; 6 months-12 years: *see page 627 for dose by weight*
    Cefzil *Tab:* 250, 500 mg; *Oral susp:* 125, 250 mg/5 ml (50, 75, 100 ml) (bubble gum) (phenylalanine)

▷ *ceftaroline fosamil* (B) administer by IV infusion after reconstitution every 12 hours x 5-14 days; *CrCl >50 mL/min:* 600 mg; *CrCl >30-<50 mL/min:* 400 mg; *CrCl >1 5-<30 mL/min:* 300 mg; *ESRD:* 200 mg
    Teflaro *Vial:* 400, 600 mg

▷ *cephalexin* (B) (G) 250-500 mg qid or 500 mg bid x 10 days
Pediatric: 25-50 mg/kg/day in 4 divided doses x 10 days; *see page 629 for dose by weight*
    Keflex *Cap:* 250, 333, 500, 750 mg; *Oral susp:* 125, 250 mg/5 ml (100, 200 ml) (strawberry)

▷ *clarithromycin* (C)(G) 500 mg or 500 mg ext-rel daily x 7 days
Pediatric: <6 months: not recommended; ≥6 months: 7.5 mg/kg bid x 7 days; *see page 630 for dose by weight*
    Biaxin *Tab:* 250, 500 mg
    Biaxin Oral Suspension *Oral susp:* 125, 250 mg/5 ml (50, 100 ml) (fruit punch)
    Biaxin XL *Tab:* 500 mg ext-rel

▷ *dicloxacillin* (B) (G) 500 mg q 6 hours x 10 days
Pediatric: 12.5-25 mg/kg/day in 4 divided doses x 10 days; *see page 632 for dose by weight*
    Dynapen *Cap:* 125, 250, 500 mg; *Oral susp:* 62.5 mg/5 ml (80, 100, 200 ml)

▷ *erythromycin base* (B)(G) 250 mg qid, or 333 mg tid, or 500 mg bid x 7-10 days
Pediatric: ≤45 kg: 30-50 mg in 2-4 divided doses x 7-10 days; ≥45 kg: same as adult
    Ery-Tab *Tab:* 250, 333, 500 mg ent-coat
    PCE *Tab:* 333, 500 mg

Comment: *erythromycin* may increase INR with concomitant *warfarin*, as well as increase serum level of *digoxin*, benzodiazepines and statins.

▶ *erythromycin ethylsuccinate* (B)(G) 400 mg tid x 7-10 days
Pediatric: 30-50 mg/kg/day in 4 divided doses x 7-10 days; may double dose with severe infection; max 100 mg/kg/day; *see page 635 for dose by weight*
    EryPed *Oral susp:* 200 mg/5 ml (100, 200 ml) (fruit); 400 mg/5 ml (60, 100, 200 ml) (banana); *Oral drops:* 200, 400 mg/5 ml (50 ml) (fruit); *Chew tab:* 200 mg wafer (fruit)
    E.E.S. *Oral susp:* 200, 400 mg/5 ml (100 ml) (fruit)
    E.E.S. Granules *Oral susp:* 200 mg/5 ml (100, 200 ml) (cherry)
    E.E.S. 400 Tablets *Tab:* 400 mg
Comment: *erythromycin* may increase INR with concomitant *warfarin*, as well as increase serum level of *digoxin*, benzodiazepines and statins.
▶ *loracarbef* (B) 200 mg bid x 10 days
Pediatric: 15 mg/kg/day in 2 divided doses x 10 days; *see page 642 for dose by weight*
Pediatric: 30 mg/kg/day in 2 divided doses x 7 days
    Lorabid *Pulvule:* 200, 400 mg; *Oral susp:* 100 mg/5 ml (50, 100 ml); 200 mg/5 ml (50, 75, 100 ml) (strawberry bubble gum)
▶ *penicillin g (benzathine)* (B) 1.2 million units IM x 1 dose
Pediatric: <60 lb: 300,000-600,000 units IM x 1 dose; ≥60 lb: 900,000 units x 1 dose
    Bicillin L-A *Cartridge-needle unit:* 600,000 units (1 ml); 1.2 million units (2 ml)
▶ *penicillin g (benzathine procaine)* (B) (G) 2.4 million units IM x 1 dose
Pediatric: <30 lb: 600,000 units IM x 1 dose; 30-60 lb: 900,000-1.2 million units IM x 1 dose
    Bicillin C-R *Cartridge-needle unit:* 600,000 units (1 ml); 1.2 million units (2 ml); 2.4 million units (4 ml)
▶ *penicillin v potassium* (B) 250-500 mg q 6 hours x 10 days
Pediatric: 50 mg/kg/day in 4 divided doses x 3 days; ≥12 years: same as adult; *see page 644 for dose by weight*
    Pen-Vee K *Tab:* 250, 500 mg; *Oral soln:* 125 mg/5 ml (100, 200 ml); 250 mg/5 ml (100, 150, 200 ml)

INCONTINENCE: FECAL

Comment: Treatment of fecal incontinence in patients who have failed conservative therapy (e.g., diet, fiber therapy, antimotility agents).
▶ *dextranomer microspheres+sodium hyaluronate*
Pediatric: <18 years: not recommended; ≥18 years: same as adult
    Pretreatment: bowel preparation using enema (required) and prophylactic antibiotics (recommended) prior to injection
    Treatment: inject slowly into the deep submucosal layer in the proximal part of the high pressure zone of the anal canal about 5 mm above the dentate line; four 1-ml injections in the following order: posterior, left lateral, anterior, right lateral; keep needle in place 15-30 seconds to minimize leakage; use a new needle for each syringe and injection site
    Posttreatment: avoid hot baths and physical activity during first 24 hours; avoid antidiarrheal drugs, sexual intercourse, and strenuous activity for 1 week; avoid anal manipulation for 1 month
    Retreatment: may repeat if needed with max 4 ml, no sooner than 4 weeks after the first injection; point of injection should be made in between initial injection sites (i.e., shifted 1/8 of a turn)
    Solesta *dex micro* 50 mg+*sod hyal* 15 mg per ml
        Syringe: 1 ml (4 w. needles)

INCONTINENCE: URINARY OVERACTIVE BLADDER, STRESS INCONTINENCE, URGE INCONTINENCE

See **Enuresis** *page* 158

▷ *estrogen* replacement (X) *see* **Menopause** *page* 295
▷ *pseudoephedrine* (C)(G) 30-60 mg tid
    Sudafed (OTC) *Tab:* 30 mg; *Liq:* 15 mg/5 ml (1, 4 oz)

VASOPRESSIN

▷ *desmopressin acetate (DDAVP)* (B)(G)
    DDAVP usual dosage 0.1-1.2 mg/day in 2-3 divided doses; 0.2 mg q HS prn for nocturnal enuresis
    Pediatric: <6 years: not recommended; ≥6 years: 0.5 mg daily or q HS prn
    Tab: 0.1*, 0.2*mg
    DDAVP Rhinal Tube
    Pediatric: <6 years: not recommended; ≥6 years: 10 mcg or 0.1 ml of soln each nostril (20 mcg total dose) q HS prn; max 40 mcg total dose
    Rhinal tube: 0.1 mg/ml (2.5 ml)

BETA-3 ADRENERGIC AGONIST

▷ *mirabegron* (C) initially 25 mg once daily; max 50 mg once daily; severe renal impairment, 25 mg once daily
    Myrbetriq *Tab:* 25, 50 mg ext-rel

MUSCARINIC RECEPTOR ANTAGONISTS

▷ *fesoterodine* (C)(G) 4 mg daily; max 8 mg/day
    Pediatric: <12 years: not recommended; ≥12 years: same as adult
    Toviaz *Tab:* 4, 8 mg ext-rel
▷ *tolterodine tartrate* (C)(G)
    Pediatric: <12 years: not recommended; ≥12 years: same as adult
    Detrol 2 mg bid; may decrease to 1 mg bid
        Tab: 1, 2 mg
    Detrol LA 2-4 mg once daily
        Cap: 2, 4 mg ext-rel

ANTISPASMODIC/ANTICHOLINERGICS AGENTS

▷ *darifenacin* (C) 7.5-15 mg daily with liquid; max 15 mg/day
    Pediatric: <12 years: not recommended; ≥12 years: same as adult
        Enablex 7.5-15 mg daily with liquid; max 15 mg/day
        Tab: 7.5, 15 mg ext-rel
▷ *dicyclomine* (B)(G) 10-20 mg qid
    Pediatric: <12 years: not recommended; ≥12 years: same as adult
        Bentyl *Tab:* 20 mg; *Cap:* 10 mg; *Syr:* 10 mg/5 ml (16 oz)
▷ *flavoxate* (B) 100-200 mg tid-qid
    Pediatric: <12 years: not recommended; ≥12 years: same as adult
        Urispas *Tab:* 100 mg
▷ *hyoscyamine* (C)(G)
        Anaspaz 1-2 tabs q 4 hours prn; max 12 tabs/day
        Pediatric: <2 years: not recommended; 2-12 years: 0.0625-0.125 mg q 4 hours prn; max 0.75 mg/day
        Tab: 0.125*mg
        Levbid 1-2 tabs q 12 hours prn; max 4 tabs/day
        Pediatric: <12 years: not recommended; ≥12 years: same as adult
        Tab: 0.375*mg ext-rel

Levsin 1-2 tabs q 4 hours prn; max 12 tabs/day
Pediatric: <6 years: not recommended; 6-12 years: 1 tab q 4 hours prn
    Tab: 0.125*mg
Levsin Drops 1-2 ml q 4 hours prn; max 60 ml/day
Pediatric: 3.4 kg: 4 drops q 4 hours prn; max 24 drops/day; 5 kg: 5 drops q 4 hours prn; max 30 drops/day; 7 kg: 6 drops q 4 hours prn; max 36 drops/day; 10 kg: 8 drops q 4 hours prn; max 40 drops/day; 2-12 years: 0.25-1 ml; max 6 ml/day
    Oral drops: 0.125 mg/ml (15 ml) (orange) (alcohol 5%)
Levsin Elixir 5-10 ml q 4 hours prn
Pediatric: <10 kg: use drops; 10-19 kg: 1.25 ml q 4 hours prn; 20-39 kg: 2.5 ml q 4 hours prn; 40-49 kg: 3.75 ml q 4 hours prn; ≥50 kg: 5 ml q 4 hours prn
    Elix: 0.125 mg/5 ml (16 oz) (orange) (alcohol 20%)
Levsinex SL 1-2 tabs q 4 hours SL <u>or</u> PO; max 12 tabs/day
Pediatric: <2 years: not recommended; 2-12 years: 1 tab q 4 hours; max 6 tabs/day; >12 years: same as adult
    Tab: 0.125 mg sublingual
Levsinex Timecaps 1-2 caps q 12 hours; may adjust to 1 cap q 8 hours
Pediatric: 2-12 years: 1 cap q 12 hours; max 2 caps/day; >12 years: same as adult
    Cap: 0.375 mg time-rel
NuLev dissolve 1-2 tabs on tongue, with <u>or</u> without water, q 4 hours prn; max 12 tabs/day
Pediatric: <2 years: not recommended; 2-12 years: dissolve 1 tab on tongue, with <u>or</u> without water, q 4 hours prn; max 6 tabs/day; ≥12 years: same as adult
    ODT: 0.125 mg (mint) (phenylalanine)
➢ *oxybutynin chloride* (B)
    Ditropan 5 mg bid-tid; max 20 mg/day
Pediatric: <5 years: not recommended; 5-12 years: 5 mg bid; max 15 mg/day; ≥16 years: same as adult
    Tab: 5*mg; *Syr:* 5 mg/5 ml
Ditropan XL initially 5 mg daily; may increase weekly in 5-mg increments as needed; max 30 mg/day
Pediatric: <6 years: not recommended; ≥6 years: initially 5 mg once daily; may increase weekly in 5-mg increments as needed; max 20 mg/day
    Tab: 5, 10, 15 mg ext-rel
GelniQUE 3 mg Pump: apply 3 pumps (84 mg) once daily to clean dry intact skin on the abdomen, upper arm, shoulders, <u>or</u> thighs; rotate sites; wash hands; avoid washing application site for 1 hour after application
Pediatric: <12 years: not recommended; ≥12 years: same as adult
    Gel: 3% (92 gm, metered pump dispenser) (alcohol)
GelniQUE 1 gm Sachet: apply 1 gm gel (1 sachet) once daily to dry intact skin on abdomen, upper arms/shoulders, <u>or</u> thighs; rotate sites; wash hands; avoid washing application site for 1 hour after application
Pediatric: <12 years: not recommended; ≥12 years: same as adult
    Gel: 10%, 1 gm/sachet (30/carton) (alcohol)
Oxytrol Transdermal Patch (OTC): apply patch to clean dry area of the abdomen, hip, <u>or</u> buttock; one patch twice weekly; rotate sites
Pediatric: <12 years: not recommended; ≥12 years: same as adult
    Transdermal patch: 3.9 mg/day
➢ *propantheline* (C) 15-30 mg tid
Pediatric: <12 years: not recommended; ≥12 years: same as adult
    Pro-Banthine *Tab:* 7.5, 15 mg
➢ *solifenacin* (C)(G) 5-10 mg daily
Pediatric: <12 years: not recommended; ≥12 years: same as adult
    VESIcare *Tab:* 5, 10 mg

▷ *trospium chloride* (C)(G)
    Pediatric: <12 years: not recommended; ≥12 years: same as adult
        Sanctura 20 mg twice daily; ≥75 years: *CrCl ≤30 mL/min:* 20 mg once daily
            Tab: 20 mg
        Sanctura XR 60 mg daily in the morning
            Cap: 60 mg ext-rel
Comment: Take *trospium chloride* on an empty stomach.

OVERFLOW INCONTINENCE: ATONIC BLADDER

▷ *bethanechol* (C) 10-30 mg tid
    Urecholine *Tab:* 5, 10, 25, 50 mg

OVERFLOW INCONTINENCE: PROSTATIC ENLARGEMENT

Alpha-1 Blockers

Comment: Educate the patient regarding the potential side effect of hypotension when taking an alpha-1 blocker, especially with first dose. Start at lowest dose and titrate upward.
▷ *terazosin* (C) initially 1 mg q HS; titrate to 10 mg q HS; max 20 mg/day
    Hytrin *Cap:* 1, 2, 5, 10 mg
▷ *doxazosin* (C) initially 1 mg q HS; may double dose every 1-2 weeks; max 8 mg/day
    Cardura *Tab:* 1*, 2*, 4*, 8*mg
    Cardura XL *Tab:* 4, 8 mg
▷ *prazosin* (C)(G) 1-15 mg q HS; max 15 mg/day
    Minipress *Tab:* 1, 2, 5 mg
▷ *tamsulosin* (C) initially 0.4 mg daily; may increase to 0.8 mg daily after 2-4 weeks if needed
    Flomax *Cap:* 0.4 mg

5-ALPHA REDUCTASE INHIBITOR

▷ *finasteride* (X)(G) 5 mg daily
    Proscar *Tab:* 5 mg

ALPHA 1A-BLOCKER

▷ *silodosin* (B)(G) take 8 mg with food once daily; *CrCl 30-50 mL/min:* take 4 mg
    Rapaflo *Cap:* 4, 8 mg

 INFLUENZA (FLU)

Comment: Egg allergy affects as many as 2% of children in the US. New data have affirmed what the American College of Allergy, Asthma and Immunology said has been known for several years: there are no special precautions needed to dispense the influenza vaccine in people with egg allergy. Based on recommendations from the clinical immunization safety assessment hypersensitivity working group of the ACIP, the members voted during the meeting this week to recommend administration of trivalent inactivated influenza vaccine to patients with a history of egg allergy. The consensus of the working group: egg allergy of any severity, including anaphylaxis, should not be a contraindication of the administration of the influenza vaccine, but rather a precaution. Both the single-dose and two-dose methods are appropriate for administering influenza vaccine to those who are allergic to eggs. No special precautions beyond those recommended for providing any vaccine to any patient are necessary for administration of influenza vaccine to persons allergic to eggs. The recommendation will be included in the ACIP draft guidelines for use of influenza vaccines for the upcoming season.

REFERENCES

Greenhawt, M., Turner, P. J., & Kelso, J. M. (2017). Allergy experts set the record straight on flu shots for patients with egg sensitivity. *Annals of Allergy, Asthma & Immunology*. doi:10.1016/j.anai.2017.10.020.

Turner, P. J., Southern, J., Andrews, N. J., Miller, E., Erlewyn-Lajeunesse, M., Doyle, C., . . . Turner, P. J. (2015). Safety of live attenuated influenza vaccine in atopic children with egg allergy. *Journal of Allergy and Clinical Immunology, 136*(2), 376–381. doi:10.1016/j.jaci.2014.12.1925

Comment: Until official guidelines are available, provider discretion should be used with appropriate precautions with individual patient consideration and informed consent. Refer to mfr's pkg insert for product maker's recommendations and precautions. With the exception of **Flucelvax**, current flu vaccine mfr pkg inserts report that flu vaccine is contraindicated with allergy to egg or chicken proteins, or egg products, and all flu vaccines are contraindicated with allergy to latex, active infection, acute respiratory disease, active neurological disorder; history of Guillain-Barre syndrome. Have epinephrine 1:1,000 on hand. Flu vaccine is contraindicated for children under 18 years-of-age who are taking *aspirin* and/or an *aspirin*-containing product due to the risk of developing Reye's syndrome. Under 1 year-of-age, administer flu vaccine in the vastus lateralis in two split doses one month apart. Over 1 year-of-age, administer flu vaccine in the deltoid. Flu vaccine formulations change annually. Administer flu vaccine 1 month before flu season. Flu vaccine delivered via nasal spray may be administered earlier.

PROPHYLAXIS (NASAL SPRAY)

▷ *trivalent, live attenuated influenza* vaccine, types A and B **(C)** 1 spray each nostril; ≥50 years not recommended

Pediatric: ≤5 years: not recommended; ≥5 years: same as adult

Never vaccinated with FluMist: 5-8 years: 2 divided doses 46-74 days apart. *Previously vaccinated with FluMist:* 5-8 years: same as adult

FluMist Nasal Spray 0.5 ml spray annually

Nasal spray: 0.5 ml (0.25 ml/spray) (10/carton) (preservative-free)

PROPHYLAXIS (INJECTABLE)

▷ *quadrivalent inactivated influenza subvirion vaccine, types a and b* (C)

Fluad 0.5 ml IM annually

Comment: **Fluad** is the first seasonal influenza vaccine with adjuvant, indicated for persona ≥65 years-of-age. Adjuvants are incorporated into some vaccine formulations to enhance or direct the immune response.

Fluarix Quadrivalent 0.5 ml IM annually

Pediatric: <3 years: not recommended; ≥3 years: same as adult

Prefilled syringe: 0.5 ml (10/carton) (preservative-free, latex-free)

▷ *trivalent inactivated influenza subvirion vaccine, types a and b*

Afluria (B) <5 years: not recommended; 5-8 years: 1-2 doses/season at least 4 weeks apart; >9 years: 1 dose/season

Comment: Contraindicated with allergy to egg or chicken protein, neomycin, polymyxin, or history of life-threatening reaction to any previous fly vaccine.

Fluarix (B) 0.5 ml IM annually

Pediatric: <3 years: not recommended; 3-9 years (previously unvaccinated or vaccinated for the first time last season with one dose of flu vaccine): 2 doses per season at least 1 month apart; 3-9 years (previously vaccinated with two doses of flu vaccine) or >9 years: 1 dose per season

Prefilled syringe: 0.5 ml single-dose (5/carton) (may contain trace amounts of hydrocortisone, gentamicin; preservative-free)

Flublok 0.5 ml IM annually; ≥49 years, not recommended

Pediatric: <18 years: not recommended; ≥18 years: same as adult

Vial: 0.5 ml single-dose (10/carton) (preservative-free, egg protein-free, antibiotic-free, latex-free)

Comment: **Flublok** is a cell culture-derived vaccine and, therefore, is an alternative to the traditional egg-based vaccines. Contains 3 times the amount of active ingredient in traditional flu vaccines **Flucelvax** 0.5 ml IM annually

Pediatric: <18 years: not recommended; ≥18 years: same as adult
Prefilled syringes: 0.5 ml (10/carton; preservative-free, latex-free)

Comment: **Flucelvax** is a cell culture-derived vaccine and, therefore, is an alternative to the traditional egg-based vaccines.

FluLaval (C) 0.5 ml IM annually
Pediatric: <6 months: not recommended; ≥6 years: same as adult
Vial: (5 ml)

FluShield 0.5 ml IM annually
Pediatric: <6 months: not recommended; *Never vaccinated:* <9 years: 2 doses at least 4 weeks apart; 9-12 years: same as adult; *Previously vaccinated:* 6-35 months: 0.25 ml IM x 1 dose; 3-8 years: same as adult

Fluzone 0.5 ml IM annually
Vial: 5 ml (thimerosal)

Fluzone Preservative-Free: Adult Dose 0.5 ml IM annually
Pediatric: <6 months: not recommended; *Not previously vaccinated:* 6 months-8 years: 0.25 ml IM; repeat in 1 month; *Previously vaccinated:* 6-35 months: 0.25 ml IM x 1 dose; >3 years: same as adult
Prefilled syringe: 0.5 ml (10/carton) (preservative-free, trace thimerosal)

Fluzone Preservative-Free: Pediatric Dose
Pediatric: <6 months: not recommended; *Not previously vaccinated:* 6 months-8 years: 0.25 ml IM; repeat in 1 month; *Previously vaccinated:* 6-35 months: 0.25 ml IM x 1 dose; ≥3 years: 0.5 ml IM (use **Fluzone for Adult**)
Prefilled syringe: 0.5 ml (10/carton; preservative-free; trace thimerosal)

Comment: Contraindicated with allergy to egg protein, or history of life-threatening reaction to any previous flu vaccine.

PROPHYLAXIS AND TREATMENT

Neuraminidase Inhibitors

Comment: Effective for influenza type A and B. Indicated for treatment of uncomplicated acute illness in patients who have been symptomatic for no more than 2 days; therefore, start within 2 days of symptom onset <u>or</u> exposure. Indicated for influenza prophylaxis in patients ≥3 months of age.

▷ *oseltamivir* phosphate (C)(G)
Prophylaxis: 75 mg daily for at least 7 days and up to 6 weeks for community outbreak
Pediatric: <1 year: not recommended; 1-12 years: <15 kg: 30 mg once daily x 10 days; 16-23 kg: 45 mg once daily x 10 days; 24-40 kg: 60 mg once daily x 10 days; >40 kg: same as adult
Treatment: 75 mg bid x 5 days; initiate treatment only if symptomatic <2 days
Pediatric: <1 year: not recommended; 1-12 years: <15 kg: 30 mg bid x 5 days; 16-23 kg: 45 mg bid x 5 days; 24-40 kg: 60 mg bid x 5 days; >40 kg: same as adult
Tamiflu *Cap:* 30, 45, 75 mg; *Oral susp:* 6 mg/ml pwdr for reconstitution (60 ml w. oral dispenser) (tutti-frutti)

Comment: **Tamiflu** is effective for influenza type A and B.
▷ *zanamivir* (C) 2 inhalations (10 mg) bid x 5 days
Pediatric: <7 years: not recommended; ≥7 years: same as adult
Relenza Inhaler *Inhaler:* 5 mg/inh blister; 4 blisters/Rotadisk (5 Rotadisks/carton w. 1 inhaler)

Comment: Relenza Inhaler is effective for influenza type A and B. Use caution with asthma and COPD.

 INSECT BITE/STING

Topical Corticosteroids *see page* 566
Parenteral Corticosteroids *see page* 570
Oral Corticosteroids *see page* 569

TOPICAL ANESTHETIC

▷ *lidocaine* 3% cream **(B)** apply bid-tid prn
   Pediatric: reduce dosage commensurate with age, body weight, and physical condition
      LidaMantle *Crm:* 3% (1 oz)
Drugs for the Management of Allergy, Cough, and Cold Symptoms *see page* 598

EPINEPHRINE

▷ *epinephrine* **(C)(G)** 1:1,000 0.3-0.5 ml SC
   Pediatric: 0.01 ml/kg SC

TETANUS PROPHYLAXIS

▷ *tetanus toxoid* vaccine **(C)(G)** 0.5 ml IM x 1 dose if previously immunized
   Vial: 5 Lf units/0.5 ml (0.5, 5 ml); *Prefilled syringe:* 5 Lf units/0.5 ml (0.5 ml) (For patients not previously immunized *see* **Tetanus** page 460)

 INSOMNIA

Tricyclic Antidepressants *see* **Depression** page 117

MELATONIN RECEPTOR AGONIST

▷ *ramelteon* **(C)(IV)** 8 mg within 30 minutes of bedtime; delayed effect if taken with a meal
   Pediatric: <12 years: not recommended; ≥12 years: same as adult
      Rozerem *Tab:* 8 mg

NON-BENZODIAZEPINES

▷ *eszopiclone* **(C)(IV)(G)** (pyrrolopyrazine) 1-3 mg; max 3 mg/day x 1 month; do not take if unable to sleep for at least 8 hours before required to be active again; delayed effect if taken with a meal
   Pediatric: <18 years: not recommended; ≥18 years: same as adult
      Lunesta *Tab:* 1, 2, 3 mg
▷ *zaleplon* **(C)(IV)** (imidazopyridine) 5-10 mg at HS <u>or</u> after going to bed if unable to sleep; do not take if unable to sleep for at least 4 hours before required to be active again; max 20 mg/day x 1 month; delayed effect if taken with a meal
   Pediatric: <12 years: not recommended; ≥12 years: same as adult
      Sonata *Cap:* 5, 10 mg (tartrazine)
Comment: Sonata is indicated for the treatment of insomnia when a middle-of-the-night awakening is followed by difficulty returning to sleep.
▷ *zolpidem* oral solution spray **(C)(IV)** (imidazopyridine hypnotic) 2 actuations (10 mg) immediately before bedtime; *Elderly, debilitated,* <u>or</u> *hepatic impairment:* 2 actuations (5 mg); max 2 actuations (10 mg)

Pediatric: <18 years: not recommended; ≥18 years: same as adult

    ZolpiMist *Oral soln spray:* 5 mg/actuation (60 metered actuations) (cherry)

Comment: The lowest dose of **zolpidem** in all forms is recommended for persons >50 years-of-age and women as drug elimination is slower than in men.

▷ *zolpidem* tabs (B)(IV)(G) (pyrazolopyrimidine hypnotic) 5-10 mg <u>or</u> 6.25-12.5 ext-rel q HS prn; max 12.5 mg/day x 1 month; do not take if unable to sleep for at least 8 hours before required to be active again; delayed effect if taken with a meal

Pediatric: <18 years: not recommended; ≥18 years: same as adult

    Ambien *Tab:* 5, 10 mg

    Ambien CR *Tab:* 6.25, 12.5 mg ext-rel

Comment: The lowest dose of **zolpidem** in all forms is recommended for persons >50 years-of-age and women as drug elimination is slower than in men.

▷ *zolpidem* sublingual tabs (C)(IV)(G) (imidazopyridine hypnotic) dissolve 1 tab under the tongue; allow to disintegrate completely before swallowing; take only once per night and only if at least 4 hours of bedtime remain before planned time for awakening

Pediatric: <18 years: not recommended; ≥18 years: same as adult

    Edluar *SL Tab:* 5, 10 mg

    Intermezzo *SL Tab:* 1.75, 3.5 mg

Comment: Intermezzo is indicated for the treatment of insomnia when a middle-of-the-night awakening is followed by difficulty returning to sleep. The lowest dose of **zolpidem** in all forms is recommended for persons >50 years-of-age and women as drug elimination is slower than in men.

OREXIN RECEPTOR ANTAGONIST

▷ *suvorexant* (C)(IV) use lowest effective dose; take 30 minutes before bedtime; do not take if unable to sleep for ≥7 hours, max 20 mg

Pediatric: <12 years: not recommended; ≥12 years: same as adult

    Belsomra *Tab:* 5, 10, 15, 20 mg (30/blister pck)

BENZODIAZEPINES

▷ *estazolam* (X)(IV)(G) initially 1 mg q HS prn; may increase to 2 mg q HS

Pediatric: <18 years: not recommended; ≥18 years: same as adult

    ProSom *Tab:* 1*, 2*mg

▷ *flurazepam* (X)(IV)(G) 30 mg q HS prn; elderly <u>or</u> debilitated, 15 mg

Pediatric: <15 years: not recommended; ≥15 years: same as adult

    Dalmane *Cap:* 15, 30 mg

▷ *temazepam* (X)(IV)(G) 7.5-30 mg q HS prn; short term, 7-10 days; max 30 mg; max 1 month

Pediatric: <18 years: not recommended; ≥18 years: same as adult

    Restoril *Cap:* 7.5, 15, 22.5, 30 mg

▷ *triazolam* (X)(IV) 0.125-0.25 mg q HS prn; short term, 7-10 days; max 0.5 mg; max 1 month

Pediatric: <18 years: not recommended; ≥18 years: same as adult

    Halcion *Tab:* 0.125, 0.25*mg

    Barbiturates

▷ *pentobarbital* (D)(II)(G)

    Nembutal 100 mg q HS prn

        Cap: 50, 100 mg

    Nembutal Suppository 120 <u>or</u> 200 mg suppository rectally q HS prn

Pediatric: 2-12 months (10-20 lb): 30 mg supp; 1-4 years (21-40 lb): 30 <u>or</u> 60 mg supp; 5-12 years (41-80 lb): 60 mg supp; 12-14 years (81-110 lb): 60 <u>or</u> 120 mg sup

        Rectal supp: 30, 60, 120, 200 mg

ORAL H1 RECEPTOR AGONIST (FIRST GENERATION ANTIHISTAMINE)

▷ *doxepin* (C)
>> **Silenor** 3-6 mg q HS prn; *Elderly, hepatic impairment, tendency to urinary reten-*
>> *tion*: initially 3 mg
>>> *Tab:* 3, 6 mg

Other Oral 1st Generation Antihistamines *see page* 598

ANALGESIC+FIRST GENERATION ANTIHISTAMINE COMBINATIONS

▷ *acetaminophen+diphenhydramine* (B)
>> **Excedrin PM** (OTC) 2 tabs q HS prn
>>> *Pediatric:* <12 years: not recommended; ≥12 years: same as adult
>>> *Tab/Geltab:* acet 500 mg+diphen 38 mg
>> **Tylenol PM** (OTC) 2 caps q HS prn
>>> *Pediatric:* <12 years: not recommended; ≥12 years: same as adult
>>> *Tab/Cap/Gel cap:* acet 500 mg+diphen 25 mg

 INTERSTITIAL CYSTITIS

Acetaminophen for IV Infusion *see Pain page* 344
Oral Prescription NSAIDs *see page* 562
Comment: Avoid peppers and spicy food, citrus, vinegar, caffeine (e.g., coffee, tea, colas), alcohol, carbonated beverages, and other GU tract irritants.

MANAGEMENT OF PAIN AND URINARY URGENCY

▷ *phenazopyridine* (B)(G) 95-200 mg q 6 hours prn; max 2 days
> *Pediatric:* <12 years: not recommended; ≥12 years: same as adult
>> **AZO Standard, Prodium, Uristat** (OTC) *Tab:* 95 mg
>> **AZO Standard Maximum Strength** (OTC) *Tab:* 97.5 mg
>> **Pyridium, Urogesic** *Tab:* 100, 200 mg *phenazopyridine* (B)(G) 190-200 mg tid;
>> max 2 days
>> **Azo Standard** (OTC) *Tab:* 95 mg
>> **Azo Standard Maximum Strength** (OTC) *Tab:* 97.5 mg
>> **Pyridium** *Tab:* 100, 200 mg ent-coat
>> **Uristat** (OTC) *Tab:* 95 mg
>> **Urogesic** *Tab:* 100, 200 mg
▷ *hyoscyamine* (C)(G)
>> **Anaspaz** 1-2 tabs q 4 hours prn; max 12 tabs/day
>> *Pediatric:* <2 years: not recommended; 2-12 years: 0.0625-0.125 mg q 4 hours prn;
>> max 0.75 mg/day; ≥12 years: same as adult
>>> *Tab:* 0.125*mg
>> **Levbid** 1-2 tabs q 12 hours prn; max 4 tabs/day
>> *Pediatric:* <12 years: not recommended; ≥12 years: same as adult
>>> *Tab:* 0.375*mg ext-rel
>> **Levsin** 1-2 tabs q 4 hours prn; max 12 tabs/day
>> *Pediatric:* <6 years: not recommended; 6-12 years: 1 tab q 4 hours prn; ≥12 years:
>> same as adult
>>> *Tab:* 0.125*mg
>> **Levsin Drops** 1-2 ml q 4 hours prn; max 60 ml/day
>> *Pediatric:* 3.4 kg: 4 drops q 4 hours prn; max 24 drops/day; 5 kg: 5 drops q 4 hours
>> prn; max 30 drops/day; 7 kg: 6 drops q 4 hours prn; max 36 drops/day; 10 kg: 8
>> drops q 4 hours prn; max 40 drops/day
>>> *Oral drops:* 0.125 mg/ml (15 ml) (orange) (alcohol 5%)

Levsin Elixir 5-10 ml q 4 hours prn
Pediatric: <10 kg: use drops; 10-19 kg: 1.25 ml q 4 hours prn; 20-39 kg: 2.5 ml q 4
hours prn; 40-49 kg: 3.75 ml q 4 hours prn; ≥50 kg: 5 ml q 4 hours prn;
  Elix: 0.125 mg/5 ml (16 oz) (orange) (alcohol 20%)
Levsinex SL 1-2 tabs q 4 hours SL or PO; max 12 tabs/day
Pediatric: <2 years: not recommended; 2-12 years: 1 tab q 4 hours; max 6 tabs/
day; ≥12 years: same as adult
  SL tab: 0.125 mg
Levsinex Timecaps 1-2 caps q 12 hours; may adjust to 1 cap q 8 hours
Pediatric: <2 years: not recommended; 2-12 years: 1 cap q 12 hours; max 2 caps/
day; ≥12 years: same as adult
  Cap: 0.375 mg time-rel
NuLev dissolve 1-2 tabs on tongue, with or without water, q 4 hours prn; max 12
tabs/day
Pediatric: <2 years: not recommended; 2-12 years: dissolve 1 tab on tongue, with or
without water, q 4 hours prn; max 6 tabs/day; ≥12 years: same as adult
  ODT: 0.125 mg (mint) (phenylalanine)
▷ *methenamine+sod phosphate monobasic+phenyl salicylate+methylene blue+hyoscy-
amine sulfate (C)* 1 cap qid
Pediatric: <6 years: not recommended; ≥6 years: individualize dose
  Uribel *Cap:* meth 118 mg+sod phos 40.8 mg+phenyl sal 36 mg+meth blue 10
  mg+hyoscy 0.12 mg
▷ *methenamine+phenyl salicylate+methylene blue+benzoic acid+atropine sulfate+-
hyoscyamine sulfate (C)(G)* 2 tabs qid
Pediatric: <6 years: not recommended; ≥6 years: same as adult
  Urised *Tab:* meth 40.8 mg+phenyl sal 18.1 mg+meth blue 5.4 mg+benz acid 4.5
  mg+atro sul 0.03 mg+hyoscy 0.03 mg
Comment: **Urised** imparts a blue-green color to urine which may stain fabrics.
▷ *oxybutynin chloride (B)*
  Ditropan 5 mg bid-tid; max 20 mg/day
  Pediatric: <5 years: not recommended; 5-12 years: 5 mg bid; max 15 mg/day; ≥12
  years: same as adult
    Tab: 5*mg; *Syr:* 5 mg/5 ml
  Ditropan XL initially 5 mg daily; may increase weekly in 5-mg increments as
  needed; max 30 mg/day
  Pediatric: <5 years: not recommended; ≥5 years: same as adult
    Tab: 5, 10, 15 mg ext-rel
▷ *pentosan (B)* 100 mg tid; reevaluate at 3 and 6 months
Pediatric: <16 years: not recommended; ≥16 years: same as adult
  Elmiron *Cap:* 100 mg

URINARY TRACT ANALGESIA

▷ *phenazopyridine (B)(G)* 95-200 mg q 6 hours prn; max 2 days
Pediatric: <12 years: not recommended; ≥12 years: same as adult
  AZO Standard, Prodium, Uristat (OTC) *Tab:* 95 mg
  AZO Standard Maximum Strength (OTC) *Tab:* 97.5 mg
  Pyridium, Urogesic *Tab:* 100, 200 mg
  Azo Standard (OTC) *Tab:* 95 mg
  Azo Standard Maximum Strength (OTC) *Tab:* 97.5 mg
  Pyridium *Tab:* 100, 200 mg ent-coat
  Uristat (OTC) *Tab:* 95 mg
  Urogesic *Tab:* 100, 200 mg

Comment: *Phenazopyridine* imparts an orange-red color to urine which may stain fabrics.

▷ *propantheline* (C) 15-30 mg tid
    Pro-Banthine *Tab:* 7.5, 15 mg
▷ *tolterodine tartrate* (C)(G) 2 mg bid; may decrease to 1 mg bid
    Detrol 2 mg bid; may decrease to 1 mg bid
      Tab: 1, 2 mg
    Detrol XL 2-4 mg daily
      Cap: 2, 4 mg ext-rel

ANTICHOLINERGIC+SEDATIVE COMBINATION

▷ *chlordiazepoxide+clidinium* (D)(IV) 1-2 caps ac and HS; max 8 caps/day
    Pediatric: <12 years: not recommended; ≥12 years: same as adult
    Librax *Cap: chlor* 5 mg+*clid* 2.5 mg

TRICYCLIC ANTIDEPRESSANTS (TCAs)

▷ *amitriptyline* (C)(G) 25-50 mg q HS
    Pediatric: <12 years: not recommended; ≥12 years: same as adult
    Tab: 10, 25, 50, 75, 100, 150 mg
▷ *imipramine* (C)(G)
    Pediatric: <12 years: not recommended; ≥12 years: same as adult
    Tofranil initially 75 mg daily (max 200 mg); adolescents initially 30-40 mg daily (max 100 mg/day); if maintenance dose exceeds 75 mg daily, may switch to **Tofranil PM** for divided <u>or</u> bedtime dose
      Tab: 10, 25, 50 mg
    Tofranil PM initially 75 mg daily 1 hour before HS; max 200 mg
      Cap: 75, 100, 125, 150

 INTERTRIGO

See Candidiasis: Skin *page 68*
Topical Antifungals see *Tinea Corporis page 462*
Topical Anti-infectives see *Skin Infection: Bacterial page 443*
Topical Corticosteroids see *page 566*
OTC hydrocortisone 1% paste or ointment
OTC Zinc Oxide paste or ointment
OTC A&D Ointment

Comment: Intertrigo is an irritant dermatitis in the intertriginous zones (skin creases and folds) characterized by inflammation and excoriation caused by skin-to-skin friction, moisture, and heat and may be itching, stinging, burning with a musty odor. Common areas at risk include breast folds, axillae, groin folds, buttocks folds, and the abdominal panniculus in obese persons, finger and toe webs. Treatment includes keeping the areas clean, moisture-free, application of a steroid cream and a protective lubricant barrier. Intertrigo may be complicated by a superimposed infection such as yeast (*Candida albicans*), dermatophytic fungi, <u>or</u> bacteria. Oral agents may be required based on severity of the skin breakdown and invasive infectious process. Apply appropriate topical anti-infective first and barrier product last. Non-medicated powders (e.g., corn starch) are contraindicated in the affected areas as they trap moisture. Exposure to light and air when possible and as appropriate facilitates integumentary healing.

IRITIS: ACUTE

▷ *loteprednol etabonate* (C) 1-2 drops qid; may increase to 1 drop hourly as needed
   Pediatric: <12 years: not recommended; ≥12 years: same as adult
      Lotemax Ophthalmic Solution *Ophth soln:* 0.3% (2.5, 5, 10, 15 ml)
▷ *prednisone acetate* (C) 1 drop q 1 hour x 24-48 hours, then 1 drop q 2 hours while
   awake x 24-48 hours, then 1 drop bid-qid until resolved
   Pediatric: <12 years: not recommended; ≥12 years: same as adult
      Pred Forte *Ophth soln:* 1% (1, 5, 10, 15 ml)

IRON OVERLOAD

IRON CHELATING AGENTS

▷ *deferasirox* (**tridentate ligand**) (C)(G) initially 20 mg/kg/day; titrate; may increase
   5-10 mg/kg q 3-6 months based on serum ferritin trends; max 30 mg/kg/day
   Pediatric: <2 years: not recommended; ≥2 years: same as adult
      Exjade *Tab for oral soln:* 125, 250, 500 mg
      Jadenu *Tab:* 90, 180, 360 mg film-coat
      Jadenu Sprinkle *Sachet:* 90, 180, 360 mg (30/carton)
Comment: *deferasirox* is an orally active chelator selective for iron. It is indicated
for the treatment of chronic iron overload due to blood transfusions (transfusional
hemosiderosis). Monitor serum ferritin monthly. Consider interrupting therapy if serum
ferritin falls below 500 mcg/L. Take *deferasirox* (**Exjade, Jadenu, Jadenu Sprinkle**) on an
empty stomach. Completely disperse tablet(s) or granules in 3.5 oz liquid if dose is ≤1
gm or 7 oz liquid if dose is ≥1 gm.
▷ *Succimer* (C) initially 10 mg/kg q 8 hours x 5 days; then, reduce frequency to every 12
   hours x 14 more days; allow at least 14 days between courses unless blood lead levels
   indicate need for prompt treatment
   Pediatric: <12 months: not recommended; ≥12 months: same as adult
      Chemet *Cap:* 100 mg
Comment: *Chemet is* indicated for the treatment of lead poisoning when blood lead level
45 mcg/dL. Treatment for more than 3 consecutive weeks is not recommended. Monitor
hydration, renal, and hepatic function.

IRRITABLE BOWEL SYNDROME WITH CONSTIPATION (IBS-C)

Bulk-Producing Agents, Laxatives, Stool Softeners see *Constipation page* 102

GUANYLATE CYCLASE-C AGONIST

Comment: Guanylate cyclase-c agonists increase intestinal fluid and intestinal transit
time may induce diarrhea and bloating and therefore, are contraindicated with known or
suspected mechanical GI obstruction.
▷ *linaclotide* (C) 290 mcg once daily; take on an empty stomach at least 30 minutes
   before the first meal of the day; swallow whole or may open cap and sprinkle on
   applesauce or in water for administration
   Pediatric: <6 years: not recommended; 6-17 years: avoid; >17 years: same as adult
      Linzess *Cap:* 145, 290 mcg
Comment: *linaclotide* and its active metabolite are negligibly absorbed systemically following oral administration and maternal use is not expected to result in fetal exposure to the
drug. There is no information regarding the presence of *plecanatide* in human milk or its
effects on the breastfed infant.

CHLORIDE CHANNEL ACTIVATOR

▷ *lubiprostone* (C) 8 mcg bid; take with food and water; *Severe hepatic impairment (Child-Pugh Class C):* 8 mcg once daily
   Pediatric: <18 years: not recommended; ≥18 years: same as adult
      Amitiza *Cap:* 8, 24 mcg

Comment: **Amitiza** increases intestinal fluid and intestinal transit time. Suspend dosing and rehydrate if severe diarrhea occurs. **Amitiza** is contraindicated with known or suspected mechanical GI obstruction. Most common adverse reactions in CIC are nausea, diarrhea, headache, abdominal pain, abdominal distension, and flatulence.

 IRRITABLE BOWEL SYNDROME WITH DIARRHEA (IBS-D)

Bulk-Producing Agents *see Constipation page* 102

CONSTIPATING AGENTS

▷ *difenoxin+atropine* (C) 2 tabs, then 1 tab after each loose stool or 1 tab q 3-4 hours as needed; max 8 tab/day x 2 days
   Pediatric: <12 years: not recommended; ≥12 years: same as adult
      Motofen *Tab:* difen 1 mg+atro 0.025 mg
▷ *diphenoxylate+atropine* (C)(G) 2 tabs or 10 ml qid
   Pediatric: <2 years: not recommended; 2-12 years: initially 0.3-0.4 mg/kg/day in 4 divided doses; ≥12 years: same as adult
      Lomotil *Tab:* difen 2.5 mg+atro 0.025 mg; *Liq:* difen 2.5 mg+atro 0.025 mg per 5 ml (2 oz)
▷ *eluxadoline* (NA)(IV) 100 mg bid; 75 mg bid if unable to tolerate 100 mg, or without a gall bladder, or mild-to-moderate hepatic impairment, or receiving concomitant OATP1B1 inhibitors
   Pediatric: <12 years: not established; ≥12 years: same as adult
      Viberzi 4 mg initially, then 2 mg after each loose stool; max 16 mg/day
         Tab: 75, 100 mg film-coat

Comment: *Eluxadoline* is a mu-opioid receptor agonist. It is contraindicated with biliary obstruction, Sphincter of Oddi disease or dysfunction, alcohol abuse or addiction, pancreatitis, pancreatic duct obstruction, severe hepatic impairment, and mechanical GI obstruction.

▷ *loperamide* (B)(G)
      Imodium (OTC) 4 mg initially, then 2 mg after each loose stool; max 16 mg/day
         Pediatric: <5 years: not recommended; ≥5 years: same as adult
            Cap: 2 mg
      Imodium A-D (OTC) 4 mg initially, then 2 mg after each loose stool; usual max 8 mg/day x 2 days
         Pediatric: <2 years: not recommended; 2-5 years (24-47 lb): 1 mg up to tid x 2 days; 6-8 years (48-59 lb): 2 mg initially, then 1 mg after each loose stool; max 4 mg/day x 2 days; 9-11 years (60-95 lb): 2 mg initially, then 1 mg after each loose stool; max 6 mg/day x 2 days; ≥12 years: same as adult
            Cplt: 2 mg; *Liq:* 1 mg/5 ml (2, 4 oz)
▷ *loperamide+simethicone* (B)(G)
      Imodium Advanced (OTC) 2 tabs chewed after loose stool, then 1 after the next loose stool; max 4 tabs/day
         Pediatric: <6 years: not recommended; 6-8 years: 1 tab chewed after loose stool, then 1/2 after next loose stool; max 2 tabs/day; 9-11 years: 1 tab chewed after loose stool, then 1/2 after next loose stool; max 3 tabs/day; ≥12 years: same as adult
            Chew tab: lop 2 mg+sim 125 mg

SEROTONIN (5-HT3) RECEPTOR ANTAGONIST

▷ *alosetron* (B)(G) initially 0.5 mg bid; may increase to 1 mg bid after 4 weeks if starting dose is tolerated but inadequate
  Pediatric: <12 years: not recommended; ≥12 years: same as adult
    Lotronex *Tab:* 0.5, 1 mg

ANTISPASMODIC+ANTICHOLINERGIC COMBINATIONS

▷ *dicyclomine* (B)(G) initially 20 mg bid-qid; may increase to 40 mg qid PO; usual IM dose 80 mg/day divided qid; do not use IM route for more than 1-2 days
  Pediatric: <12 years: not recommended; ≥12 years: same as adult
    Bentyl *Tab:* 20 mg; *Cap:* 10 mg; *Syr:* 10 mg/5 ml (16 oz); *Vial:* 10 mg/ml (10 ml); *Amp:* 10 mg/ml (2 ml)
▷ *methscopolamine bromide* (B) 1 tab q 6 hours prn
  Pediatric: <12 years: not recommended; ≥12 years: same as adult
    Pamine *Tab:* 2.5 mg
    Pamine Forte *Tab:* 5 mg

ANTICHOLINERGICS

▷ *hyoscyamine* (C)(G)
    Anaspaz 1-2 tabs q 4 hours prn; max 12 tabs/day
    Pediatric: <2 years: not recommended; 2-12 years: 0.0625-0.125 mg q 4 hours prn; max 0.75 mg/day; ≥12 years: same as adult
      Tab: 0.125*mg
    Levbid 1-2 tabs q 12 hours prn; max 4 tabs/day
    Pediatric: <12 years: not recommended; ≥12 years: same as adult
      Tab: 0.375*mg ext-rel
    Levsin 1-2 tabs q 4 hours prn; max 12 tabs/day
    Pediatric: <6 years: not recommended; 6-12 years: 1 tab q 4 hours prn; >12 years: same as adult
      Tab: 0.125*mg
    Levsinex SL 1-2 tabs q 4 hours SL or PO; max 12 tabs/day
    Pediatric: <2 years: not recommended; 2-12 years: 1 tab q 4 hours; max 6 tabs/day; >12 years: same as adult
      Tab: 0.125 mg sublingual
    Levsinex Timecaps 1-2 caps q 12 hours; may adjust to 1 cap q 8 hours
    Pediatric: <2 years: not recommended; 2-12 years: 1 cap q 12 hours; max 2 caps/day; >12 years: same as adult
      Cap: 0.375 mg time-rel
    NuLev dissolve 1-2 tabs on tongue, with or without water, q 4 hours prn; max 12 tabs/day
    Pediatric: <2 years: not recommended; 2-12 years: dissolve 1 tab on tongue, with or without water, q 4 hours prn; max 6 tabs/day; >12 years: same as adult
      ODT: 0.125 mg (mint; phenylalanine)
▷ *simethicone* (C)(G) 0.3 ml qid pc and HS
    Mylicon Drops (OTC) *Oral drops:* 40 mg/0.6 ml (30 ml)
▷ *phenobarbital+hyoscyamine+atropine+scopolamine* (C)(IV)(G)
    Donnatal 1-2 tabs ac and HS
    Pediatric: <12 years: not recommended; ≥12 years: same as adult
      Tab: pheno 16.2 mg+hyo 0.1037 mg+atro 0.0194 mg+scop 0.0065 mg
    Donnatal Elixir 1-2 tsp ac and HS
    Pediatric: 20 lb: 1 ml q 4 hours or 1.5 ml q 6 hours; 30 lb: 1.5 ml q 4 hours or 2 ml q 6 hours; 50 lb: 1/2 tsp q 4 hours or 3/4 tsp q 6 hours; 75 lb: 3/4 tsp q 4 hours or 1 tsp q 6 hours; 100 lb: 1 tsp q 4 hours or 1 tsp q 6 hours

Elix: pheno 16.2 mg+*hyo* 0.1037 mg+*atro* 0.0194 mg+*scop* 0.0065 mg per 5 ml
(4, 16 oz)

Donnatal Extentabs 1 tab q 12 hours
Pediatric: <12 years: not recommended; ≥12 years: same as adult
Tab: pheno 48.6 mg+*hyo* 0.3111 mg+*atro* 0.0582 mg+*scop* 0.0195 mg ext-rel

ANTICHOLINERGIC+SEDATIVE COMBINATION

➤ *chlordiazepoxide+clidinium* (D)(IV) 1-2 caps ac and HS: max 8 caps/day
Pediatric: <12 years: not recommended; ≥12 years: same as adult
Librax *Cap: chlor* 5 mg+*clid* 2.5 mg

TRICYCLIC ANTIDEPRESSANTS (TCAs)

➤ *amitriptyline* (C)(G) 25-50 mg q HS
Pediatric: <12 years: not recommended; ≥12 years: same as adult
Tab: 10, 25, 50, 75, 100, 150 mg
➤ *imipramine* (C)(G) 25-50 mg tid
Pediatric: <12 years: not recommended; ≥12 years: same as adult
Tofranil initially 75 mg daily (max 200 mg); adolescents initially 30-40 mg daily
(max 100 mg/day); if maintenance dose exceeds 75 mg daily, may switch to
Tofranil PM for divided <u>or</u> bedtime dose
Tab: 10, 25, 50 mg
Tofranil PM initially 75 mg daily 1 hour before HS; max 200 mg
Cap: 75, 100, 125, 150
Tofranil Injection 50 mg IM; lower dose for adolescents; switch to oral form as
soon as possible
Amp: 25 mg/2 ml (2 ml)
➤ *nortriptyline* (D)(G) initially 25 mg tid-qid; max 150 mg/day
Pediatric: <12 years: not recommended; ≥12 years: same as adult
Pamelor *Cap:* 10, 25, 50, 75 mg; *Oral soln:* 10 mg/5 ml (16 oz)
➤ *protriptyline* (C) initially 5 mg tid; usual dose 15-40 mg/day in 3-4 divided doses; max
60 mg/day
Pediatric: <12 years: not recommended; ≥12 years: same as adult
Vivactil *Tab:* 5, 10 mg
➤ *trimipramine* (C) initially 75 mg/day in divided doses; max 200 mg/day
Pediatric: <12 years: not recommended; ≥12 years: same as adult
Surmontil *Cap:* 25, 50, 100 mg

JAPANESE ENCEPHALITIS

Comment: Japanese encephalitis is a viral disease spread by the bite of an infected
mosquito. It is not spread from person-to-person. Currently there is no cure. A person
with encephalitis can experience fever, neck stiffness, seizures, and coma. About 1
person in 4 with encephalitis dies. Up to half of those who don't die have permanent
disability. There is one vaccine for Japanese encephalitis, currently licensed in the
UK, for use in adults and children >2 months-of-age. The **live** attenuated vaccine
is administered in two doses for full protection, with the second dose administered
28 days after the first. The second dose should be given at least a week before travel.
Children younger than 3 years of age get a smaller dose than patients who are 3
<u>or</u> older. A booster dose might be recommended for anyone 17 <u>or</u> older who was
vaccinated more than a year ago and is still at risk of exposure. There is no information
yet on the need for a booster dose for children. The vaccine is usually available through
the local health department.

JUVENILE IDIOPATHIC ARTHRITIS (JIA), POLYARTICULAR JUVENILE IDIOPATHIC ARTHRITIS (PJIA), SYSTEMIC JUVENILE IDIOPATHIC ARTHRITIS (SJIA)

Acetaminophen for IV Infusion *see Pain page 344*
NSAIDs *see page 562*
Opioid Analgesics *see Pain page 345*
Topical and Transdermal NSAIDs *see Pain page 344*
Parenteral Corticosteroids *see page 570*
Oral Corticosteroids *see page 569*
Topical Analgesic and Anesthetic Agents *see page 560*

TOPICAL ANALGESICS

▷ *capsaicin* (B)(G) apply tid or qid prn to intact skin
    Pediatric: <2 years: not recommended; ≥2 years: same as adult
        Axsain *Crm:* 0.075% (1, 2 oz)
        Capsin *Lotn:* 0.025, 0.075% (59 ml)
        Capzasin-P (OTC) *Crm:* 0.025% (1.5 oz); *Lotn:* 0.025% (2 oz)
        Dolorac *Crm:* 0.025% (28 gm)
        Double Cap (OTC) *Crm:* 0.05% (2 oz)
        R-Gel *Gel:* 0.025% (15, 30 gm)
        Zostrix (OTC) *Crm:* 0.025% (0.7, 1.5, 3 oz)
        Zostrix HP (OTC) *Emol crm:* 0.075% (1, 2 oz)
Comment: Provides some relief by 1-2 weeks; optimal benefit may take 4-6 weeks.

ORAL SALICYLATES

▷ *indomethacin* (C) initially 25 mg bid or tid, increase as needed at weekly intervals by 25-50 mg/day; max 200 mg/day
    Pediatric: <14 years: usually not recommended; >2 years, if risk warranted: 1-2 mg/kg/day in divided doses; max 3-4 mg/kg/day (or 150-200 mg/day, whichever is less; <14 years: ER cap not recommended
    Cap: 25, 50 mg; *Susp:* 25 mg/5 ml (pineapple-coconut, mint) (alcohol 1%); *Supp:* 50 mg; *ER Cap:* 75 mg ext-rel
Comment: *indomethacin* is indicated only for acute painful flares. Administer with food and/or antacids. Use lowest effective dose for shortest duration.

▷ *methotrexate* (X) 7.5 mg x 1 dose per week or 2.5 mg x 3 at 12 hour intervals once a week; max 20 mg/week; therapeutic response begins in 3-6 weeks; administer *methotrexate* injection SC only into the abdomen or thigh
    Pediatric: <2 years: not recommended; ≥2 years: 10 mg/m^2 once weekly; max 20 mg/m^2
        Rasuvo *Autoinjector:* 7.5 mg/0.15 ml, 10 mg/0.20 ml, 12.5 mg/0.25 ml, 15 mg/0.30 ml, 17.5 mg/0.35 ml, 20 mg/0.40 ml, 22.5 mg/0.45 ml, 25 mg/0.50 ml, 27.5 mg/0.55 ml, 30 mg/0.60 ml (solution concentration for SC injection is 50 mg/ml)
        Rheumatrex *Tab:* 2.5*mg (5, 7.5, 10, 12.5, 15 mg/week, 4/card unit dose pack)
        Trexall *Tab:* 5*, 7.5*, 10*, 15*mg (5, 7.5, 10, 12.5, 15 mg/week, 4/card unit dose pack)
Comment: *methotrexate* (MTX) is contraindicated with immunodeficiency, blood dyscrasias, alcoholism, and chronic liver disease.

INTERLEUKIN-6 RECEPTOR ANTAGONIST

▷ *tocilizumab* (B) *IV Infusion:* administer over 1 hour; do not administer as bolus or IV push; *Adults, PJIA, and SJIA,* ≥30 kg: dilute to 100 mL in 0.9% or 0.45% NaCl. *PJIA and SJIA,* <30 kg: dilute to 50 mL in 0.9% or 0.45% NaCl.

Adults: IV Infusion: Whether used in combination with DMARDs <u>or</u> as mono-therapy, the recommended IV infusion starting dose is 4 mg/kg IV every 4 weeks followed by an increase to 8 mg/kg IV every 4 weeks based on clinical response; Max 800 mg per infusion in RA patients; *SC Administration:* ≥*100 kg:* 162 mg SC once weekly on the same day; <*100 kg:* 162 mg SC every other week on the same day followed by an increase according to clinical response

Pediatric: <2 years: not recommended; ≥2 years: weight-based dosing according to diagnosis: *PJIA:* ≥*30 kg:* 8 mg/kg SC every 4 weeks; <*30 kg:* 10 mg/kg SC every 4 weeks; *SJIA:* ≥*30 kg:* 8 mg/kg SC every 2 weeks; <*30 kg:* 12 mg/kg SC every 2 weeks

Actemra *Vial:* 80 mg/4 ml, 200 mg/10 ml, 400 mg/20 ml, single-use, for IV infusion after dilution; *Prefilled syringe:* 162 mg (0.9 ml, single-dose)

Comment: *tocilizumab* is an interleukin-6 receptor-α inhibitor indicated for use in moderate-to-severe rheumatoid arthritis (RA) that has not responded to conventional therapy, and also for some subtypes of juvenile idiopathic arthritis (JIA). **Actemra** may be used alone <u>or</u> in combination with **methotrexate** and in RA, other DMARDs may be used. Monitor patient for dose related laboratory changes including elevated LFTs, neutropenia, and thrombocytopenia. **Actemra** should not be initiated in patients with an absolute neutrophil count (ANC) below 2000 per mm³, platelet count below 100,000 per mm³, <u>or</u> who have ALT <u>or</u> AST above 1.5 times the upper limit of normal (ULN).

TUMOR NECROSIS FACTOR (TNF) BLOCKER

▷ *adalimumab-adbm* (B) ≥ *30 kg (66 lbs):* 40 mg every other week; inject into thigh or abdomen; rotate sites

Pediatric: <30 kg, <66 lbs: not recommended; ≥30 kg, ≥66 lbs: same as adult

Cyltezo *Prefilled syringe:* 40 mg/0.8 ml single-dose (preservative-free)

Comment: **Cyltezo** is biosimilar to **Humira** (*adalimumab*).

 JUVENILE RHEUMATOID ARTHRITIS (JRA)

Juvenile Idiopathic Arthritis (JIA), Polyarticular Juvenile Idiopathic Arthritis (PJIA), Systemic Juvenile Idiopathic Arthritis (SJIA) *see page* 280
Acetaminophen for IV Infusion *see Pain page* 344
NSAIDs *see page* 562
Opioid Analgesics *see Pain page* 345
Topical and Transdermal NSAIDs *see Pain page* 344
Parenteral Corticosteroids *see page* 570
Oral Corticosteroids *see page* 569

TOPICAL ANALGESICS

▷ *capsaicin* (B)(G) apply tid-qid prn to intact skin
Pediatric: <2 years: not recommended; ≥2 years: same as adult
Axsain *Crm:* 0.075% (1, 2 oz)
Capsin *Lotn:* 0.025, 0.075% (59 ml)
Capzasin-P (OTC) *Crm:* 0.025% (1.5 oz); *Lotn:* 0.025% (2 oz)
Dolorac *Crm:* 0.025% (28 gm)
Double Cap (OTC) *Crm:* 0.05% (2 oz)
R-Gel *Gel:* 0.025% (15, 30 gm)
Zostrix (OTC) *Crm:* 0.025% (0.7, 1.5, 3 oz)
Zostrix HP (OTC) *Emol crm:* 0.075% (1, 2 oz)
Comment: Provides some relief by 1-2 weeks; optimal benefit may take 4-6 weeks.

ORAL SALICYLATE

▷ *indomethacin* (C) initially 25 mg bid-tid, increase as needed at weekly intervals by 25-50 mg/day; max 200 mg/day

Pediatric: <14 years: usually not recommended; ≥2 years, if risk warranted: 1-2 mg/kg/day in divided doses; max 3-4 mg/kg/day (or total 150-200 mg/day, whichever is less); ≤14 years: ER cap not recommended

Cap: 25, 50 mg; Susp: 25 mg/5 ml (pineapple-coconut, mint; alcohol 1%); Supp: 50 mg; ER Cap: 75 mg ext-rel

Comment: *Indomethacin* is indicated only for acute painful flares. Administer with food and/or antacids. Use lowest effective dose for shortest duration.

▷ *methotrexate* (X) 7.5 mg x 1 dose per week or 2.5 mg x 3 at 12-hour intervals once a week; max 20 mg/week; therapeutic response begins in 3-6 weeks; administer methotrexate injection SC only into the abdomen or thigh

Pediatric: <2 years: not recommended; ≥2 years: 10 mg/m^2 once weekly; max 20 mg/m^2

Rasuvo *Autoinjector:* 7.5 mg/0.15 ml, 10 mg/0.20 ml, 12.5 mg/0.25 ml, 15 mg/0.30 ml, 17.5 mg/0.35 ml, 20 mg/0.40 ml, 22.5 mg/0.45 ml, 25 mg/0.50 ml, 27.5 mg/0.55 ml, 30 mg/0.60 ml (solution concentration for SC injection is 50 mg/ml)

Rheumatrex *Tab:* 2.5*mg (5, 7.5, 10, 12.5, 15 mg/week, 4/card unit-of-use dose pack)

Trexall *Tab:* 5*, 7.5*, 10*, 15*mg (5, 7.5, 10, 12.5, 15 mg/week, 4/card unit-of-use dose pack)

Comment: *methotrexate* (MTX) is contraindicated with immunodeficiency, blood dyscrasias, alcoholism, and chronic liver disease.

◯ KERATITIS/KERATOCONJUNCTIVITIS: HERPES SIMPLEX

▷ *ganciclovir* (C) instill 1 drop 5 x/day (every 3 hours) while awake until corneal ulcer heals; then 1 drop tid x 7 days

Pediatric: <2 years: not recommended; ≥2 years: same as adult

Zirgan *Ophth gel:* 0.15% (5 gm) (benzalkonium chloride)

▷ *idoxuridine* (C) instill 1 drop q 1 hour during day and every other hour at night or 1 drop every minute for 5 minutes and repeat q 4 hours during day and night

Herplex *Ophth soln:* 0.1% (15 ml)

▷ *trifluridine* (C) instill 1 drop q 2 hours while awake (max 9 drops/day until reepithelialization; then 1 drop q 4 hours x 7 more days (at least 5 drops/day); max 21 days

Pediatric: <6 years: not recommended; ≥6 years: same as adult

Viroptic *Ophth soln:* 1% (7.5 ml) (thimerosal)

▷ *vidarabine* (C) apply 1/2 inch in lower conjunctival sac 5 x/day q 3 hours until reepithelialization occurs, then bid x 7 more days

Pediatric: <2 years: not recommended; ≥2 years: same as adult

Vira-A *Ophth oint:* 3% (3.5 gm)

◯ KERATITIS/KERATOCONJUNCTIVITIS: VERNAL

OPHTHALMIC MAST CELL STABILIZERS

Comment: Contact lens wear is contraindicated

▷ *cromolyn sodium* (B) 1-2 drops 4-6 x/day

Pediatric: <4 years: not recommended; ≥4 years: same as adult

Crolom, Opticrom *Ophth soln:* 4% (10 ml) (benzalkonium chloride)

▷ *lodoxamide tromethamine* (B) 1-2 drops qid; max 3 months

Pediatric: <2 years: not recommended; ≥2 years: same as adult

Alomide *Ophth susp:* 0.1% (10 ml)

LABYRINTHITIS

▷ *meclizine* (B) 25 mg tid
Pediatric: <12 years: not recommended; ≥12 years: same as adult
Antivert *Tab:* 12.5, 25, 50*mg
Bonine (OTC) *Cap:* 15, 25, 30 mg; *Tab:* 12.5, 25, 50 mg; *Chew tab/Film-coat tab:* 25 mg
Dramamine II (OTC) *Tab:* 25*mg
Zentrip *Strip:* 25 mg orally disintegrating
▷ *promethazine* (C)(G) 25 mg tid
Pediatric: <2 years: not recommended; ≥2 years: 0.5 mg/lb or 6.25-25 mg tid
Phenergan *Tab:* 12.5*, 25*, 50 mg; *Plain syr:* 6.25 mg/5 ml; *Fortis syr:* 25 mg/5 ml; *Rectal supp:* 12.5, 25, 50 mg

Comment: *promethazine* is contraindicated in children with uncomplicated nausea, dehydration, Reye's syndrome, history of sleep apnea, asthma, and lower respiratory disorders in children. *promethazine* lowers the seizure threshold in children, may cause cholestatic jaundice, anticholinergic effects, extrapyramidal effects, and potentially fatal respiratory depression.

▷ *scopolamine* (C)
Transderm Scop 1 patch behind ear at least 4 hours before travel; each patch is effective for 3 days
Transdermal patch: 1.5 mg (4/carton)

 LACTOSE INTOLERANCE

▷ *lactase* enzyme 9,000 FCC units taken with dairy food; adjust based on abatement of symptoms; usual max 18,000 units/dose
Pediatric: same as adult
Lactaid Drops (OTC) 5-7 drops to each quart of milk and shake gently; may increase to 10-15 drops if needed; hydrolyzes 70%-99% of lactose at refrigerator temperature in 24 hours
Oral drops: 1,250 units/5 gtts (7 ml w. dropper)
Lactaid Extra (OTC) *Cplt:* 4,500 FCC units
Lactaid Fast ACT (OTC) *Cplt:* 9,000 FCC units; *Chew tab:* 9,000 FCC units (vanilla twist)
Lactaid Original (OTC) *Cplt:* 3,000 FCC units
Lactaid Ultra (OTC) *Cplt:* 9,000 FCC units; *Chew tab:* 9,000 FCC units (vanilla twist)

 LARVA MIGRANS: CUTANEOUS, VISCERAL

▷ *thiabendazole* (C) Adult and pediatric dosing schedules are the same; dosing is bid, is based on weight in pounds, and must be taken with meals.
Cutaneous Larva Migrans: treat bid x 2 days
Visceral Larva Migrans: treat bid x 7 days
<30 lbs: consult mfr pkg insert; 30 lbs: 250 mg bid; 50 lbs: 500 mg bid; 75 lbs: 750 mg bid; 100 lbs: 1000 mg bid; 125 lbs: 1250 mg bid; ≥150 lbs: 1500 mg bid; max 3000 mg/day.
Mintezol *Chew tab:* 500*mg (orange); *Oral susp:* 500 mg/5 ml (120 ml) (orange)
Comment: *thiabendazole* is not for prophylaxis. May impair mental alertness. May not be available in the US.

LEAD POISONING

Comment: Chelation therapy for lead poisoning requires maintenance of adequate hydration, close monitoring of renal and hepatic function, and monitoring for neutropenia; discontinue therapy at first sign of toxicity. Contraindicated with severe renal disease or anuria.

CHELATING AGENTS

▷ *deferoxamine mesylate* (C) initially 1 gm IM, followed by 500 mg IM every 4 hours x 2 doses; then repeat every 4-12 hours if needed; max 6 gm/day
Pediatric: <3 months: not recommended; ≥3 months: same as adult
Desferal *Vial:* 250 mg/ml after reconstitution (500 mg)

▷ *edetate calcium disodium (EDTA)* (B) administer IM or IV; use IM route of administration for children and overt lead encephalopathy
Pediatric: same as adult; *Serum lead level:* 20-70 mcg/dL: 1 gm/m² per day; *IV:* infuse over 8-12 hours; *IM:* divided doses q 8-12 hours; Treat for 5 days; then stop for 2-4 days; may repeat if serum lead level is ≥70 mcg/dL
Calcium Disodium Versenate *Amp:* 200 mg/ml (5 ml)

▷ *succimer* (C) may swallow caps whole or put contents onto a small amount of soft food or a spoon and swallow, followed by a fruit drink
Pediatric: <12 months: not recommended; ≥12 months: same as adult; *Serum lead level:* >45 mcg/dL: initially 10 mg/kg (or 350 mg/m²) every 8 hours for 5 days; then reduce frequency to every 12 hours for 14 more days; allow at least 14 days between courses unless serum lead levels indicate a need for more prompt treatment; for more than 3 consecutive weeks not recommended
Chemet *Cap:* 100 mg

 LEG CRAMPS: NOCTURNAL, RECUMBENCY

▷ *quinine sulfate* (C)(G) 1 tab or cap q HS
Pediatric: <16 years: not recommended; ≥16 years: same as adult
Qualaquin *Tab:* 260 mg; *Cap:* 260, 300, 325 mg
Comment: If **hypokalemia** is the cause of leg cramps, treat with potassium supplementation (*see page 257*).

 LEISHMANIASIS: CUTANEOUS, MUCOSAL, VISCERAL

Comment: The leishmanial parasite species addressed in this section are: **cutaneous leishmaniasis** (due to *Leishmania braziliensis, Leishmania guyanensis, Leishmania panamensis*), **mucosal leishmaniasis** (due to *Leishmania braziliensis*), and **visceral leishmaniasis** (due to *Leishmania donovani*). The weight-based treatment for adults and adolescents is the same for each of the species, the anti-leishmanial drug *miltefosone* (Impavido). Contraindications to this drug include pregnancy, lactation, and Sjogren-Larsson-Syndrome. The contraindication in pregnancy is due to embryo-fetal toxicity, teratogenicity, and fetal death. Obtain a serum or urine pregnancy test for females of reproductive potential and advise females to use effective contraception during therapy and for 5 months following treatment. Breastfeeding is contraindicated while taking this drug and for 5 months following termination of breastfeeding. Potential ASEs include loss of appetite, abdominal pain, nausea, vomiting, diarrhea, headache, dizziness, pruritis, somnolence, elevated liver transaminases, bilirubin, and serum creatinine and thrombocytopenia. *miltefosine* is associated with impaired fertility in females and males in animal studies. To report a suspected adverse reaction to this drug, call 888-550-6060 or the FDA at 800-FDA-1088 or visit www.fda.gov/medwatch

➤ *miltefosine* (D)(G) 30-44 kg: one cap bid x 28 consecutive days; ≥45 kg: one cap tid x 28 consecutive days; take with a full meal
Pediatric: <12 years, <30 kg (60 lbs): not established; ≥12 years, ≥30 kg (≥60 lbs): same as adult
Impavido *Cap:* 50 mg

 LENTIGINES: BENIGN, SENILE

Comment: Wash affected area with a soap-free cleanser; pat dry and wait 20-30 minutes; then apply agent sparingly to affected area; use only once daily in PM. Avoid eyes, ears, nostrils, mouth, and healthy skin. Avoid sun exposure. Cautious use of concomitant astringents, alcohol-based products, sulfur-containing products, salicylic acid-containing products, soap, and other topical agents.

TOPICAL RETINOIDS

➤ *tazarotene* (X)(G) apply daily at HS
Pediatric: <12 years: not recommended; ≥12 years: same as adult
Avage Cream *Crm:* 0.1% (30 gm)
Tazorac Cream *Crm:* 0.05, 0.1% (15, 30, 60 gm)
Tazorac Gel *Gel:* 0.05, 0.1% (30, 100 gm)
➤ *tretinoin* (C)(G) apply daily at HS
Pediatric: <12 years: not recommended; ≥12 years: same as adult
Avita *Crm:* 0.025% (20, 45 gm); *Gel:* 0.025% (20, 45 gm)
Renova *Crm:* 0.02% (40 gm); 0.05% (40, 60 gm)
Retin-A Cream *Crm:* 0.025, 0.05, 0.1% (20, 45 gm)
Retin-A Gel *Gel:* 0.01, 0.025% (15, 45 gm) (alcohol 90%)
Retin-A Liquid *Liq:* 0.05% (28 ml; alcohol 55%)
Retin-A Micro *Microspheres:* 0.04, 0.1% (20, 45 gm)
Retin-A Micro Gel *Gel:* 0.04, 0.1% (20, 45 gm)

 LISTERIOSIS *(LISTERIA MONOCYTOGENES)*

Comment: *L. monocytogenes* is a potentially lethal foodborne pathogen that is a common contaminant of food and food preparation equipment, and has been isolated in soil, farm environments, produce, raw foods, dairy products, and the feces of asymptomatic people. IV *ampicillin* is the mainstay of treatment, but penicillin may be as effective. Some experts recommend combination antibiotic therapy for neuro-invasive *L. monocytogenes*. The most common antimicrobial combination is IV *ampicillin* and IV *gentamycin* (which is usually discontinued when the patient shows signs of improvement to limit the potential for toxicity). If the patient is penicillin-allergic, IV *trimethoprim-sulfamethoxazole* (TMP-SMX) as mono therapy x 28 days. Patients with bacteremia but without CNS involvement may be treated with combination (*ampicillin+gentamycin*) therapy for 14 days, but patients with meningitis require a full 21 day combination course of antibiotics. Endocarditis, encephalitis, and brain abscesses may require a longer duration of high dose antimicrobials. Cephalosporins are ineffective. Supportive care and standard isolation precautions are required.

REFERENCES

Kasper, D. L., & Fauci, A. S. (2017). Listeria monocytogenes infections. In: *Harrison's Infectious Diseases* (3rd ed.). New York: McGraw Hill Education.

McNeill, C., Sisson, W., & Jarrett, A. (2017). Listeriosis: A Resurfacing Menace. *The Journal for Nurse Practitioners, 13*(10), 647–654.

▷ *ampicillin (B)(G)* 2 gm IV infusion q 4 hours (in combination with IV gentamycin q 8 hours)
  Pediatric: 50-100 mg/kg (max 3 gm) IV infusion q 6 hours
      Unasyn *Vial:* 1.5, 3 gm
▷ *gentamicin (C)(G)* 1-2 mg/kg q 8 hours (in combination with IV ampicillin q 4 hours; monitor plasma levels; dilution not less than 1 mg/ml in D5W *or* NS; administer dose over 30 min-2 hours
  Pediatric: 2 mg/kg/dose q 8 hours; monitor plasma levels; dilution not less than 1 mg/ml in D5W *or* NS; administer dose over 30 min-2 hours
      Geramycin *Vial:* 20, 80 mg/2 ml (2 ml) for dilution (not less than 1 mg/ml) and IV infusion (over 30 min-2 hours
▷ *penicillin g potassium (B)(G)* 4 million units via IV infusion q 4 hours
  Pediatric: 65,000 units/kg/dose via IV infusion q 4 hours; max 4 million units/dose; infuse dose over 1-2 hours
      Vial: 5, 20 MU pwdr for reconstitution (in D5W *or* NS) and IV infusion; *Pre-mixed bag:* 1, 2, 3 MU (50 ml); infuse dose over 1-2 hours
▷ *trimethoprim-sulfamethoxazole (TMP-SMX) (C)(G)* TMP 5 mg/kg IV infusion q 6 hours; max TMP 160 mg/dose
  Pediatric: <2 months: contraindicated: ≥2 months: 2-5 mg/kg/dose q 8 hours; max TMP 160 mg/dose
Comment: TMP-SMX is contraindicated in the first trimester of pregnancy, the final month of pregnancy, and in infants <8 weeks of age.

LIVER FLUKES

TREMATODICIDE

Comment: *praziquantel* is a trematodicide indicated for the treatment of infections due to all species of Schistosoma (e.g., *Schistosoma mekongi, Schistosoma japonicum, Schistosoma mansoni,* and *Schistosoma hematobium*) and infections due to liver flukes (i.e., *Clonorchis sinensis, Opisthorchis viverrini*). *praziquantel* induces a rapid contraction of schistosomes by a specific effect on the permeability of the cell membrane. The drug further causes vacuolization and disintegration of the schistosome tegument.

▷ *praziquantel (B)* 25 mg/kg tid as a one-day treatment; take the 3 doses at intervals of not less than 4 hours and not more than 6 hours; swallow whole with water during meals; holding the tablets in the mouth leaves a bitter taste which can trigger gagging or vomiting.
  Pediatric: <4 years: not established; >4 years: same as adult
      Biltricide *Tab:* 600mg*** film-coat (3 scores, 4 segments, 150 mg/segment)
Comment: Concomitant administration with strong Cytochrome P450 (P450) inducers, such as *rifampin*, is contraindicated since therapeutically effective blood levels of *praziquantel* may not be achieved. In patients receiving *rifampin* who need immediate treatment for schistosomiasis, alternative agents for schistosomiasis should be considered. However, if treatment with *praziquantel* is necessary, *rifampin* should be discontinued 4 weeks before administration of *praziquantel*. Treatment with *rifampin* can then be restarted one day after completion of *praziquantel* treatment. Concomitant administration of other P450 inducers (e.g., antiepileptic drugs such as *phenytoin, phenobarbital, carbamazepine*) and *dexamethasone*, may also reduce plasma levels of *praziquantel*. Concomitant administration of P450 inhibitors (e.g., *cimetidine, ketoconazole, itraconazole, erythromycin*) may increase plasma levels of *praziquantel*. Patients should be warned not to drive a car or operate machinery on the day of **Biltricide** treatment and the following day. There are no adequate or well-controlled

studies in pregnant women. This drug should be used during pregnancy only if clearly needed. *praziquantel* appears in the milk of nursing women at a concentration of about 1/4 that of maternal serum. It is not known whether a pharmacological effect is likely to occur in children. Women should not nurse on the day of **Biltricide** treatment and during the subsequent 72 hours.

 LOW BACK STRAIN

Acetaminophen for IV Infusion *see Pain page* 344
NSAIDs *see page* 562
Opioid Analgesics *see Pain page* 345
Topical and Transdermal NSAIDs *see Pain page* 344
Muscle Relaxants *see page* 307
Parenteral Corticosteroids *see page* 570
Oral Corticosteroids *see page* 569
Topical Analgesic and Anesthetic Agents *see page* 560

 LOW LIBIDO, HYPOACTIVE SEXUAL DESIRE DISORDER (HSDD)

5-HT1A AGONIST/5-HT2A

➤ *flibanserin* 1 tab once daily at bedtime; discontinue if no improvement in 8 weeks
Pediatric: <18 years: not recommended; ≥18 years: same as adult
   Addyi *Tab:* 100 mg
Comment: **Addyi** is for use in premenopausal women. **Addyi** is not for use in men, postmenopausal women, and is not recommended in pregnancy, or lactation. Potential ASEs include dry mouth, nausea, hypotension, dizziness, syncope, fatigue, somnolence, and insomnia.

 LYME DISEASE (*ERYTHEMA CHRONICUM MIGRANS*)

Comment: The bite of the deer tick (*Ioxodes scapularis*) carries the *Borrelia burgdorferi* organism causing Lyme disease. Proper removal of the tick, and early diagnosis and treatment are essential to effective management of this disease.

STAGE 1

➤ *amoxicillin* (B)(G) 500-875 mg bid or 250-500 mg tid x 10 days
Pediatric: <40 kg (88 lb): 20-40 mg/kg/day in 3 divided doses x 10 days or 25-45 mg/kg/day in 2 divided doses x 10 days; ≥40 kg: same as adult; *see page* 616 *for dose by weight*
   Amoxil *Cap:* 250, 500 mg; *Tab:* 875*mg; *Chew tab:* 125, 200, 250, 400 mg (cherry-banana-peppermint) (phenylalanine); *Oral susp:* 125, 250 mg/5 ml (80, 100, 150 ml) (strawberry); 200, 400 mg/5 ml (50, 75, 100 ml) (bubble gum); *Oral drops:* 50 mg/ml (30 ml) (bubble gum)
   Moxatag *Tab:* 775 mg ext-rel
   Trimox *Tab:* 125, 250 mg; *Cap:* 250, 500 mg; *Oral susp:* 125, 250 mg/5 ml (80, 100, 150 ml) (raspberry-strawberry)
➤ *clarithromycin* (C)(G) 500 mg bid or 500 mg ext-rel daily x 14-21 days
Pediatric: <6 months: not recommended; ≥6 months: 7.5 mg/kg bid x 7 days; *see page* 630 *for dose by weight*
   Biaxin *Tab:* 250, 500 mg

Biaxin Oral Suspension *Oral susp:* 125, 250 mg/5 ml (50, 100 ml)
Biaxin XL *Tab:* 500 mg ext-rel

▷ *doxycycline* (D)(G) 100 mg bid x 14-21 days
Pediatric: <8 years: not recommended; ≥8 years, ≤100 lb: 2 mg/lb on first day in 2 divided doses, followed by 1 mg/lb/day in 1-2 divided doses; ≥8 years, >100 lb: same as adult; *see page 633 for dose by weight*

Acticlate *Tab:* 75, 150**mg
Adoxa *Tab:* 50, 75, 100, 150 mg ent-coat
Doryx *Tab:* 50, 75, 100, 150, 200 mg del-rel
Doxteric *Tab:* 50 mg del-rel
Monodox *Cap:* 50, 75, 100 mg
Oracea *Cap:* 40 mg del-rel
Vibramycin *Tab:* 100 mg; *Cap:* 50, 100 mg; *Syr:* 50 mg/5 ml (raspberry-apple) (sulfites); *Oral susp:* 25 mg/5 ml (raspberry)
Vibra-Tab *Tab:* 100 mg film-coat

Comment: *doxycycline* is contraindicated <8 years-of-age, in pregnancy, and lactation (discolors developing tooth enamel). A side effect may be photosensitivity (photophobia). Do not take with antacids, calcium supplements, milk or other dairy, or within 2 hours of taking another drug.

▷ *minocycline* (D)(G) 200 mg on first day; then 100 mg q 12 hours x 9 more days
Pediatric: ≤8 years: not recommended; ≥8 years, <100 lb: 2 mg/lb on first day in 2 divided doses, followed by 1 mg/lb q 12 hours x 9 more days; ≥8 years, >100 lb: same as adult

Dynacin *Cap:* 50, 100 mg
Minocin *Cap:* 50, 75, 100 mg; *Oral susp:* 50 mg/5 ml (60 ml) (custard) (sulfites, alcohol 5%)

Comment: *minocycline* is contraindicated <8 years-of-age, in pregnancy, and lactation (discolors developing tooth enamel). A side effect may be photo-sensitivity (photophobia). Do not give with antacids, calcium supplements, milk or other dairy, or within two hours of taking another drug.

▷ *tetracycline* (D)(G) 250-500 mg qid ac x 21 days
Pediatric: <8 years: not recommended; ≥8 years, ≤100 lb: 25-50 mg/kg/day in 2-4 divided doses x 7 days; ≥8 years, >100 lb: same as adult; *see page 646 for dose by weight*

Achromycin V *Cap:* 250, 500 mg
Sumycin *Tab:* 250, 500 mg; *Cap:* 250, 500 mg; *Oral susp:* 125 mg/5 ml (100, 200 ml) (fruit) (sulfites)

Comment: *tetracycline* is contraindicated <8 years-of-age, in pregnancy, and lactation (discolors developing tooth enamel). A side effect may be photo-sensitivity (photophobia). Do not give with antacids, calcium supplements, milk or other dairy, or within two hours of taking another drug.

 LYMPHADENITIS

Comment: Therapy should continue for no less than 5 days after resolution of symptoms.

▷ *amoxicillin+clavulanate* (B)(G)
Augmentin 500 mg tid <u>or</u> 875 mg bid x 7-10 days
Pediatric: 40-45 mg/kg/day divided tid x 10 days <u>or</u> 90 mg/kg/day divided bid x 10 days *see pages 618-619 for dose by weight*
Tab: 250, 500, 875 mg; *Chew tab:* 125, 250 mg (lemon-lime); 200, 400 mg (cherry-banana) (phenylalanine); *Oral susp:* 125 mg/5 ml (banana),

250 mg/5 ml (75, 100, 150 ml) (orange); 200, 400 mg/5 ml (50, 75, 100 ml) (orange) (phenylalanine)

Augmentin ES-600 not recommended for adults

Pediatric: <3 months: not recommended; ≥3 months, <40 kg: 90 mg/kg/day in 2 divided doses x 7-10 days; ≥40 kg: not recommended

Oral susp: 42.9 mg/5 ml (50, 75, 100, 125, 150, 200 ml) (strawberry cream) (phenylalanine)

Augmentin XR 2 tabs q 12 hours x 7-10 days

Pediatric: <16 years: use other forms; ≥16 years: same as adult

Tab: 1000*mg ext-rel

➤ *cephalexin* (B)(G) 500 mg bid x 10 days

Pediatric: 25-50 mg/kg/day in 4 divided doses x 10 days; *see page 629 for dose by weight*

Keflex *Cap:* 250, 333, 500, 750 mg; *Oral susp:* 125, 250 mg/5 ml (100, 200 ml) (strawberry)

➤ *dicloxacillin* (B) 500 mg qid x 10 days

Pediatric: 12.5-25 mg/kg/day in 4 divided doses x 10 days; *see page 632 for dose by weight*

Dynapen *Cap:* 125, 250, 500 mg; *Oral susp:* 62.5 mg/5 ml (80, 100, 200 ml)

LYMPHOGRANULOMA VENEREUM

Comment: The following treatment regimens are published in the **2015 CDC Sexually Transmitted Diseases Treatment Guidelines**. This section contains treatment regimens for adults only; consult a specialist for treatment of patients less than 18 years of age. Treatment regimens are presented in alphabetical order by generic drug name, followed by brands and dose forms. Treat all sexual contacts. Persons with both LGV and HIV infection should receive the same treatment regimens as those who are HIV-negative; however, prolonged treatment may be required and delay in resolution of symptoms may occur.

RECOMMENDED REGIMEN
Regimen 1

➤ *doxycycline* 100 mg bid x 21 days

ALTERNATIVE REGIMEN
Regimen 1

➤ *erythromycin base* 500 mg qid x 21 days **or** *erythromycin ethylsuccinate* 400 mg qid x 21 days

RECOMMENDED REGIMENS FOR THE MANAGEMENT OF SEXUAL CONTACTS

Comment: LGV is caused by *C. trachomatis* serovars L1, L2, **or** L3. Persons who have had sexual contact with a patient who has LGV within 60 days before onset of the patient's symptoms should be examined, tested for urethral **or** cervical chlamydial infection, and treated with a chlamydia regimen.

Regimen 1

➤ *azithromycin* 1 gm in a single dose

Regimen 2

➤ *doxycycline* 100 mg bid x 7 days

DRUG BRANDS AND DOSE FORMS

▷ *azithromycin* (B)(G)

> **Zithromax** *Tab:* 250, 500, 600 mg; *Oral susp:* 100 mg/5 ml (15 ml); 200 mg/5 ml (15, 22.5, 30 ml) (cherry); *Pkt:* 1 gm for reconstitution (cherry-banana)
> **Zithromax Tri-pak** *Tab:* 3 x 500 mg tabs/pck
> **Zithromax Z-pak** *Tab:* 6 x 250 mg tabs/pck
> **Zmax** *Oral susp:* 2 gm ext-rel for reconstitution (cherry-banana) (148 mg Na⁺)

▷ *doxycycline* (D)(G)

> **Acticlate** *Tab:* 75, 150**mg
> **Adoxa** *Tab:* 50, 75, 100, 150 mg ent-coat
> **Doryx** *Tab:* 50, 75, 100, 150, 200 mg del-rel
> **Doxteric** *Tab:* 50 mg del-rel
> **Monodox** *Cap:* 50, 75, 100 mg
> **Oracea** *Cap:* 40 mg del-rel
> **Vibramycin** *Tab:* 100 mg; *Cap:* 50, 100 mg; *Syr:* 50 mg/5 ml (raspberry-apple) (sulfites); *Oral susp:* 25 mg/5 ml (raspberry)
> **Vibra-Tab** *Tab:* 100 mg film-coat

▷ *erythromycin base* (B)(G)

> **Ery-Tab** *Tab:* 250, 333, 500 mg ent-coat
> **PCE** *Tab:* 333, 500 mg

Comment: *erythromycin* may increase INR with concomitant *warfarin*, as well as increase serum level of *digoxin, benzodiazepines*, and *statins*.

▷ *erythromycin ethylsuccinate* (B)(G)

> **EryPed** *Oral susp:* 200 mg/5 ml (100, 200 ml) (fruit); 400 mg/5 ml (60, 100, 200 ml) (banana); *Oral drops:* 200, 400 mg/5 ml (50 ml) (fruit); *Chew tab:* 200 mg wafer (fruit)
> **E.E.S.** *Oral susp:* 200, 400 mg/5 ml (100 ml) (fruit)
> **E.E.S. Granules** *Oral susp:* 200 mg/5 ml (100, 200 ml) (cherry)
> **E.E.S. 400 Tablets** *Tab:* 400 mg

Comment: *erythromycin* may increase INR with concomitant *warfarin*, as well as increase serum level of *digoxin*, benzodiazepines and statins.

◯ MALARIA (*PLASMODIUM FALCIPARUM, PLASMODIUM VIVAX*)

▷ *doxycycline* (D)(G) 100 mg daily; initiate 1-2 days prior to travel; take during travel; continue for 4 weeks after leaving the endemic area
Pediatric: ≤8 years: not recommended; ≥8 years, ≤100 lb: 1 mg/lb/day prior to travel; take during travel; continue for 4 weeks after leaving the endemic area; ≥8 years, ≥100 lb: same as adult; *see page 633 for dose by weight*

> **Acticlate** *Tab:* 75, 150**mg
> **Adoxa** *Tab:* 50, 75, 100, 150 mg ent-coat
> **Doryx** *Tab:* 50, 75, 100, 150, 200 mg del-rel
> **Doxteric** *Tab:* 50 mg del-rel
> **Monodox** *Cap:* 50, 75, 100 mg
> **Oracea** *Cap:* 40 mg del-rel
> **Vibramycin** *Tab:* 100 mg; *Cap:* 50, 100 mg; *Syr:* 50 mg/5 ml (raspberry-apple) (sulfites); *Oral susp:* 25 mg/5 ml (raspberry)
> **Vibra-Tab** *Tab:* 100 mg film-coat

Comment: *doxycycline* is contraindicated <8 years-of-age, in pregnancy, and lactation (discolors developing tooth enamel). A side effect may be photosensitivity (photophobia). Do not take with antacids, calcium supplements, milk or other dairy, or within 2 hours of taking another drug.

▷ *minocycline* (D)(G) 100 mg daily; initiate 1-2 days prior to travel; take during travel; continue for 4 weeks after leaving the endemic area
Pediatric: <8 years: not recommended; ≥8 years, ≤100 lb: 2 mg/lb on first day in 2 divided doses, followed by 1 mg/lb q 12 hours x 9 more days; ≥8 years, >100 lb: same as adult
   Dynacin *Cap:* 50, 100 mg
   Minocin *Cap:* 50, 75, 100 mg; *Oral susp:* 50 mg/5 ml (60 ml) (custard) (sulfites, alcohol 5%)

Comment: *minocycline* is contraindicated <8 years-of-age, in pregnancy, and lactation (discolors developing tooth enamel). A side effect may be photo-sensitivity (photophobia). Do not give with antacids, calcium supplements, milk or other dairy, or within 2 hours of taking another drug.

▷ *tetracycline* (D) 250 mg daily; initiate 1-2 days prior to travel; take during travel; continue for 4 weeks after leaving the endemic area
Pediatric: <8 years: not recommended; ≥8 years, ≤100 lb: 25-50 mg/kg/day in 4 divided doses x 10 days; ≥8 years, >100 lb: same as adult; *see page 646 for dose by weight*
   Achromycin V *Cap:* 250, 500 mg
   Sumycin *Tab:* 250, 500 mg; *Cap:* 250, 500 mg; *Oral susp:* 125 mg/5 ml (100, 200 ml) (fruit) (sulfites)

Comment: *tetracycline* is contraindicated <8 years-of-age, in pregnancy, and lactation (discolors developing tooth enamel). A side effect may be photosen-sensitivity (photophobia). Do not give with antacids, calcium supplements, milk or other dairy, or within 2 hours of taking another drug.

ANTIMALARIALS

▷ *quinine sulfate* (C)(G) 1 tab or cap every 8 hours x 7 days
Pediatric: <16 years: not recommended; ≥16 years: same as adult
     Tab: 260 mg; *Cap:* 260, 300, 325 mg
   Qualaquin *Cap:* 324 mg

Comment: *Qualaquin* is indicated in the treatment of uncomplicated *P. falciparum* malaria (including chloroquine-resistant strains).

▷ *atovaquone* (C)(G) take as a single dose with food or a milky drink at the same time each day; repeat dose if vomited within 1 hour; *Prophylaxis:* 1,500 mg once daily; *Treatment:* 750 mg bid x 21 days
   Mepron *Susp:* 750 mg/5 ml

▷ *atovaquone+proguanil* (C)(G) take as a single dose with food or a milky drink at the same time each day; repeat dose if vomited within 1 hour; *Prophylaxis:* 1 tab daily starting 1-2 days before entering endemic area, during stay, and for 7 days after return; *Treatment (acute, uncomplicated):* 4 tabs daily x 3 days
Pediatric: <5 kg: not recommended; 5-40 kg:
Prophylaxis: daily dose starting 1-2 days before entering endemic area, during stay, and for 7 days after return; 5-20 kg: 1 ped tab; 21-30 kg: 2 ped tabs; 31-40 kg: 3 ped tabs; ≥40 kg: same as adult; *Treatment (acute, uncomplicated):* daily dose x 3 days; 5-8 kg: 2 ped tabs; 9-10 kg: 3 ped tabs; 11-20 kg: 1 adult tab; 21-30 kg: 2 adult tabs; 31-40 kg: 3 adult tabs; >40 kg: same as adult
   Malarone *Tab: atov* 250 mg+*prog* 100 mg
   Malarone Pediatric *Tab: atov* 62.5 mg+*prog* 25 mg

Comment: *atovaquone* is antagonized by *tetracycline* and *metoclopramide*. Concomitant *rifampin* is not recommended (may elevate LFTs).

▷ *chloroquine* (C)(G) *Prophylaxis:* 500 mg once weekly (on the same day of each week); start 2 weeks prior to exposure, continue while in the endemic area, and continue 4 weeks after departure; *Treatment:* initially 1 gm; then 500 mg 6 hours, 24 hours, and 48 hours after initial dose or initially 200-250 mg IM; may repeat in 6 hours; max 1 gm in first 24 hours; continue to 1.875 gm in 3 days

Pediatric: Suppression: 8.35 mg/kg (max 500 mg) weekly (on the same day of each week); *Treatment:* initially 16.7 mg/kg (max 1 gm); then 8.35 mg/kg (max 500 mg) 6 hours, 24 hours, and 48 hours after initial dose, <u>or</u> initially 6.25 mg/kg IM; may repeat in 6 hours; max 12.5 mg/kg/day

Aralen *Tab:* 500 mg; *Amp:* 50 mg/ml (5 ml)

▷ **hydroxychloroquine (C)(G)** *Prophylaxis:* 400 mg once weekly (on the same day of each week); start 2 weeks prior to exposure, continue while in the endemic area, and continue 8 weeks after departure; *Treatment:* initially 800 mg; then 400 mg 6 hours, 24 hours, and 48 hours after initial dose

Pediatric: Suppression: 6.45 mg/kg (max 400 mg) weekly (on the same day of each week) beginning 2 weeks prior to arrival, continuing while in endemic area, and continuing 4 weeks after departure; *Treatment:* initially 12.9 mg/kg (max 800 mg); then 6.45 mg/kg (max 400 mg) 6 hours, 24 hours, and 48 hours after initial dose hours after initial dose

Plaquenil *Tab:* 200 mg

▷ **mefloquine (C)** *Prophylaxis:* 250 mg once weekly (on the same day of each week); start 1 week prior to exposure, continue while in the endemic area, and continue for 4 weeks after departure; *Treatment:* 1,250 mg as a single dose

Pediatric: <6 months: not recommended; *Prophylaxis:* ≥6 months: 3-5 mg/kg (max 250 mg) weekly (on the same day of each week); start 1 week prior to exposure, continue while in the endemic area, and continue for 4 weeks after departure; *Treatment:* ≥6 months: 25-50 mg/kg as a single dose; max 250 mg

Lariam *Tab:* 250*mg

Comment: *mefloquine* is contraindicated with active <u>or</u> recent history of depression, generalized anxiety disorder, psychosis, schizophrenia <u>or</u> any other psychiatric disorder <u>or</u> history of convulsions.

⬤ MASTITIS (BREAST ABSCESS)

ANTI-INFECTIVES

▷ **amoxicillin+clavulanate (B)(G)**

Augmentin 500 mg tid <u>or</u> 875 mg bid x 7-10 days

Pediatric: 40-45 mg/kg/day divided tid x 10 days <u>or</u> 90 mg/kg/day divided bid x 10 days *see pages 618-619 for dose by weight*

Tab: 250, 500, 875 mg; *Chew tab:* 125, 250 mg (lemon-lime); 200, 400 mg (cherry-banana) (phenylalanine); *Oral susp:* 125 mg/5 ml (banana), 250 mg/5 ml (75, 100, 150 ml) (orange); 200, 400 mg/5 ml (50, 75, 100 ml) (orange) (phenylalanine)

Augmentin ES-600 not recommended for adults

Pediatric: <3 months: not recommended; ≥3 months, <40 kg: 90 mg/kg/day in 2 divided doses x 7-10 days; ≥40 kg: not recommended

Oral susp: 42.9 mg/5 ml (50, 75, 100, 125, 150, 200 ml) (strawberry cream) (phenylalanine)

Augmentin XR 2 tabs q 12 hours x 7-10 days

Pediatric: <16 years: use other forms; ≥16 years: same as adult

Tab: 1000*mg ext-rel

▷ **cefaclor (B)(G)** 250-500 mg q 8 hours x 10 days; max 2 gm/day

Pediatric: <1 month: not recommended; 20-40 mg/kg bid <u>or</u> q 12 hours x 10 days; max 1 gm/day; *see page 622 for dose by weight*

Tab: 500 mg; *Cap:* 250, 500 mg; *Susp:* 125 mg/5 ml (75, 150 ml) (strawberry); 187 mg/5 ml (50, 100 ml) (strawberry); 250 mg/5 ml (75, 150 ml) (strawberry); 375 mg/5 ml (50, 100 ml) (strawberry)

Pediatric: <16 years: ext-rel not recommended; ≥12 years: same as adult
    Cefaclor Extended Release *Tab:* 375, 500 mg ext-rel

▷ *ceftriaxone* (B)(G) 1-2 gm IM daily continued 2 days after signs of infection have disappeared; max 4 gm/day
Pediatric: 50 mg/kg IM daily continued 2 days after signs of infection have disappeared
    Rocephin *Vial:* 250, 500 mg; 1, 2 gm

▷ *cephalexin* (B)(G) 500 mg bid x 10 days
Pediatric: 25-50 mg/kg/day in 4 divided doses x 10 days; *see page* 629 *for dose by weight*
    Keflex *Cap:* 250, 333, 500, 750 mg; *Oral susp:* 125, 250 mg/5 ml (100, 200 ml) (strawberry)

▷ *clindamycin* (B)(G) 300 mg tid x 10 days
Pediatric: <12 years: not recommended; ≥12 years: same as adult
    Cleocin *Cap:* 75 (tartrazine), 150 (tartrazine), 300 mg
    Cleocin Pediatric Granules *Oral susp:* 75 mg/5 ml (100 ml) (cherry)

▷ *erythromycin base* (B)(G) 250-500 mg qid x 10 days
Pediatric: <45 kg: 30-40 mg/kg/day in 4 divided doses x 10 days; ≥45 kg: same as adult
    Ery-Tab *Tab:* 250, 333, 500 mg ent-coat
    PCE *Tab:* 333, 500 mg

Comment: *erythromycin* may increase INR with concomitant *warfarin*, as well as increase serum level of *digoxin, benzodiazepines*, and *statins*.

MELASMA/CHLOASMA

SKIN DEPIGMENTING AGENTS

▷ *hydroquinone* (C) apply a thin film to clean dry affected areas bid; discontinue if lightening does not occur after 2 months
Pediatric: <12 years: not recommended; ≥12 years: same as adult
    Lustra *Crm:* hydro 4% (1, 2 oz) (sulfites)
    Lustra AF *Crm:* hydro 4% (1, 2 oz) (sunscreens, sulfites)

▷ *hydroquinone+fluocinolone acetonide+tretinoin* (C) apply a thin film to clean dry affected areas once daily at least 30 minutes before bedtime
Pediatric: <12 years: not recommended; ≥12 years: same as adult
    Tri-Luma *Crm:* hydro 4%+*fluo acet* 0.01%+*tret* 0.05% (30 gm) (sulfites, parabens)

MENIERE'S DISEASE

▷ *diazepam* (D)(IV)(G) initially 1-2.5 mg tid-qid; may increase gradually
Pediatric: <6 months: not recommended; ≥6 months: same as adult
    Diastat *Rectal gel delivery system:* 2.5 mg
    Diastat AcuDial *Rectal gel delivery system:* 10, 20 mg
    Valium *Tab:* 2*, 5*, 10*mg
    Valium Intensol Oral Solution *Conc oral soln:* 5 mg/ml (30 ml w. dropper) (alcohol 19%)
    Valium Oral Solution *Oral soln:* 5 mg/5 ml (500 ml) (wintergreen-spice)

▷ *dimenhydrinate* (B) 50 mg q 4-6 hours
Pediatric: <2 years: not recommended; 2-6 years: 12.5-25 mg q 6-8 hours; max 75 mg/day; >6-11 years: 25-50 mg q 6-8 hours; max 150 mg/day; >11 years: same as adult
    Dramamine (OTC) *Tab:* 50*mg; *Chew tab:* 50 mg (phenylalanine, tartrazine); *Liq:* 12.5 mg/5 ml (4 oz)

▷ *diphenhydramine* (B)(OTC)(G) 25-50 mg q 6-8 hours; max 100 mg/day
Pediatric: <2 years: not recommended; 2-6 years: 6.25 mg q 4-6 hours; max 37.5 mg/day; >6-12 years: 12.5-25 mg q 4-6 hours; max 150 mg/day; >12 years: same as adult

Benadryl (OTC) *Chew tab:* 12.5 mg (grape; phenylalanine); *Liq:* 12.5 mg/5 ml (4, 8 oz); *Cap:* 25 mg; *Tab:* 25 mg; *dye-free softgel:* 25 mg; Dye-free liq: 12.5 mg/5 ml (4, 8 oz)

▷ *meclizine* **(B)(G)** 25-100/day in divided doses
  Pediatric: <12 years: not recommended; ≥12 years: same as adult
    Antivert *Tab:* 12.5, 25, 50*mg; *Amp:* 50 mg/ml (1 ml); *Vial:* 50 mg/ml (1 ml single-use); 50 mg/ml (10 ml multi-dose)
    Bonine (OTC) *Cap:* 15, 25, 30 mg; *Tab:* 12.5, 25, 50 mg; *Chew tab/Film-coat tab:* 25 mg
    Dramamine II 25 mg bid; max 50 mg/day
      Tab: 25*mg
    Zentrip *Strip:* 25 mg orally disintegrating

▷ *promethazine* **(C)** 12.5-25 q 4-6 hours PO or rectally
  Pediatric: <2 years: not recommended; ≥2 years: 0.5 mg/lb or 6.25-25 mg q 4-6 hours PO or rectally
    Phenergan *Tab:* 12.5*, 25*, 50 mg; *Plain syr:* 6.25 mg/5 ml; *Fortis syr:* 25 mg/5 ml; *Rectal supp:* 12.5, 25, 50 mg

Comment: *promethazine* is contraindicated in children with uncomplicated nausea, dehydration, Reye's syndrome, history of sleep apnea, asthma, and lower respiratory disorders in children. **Promethazine** lowers the seizure threshold in children, may cause cholestatic jaundice, anticholinergic effects, extrapyramidal effects, and potentially fatal respiratory depression.

▷ *scopolamine* transdermal patch **(C)** 1 patch behind ear; each patch is effective for 3 days; change patch every 4th day; alternate sites
  Pediatric: <12 years: not recommended; ≥12 years: same as adult
    Transderm Scop *Patch:* 1.5 mg (4/carton)

MENINGITIS (*NEISSERIA MENINGITIDIS*)

PROPHYLAXIS

Comment: Meningitis vaccine is a 3-dose series (0, 2, 6 month schedule) indicated for persons age ≥10-25 years. Have epinephrine 1:1,000 readily available and monitor for 15 minutes post-dose of meningitis vaccine.

▷ *Meningococcal group b vaccine [recombinant, absorbed]* administer first dose IM in the deltoid; administer second dose 2 months later; administer the third dose 6 months from the first dose;
  Pediatric: <10 years: not established; ≥10 years: same as adult
    Bexsero *Susp for IM inj:* 0.5 ml single-dose prefilled syringes (1, 10/carton)
    Trumenba *Susp for IM inj:* 0.5 ml single-dose prefilled syringes (5, 10/carton)

▷ *Neisseria meningitides oligosaccharide conjugate* quadrivalent meningococcal vaccine **(B)** contains *Corynebacterium diphtheria* CRM197 protein; 10 mcg of Group A + 5 mcg each of Group C, Y, and W-135 + 32.7-64.1 mcg of diphtheria CRM 197 protein per 0.5 m.
  Pediatric: <11 years: not recommended; ≥11-55 years: 0.5 ml IM x 1 dose in the deltoid
    Menveo *Vial multi-dose:* 5 doses/vial (MenA conjugate component pwdr for reconstitution + 1 vial liquid MenCWY conjugate component for reconstitution) (preservative-free)

▷ *Neisseria meningitidis polysaccharides* vaccine **(C)** 0.5 ml SC x 1 dose; if at high risk, may revaccinate after 3-5 years; age ≥55 years contact mfr
    Menactra (A/C/Y/W-135)
    Pediatric: <2 years: see mfr pkg insert; ≥2 years: same as adult; if at high risk, may revaccinate children first vaccinated ≤4 years-of-age after 2-3 years

Vial (single-dose): 4 mcg each of group A, C, Y, and W-135 per 0.5 ml (pwdr for SC inj after reconstitution) (preservative-free diluent); *Vial (multi-dose):* 4 mcg each of group A, C, Y, and W-130 per 0.5 ml [pwdr for SC inj after reconstitution (5 doses/vial) (preservative-free)]

Comment: Latex allergy is a contraindication to **Menactra**.

Menomune-A/C/Y/W-135

Pediatric: <2 years: not recommended (except ≥3 months of age as short-term protection against group A); ≥2 years: same as adult; if at high risk, may revaccinate children first vaccinated ≤4 years of age after 2-3 years (older children after 3-5 years)

Vial (single-dose): 50 mcg each of group A, C, Y, and W-135 per 0.5 ml (pwdr for SC inj after reconstitution; preservative-free diluent); *Vial (multi-dose):* 50 mcg each of group A, C, Y, and W-130 per 0.5 ml [pwdr for SC inj after reconstitution (10 doses/vial) (thimerosal-preserved diluent)]

Comment: Use precaution with latex allergy.

MENOPAUSE

Comment: *Estrogen* replacement lowers LDL and raises HDL. *Estrogen* replacement is indicated for osteoporosis prevention. However, exogenous *estrogen* administration increases risk for endometrial cancer, MI, stroke, invasive breast cancer, pulmonary embolism, and DVT. *estrogen* replacement is contraindicated in known or suspected pregnancy, known or suspected cancer of the breast, known or suspected *estrogen*-dependent neoplasia, undiagnosed genital bleeding, and active thrombophlebitis or thromboembolic disorders. HRT should be used with extreme caution, and only after a thorough risk/benefit assessment, in patients with cardiovascular or peripheral vascular disease. The US Preventive Services Task Force (USPSTF) recommends against using hormone replacement therapy (HRT) for primary prevention of chronic conditions among postmenopausal women. The harms associated with combined use of estrogen and a progestin, such as increased risks of invasive breast cancer, venous thromboembolism and coronary heart disease, far outweigh the benefits.

However, In an update of their 2012 Hormone Therapy Position Statement, the North American Menopause Society (NAMS) suggests the benefits of hormone therapy, particularly for vasomotor symptoms, outweigh the risks among women under age 60, within a decade of the onset of menopause without other contraindications, who also have an increased risk of fracture or bone loss. Current FDA-approved indications for hormone therapy include the treatment of vasomotor symptoms, prevention of bone loss, genitourinary symptoms, and premature hypoestrogenism caused by castration, hypogonadism, or primary ovarian insufficiency. The work group suggested there are notably higher risks with initiation of hormone therapy after a decade of the onset of menopause, or among women who are over the age of 60, citing an increased absolute risk for cardiovascular harms including stroke, coronary heart disease, venous thromboembolism, and dementia. The statement also noted that for women who exclusively have genitourinary syndrome symptoms, such as urinary, vulvar, and vaginal-related symptoms alone, low-dose vaginal estrogen therapy, such as creams, rings, and tablets that contain estradiol or conjugated equine estrogens are considered "generally safe," but should be more closely considered among women with breast cancer. Patients who require longer durations of hormone therapy, such as to treat persistent vasomotor symptoms or continued bone loss, should determine the benefit-risk profile with her healthcare provider in addition to reassessment during treatment, the statement recommended. The full 2017 position statement appears in *Menopause: The Journal of the North American Menopause Society*.

REFERENCES

Langer, R. D., Simon, J. A., Pines, A., Lobo, R. A., Hodis, H. N., Pickar, J. H., . . . Utian, W. H. (2017). Menopausal hormone therapy for primary prevention. *Menopause, 24*(10), 1101–1112. doi:10.1097/gme.0000000000000983

Monaco, K. HRT Benefits Outweigh Risks for Certain Menopausal Women—Menopause Society statement aims to clear up confusion. https://www.medpagetoday.com/Endocrinology/Menopause/66158?xid=NL_MPT_IRXHealthWomen_2017-12-27&eun=g766320d0r

The 2017 hormone therapy position statement of The North American Menopause Society. (2017). *Menopause, 24*(7), 728–753. doi:10.1097/gme.0000000000000921

VAGINAL RINGS

▷ *estradiol, acetate* (X)

    Femring Vaginal Ring insert high into vagina; replace every 90 days

▷ *estradiol, micronized* (X)

    Estring Vaginal Ring insert high into vagina; replace every 90 days

       Vag ring: 7.5 mcg/24 hours (1/pck)

REGIMENS FOR PATIENTS WITH INTACT UTERUS

Vaginal Preparations (With Uterus)

Comment: Vaginal preparations provide relief from vaginal and urinary symptoms only (i.e., atrophic vaginitis, dyspareunia, dysuria, and urinary frequency).

▷ *estradiol* (X)(G)

    Vagifem Tabs insert one 10 mcg or 25 mcg vaginal tablet once daily x 2 weeks; then twice weekly for 2 weeks (e.g., tues/fri); consider the addition of a progestin

       Vag tab: 10, 25 mcg (8, 18/blister pck with applicator)

    Yuvafem Vaginal Tablet 1 tab intravaginally daily x 2 weeks; then 1 tab intravaginally twice weekly

       Vag tab: 10 mcg (15 tabs w. applicators)

▷ *estradiol, micronized* (X) **Estrace Vaginal Cream** 2-4 gm daily x 1-2 weeks, then gradually reduced to 1/2 initial dose x 1-2 weeks, then maintenance dose of 1 gm 1-3 x/week

       Vag crm: 0.01% (12, 42.5 gm w. calib applicator)

▷ *estrogen, conjugated equine* (X)

    Premarin Vaginal Cream 0.5-2 gm/day intravaginally; cyclically (3 weeks on, 1 week off)

       Vag crm: 1.5 oz w. applicator marked in 1/2 gm increments to max of 2 gm

Transdermal Systems (With Uterus)

Comment: Alternate sites. Do not apply patches on or near breasts.

▷ *estradiol* (X)(G)

    Climara initially 0.025 mg/day patch once/week to trunk (3 weeks on and 1 week off)

       Transdermal patch: 0.025, 0.0375, 0.05, 0.075, 0.1 mg/day (4/pck)

    Esclim apply twice weekly x 3 weeks, then 1 week off; use with an oral progestin to prevent endometrial hyperplasia

       Transdermal patch: 0.025, 0.0375, 0.05, 0.075, 0.1 mg/day (8, 48/pck)

    Vivelle initially one 0.0375 mg/day patch twice weekly to trunk area; use with an oral progestin to prevent endometrial hyperplasia

       Transdermal patch: 0.025, 0.0375, 0.05, 0.075, 0.1 mg/day (8, 48/pck)

    Vivelle-Dot initially one 0.05 mg/day patch twice weekly to lower-abdomen, below the waist; use with an oral progestin to prevent endometrial-hyperplasia

       Transdermal patch: 0.025, 0.0375, 0.05, 0.075, 0.1 mg/day (8, 24/pck)

➢ *estradiol+levonorgestrel* (X) apply 1 patch weekly to lower abdomen; avoid waistline; alternate sites

Climara Pro *Transdermal patch: estra* 0.045 mg+*levo* 0.015 mg per day (4/pck)
➢ *estradiol+norethindrone* (X)

CombiPatch apply twice weekly <u>or</u> q 3-4 days

Transdermal patch: 9 cm^2: *estra* 0.05 mg+*noreth* 0.14 mg; 16 cm^2: *estra* 0.05 mg+*noreth* 0.25 mg

Comment: May cause irregular bleeding in first 6 months of therapy, but usually decreases over time (often to amenorrhea).

ORAL AGENTS (WITH UTERUS)

➢ *estradiol* (X)(G)

Estrace 1-2 mg daily cyclically (3 weeks on and 1 week off)

Tab: 0.5, 1, 2*mg (tartrazine)
➢ *estradiol+drospirenone* (X)

Angeliq 1 tab daily

Tab: **Angeliq 0.5/0.25** *estra* 0.5 mg+*dros* 0.25 mg

Angeliq 1/0.5 *estra* 1 mg+*dros* 0.5 mg
➢ *estradiol+norethindrone* (X) 1 tab daily

Activella (G) *Tab: estra* 1 mg+*noreth* 0.5 mg

FemHRT (G) 1/5 *Tab: estra* 5 mcg+*noreth* 1 mg

Fyavolv (G) *Tab: estra* 0.25 mg+*noreth* 1 mg; *Tab: estra* 0.5 mg+*noreth* 1 mg

Mimvey LO *Tab: estra* 0.5 mg+*noreth* 0.1 mg
➢ *estradiol+norgestimate* (X) 1 x *estradiol* 1 mg tab once daily x 3 days, then 1 x *estradiol* 1 mg+*norgestimate* 0.09 mg tab daily x 3 days; repeat this pattern continuously

Ortho-Prefest *Tab: estra* 1 mg+*norgest* 0.09 mg (30/blister pck)
➢ *estrogen, conjugated+medroxyprogesterone* (X)

Prempro 1 tab daily

Tab: **Prempro 0.3/1.5** estro, conj 0.3 mg+medroxy 1.5 mg

Prempro 0.45/1.5 estro, conj 0.45 mg+medroxy 1.5 mg

Prempro 0.625/2.5 estro, conj 0.625 mg+medroxy 2.5 mg

Prempro 0.625/5 estro, conj 0.625 mg+medroxy 5 mg

Premphase 0.625 *estrogen* on days 1-14, then 0.625 mg *estrogen*+5 mg *medroxyprogesterone* on days 15-28

Tab (in dial dispenser): estro, conj 0.625 mg (14 maroon tabs) + medroxy 5 mg (14 blue tabs)
➢ *estrogen, esterified (plant derived)* (X)

Menest 0.3-2.5 mg daily cyclically, 3 weeks on and 1 week off (with progestins in the latter part of the cycle to prevent endometrial hyperplasia)

Tab: 0.3, 0.625, 1.25, 2.5 mg
➢ *estrogen, esterified+methyltestosterone* (X)

Estratest 1 tab daily cyclically, 3 weeks on and 1 week off

Tab: estro ester 1.25 mg+*meth* 2.5 mg

Estratest HS 1-2 tabs daily cyclically, 3 weeks on and 1 week off

Tab: estro ester 0.625 mg+*meth* 1.25 mg
➢ *ethinyl estradiol* (X) 0.02-0.05 mg q 1-2 days cyclically, 3 weeks on and 1 week off (with progestins in the latter part of the cycle to prevent endometrial hyperplasia)

Estinyl *Tab:* 0.02 (tartrazine), 0.05 mg
➢ *estropipate, piperazine estrone sulfate* (X)(G)

Ogen 0.625-1.25 mg daily cyclically (3 weeks on and 1 week off)

Tab: 0.625, 1.25, 2.5 mg

Ortho-Est 0.75-6 mg daily cyclically (3 weeks on and 1 week off)

Tab: 0.625, 1.25 mg

▷ *medroxyprogesterone* (X) 5-10 mg daily for 12 sequential days of each 28-day cycle to prevent endometrial hyperplasia in the postmenopausal women with an intact uterus receiving conjugated estrogens
   Provera *Tab:* 2.5, 5, 10 mg
▷ *norethindrone acetate* (X) 2.5-10 mg daily x 5-10 days during second half of menstrual cycle
   Aygestin *Tab:* 5*mg
▷ *progesterone, micronized* (X)(G)
   Prometrium 200 mg daily in the PM for 12 sequential days of each 28-day cycle to prevent endometrial hyperplasia in the postmenopausal woman with an intact uterus receiving conjugated estrogens
      Cap: 100, 200 mg (peanut oil)

ESTROGENS, CONJUGATED+ESTROGEN AGONIST-ANTAGONIST

▷ *estrogen, conjugated+bazedoxifene* (X)
   Duavee 1 tab daily
      Tab: conj estra 0.45 mg+*baze* 20 mg

REGIMENS FOR PATIENTS WITHOUT UTERUS
Oral Agents (Without Uterus)

▷ *estradiol* (X)(G)
   Estrace 1-2 mg daily
      Tab: 0.5*, 1*, 2*mg (tartrazine)
▷ *estrogen, conjugated (equine)* (X)
   Premarin 1 tab daily
      Tab: 0.3, 0.45, 0.625, 0.9, 1.25, 2.5 mg
▷ *estrogen, conjugated (synthetic)* (X) 1 tab daily; may titrate up to max 1.25 mg/day
   Cenestin *Tab:* 0.3, 0.625, 0.9, 1.25 mg
   Enjuvia *Tab:* 0.3, 0.45, 0.625 mg
▷ *estrogen, esterified (plant derived)* (X) 1 tab daily
   Estratab *Tab:* 0.3, 0.625, 2.5 mg
   Menest *Tab:* 0.3, 0.625, 1.25, 2.5 mg
▷ *ethinyl estradiol* (X) 0.02-0.05 mg q 1-2 days
   Estinyl *Tab:* 0.02 (tartrazine), 0.05 mg

Vaginal Preparations (Without Uterus)

Comment: Vaginal preparations provide relief from vaginal and urinary symptoms only (i.e., atrophic vaginitis, dyspareunia, dysuria, and urinary frequency).
▷ *estradiol* (X)(G)
   Vagifem Tabs insert one 10 mcg or 25 mcg vaginal tablet once daily x 2 weeks; then twice weekly for 2 weeks (e.g., tues/fri); consider the addition of a progestin
      Vag tab: 10, 25 mcg (8, 18/blister pck with applicator)
   Yuvafem Vaginal Tablet 1 tab intravaginally daily x 2 weeks; then 1 tab intravaginally twice weekly
      Vag tab: 10 mcg (15 tabs w. applicators)

Topical Agents (Without Uterus)

▷ *estradiol* (X)
   Estrasorb apply 3.48 gm (2 pouches) every morning; apply one pouch to each leg from the upper thigh to the calf; rub in for 3 minutes; rub excess on hands onto buttocks
      Emul: 0.025 mg/day/pouch (2.5 mg/gm; 1.74 gm/pouch)

EstroGel apply 1.25 gm (one compression) to one arm from wrist to shoulder once daily at the same time each day

Gel: 0.06% per compression (93 gm)

Transdermal Systems (Without Uterus)

Comment: Do not apply patches on *or* near breasts. Alternate sites.

▷ *estradiol* (X)

Alora initially 0.05 mg/day apply patch twice weekly to lower abdomen, upper quadrant of buttocks *or* outer aspect of hip

Transdermal patch: 0.025, 0.05, 0.075, 0.1 mg/day (8, 24/pck)

Climara initially 0.025 mg/day patch once/week to trunk

Transdermal patch: 0.025, 0.0375, 0.05, 0.075, 0.1 mg/day (4, 8, 24/pck)

Esclim initially 0.025 mg/day apply patch twice weekly to buttocks, femoral triangle, *or* upper arm

Transdermal patch: 0.025, 0.0375, 0.05, 0.075, 0.1 mg/day (8/pck)

Estraderm initially apply one 0.05 mg/day patch twice weekly to trunk

Transdermal patch: 0.05, 0.1 mg/day (8, 24/pck)

Menostar apply one patch weekly to lower abdomen, below the waist; avoid the breasts; alternate sites

Transdermal patch: 14 mcg/day (4/pck)

Minivelle initially one 0.0375 mg/day patch twice weekly to trunk area; adjust after one month of therapy

Transdermal patch: 0.025, 0.0375, 0.05, 0.075, 0.1 mg/day (8/pck)

Vivelle initially one 0.0375 mg/day patch twice weekly to trunk area; adjust after one month of therapy

Transdermal patch: 0.025, 0.0375, 0.05, 0.075, 0.1 mg/day (8, 48/pck)

Vivelle-Dot initially apply one 0.05 mg/day patch twice weekly to lower abdomen, below the waist; adjust after one month of therapy

Transdermal patch: 0.025, 0.0375, 0.05, 0.075, 0.1 mg/day (8, 24/pck)

Comment: The *estrogens* in **Alora**, **Climara**, **Estraderm**, and **Vivelle-Dot** are plant derived.

MENOMETRORRHAGIA: IRREGULAR HEAVY MENSTRUAL BLEEDING AND MENORRHAGIA: HEAVY CYCLICAL MENSTRUAL BLEEDING

ANTIFIBROLYTIC AGENT

▷ *tranexamic acid* (B)(G) 1,300 mg tid; treat for up to 5 days during menses; *Normal renal function (SCr ≤1.4 mg/dL):* 1,300 mg tid; *SCr ≥1.4-2.8 mg/dL:* 1,300 mg bid; *SCr ≥2.8-5.7 mg/dL:* 1,300 mg once daily; *SCr ≥5.7 mg/dL:* 650 mg once daily

Pediatric: <18 years: not recommended; ≥18 years: same as adult

Lysteda *Tab:* 650 mg

Injectible Progesterone Only Contraceptives

▷ *medroxyprogesterone* (X)(G)

Depo-Provera 150 mg deep IM q 3 months

Vial: 150 mg/ml (1 ml)

Prefilled syringe: 150 mg/ml

Depo-SubQ 104 mg SC q 3 months

Prefilled syringe: 104 mg/ml (0.65 ml; parabens)

Comment: Administer first dose within 5 days of onset of normal menses, within 5 days postpartum if not breastfeeding, *or* at 6 weeks postpartum if breastfeeding exclusively. Do not use for >2 years unless other methods are inadequate.

Combined Oral Contraceptives *see page* 548
Intrauterine Devices *see page* 559

 METHAMPHETAMINE-INDUCED PSYCHOSIS

ANTIPSYCHOSIS AGENTS

For more antipsychotics, see **Appendix Q: Antipsychosis Drugs** *pages* 581
Tardive Dyskinesia *see page* 456

Comment: First-generation antipsychotics (e.g., *haloperidol* or *fluphenazine*) should be used sparingly and cautiously in patients with methamphetamine-induced psychosis because of the risk of developing extrapyramidal symptoms (EPS) and because these patients are prone to develop motor complications as a result of methamphetamine abuse. Second-generation antipsychotics (e.g., *risperidone* and *olanzapine*) may be more appropriate because of the lower risks of EPS. The presence of high norepinephrine levels in some patients with recurrent methamphetamine psychosis suggests that drugs that block norepinephrine receptors (e.g., *prazosin* or *propranolol*) might be of therapeutic benefit although they have not been studied in controlled trials.

REFERENCE
Zarrabi, H., Khalkhali, M., Hamidi, A., Ahmadi, R., & Zavarmousavi, M. (2016). Clinical features, course and treatment of methamphetamine-induced psychosis in psychiatric inpatients. *BMC Psychiatry, 16*(44).

▷ *aripiprazole* (C)(G) initially 15 mg once daily; may increase to max 30 mg/day
Pediatric: <10 years: not recommended; ≥10-17 years: initially 2 mg/day in a single dose for 2 days; then increase to 5 mg/day in a single dose for 2 days; then increase to target dose of 10 mg/day in a single dose; may increase by 5 mg/day at weekly intervals as needed to max 30 mg/day
   Abilify *Tab:* 2, 5, 10, 15, 20, 30 mg
   Abilify Discmelt *Tab:* 15 mg orally-disint (vanilla) (phenylalanine)
   Abilify Maintena *Vial:* 300, 400 mg ext-rel pwdr for IM injection after reconstitution; 300, 400 mg single-dose prefilled dual-chamber syringes w. supplies
▷ *aripiprazole lauroxil* (C) administer by IM injection in the deltoid (441 mg dose only) or gluteal (441 mg, 662 mg, 882 mg or 1064 mg) muscle by a qualified healthcare professional; initiate at a dose of 441 mg, 662 mg or 882 mg administered monthly, or 882 mg every 6 weeks, or 1064 mg every 2 months;
Pediatric: <18 years: not recommended; ≥18 years: same as adult
   Aristada *Prefilled syringe:* 441, 662, 882, 1064 mg single-use, ext-rel susp

Comment: **Aristada** is an atypical antipsychotic available in 4 doses with 3 dosing duration options for flexible dosing. For patients naïve to *aripiprazole*, establish tolerability with oral *aripiprazole* prior to initiating treatment with **Aristada**. **Aristada** can be initiated at any of the 4 doses at the appropriate dosing duration option. In conjunction with the first injection, administer treatment with oral *aripiprazole* for 21 consecutive days for all 4 dose sizes. The most common adverse event associated with **Aristada** is akathisia. Patients are also at increased risk for developing neuroleptic malignant syndrome, tardive dyskinesia, pathological gambling or other compulsive behaviors, orthostatic hypotension, hyperglycemic, dyslipidemia, and weight gain. Hypersensitive reactions can occur and range from pruritus or urticaria to anaphylaxis. Stroke, transient ischemic attacks, and falls have been reported in elderly patients with dementia-related psychosis who were treated with *apriprazole*. **Aristada** is not for treatment of people who have lost touch with reality (psychosis) due to confusion and memory loss (dementia). May cause extrapyramidal and/or withdrawal symptoms in neonates exposed in utero in the third trimester of pregnancy. **Aripiprazole** is present in human breast milk; however, there are insufficient data to assess the amount in human milk or the effects on the breast-fed infant. The development and health benefits of breastfeeding should be considered along with the mother's clinical need for **Aristada** and any potential adverse effects on the breastfed infant from **Aristada** or from the underlying maternal condition. For more information or to report ASEs, contact the National Pregnancy Registry for Atypical Antipsychotics at 1-866-961-2388 or visit http://womensmentalhealth.org/clinical-and-research-programs/pregnancyregistry/. Limited published data on aripiprazole use in pregnant women are not sufficient to inform any drug-associated risks for birth defects or miscarriage. To report suspected adverse reactions, contact Alkermes at 1-866-274-7823 or FDA at 1-800-FDA-1088 or www.fda.gov/medwatch

▷ *fluphenazine hcl* [Prolixin] (C)(G)
   Pediatric: <18 years: not studied
         Tab: 1, 2.5, 5, 10 mg; *Elixer:* 2.5 mg/5 ml; *Conc:* 5 mg/ml; *Vial:* 2.5 mg/ml for injection

▷ *fluphenazine decanoate* [Prolixin Decanoate] (C)(G)
   Pediatric: <18 years: not studied
         Vial: 2.5 mg/ml (5 ml)

Comment: Previously, *fluphenazine* was marketed as **Prolixin**, but is currently only available in generic form. Optimal dose and frequency of administration of *fluphenazine* must be determined for each patient, since dosage requirements have been found to vary with clinical circumstances as well as with individual response; dosage should not exceed 100 mg; if doses > 50 mg are deemed necessary, the next dose and succeeding doses should be increased cautiously in increments of 12.5 mg. *fluphenazine decanoate injection* and *fluphenazine enanthate injection* are long-acting parenteral antipsychotic forms intended for use in the management of patients requiring prolonged parenteral neuroleptic therapy. *fluphenazine* has activity at all levels of the central nervous system (CNS) as well as on multiple organ systems. The mechanism whereby its therapeutic action is exerted is unknown. *fluphenazine* differs from other phenothiazine derivatives in several respects: it is more potent on a milligram basis, it has less potentiating effect on CNS depressants and anesthetics than do some of the phenothiazines and appears to be less sedating, and it is less likely than some of the older phenothiazines to produce hypotension (nevertheless, appropriate cautions should be observed. Neuroleptic Malignant Syndrome (NMS), a potentially fatal symptom complex, is associated with all antipsychotic drugs. Clinical manifestations of NMS are hyperpyrexia, muscle rigidity, altered mental status and evidence of autonomic instability (irregular pulse or blood pressure, tachycardia, diaphoresis, and cardiac dysrhythmias). Anticholinergic effects may be potentiated with concomitant *atropine* and *fluphenazine.* Safety and efficacy in children have not been established. Safety during pregnancy has not been established; therefore, the possible hazards should be weighed against the potential benefits when administering this drug to pregnant patients.

▷ *haloperidol* (C)(G)
   Oral route of administration: Moderate Symptomology: 0.5 to 2 mg orally 2 to 3 times a day; *Severe symptomology:* 3 to 5 mg orally 2 to 3 times a day; initial doses of up to 100 mg/day have been necessary in some severely resistant cases;
   Maintenance: after achieving a satisfactory response, the dose should be adjusted as practical to achieve optimum control
   Parenteral route of administration: Prompt control of acute agitation: 2 to 5 mg IM every 4 to 8 hours; *Maintenance:* frequency of IM administration should be determined by patient response and may be given as often as every hour; max: 20 mg/day
         Haldol *Tab:* 0.5*, 1*, 2*, 5*, 10*, 20*mg
         Haldol Lactate *Vial:* 5 mg for IM injection, single-dose

▷ *mesoridazine* (C) initially 25 mg tid; max 300 mg/day
  Serentil *Tab:* 10, 25, 50, 100 mg; *Conc:* 25 mg/ml (118 ml)
▷ *olanzapine* (C) initially 2.5-10 mg daily; increase to 10 mg/day within a few days; then
  by 5 mg/day at weekly intervals; max 20 mg/day
  Zyprexa *Tab:* 2.5, 5, 7.5, 10 mg
  Zyprexa Zydis *ODT:* 5, 10, 15, 20 mg (phenylalanine)
▷ *quetiapine fumarate* (C)(G)
  SeroQUEL initially 25 mg bid, titrate q 2nd or 3rd day in increments of 25-50 mg
  bid-tid; usual maintenance 400-600 mg/day in 2-3 divided doses
    Tab: 25, 50, 100, 200, 300, 400 mg
  SeroQUEL XR administer once daily in the PM; *Day 1:* 50 mg; *Day 2:* 100 mg;
  Day 3: 200 mg; *Day 4:* 300 mg; usual range 400-600 mg/day
    Tab: 50, 150, 200, 300, 400 mg ext-rel
▷ *risperidone* (C) 0.5 mg bid x 1 day; adjust in increments of 0.5 mg bid; usual range
  0.5-5 mg/day
  Risperdal *Tab:* 1, 2, 3, 4 mg; *Oral soln:* 1 mg/ml (100 ml)
  Risperdal M-Tab *Tab:* 0.5, 1, 2 mg
▷ *thioridazine* (C)(G) 10-25 mg bid
  Mellaril *Tab:* 10, 15, 25, 50, 100, 150, 200 mg; *Oral susp:* 25 mg/5 ml, 100 mg/5 ml;
  Oral conc: 30 mg/ml, 100 mg/ml (4 oz)

◯ MITRAL VALVE PROLAPSE (MVP)

▷ *propranolol* (C)(G)
  Inderal 10-30 mg tid-qid
    Tab: 10*, 20*, 40*, 60*, 80*mg
  Inderal LA initially 80 mg daily in a single dose; increase q 3-7 days; usual range
  120-160 mg/day; max 320 mg/day in a single dose
    Cap: 60, 80, 120, 160 mg sust-rel
  InnoPran XL initially 80 mg q HS; max 120 mg/day
    Cap: 80, 120 mg ext-rel

◯ MONONUCLEOSIS (MONO)

Opioid Analgesics *see Pain page* 345
Parenteral Corticosteroids *see page* 570
Oral Corticosteroids *see page* 569

▷ *prednisone* (C) initially 40-80 mg/day, then taper off over 5-7 days
Comment: Corticosteroids are recommended in patients with significant pharyngeal edema.

◯ MOTION SICKNESS

▷ *dimenhydrinate* (B)(OTC) 50-100 mg q 4-6 hours; start 1 hour before travel; max 400
  mg/day
  Pediatric: <2 years: not recommended; 2-6 years: 12.5-25 mg; max 75 mg/day; start
  1 hour before travel; may repeat q 6-8 hours; 6-11 years: 25-50 mg; max 150 mg/day;
  start 1 hour before travel; may repeat q 6-8 hours; ≥12 years: same as adult
  Dramamine *Tab:* 50*mg; *Chew tab:* 50 mg (phenylalanine, tartrazine); *Liq:* 12.5
  mg/5 ml (4 oz)
▷ *meclizine* (B)(G) 25-50 mg 1 hour before travel; may repeat q 24 hours as needed;
  max 50 mg/day
  Pediatric: <12 years: not recommended; ≥12 years: same as adult
  Antivert *Tab:* 12.5, 25, 50*mg

> **Bonine (OTC)** *Cap:* 15, 25, 50 mg; *Tab:* 12.5, 25, 50 mg;
> *Chew tab/Film-coat tab:* 25 mg
> **Dramamine II (OTC)** *Tab:* 25 mg
> **Zentrip** *Strip:* 25 mg orally-disint

➤ *prochlorperazine* (C)(G)
Pediatric: <12 years: not recommended; ≥12 years: same as adult
Compazine 5-10 mg q 4 hours as needed
Tab: 5 mg; *Syr:* 5 mg/5 ml (4 oz; fruit); *Rectal supp:* 2.5, 5, 25 mg
Compazine Spansule 15 mg q AM <u>or</u> 10 mg q 12 hours
Spansules: 10, 15 mg sust-rel

➤ *promethazine* (C)(G) 25 mg 30-60 minutes before travel; may repeat in 8-12 hours
Pediatric: <2 years: not recommended; ≥2 years: 12.5-25 mg 30-60 minutes before travel; may repeat in 8-12 hours
Phenergan *Tab:* 12.5*, 25*, 50 mg; *Plain syr:* 6.25 mg/5 ml; *Fortis syr:* 25 mg/5 ml;
Rectal supp: 12.5, 25, 50 mg

Comment: *promethazine* is contraindicated in children with uncomplicated nausea, dehydration, Reye's syndrome, history of sleep apnea, asthma, and lower respiratory disorders in children. *Promethazine* lowers the seizure threshold in children, may cause cholestatic jaundice, anticholinergic effects, extrapyramidal effects, and potentially fatal respiratory depression.

➤ *scopolamine* (C)
Pediatric: <12 years: not recommended; ≥12 years: same as adult
Scopace 0.4-0.8 mg 1 hour before travel; may repeat in 8 hours
Tab: 0.4 mg
Transderm Scop 1 patch behind ear at least 4 hours before travel; each patch is effective for 3 days
Transdermal patch: 1.5 mg (4/carton)

MULTIPLE SCLEROSIS (MS)

NICOTINIC ACID RECEPTOR AGONIST

➤ *dimethyl fumarate* (C) initially 120 mg bid x 7 days; then maintenance 240 mg bid
Pediatric: <18 years: not recommended; ≥18 years: same as adult
Tecfidera *Cap:* 120, 240 mg del-rel; *Starter Pack:* 14 x 120 mg, 46 x 240 mg

Comment: The mechanism by which *dimethyl fumarate* (DMF) exerts its therapeutic effect in multiple sclerosis is unknown. DMF and the metabolite, *mono-methyl fumarate* (MMF), have been shown to activate the nuclear factor (erythroid-derived 2)-like 2 (Nrf2) pathway in vitro and in vivo in animals and humans. The Nrf2 pathway is involved in the cellular response to oxidative stress. MMF has been identified as a nicotinic acid receptor agonist in vitro.

SELECTIVE IMMUNOMODULATORY AGENTS

Comment: Selective immunosuppressive agents are drugs that suppress the immune system due to a selective point of action. They are used to reduce the risk of rejection in organ transplants, in autoimmune diseases, and can be used as cancer chemotherapy. As immunosuppressive agents lower the immunity, there is increased risk of infection.

➤ *daclizumab* (C) administer 150 mg by SC injection once monthly (A higher dosage of 300 mg once monthly not shown in clinical studies to provide additional clinical benefit) in the back of upper arm, abdomen, <u>or</u> thigh; allow at least 30 minutes for the prefilled syringe to reach room temperature; if a dose is missed, administer as soon as possible; however, if >2 weeks have elapsed, omit missed dose and resume regular dosing schedule

Pediatric: <17 years: not established/not recommended; ≥17 years: same as adult

Zinbryta *Prefilled syringe/Prefilled autoinjector:* 150 mg/ml, single-dose

Comment: *daclizumab* is a humanized anti-interleukin-2 (IL-2) receptor mono-clonal antibody indicated for the management of relapsing forms of MS (e.g., relapsing-remitting MS [RRMS]). Because of potentially life-threatening adverse effects (e.g., hepatotoxicity, immune-mediated disorders), *daclizumab* is generally reserved for patients with inadequate response to ≥2 MS drugs. *daclizumab* is contraindicated in patients with preexisting hepatic disease or impairment (e.g., ALT or AST ≥2 times the ULN) and history of autoimmune hepatitis or other autoimmune condition involving the liver. Evaluate serum aminotransferase (ALT/AST) and total bilirubin concentrations prior to initiating therapy, then monthly before each dose is administered and for 6 months after discontinuance of therapy. Interrupt therapy in patients with ALT or AST >5 times the ULN, total bilirubin >2 times the ULN, or ALT or AST ≥3 times but <5 times the ULN *with* total bilirubin >1.5 times but <2 times the ULN. No dosage adjustment is required for renal impairment. Prior to initiating therapy with **Zinbryta**, screen for hepatitis B and C, complete any necessary immunizations with live vaccines, and evaluate for tuberculosis infection in patients at high risk and treat appropriately. Depression-related events, including suicidal ideation and suicide attempt, have been reported. No adequate data in pregnant women; limited data from clinical trials do not suggest an increased risk of adverse fetal or maternal outcomes. There are no data on the presence of *semaglutide* in human milk or the effects on the breastfed infant. *daclizumab* is available only through the Zinbryta REMS Program. Clinicians, pharmacies, and patients must be enrolled and meet all conditions of this program before they can prescribe, dispense, or receive the drug. To report suspected adverse reactions, contact Biogen at 1800-456-2255 or FDA at 1-800-FDA-1088 or www.fda.gov/medwatch.

POTASSIUM CHANNEL BLOCKER

▷ *dalfampridine* (C)(G) 10 mg q 12 hours

Pediatric: <18 years: not recommended; ≥18 years: same as adult

Ampyra *Tab:* 10 mg ext-rel

Comment: *dalfampridine* is indicated to improve walking speed.

PYRIMIDINE SYNTHESIS INHIBITOR (DMARD)

▷ *teriflunomide* (X) 7 mg or 14 mg once daily

Pediatric: <12 years: not recommended; ≥12 years: same as adult

Aubagio *Tab:* 7, 14 mg

Comment: Contraindicated with severe hepatic impairment and women of childbearing potential not using reliable contraception. Co-administer *teriflunomide* with the DMARD *leflunomide* (**Arava**).

IMMUNOMODULATORS

Comment: The role of immunomodulators in the treatment of MS is to slow the progression of physical disability and to decrease frequency of clinical exacerbations.

▷ *alemtuzumab* (C) administer two treatment courses:

First treatment course: 12 mg/day x 5 days (total 60 mg); *Second treatment course:* 12 months later, administer 12 mg/day x 3 days (total 36 mg); complete all immunizations 6 weeks prior to the first treatment; premedicate with 1000 mg methylprednisolone or equivalent immediately prior to the first 3 treatment days in each treatment course

Pediatric: <18 years: not recommended; ≥18 years: same as adult

Lemtrada *Vial:* 12 mg/1.2 ml soln for IV infusion, single-use vial

Comment: **Lemtrada** is indicated for the treatment of patients with relapsing forms of MS. Because of its safety profile, the use of **Lemtrada** should generally be reserved for patients who have had an inadequate response to two or more drugs indicated for the treatment of MS. **Lemtrada REMS** is a restricted distribution program, which allows early detection and management of some of the serious risks associated with its use.

▷ *fingolimod* **(C)** 0.5 mg once daily
   Pediatric: <18 years: not recommended; ≥18 years: same as adult
      Gilenya *Cap:* 0.5 mg

Comment: First-dose monitoring for bradycardia. In the first 2 weeks, first-dose monitoring is recommended after an interruption of 1 day or more. During weeks 3 and 4, first-dose monitoring is recommended after an interruption of more than 7 days.

▷ *glatiramer acetate* **(B)(G)** 20-40 mg SC daily
   Pediatric: <18 years: not recommended; ≥18 years: same as adult
      Copaxone *Prefilled syringe:* 20, 40 mg/ml (mannitol, preservative-free)

▷ *interferon beta-1a* **(C)**
   Pediatric: <18 years: not recommended; ≥18 years: same as adult
      Avonex 30 mcg IM weekly; rotate sites; may titrate to reduce flu-like symptoms; may use concurrent analgesics/antipyretics on treatment days; *Titration Schedule:* 7.5 mcg week 1; 15 mcg week 2; 22.5 mcg week 3; 30 mcg week 4 and ongoing
         Vial: 30 mcg/vial pwdr for reconstitution (single-dose w. diluent, 4 vials/kit) (albumin [human], preservative-free); *Prefilled syringe:* 30 mcg single-dose (0.5 ml) (4/dose pck)
      Rebif, administer SC 3x/week (at least 48 hours apart and preferably in the late afternoon or evening); increase over 4 weeks to usual dose 22-44 mcg 3x/week; *Titration Schedule (22 mcg prescribed dose):* 4.4 mcg week 1 and 2; 11 mcg week 3 and 4; 22 mcg week 5 and ongoing; *Titration Schedule (44 mcg prescribed dose):* 8.8 mcg week 1 and 2; 22 mcg week 3 and 4; 44 mcg week 5 and ongoing
         Prefilled syringe: 22, 44 mcg/0.5 ml w. needle (12/carton) (albumin [human], preservative-free); (titration pack, 6 doses of 8.8 mcg [0.2 ml] w. needle per carton) (albumin [human], preservative-free)

Comment: Only prefilled syringes (**Rebif**) can be used to titrate to the 22 mcg prescribed dose. Prefilled syringes or autoinjectors (**Rebif Rebidose**) can be used to titrate to the 44 mcg prescribed dose.

      Rebif Rebidose administer SC 3x/week (at least 48 hours apart and preferably in the late afternoon or evening) after titration to 22 mcg or 44 mcg
         Titration Schedule: *see* **Rebif**.
         Prefilled autoinjector: 22, 44 mcg/0.5 ml (0.5 ml, 12/carton) (titration pack, 6 doses of 8.8 mcg [0.2 ml] per carton (albumin [human], preservative-free)

Comment: Only prefilled syringes (**Rebif**) can be used to titrate to the 22 mcg prescribed dose. Prefilled syringes or autoinjectors (**Rebif Rebidose**) can be used to titrate to the 44 mcg prescribed dose.

▷ *interferon beta-1b* **(C)**
   Pediatric: <18 years: not recommended; ≥18 years: same as adult
      Actimmune *BSA ≤0.5m²:* 1.5 mcg/kg SC in a single dose 3x weekly; *BSA ≥0.5m²:* 50 mcg/m² SC in a single dose 3x weekly *Vial:* 100 mcg/0.5 ml single-dose for SC injection
      Betaseron, Extavia 0.0625 mg (0.25 ml) SC every other day; increase over 6 weeks to 0.25 mg (1 ml) SC every other day
         Vial: 0.3 mg/vial pwdr for reconstitution (single-dose w. prefilled diluents syringes) (albumin [human], mannitol, preservative-free)

▷ *natalizumab* **(C)** administer 300 mg by IV infusion over 1 hour every 4 weeks; monitor during infusion and for 1 hour postinfusion

Pediatric: <18 years: not recommended; ≥18 years: same as adult
    Tysabri *Vial:* 300 mg/15 ml (15 ml)

CD20-DIRECTED CYTOLYTIC MONOCLONAL ANTIBODY

▷ *ocrelizumab* pre-medicate with corticosteroid and antihistamine, and consider anti-pyretic, prior to each infusion; initially administer 300 mg by IV infusion followed by another 300 mg infusion 2 weeks later; then administer 600 mg every 6 months; see mfr lit for infusion rates and dose modifications
Pediatric: <18 years: not recommended; ≥18 years: same as adult
    Ocrevus *Vial:* 30 mg/ml (10 ml, single-dose) for dilution (preservative-free)
Comment: The precise mechanism of action is unknown; however, it is thought to involve binding to CD20, a cell surface antigen present on pre-B and mature B lymphocytes which results in antibody-dependent cellular cytolysis and complement-mediated lysis. **Ocrevus** is contraindicated with active HBV infection. Screen for HBV infection (HBsAg/anti-HB) prior to initiation. Concomitant live or attenuated vaccine not recommended during treatment and until B-cell repletion. Administer these at least 6 weeks prior to initiation of treatment. Additive immunosuppressive effects with other immunosupressants. Monitor for infusion reaction (pruritis, rash, urticaria, erythema, throat irritation, bronchospasm). Delay treatment with active infection. Withhold at first sign/symptom of progressive multifocal leukoencephalopathy (PMI) or HBV reactivation. Females of reproductive potential should use effective contraception during treatment and for 6 months after the last dose of **Ocrevus**. It is not known whether *ocrelizumab* is excreted in human breast milk or has any effect on the breastfed infant.

PSEUDOBULBAR AFFECT (PBA)

Comment: Pseudobulbar affect (PBA), emotional lability, labile affect, or emotional incontinence refers by to a neurologic disorder characterized by involuntary crying or uncontrollable episodes of crying and/or laughing, or other emotional outbursts. PBA occurs secondary to a neurologic disease or brain injury such as traumatic brain injury (TBI), stroke, Parkinson's disease, multiple sclerosis, and amyotrophic lateral sclerosis (ALS, or Lou Gehrig disease).

▷ *dextromethorphan+quinidine* (C)(G) 1 cap once daily x 7 days; then starting on day 8, 1 cap bid
Pediatric: <12 years: not recommended; ≥12 years: same as adult
    Nuedexta *Cap:* dextro 20 mg+quini 10 mg
Comment: *dextromethorphan hydrobromide* is an uncompetitive NMDA receptor antagonist and sigma-1 agonist. *quinidine sulfate* is a CYP450 2D6 inhibitor. **Nuedexta** is contraindicated with an MAOI or within 14 days of stopping an MAOI, with prolonged QT interval, congenital long QT syndrome, history suggestive of torsades de pointes, or heart failure, complete atrioventricular (AV) block without implanted pacemaker or patients at high risk of complete AV block, and concomitant drugs that both prolong QT interval and are metabolized by CYP2D6 (e.g., *thioridazine* or *pimozide*). Discontinue **Nuedexta** if the following occurs: hepatitis or thrombocytopenia or any other hypersensitivity reaction. Monitor ECG in patients with left ventricular hypertrophy (LVH) or left ventricular dysfunction (LVD). *desipramine* exposure increases **Nuedexta** 8-fold; reduce *desipramine* dose and adjust based on clinical response. Use of **Nuedexta** with selective serotonin reuptake inhibitors (SSRIs) or tricyclic antidepressants (TCAs) increases the risk of serotonin syndrome. *paroxetine* exposure increases **Nuedexta** 2-fold; therefore, reduce *paroxetine* dose and adjust based on clinical response (*digoxin* exposure may increase *digoxin* substrate plasma

concentration. **Nuedexta** is not recommended in pregnancy <u>or</u> breastfeeding. Safety and effectiveness of **Nuedexta** in children have not been established. To report suspected adverse reactions, contact Avanir Pharmaceuticals at 1-866-388-5041 <u>or</u> FDA at 1-800-FDA-1088 <u>or</u> www.fda.gov/medwatch

 MUMPS (*INFECTIOUS PAROTITIS*)

see **Childhood Immunizations** *page* 546
Parenteral Corticosteroids *see page* 570
Oral Corticosteroids *see page* 569
Antipyretics *see Fever page* 165

PROPHYLAXIS VACCINE

▷ *measles, mumps, rubella, live, attenuated, neomycin vaccine* (C)
   MMR II 25 mcg SC (preservative-free)
   Comment: Contraindications: hypersensitivity to *neomycin* <u>or</u> eggs, primary <u>or</u> acquired immune deficiency, immunosuppressant therapy, bone marrow <u>or</u> lymphatic malignancy, and pregnancy (within 3 months after vaccination).

 MUSCLE STRAIN

Acetaminophen for IV Infusion *see Pain page* 344
Parenteral Corticosteroids *see page* 570
Oral Corticosteroids *see page* 569
Opioid Analgesics *see Pain page* 345

Comment: Usual length of treatment for acute injury is approximately 5 days.

SKELETAL MUSCLE RELAXANTS

▷ *baclofen* (C)(G) 5 mg tid; titrate up by 5 mg every 3 days to 20 mg tid; max 80 mg/day
   Pediatric: <12 years: not recommended; ≥12 years: same as adult
   Lioresal *Tab:* 10*, 20*mg
   Comment: *baclofen* is indicated for muscle spasm pain and chronic spasticity associated with multiple sclerosis and spinal cord injury <u>or</u> disease. Potential for seizures <u>or</u> hallucinations on abrupt withdrawal.
▷ *carisoprodol* (C)(G) 1 tab tid <u>or</u> qid
   Pediatric: <12 years: not recommended; ≥12 years: same as adult
   Soma *Tab:* 350 mg
▷ *chlorzoxazone* (G) 1 caplet qid; max 750 mg qid
   Pediatric: <12 years: not recommended; ≥12 years: same as adult
   Parafon Forte DSC *Cplt:* 500*mg
▷ *cyclobenzaprine* (B)(G) 10 mg tid; usual range 20-40 mg/day in divided doses; max 60 mg/day x 2-3 weeks <u>or</u> 15 mg ext-rel once daily; max 30 mg ext-rel/day x 2-3 weeks
   Pediatric: <15 years: not recommended; ≥15 years: same as adult
   Amrix *Cap:* 15, 30 mg ext-rel
   Fexmid *Tab:* 7.5 mg
   Flexeril *Tab:* 5, 10 mg
▷ *dantrolene* (C) 25md daily x 7 days; then 25 mg tid x 7 days; then 50 mg tid x 7 days; max 100 mg qid
   Pediatric: 0.5 mg/kg daily x 7 days; then 0.5 mg/kg tid x 7 days; then 1 mg/kg tid x 7 days; then 2 mg/kg tid; max 100 mg qid
   Dantrium *Tab:* 25, 50, 100 mg

Comment: *dantrolene* is indicated for chronic spasticity associated with multiple sclerosis and spinal cord injury or disease.

▷ *diazepam* (C)(IV) 2-10 mg bid-qid; may increase gradually
Pediatric: <6 months: not recommended; ≥6 months: initially 1-2.5 mg bid-qid; may increase gradually
  Diastat *Rectal gel delivery system:* 2.5 mg
  Diastat AcuDial *Rectal gel delivery system:* 10, 20 mg
  Valium *Tab:* 2, 5, 10 mg
  Valium Intensol Oral Solution *Conc oral soln:* 5 mg/ml (30 ml w. dropper) (alcohol 19%)
  Valium Oral Solution *Oral soln:* 5 mg/5 ml (500 ml) (wintergreen spice)

▷ *metaxalone* (B) 1 tab tid-qid
Pediatric: <12 years: not recommended; ≥12 years: same as adult
  Skelaxin *Tab:* 800*mg

▷ *methocarbamol* (C)(G) initially 1.5 gm qid x 2-3 days; maintenance, 750 mg every 4 hours or 1.5 gm 3x daily; max 8 gm/day
Pediatric: <16 years: not recommended; ≥16 years: same as adult
  Robaxin *Tab:* 500 mg
  Robaxin 750 *Tab:* 750 mg
  Robaxin Injection 10 ml IM or IV; max 30 ml/day; max 3 days; max 5 ml/gluteal injection q 8 hours; max IV rate 3 ml/min
  Vial: 100 mg/ml (10 ml)

▷ *nabumetone* (C)
Pediatric: <12 years: not recommended; ≥12 years: same as adult
  Relafen *Tab:* 500, 750 mg
  Relafen 500 *Tab:* 500 mg

▷ *orphenadrine citrate* (C)(G) 1 tab bid
Pediatric: <12 years: not recommended; ≥12 years: same as adult
  Norflex *Tab:* 100 mg sust-rel

▷ *tizanidine* (C) 1-4 mg q 6-8 hours; max 36 mg/day
Pediatric: <12 years: not recommended; ≥12 years: same as adult
  Zanaflex *Tab:* 2*, 4**mg; *Cap:* 2, 4, 6 mg

SKELETAL MUSCLE RELAXANT+NSAID COMBINATIONS

Comment: *aspirin*-containing medications are contraindicated with history of allergic-type reaction to *aspirin*, children and adolescents with *Varicella* or other viral illness, and 3rd trimester of pregnancy.

▷ *carisoprodol+aspirin* (C)(III)(G) 1-2 tabs qid
Pediatric: <12 years: not recommended; ≥12 years: same as adult
  Soma Compound *Tab:* caris 200 mg+asp 325 mg (sulfites)

▷ *meprobamate+aspirin* (D)(IV) 1-2 tabs tid or qid
Pediatric: <12 years: not recommended; ≥12 years: same as adult
  Equagesic *Tab:* mepro 200 mg+asp 325*mg

Comment: *aspirin*-containing medications are contraindicated with history of allergic-type reaction to *aspirin*, children and adolescents with *varicella* or other viral illness, and 3rd trimester of pregnancy.

SKELETAL MUSCLE RELAXANT+NSAID+CAFFEINE COMBINATIONS

▷ *orphenadrine+aspirin+caffeine* (D)(G)
Pediatric: <12 years: not recommended; ≥12 years: same as adult
  Norgesic 1-2 tabs tid-qid
    Tab: orphen 25 mg+asp 385 mg+caf 30 mg

Norgesic Forte 1 tab tid or qid; max 4 tabs/day
Tab: orphen 50 mg+*asp* 770 mg+*caf* 60*mg
Comment: *aspirin*-containing medications are contraindicated with history of allergic-type reaction to **aspirin**, children and adolescents with *Varicella* or other viral illness, and 3rd trimester of pregnancy.

SKELETAL MUSCLE RELAXANT+NSAID+CODEINE COMBINATIONS

➤ *carisoprodol+aspirin+codeine* (D)(III)(G) 1-2 tabs qid prn
  Pediatric: <12 years: contraindicated; 12-<18: use extreme caution; not recommended for children and adolescents with obesity, asthma, obstructive sleep apnea, or other chronic breathing problem, or for post-tonsillectomy/adenoidectomy pain; ≥18 years: same as adult
  Soma Compound w. Codeine
  Tab: caris 200 mg+*asp* 325 mg+*cod* 16 mg (sulfites)
Comment: **Codeine** is known to be excreted in breast milk. <12 years: not recommended; 12-<18: use extreme caution; not recommended for children and adolescents with asthma or other chronic breathing problem. The FDA and the European Medicines Agency (EMA) are investigating the safety of using **codeine** containing medications to treat pain, cough and colds, in children 12-<18 years because of the potential for serious side effects, including slowed or difficult breathing. *aspirin*-containing medications are contraindicated with history of allergic-type reaction to **aspirin**, children and adolescents with *Varicella* or other viral illness, and 3rd trimester of pregnancy.

TOPICAL AND TRANSDERMAL NSAIDs

➤ *capsaicin* (B)(G) apply tid-qid prn to intact skin
  Pediatric: <2 years: not recommended; ≥2 years: apply sparingly tid-qid prn
  Axsain *Crm:* 0.075% (1, 2 oz)
  Capsin *Lotn:* 0.025, 0.075% (59 ml)
  Capzasin-P (OTC) *Crm:* 0.025% (1.5 oz); *Lotn:* 0.025% (2 oz)
  Dolorac *Crm:* 0.025% (28 gm)
  Double Cap (OTC) *Crm:* 0.05% (2 oz)
  R-Gel *Gel:* 0.025% (15, 30 gm)
  Zostrix (OTC) *Crm:* 0.025% (0.7, 1.5, 3 oz)
  Zostrix HP (OTC) *Emol crm:* 0.075% (1, 2 oz)
➤ *capsaicin* 8% patch (B) apply up to 4 patches for one 60-minute application to clean dry skin; may prep area with topical anesthetic; wear nonlatex gloves; patches may be cut to size/shape; treatment may be repeated every 3 months; remove with cleansing gel after treatment
  Pediatric: <18 years: not recommended; ≥18 years: same as adult
  Qutenza *Patch:* 8% 1640 mcg/cm (179 mg; 1 or 2 patches, each w. 1-50 gm tube cleansing gel/carton)
➤ *diclofenac epolamine transdermal patch* (C; D ≥30 wks) apply one patch to affected area bid; remove during bathing; avoid non-intact skin
  Pediatric: <12 years: not recommended; ≥12 years: same as adult
  Flector Patch *Patch:* 180 mg/patch (30/carton)

ORAL NSAIDs

For an expanded list of NSAIDs see page 562
➤ *diclofenac* (C)
  Pediatric: <18 years: not recommended; ≥18 years: same as adult
  Zorvolex take on empty stomach; 35 mg tid; *Hepatic impairment:* use lowest dose
  Gelcap: 18, 35 mg

▷ *diclofenac sodium* (C)
  Pediatric: <18 years: not recommended; ≥18 years: same as adult
    Voltaren 50 mg bid-qid <u>or</u> 75 mg bid <u>or</u> 25 mg qid with an additional 25 mg at HS if necessary
      Tab: 25, 50, 75 mg ent-coat
    Voltaren XR 100 mg once daily; rarely, 100 mg bid may be used
      Tab: 100 mg ext-rel

ORAL NSAIDs+PPI COMBINATIONS

▷ *esomeprazole+naproxen* (C)(G) 1 tab bid; use lowest effective dose for the shortest duration swallow whole; take at least 30 minutes before a meal
  Pediatric: <18 years: not recommended; ≥18 years: same as adult
    Vimovo *Tab:* nap 375 mg+eso 20 mg ext-rel; *nap* 500 mg+*eso* 20 mg ext-rel
    Comment: **Vimovo** is indicated to improve signs/symptoms, and risk of gastric ulcer in patients at risk of developing NSAID-associated gastric ulcer.

COX-2 INHIBITORS

Comment: Cox-2 inhibitors are contraindicated with history of asthma, urticaria, and allergic-type reactions to *aspirin*, other NSAIDs, and sulfonamides, 3rd trimester of pregnancy, and coronary artery bypass graft (CABG) surgery.

▷ *celecoxib* (C)(G) 100-400 mg daily bid; max 800 mg/day
  Pediatric: <18 years: not recommended; ≥18 years: same as adult
    Celebrex *Cap:* 50, 100, 200, 400 mg

▷ *meloxicam* (C)(G)
    Mobic <2 years, <60 kg: not recommended; ≥2, >60 kg: 0.125 mg/kg; max 7.5 mg once daily; ≥18 years: initially 7.5 mg once daily; max 15 mg once daily; *Hemodialysis:* max 7.5 mg/day
      Tab: 7.5, 15 mg; *Oral susp:* 7.5 mg/5 ml (100 ml) (raspberry)
    Vivlodex <18 years: not established; ≥18 years: initially 5 mg qd; may increase to max 10 mg/day; *Hemodialysis:* max 5 mg/day
      Cap: 5, 10 mg

TOPICAL AND TRANSDERMAL NSAIDs

▷ *capsaicin* (B)(G) apply tid-qid prn to intact skin
  Pediatric: <2 years: not recommended; ≥2 years: apply sparingly tid-qid prn
    Axsain *Crm:* 0.075% (1, 2 oz)
    Capsin *Lotn:* 0.025, 0.075% (59 ml)
    Capzasin-P (OTC) *Crm:* 0.025% (1.5 oz); *Lotn:* 0.025% (2 oz)
    Dolorac *Crm:* 0.025% (28 gm)
    Double Cap (OTC) *Crm:* 0.05% (2 oz)
    R-Gel *Gel:* 0.025% (15, 30 gm)
    Zostrix (OTC) *Crm:* 0.025% (0.7, 1.5, 3 oz)
    Zostrix HP (OTC) *Emol crm:* 0.075% (1, 2 oz)

▷ *capsaicin* 8% patch (B) apply up to 4 patches for one 60-minute application to clean dry skin; may prep area with topical anesthetic; wear nonlatex gloves; patches may be cut to size/shape; treatment may be repeated every 3 months; remove with cleansing gel after treatment
  Pediatric: <18 years: not recommended; ≥18 years: same as adult
    Qutenza *Patch:* 8% 1640 mcg/cm (179 mg; 1 <u>or</u> 2 patches, each w. 1-50 gm tube cleansing gel/carton)

▷ *diclofenac epolamine transdermal patch* (C; D ≥30 wks) apply one patch to affected area bid; remove during bathing; avoid nonintact skin
  Pediatric: <12 years: not recommended; ≥12 years: same as adult
    Flector Patch *Patch:* 180 mg/patch (30/carton)

▷ *diclofenac sodium* (C; D ≥30 wks)(G) apply gel qid prn; avoid non-intact skin
  Pediatric: <12 years: not recommended; ≥12 years: same as adult
    Voltaren Gel *Gel:* 1% (100 gm)

TOPICAL AND TRANSDERMAL LIDOCAINE

▷ *lidocaine* transdermal patch (C)(G) apply one patch to affected area for 12 hours
  (then off for 12 hours); remove during bathing; avoid non-intact skin
  Pediatric: <12 years: not recommended; ≥12 years: same as adult
    Lidoderm *Patch:* 5% (10 cm x 14 cm; 30/carton)

 NARCOLEPSY

STIMULANTS

▷ *amphetamine sulfate* (C)(II) administer first dose on awakening, and additional doses
  at 4- to 6-hour intervals; usual range 5-60 mg/day
  Pediatric: <6 years: not recommended; 6-12 years: 5 mg daily in the AM; may increase by 5 mg/day at weekly intervals; ≥12-18 years: initially 10 mg in the AM; may
  increase by 10 mg daily at weekly intervals; >18 years: same as adult
    Evekeo initially 10 mg once <u>or</u> twice daily at the same time(s) each day; may
    increase by 10 mg/day at weekly intervals; max 40 mg/day
      Tab: 5, 10 mg
▷ *armodafinil* (C)(IV)(G) *OSAHS:* 50-250 mg once daily in the AM; *SWSD:* 150 mg 1
  hour before starting shift; reduce dose with severe hepatic impairment
  Pediatric: <17 years: not recommended; ≥17 years: same as adult
    Nuvigil *Tab:* 50, 150, 200, 250 mg
▷ *modafinil* (C)(IV)(G) 100-200 mg q AM; max 400 mg/day
  Pediatric: <17 years: not recommended; ≥17 years: same as adult
    Provigil *Tab:* 100, 200*mg
Comment: **Provigil** also promotes wakefulness in patients with shift work sleep disorder and
excessive sleepiness due to obstructive sleep apnea/hypopnea syndrome.
▷ *sodium oxybate* (B)(G) take dose at bedtime while in bed and repeat 2.5-4 hours later;
  titrate to effect; initially 4.5 gm/night in 2 divided doses; may increase by 1.5 gm/
  night in 2 divided doses; max 9 gm/night
  Pediatric: <16 years: not recommended; ≥16 years: same as adult
    Xyrem *Oral soln:* 100, 200*mg
Comment: **Xyrem** is used to reduce the number of cataplexy attacks (sudden loss of
muscle strength) and reduce daytime sleepiness in patients with narcolepsy. Contraindicated with *alcohol* <u>or</u> CNS depressant (may impair consciousness; may lead to
respiratory depression, coma, <u>or</u> death). Prepare both doses prior to bedtime and do not
attempt to get out of bed after taking the first dose. Place both doses within reach at the
bedside. Set the bedside clock to awaken for the second dose. Dilute each dose in 60 ml
(1/4 cup, 4 tbsp) water in child resistant dosing containers. Food significantly reduces
the bioavailability of *sodium oxybate*; take at least 2 hours after ingesting food.

STIMULANTS

▷ *dextroamphetamine sulfate* (C)(II)(G) initially start with 10 mg daily; increase by
  10 mg at weekly intervals if needed; may switch to daily dose with sust-rel spansules
  when titrated
  Pediatric: <3 years: not recommended; 3-5 years: 2.5 mg daily; may increase by
  2.5 mg daily at weekly intervals if needed; 6-12 years: initially 5 mg daily-bid; may
  increase by 5 mg/day at weekly intervals; usual max 40 mg/day; >12 years: initially 10
  mg daily; may increase by mg/day at weekly intervals; max 40 mg/day 10
    Dexedrine *Tab:* 5*mg (tartrazine)

Dexedrine Spansule *Cap:* 5, 10, 15 mg sust-rel

Dextrostat *Tab:* 5, 10 mg (tartrazine)

▷ *dextroamphetamine saccharate+dextroamphetamine sulfate+amphetamine aspartate+amphetamine sulfate* (C)(II)(G)

Adderall initially 10 mg daily; may increase weekly by 10 mg/day; usual max 60 mg/day in 2-3 divided doses; first dose on awakening and then q 4-6 hours prn
Pediatric: <6 years: not indicated; 6-12 years: initially 5 mg daily; may increase weekly by 5 mg/day; usual max 40 mg/day in 2-3 divided doses; >12 years: same as adult
Tab: 5**, 7.5**, 10**, 12.5**, 15**, 20**, 30**mg

Adderall XR
Pediatric: <6 years: not recommended; 6-12 years: initially 10 mg daily in the AM; may increase by 10 mg weekly; max 30 mg/day; 13-17 years: initially 10 mg daily; may increase to 20 mg/day after 1 week; max 30 mg/day; Do not crush or chew; may sprinkle on apple sauce
Cap: 5, 10, 15, 20, 25, 30 mg ext-rel

Comment: **Adderall** is also indicated to improve wakefulness in patients with shift-work sleep disorder and excessive sleepiness due to obstructive sleep apnea/hypopnea syndrome.

▷ *dexmethylphenidate* (C)(II)(G) take once daily in the AM
Pediatric: <6 years: not recommended; ≥6 years: same as adult

Focalin initially 2.5 mg bid; allow at least 4 hours between doses; may increase at 1 week intervals; max 40 mg/day
Tab: 2.5, 5, 10*mg (dye-free)
Focalin XR 20-40 mg q AM; max 40 mg/day
Tab: 5, 10, 15, 20, 30, 40 mg ext-rel (dye-free)

▷ *methylphenidate (regular-acting)* (C)(II)(G)
Pediatric: <6 years: not recommended; ≥6 years: initially 5 mg bid ac (before breakfast and lunch); may gradually increase by 5-10 mg at weekly intervals as needed; max 60 mg/day

Methylin, Methylin Chewable, Methylin Oral Solution usual dose 20-30 mg/day in 2-3 divided doses 30-45 minutes before a meal; may increase to 60 mg/day
Ritalin 10-60 mg/day in 2-3 divided doses 30-45 minutes ac; max 60 mg/day
Tab: 5, 10*, 20*mg

▷ *methylphenidate (long-acting)* (C)(II)

Concerta initially 18 mg q AM; may increase in 18 mg increments as needed; max 54 mg/day; do not crush or chew
Tab: 18, 27, 36, 54 mg sust-rel

Metadate CD (G) 1 cap daily in the AM; may sprinkle on food; do not crush or chew
Pediatric: <6 years: not recommended; ≥6 years: initially 20 mg daily; may gradually increase by 20 mg/day at weekly intervals as needed; max 60 mg/day
Cap: 10, 20, 30, 40, 50, 60 mg immed- and ext-rel beads

Metadate ER 1 tab daily in the AM; do not crush or chew
Pediatric: <6 years: not recommended; ≥6 years: use in place of regular-acting *methylphenidate* when the 8-hour dose of **Metadate-ER** corresponds to the titrated 8-hour dose of regular-acting *methylphenidate*
Tab: 10, 20 mg ext-rel (dye-free)

Ritalin LA 1 cap daily in the AM
Pediatric: <6 years: not recommended; ≥6 years: use in place of regular-acting *methylphenidate* when the 8-hour dose of **Ritalin LA** corresponds to the titrated 8-hour dose of regular-acting *methylphenidate*; max 60 mg/day

    Cap: 10, 20, 30, 40 mg ext-rel (immed- and ext-rel beads)
    Ritalin SR 1 cap daily in the AM
    Pediatric: <6 years: not recommended; ≥6 years: use in place of regular-acting
    methylphenidate when the 8-hour dose of **Ritalin SR** corresponds to the titrated
    8-hour dose of regular-acting ***methylphenidate***; max 60 mg/day
      Tab: 20 mg sust-rel (dye-free)
➤ *methylphenidate (transdermal patch)* (C)(II)(G) 1 patch daily in the AM
    Pediatric: <6 years: not recommended; ≥6 years: initially 10 mg patch daily in the
    AM; may increase by 5-10 mg/week; max 60 mg/day
      Transdermal patch: 10, 15, 20, 30 mg
➤ *pemoline* (B)(IV) 18.75-112.5 mg/day; usually start with 37.5 mg in AM; increase
    weekly by 18.75 mg/day if needed; max 112.5 gm/day
    Pediatric: <6 years: not recommended; ≥6 years: same as adult
      Cylert *Tab:* 18.75*, 37.5*, 75*mg
      Cylert Chewable *Chew tab:* 37.5*mg
Comment: Monitor baseline serum ALT and repeat every 2 weeks thereafter.

NAUSEA/VOMITING: POST-ANESTHESIA

Rx ANTIEMETICS

➤ *ondansetron* (C)(G) 8 mg q 8 hours x 2 doses; then 8 mg q 12 hours
    Pediatric: <4 years: not recommended; 4-11 years: 4 mg q 4 hours x 3 doses; then 4
    mg q 8 hours
      Zofran *Tab:* 4, 8, 24 mg
      Zofran ODT *ODT:* 4, 8 mg (strawberry) (phenylalanine)
      Zofran Oral Solution *Oral soln:* 4 mg/5 ml (50 ml) (strawberry) (phenyl-alanine);
        Parenteral form: see mfr pkg insert
      Zofran Injection *Vial:* 2 mg/ml (2 ml single-dose); 2 mg/ml (20 ml multi-dose);
        32 mg/50 ml (50 ml multi-dose); *Prefilled syringe:* 4 mg/2 ml, single-use (24/
        carton)
      Zuplenz Oral Soluble Film: 4, 8 mg oral-dis (10/carton) (peppermint)
➤ *palonosetron* (B)(G) administer 0.25 mg IV over 30 seconds; max 1 dose/week
    Pediatric: <1 month: not recommended; 1 month to 17 years: 20 mcg/kg; max 1.5 mg/
    single dose; infuse over 15 minutes beginning 30 minutes
      Aloxi *Vial (single-use):* 0.075 mg/1.5 ml; 0.25 mg/5 ml (mannitol)
➤ *promethazine* (C)(G) 25 mg PO or rectally q 4-6 hours prn
    Pediatric: <2 years: not recommended; ≥2 years: 0.5 mg/lb or 6.25-25 mg q 4-6 hours
    prn
      Phenergan *Tab:* 12.5*, 25*, 50 mg; *Plain syr:* 6.25 mg/5 ml; *Fortis syr:* 25 mg/5 ml;
      Rectal supp: 12.5, 25, 50 mg
Comment: *promethazine* is contraindicated in children with uncomplicated nausea,
dehydration, Reye's syndrome, history of sleep apnea, asthma, and lower respiratory
disorders in children. *Promethazine* lowers the seizure threshold in children, may cause
cholestatic jaundice, anticholinergic effects, extrapyramidal effects, and potentially fatal
respiratory depression.

NERVE AGENT POISONING

➤ *atropine sulfate* (G) 2 mg IM
    Pediatric: <15 lb: not recommended; ≥15-40 lb: 0.5 mg IM; ≥40-90 lb: 1 mg IM; >90
    lb: same as adult
      AtroPen *Pen (single-use):* 0.5, 1, 2 mg (0.5 ml)

NON-24 SLEEP-WAKE DISORDER

Comment: For other drug options (stimulants, sedative hypnotics), *see* **Insomnia** *page* 231, or **Sleepiness: Excessive, Shift Work Sleep Disorder** *page* 447

MELATONIN RECEPTOR AGONIST

▷ *tasimelteon* (C) take 1 gelcap before bedtime at the same time every night; do not take with food
  Pediatric: <12 years: not established; ≥12 years: same as adult
    Hetlioz *Gel cap:* 20 mg

OREXIN RECEPTOR ANTAGONIST

▷ *suvorexant* (C)(IV) use lowest effective dose; take 30 minutes before bedtime; do not take if unable to sleep for ≥7 hours; max 20 mg
  Pediatric: <12 years: not recommended; ≥12 years: same as adult
    Belsomra *Tab:* 5, 10, 15, 20 mg (30/blister pck)

 OBESITY

Comment: Target BMI is 25-30 (≤27 preferred). Approximately 17% of children and adolescents in the US aged 2 to 19 years are obese. Almost 32% of children and adolescents are either overweight or obese, and the proportion of children with severe obesity continues to rise. Obesity in childhood increases the risk of having obesity as an adult and children with obesity are about 5 times more likely to have obesity as adults than children without obesity. The immediate consequences of childhood obesity include increased incidence of psychological issues, asthma, obstructive sleep apnea, orthopedic problems, high blood pressure, elevated lipid levels, and insulin resistance. The US Preventive Services Task Force (USPSTF) recommends that clinicians screen for obesity in children and adolescents 6 years and older and offer or refer them to comprehensive, intensive behavioral interventions (at least 26 hours of contact) to promote improvements in weight status.

REFERENCE

US Preventive Services Task Force. (2017). Screening for obesity in children and adolescents. US preventive services task force recommendation statement. *Journal of the American Medical Association, 317*(23), 2417–2426. doi:10.1001/jama.2017.6803

STIMULANTS

▷ *amphetamine sulfate* (C)(II)
  Pediatric: <12 years: not recommended; ≥12 years: same as adult
    Evekeo initially 5 mg 30-60 minutes before meals; usually up to 30 mg/day
      Tab: 5, 10 mg

LIPASE INHIBITOR

▷ *orlistat* (X)(G) 1 cap tid 1 hour before or during each main meal containing fat
  Pediatric: <12 years: not recommended; ≥12 years: same as adult
    Alli (OTC) *Cap:* 60 mg
    Xenical *Cap:* 120 mg
  Comment: For use when BMI >30 kg/m² or BMI >27 kg/m² in the presence of other risk factors (i.e., HTN, DM, dyslipidemia).

ANOREXIGENICS

Sympathomimetics

Comment: ASEs of sympathomimetics include hypertension, tachycardia, restlessness, insomnia, and dry mouth.

▷ *benzphetamine* (X)(III) initially 25-50 mg daily in the mid-morning or mid-afternoon; may increase to bid-tid as needed
Pediatric: <12 years: not recommended; ≥12 years: same as adult
   Didrex *Tab:* 50*mg

▷ *naltrexone+bupropion* (X)(G) swallow whole; avoid high-fat meals; initially 10 mg bid; evaluate weight loss after 12 weeks; discontinue if less than 5% weight loss
Pediatric: <18 years: not recommended; ≥18 years: same as adult
   Contrave *Tab:* nal 8 mg+*bup* 900 mg ext-rel

▷ *methamphetamine* (C)(II) 10-15 mg q AM
Pediatric: <12 years: not recommended; ≥12 years: same as adult
   Desoxyn *Tab:* 5, 10, 15 mg sust-rel

▷ *phendimetrazine* (C)(III)
Pediatric: <12 years: not recommended; ≥12 years: same as adult
   Bontril PDM 35 mg bid-tid 1 hour ac; may reduce to 17.5 mg (1/2 tab)/dose; max 210 mg/day in 3 divided doses
      Tab: 35*mg
   Bontril Slow-Release 105 mg in the AM 30-60 minutes before breakfast
      Cap: 105 mg slow-rel

▷ *phentermine* (X)(IV)(G)
Pediatric: <16 years: not recommended; ≥16 years: same as adult
   Adipex-P 1 cap or tab before breakfast or 1/2 tab bid ac
      Cap: 37.5 mg; *Tab:* 37.5*mg
   Fastin 1 cap before breakfast
      Cap: 30 mg
   Ionamin 1 cap before breakfast or 10-14 hours prior to HS
      Cap: 15, 30 mg
   Suprenza ODT (X)(IV) dissolve 1 tab on top of tongue once daily in the morning, with or without food; use lowest effective dose
      Tab: 15, 30, 37.5 mg orally-disint

Comment: Contraindicated with history of cardiovascular disease (e.g., coronary artery disease, stroke, arrhythmias, congestive heart failure, uncontrolled hypertension, during or within 14 days following the administration of an MAOI, hyperthyroidism, glaucoma, agitated states, history of drug abuse, pregnancy, nursing).

Sympathomimetic+Antiepileptic Combination

▷ *phentermine+topiramate ext-rel* (X)(IV)(G) initially 3.75/23 daily in the AM x 14 days; then increase to 7.5/46 and evaluate weight loss on this dose after 12 weeks; if ≤3% weight loss from baseline, discontinue or increase dose to 11.25/69 x 14 days; then increase to 15/92 and evaluate weight loss on this dose after 12 weeks; if ≤5% weight loss from baseline, discontinue by taking a dose every other day for at least one week prior to stopping; max 7.5/46 for moderate to severe renal impairment or moderate hepatic impairment.
Pediatric: <16 years: not established; ≥16 years: same as adult
   Qsymia
      Cap: Qsymia 3.75/23 *phen* 3.75 mg+*topir* 23 mg ext-rel
         Qsymia 7.5/46 *phen* 7.5 mg+*topir* 46 mg ext-rel
         Qsymia 11.25/69 *phen* 11.25 mg+*topir* 69 mg ext-rel
         Qsymia 15/92 *phen* 15 mg+*topir* 92 mg ext-rel

Comment: Side effects include hypertension, tachycardia, restlessness, insomnia, and dry mouth. Contraindicated with glaucoma, hyperthyroidism, and within 14 days of taking an MAOI. **Qsymia 3.75/23** and **Qsymia 11.25/69** are for titration purposes only.

Serotonin 2C Receptor Agonist

▷ *lorcaserin* **(X)(G)** 10 mg bid; discontinue if 5% weight loss is not achieved by week 12
  Pediatric: <18 years: not recommended; ≥18 years: same as adult
    Belviq *Tab:* 10 mg film-coat
Comment: **Belviq** is indicated as an adjunct to a reduced-calorie diet and increased physical activity for chronic weight management in adults with an initial body mass index (BMI) of 30 kg/m² or greater (obese) or 27 kg/m² or greater (over weight) in the presence of at least one weight-related comorbid condition (e.g., hypertension, dyslipidemia, type 2 diabetes). Serotonin 2C receptor agonists interact with serotonergic drugs (selective serotonin reuptake inhibitors (SSRIs), serotonin-norepinephrine reuptake inhibitors (SNRIs), monoamine oxidase inhibitors (MAOIs), triptans, *bupropion*, *dextromethorphan*, *St. John's wort*); therefore, use with extreme caution due to the risk of serotonin syndrome.

GLUCAGON-LIKE PEPTIDE-1 (GLP-1) RECEPTOR AGONIST

▷ *liraglutide* **(C)** administer SC in the upper arm, abdomen, or thigh once daily; escalate dose gradually over 5 weeks to 3 mg SC daily; *Week 1:* 0.6 mg SC daily; *Week 2:* 1.2 mg SC daily; *Week 3:* 1.8 mg SC daily; *Week 4:* 2.4 mg SC daily; *Week 5:* 3 mg SC daily;
  Pediatric: <18 years: not recommended
    Saxenda Soln for SC inj: 6 mg/ml multi-dose prefilled pen (3 ml; 3, 5 pens/carton)
Comment: **Saxenda** is indicated as an adjunct to a reduced-calorie diet and increased physical activity for chronic weight management in adults with an initial body mass index (BMI) of 30 kg/m² or greater (obese) or 27 kg/m² or greater over weight) in the presence of at least one weight-related comorbid condition (e.g., hypertension, dyslipidemia, type 2 diabetes). Not indicated for treatment of T2DM. Do not use with **Victoza**, other GLP-1 receptor agonists, or insulin. Contraindicated with personal or family history of medullary thyroid carcinoma (MTC) and multiple endocrine neoplasia syndrome (MENS) type 2. Monitor for signs/symptoms pancreatitis. Discontinue if gastroparesis, renal, or hepatic impairment.

 OBSESSIVE-COMPULSIVE DISORDER (OCD)

SELECTIVE SEROTONIN REUPTAKE INHIBITORS (SSRIs)

Comment: Co-administration of SSRIs with TCAs requires extreme caution. Concomitant use of MAOIs and SSRIs is absolutely contraindicated. Avoid other serotonergic drugs. A potentially fatal adverse event is *Serotonin Syndrome*, caused by serotonin excess. Milder symptoms require HCP intervention to avert severe symptoms which can be rapidly fatal without urgent/emergent medical care. Symptoms include restlessness, agitation, confusion, hallucinations, tachycardia, hypertension, dilated pupils, muscle twitching, muscle rigidity, loss of muscle coordination, diaphoresis, diarrhea, headache, shivering, piloerection, hyperpyrexia, cardiac arrhythmias, seizures, loss of consciousness, coma, death. Abrupt withdrawal or interruption of treatment with an antidepressant medication is sometimes associated with an *Antidepressant Discontinuation Syndrome* which may be mediated by gradually tapering the drug over a period of two weeks or longer, depending on the dose strength and length of treatment. Common symptoms of the *Serotonin Discontinuation Syndrome* include flu-like symptoms (nausea, vomiting, diarrhea, headaches, sweating), sleep disturbances (insomnia, nightmares, constant sleepiness), mood disturbances (dysphoria, anxiety, agitation), cognitive disturbances (mental confusion, hyperarousal), sensory and movement disturbances (imbalance, tremors, vertigo, dizziness, electric-shock-like sensations in the brain, often described by sufferers as "brain zaps."

▷ *fluoxetine* (C)(G)

Prozac initially 20 mg daily; may increase after 1 week; doses >20 mg/day may be divided into AM and noon doses; max 80 mg/day

Pediatric: <8 years: not recommended; 8-17 years: initially 10 mg/day; may increase after 2 weeks to 20 mg/day; range 20-60 mg/day; range for lower weight children 20-30 mg/day; >17: same as adult

Cap: 10, 20, 40 mg; *Tab:* 30*, 60*mg; *Oral soln:* 20 mg/5 ml (4 oz) (mint)

Prozac Weekly following daily *fluoxetine* therapy at 20 mg/day for 13 weeks, may initiate **Prozac Weekly** 7 days after the last 20 mg *fluoxetine* dose

Pediatric: <12 years: not recommended; ≥12 years: same as adult

Cap: 90 mg ent-coat del-rel pellets

▷ *fluvoxamine* (C)(G)

Luvox initially 50 mg q HS; adjust in 50 mg increments at 4-7 day intervals; range 100-300 mg/day; over 100 mg/day, divide into 2 doses giving the larger dose at HS

Pediatric: <8 years: not recommended; 8-17 years: initially 25 mg q HS; a just in 25 mg increments q 4-7 days; usual range 50-200 mg/day; over 50 mg/day, divide into 2 doses giving the larger dose at HS

Tab: 25, 50*, 100*mg

Luvox CR initially 100 mg once daily at HS; may increase by 50 mg increments at 1 week intervals; max 300 mg/day; swallow whole; do not crush or chew

Pediatric: <18 years: not recommended; ≥18 years: same as adult

Cap: 100, 150 mg ext-rel

▷ *paroxetine maleate* (D)(G)

Pediatric: <12 years: not recommended; ≥12 years: same as adult

Paxil initially 20 mg daily in AM; may increase by 10 mg/day at weekly intervals as needed; max 60 mg/day

Tab: 10*, 20*, 30, 40 mg

Paxil CR initially 25 mg daily in AM; may increase by 12.5 mg at weekly intervals as needed; max 62.5 mg/day

Tab: 12.5, 25, 37.5 mg cont-rel ent-coat

Paxil Suspension initially 20 mg daily in AM; may increase by 10 mg/day at weekly intervals as needed; max 60 mg/day

Oral susp: 10 mg/5 ml (250 ml) (orange)

▷ *paroxetine mesylate* (D)(G) initially 7.5 mg daily in AM; may increase by 10 mg/day at weekly intervals as needed; max 60 mg/day

Pediatric: <12 years: not recommended; ≥12 years: same as adult

Brisdelle *Cap:* 7.5 mg

▷ *sertraline* (C) initially 50 mg daily; increase at 1 week intervals if needed; max 200 mg daily

Pediatric: <6 years: not recommended; 6-12 years: initially 25 mg daily; max 200 mg/day; 13-17 years: initially 50 mg daily; max 200 mg/day; >17 years: same as adult

Zoloft *Tab:* 15*, 50*, 100*mg; *Oral conc:* 20 mg per ml (60 ml [dilute just before administering in 4 oz water, ginger ale, lemon-lime soda, lemonade, or orange juice]) (alcohol 12%)

TRICYCLIC ANTIDEPRESSANTS (TCAs)

▷ *clomipramine* (C)(G) initially 25 mg daily in divided doses; gradually increase to 100 mg during first 2 weeks; max 250 mg/day; total maintenance dose may be given at HS

Pediatric: <10 years: not recommended; ≥10 years: initially 25 mg daily in divided doses; gradually increase; max 3 mg/kg or 100 mg, whichever is smaller

Anafranil *Cap:* 25, 50, 75 mg

▷ *imipramine* (C)(G)
  Tofranil initially 75 mg/day; max 200 mg/day
  Pediatric: adolescents initially 30-40 mg/day; max 100 mg/day
    Tab: 10, 25, 50 mg
  Tofranil PM initially 75 mg/day; max 200 mg/day
  Pediatric: <12 years: not recommended; ≥12 years: same as adult
    Cap: 75, 100, 125, 150 mg

 ONYCHOMYCOSIS (FUNGAL NAIL)

ORAL AGENTS

▷ *griseofulvin, microsize* (C)(G) 1 gm daily for at least 4 months for fingernails and at
  least 6 months for toenails
  Pediatric: 5 mg/lb/day; *see page 640 for dose by weight*
    Grifulvin V *Tab:* 250, 500 mg; *Oral susp:* 125 mg/5 ml (120 ml; alcohol 0.02%)
▷ *griseofulvin, ultramicrosize* (C) 750 mg in a single or divided doses for at least 4
  months for fingernails and at least 6 months for toenails
  Pediatric: <2 years: not recommended; ≥2 years: 3.3 mg/lb in a single or divided
  doses
    Gris-PEG *Tab:* 125, 250 mg
▷ *itraconazole* (C)(G) 200 mg daily x 12 consecutive weeks for toenails; 200 mg bid x 1
  week, off 3 weeks, then 200 mg bid x 1 additional week for fingernails
  Pediatric: <12 years: not recommended; ≥12 years: same as adult
    Sporanox *Cap:* 100 mg; *Soln:* 10 mg/ml (150 ml) (cherry-caramel)
    Pulse Pack: 100 mg caps (7/pck)
▷ *terbinafine* (B)(G) 250 mg daily x 6 weeks for fingernails; 250 mg daily x 12 weeks for
  toenails
  Pediatric: <12 years: not recommended; ≥12 years: same as adult
    Lamisil *Tab:* 250 mg

TOPICAL AGENTS

Comment: File and trim nail while nail is free from drug. Remove unattached
infected nail as frequently as monthly. For use with mild to moderate onychomycosis
of the fingernails and toenails, without lunula involvement due to *Trichophyton
rubrum* immunocompetent patients as part of a comprehensive treatment program.
For use on nails and adjacent skin only. Apply evenly to entire onycholytic nail and
surrounding 5 mm of skin daily, preferably at HS or 8 hours before washing; apply to
nail bed, hyponychium, and under surface of nail plate when it is free of the nail bed;
apply over previous coats, then remove with alcohol once per week; treat for up to 48
weeks.
▷ *ciclopirox* (B)
  Pediatric: <12 years: not established; ≥12 years: same as adult
    Penlac Nail Lacquer *Topical soln (lacquer):* 8% (6.6 ml w. applicator)
▷ *efinaconazole* (C)
  Pediatric: <12 years: not established; ≥12 years: same as adult
    Jublia *Topical soln:* 5% (10 ml w. brush applicator)
▷ *tavaborole* (C)
  Pediatric: <12 years: not established; ≥12 years: same as adult
    Kerydin *Topical soln:* 10% (10 ml w. dropper)

OPHTHALMIA NEONATORUM: CHLAMYDIAL

PROPHYLAXIS

▷ *erythromycin* ophthalmic ointment 0.5-1 cm ribbon into lower conjunctival sac of each eye x 1 application

Ilotycin Ophthalmic Ointment *Ophth oint:* 5 mg/gm (1/8 oz)

Comment: The following treatment regimens are published in the **2015 CDC Sexually Transmitted Diseases Treatment Guidelines**. Treatment regimens are presented by generic drug name first, followed by information about brands and dose forms.

RECOMMENDED TREATMENT REGIMENS

Comment: The following treatment regimens are published in the **2015 CDC Sexually Transmitted Diseases Treatment Guidelines**.

Regimen 1

▷ *erythromycin base* 50 mg/kg/day in 4 doses x 14 days

Regimen 2

▷ *erythromycin ethylsuccinate* 50 mg/kg/day in 4 doses x 14 days; *see page 629 for dose by weight*

DRUG BRANDS AND DOSE FORMS

▷ *erythromycin base* (B)(G)

Ery-Tab *Tab:* 250, 333, 500 mg ent-coat

PCE *Tab:* 333, 500 mg

Comment: *erythromycin* may increase INR with concomitant *warfarin*, as well as increase serum level of *digoxin, benzodiazepines*, and *statins*.

▷ *erythromycin ethylsuccinate* (B)(G)

EryPed *Oral susp:* 200 mg/5 ml (100, 200 ml) (fruit); 400 mg/5 ml (60, 100, 200 ml) (banana); *Oral drops:* 200, 400 mg/5 ml (50 ml) (fruit); *Chew tab:* 200 mg wafer (fruit)

E.E.S. *Oral susp:* 200, 400 mg/5 ml (100 ml) (fruit)

E.E.S. Granules *Oral susp:* 200 mg/5 ml (100, 200 ml) (cherry)

Comment: *erythromycin* may increase INR with concomitant *warfarin*, as well as increase serum level of *digoxin, benzodiazepines*, and *statins*.

 OPHTHALMIA NEONATORUM: GONOCOCCAL

Comment: The following prophylaxis and treatment regimens for gonococcal conjunctivitis is published in the **2015 CDC Sexually Transmitted Diseases Treatment Guidelines**.

PROPHYLAXIS

▷ *erythromycin 0.5%* ophthalmic ointment 0.5-1 cm ribbon into lower conjunctival sac of each eye x 1 application

Ilotycin Ophthalmic Ointment *Ophth oint:* 5 mg/gm (1/8 oz)

TREATMENT

▷ *ceftriaxone* (B)(G) 25-50 mg/kg IV <u>or</u> IM in a single dose, not to exceed 125 mg

Rocephin *Vial:* 250, 500 mg; 1, 2 gm

OPIOID DEPENDENCE, OPIOID USE DISORDER, OPIOID WITHDRAWAL SYNDROME

Comment: Safety labeling for all immediate-release (IR) opioids has been issued by the FDA. The Black Boxed Warning (BBW) includes serious risks of misuse, abuse, addiction, overdose, and death. The dosing section offers clear steps regarding administration and patient monitoring including initial dose, dose changes, and the abrupt cessation of treatment in physical dependence. Chronic maternal use of opioids during pregnancy can lead to potentially life-threatening neonatal opioid withdrawal. The American Pain Society (APS) has released new evidence-based clinical practice guidelines that include 32 recommendations related to post-op pain management in adults and children. The Transmucosal Immediate Release Fentanyl (TIRF) Risk Evaluation and Mitigation Strategy (REMS) program is an FDA-required program designed to ensure informed risk-benefit decisions before initiating treatment, and while patients are treated to ensure appropriate use of TIRF medicines. The purpose of the TIRF REMS Access program is to mitigate the risk of misuse, abuse, addiction, overdose and serious complications due to medication errors with the use of TIRF medicines. You must enroll in the TIRF REMS Access program to prescribe, dispense, or distribute TIRF medicines. To register, call the TIRF REMS Access program at 1-866-822-1483 or register online at https://www.tirfremsaccess.com/TirfUI/rems/home.action

OPIOID AGONISTS

Methadone Detoxification and Methadone Maintenance

Comment: *methadone* is not indicated as an as-needed (prn) analgesic. For use in chronic moderately severe-to-severe pain management (e.g., hospice care).

▷ *methadone* (C)(II)(G) A single dose of 20 to 30 mg may be sufficient to suppress withdrawal syndrome; *Narcotic Detoxification:* 15-40 mg daily in decreasing doses not to exceed 21 days; *Narcotic Maintenance:* >21 days; see mfr pkg insert; clinical stability is most commonly achieved at doses between 80 to 120 mg/day; monitor patients with periodic ECGs (e.g., risk of lethal QT interval prolongation, *torsades de pointes*)
  Pediatric: <12: not recommended; ≥12 years: same as adult
    Dolophine *Tab:* 5, 10 mg; *Dispersible tab:* 40 mg (dissolve in 120 ml orange juice or other citrus drink); *Oral soln:* 5, 10 mg/ml; *Oral conc:* 10 mg/ml; *Syr:* 10 mg/30 ml; *Vial:* 10 mg/ml (200 mg/20 ml multi-dose) for injection

Comment: *methadone* administration is allowed only by approved providers with strict state and federal regulations (as stipulated in 42 CFR 8.12). Black Box Warning (BBW): **Dolophine** exposes users to risks of addiction, abuse, and misuse, which can lead to overdose and death. Assess each patient's risk and monitor regularly for development of these behaviors and conditions. Serious, life-threatening, or fatal respiratory depression may occur. The peak respiratory depressant effect of *methadone* occurs later, and persists longer than the peak analgesic effect. Accidental ingestion, especially by children, can result in fatal overdose. QT interval prolongation and serious arrhythmia (*torsades de pointes*) have occurred during treatment with *methadone*. Closely monitor patients with risk factors for development of prolonged QT interval, a history of cardiac conduction abnormalities, and those taking medications affecting cardiac conduction. Neonatal Opioid Withdrawal Syndrome (NOWS) is an expected and treatable outcome of use of methadone use during pregnancy. NOWS may be life-threatening if not recognized and treated in the neonate. The balance between the risks of NOWS and the benefits of maternal *methadone* use should be considered and the patient advised of the risk of NOWS so that appropriate planning for management of the neonate can occur.

methadone has been detected in human milk. Concomitant use with CYP3A4, 2B6, 2C19, 2C9 or 2D6 inhibitors or discontinuation of concomitantly used CYP3A4 2B6, 2C19, or 2C9 inducers can result in a fatal overdose of methadone. Concomitant use of opioids with benzodiazepines or other central nervous system (CNS) depressants, including alcohol, may result in profound sedation, respiratory depression, coma, and death.

OPIOID ANTAGONIST

▷ *naltrexone* (C)
  Pediatric: <12 years: not established; ≥12 years: same as adult
    ReVia 50 mg daily
      Tab: 50 mg
    Vivitrol 380 mg IM once monthly; alternate buttocks
      Vial: 380 mg

OPIOID PARTIAL AGONIST-ANTAGONIST

Comment: **Belbuca, Butrans, Probuphine, Sublocade, and Subutex** maintenance are allowed only by approved providers with strict state and federal regulations. These drugs are potentiated by CYP3A4 inhibitors (e.g, azole antifungals, macrolides, HIV protease inhibitors) and antagonized by CYP3A4 inducers (monitor for opioid withdrawal). Concomitant NNRTIs (e.g., *efavirenz, nevirapine, etravirine, delavirdine*) or PIs (e.g., *atazanavir* with or without *ritonavir*): monitor. Risk of respiratory or CNS depression with concomitant opioid analgesics, general anesthetics, benzodiazepines, phenothiazines, other tranquilizers, sedative/hypnotics, alcohol, or other CNS depressants. Risk of serotonin syndrome with concomitant SSRIs, SNRIs, TCAs, 5-HT3 receptor antagonists, *mirtazapine, trazodone, tramadol,* MAO inhibitors.

▷ *buprenorphine* (C)(III)
    Belbuca apply buccal film to inside of cheek; do not chew or swallow; *Opioid naïve:* initially 75 mcg once daily-q 12 hours x at least 4 days; then, increase to 150 mcg q 12 hours; may increase in increments of 150 mcg q 12 hours no sooner than every 4 days; max 900 mcg q 12 hours; see mfr pkg insert for conversion from other opioids; *Severe hepatic impairment or oral mucositis:* reduce initial and titration doses by half
    Pediatric: <12 years: not established; ≥12 years: same as adult
      Buccal film: 75, 150, 300, 450, 600, 750, 900 mcg (60/pck) (peppermint)
    Butrans Transdermal System apply one patch to clean, dry, hairless, intact skin on the upper outer arm, upper chest, upper back, or side of chest every 7 days; rotate sites and do not re-use a site for at least 21 days; *Opioid naïve or oral morphine <30 mg/day or equivalent:* one 5 mcg/hour patch; *Converting from oral morphine equivalents 30-80 mg/day:* taper current opioids for up to 7 days to ≤30 mg/day oral morphine equivalents before starting; then initiate with 10 mcg/hour patch; may use a short-acting analgesic until efficacy is attained; increase dose only after exposure to previous dose x at least 72 hours; max one 20 mcg/hour patch/week; *Conversion from higher opioid doses:* not recommended
    Pediatric: <12 years: not established; ≥12 years: same as adult
      Transdermal patch: 5, 7.5, 10, 15, 20 mcg/hour (4/pck)
    Probuphine initiate when stable on *buprenorphine* ≤8 mg/day; insertion site is the inner side of the upper arm; 4 implants are intended to be in place for 6 months; remove the implants by the end of the 6th month and insert four new implants on the same day in the contralateral arm; if a new implant is not inserted on the same day as removal of a previous implant, maintain the patient on the previous dose of transmucosal *buprenorphine* (i.e., the dose from which the patient was transferred to **Probuphine** treatment).

Pediatric: <16 years: not established; ≥16 years: same as adult

Subdermal implant: 74.2 mg of **buprenorphine** (equivalent to 80 mg of *bu-prenorphine hydrochloride*)

Comment: Healthcare providers who prescribe, perform insertions and/or perform removals of **Probuphine** must successfully complete a live training program, and demonstrate procedural competency prior to inserting or removing the implants. Further information: visit www.ProbuphineREMS.com or call 1-844-859-6341

Subutex (G) 8 mg in a single dose on day 1; then 16 mg in a single dose on day 2; target dose is 16 mg/day in a single dose; dissolve under tongue; do not chew or swallow whole

Pediatric: <12 years: not established; ≥12 years: same as adult

SL tab (lemon-lime) or *SL film (lime):* 2, 8 mg (30/pck)

Sublocade verify that patient is clinically stable on transmucosal **buprenorphine** before initiating **Sublocade**; doses must be prepared by an authorized healthcare provider and administered once monthly only by SC injection in the abdominal region; initially, 300 mg SC once monthly x the first 2 months, followed by 100 mg SC once monthly maintenance dose; increasing the maintenance dose to 300 mg once monthly may be considered for patients in which the benefits outweigh the risks

Pediatric: <12 years: not established; ≥12 years: same as adult

Prefilled syringe: 100 mg/0.5 ml, 300 mg/1.5 ml sust-rel single-dose w. 19 gauge 5/8-inch needle

Comment: Serious harm or death could result if **Sublocade** is administered intravenously. Neonatal opioid withdrawal syndrome (NOWS) is an expected and treatable outcome of prolonged use of opioids during pregnancy. (Not recommended with moderate-to-severe hepatic impairment. Monitor liver function tests prior to and during treatment. If diagnosed with adrenal insufficiency, treat with physiologic replacement of corticosteroids, and wean patient off of the opioid. **Sublocade** is only available through the restricted SUBLOCADE REMS Program. Healthcare settings and pharmacies that order and dispense **Sublocade** must be certified in this program. To report suspected adverse reactions, contact Indivior Inc. at 1877-782-6966 or FDA at 1-800-FDA-1088 or www.fda.gov/medwatch

OPIOID PARTIAL AGONIST-ANTAGONIST+OPIOID ANTAGONIST

Comment: Bunabail, Suboxone, Sucartonone, Troxyca ER, and **Zubsolv** maintenance are allowed only by approved providers with strict state and federal regulations.

▷ *buprenorphine+naloxone* (C)(III)

Bunavail administer one buccal film once daily at the same time each day; target dose is 8.4/1.4 once daily; place the side of the **Bunavail** film with the text (BN2, BN4, or BN6) against the inside of the cheek; press and hold the film in place for 5 seconds; maintenance is usually 2.1/0.3 to 12.6/2.1 once daily

Pediatric: <16 years: not recommended; ≥16 years: same as adult

SL film:

Bunavail 2.1/0.3 *bup* 2.1 mg+*nal* 0.3 mg (30/carton)
Bunavail 4.2/0.7 *bup* 4.2 mg+*nal* 0.7 mg (30/carton)
Bunavail 6.3/1 *bup* 6.3 mg+*nal* 1 mg (30/carton)

Comment: A **Bunavail** 4.2/0.7 buccal film provides equivalent **buprenorphine** exposure to a **Sucartonone** 8/2 sublingual tablet.

Suboxone (G) adjust dose in increments/decrements of 2/0.5 or 4/1 once daily **buprenorphine+naloxone**, based on the patient's daily dose of **buprenorphine**, to a level that suppresses opioid withdrawal signs and symptoms; *Recommended target*

dosage: 16/4 as a single daily dose; *Maintenance dose:* generally in the range of 4/1 to 24/6 per day; higher once daily doses have not been demonstrated to provide any clinical advantage

Pediatric: <12 years: not established; ≥12 years: same as adult

>   Suboxone
>>   *SL tab, SL film:* **Suboxone 2/0.5** bup 2 mg+nal 0.5 mg (30/bottle) (lime)
>>   **Suboxone 8/2** bup 8 mg+nal 2 mg (30/bottle) (lime)

Sucartonone adjust in 2-4 mg of *buprenorphine*/day in a single dose; usual range is 4-24 mg/day in a single dose; target dose is 6 mg/day in a single dose; dissolve under tongue; do not chew <u>or</u> swallow whole

Pediatric: <16 years: not recommended; ≥16 years: same as adult

>   Sucartonone
>>   *SL film:* **Sucartonone 2/0.5** bup 2 mg+nal 0.5 mg (30/pck) (lime)
>>   **Sucartonone 4/1** bup 4 mg+nal 1 mg (30/pck) (lime)
>>   **Sucartonone 8/2** bup 8 mg+nal 2 mg (30/pck) (lime)
>>   **Sucartonone 12/3** bup 12 mg+nal 3 mg (30/pck) (lime)

Zubsolv initial induction with buprenorphine sublingual tabs; administer as a single dose once daily; titrate dose in increments of 1.4/0.36 <u>or</u> 2.9/0.72 per day; recommended target dose is 11.4/2.9 per day; usual max 17.2/4.2 per day

Pediatric: <16 years: not recommended; ≥16 years: same as adult

>   Zubsolv
>>   *SL tab:* **Zubsolv 1.4/0.36** bup 1.4 mg+nal 0.36 mg
>>   **Zubsolv 2.9/0.72** bup 2.9 mg+nal 0.71 mg
>>   **Zubsolv 5.7/1.4** bup 5.7 mg+nal 1.4 mg
>>   **Zubsolv 8.6/2.1** bup 8.6 mg+nal 2.1 mg
>>   **Zubsolv 11.4/2.9** bup 11.4 mg+nal 2.9 mg

Comment: One **Subutex 5.7/1.4** SL tab is bioequivalent to one **Sucartonone 8/2** SL film.

▶   *oxycodone+naloxone* **(C)(II)** *Opioid-naïve and opioid non-tolerant:* initially 10/1.2 q 12 hours; *Opioid tolerant:* single doses greater than 40/4.8, <u>or</u> a total daily dose greater than 80/9.6 are only for use in patients for whom tolerance to an opioid of comparable potency has been established; swallow whole, <u>or</u> sprinkle contents on applesauce and swallow immediately without chewing

Pediatric: <18 years: not recommended; ≥18 years: same as adult

>   Troxyca ER
>>   *Cap:* **Troxyca ER 10/1.2** oxy 10 mg+nalox 1.2 mg ext-rel
>>   **Troxyca ER 20/1.2** oxy 20 mg+nalox 2.4 mg ext-rel
>>   **Troxyca ER 30/1.2** oxy 30 mg+nalox 3.6 mg ext-rel
>>   **Troxyca ER 40/1.2** oxy 40 mg+nalox 4.8 mg ext-rel
>>   **Troxyca ER 60/1.2** oxy 60 mg+nalox 7.2 mg ext-rel
>>   **Troxyca ER 80/1.2** oxy 80 mg+nalox 9.6 mg ext-rel

Comment: Opioid tolerant patients are those taking, for one week <u>or</u> longer, at least 60 mg oral *morphine* per day, 25 mcg transdermal *fentanyl* per hour, 30 mg oral *oxycodone* per day, 8 mg oral *hydromorphone* per day, 25 mg oral *oxymorphone* per day, 60 mg oral *hydrocodone* per day, <u>or</u> an equianalgesic dose of another opioid.

OPIOID-INDUCED CONSTIPATION (OIC)

▶   *lubiprostone* **(C)** swallow whole; take with food and water; initially 24 mcg bid; *Moderate hepatic impairment (Child Pugh Class B):* 16 mg bid; *Severe hepatic impairment (Child Pugh Class C):* 8 mg bid

Pediatric: <12 years: not recommended; ≥12 years: same as adult

>   Amitiza *Cap:* 8, 24 mg

▷ *methylnaltrexone bromide* (C) one oral dose or one weight-based SC dose every other day as needed; max one dose per 24 hours; administer SC inject into the upper arm, abdomen, or thigh; rotate sites

Chronic Non-cancer Pain: 450 mg po once daily in the morning (take with water on an empty stomach at least 30 minutes before the first meal of the day) or 12 mg SC once daily in the morning; *Severe Hepatic Impairment:* <38 kg: 0.075 mg/kg; 38-<62 kg: 4 mg (0.2 ml); 62-114 kg: 6 mg (0.3 ml); >114 kg: 0.075 mg/kg

Advanced Illness, Receiving Palliative Care: <38 kg: 0.15 mg/kg; 38-<62 kg: 8 mg (0.4 ml); 62-114 kg: 12 mg (0.6 ml); >114 kg: 0.15 mg/kg; *Moderate and Severe Renal Impairment (CrCl<60 mL/min):* <38 kg: 0.075 mg/kg; 38-<62 kg: 4 mg (0.2 ml); 62-114 kg: 6 mg (0.3 ml); >114 kg: 0.075 mg/kg

Pediatric: <18 years: not established; ≥18 years: same as adult

  Relistor *Tab:* 150 mg film-coat; *Vial:* 12 mg single-dose (0.6 ml, 7/carton)
  Prefilled syr: 8 mg (0.4 ml), 12 mg (0.6 ml) (7/carton)

Comment: *methylnaltrexone* is a selective antagonist of opioid binding at the mu-opioid receptor. As a quaternary amine, the ability of *methylnaltrexone* to cross the blood-brain barrier is restricted. This allows *methylnaltrexone* to function as a peripherally-acting mu-opioid receptor antagonist in tissues such as the gastrointestinal tract, thereby decreasing the constipating effects of opioids without impacting opioid-mediated analgesic effects on the central nervous system. The pre-filled syringe is only for patients who require a **Relistor** injection dose of 8 mg or 12 mg. Use the vial for patients who require other doses. **Relistor** is contraindicated with known or suspected GI obstruction and patients at increased risk of recurrent obstruction, due to the potential for gastrointestinal perforation. Be within close proximity to toilet facilities once **Relistor** is administered. Discontinue all maintenance laxative therapy prior to initiation. Laxative(s) can be used as needed if there is a suboptimal response after three days. Discontinue if treatment with the opioid pain medication is also discontinued. Safety and effectiveness of **Relistor** have not been established in pediatric patients. Avoid concomitant use with other opioid antagonists because of the potential for additive effects of opioid receptor antagonism and increased risk of opioid withdrawal symptoms (sweating, chills, diarrhea, abdominal pain, anxiety, and yawning). Advise females of reproductive potential, who become pregnant or are planning to become pregnant, that the use of **Relistor** during pregnancy may precipitate opioid withdrawal in a fetus due to the undeveloped blood-brain barrier. Breastfeeding is not recommended during treatment.

▷ *naldemedine* (C) <12 years: not established; ≥12 years: take one tab once daily; take with or without food; discontinue if opioid pain therapy discontinued

Pediatric: <12 years: not established; ≥12 years: same as adult

  Symproic *Tab:* 0.2 mg

Comment: **Symproic** is contraindicated with known or suspected GI obstruction and patients at increased risk for recurrent obstruction. Avoid with severe hepatic impairment (Child-Pugh Class C). Not recommended in pregnancy and breastfeeding (during and 3 days after final dose). There is risk of perforation in persons with conditions associated with reduction in structural integrity the GI tract wall (e.g., peptic ulcer disease [PUD], Ogilvie's syndrome, diverticulitis disease, infiltrative GI tract malignancies, or peritoneal metastases).

▷ *naloxegol* (C) swallow whole; take on an empty stomach; initially 25 mg once daily in the AM; discontinue other laxatives; *CrCl <60 mL/min:* 12.5 mg

Pediatric: <12 years: not established; ≥12 years: same as adult

  Movantik *Tab:* 12.5, 25 mg

Comment: **Movantik** is an opioid antagonist indicated for the treatment of opioid-induced constipation (OIC) in adult patients with chronic non-cancer pain, including patients with chronic pain related to prior cancer or its treatment who do not require frequent (e.g., weekly) opioid dosage escalation. Alteration in analgesic dosing regimen prior to starting **Movantik** is not required. Patients receiving opioids for less than 4 weeks may be less responsive to **Movantik**. Take on an empty stomach at least 1 hour prior to the first meal of the day or 2 hours after the meal. For patients who are unable to swallow the **Movantik** tablet whole, the tablet can be crushed and given orally or administered via nasogastric tube (see full prescribing information). Avoid consumption of grapefruit or grapefruit juice. Discontinue if treatment with the opioid pain medication is also discontinued.

OPIOID-INDUCED NAUSEA/VOMITING (OINV)

Comment: Opioid analgesics bind to μ (mu), κ (kappa), or δ (delta) opioid receptors in the brain, spinal cord, and digestive tract. However, opioids cause adverse effects that may interfere with their therapeutic use. Opioid-induced nausea/vomiting (OINV) treatment options include serotonin receptor antagonists, dopamine receptor antagonists, and neurokinin-1 receptor antagonists.

SEROTONIN RECEPTOR ANTAGONISTS

▷ *dolasetron* (B) administer 100 mg IV over 30 seconds; max 100 mg/dose
  Pediatric: <2 years: not recommended; 2-16 years: 1.8 mg/kg; >16 years: same as adult
    Anzemet *Tab:* 50, 100 mg; *Amp:* 12.5 mg/0.625 ml; *Prefilled carpuject syringe:* 12.5 mg (0.625 ml); *Vial:* 100 mg/5 ml (single-use); *Vial:* 500 mg/25 ml (multi-dose)
▷ *granisetron*
    Kytril (B) administer IV over 30 seconds, 30 min; max 1 dose/week
    Pediatric: <2 years: not recommended; ≥2 years: 10 mcg/kg
      Tab: 1 mg; *Oral soln:* 2 mg/10 ml (30 ml; orange); *Vial:* 1 mg/ml (1 ml single-dose) (preservative-free); 1 mg/ml (4 ml multi-dose) (benzyl alcohol)
    Sancuso (B) apply 1 patch 24-48 hours before chemo; remove 24 hours (minimum) to 7 days (maximum) after completion of treatment
    Pediatric: <12 years: not recommended; ≥12 years: same as adult
      Transdermal patch: 3.1 mg/day
▷ *ondansetron* (C)(G) 8 mg q 8 hours x 2 doses; then 8 mg q 12 hours
  Pediatric: <4 years: not recommended; 4-11 years: 4 mg q 4 hours x 3 doses; then 4 mg q 8 hours
    Zofran *Tab:* 4, 8, 24 mg
    Zofran ODT *ODT:* 4, 8 mg (phenylalanine)
    Zofran Oral Solution *Oral soln:* 4 mg/5 ml (50 ml) (strawberry) (phenylalanine); *Parenteral form:* see mfr pkg insert
    Zofran Injection *Vial:* 2 mg/ml (2 ml single-dose); 2 mg/ml (20 ml multi-dose); 32 mg/50 ml (50 ml multi-dose); *Prefilled syringe:* 4 mg/2 ml, single-use (24/carton)
    Zuplenz Oral Soluble Film: 4, 8 mg oral-dis (10/carton) (peppermint)
▷ *palonosetron* (B)(G) administer 0.25 mg IV over 30 seconds; max 1 dose/week
  Pediatric: <1 month: not recommended; 1 month to 17 years: 20 mcg/kg; max 1.5 mg/ single dose; infuse over 15 minutes
    Aloxi *Vial (single-use):* 0.075 mg/1.5 ml; 0.25 mg/5 ml (mannitol)

DOPAMINE RECEPTOR ANTAGONISTS

▷ *prochlorperazine* (C)(G)
    Compazine 5-10 mg tid-qid prn; usual max 40 mg/day
    Pediatric: <2 years or <20 lb: not recommended; 20-29 lb: 2.5 mg daily bid prn; max 7.5 mg/day; 30-39 lb: 2.5 mg bid-tid prn; max 10 mg/day; 40-85 lb: 2.5 mg tid or 5 mg bid prn; max 15 mg/day
      Tab: 5, 10 mg; *Syr:* 5 mg/5 ml (4 oz) (fruit)

Compazine Suppository 25 mg rectally bid prn; usual max 50 mg/day
Pediatric: <2 years <u>or</u> <20 lb: not recommended; 20-29 lb: 2.5 mg daily-bid prn; max 7.5; mg/day; 30-39 lb: 2.5 mg bid-tid prn; max 10 mg/day; 40-85 lb: 2.5 mg tid <u>or</u> 5 mg bid prn; max 15 mg/day
  Rectal supp: 2.5, 5, 25 mg
Compazine Injectable 5-10 mg tid <u>or</u> qid prn
Pediatric: <2 years <u>or</u> <20 lb: not recommended; ≥2 years <u>or</u> ≥20 lb: 0.06 mg/kg x 1 dose
  Vial: 5 mg/ml (2, 10 ml)
Compazine Spansule 15 mg q AM prn <u>or</u> 10 mg q 12 hours prn usual max 40 mg/day
Pediatric: <12 years: not recommended; ≥12 years: same as adult
  Spansule: 10, 15 mg sust-rel

NEUROKININ-1 RECEPTOR ANTAGONISTS

▷ *aprepitant* (B)(G) administer with 5HT-3 receptor antagonist; *Day 1:* 125 mg; *Day 2* and *3:* 80 mg in the morning
Pediatric: <6 months: years: not recommended; ≥6 months: use oral suspension (see mfr pkg insert for dose by weight
  Emend *Cap:* 40, 80, 125 mg (2 x 80 mg bi-fold pck; 1 x 25 mg/2 x 80 mg tri-fold pck); *Oral susp:* 125 mg pwdr for oral suspension, single-dose pouch w. dispenser; *Vial:* 150 mg pwdr for reconstitution and IV infusion

 OPIOID OVERDOSE

OPIOID ANTAGONISTS

▷ *nalmefene* (B) initially 0.25 mcg/kg IV, IM, <u>or</u> SC, then incremental doses of 0.25 mcg/kg at 2-5 minute intervals; cumulative max 1 mcg/kg; if opioid dependency suspected use 0.1 mg/70 kg initially and then proceed as usual if no response in 2 minutes
Pediatric: not recommended
  Revex *Amp:* 100 mcg/ml (1 ml); 1 mg/ml (2 ml)
▷ *naloxone* (B)(G) 0.4-2 mg; repeat in 2-3 minutes if no response
Pediatric: 0.01 mg/kg initially, repeat in 2-3 minutes at 0.1 mg/kg if response inadequate
  Evzio *Prefilled autoinjector:* 0.4 mg/0.4, 2 mg/0.4 ml IM/SC only
Comment: Evzio 2 mg/0.4 ml comes with 2 autoinjectors and one trainer. This strength is indicated for the emergency treatment of known <u>or</u> suspected opioid overdose manifested by CNS depression.
If the electronic voice instruction system does not operate properly, **Evzio** will still deliver the intended dose of *naloxone* when used according to the printed instructions on the flat surface of the autoinjector label. **Evzio** cannot be administered IV. Due to the short duration of action of naloxone, as compared to opioids which are longer acting, monitoring of the patient is critical as the opioid reversal effects of naloxone may wear off before the effects of the opioid.
  Narcan *Vial/Amp:* 0.4 mg/ml (1 ml), 1 mg/ml (2 ml); *Prefilled syringe:* 0.4 mg/ml (1 ml), 1 mg/ml (2 ml) IV, IM, <u>or</u> SC (parabens-free)
  Narcan Nasal Spray position supine with head tilted back; 1 spray in one nostril; if an additional dose is needed, spray into the opposite nostril
    Nasal spray: 4 mg/0.1 ml, single-dose (2 blister pcks, each w a single nasal spray/carton)

ORGAN TRANSPLANT REJECTION PROPHYLAXIS

SELECTIVE IMMUNOMODULATORY AGENTS

Comment: Selective immunosuppressive agents are drugs that suppress the immune system due to a selective point of action. They are used to reduce the risk of rejection in organ transplants, in autoimmune diseases, and can be use as cancer chemotherapy. As immunosuppressive agents lower the immunity, there is increased risk of infection.

Humanized Anti-interleukin-2 (IL-2) Receptor Monoclonal Antibody

➢ *daclizumab* (C) administer 150 mg by SC injection once monthly (A higher dosage of 300 mg once monthly not shown in clinical studies to provide additional clinical benefit) in the back of upper arm, abdomen, or thigh; allow at least 30 minutes for the prefilled syringe to reach room temperature; if a dose is missed, administer as soon as possible; however, if >2 weeks have elapsed, omit missed dose and resume regular dosing schedule

Pediatric: <17 years: not established/not recommended; ≥17 years: same as adult

 Zinbryta *Prefilled syringe/Prefilled autoinjector:* 150 mg/ml, single-dose

Comment: *daclizumab* is indicated for the management of relapsing forms of MS (e.g., relapsing-remitting MS [RRMS]) and organ transplant rejection prophylaxis. *daclizumab* is contraindicated in patients with preexisting hepatic disease or impairment (e.g., ALT or AST ≥2 times the ULN) and history of autoimmune hepatitis or other autoimmune condition involving the liver. Evaluate serum aminotransferase (ALT/ AST) and total bilirubin concentrations prior to initiating therapy, then monthly before each dose is administered and for 6 months after discontinuance of therapy. Interrupt therapy in patients with ALT or AST >5 times the ULN, total bilirubin >2 times the ULN, or ALT or AST ≥3 times but <5 times the ULN *with* total bilirubin >1.5 times but <2 times the ULN. No dosage adjustment is required for renal impairment. Prior to initiating therapy with **Zinbryta**, screen for hepatitis B and C, complete any necessary immunizations with live vaccines, and evaluate for tuberculosis infection in patients at high risk and treat appropriately. Depression-related events, including suicidal ideation and suicide attempt, have been reported. No adequate data in pregnant women; limited data from clinical trials do not suggest an increased risk of adverse fetal or maternal outcomes. There are no data on the presence of *semaglutide* in human milk or the effects on the breastfed infant. *daclizumab* is available only through the Zinbryta REMS Program. Clinicians, pharmacies, and patients must be enrolled and meet all conditions of this program before they can prescribe, dispense, or receive the drug. To report suspected adverse reactions, contact Biogen at 1-800-456-2255 or FDA at 1-800-FDA-1088 or www.fda.gov/medwatch.

Mammalian Target of Rapamycin (mTOR) Inhibitors (mTORi)

Comment: The most frequently occurring adverse events associated with mTOR inhibitors (≥30%) include aphthous stomatitis, rash, anemia, fatigue, hyperglycemia, hypertriglyceridemia, hypercholesterolemia, decreased appetite, nausea, diarrhea, abdominal pain, headache, peripheral edema, hypertension, increased serum creatinine, fever, urinary tract infection, arthralgia, pain, thrombocytopenia, and interstitial lung disease. There are no adequate and well-controlled studies in pregnant females. Effective contraception must be initiated before mTORi therapy, continued during therapy, and for 12 weeks after therapy has been stopped. It is not known whether *serolimus*-based drugs are excreted in human milk. The pharmacokinetic and safety profiles in breastfed infants are not known; therefore, a decision should be made whether to discontinue nursing or to discontinue the drug, taking into account the importance of the drug to the mother.

▷ *everolimus* (C) administer consistently with <u>or</u> without food at the same time time as *cyclosporine* <u>or</u> *tacrolimus*; monitor *everolimus* concentrations: adjust just maintenance dose to achieve trough concentrations within the 3-8 ng/mL target range (using LC/MS/MS assay method); *Mild hepatic impairment:* reduce initial daily dose by one-third; *Moderate <u>or</u> severe hepatic impairment:* reduce initial daily dose by one-half *Kidney Transplant:* indicated for patients at low-moderate immunologic risk; use in combination with *basiliximab, cyclosporine* (reduced doses), and *corticosteroids;* starting dose is 0.75 mg bid; initiate as soon as possible after transplantation *Liver Transplant:* use in combination with *tacrolimus* (reduced doses) and *corticosteroids*; starting dose is 1.0 mg bid; initiate 30 days after transplantation

Pediatric: <18 years: not established/not recommended; ≥18 years: same as adult

Zortress *Tab:* 0.25, 0.5, 0.75 mg

Comment: To report suspected adverse reactions, contact Novartis Pharmaceuticals Corporation at 1-888-669-6682 <u>or</u> FDA at 1-800-FDA1088 <u>or</u> www.fda.gov/medwatch

▷ *serolimus* (C)

Generic: (for prescribing information, *see* **Rapamune**)

Tab: 1, 2 mg

Rapamune administer consistently with <u>or</u> without food at the same time as *cyclosporine (CsA) Low to moderate-immunologic risk: Day 1:* 6 mg as a single loading dose; *Day 2:* initiate 2 mg once daily maintenance; use initially with *cyclosporine* (CsA) and *corticosteroids*; initiate CsA withdrawal over 4-8 weeks beginning 2-4 months post-transplantation *High-immunologic risk: Day 1:* up to 15 mg as a single loading dose; *Day 2:* initiate 5 mg once daily maintenance; use with CsA for the first 12 months post-transplantation

Pediatric: <13 years: not established/not recommended; ≥13 years: same as

Tab: 0.5, 1, 2, mg; *Oral soln:* 60 mg/60 ml in amber glass bottle, one oral syringe adapter for fitting into the neck of the bottle, sufficient disposable amber oral syringes and caps for daily dosing, and a carrying case; bottles should be stored protected from light and refrigerated at 2°C to 8°C (36°F to 46°F); once the bottle is opened, the contents should be used within one month; If necessary, bottles may be stored the bottles at room temperatures up to 25°C (77°F) for a short period of time (not more than 15 days)

Comment: To report suspected adverse reactions, contact Pfizer at 1-800-438-1985 <u>or</u> FDA at 1-800-FDA-1088 <u>or</u> www.fda.gov/medwatch

---

 OSGOOD-SCHLATTER DISEASE

Acetaminophen for IV Infusion *see Pain page* 344
NSAIDs *see page* 562
Opioid Analgesics *see Pain page* 345
Topical and Transdermal NSAIDs *see Pain page* 344
Parenteral Corticosteroids *see page* 570
Oral Corticosteroids *see page* 569
Topical Analgesic and Anesthetic Agents *see page* 560

 OSTEOARTHRITIS, ANKYLOSING SPONDYLITIS

Acetaminophen for IV Infusion *see Pain page* 344
NSAIDs *see page* 562
Opioid Analgesics *see Pain page* 345
Topical and Transdermal NSAIDs *see Pain page* 344
Parenteral Corticosteroids *see page* 570
Oral Corticosteroids *see page* 569
Topical Analgesic and Anesthetic Agents *see page* 560

TOPICAL ANALGESICS

▷ *capsaicin* (B)(G) apply tid to qid prn to intact skin
Pediatric: <2 years: not recommended; ≥2 years: same as adult
  Axsain *Crm:* 0.075% (1, 2 oz)
  Capsin *Lotn:* 0.025, 0.075% (59 ml)
  Capzasin-P (OTC) *Crm:* 0.025% (1.5 oz); *Lotn:* 0.025% (2 oz)
  Dolorac *Crm:* 0.025% (28 gm)
  Double Cap (OTC) *Crm:* 0.05% (2 oz)
  R-Gel *Gel:* 0.025% (15, 30 gm)
  Zostrix (OTC) *Crm:* 0.025% (0.7, 1.5, 3 oz)
  Zostrix HP (OTC) *Emol crm:* 0.075% (1, 2 oz)
Comment: Provides some relief by 1-2 weeks; optimal benefit may take 4-6 weeks.

ORAL SALICYLATE

▷ *indomethacin* (C) initially 25 mg bid to tid, increase as needed at weekly intervals by
25-50 mg/day; max 200 mg/day
Pediatric: <14 years: usually not recommended; >2 years, if risk warranted: 1-2 mg/
kg/day in divided doses; max 3-4 mg/kg/day (or 150-200 mg/day, whichever is less);
<14 years: ER cap not recommended
  Cap: 25, 50 mg; *Susp;* 25 mg/5 ml (pineapple-coconut, mint) (alcohol 1%);
  Supp: 50 mg; *ER Cap:* 75 mg ext-rel
Comment: *indomethacin* is indicated only for acute painful flares. Administer with food
and/or antacids. Use lowest effective dose for shortest duration.

ORAL NSAIDs

See more Oral NSAIDs page 562

▷ *diclofenac* (C)
Pediatric: <18 years: not recommended; ≥18 years: same as adult
  Zorvolex take on empty stomach; 35 mg tid; *Hepatic impairment:* use lowest dose
  Gelcap: 18, 35 mg
▷ *diclofenac sodium* (C)
Pediatric: <18 years: not recommended; ≥18 years: same as adult
  Voltaren 50 mg bid to qid or 75 mg bid or 25 mg qid with an additional 25 mg at
  HS if necessary
  Tab: 25, 50, 75 mg ent-coat
  Voltaren XR 100 mg once daily; rarely, 100 mg bid may be used
  Tab: 100 mg ext-rel

ORAL NSAIDs+PPI

▷ *esomeprazole+naproxen* (C)(G) 1 tab bid; use lowest effective dose for the shortest
duration swallow whole; take at least 30 minutes before a meal
Pediatric: <18 years: not recommended; ≥18 years: same as adult
  Vimovo *Tab:* nap 375 mg+eso 20 mg ext-rel; nap 500 mg+eso 20 mg ext-rel
Comment: **Vimovo** is indicated to improve signs/symptoms, and risk of gastric ulcer in
patients at risk of developing NSAID-associated gastric ulcer.

COX-2 INHIBITORS

Comment: Cox-2 inhibitors are contraindicated with history of asthma, urticaria, and
allergic-type reactions to *aspirin*, other NSAIDs, and sulfonamides, 3rd trimester of
pregnancy, and coronary artery bypass graft (CABG) surgery.

▷ *celecoxib* (C)(G) 100-400 mg daily bid; max 800 mg/day
  Pediatric: <18 years: not recommended; ≥18 years: same as adult
    Celebrex *Cap:* 50, 100, 200, 400 mg
▷ *meloxicam* (C)(G)
    Mobic <2 years, <60 kg: not recommended; ≥2, >60 kg: 0.125 mg/kg; max 7.5 mg once daily; ≥18 years: initially 7.5 mg once daily; max 15 mg once daily; *Hemodialysis:* max 7.5 mg/day
      Tab: 7.5, 15 mg; *Oral susp:* 7.5 mg/5 ml (100 ml) (raspberry)
    Vivlodex <18 years: not established; ≥18 years: initially 5 mg qd; may increase to max 10 mg/day; *Hemodialysis:* max 5 mg/day
      Cap: 5, 10 mg

INTRA-ARTICULAR INJECTIONS

▷ *sodium hyaluronate* (B) using strict aseptic technique, administer by intra-articular injection (into the synovial space) once weekly for the prescribed number of weeks (see mfr pkg insert); after preparing the injection site and attaining local analgesia, remove joint synovial fluid or effusion prior to injection
  Pediatric: <12 years: not recommended; ≥12 years: same as adult
    Gelsyn-3 *Syringe:* 8.4 mg/ml (2 ml) prefilled
    Hyalgan *Vial:* 20 mg (2 ml); Prefilled syringe: 20 mg (2 ml)
    Hylan *Syringe:* 48 mg/6 ml (6 ml) prefilled
    Synvisc One *Syringe:* 46 mg/6 ml (6 ml) prefilled

TUMOR NECROSIS FACTOR (TNF) ALPHA BLOCKERS FOR ANKYLOSING SPONDYLITIS

▷ *adalimumab-adbm* (B) initially 80 SC; then, 40 mg SC every other week starting one week after initial dose; inject into thigh <u>or</u> abdomen; rotate sites
  Pediatric: <18 years: not recommended; ≥18 years: same as adult
    Cyltezo *Prefilled syringe:* 40 mg/0.8 ml single-dose (preservative-free)
Comment: **Cyltezo** is biosimilar to **Humira** (*adalimumab*).
▷ *infliximab (tumor necrosis factor-alpha blocker)* must be refrigerated at 2ºC to 8ºC (36ºF to 46ºF); administer dose intravenously over a period of not less than 2 hours; do not use beyond the expiration date as this product contains no preservative; 5 mg/kg at 0, 2 and 6 weeks, then every 8 weeks.
  Pediatric: <6 years: not studied; ≥6-17 years: mg/kg at 0, 2 and 6 weeks, then every 8 weeks; ≥18 years: same as adult
    Remicade *Vial:* 100 mg for reconstitution to 10 ml administration volume, single-dose (preservative-free)
Comment: **Remicade** is indicated to reduce signs and symptoms, and induce and maintain clinical remission, in adults and children ≥6 years-of-age with moderately to severely active disease who have had an inadequate response to conventional therapy <u>and</u> reduce the number of draining enterocutaneous and rectovaginal fistulas, and maintain fistula closure, in adults with fistulizing disease. Common adverse effects associated with **Remicade** included abdominal pain, headache, pharyngitis, sinusitis, and upper respiratory infections. In addition, **Remicade** might increase the risk for serious infections, including tuberculosis, bacterial sepsis, and invasive fungal infections. Available data from published literature on the use of *infliximab* products during pregnancy have not reported a clear association with *infliximab* products and adverse pregnancy outcomes. *infliximab* products cross the placenta and infants exposed *in utero* should not be administered live vaccines for at least 6 months after birth. Otherwise, the infant may be at increased risk of infection, including disseminated infection which can become fatal. Available information is insufficient to inform the

amount of *infliximab* products present in human milk or effects on the breastfed infant. To report suspected adverse reactions, contact Merck Sharp & Dohme Corp., a subsidiary of Merck & Co. at 1-877-888-4231 or FDA at 1-800-FDA1088 or www.fda.gov/medwatch

▷ *infliximab-abda (tumor necrosis factor-alpha blocker)* (B)

Renflexis: see *infliximab* (Remicade) above for full prescribing information

Comment: Renflexis is a biosimilar to Remicade for the treatment of immune-disorders including Crohn's disease, ulcerative colitis, rheumatoid arthritis, ankylosing spondylitis, psoriatic arthritis and plaque psoriasis. Renflexis was approved under the FDA category for biosimilars and demonstrated no clinically meaningful differences for use, dosing regimens, strengths, dosage forms, and routes of administration from the FDA-approved biological product Remicade.

▷ *infliximab-dyyb (tumor necrosis factor-alpha blocker)* (B)

Inflectra: see *infliximab* (Remicade) above for full prescribing information

Comment: Inflectra is a biosimilar to Remicade for the treatment of immune-disorders including Crohn's disease, ulcerative colitis, rheumatoid arthritis, ankylosing spondylitis, psoriatic arthritis and plaque psoriasis. Inflectra was approved under the FDA category for biosimilars and demonstrated no clinically meaningful differences for use, dosing regimens, strengths, dosage forms, and routes of administration from the FDA-approved biological product Remicade.

▷ *infliximab-qbtx (tumor necrosis factor-alpha blocker)* (B)

Ifixi: see *infliximab* (Remicade) above for full prescribing information

Comment: Ifixi is a biosimilar to Remicade for the treatment of immune disorders including Crohn's disease, ulcerative colitis, rheumatoid arthritis, ankylosing spondylitis, psoriatic arthritis and plaque psoriasis. Ifixi was approved under the FDA category for biosimilars and demonstrated no clinically meaningful differences for use, dosing regimens, strengths, dosage forms, and routes of administration from the FDA-approved biological product Remicade.

 OSTEOPOROSIS

Comment: Indications for bone density screening include: Postmenopausal women not receiving HRT, maternal history of hip fracture, personal history of fragility fracture, presence of high serum markers of bone resorption, smoker, height >67 inches, weight <125 lb, taking a steroid, GnRH agonist, or antiseizure drug, immobilization, hyperthyroidism, posttransplantation, malabsorption syndrome, hyperparathyroidism, prolactinemia. The mnemonic ABONE [Age >65, Bulk (weight <140 lbs at menopause), and Never Estrogens (for more than 6 months)], represents other indications for bone density screening. Foods high in calcium include almonds, broccoli, baked beans, salmon, sardines, buttermilk, turnip greens, collard greens, spinach, pumpkin, rhubarb, and bran. Recommended Daily Calcium Intake: 1-3 years: 700 mg; 4-8 years: 1000 mg; 9-18 years: 1300 mg; 19-50 years: 1000 mg: 51-70 years (males): 1000 mg; ≥51 years (females): 1200 mg; pregnancy or nursing: 1000-1300 mg Recommended Daily Vitamin D Intake: >1 year: 600 IU; 50+ years: 800-1000 IU. Prior to initiating, or concomitant prescribing, corticosteroids in patients at risk for, or diagnosed with, osteoporosis, referral to the following ACR guidelines is recommended: ACR Guidelines on Prevention & Treatment of Glucocorticoid-induced Osteoporosis [press release, June 7, 2017]. Atlanta, GA. American College of Rheumatology https://www.rheumatology.org/About-Us/Newsroom/Press-Releases/ID/812/ACR-Releases-Guideline-on-Prevention-Treatment-of-Glucocorticoid-Induced-Osteoporosis

ESTROGEN REPLACEMENT THERAPY

Comment: *estrogen* plus progesterone is indicated for postmenopausal women with an intact uterus. *estrogen* monotherapy is indicated in women without a uterus. The following list is not inclusive; for more estrogen replacement therapies *see Menopause page* 295)

▷ *estradiol* (X)

> **Alora** initially 0.05 mg/day apply patch twice weekly to lower abdomen, upper quadrant of buttocks <u>or</u> outer aspect of hip
> *Transdermal patch:* 0.025, 0.05, 0.075, 0.1 mg/day (8, 24/pck)
>
> **Climara** initially 0.025 mg/day patch once/week to trunk
> *Transdermal patch:* 0.025, 0.0375, 0.05, 0.075, 0.1 mg/day (4, 8, 24/pck)
>
> **Estrace** 1-2 mg daily cyclically (3 weeks on and 1 week off)
> *Tab:* 0.5, 1, 2*mg (tartrazine)
>
> **Estraderm** initially apply one 0.05 mg/day patch twice weekly to trunk
> *Transdermal patch:* 0.05, 0.1 mg/day (8, 24/pck)
>
> **Menostar** apply one patch weekly to lower abdomen, below the waist; avoid the breasts; alternate sites; *Transdermal patch:* 14 mcg/day (4/pck)
>
> **Minivelle** initially one 0.0375 mg/day patch twice weekly to trunk area; adjust after one month of therapy
> *Transdermal patch:* 0.025, 0.0375, 0.05, 0.075, 0.1 mg/day (8/pck)
>
> **Vivelle** initially one 0.0375 mg/day patch twice weekly to trunk area; use with an oral progestin to prevent endometrial hyperplasia
> *Transdermal patch:* 0.025, 0.0375, 0.05, 0.075, 0.1 mg/day (8, 48/pck)
>
> **Vivelle-Dot** initially one 0.05 mg/day patch twice weekly to lower abdomen, below the waist; use with an oral progestin to prevent endometrial hyperplasia
> *Transdermal patch:* 0.025, 0.0375, 0.05, 0.075, 0.1 mg/day (8, 24/pck)

▷ *estradiol+levonorgestrel* (X) apply 1 patch weekly to lower abdomen; avoid waistline; alternate sites

> **Climara Pro** *Transdermal patch:* estra 0.045 mg+*levo* 0.015 mg per day (4/pck)

▷ *estradiol+norethindrone* (X) 1 tab daily

> **Activella (G)** *Tab:* estra 1 mg+*noreth* 0.5 mg
> **FemHRT 1/5** *Tab:* estra 5 mcg+*noreth* 1 mg

▷ *estradiol+norgestimate* (X) one x 1 mg *estradiol* tab daily x 3 days, then 1 x *estradiol* 1 mg+**norgestimate** 0.09 mg tab once daily x 3 days; repeat this pattern continuously

> **Ortho-Prefest** *Tab:* estra 1 mg+*norgest* 0.09 mg (30/blister pck)

▷ *estrogen, conjugated (equine)* (X)

> **Premarin** 1 tab daily
> *Tab:* 0.3, 0.45, 0.625, 0.9, 1.25, 2.5 mg

▷ *estropipate, piperazine estrone sulfate* (X)(G)

> **Ogen** 0.625-1.25 mg daily cyclically (3 weeks on and 1 week off)
> *Tab:* 0.625, 1.25, 2.5 mg
>
> **Ortho-Est** 0.75-6 mg daily cyclically (3 weeks on and 1 week off)
> *Tab:* 0.625, 1.25 mg

ESTROGENS, CONJUGATED+ESTROGEN AGONIST-ANTAGONIST COMBINATION

▷ *estrogen, conjugated+bazedoxifene* (X)

> **Duavee** 1 tab daily
> *Tab:* estra, conj 0.45 mg+baze 20 mg

CALCIUM SUPPLEMENTS

Comment: Take *calcium* supplements after meals to avoid gastric upset. Dosages of calcium over 2000 mg/day have not been shown to have any additional benefit. *calcium* decreases *tetracycline* absorption. *calcium* absorption is decreased by corticosteroids.

▷ *calcitonin-salmon* (C)

> **Fortical** 200 IU intranasally daily; alternate nostrils each day
> > *Nasal spray:* 200 IU/actuation (30 doses, 3.7 ml)
>
> **Miacalcin Nasal spray** 200 IU spray in one nostril once daily; alternate nostrils each day
> > *Nasal spray:* 200 IU/actuation (30 doses, 3.7 ml)
>
> **Miacalcin Injection** 100 units SC <u>or</u> IM every other day
> > *Vial:* 200 units/ml (2 ml)

Comment: Supplement diet with calcium (1 gm/day) and vitamin D (400 IU/day).

▷ *calcium carbonate* (C)(OTC)(G)

> **Rolaids** chew 2 tabs bid; max 14 tabs/day
> > *Chew tab:* 550 mg
>
> **Rolaids Extra Strength** chew 2 tabs bid; max 8 tabs/day
> > *Chew tab:* 1000 mg
>
> **Tums** chew 2 tabs bid; max 16 tabs/day
> > *Chew tab:* 500 mg
>
> **Tums Extra Strength** chew 2 tabs bid; max 10 tabs/day
> > *Chew tab:* 750 mg
>
> **Tum Sultra** chew 2 tabs bid; max 8 tabs/day
> > *Chew tab:* 1000 mg
>
> **Os-Cal 500 (OTC)** 1-2 tab bid to tid
> > *Chew tab: elemental calcium carbonate* 500 mg

▷ *calcium carbonate+vitamin D* (C)(G)

> **Os-Cal 250+D (OTC)** 1-2 tab tid
> > *Tab:* calc carb 250 mg+vit d 125 IU
>
> **Os-Cal 500+D (OTC)** 1-2 tab bid-tid
> > *Tab:* calc carb 500 mg+vit d 125 IU
>
> **Viactiv (OTC)** 1 tab tid
> > *Chew tab:* calc carb 500 mg+vit d 100 IU+vit k 40 mcg

▷ *calcium citrate* (C)(G)

> **Citracal (OTC)** 1-2 tabs bid
> > *Tab:* calc cit 200 mg

▷ *calcium citrate+vitamin D* (C)(G)

> **Citracal+D (OTC)** 1-2 cplts bid
> > *Cplt:* calc cit 315 mg+vit d 200 IU
>
> **Citracal 250+D (OTC)** 1-2 tabs bid
> > *Tab:* calc cit 250 mg+vit d 62.3 IU

VITAMIN D ANALOGS

Comment: Concurrent *vitamin D* supplementation is contraindicated for patients taking *calcitriol* <u>or</u> *doxercalciferol* due to the risk of *vitamin D* toxicity.

▷ *calcitriol* (C) *Predialysis:* initially 0.25 mcg daily; may increase to 0.5 mcg daily; *Dialysis:* initially 0.25 mcg daily; may increase by 0.25 mcg/day at 4-8 week intervals; usual maintenance 0.5-1 mcg/day; *Hypoparathyroidism:* initially 0.25 mcg q AM; may increase by 0.25 mcg/day at 4- to 8-week intervals; usual maintenance 0.5-2 mcg/day
Pediatric: Predialysis: <3 years: 10-15 ng/kg/day; ≥3 years: initially 0.25 mcg daily; may increase to 0.5 mcg/day; *Dialysis:* not recommended; *Hypoparathyroidism:* initially 0.25 mcg daily; may increase by 0.25 mcg/day at 2-4 week intervals; usual maintenance (1-5 years) 0.25-0.75 mcg/day, (≥6 years) 0.5-2 mcg/day

> **Rocaltrol** *Cap:* 0.25, 0.5 mcg
> **Rocaltrol Solution** *Soln:* 1 mcg/ml (15 ml, single-use dispensers)

▷ *doxercalciferol* (C) initially 0.25 mcg q AM; may increase by 0.25 mcg/day at 4-8 week intervals; usual maintenance 0.5-2 mcg/day

Pediatric: initially 0.25 mcg daily; may increase by 0.25 mcg; 0.25 mcg/day at 2-4 week intervals; usual maintenance (1-5 years) 0.25-0.75 mcg/day, (≥6 years) 0.5-2 mcg/day

> Hectorol *Cap:* 0.25, 0.5 mcg

BISPHOSPHONATES (CALCIUM MODIFIERS)

Comment: Bisphosphonates should be swallowed whole in the AM with 6-8 oz of plain water 30 minutes before first meal, beverage, <u>or</u> other medications of the day. Monitor serum alkaline phosphatase. Contraindications include abnormalities of the esophagus which delay esophageal emptying such as stricture <u>or</u> achalasia, inability to stand <u>or</u> sit upright for at least 30 minutes postdose, patients at risk of aspiration, and hypocalcemia. Co-administration of bisphosphonates and *calcium*, antacids, <u>or</u> oral medications containing multivalent cations will interfere with absorption of the bisphosphonate. Therefore, instruct patients to wait at least half hour after taking the bisphosphonate before taking any other oral medications.

▷ *alendronate (as sodium)* **(C)(G)** take once weekly, in the AM, 30 minutes before the first food, beverage, <u>or</u> medication of the day; do not lie down (remain upright) for at least 30 minutes and after the first food of the day; *CrCl <35 mL/min:* not recommended
Pediatric: <12 years: not recommended; ≥12 years: same as adult

> **Binosto** dissolve the effervescent tab in 4 oz (120 ml) of plain, room temperature, water (not mineral <u>or</u> flavored); wait 5 minutes after the effervescence has subsided, then stir for 10 seconds, then drink
>> *Tab:* 70 mg effervescent for buffered solution (4, 12/carton) (strawberry)
> **Fosamax (G)** swallow tab whole; dosing regimens are the same for men and postmenopausal women; *Prevention:* 5 mg once daily <u>or</u> 35 mg once weekly; *Treatment:* 10 mg once daily <u>or</u> 70 mg once weekly
>> *Tab:* 5, 10, 35, 40, 70 mg

▷ *alendronate+cholecalciferol (vit d3)* **(C)(G)** take 1 tab once weekly, in the AM, with plain water (not mineral) 30 minutes before the first food, beverage, <u>or</u> medication of the day; do not lie down (remain upright) for at least 30 minutes and after the first food of the day
Pediatric: <12 years: not recommended; ≥12 years: same as adult

> **Fosamax Plus D**
>> *Tab:* **Fosamax Plus D 70/2800** *alen* 70 mg+*chole* 2800 IU
> **Fosamax Plus D 70/5600** *alen* 70 mg+*chole* 5600 IU

▷ *ibandronate (as monosodium monohydrate)* **(C)(G)**
Pediatric: <12 years: not recommended; ≥12 years: same as adult

> **Boniva** take 2.5 mg once daily <u>or</u> 150 mg once monthly on the same day; take in the AM, with plain water (not mineral) 60 minutes before the first food, beverage, <u>or</u> medication of the day; do not lie down (remain upright) for at least 30 minutes and after the first food of the day
>> *Tab:* 2.5, 150 mg
> **Boniva Injection** administer 3 mg every 3 months by IV bolus over 15-30 seconds; if dose is missed, administer as soon as possible; then every 3 months from the date of the last dose
>> *Prefilled syringe:* 3 mg/3 ml (5 ml)
> Comment: **Boniva Injection** must be administered by a health care professional.

▷ *risedronate (as sodium)* **(C)(G)** take in the AM; swallow whole with a full glass of plain water (not mineral); do not lie down (remain upright) for 30 minutes afterward
Pediatric: <12 years: not recommended; ≥12 years: same as adult

> **Actonel** take at least 30 minutes before any food <u>or</u> drink; *Women:* 5 mg once daily <u>or</u> 35 mg once weekly <u>or</u> 75 mg on two consecutive days monthly <u>or</u> 150 mg once monthly; *Men:* 35 mg once weekly
>> *Tab:* 5, 30, 35, 75, 150 mg

Atelvia 35 mg once weekly immediately after breakfast
Tab: 35 mg del-rel
▷ *risedronate+calcium* (C) 1 x 5 mg *risedronate* tab weekly plus 1 x 500 mg *calcium* tab on days 2-7 weekly
Actonel with Calcium *Tab: risedronate* 5 mg and *Tab: calcium* 500 mg (4 *risedronate* tabs + 30 *calcium* tabs/pck)
▷ *zoledronic acid* (D)(G)
Pediatric: <12 years: not recommended; ≥12 years: same as adult
Reclast administer 5 mg via IV infusion over at least 15 minutes mg once a year (for osteoporosis) or once every 2 years (for osteopenia or prophylaxis)
Bottle: 5 mg/100 ml (single-dose)
Comment: **Reclast** is indicated for the treatment of postmenopausal osteoporosis in women who are at high risk for fracture and to increase bone mass in men with primary or hypogonadal osteoporosis who are at high risk for fracture. Administered by a health care professional. Contraindicated in hypocalcemia.
Zometa *Bottle:* 4 mg/5 ml administer 4 mg via IV infusion over at least 15 minutes every 3-4 weeks; optimal duration of treatment not known
Vial: 4 mg/5 ml (single-dose)
Comment: **Zometa** is indicated for the treatment of hypercalcemia of malignancy. The safety and efficacy of **Zometa** in the treatment of hypercalcemia associated with hyperparathyroidism or with other nontumor-related conditions has not been established.

SELECTIVE ESTROGEN RECEPTOR MODULATOR (SERMs)

▷ *raloxifene* (X)(G) 60 mg once daily
Evista *Tab:* 60 mg
Comment: Contraindicated in women who have history of, or current, venous thrombotic event.

HUMAN PARATHYROID HORMONE

▷ *teriparatide* (C) 20 mcg SC daily in the thigh or abdomen; may treat for up to 2 years
Pediatric: <12 years: not recommended; ≥12 years: same as adult
Forteo Multidose Pen *Multi-dose pen:* 250 mcg/ml (3 ml)
Comment: **Forteo** is indicated for the treatment of postmenopausal osteoporosis in women who are at high risk for fracture and to increase bone mass in men with primary or hypogonadal osteoporosis who are at high risk for fracture.

HUMAN PARATHYROID HORMONE RELATED PEPTIDE (PTHrP [1-34]) ANALOG

▷ *abaloparatide* 80 mcg (40 mcl) SC once daily
Tymlos *Pen:* 80 mcg/40 mcl (1.56 ml, 2,000 mcg/ml) (30 doses) preassembled, single-patient use, disposable w. glass cartridge
Comment: **Tymlos** is a bone building agent for the treatment of postmenopausal women with osteoporosis at high risk for fracture. **Tymlos** is not indicated for use in females of reproductive potential. There are no human data with use in pregnant women to inform any drug associated risks and animal reproduction studies with *abaloparatide* have not been conducted. There is no information on the presence of *abaloparatide* in human milk, the effects on the breastfed infant, or the effects on milk production; however, breastfeeding is not recommended while using **Tymlos**. **Tymlos** is not recommended for use in pediatric patients with open epiphyses or hereditary disorders predisposing to osteosarcoma because of an increased baseline risk of osteosarcoma. **Tymlos** may cause hypercalciuria. It is unknown whether **Tymlos** may exacerbate urolithiasis in patients with active or a history of urolithiasis. If active urolithiasis or pre-existing hypercalciuria

is suspected, measurement of urinary calcium excretion should be considered. No dosage adjustment is required for patients any degree of renal impairment. Currently, there are no specific drug-drug interaction studies.

BIOENGINEERED REPLICA OF HUMAN PARATHYROID HORMONE

▷ *bioengineered replica of human parathyroid hormone* (C) initially inject mg IM into the thigh once daily; when initiating, decrease dose of active *vitamin D* by 50% if serum *calcium* is above 7.5 mg/dL; monitor serum *calcium* levels every 3 to 7 days after starting or adjusting dose and when adjusting either active *vitamin D* or *calcium* supplements dose

Pediatric: <18 years: not recommended; ≥18 years: same as adult

Natpara *Soln for inj:* 25, 50, 75, 100 mcg (2/pkg) multi-dose, dual-chamber glass cartridge containing a sterile powder and diluent

Comment: **Natpara** is indicated as adjunct to *calcium* and *vitamin D* in patients with parathyroidism.

OSTEOCLAST INHIBITOR (RANK LIGAND [RANKL] INHIBITOR)

▷ *denosumab* (X)

Pediatric: <18 years: not established; treatment with **Prolia** may impair bone growth in children with open growth plates and may inhibit eruption of dentition. ≥18 years: same as adult

Prolia for SC route only; should not be administered intravenously, intramuscularly, or intradermally; 60 mcg SC once every 6 months in the upper arm, abdomen, or upper thigh

Vial/Pen: 60 mg/ml (1 ml) single-dose

Comment: **Prolia** is indicated for the treatment of postmenopausal osteoporosis in females who are at high risk for fracture defined as a history of osteoporotic fracture or multiple risk factors for fracture or patients who have failed or are intolerant to other therapy and treatment to increase bone mass in women at high risk for fracture receiving adjuvant aromatase inhibitor therapy for breast cancer.

Prolia is also indicated for treatment to increase bone mass in men at high risk for fracture receiving androgen deprivation therapy for non-metastatic prostate cancer. **Prolia** must be administered by a health care professional. *denosumab* contraindicated with hypocalcemia. Instruct patients to take *calcium* 1,000 mg daily and at least 400 IU *vitamin D* daily. There is no information regarding the presence of *denosumab* in human milk or effects on the breastfed invent. To report suspected adverse reactions, contact Amgen Inc. at 1-800-77-AMGEN (1-800-772-6436) or FDA at 1-800-FDA-1088 or www.fda.gov/medwatch.

Xgeva *Multiple Myeloma and Bone Metastasis from Solid Tumors: admin*ister 120 mg SC every 4 weeks; *Giant Cell Tumor of Bone:* administer 120 mg SC 4 every weeks with additional 120 mg doses on Days 8 and 15 of the first month of therapy and administer calcium and vitamin D as necessary to treat or prevent hypocalcemia; *Hypercalcemia of Malignancy:* administer 120 mg every 4 weeks with additional 120 mg doses Days 8 and 15 of the first month of therapy

Pediatric: recommended only for treatment of skeletally mature adolescents with giant cell tumor of bone

Vial: 120 mg/1.7 ml (70 mg/ml) solution in a single-dose

Comment: **Xgeva** is indicated for prevention of skeletal-related events in patients with multiple myeloma and in patients with bone metastases from solid tumors, treatment of adults and skeletally mature adolescents with giant cell tumor of bone that is un-resectable or where surgical resection is likely to result in severe morbidity, and treatment of hypercalcemia of malignancy refractory to bisphosphonate therapy.

CrCl < 30 mL/min or receiving dialysis are at risk for hypocalcemia. Adequately supplement with calcium and vitamin D. There is no information regarding the presence of *denosumab* in human milk or effects on the breastfed invent. To report suspected adverse reactions, contact Amgen Inc at 1-800-77-AMGEN (1-800-772-6436) or FDA at 1-800-FDA-1088 or www.fda.gov/medwatch.

OTITIS EXTERNA

OTIC ANALGESIC

▷ *antipyrine+benzocaine+zinc acetate dihydrate* (C) fill ear canal with solution; then insert a cotton pluge into meatus; may repeat every 1-2 hours prn
  Pediatric: same as adult
  Otozin *Otic soln: antipyr* 5.4%+*benz* 1%+*zinc*1% per ml (10 ml w. dropper)

OTIC ANTI-INFECTIVE

▷ *chloroxylenol+pramoxine* (C) 4-5 drops tid x 5-10 days
  Pediatric: <1 year: not recommended; 1-12 years: 5 drops bid x 10 days; ≥12 years: same as adult
  PramOtic *Otic drops: chlorox+pramox* (5 ml w. dropper)
▷ *finafloxacin* (C) otic 4-5 drops tid x 5-10 days
  Pediatric: <1 year: not recommended; ≥1 year: same as adult
  Xtoro *Otic soln:* 0.3% (5, 8 ml)
▷ *ofloxacin* (C)(G) 10 drops bid x 10 days
  Pediatric: <1 year: not recommended; 1-12 years: 5 drops bid x 10 days; ≥12 years: same as adult
  Floxin Otic *Otic soln:* 0.3% (5, 10 ml w. dropper; 0.25 ml, 5 drop singles, 20/carton)
Comment: **Floxin Otic** is indicated for adult patients with perforated tympanic membranes and pediatric patients with PE tubes.

OTIC ANTI-INFECTIVE+CORTICOSTEROID COMBINATIONS

▷ *chloroxylenol+pramoxine+hydrocortisone* (C) drops 4 drops tid-qid x 5-10 days
  Pediatric: 3 drops tid-qid x 5-10 days
  Cortane B, Cortane B Aqueous *Otic soln: chlo* 1 mg+*pram* 10 mg+*hydro* 10 mg per ml (10 ml w. dropper)
Comment: **Cortane B Aqueous** may be used to saturate a cotton wick.
▷ *ciprofloxacin+hydrocortisone* (C) susp 3 drops bid x 7 days
  Pediatric: <1 year: not recommended; ≥1 year: same as adult
  Cipro HC Otic *Otic susp: cipro* 0.2%+*hydro* 1% (10 ml w. dropper)
▷ *ciprofloxacin+dexamethasone* (C) 4 drops bid x 7 days
  Pediatric: <6 months: not recommended; ≥6 months: same as adult
  Ciprodex *Otic susp: cipro* 0.3%+*dexa* 1% (7.5 ml)
Comment: **Ciprodex** is indicated for the treatment of otitis media in pediatric patients with tympanostomy tubes.
▷ *colistin+neomycin+hydrocortisone+thonzonium* (C) 5 drops tid or qid x 5-10 days
  Pediatric: 4 drops tid-qid x 5-10 days
  Coly-Mycin S *Otic susp:* 5, 10 ml
  Cortisporin-TC Otic *Otic susp: colis* 3 mg+*neo* 3.3 mg+*hydro* 10 mg+*thon* 0.5 mg per ml (10 ml w. dropper) (thimerosal)
▷ *polymyxin b+neomycin+hydrocortisone* (C) 4 drops tid-qid; max 10 days
  Pediatric: 3 drops tid-qid; max 10 days

Cortisporin Otic Suspension *Otic susp: poly b* 10,000 u+*neo* 3.5 mg+*hydro* 10 mg per 5 ml (10 ml w. dropper)
Cortisporin Otic Solution *Otic soln: poly b* 10000 u+*neo* 3.5 mg+*hydro* 10 mg per 5 ml (10 ml w. dropper)

OTIC ASTRINGENTS

▷ *acetic acid 2% in aluminum sulfate* (C) 4-6 drops q 2-3 hours
  Pediatric: same as adult
    Domeboro Otic *Otic soln:* 60 ml w. dropper
▷ *acetic acid+propylene glycol+benzethonium chloride+sodium acetate* (C) 3-5 drops q 4-6 hours
  Pediatric: same as adult
    VoSol *Otic soln: acet* 2% (15, 30 ml)
▷ *acetic acid+propylene glycol+hydrocortisone+benzethonium chloride+sodium acetate* (C) 3-5 drops q 4-6 hours
  Pediatric: same as adult
    VoSol HC *Otic soln: acet* 2%+*hydro* 1% (10 ml)

OTIC ANESTHETIC+ANALGESIC COMBINATIONS

▷ *antipyrine+benzocaine+glycerine* (C) fill ear canal and insert cotton plug; may repeat q 1-2 hours as needed
  Pediatric: same as adult
    A/B Otic *Otic soln:* 15 ml w. dropper
▷ *benzocaine* (C) 4-5 drops q 1-2 hours
  Pediatric: <1 year: not recommended; ≥1 year: same as adult
    Americaine Otic *Otic soln:* 20% (15 ml w. dropper)
    Benzotic *Otic soln:* 20% (15 ml w. dropper)

SYSTEMIC ANTI-INFECTIVES

Comment: Used for severe disease or with culture.
▷ *amoxicillin+clavulanate* (B)(G)
    Augmentin 500 mg tid or 875 mg bid x 7-10 days
    Pediatric: 40-45 mg/kg/day divided tid x 10 days or 90 mg/kg/day divided bid x 10 days *see pages 618-619 for dose by weight*
      Tab: 250, 500, 875 mg; *Chew tab:* 125, 250 mg (lemon-lime); 200, 400 mg (cherry-banana) (phenylalanine); *Oral susp:* 125 mg/5 ml (banana), 250 mg/5 ml (75, 100, 150 ml) (orange); 200, 400 mg/5 ml (50, 75, 100 ml) (orange) (phenylalanine)
    Augmentin ES-600 not recommended for adults
    Pediatric: <3 months: not recommended; ≥3 months, <40 kg: 90 mg/kg/day in 2 divided doses x 7-10 days; ≥40 kg: not recommended
      Oral susp: 42.9 mg/5 ml (50, 75, 100, 125, 150, 200 ml) (strawberry cream) (phenylalanine)
    Augmentin XR 2 tabs q 12 hours x 7-10 days
    Pediatric: <16 years: use other forms; ≥16 years: same as adult
      Tab: 1000*mg ext-rel
▷ *cefaclor* (B)(G) 250-500 mg q 8 hours x 7-10 days
  Pediatric: <1 month: not recommended; 20-40 mg/kg bid or q 12 hours x 10 days; max 1 gm/day; *see page 622 for dose by weight*
    Tab: 500 mg; *Cap:* 250, 500 mg; *Susp:* 125 mg/5 ml (75, 150 ml) (strawberry); 187 mg/5 ml (50, 100 ml) (strawberry); 250 mg/5 ml (75, 150 ml) (strawberry); 375 mg/5 ml (50, 100 ml) (strawberry)
    Cefaclor Extended Release

Pediatric: <16 years: ext-rel not recommended; ≥16 years: same as adult
Tab: 375, 500 mg ext-rel
▷ *dicloxacillin* (B) 500 mg qid x 7-10 days
Pediatric: 12.5-25 mg/kg/day in 4 divided doses x 7-10 days; *see page 632 for dose by weight*
Dynapen *Cap:* 125, 250, 500 mg; *Oral susp:* 62.5 mg/5 ml (80, 100, 200 ml)
▷ *trimethoprim+sulfamethoxazole (TMP-SMX)* (C)(G)
Pediatric: <2 months: not recommended; ≥2 months: 40 mg/kg/day of *sulfamethoxazole* in 2 doses bid x 10 days; *see page 648 for dose by weight*
Bactrim, Septra 2 tabs bid x 10 days
Tab: trim 80 mg+sulfa 400 mg*
Bactrim DS, Septra DS 1 tab bid x 10 days
Tab: trim 160 mg+sulfa 800 mg*
Bactrim Pediatric Suspension, Septra Pediatric Suspension
Oral susp: trim 40 mg+sulfa 200 mg per 5 ml (100 ml) (cherry) (alcohol 0.3%)

⊙ OTITIS MEDIA: ACUTE

OTIC ANALGESIC

▷ *antipyrine+benzocaine+zinc acetate dihydrate* otic (C) fill ear canal with solution; then insert cotton plug into meatus; may repeat every 1-2 hours prn
Pediatric: same as adult
Otozin *Otic soln:* antipyr 5.4%+benz 1%+zinc1% per ml (10 ml w. dropper)

SYSTEMIC ANTI-INFECTIVES

▷ *amoxicillin* (B)(G) 500-875 mg bid or 250-500 mg tid x 10 days
Pediatric: <40 kg (88 lb): 20-40 mg/kg/day in 3 divided doses x 10 days or 25-45 mg/kg/day in 2 divided doses x 10 days; *see page 616 for dose by weight*
Amoxil *Cap:* 250, 500 mg; *Tab:* 875*mg; *Chew tab:* 125, 200, 250, 400 mg (cherry-banana-peppermint) (phenylalanine); *Oral susp:* 125, 250 mg/5 ml (80, 100, 150 ml) (strawberry); 200, 400 mg/5 ml (50, 75, 100 ml) (bubble gum); *Oral drops:* 50 mg/ml (30 ml) (bubble gum)
Moxatag *Tab:* 775 mg ext-rel
Trimox *Tab:* 125, 250 mg; *Cap:* 250, 500 mg; *Oral susp:* 125, 250 mg/5 ml (80, 100, 150 ml) (raspberry-strawberry)
Comment: Consider 80-90 mg/kg/day in 3 divided doses for resistant for cases
▷ *amoxicillin+clavulanate* (B)(G)
Augmentin 500 mg tid or 875 mg bid x 7-10 days
Pediatric: 40-45 mg/kg/day divided tid x 10 days or 90 mg/kg/day divided bid x 10 days *see pages 618-619 for dose by weight*
Tab: 250, 500, 875 mg; *Chew tab:* 125, 250 mg (lemon-lime); 200, 400 mg (cherry-banana) (phenylalanine); *Oral susp:* 125 mg/5 ml (banana), 250 mg/5 ml (75, 100, 150 ml) (orange); 200, 400 mg/5 ml (50, 75, 100 ml) (orange) (phenylalanine)
Augmentin ES-600 not recommended for adults
Pediatric: <3 months: not recommended; ≥3 months, <40 kg: 90 mg/kg/day in 2 divided doses x 7-10 days; ≥40 kg: not recommended
Oral susp: 42.9 mg/5 ml (50, 75, 100, 125, 150, 200 ml) (strawberry cream) (phenylalanine)
Augmentin XR 2 tabs q 12 hours x 7-10 days
Pediatric: <16 years: use other forms; ≥16 years: same as adult
Tab: 1000*mg ext-rel

▷ **ampicillin (B)** 250-500 mg qid x 10 days
Pediatric: 50-100 mg/kg/day in 4 divided doses x 10 days; *see page* 620 *for dose by weight*
   Omnipen, Principen *Cap:* 250, 500 mg; *Oral susp:* 125, 250 mg/5 ml (100, 150, 200 ml) (fruit)

▷ **azithromycin (B)(G)** 500 mg x 1 dose on day 1, then 250 mg daily on days 2-5 or 500 mg daily x 3 days or **Zmax** 2 gm in a single dose
Pediatric: 12 mg/kg/day x 5 days; max 500 mg/day; *see page* 621 *for dose by weight*
   Zithromax *Tab:* 250, 500, 600 mg; *Oral susp:* 100 mg/5 ml (15 ml); 200 mg/5 ml (15, 22.5, 30 ml) (cherry); *Pkt:* 1 gm for reconstitution (cherry-banana)
   Zithromax Tri-pak *Tab:* 3 x 500 mg tabs/pck
   Zithromax Z-pak *Tab:* 6 x 250 mg tabs/pck
   Zmax *Oral susp:* 2 gm ext-rel for reconstitution (cherry-banana) (148 mg Na$^+$)

▷ **cefaclor (B)(G)** 250-500 mg q 8 hours x 7-10 days
Pediatric: <1 month: not recommended; 20-40 mg/kg bid or q 12 hours x 10 days; max 1 gm/day; *see page* 622 *for dose by weight*
   Tab: 500 mg; *Cap:* 250, 500 mg; *Susp:* 125 mg/5 ml (75, 150 ml) (strawberry); 187 mg/5 ml (50, 100 ml) (strawberry); 250 mg/5 ml (75, 150 ml) (strawberry); 375 mg/5 ml (50, 100 ml) (strawberry)
   Cefaclor Extended Release
   Pediatric: <16 years: ext-rel not recommended
   Tab: 375, 500 mg ext-rel

▷ **cefdinir (B)** 300 mg bid or 600 mg daily x 5-10 days
Pediatric: <6 months: not recommended; 6 months-12 years: 14 mg/kg/day in 1-2 divided doses x 10 days; *>12 years: same as adult; see page* 624 *for dose by weight*
   Omnicef *Cap:* 300 mg; *Oral susp:* 125 mg/5 ml (60, 100 ml) (strawberry)

▷ **cefixime (B)(G)**
Pediatric: <6 months: not recommended; 6 months-12 years, <50 kg: 8 mg/kg/day in 1-2 divided doses x 10 days; >12 years, ≥50 kg: same as adult; *see page* 625 *for dose by weight*
   Suprax *Tab:* 400 mg; *Cap:* 400 mg; *Oral susp:* 100, 200, 500 mg/5 ml (50, 75, 100 ml) (strawberry)

▷ **cefpodoxime proxetil (B)** 100 mg bid x 5 days
Pediatric: <2 months: not recommended; 2 months-12 years: 10 mg/kg/day (max 400 mg/dose) or 5 mg/kg/day bid (max 200 mg/dose) x 5 days; >12 years: same as adult; *see page* 626 *for dose by weight*
   Vantin *Tab:* 100, 200 mg; *Oral susp:* 50, 100 mg/5 ml (50, 75, 100 ml) (lemon creme)

▷ **cefprozil (B)** 250-500 mg bid or 500 mg daily x 10 days
Pediatric: <2 years: same as adult; 2-12 years: 7.5 mg/kg bid x 10 days; *see page* 627 *for dose by weight;* >12 years: same as adult
   Cefzil *Tab:* 250, 500 mg; *Oral susp:* 125, 250 mg/5 ml (50, 75, 100 ml) (bubble gum) (phenylalanine)

▷ **ceftibuten (B)** 400 mg daily x 10 days
Pediatric: 9 mg/kg daily x 10 days; max 400 mg/day; *see page* 628 *for dose by weight*
   Cedax *Cap:* 400 mg; *Oral susp:* 90 mg/5 ml (30, 60, 90, 120 ml); 180 mg/5 ml (30, 60, 120 ml) (cherry)

▷ **ceftriaxone (B)(G)** 1-2 gm IM x 1 dose; max 4 g
Pediatric: 50 mg/kg IM x 1 dose
   Rocephin *Vial:* 250, 500 mg; 1, 2 gm

▷ **cephalexin (B)(G)** 250 mg qid x 10 days
Pediatric: 25-50 mg/kg/day in 4 doses x 10 days; *see page* 629 *for dose by weight*
   Keflex *Cap:* 250, 333, 500, 750 mg; *Oral susp:* 125, 250 mg/5 ml (100, 200 ml) (strawberry)

▷ *clarithromycin* (C)(G) 500 mg bid or 500 mg ext-rel daily
   Pediatric: <6 months: not recommended; ≥6 months: 7.5 mg/kg divided bid x 7 days; *see page 630 for dose by weight*
      Biaxin *Tab:* 250, 500 mg
      Biaxin Oral Suspension *Oral susp:* 125, 250 mg/5 ml (50, 100 ml) (fruit-punch)
      Biaxin XL *Tab:* 500 mg ext-rel
▷ *erythromycin+sulfisoxazole* (C)(G)
   Pediatric: <2 months: not recommended; ≥2 months: 50 mg/kg/day in 3 divided doses x 10 days; *see page 637 for dose by weight*
      Eryzole *Oral susp: eryth* 200 mg+*sulfa* 600 mg per 5 ml (100, 150, 200, 250 ml)
      Pediazole *Oral susp: eryth* 200 mg+*sulfa* 600 mg per 5 ml (100, 150, 200 ml) (strawberry-banana)
Comment: *erythromycin* may increase INR with concomitant *warfarin*, as well as increase serum level of *digoxin, benzodiazepines,* and *statins.*
▷ *loracarbef* (B) 400 mg bid x 10 days
   Pediatric: 30 mg/kg/day in divided bid x 7 days; *see page 642 for dose by weight*
      Lorabid *Pulvule:* 200, 400 mg; *Oral susp:* 100 mg/5 ml (50, 100 ml); 200 mg/5 ml (50, 75, 100 ml) (strawberry bubble gum)
▷ *trimethoprim+sulfamethoxazole (TMP-SMX])* (C)(G)
   Pediatric: <2 months: not recommended; >2 months: 40 mg/kg/day of *sulfamethoxazole* in divided doses bid x 10 days; *see page 648 for dose by weight*
      Bactrim, Septra 2 tabs bid x 10 days
         Tab: trim 80 mg+*sulfa* 400 mg*
      Bactrim DS, Septra DS 1 tab bid x 10 days
         Tab: trim 160 mg+*sulfa* 800 mg*
      Bactrim Pediatric Suspension, Septra Pediatric Suspension
         Oral susp: trim 40 mg+*sulfa* 200 mg per 5 ml (100 ml) (cherry) (alcohol 0.3%)

OTIC ANTI-INFECTIVE

▷ *ofloxacin* (C)(G) 10 drops bid x 14 days
      Pediatric: <6 months: not recommended; 6 months-12 years: 5 drops bid x 14 days; >12 years: same as adult
      Floxin Otic *Otic soln:* 0.3% (5, 10 ml w. dropper)

OTIC ANTI-INFECTIVE+CORTICOSTEROID COMBINATIONS

Comment: *neomycin* may cause ototoxicity. Do not use with known or suspected tympanic membrane rupture.
▷ *chloroxylenol+pramoxine+hydrocortisone* (C) 4 drops tid-qid x 5-10 days
   Pediatric: 3 drops tid-qid x 5-10 days
      Cortane Ear Drops, *Otic drops:* 10 ml
▷ *ciprofloxacin+hydrocortisone* (C) otic susp 3 drops bid x 7 days
   Pediatric: <1 year: not recommended; ≥1 year: same as adult
      Cipro HC *Otic susp: cipro* 0.3%+*dexa* 0.1% (10 ml)
▷ *ciprofloxacin+dexamethasone* (C) otic susp 4 drops bid x 7 days
   Pediatric: <6 months: not recommended; ≥6 months: same as adult
      Ciprodex *Otic susp: cipro* 0.3%+*dexa* 1% (7.5 ml)
      Comment: **Ciprodex** is indicated for the treatment of otitis media in pediatric patients with tympanostomy tubes (PE tubes).
▷ *colistin+neomycin+hydrocortisone+thonzonium* (C) 5 drops tid-qid x 5-10 days
   Pediatric: 4 drops tid-qid x 5-10 days
      Coly-Mycin S *Otic susp:* 5, 10 ml
▷ *polymyxin b+neomycin+hydrocortisone* (C)(G) 4 drops tid-qid; max 10 days
   Pediatric: 3 drops tid-qid; max 10 days

Cortisporin *Otic susp:* 10 ml w. dropper; *Otic soln:* 10 ml w. dropper
PediOtic *Otic susp:* 7.5 ml w. dropper
 polymyxin b+neomycin+hydrocortisone+surfactant (C) 4 drops tid-qid
Pediatric: 3 drops tid-qid; max 10 days
Cortisporin-TC *Otic susp:* 10 ml w. dropper

OTIC ANESTHETIC+ANALGESIC COMBINATIONS

▷ *antipyrine+benzocaine+glycerine* (C) fill ear canal and insert cotton plug; may repeat
q 1-2 hours as needed
Pediatric: same as adult
A/B Otic *Otic soln:* antipy 5.4%+benzo 1.4% 15 ml w. dropper
▷ *benzocaine* (C)(OTC) 4-5 drops q 1-2 hours
Pediatric: <1 year: not recommended; ≥1 year: same as adult
Otic drops: 20% (15 ml dropper-top bottle)
Americaine Otic *Otic soln:* 15 ml w. dropper
Benzotic *Otic soln:* 20% (15 ml w. dropper)

OTITIS MEDIA: SEROUS

Anti-infectives *see Otitis Media: Acute page* 339
Antihistamines and Decongestants *see Drugs for the Management of Allergy, Cough, and Cold Symptoms page* 598
Oral Corticosteroids *see page* 569

PAGET'S DISEASE: BONE

Comment: Calcium decreases *tetracycline* absorption. *calcium* absorption is decreased by corticosteroids. *calcium* absorption is decreased by foods such as rhubarb, spinach, and bran.

BISPHOSPHONATES (CALCIUM MODIFIERS)

Comment: Bisphosphonates should be swallowed whole in the AM with 6-8 oz of plain water 30 minutes before first meal, beverage, <u>or</u> other medications of the day. Monitor serum alkaline phosphatase. Contraindications include abnormalities of the esophagus which delay esophageal emptying such as stricture <u>or</u> achalasia, inability to stand <u>or</u> sit upright for at least 30 minutes post-dose, patients at risk of aspiration, and hypocalcemia. Co-administration of bisphosphonates and calcium, antacids, <u>or</u> oral medications containing multivalent cations will interfere with absorption of the bisphosphonate. Therefore, instruct patients to wait at least half hour after taking the bisphosphonate before taking any other oral medications.
 alendronate (as sodium) (C)(G) take once weekly, in the AM, 30 minutes before the first food, beverage, <u>or</u> medication of the day; do not lie down (remain upright) for at least 30 minutes and after the first food of the day; not recommended with *CrCl <35 mL/min.*
Pediatric: <12 years: not recommended; ≥12 years: same as adult
Binosto dissolve the effervescent tab in 4 oz (120 ml) of plain, room temperature, water (not mineral <u>or</u> flavored); wait 5 minutes after the effervescence has subsided, then stir for 10 seconds, then drink
Tab: 70 mg effervescent for buffered solution (4, 12/carton) (strawberry)
Fosamax (G) swallow tab whole; dosing regimens are the same for men and post-menopausal women; *Prevention:* 5 mg once daily <u>or</u> 35 mg once weekly; *Treatment:* 10 mg once daily <u>or</u> 70 mg once weekly
Tab: 5, 10, 35, 40, 70 mg

➤ *alendronate+cholecalciferol (vit d3)* (C)(G) take 1 tab once weekly, in the AM, with plain water (not mineral) 30 minutes before the first food, beverage, or medication of the day; do not lie down (remain upright) for at least 30 minutes and after the first food of the day
Pediatric: <12 years: not recommended; ≥12 years: same as adult
  Fosamax Plus D
    Tab: **Fosamax Plus D 70/2800** *alen* 70 mg+*chole* 2800 IU
    Fosamax Plus D 70/5600 *alen* 70 mg+*chole* 5600 IU

➤ *ibandronate (as monosodium monohydrate)* (C)(G)
Pediatric: <12 years: not recommended; ≥12 years: same as adult
  Boniva take 2.5 mg once daily or 150 mg once monthly on the same day; take in the AM, with plain water (not mineral) 60 minutes before the first food, beverage, or medication of the day; do not lie down (remain upright) for at least 30 minutes and after the first food of the day
    Tab: 2.5, 150 mg
  Boniva Injection administer 3 mg every 3 months by IV bolus over 15-30 seconds; if dose is missed, administer as soon as possible, then every 3 months from the date of the last dose
    Prefilled syringe: 3 mg/3 ml (5 ml)
Comment: **Boniva Injection** must be administered by a qualified health care professional.

➤ *risedronate (as sodium)* (C)(G) take in the AM; swallow whole with a full glass of plain water (not mineral) do not lie down (remain upright) for 30 minutes afterward
Pediatric: <12 years: not recommended; ≥12 years: same as adult
  Actonel take at least 30 minutes before any food or drink; *Women:* 5 mg once daily or 35 mg once weekly or 75 mg on two consecutive days monthly or 150 mg once monthly; *Men:* 35 mg once weekly
    Tab: 5, 30, 35, 75, 150 mg
  Atelvia 35 mg once weekly immediately after breakfast
    Tab: 35 mg del-rel

➤ *risedronate+calcium* (C) 1 x 5 mg *risedronate* tab weekly and 1 x 500 mg *calcium* tab on days 2-7 weekly
  Actonel with Calcium *Tab:* *risedronate* 5 mg and *Tab:* *calcium* 500 mg
  (4 *risedronate* tabs + 30 *calcium* tabs/pck)

➤ *zoledronic acid* (D)(G)
Pediatric: <12 years: not recommended; ≥12 years: same as adult
  Reclast administer 5 mg via IV infusion over at least 15 minutes mg once a year (for osteoporosis) or once every 2 years (for osteopenia or prophylaxis)
    Bottle: 5 mg/100 ml (single-dose)
Comment: **Reclast** is indicated for the treatment of postmenopausal osteoporosis in women who are at high risk for fracture and to increase bone mass in men with primary or hypogonadal osteoporosis who are at high risk for fracture. Administered by a qualified health care professional. Contraindicated in hypocalcemia.
  Zometa administer 4 mg via IV infusion over at least 15 minutes every 3-4 weeks; optimal duration of treatment not known
    Bottle: 4 mg/5 ml; *Vial:* 4 mg/5 ml (single-dose)
Comment: **Zometa** is indicated for the treatment of hypercalcemia of malignancy. The safety and efficacy of **Zometa** in the treatment of hypercalcemia associated with hyperparathyroidism or with other non-tumor-related conditions has not been established.

 PAIN

Antidepressants *see Depression page* 117
Skeletal Muscle Relaxants *see Muscle Strain page* 307

ACETAMINOPHEN FOR IV INFUSION

▷ *acetaminophen* injectable (B) administer by IV infusion over 15 minutes; 1,000 mg q 6 hours prn or 650 mg q 4 hours prn; max 4,000 mg/day

Pediatric: <2 years: not recommended; 2-13 years <50 kg: 15 mg/kg q 6 hours prn or 2.5 mg/kg q 4 hours prn; max 750 mg/single dose; max 75 mg/kg per day; >13 years: same as adult

   Ofirmev *Vial:* 10 mg/ml (100 ml) (preservative-free)

Comment: The **Ofirmev** vial is intended for single-use. If any portion is withdrawn from the vial, use within 6 hours. Discard the unused portion. For pediatric patients, withdraw the intended dose and administer via syringe pump. Do not admix **Ofirmev** with any other drugs. **Ofirmev** is physically incompatible with *diazepam* and *chlorpromazine hydrochloride.*

IBUPROFEN FOR IV INFUSION

▷ *ibuprofen* (B) dilute dose in 0.9% NS, D5W, or Lactated Ringers (LR) solution; administer by IV infusion over at least 10 minutes; do not administer via IV bolus or IM; 400-800 mg q 6 hours prn; maximum 3,200 mg/day

Pediatric: <6 months; not recommended; 6 months-<12 years: 10 mg/kg q 4-6 hours prn; max 400 mg/dose; max 40 mg/kg or 2,400 mg/24 hours, whichever is less; 12-17 years: 400 mg q 4-6 hours prn; max 2,400 mg/24 hours

   Caldolor *Vial:* 800 mg/8 ml single-dose

Comment: Prepare **Caldolor** solution for IV administration as follows: 100 mg dose: dilute 1 ml of **Caldolor** in at least 100 ml of diluent (IVF); 200 mg dose: dilute 2 ml of **Caldolor** in at least 100 ml of diluent; 400 mg dose: dilute 4 ml of **Caldolor** in at least 100 ml of diluent; 800 mg dose: dilute 8 ml of **Caldolor** in at least 200 ml of diluent. **Caldolor** is also indicated for management of fever. For adults with fever, 400 mg via IV infusion, followed by 400 mg q 4-6 hours or 100-200 mg q 4 hours prn.

OCULAR PAIN

▷ *difluprednate* (C) apply 1 drop to affected eye qid; for postop ocular pain, begin treatment 24 hours postop and continue x 2 weeks; then bid daily x 1 week; then taper

Pediatric: <12 years: not recommended; ≥12 years: same as adult

   Durezol *Ophth emul:* 0.05% (5 ml)

Comment: **Durezol** is an ophthalmic steroid.

▷ *nepafenac* (C) apply 1 drop to affected eye tid; for postop ocular pain, begin treatment 24 hours before surgery and continue day of surgery and for two weeks post-op

Pediatric: <10 years: not recommended; ≥10 years: same as adult

   Nevanac *Ophth susp:* 0.1% (3 ml) (benzalkonium chloride)

Comment: **Nevanac** is an ophthalmic NSAID.

TOPICAL AND TRANSDERMAL NSAIDs

▷ *capsaicin* (B)(G) apply tid-qid prn to intact skin

Pediatric: <2 years: not recommended; ≥2 years: apply sparingly tid-qid prn

   Axsain *Crm:* 0.075% (1, 2 oz)
   Capsin (OTC) *Lotn:* 0.025, 0.075% (59 ml)
   Capzasin-P (OTC) *Crm:* 0.025% (1.5 oz); *Lotn:* 0.025% (2 oz)
   Dolorac *Crm:* 0.025% (28 gm)
   Double Cap (OTC) *Crm:* 0.05% (2 oz)
   R-Gel *Gel:* 0.025% (15, 30 gm)
   Zostrix (OTC) *Crm:* 0.025% (0.7, 1.5, 3 oz)
   Zostrix HP (OTC) *Emol crm:* 0.075% (1, 2 oz)

▷ *capsaicin* 8% patch **(B)** apply up to 4 patches for one 60-minute application to clean dry skin; may prep area with topical anesthetic; wear nonlatex gloves; patches may be cut to size/shape; treatment may be repeated every 3 months; remove with cleansing gel after treatment

Pediatric: <18 years: not recommended; ≥18 years: same as adult

> **Qutenza** *Patch:* 8% 1640 mcg/cm (179 mg) (1 or 2 patches, each w. 1-50 gm tube cleansing gel/carton)

▷ *diclofenac epolamine transdermal patch* **(C; D ≥30 wks)** apply one patch to affected area bid; remove during bathing; avoid non-intact skin

Pediatric: <12 years: not recommended; ≥12 years: same as adult

> **Flector Patch** *Patch:* 180 mg/patch (30/carton)

▷ *diclofenac sodium* **(C; D ≥30 wks)(G)**

Comment: *diclofenac* is contraindicated with *aspirin* allergy and should be avoided in late pregnancy (≥30 weeks) because it may cause premature closure of the ductus arteriosus.

Pediatric: <12 years: not established; ≥12 years: same as adult

> **Pennsaid 1.5%** in 10 drop increments, dispense and rub into front, side, and back of knee: usually; 40 drops (40 mg) qid
>
> *Topical soln:* 1.5% (150 ml)
>
> **Pennsaid 2%** apply 2 pump actuations (40 mg) and rub into front, side, and back of knee bid
>
> *Topical soln:* 2% (20 mg/pump actuation, 112 gm)

Comment: **Pennsaid** is indicated for the treatment of pain associated with osteoarthritis of the knee.

> **Voltaren Gel** apply qid; avoid nonintact skin
>
> *Gel:* 1% (100 gm)

TOPICAL AND TRANSDERMAL LIDOCAINE

▷ *lidocaine* transdermal patch **(C)(G)** apply one patch to affected area for 12 hours (then off for 12 hours); remove during bathing; avoid non-intact skin; do not re-use

Pediatric: <12 years: not recommended; ≥12 years: same as adult

> **Lidoderm** *Patch:* 5% (10 cm x 14 cm, 30/carton)

OPIOID ANALGESICS

Comment: According to the American Society of Interventional Pain Physicians (ASIPP), presumptive urine drug testing (UDT) should be performed when opioid therapy for chronic pain is initiated, along with subsequent use as adherence monitoring, using in-office point of service testing, to identify patients who are non-compliant or abusing prescription drugs or illicit drugs.

REFERENCE

Manchikanti, L., Kaye, A. M., Knezevic, N. N., McAnally, H., Slavin, K., Trescot, A.M., . . . Hirsch, J. A. (2017). Responsible, safe, and effective prescription of opioids for chronic non-cancer pain: American Society of Interventional Pain Physicians (ASIPP) guidelines. *Pain Physician, 20*(2S), S3-S92.

▷ *butalbital+acetaminophen* **(C)(G)** 1 tab q 4 hours prn; max 6 tabs/day

Pediatric: <12 years: not recommended; ≥12 years: same as adult

> *Tab: but* 50 mg+*acet* 325 mg
>
> **Phrenilin** 1-2 tabs q 4 hours prn; max 6 tabs/day
>
> *Tab: but* 50 mg+*acet* 325 mg
>
> **Phrenilin Forte** 1 tab or cap q 4 hours prn; max 6 caps/day
>
> *Cap: but* 50 mg+*acet* 325 mg; *Tab: but* 50 mg+*acet* 325 mg

▷ *butalbital+acetaminophen+caffeine* (C)(G)
  Pediatric: <12: not recommended; ≥12 years: same as adult
    Fioricet 1-2 tabs q 4 hours prn; max 6/day
      Tab: but 50 mg+*acet* 325 mg+*caf* 40 mg
    Zebutal 1 cap q 4 hours prn; max 5/day
      Cap: but 50 mg+*acet* 325 mg+*caf* 40 mg
▷ *butalbital+aspirin+caffeine* (C)(III)(G)
  Pediatric: <12 years: not recommended; ≥12 year: same as adult
    Fiorinal 1-2 tabs or caps q 4 hours prn; max 6 caps/day
      Tab/Cap: but 50 mg+*asp* 325 mg+*caf* 40 mg
Comment: *aspirin*-containing medications are contraindicated with history of allergic-type reaction to *aspirin*, children and adolescents with *Varicella* or other viral illness, and 3rd trimester of pregnancy.
▷ *butalbital+aspirin+codeine+caffeine* (C)(III)(G)
  Pediatric: <18 years: not recommended; ≥18 year: same as adult
    Fiorinal with Codeine 1-2 caps q 4 hours prn; max 6 caps/day
      Cap: but 50 mg+*asp* 325 mg+*cod* 30 mg+*caf* 40 mg
Comment: *Codeine* is known to be excreted in breast milk. <12 years: not recommended; 12-<18: use extreme caution; not recommended for children and adolescents with asthma or other chronic breathing problem. The FDA and the European Medicines Agency (EMA) are investigating the safety of using *codeine* containing medications to treat pain, cough and colds, in children 12-<18 years because of the potential for serious side effects, including slowed or difficult breathing. *aspirin*-containing medications are contraindicated with history of allergic-type reaction to *aspirin*, children and adolescents with *Varicella* or other viral illness, and 3rd trimester of pregnancy.
▷ *codeine sulfate* (C)(III)(G) 15-60 q 4-6 hours prn; max 60 mg/day
  Pediatric: <18 years: not recommended; ≥18 year: same as adult
    Tab: 15, 30, 60 mg
Comment: *codeine* is known to be excreted in breast milk. <12 years: not recommended; 12-<18: use extreme caution; not recommended for children and adolescents with asthma or other chronic breathing problem. The FDA and the European Medicines Agency (EMA) are investigating the safety of using *codeine* containing medications to treat pain, cough and colds, in children 12-<18 years because of the potential for serious side effects, including slowed or difficult breathing.
▷ *codeine+acetaminophen* (C)(III)(G) 15-60 mg of *codeine* q 4 hours prn; max 360 mg of *codeine*/day
  Pediatric: <18 years: not recommended; ≥18 year: same as adult
    Tab: **Tylenol #1** *cod* 7.5 mg+*acet* 300 mg (sulfites)
         Tylenol #2 *cod* 15 mg+*acet* 300 mg (sulfites)
         Tylenol #3 *cod* 30 mg+*acet* 300 mg (sulfites)
         Tylenol #4 *cod* 60 mg+*acet* 300 mg (sulfites)
         Tylenol with Codeine Elixir (C)(III)
    Elix: cod 12 mg+*acet* 120 mg per 5 ml (cherry) (alcohol)
Comment: *Codeine* is known to be excreted in breast milk. <12 years: not recommended; 12-<18: use extreme caution; not recommended for children and adolescents with asthma or other chronic breathing problem. The FDA and the European Medicines Agency (EMA) are investigating the safety of using *codeine* containing medications to treat pain, cough and colds, in children 12-<18 years because of the potential for serious side effects, including slowed or difficult breathing.
▷ *dihydrocodeine+acetaminophen+caffeine* (C)(III)(G)
  Pediatric: <18 years: not recommended; ≥18 years: same as adult
    Panlor DC 1-2 caps q 4-6 hours prn; max 10 caps/day
      Cap: dihydro 16 mg+*acet* 325 mg+*caf* 30 mg

Panlor SS 1 tab q 4 hours prn; max 5 tabs/day
Tab: dihydro 32 mg+*acet* 325 mg+*caf* 60*mg

Comment: *Codeine* is known to be excreted in breast milk. <12 years: not recommended;
12-<18: use extreme caution; not recommended for children and adolescents with asthma
or other chronic breathing problem. The FDA and the European Medicines Agency
(EMA) are investigating the safety of using *codeine* containing medications to treat pain,
cough and colds, in children 12-<18 years because of the potential for serious side effects,
including slowed or difficult breathing.

▷ *dihydrocodeine+aspirin+caffeine* (D)(III)(G) 1-2 caps q 4 hours prn
Pediatric: <18 years: not recommended; ≥18 years: same as adult
Synalgos-DC
Cap: dihydro 16 mg+*asp* 356.4 mg+*caf* 30 mg

Comment: *Codeine* is known to be excreted in breast milk. <12 years: not recommended;
12-<18: use extreme caution; not recommended for children and adolescents with asthma
or other chronic breathing problem. The FDA and the European Medicines Agency
(EMA) are investigating the safety of using *codeine* containing medications to treat pain,
cough and colds, in children 12-<18 years because of the potential for serious side effects,
including slowed or difficult breathing. *aspirin*-containing medications are contraindicated
with history of allergic-type reaction to *aspirin*, children and adolescents with *Varicella* or
other viral illness, and 3rd trimester of pregnancy.

▷ *hydrocodone bitartrate* (C)(II)
Pediatric: <18 years: not recommended; ≥18 years: same as adult
Hysingla ER swallow whole; 1 tab once daily at the same time each day
Tab: 20, 30, 40, 60, 80, 100, 120 mg ext-rel
Vantrela ER swallow whole; 1 tab once daily at the same time each day
Tab: 15, 30, 45, 60, 90 mg ext-rel
Zohydro ER swallow whole; *Opioid naïve:* 10 mg q 12 hours; may increase by 10 mg q
12 hours every 3-7 days; when discontinuing, titrate downward every 2-4 days
Cap: 10, 15, 20, 30, 40, 50 mg ext-rel

▷ *hydrocodone bitartrate+acetaminophen* (C)(II)(G)
Pediatric: <18: not recommended; ≥18 years: same as adult
Hycet 3 tsp (15 ml) q 4-6 hours prn; max 18 tsp/day
Liq: hydro 7.5 mg+*acet* 325 mg per 15 ml
Lorcet 1-2 caps q 4-6 hours prn; max 8 caps/day
Cap: hydro 5 mg+*acet* 325 mg
Lorcet 10/650 1 tab q 4-6 hours prn; max 6 tabs/day
Tab: hydro 10 mg+*acet* 325 mg
Lorcet-HD 1 cap q 4-6 hours prn; max 6 tabs/day
Cap: hydro 5 mg+*acet* 325 mg
Lorcet Plus 1 tab q 4-6 hours prn; max 6 tabs/day
Tab: hydro 7.5 mg+*acet* 325 mg
Lortab 2.5/500 1-2 tabs q 4-6 hours prn; max 8 tabs/day
Tab: hydro 2.5 mg+*acet* 325*mg
Lortab 5/500 1-2 tabs q 4-6 hours prn; max 8 tabs/day
Tab: hydro 5 mg+*acet* 325*mg
Lortab 7.5/500 1 tab q 4-6 hours prn; max 6 tabs/day
Tab: hydro 7.5 mg+*acet* 325*mg
Lortab 10/500 1 tab q 4-6 hours prn; max 6 tabs/day
Tab: hydro 10 mg+*acet* 325*mg
Lortab Elixir 3 tsp q 4-6 hours prn; max 18 tsp/day
Liq: hydro 7.5 mg+*acet* 300 mg per 15 ml (tropical fruit punch) (alcohol)
Maxidone 1 tab q 4-6 hours prn; max 5 tabs/day
Tab: hydro 10 mg+*acet* 325*mg

    Norco 5/325 1 tab q 4-6 hours prn; max 8 tabs/day
      Tab: hydro 5 mg+*acet* 325*mg
    Norco 7.5/325 1 tab q 4-6 hours prn; max 6 tabs/day
      Tab: hydro 7.5 mg+*acet* 325*mg
    Norco 10/325 1 tab q 4-6 hours prn; max 6 tabs/day
      Tab: hydro 10 mg+*acet* 325*mg
    Vicodin 1-2 tabs q 4-6 hours prn; max 8 tabs/day
      Tab: hydro 5 mg+*acet* 300*mg
    Vicodin ES 1 tab q 4-6 hours prn; max 6 tabs/day
      Tab: hydro 7.5 mg+*acet* 300*mg
    Vicodin HP 1 tab q 4-6 hours prn; max 6 tabs/day
      Tab: hydro 10 mg+*acet* 300*mg
    Xodol 5/300 1-2 tabs q 4-6 hours prn; max 8 caps/day
      Tab: hydro 5 mg+*acet* 300*mg
    Xodol 7.5/300 1 tab q 4-6 hours prn; max 6 caps/day
      Tab: hydro 7.5 mg+*acet* 300*mg
    Xodol 10/300 1 tab q 4-6 hours prn; max 6 caps/day
      Tab: hydro 10 mg+*acet* 300*mg
    Zamicet 10/325 1-2 tabs q 4-6 hours prn; max 8 caps/day
      Liq: hydro 10 mg+*acet* 325 mg per 15 ml
    Zydone 5/400 1-2 tabs q 4-6 hours prn; max 8 caps/day
      Tab: hydro 5 mg+*acet* 400 mg
    Zydone 7.5/400 1 tab q 4-6 hours prn; max 6 caps/day
      Tab: hydro 7.5 mg+*acet* 400 mg
    Zydone 10/400 1 tab q 4-6 hours prn; max 6 caps/day
▶ *hydrocodone+ibuprofen* **(C; not for use in 3rd)(II)(G)**
  Pediatric: <18: not recommended; ≥18 years: same as adult
    Ibudone 5/200 1 tab q 4-6 hours prn; max 5 tabs/day
      Tab: hydro 5 mg+*ibup* 200 mg
    Ibudone 10/200 1 tab q 4-6 hours prn; max 5 tabs/day
      Tab: hydro 10 mg+*ibup* 200 mg
    Reprexain 1 tab q 4-6 hours prn; max 5 tabs/day
      Tab: hydro 5 mg+*ibup* 200 mg
    Vicoprofen 1 tab q 4-6 hours prn; max 5 tabs/day
      Tab: hydro 7.5 mg+*ibup* 200 mg
▶ *hydromorphone* **(C)(II)(G)**
  Pediatric: <18: not recommended; ≥18 years: same as adult
    Dilaudid initially 2-4 mg q 4-6 hours prn
      Tab: 2, 4, 8 mg (sulfites)
    Dilaudid Oral Liquid 2.5-10 mg q 3-6 hours prn
      Liq: 5 mg/5 ml (sulfites)
    Dilaudid Rectal Suppository 2.5-10 mg q 6-8 hours prn
      Rectal supp: 3 mg
    Dilaudid Injection initially 1-2 mg SC <u>or</u> IM q 4-6 hours prn
      Amp: 1, 2, 4 mg/ml (1 ml)
    Dilaudid-HP Injection initially 1-2 mg SC <u>or</u> IM q 4-6 hours prn
      Amp: 10 mg/ml (1 ml)
    Exalgo initially 8-64 mg once daily
      Tab: 8, 12, 16, 32 mg ext-rel (sulfites)
▶ *meperidine* **(C; D in 2nd, 3rd)(II)(G)** 50-150 mg q 3-4 hours prn
  Pediatric: 0.5-0.8 mg/lb q 3-4 hours prn; max adult dose
    Demerol *Tab:* 50, 100 mg; *Syr:* 50 mg/5 ml (banana) (alcohol-free)

▷ *meperidine+promethazine* (C; D in 2nd, 3rd)(II)(G)
  Pediatric: <18: not recommended; ≥18 years: same as adult
    Mepergan 1-2 tsp q 3-4 hours prn
      Syr: mep 25 mg+*prom* 25 mg per ml
    Mepergan Fortis 1-2 tsp q 4-6 hours prn
      Tab: mep 50 mg+*prom* 25 mg
▷ *methadone* (C)(II)(G) 2.5-10 mg PO, SC, or IM q 3-4 hours; for use only in chronic
  moderately severe-to-severe pain management (e.g., hospice care). For opioid naïve
  patients, initiate **Dolophine** tablets with 2.5 mg every 8 to 12 hours; unlike other
  opioid analgesics, *methadone* is not indicated as an as-needed (prn) analgesic, per se;
  titrate slowly with dose increases no more frequent than every 3 to 5 days; to convert
  to **Dolophine** tablets from another opioid, use available conversion factors to obtain
  estimated dose (see mfr pkg insert); do not abruptly discontinue **Dolophine** in a
  physically dependent patient
  Pediatric: <18: not recommended; ≥18 years: same as adult
    Dolophine *Tab:* 5, 10 mg; *Dispersible tab:* 40 mg (dissolve in 120 ml orange
    juice or other citrus drink); *Oral soln:* 5, 10 mg/ml; *Oral conc:* 10 mg/ml; *Syr:*
    10 mg/30 ml; *Vial:* 10 mg/ml (200 mg/20 ml multi-dose) for injection
Comment: *methadone* administration is allowed only by approved providers with strict
state and federal regulations (as stipulated in 42 CFR 8.12). Black Box Warning (BBW):
Dolophine exposes users to risks of addiction, abuse, and misuse, which can lead to
overdose and death. Assess each patient's risk and monitor regularly for development of
these behaviors and conditions. Serious, life-threatening, or fatal respiratory depression
may occur. The peak respiratory depressant effect of *methadone* occurs later, and persists
longer than the peak analgesic effect. Accidental ingestion, especially by children, can
result in fatal overdose. QT interval prolongation and serious arrhythmias (*torsades de
pointes*) have occurred during treatment with *methadone*. Closely monitor patients with
risk factors for development of prolonged QT interval, a history of cardiac conduction
abnormalities, and those taking medications affecting cardiac conduction. Neonatal
Opioid Withdrawal Syndrome (NOWS) is an expected and treatable outcome of use
of methadone use during pregnancy. NOWS may be life-threatening if not recognized
and treated in the neonate. The balance between the risks of NOWS and the benefits
of maternal *methadone* use should be considered and the patient advised of the risk
of NOWS so that appropriate planning for management of the neonate can occur.
methadone has been detected in human milk. Concomitant use with CYP3A4, 2B6, 2C19,
2C9 or 2D6 inhibitors or discontinuation of concomitantly used CYP3A4 2B6, 2C19, or
2C9 inducers can result in a fatal overdose of *methadone*. Concomitant use of opioids
with benzodiazepines or other central nervous system (CNS) depressants, including
alcohol, may result in profound sedation, respiratory depression, coma, and death.
▷ *morphine sulfate (immed-release)* (C)(II)(G) usually 15-30 mg q 4 hours prn; solution, usually 10-20 mg q 4 hours prn
  Pediatric: <18: not recommended; ≥18 years: same as adult
    Tab: 15*, 30*mg; *Oral soln:* 10 mg/5 ml, 20 mg/5 ml (100, 500 ml), 100 mg/5 ml
    (30, 120 ml)
▷ *morphine sulfate (immed- and sust-rel)* (C)(II)
Comment: Dosage dependent upon previous opioid dosage; see mfr pkg insert for
conversion guidelines; not for prn use; swallow whole or sprinkle contents of caps on
applesauce (do not crush, chew, or dissolve). Generic *morphine sulfate* is available in the
following forms: *Tab:* 15*, 30*mg; *Oral soln:* 10, 20 mg/5 ml (100 ml); 100 mg/5 ml (30,
120 ml w. oral syringe)
  Pediatric: <18 years: not recommended; ≥18 years: same as adult
    Arymo ER swallow whole; 1 tab once daily at the same time each day
      Tab: 15, 30, 60 mg ext-rel

Duramorph administer per anesthesia
IV/Intrathecal/Epidural: 0.5, 1 mg/ml
Infumorph administer per anesthesia
Intrathecal/Epidural: 10, 20 mg/ml
Kadian (G) 1 cap every 12-24 hours
Cap: 10, 20, 30, 50, 60, 80, 100, 200 mg sust-rel
MS Contin (G) 1 tab every 24 hours
Tab: 15, 30, 60, 100, 200 mg sust-rel
MSIR 5-30 mg q 4 hours prn
Tab: 15*, 30*mg; *Cap:* 15, 30 mg
MSIR Oral Solution 5-30 mg q 4 hours prn
Oral soln: 10, 20 mg/5 ml (120 ml)
MSIR Oral Solution Concentrate 5-30 mg q 4 hours prn
Oral conc: 20 mg/ml (30, 120 ml w. dropper)
Oramorph SR 1 cap every 12-24 hours
Tab: 15, 30, 60, 100 mg sust-rel
Roxanol Oral Solution 10-30 mg q 4 hours prn
Oral soln: 20 mg/ml (1, 4, 8 oz)
Roxanol Rescudose
Oral soln: 10 mg/2.5 ml (25 single-dose)
▷ *morphine sulfate (ext-rel)* (C)(II)
Pediatric: <18 years: not recommended; ≥18 years: same as adult
MorphaBond ER *Tab:* 15, 30, 60, 100 mg ext-rel
Comment: **MorphaBond** may be prescribed only by a qualified Healthcare providers knowledgeable in use of potent opioids for management of chronic pain. Do not abruptly discontinue in a physically dependent patient. Instruct patients to swallow **MorphaBond ER** tablets intact and not to cut, break, crush, chew, or dissolve **MorphaBond ER** to avoid the risk of release and absorption of potentially fatal dose of morphine. **MorphaBond 100** mg tablets, a single dose greater than 60 mg, or a total daily dose >120 mg, are only for use in patients in whom tolerance to an opioid of comparable potency has been established. Patients considered opioid-tolerant are those taking, for one week or longer, at least 60 mg oral *morphine* per day, 25 mcg transdermal *fentanyl* per hour, 30 mg oral *oxycodone* per day, 8 mg oral *hydromorphone* per day, 25 mg oral *oxymorphone* per day, 60 mg oral *hydrocodone* per day, or an equianalgesic dose of another opioid. Use the lowest effective dosage for the shortest duration consistent with individual patient treatment goals. Individualize dosing based on the severity of pain, patient response, prior analgesic experience, and risk factors for addiction, abuse, and misuse
▷ *morphine sulfate+naltrexone* (C)(II)
Pediatric: <18 years: not recommended; ≥18 years: same as adult
Embeda 1 cap q 12-24 hours
Cap: **Embeda 20/0.8** *morph* 20 mg+*nal* 0.8 mg ext-rel
Embeda 30/1.2 *morph* 30 mg+*nal* 1.2 mg ext-rel
Embeda 50/2 *morph* 50 mg+*nal* 2 mg ext-rel
Embeda 60/2.4 *morph* 60 mg+*nal* 2.4 mg ext-rel
Embeda 80/3.2 *morph* 80 mg+*nal* 3.2 mg ext-rel
Embeda 100/4 *morph* 100 mg+*nal* 4 mg ext-rel
Comment: **Embeda** is not for prn use; for use in opioid-tolerant patients only; swallow whole or sprinkle contents of caps on applesauce (do not crush, chew, or dissolve); do not administer via NG or gastric tube (PEG tube).
▷ *oxycodone* (B)(II) 5-15 mg q 4-6 hours prn
Comment: Concomitant use of CYP3A4 inhibitors may increase opioid effects and CYP3A4 inducers may decrease effects or possibly cause development of an abstinence

syndrome (withdrawal symptoms) in patients who are physically *oxycodone* dependent/addicted.

> *Pediatric:* <18 years: not recommended; ≥18 years: same as adult

> **Oxaydo** *Tab:* 5, 7.5 mg

Comment: **Oxaydo** is the first and only immediate-release oral *oxycodone* that discourages intranasal abuse. **Oxaydo** is formulated with sodium lauryl sulfate, an inactive ingredient that may cause nasal burning and throat irritation when snorted and, thus potentially reducing abuse liability. There is no generic equivalent.

> **Oxecta** *Tab:* 5, 7.5 mg
> **Oxycodone Oral Solution (G)** *Oral soln:* 5 mg/5 ml (15, 30 ml)
> **OxyIR (G)** *Cap:* 5 mg
> **RoxyBond** *Tab:* 5, 15, 30 mg

Comment: The FDA recently approved **RoxyBond** immediate-release tablets for the management of severe pain that does not respond to alternative treatment and requires an opioid analgesic. **RoxyBond** is the first immediate-release opioid analgesic to received FDA approval with a label describing its abuse-deterrent properties under the FDA 2015 Guidance for Industry: Abuse-Deterrent Opioids Evaluation and Labeling. The drug is formulated with inactive ingredients making it more difficult to misuse and abuse. When compared with another approved immediate-release tablet, **RoxyBond** was shown to be more resistant to cutting, crushing, grinding, or breaking, and more resistant to extraction. Adverse events associated with **RoxyBond** include nausea, constipation, vomiting, headache, pruritus, insomnia, dizziness, asthenia, somnolence, and addiction.

> **Roxycodone** *Tab:* 5, 15*, 30*mg; *Oral soln:* 5 mg/ml
> **Roxycodone Intensol** *Oral soln:* 20 mg/ml

▷ *oxycodone cont-rel* (B)(II)(G) dosage dependent upon previous opioid dosages; see mfr pkg insert: <11 years: not recommended; 11-16 years: the child's pain must be severe enough to require around-the-clock, long-term treatment not managed well by other treatments; must already be taking and tolerating minimum opium dose equal to *oxycodone* 20 mg/day x 5 consecutive days; >16 year: same as adult; no previous treatment with *oxycodone* required

> **OxyContin** dose q 12 hours
> > *Tab:* 10, 15, 20, 30, 40, 60, 80 mg cont-rel
> **OxyFast** dose q 6 hours
> > *Oral conc:* 20 mg/ml (30 ml w. dropper)
> **Xtampza ER** dose q 12 hours
> > *Cap:* 10, 15, 20, 30, 40 mg ext-rel

Comment: May open the **Xtampza ER** capsule and sprinkle in water or on soft food.

▷ *oxycodone+acetaminophen* (C)(II)(G)

> Comment: Maximum 4 gm acetaminophen per day.
> *Pediatric:* not recommended

> **Magnacet 2.5/400** 1 tab q 6 hours prn; max 10 tabs/day
> > *Tab: oxy* 2.5 mg+*acet* 325 mg
> **Magnacet 5/400** 1 tab q 6 hours prn; max 10 tabs/day
> > *Tab: oxy* 5 mg+*acet* 325 mg
> **Magnacet 7.5/400** 1 tab q 6 hours prn; max 8 tabs/day
> > *Tab: oxy* 7.5 mg+*acet* 325 mg
> **Magnacet 10/400** 1 tab q 6 hours prn; max 6 tabs/day
> > *Tab: oxy* 10 mg+*acet* 325 mg
> **Percocet 2.5/325** 1 tab q 6 hours prn; max 4 gm acet/day
> > *Tab: oxy* 2.5 mg+*acet* 325 mg
> **Percocet 5/325** 1 tab q 6 hours prn; max 4 gm acet/day
> > *Tab: oxy* 5 mg+*acet* 325*mg

    Percocet 7.5/325 1 tab q 6 hours prn; max 4 gm acet/day
        Tab: oxy 7.5 mg+*acet* 325 mg
    Percocet 7.5/500 1 tabs q 6 hours prn; max 4 gm acet/day
        Tab: oxy 7.5 mg+*acet* 325 mg
    Percocet 10/325 1 tabs q 6 hours prn; max 4 gm acet/day
        Tab: oxy 10 mg+*acet* 325 mg
    Percocet 10/650 1 tab q 6 hours prn; max 4 gm acet/day
        Tab: oxy 10 mg+*acet* 325 mg
    Roxicet 5/325 1 tab/tsp q 6 hours prn
        Tab: oxy 5 mg+*acet* 325 mg; *Oral soln: oxy* 5 mg+*acet* 325 mg per 5 ml
    Roxicet 5/500 1 caplet q 6 hours prn
        Cplt: oxy 5 mg+*acet* 325 mg
    Roxicet Oral Solution 1 tsp q 6 hours prn
        Oral soln: oxy 5 mg+*acet* 325 mg per 5 ml (alcohol 0.4%)
    Tylox 1 cap q 6 hours prn
        Cap: oxy 5 mg+*acet* 325 mg
    Xartemis XR 2 tabs q 12 hours prn
        Tab: oxy 7.5 mg+*acet* 325 mg
▷ *oxycodone+aspirin* (D)(II)(G)
    Percodan 1 tab q 6 hours prn
        Pediatric: not recommended
        Tab: oxy 4.8355 mg+*asp* 325*mg
    Percodan-Demi 1-2 tabs q 6 hours prn
        Pediatric: 6-12 years: 1/4 tab q 6 hours prn; >12-18 years: 1/2 tab q 6 hours prn
        Tab: oxy 2.25 mg+*asp* 325 mg
Comment: *aspirin*-containing medications are contraindicated with history of allergic-type reaction to *aspirin*, children and adolescents with *Varicella* or other viral illness, and 3rd trimester of pregnancy.
▷ *oxycodone+ibuprofen* (C)(II)(G)
    Pediatric: <14 years: not recommended; ≥14 years: same as adult
    Combunox 1 tab q 6 hours prn
        Tab: oxy 5 mg+*ibu* 400*mg
▷ *oxycodone+naloxone* (C)(II) 1 tab q 3-4 hours prn
    Pediatric: <12 years: not recommended; ≥12 years: same as adult
    Targiniq
        Tab: **Targiniq 10/5** *oxy* 10 mg+*nal* 5 mg
            Targiniq 20/10 *oxy* 20 mg+*nal* 10 mg
            Targiniq 40/20 *oxy* 40 mg+*nal* 20 mg
▷ *oxymorphone* (C)(II)(G)
    Pediatric: <18 years: not recommended; ≥18 years: same as adult
    Numorphan 1 supp q 4-6 hours prn
        Rectal supp: 5 mg; *Vial:* 1 mg/ml (1 ml), *Amp:* 1.5 mg/ml (10 ml);
Comment: Store in refrigerator in original package. 1 mg of **Numorphan** is approximately equivalent in analgesic activity to 10 mg of *morphine sulfate*.
    Opana 1-1 tab q 4-6 hours prn
        Tab: 5, 10 mg
    Opana ER 1 tab q 12 hours prn
        Tab: 5, 7.5, 10, 15, 20, 30, 40 mg ext-rel crush-resist
    Opana Injection initially 0.5 mg IV <u>or</u> IM; 1 x 1 mg IM <u>or</u> IV q 4-6 hours prn
        Amp: 1 mg/ml (1 ml) (paraben/sodium dithionite-free)
▷ *pentazocine+aspirin* (D)(IV) 2 cplts tid <u>or</u> qid prn
    Pediatric: <12 years: not recommended; ≥12 years: same as adult

      Talwin Compound *Cplt: pent* 12.5 mg+*asp* 325 mg

Comment: *aspirin*-containing medications are contraindicated with history of allergic-type reaction to *aspirin*, children and adolescents with *Varicella* or other viral illness, and 3rd trimester of pregnancy.

▷ *pentazocine+naloxone* (C)(IV) 1 tab q 3-4 hours prn

    Pediatric: <12 years: not recommended; ≥12 years: same as adult

      Talwin NX *Tab: pent* 50 mg+*nal* 0.5*mg

▷ *pentazocine lactate* (C)(IV) 30 mg IM, SC, or IV q 3-4 hours; max 360 mg/day

    Pediatric: <1 year: not recommended; ≥1 year: 0.5 mg/kg IM

      Talwin Injectable *Amp: pent* 30 mg/ml (1, 1.5, 2 ml)

▷ *propoxyphene napsylate+acetaminophen* (C)(IV)(G)

Comment: Max 4 gm acetaminophen per day.

    Pediatric: <12 years: not recommended; ≥12 years: same as adult

      Balacet 325 1 tab q 4 hours prn; max 6 tabs/day

        Tab: prop 100 mg+*acet* 325 mg

▷ *tramadol* (C)(IV)(G)

Comment: *tramadol* is known to be excreted in breast milk. The FDA and the European Medicines Agency (EMA) are investigating the safety of using *tramadol*-containing medications to treat pain in children 12-18 years because of the potential for serious side effects, including slowed or difficult breathing.

      Rybix ODT initially 100 mg once daily; may increase by 100 mg every 5 days; max 300 mg/day; *CrCl <30 mL/min or severe hepatic impairment:* not recommended; *Cirrhosis:* max 50 mg q 12 hours

    Pediatric: <12 years: contraindicated; 12-<18: use extreme caution; not recommended for children and adolescents with obesity, asthma, obstructive sleep apnea, or other chronic breathing problem, or for post-tonsillectomy/adenoidectomy pain; ≥18 years: same as adult

      ODT: 50 mg (mint) (phenylalanine)

      Ryzolt initially 100 mg once daily; may increase by 100 mg every 5 days; max 300 mg/day; *CrCl <30 mL/min or severe hepatic impairment:* not recommended

    Pediatric: <12 years: contraindicated; 12-<18: use extreme caution; not recommended for children and adolescents with obesity, asthma, obstructive sleep apnea, or other chronic breathing problem, or for post-tonsillectomy/adenoidectomy pain; ≥18 years: same as adult

      Tab: 100, 200, 300 mg ext-rel

      Ultram 50-100 mg q 4-6 hours prn; max 400 mg/day; *CrCl <30 mL/min:* max 100 mg q 12 hours; *Cirrhosis:* max 50 mg q 12 hours

    Pediatric: <12 years: contraindicated; 12-<18: use extreme caution; not recommended for children and adolescents with obesity, asthma, obstructive sleep apnea, or other chronic breathing problem, or for post-tonsillectomy/adenoidectomy pain; ≥18 years: same as adult

      Tab: 50*mg

      Ultram ER initially 100 mg once daily; may increase by 100 mg every 5 days; max 300 mg/day; *CrCl <30 mL/min or severe hepatic impairment:* not recommended

    Pediatric: <12 years: contraindicated; 12-<18: use extreme caution; not recommended for children and adolescents with obesity, asthma, obstructive sleep apnea, or other chronic breathing problem, or for post-tonsillectomy/adenoidectomy pain; ≥18 years: same as adult

      Tab: 100, 200, 300 mg ext-rel

▷ *tramadol+acetaminophen* (C)(IV)(G) 2 tabs q 4-6 hours; max 8 tabs/day; 5 days; *CrCl <30 mL/min:* max 2 tabs q 12 hours; max 4 tabs/day x 5 days

    Pediatric: <12 years: contraindicated; 12-<18: use extreme caution; not recommended for children and adolescents with obesity, asthma, obstructive sleep apnea, or other chronic breathing problem, <u>or</u> for post-tonsillectomy/adenoidectomy pain; ≥18 years: same as adult

> **Ultracet** *Tab: tram 37.5+acet 325 mg*

Comment: *tramadol* is known to be excreted in breast milk. The FDA and the European Medicines Agency (EMA) are investigating the safety of using *tramadol*-containing medications to treat pain in children 12-18 years because of the potential for serious side effects, including slowed <u>or</u> difficult breathing.

▷ *buprenorphine* (C)(III) change patch every 7 days; do not increase the dose until previous dose has been worn for at least 72 hours; after removal, do not re-use the site for at least 3 weeks; do not expose the patch to heat

Pediatric: <16 years: not recommended; ≥16 years: same as adult

> **Butrans Transdermal System**
> *Transdermal patch:* 5, 10, 20 mcg/hour (4/pck)

▷ *fentanyl* transdermal system (C)(II) apply to clean, dry, non-irritated, intact, skin; hold in place for 30 seconds; start at lowest dose and titrate upward; *Opioid-naïve:* change patch every 3 days (72 hours)

Pediatric: <18 years <u>or</u> <110 lb: not recommended; ≥18 years <u>or</u> ≥110 lb: same as adult

> **Duragesic** *Transdermal patch:* 12, 25, 37.5, 50, 62.5, 75, 87.5, 100 mcg/hour (5/pck)

▷ *fentanyl iontophoretic transdermal system*

> **Ionsys** is a transdermal patient-controlled device that sticks to the arm <u>or</u> chest; it is activated when the patient pushes the button

> **Comment:** **Ionsys** is for in-hospital use only and should be discontinued prior to hospital discharge. It is indicated for post-op pain relief.

TRANSMUCOSAL (SUB-LINGUAL, BUCCAL) OPIOIDS

Comment: For chronic severe pain. For management of breakthrough pain in patients with cancer who are already receiving and who are tolerant to opioid therapy. Opioid-tolerant patients are those taking oral *morphine* ≥60 mg/day, transdermal *fentanyl* ≥25 mcg/hour, *oxycodone* ≥30 mg/day, oral *hydromorphone* ≥8 mg/day, <u>or</u> an equianalgesic dose of another opioid, for ≥1 week

ORAL OPIOID PARTIAL AGONIST-ANTAGONIST

▷ *buprenorphine* (C)

Pediatric: <16 years: not recommended; ≥16 year: same as adult

> **Subutex** 8 mg in a single dose on day 1; then 16 mg in a single dose on day 2; target dose is 16 mg/day in a single dose; dissolve under tongue; do not chew <u>or</u> swallow whole
> *SL tab (lemon-lime)* <u>or</u> *SL film (lime):* 2, 8 mg (30/pck)

▷ *fentanyl* buccal soluble film (C)(II) dissolve 1 film on moistened area inside cheek; initially 200 mcg; no more than 4 doses/day at least 2 hours apart; max 1200 mcg/dose; do not cut film

Pediatric: <18 years: not recommended; ≥18 years: same as adult

> **Onsolis** *Buccal film:* 200, 400, 600, 800, 1200 mcg (30 films/pck)

▷ *fentanyl citrate* transmucosal unit (C)(II)(G) initially one 200 mcg unit placed between cheek and lower gum; move from side to side; suck (not chew); use 6 units before titrating; titrate dose as needed; max 4 units/day

Pediatric: <18 years: not recommended; ≥18 years: same as adult

> **Actiq** *Unit:* 200, 400, 600, 800, 1200, 1600 mcg (24 units/pck)
> **Fentora** *Unit:* 100, 200, 400, 600, 800 mcg (24 units/pck)

▷ *fentanyl* sublingual tab (C)(II) initially one 100 mcg dose; if inadequate after 30 minutes, may repeat; titrate in increments of 100 mcg; max 2 doses per episode, up to 4 episodes per day; wait at least 2 hours before treating another episode; *Maintenance:* use only one tablet of appropriate strength; do not chew, suck, <u>or</u> swallow tablets; do

not convert from other *fentanyl* products on a mcg-per-mcg basis <u>or</u> interchange with other *fentanyl* products
Pediatric: <18 years: not recommended; ≥18 years: same as adult
> **Abstral** *SL tab:* 100, 200, 300, 400, 600, 800 mcg (32 tabs/pck)

▷ *fentanyl sublingual spray* (C)(II)
Pediatric: <18 years: not recommended; ≥18 years: same as adult
> **Subsys** 100, 200, 400, 600, 800 mcg/S L spray
> Comment: **Subsys** is not bioequivalent with other *fentanyl* products. Do not convert patients from other *fentanyl* products to **Subsys** on a mcg-per-mcg basis. There are no conversion directions available for patients on any other *fentanyl* products other than **Actiq**. (Note: This includes oral, transdermal, <u>or</u> parenteral formulations of *fentanyl*.)

PARENTERAL OPIOID AGONIST-ANTAGONISTS

▷ *nalbuphine* (B)(G) 10 mg/70 kg IM, SC, <u>or</u> IV q 3-6 hours prn
Pediatric: <18 years: not recommended; ≥18 years: same as adult
> **Nubain** *Amp:* 10, 20 mg/ml (1 ml) (sulfite-free, parabens-free)

▷ *pentazocine+naloxone* (C)(IV) 1-2 tabs q 3-4 hours prn; max 12 tabs/day
Pediatric: <12 years: not recommended; ≥12 year: same as adult
> **Talwin-NX** *Tab:* pent 50 mg+nal 0.5*mg

TRANSMUCOSAL (INTRA-NASAL) OPIOIDS

▷ *butorphanol tartrate* nasal spray (C)(IV) initially 1 spray (1 mg) in one nostril and may repeat after 60-90 minutes (*Elderly* 90-120 minutes) in opposite nostril if needed <u>or</u> 1 spray in each nostril and may repeat q 3-4 hours prn
Pediatric: <18 years: not recommended; ≥18 years: same as adult
> **Butorphanol Nasal Spray** *Nasal spray:* 1 mg/actuation (10 mg/ml, 2.5 ml)
> **Stadol Nasal Spray** *Nasal spray:* 1 mg/actuation (10 mg/ml, 2.5 ml)

▷ *fentanyl* nasal spray (C)(II) initially 1 spray (100 mcg) in one nostril and may repeat after 2 hours; when adequate analgesia is achieved, use that dose for subsequent breakthrough episodes
Titration steps: 100 mcg using 1 x 100 mcg spray; 200 mcg using 2 x 100 mcg spray (1 in each nostril); 400 mcg using 1 x 400 mcg spray; 800 mcg using 2 x 400 mcg (1 in each nostril); max 800 mcg; limit to ≤4 doses per day
Pediatric: <18 years: not recommended; ≥18 years: same as adult
> **Lazanda Nasal Spray** *Nasal spray:* 100, 400 mcg/100 mcl (8 sprays/bottle)

Comment: **Lazanda Nasal Spray** is available by restricted distribution program. To enroll, call 855-841-4234 <u>or</u> visit https://www.fda.gov/downloads/drugs/drugsafety/postmarketdrugsafetyinformationforpatientsandproviders/ucm261983.pdf. **Lazanda Nasal Spray** is indicated for the management of breakthrough pain in cancer patients who are already receiving and who are tolerant to opioid therapy for their underlying persistent cancer pain. Patients considered opioid tolerant are those who are taking at least 60 mg of oral morphine/day, 25 mcg of transdermal *fentanyl*/hour, 30 mg oral *oxycodone*/day, 8 mg oral *hydromorphone*/day, 25 mg oral *oxymorphone*/day, <u>or</u> an equianalgesic dose of another opioid for a week <u>or</u> longer. Patients must remain on around-the-clock opioids when using **Lazanda Nasal Spray**. As such, it is contraindicated in the management of acute <u>or</u> post-op pain, including headache/migraine, <u>or</u> dental pain.

INTRATHECAL OPIOIDS

▷ *ziconotide* intrathecal (IT) infusion (C) initially no more than 2.4 mcg/day (0.1 mcg/hour) and titrate to upward by up to 2.4 mcg/day (0.1 mcg/day at intervals of no more than 2-3 times per week, up to a recommended maximum of 19.2 mcg/day

(0.8 mcg/hour) by Day 21; dose increases in increments of less than 2.4 mcg/day (0.1 mcg/hour) and increases in dose less frequently than 2-3 times per week may be used.
Pediatric: <12 years: not recommended; ≥12 years: same as adult

Prialt *Vial:* 25 mcg/ml (20 ml), 100 mcg/ml (1, 2, 5 ml)

Comment: Patients with a pre-existing history of psychosis should not be treated with *ziconotide*. Contraindications to the use of IT analgesia include conditions such as the presence of infection at the microinfusion injection site, uncontrolled bleeding diathesis, and spinal canal obstruction that impairs circulation of CSF.

 PANCREATIC ENZYME INSUFFICIENCY

Comment: Seen in chronic pancreatitis, postpancreatectomy, cystic fibrosis, steatorrhea, post-GI tract bypass surgery, and ductal obstruction from neoplasia. May sprinkle cap; however, do not crush or chew cap or tab. May mix with applesauce or other acidic food; follow with water or juice. Do not let any drug remain in mouth. Take dose just prior to each meal or snack. Base dose on lipase units; adjust per diet and clinical response (i.e., steatorrhea). Pancrelipase products are interchangeable. Contraindicated with pork protein hypersensitivity.

PANCRELIPASE PRODUCTS

▷ *pancreatic enzymes* (C)

 Creon 500 units/kg per meal; max 2,500 units/kg per meal or <10,000 units/kg per day or <4,000 units/gm fat ingested per day

 Pediatric: <12 months: 2,000-4,000 units per 120 ml formula or per breast-feeding (do not mix directly into formula or breast milk; 12 months to 4 years: 1,000 units/kg per meal; max 2,500 units/kg per meal <10,000 units/kg per day; >4 years: same as adult

  Cap: **Creon 3000** *lip* 3,000 units+*pro* 9,500 units+*amyl* 15,000 units del-rel
   Creon 6000 *lip* 6,000 units+*pro* 19,000 units+*amyl* 30,000 units del-rel
   Creon 12000 *lip* 12,000 units+*pro* 38,000 units+amyl 60,000 units del-rel
   Creon 24000 *lip* 24,000 units+*pro* 76,000 units+*amyl* 120,000 units del-rel
   Creon 36000 *lip* 36,000 units+*pro* 114,000 units+*amyl* 180,000 units del-rel

 Cotazym 1-3 tabs just prior to each meal or snack
 Pediatric: <12 years: not recommended; ≥12 years: same as adult

  Tab: **Cotazym** *lip* 1,000 units+*pro* 12,500 units+*amyl* 12,500 units del-rel
   Cotazym-S *lip* 5,000 units+*pro* 20,000 units+*amyl* 20,000 units del-rel

 Donnazyme 1-3 caps just prior to each meal or snack
 Pediatric: <12 years: not recommended; ≥12 years: same as adult

  Cap: **Donnazyme** *lip* 5,000 units+*pro* 20,000 units+*amyl* 20,000 units del-rel

 Ku-Zyme 1-2 caps just prior to each meal or snack
 Pediatric: <12 years: not recommended; ≥12 years: same as adult

  Cap: **Ku-Zyme:** *lip* 12,000 units+*pro* 15,000 units+*amyl* 15,000 units del-rel

 Kutrase 1-2 caps just prior to each meal or snack
 Pediatric: <12 years: not recommended; ≥12 years: same as adult

  Cap: **Kutrase:** *lip* 12,000 units+*pro* 30,000 units+*amyl* 30,000 units del-rel

 Pancreaze 2,500 lipase units/kg per meal or <10,000 lipase units/kg per day or <4,000 lipase units/gm fat ingested per day

 Pediatric: <12 months: 2,000-4,000 lipase units per 120 ml formula or per breastfeeding; >12 months to <4 years 1,000 lipase units/kg per meal; >4 years: 500 lipase units/kg per meal; max: adult dose

  Cap: **Pancreaze 4200** *lip* 4,200 units+*pro* 10,000 units+*amyl* 17,500 units ec-microtabs
   Pancreaze 10500 *lip* 10,500 units+*pro* 25,000 units+*amyl* 43,750 units ec-microtabs

> **Pancreaze 16800** *lip* 16,800 units+*pro* 40,000 units+*amyl* 70,000 units ec-microtabs
>
> **Pancreaze 21000** *lip* 21,000 units+*pro* 37,000 units+*amyl* 61,000 units ec-microtabs

Pertyze *12 months to 4 years and ≥8 kg:* initially 1,000 lipase units/kg per meal; *≥4 years and ≥16 kg:* initially 500 lipase units/kg per meal; *Both:* 2,500 lipase units/kg per meal or <10,000 units/kg per day or <4,000 lipase units/gm fat ingested per day

> *Cap:* **Pertyze 8000** *lip* 8,000 units+*pro* 28,750 units+*amyl* 30,250 units del-rel
>
> **Pertyze 16000** *lip* 16,000 units+*pro* 57,500 units+*amyl* 65,000 units del-rel

Ultrase 1-3 tabs just prior to each meal or snack

> *Pediatric:* same as adult
>
> *Cap:* **Ultrase** *lip* 4,500 units+*pro* 20,000 units+*amyl* 25,000 units del-rel
>
> **Ultrase MT** *lip* 12,000 units+*pro* 39,000 units+*amyl* 39,000 units del-rel
>
> **Ultrase MT 18** *lip* 18,000 units+*pro* 58,500 units+*amyl* 58,500 units del-rel
>
> **Ultrase MT 20** *lip* 20,000 units+*pro* 65,000 units+*amyl* 65,000 units del-rel

Viokace initially 500 lip units/kg per meal; max 2,500 lipase units/kg per meal, or <10,000 lipase units/kg per meal, or <4,000 units/gm fat ingested per day

> *Pediatric:* same as adult
>
> *Tab:* **Viokace 8** *lip* 8,000 units+*pro* 30,000 units+*amyl* 30,000 units
>
> **Viokace 16** *lip* 16,000 units+*pro* 60,000 units *amyl* 60,000 units

Viokace 0440 *lip* 10,440 units+*pro* 39,150 units *amyl* 39,150 units

Viokace 20880 *lip* 20,880 units+*pro* 78,300 units *amyl* 78,300 units

Comment: Viokace 10440 and Viokase 20880 should be taken with a daily proton pump inhibitor.

> **Viokace Powder** 1/4 tsp (0.7 gm) with meals
>
> **Viokace Powder** *lip* 16,800 units+*pro* 70,000 units+*amyl* 70,000 units per 1/4 tsp (8 oz)

Zenpep 500 units/kg per meal; max 2,500 units/kg per meal or <10,000 units/kg per day or <4,000 units/gm fat ingested per day

> *Pediatric:* <12 months: 2,000-4,000 units per 120 ml formula or per breast feeding (do not mix directly into formula or breast milk); 12 months-4 years: 1,000 units/kg per meal; max 2,500 units/kg per meal <10,000 units/kg per day; >4 years: same as adult
>
> *Cap:* **Zenpep 5000** *lip* 5,000 units+*pro* 17,000 units+*amyl* 27,000 units del-rel
>
> **Zenpep 10000** *lip* 10,000 units+*pro* 34,000 units+*amyl* 55,000 units del-rel
>
> **Zenpep 15000** *lip* 15,000 units+*pro* 51,000 units+*amyl* 82,000 units del-rel
>
> **Zenpep 20000** *lip* 20,000 units+*pro* 68,000 units+*amyl* 109,000 units del-rel

Zymase 1-3 caps just prior to each meal or snack

> *Pediatric:* <12 years: not recommended; ≥12 years: same as adult
>
> *Cap:* **Zymase** *lip* 12,000 units+*prot* 24,000 units+*amyl* 24,000 units del-rel

PANIC DISORDER

Comment: If possible when considering a benzodiazepine to treat anxiety, a short-acting benzodiazepines should be used only prn to avert intense anxiety and panic for the least time necessary while a different non-addictive anti-anxiety regimen (e.g., SSRI, SNRI, TCA, *buspirone*, beta-blocker) is established and effective treatment goals achieved. Co-administration of SSRIs with TCAs requires extreme caution. Concomitant use of MAOIs and SSRIs is absolutely contraindicated. Avoid other serotonergic drugs. A potentially fatal adverse event is **serotonin syndrome**, caused by serotonin excess. Milder symptoms require HCP intervention to avert severe symptoms which can be rapidly fatal without urgent/emergent medical care. Symptoms include restlessness, agitation, confusion, hallucinations, tachycardia, hypertension, dilated pupils, muscle twitching, muscle rigidity, loss of muscle coordination, diaphoresis, diarrhea, headache, shivering, piloerection, hyperpyrexia, cardiac arrhythmias, seizures, loss of consciousness, coma, death. Abrupt withdrawal or interruption of treatment with an antidepressant medication is sometimes associated with an **antidepressant discontinuation syndrome** which may be mediated by gradually tapering the drug over a period of two weeks or longer, depending on the dose strength and length of treatment. Common symptoms of the *serotonin discontinuation syndrome* include flu-like symptoms (nausea, vomiting, diarrhea, headaches, sweating), sleep disturbances (insomnia, nightmares, constant sleepiness), mood disturbances (dysphoria, anxiety, agitation), cognitive disturbances (mental confusion, hyperarousal), sensory and movement disturbances (imbalance, tremors, vertigo, dizziness, electric-shock-like sensations in the brain, often described by sufferers as "brain zaps."

SELECTIVE SEROTONIN REUPTAKE INHIBITORS (SSRIs)

▷ *escitalopram* (C)(G) initially 10 mg daily; may increase to 20 mg daily after 1 week;
   Elderly or hepatic impairment: 10 mg once daily
   Pediatric: <12 years: <12 years: not recommended; ≥12 years: same as adult; 12-17 years: initially 10 mg once daily; may increase to 20 mg once daily after 3 weeks
      Lexapro *Tab:* 5, 10*, 20*mg
      Lexapro Oral Solution *Oral soln:* 1 mg/ml (240 ml) (peppermint) (parabens)
▷ *fluoxetine* (C)(G)
      Prozac initially 20 mg daily; may increase after 1 week; doses >20 mg/day should be divided into AM and noon doses; max 80 mg/day
      Pediatric: <8 years: not recommended; 8-17 years: initially 10 mg/day; may increase after 2 weeks to 20 mg/day; range 20-60 mg/day; range for lower weight children 20-30 mg/day; >17 years: same as adult
         Cap: 10, 20, 40 mg; *Tab:* 30*, 60*mg; *Oral soln:* 20 mg/5 ml (4 oz) (mint)
      Prozac Weekly following daily *fluoxetine* therapy at 20 mg/day for 13 weeks, may initiate **Prozac Weekly** 7 days after the last 20 mg *fluoxetine* dose
      Pediatric: <12 years: not recommended; ≥12 years: same as adult
         Cap: 90 mg ent-coat del-rel pellets
▷ *paroxetine maleate* (D)(G)
   Pediatric: <12 years: not recommended; ≥12 years: same as adult
      Paxil initially 20 mg daily in AM; may increase by 10 mg/day at weekly intervals as needed; max 60 mg/day
         Tab: 10*, 20*, 30, 40 mg
      Paxil CR initially 25 mg daily in AM; may increase by 12.5 mg at weekly intervals as needed; max 62.5 mg/day
         Tab: 12.5, 25, 37.5 mg cont-rel ent-coat
      Paxil Suspension initially 20 mg daily in AM; may increase by 10 mg/day at weekly intervals as needed; max 60 mg/day
         Oral susp: 10 mg/5 ml (250 ml) (orange)
▷ *paroxetine mesylate* (D)(G) initially 7.5 mg daily in AM; may increase by 10 mg/day at weekly intervals as needed; max 60 mg/day
   Pediatric: <12 years: not recommended; ≥12 years: same as adult
      Brisdelle *Cap:* 7.5 mg
▷ *sertraline* (C) initially 50 mg daily; increase at 1 week intervals if needed; max 200 mg daily
   Pediatric: <6 years: not recommended; 6-12 years: initially 25 mg daily; max 200 mg/day; 13-17 years: initially 50 mg daily; max 200 mg/day; ≥17 years: same as adult
      Zoloft *Tab:* 15*, 50*, 100*mg; *Oral conc:* 20 mg per ml (60 ml, dilute just before administering in 4 oz water, ginger ale, lemon-lime soda, lemonade, or orange juice) (alcohol 12%)

SEROTONIN-NOREPINEPHRINE REUPTAKE INHIBITORS (SNRIs)

▷ *desvenlafaxine* (C)(G) swallow whole; initially 50 mg once daily; max 120 mg/day
  Pediatric: <12 years: not recommended; ≥12 years: same as adult
    Pristiq *Tab:* 50, 100 mg ext-rel
▷ *venlafaxine* (C)(G)
    Effexor initially 75 mg/day in 2-3 doses; may increase at 4 day intervals in 75 mg
    increments to 150 mg/day; max 375 mg/day
    Pediatric: <18 years: not recommended; ≥18 years: same as adult
      Tab: 25, 37.5, 50, 75, 100 mg
    Effexor XR initially 75 mg q AM; may start at 37.5 mg daily x 4-7 days, then increase by
    increments of up to 75 mg/day at intervals of at least 4 days; usual max 375 mg/day
    Pediatric: <18 years: not recommended; ≥18 years: same as adult
      Cap: 37.5, 75, 150 mg ext-rel

TRICYCLIC ANTIDEPRESSANTS (TCAs)

▷ *doxepin* (C)(G)
  Pediatric: <12 years: not recommended; ≥12 years: same as adult
    Cap: 10, 25, 50, 75, 100, 150 mg; *Oral conc:* 10 mg/ml (4 oz w. dropper)
▷ *imipramine* (C)(G)
  Pediatric: <12 years: not recommended; ≥12 years: same as adult
    Tofranil initially 75 mg daily (max 200 mg); *Adolescents:* initially 30-40 mg daily
    (max 100 mg/day); if maintenance dose exceeds 75 mg daily, may switch to **Tofra-**
    nil PM for divided <u>or</u> bedtime dose
      Tab: 10, 25, 50 mg
    Tofranil PM initially 75 mg daily 1 hour before HS; max 200 mg
      Cap: 75, 100, 125, 150
    Tofranil Injection 50 mg IM; lower dose for adolescents; switch to oral form as
    soon as possible
      Amp: 25 mg/2 ml (2 ml)

FIRST GENERATION ANTIHISTAMINE

▷ *hydroxyzine* (C)(G) 50-100 mg qid; max 600 mg/day
  Pediatric: <6 years: 50 mg/day divided qid; ≥6 years: 50-100 mg/day divided qid
    Atarax *Tab:* 10, 25, 50, 100 mg; *Syr:* 10 mg/5 ml (alcohol 0.5%)
    Vistaril *Cap:* 25, 50, 100 mg; *Oral susp:* 25 mg/5 ml (4 oz) (lemon)
Comment: *hydroxyzine* is contraindicated in early pregnancy and in patients with a
prolonged QT interval. It is not known whether this drug is excreted in human milk;
therefore, *hydroxyzine* should not be given to nursing mothers.

AZAPIRONES

▷ *buspirone* (B) initially 7.5 mg bid; may increase by 5 mg/day q 2-3 days; max 60 mg/
  day
  Pediatric: <6 years: not recommended; 6-17 years: same as adult
    BuSpar *Tab:* 5, 10, 15*, 30*mg

BENZODIAZEPINES
Short Acting

▷ *alprazolam* (D)(IV)(G)
  Pediatric: <18 years: not recommended; ≥18 years: same as adult
    Niravam initially 0.25-0.5 mg tid; may titrate every 3-4 days; max 4 mg/day
      Tab: 0.25*, 0.5*, 1*, 2*mg orally-disint

Xanax initially 0.25-0.5 mg tid; may titrate every 3-4 days; max 4 mg/day
Tab: 0.25*, 0.5*, 1*, 2*mg

Xanax XR initially 0.5-1 mg once daily, preferably in the AM; increase at intervals of at least 3-4 days by up to 1 mg/day. Taper no faster than 0.5 mg every 3 days; max 10 mg/day. When switching from immediate-release *alprazolam*, give total daily dose of immediate-release once daily.
Tab: 0.5, 1, 2, 3 mg ext-rel

➢ *oxazepam* (C)(IV)(G) 10-15 mg tid-qid for moderate symptoms; 15-30 mg tid-qid for severe symptoms
Pediatric: <12 years: not recommended; ≥12 years: same as adult
Tab: 15 mg; *Cap:* 10, 15, 30 mg

Intermediate-Acting

➢ *lorazepam* (D)(IV)(G) 1-10 mg/day in 2-3 divided doses
Pediatric: <12 years: not recommended; ≥12 years: same as adult
Ativan *Tab:* 0.5, 1*, 2*mg
Lorazepam Intensol *Oral conc:* 2 mg/ml (30 ml w. graduated dropper)

Long-Acting

➢ *chlordiazepoxide* (D)(IV)(G)
Pediatric: <6 years: not recommended; ≥6 years: 5 mg bid-qid; increase to 10 mg bid-tid
Librium 5-10 mg tid-qid for moderate symptoms; 20-25 mg tid-qid for severe symptoms
Cap: 5, 10, 25 mg
Librium Injectable 50-100 mg IM or IV; then 25-50 mg IM tid-qid prn; max 300 mg/day
Inj: 100 mg

➢ *chlordiazepoxide+clidinium* (D)(IV) 1-2 caps tid-qid: max 8 caps/day
Pediatric: <12 years: not recommended; ≥12 years: same as adult
Librax *Cap: chlor* 5 mg+*clid* 2.5 mg

➢ *clonazepam* (D)(IV)(G) initially 0.25 mg bid; increase to 1 mg/day after 3 days
Pediatric: <18 years: not recommended; ≥18 years: same as adult
Klonopin *Tab:* 0.5*, 1, 2 mg
Klonopin Wafers dissolve in mouth with or without water
Wafer: 0.125, 0.25, 0.5, 1, 2 mg orally-disint

➢ *clorazepate* (D)(IV)(G) 30 mg/day in divided doses; max 60 mg/day
Pediatric: <9 years: not recommended; ≥9 years: same as adult
Tranxene *Tab:* 3.75, 7.5, 15 mg
Tranxene SD do not use for initial therapy
Tab: 22.5 mg ext-rel
Tranxene SD Half Strength do not use for initial therapy
Tab: 11.25 mg ext-rel
Tranxene T-Tab *Tab:* 3.75*, 7.5*, 15*mg

➢ *diazepam* (D)(IV)(G) 2-10 mg bid to qid
Pediatric: <12 years: not recommended; ≥12 years: same as adult
Diastat *Rectal gel delivery system:* 2.5 mg
Diastat AcuDial *Rectal gel delivery system:* 10, 20 mg
Valium *Tab:* 2*, 5*, 10*mg
Valium Injectable *Vial:* 5 mg/ml (10 ml); *Amp:* 5 mg/ml (2 ml); *Prefilled syringe:* 5 mg/ml (5 ml)
Valium Intensol Oral Solution *Conc oral soln:* 5 mg/ml (30 ml w. dropper) (alcohol 19%)
Valium Oral Solution *Oral soln:* 5 mg/5 ml (500 ml) (wintergreen spice)

PHENOTHIAZINES

▷ *prochlorperazine* (C)(G)
  Pediatric: <12 years: not recommended; ≥12 years: same as adult
    Compazine 5 mg tid-qid
      Tab: 5 mg; *Syr:* 5 mg/5 ml (4 oz) (fruit); *Rectal supp:* 2.5, 5, 25 mg
    Compazine Spansule 15 mg q AM or 10 mg q 12 hours
      Spansule: 10, 15 mg sust-rel
▷ *trifluoperazine* (C)(G) 1-2 mg bid; max 6 mg/day; max 12 weeks
  Pediatric: <12 years: not recommended; ≥12 years: same as adult
    Stelazine *Tab:* 1, 2, 5, 10 mg

 PARKINSON'S DISEASE

Parkinson's Disease-associated Dementia, *see Dementia page* 114
Comment: When administering *carbidopa* and *levodopa* separately, administer each at the same time. Titrate daily dose ratio of 1:10 *carbidopa* to *levodopa*. Max daily *carbidopa* 200 mg. Most patients will require *levodopa* 400 to 1600 mg/day in divided doses every 4 to 8 hours. After titrating both drugs to the desired effects without intolerable side effects, switch to a *carbidopa+levodopa* combination form.

DOPAMINE PRECURSOR

▷ *levodopa* (C)(G)
  Tab: 125, 150, 200 mg

DECARBOXYLASE INHIBITOR

▷ *carbidopa* (C)(G)
  Lodosyn *Tab:* 25 mg

DOPAMINE RECEPTOR AGONISTS

▷ *amantadine* (C)
Comment: *amantadine* is a chrono-synchronous amantadine therapy for the treatment of levodopa-induced dyskinesia (LID) in patients with Parkinson's disease.
    Gocovri take once daily at bedtime; initially 137 mg; after 1 week, increase to the recommended daily dosage of 274 mg; swallow whole; may sprinkle contents on soft food; take with <u>or</u> without food; avoid use with alcohol; a lower dosage is recommended for patients with moderate <u>or</u> severe renal impairment; Contraindicated in patients with end-stage renal disease
      Cap: 68.5, 137 mg ext-rel
    Symadine (G) initially 100 mg bid; may increase after 1-2 weeks by 100 mg/day; max 400 mg/day in divided doses; for extrapyramidal effects, 100 mg bid; max 300 mg/day in divided doses
      Cap: 100 mg
    Symmetrel (G) initially 100 mg bid; may increase after 1-2 weeks by 100 mg/day; max 400 mg/day in divided doses; for extrapyramidal effects, 100 mg bid; max 300 mg/day in divided doses
      Cap: 100 mg; *Syr:* 50 mg/5 ml (16 oz) (raspberry)
▷ *bromocriptine* (B)(G) initially 1.25 mg bid to 2.5 mg tid with meals; increase as needed every 2-4 weeks by 2.5 mg/day; max 100 mg/day
    Parlodel *Tab:* 2.5*mg; *Cap:* 5 mg
▷ *pramipexole* (C)(G) initially 0.125 mg tid; increase at intervals q 5-7 days; max 1.5 mg tid
    Mirapex *Tab:* 0.125, 0.25*, 0.5*, 1*, 1.5*mg

> *ropinirole* (C) initially 0.25 mg tid for first week; then 0.5 mg tid for second week; then 0.75 mg tid for third week; then 1 mg tid for fourth week; may increase by 1.5 mg/day at 1 week intervals to 9 mg/day; then increase up to 3 mg/day at 1 week intervals; max 24 mg/day

> **Requip** *Tab:* 0.25, 0.5, 1, 2, 4, 5 mg

> *rotigotine* transdermal patch (C) apply to clean, dry, intact skin on abdomen, thigh, hip, flank, shoulder, or upper arm; rotate sites and allow 14 days before re-using site; if hairy, shave site at least 3 days before application to site; avoid abrupt cessation; taper by 2 mg/24 hr every other day; *Early stage:* initially 2 mg/24 hr patch once daily; may increase weekly by 2 mg/24 hr if needed; max 6 mg/24 hr once daily; *Advanced stage:* initially 4 mg/24 hr patch once daily; may increase weekly by 2 mg/24 hr if needed; max 8 mg/24 hr once daily

> **Neupro** *Trans patch:* 1 mg/24 hr, 2 mg/24 hr, 3 mg/24 hr, 4 mg/24 hr, 6 mg/24 hr, 8 mg/24 hr (30/carton) (sulfites)

DOPA-DECARBOXYLASE INHIBITORS

Comment: Contraindicated in narrow-angle glaucoma. Use with caution with sympathomimetics and antihypertensive agents.

> *carbidopa+levodopa* (C)(G) usually 400-1600 mg *levodopa*/day

Pediatric: <18 years: not established; ≥18 years: same as adult

> **Duopa** *Ent susp:* *carb* 4.63 mg+*levo* 20 mg single-use cassettes for use w. CADD Legacy 1400 Pump

> **Sinemet 10/100** initially 1 tab tid-qid; increase if needed daily or every other day up to qid

> *Tab: carb* 10 mg+*levo* 100 mg*

> **Sinemet 25/100** initially 1 tab bid-tid; increase if needed daily or every other day up to qid

> *Tab: carb* 25 mg+*levo* 100 mg*

> **Sinemet 25/250** 1 tab tid-qid

> *Tab: carb* 25 mg+*levo* 250 mg*

> **Sinemet CR 25/100** initially one 25/100 tab bid; allow 3 days between dosage adjustments

> *Tab: carb* 25 mg+*levo* 100 mg cont-rel

> **Sinemet CR 50/200** initially one 50/200 tab bid; allow 3 days between dosage adjustments

> *Tab: carb* 50 mg+*levo* 200 mg cont-rel*

DOPA-DECARBOXYLASE INHIBITOR+DOPAMINE PRECURSOR+COMT INHIBITOR COMBINATION

> *carbidopa+levodopa+entacapone* (C) titrate individually with separate components; then switch to corresponding strength *levodopa* and *carbidopa*; max 8 tabs/day

> *Tab:* **Stalevo 50** *carb* 12.5 mg+*levo* 50 mg+*enta* 200 mg

> **Stalevo 75** *carb* 12.5 mg+*levo* 75 mg+*enta* 200 mg

> **Stalevo 100** *carb* 12.5 mg+*levo* 100 mg+*enta* 200 mg

> **Stalevo 125** *carb* 12.5 mg+*levo* 125 mg+*enta* 200 mg

> **Stalevo 150** *carb* 12.5 mg+*levo* 150 mg+*enta* 200 mg

> **Stalevo 200** *carb* 12.5 mg+*levo* 200 mg+*enta* 200 mg

MONOAMINE OXIDASE INHIBITORS (MAOIs)

> *rasagiline* (C)(G) usual maintenance: 0.5-1 mg/day; max: 1 mg/day; initial dose for patients on concomitant *levodopa*: 0.5 mg daily; initial dose for patients not on concomitant *levodopa*: 1 mg daily

> **Azilect** *Tab:* 0.5, 1 mg

Comment: **Azelect** is indicated as monotherapy or as adjunct to *levodopa*. With mild hepatic dysfunction (Child-Pugh 5-6), limit **Azelect** dose to 0.5 mg daily. With moderate to severe hepatic dysfunction (Child-Pugh 7-15), **Azelect** is not recommended. Contraindications include co-administration with *meperidine, methadone, mirtazapine, propoxyphene, tramadol, dextromethorphan, St. John's wort, cyclobenzaprine, methylphenidate, dexmethylphenidate*, or other MAOIs.

▷ *selegiline* (C)(G) 5 mg at breakfast and at lunch; max 10 mg/day
   Tab/Cap: 5 mg
▷ *selegiline* (C)(G) 1.25 mg daily; max 2.5 mg/day
   Zelapar *ODT:* 1.25 mg orally-disint (phenylalanine)

COMT INHIBITORS

▷ *entacapone* (C) 1 tab with each dose of *levodopa* or *carbidopa*; max 8 tabs/day
   Comtan *Tab:* 200 mg
   Comment: **Comtan** is an adjunct to *levodopa+carbidopa* in patients with end-of-dose wearing off.
▷ *tolcapone* (C) 100-200 mg tid; max 600 mg/day
   Tasmar *Tab:* 100, 200 mg
   Comment: Monitor LFTs every 2 weeks. Withdraw **Tasmar** if no substantial improvement in the first 3 weeks of treatment.

CENTRALLY ACTING ANTICHOLINERGICS

▷ *benztropine mesylate* (C) initially 0.5-1 mg q HS, increase if needed; for extrapyramidal disorders 1-4 mg once daily-bid; max 6 mg/day
   Cogentin *Tab:* 0.5*, 1*, 2*mg
▷ *biperiden hydrochloride* (C) initially 1 tab tid or qid, then increase as needed; max 8 tabs/day
   Akineton *Tab:* 2 mg
▷ *procyclidine* (C) initially 2.5 mg tid; may increase as needed to 5 mg tid-qid every 3-5 days; max 15 mg/day
   Kemadrin *Tab:* 5 mg
▷ *trihexyphenidyl* (C)(G) initially 1 mg; increase as needed by 2 mg every 3-5 days; max 15 mg/day
   Artane *Tab:* 2*, 5*mg

PSEUDOBULBAR AFFECT (PBA)

Comment: Pseudobulbar affect (PBA), emotional lability, labile affect, or emotional incontinence refers to a neurologic disorder characterized by involuntary crying or uncontrollable episodes of crying and/or laughing, or other emotional outbursts. PBA occurs secondary to a neurologic disease or brain injury such as traumatic brain injury (TBI), stroke, Parkinson's disease, multiple sclerosis, and amyotrophic lateral sclerosis (ALS, or Lou Gehrig disease).

▷ *dextromethorphan+quinidine* (C)(G) 1 cap once daily x 7 days; then starting on day 8, 1 cap bid
   Pediatric: <12 years: not recommended; ≥12 years: same as adult
   Nuedexta *Cap:* dextro 20 mg+quini 10 mg
Comment: *dextromethorphan hydrobromide* is an uncompetitive NMDA receptor antagonist and sigma-1 agonist. *quinidine sulfate* is a CYP450 2D6 inhibitor. **Nuedexta** is contraindicated with an MAOI or within 14 days of stopping an MAOI, with prolonged QT interval, congenital long QT syndrome, history suggestive of torsades de pointes, or heart failure, complete atrioventricular (AV) block without implanted pacemaker or patients at high risk of complete AV block, and concomitant drugs that both prolong QT interval and are metabolized by CYP2D6 (e.g., *thioridazine* or

pimozide). Discontinue **Nuedexta** if the following occurs: hepatitis or thrombocytopenia or any other hypersensitivity reaction. Monitor ECG in patients with left ventricular hypertrophy (LVH) or left ventricular dysfunction (LVD). *desipramine* exposure increases **Nuedexta** 8-fold; reduce *desipramine* dose and adjust based on clinical response. Use of **Nuedexta** with selective serotonin reuptake inhibitors (SSRIs) or tricyclic antidepressants (TCAs) increases the risk of serotonin syndrome. *paroxetine* exposure increases **Nuedexta** 2-fold; therefore, reduce **paroxetine** dose and adjust based on clinical response (*digoxin* exposure may increase *digoxin* substrate plasma concentration. **Nuedexta** is not recommended in pregnancy or breastfeeding. Safety and effectiveness of **Nuedexta** in children have not been established. To report suspected adverse reactions, contact Avanir Pharmaceuticals at 1-866-388-5041 or FDA at 1-800-FDA-1088 or www.fda.gov/medwatch

PARONYCHIA (PERIUNGUAL ABSCESS)

▷ *cephalexin* (B)(G) 500 mg bid x 10 days
Pediatric: 25-50 mg/day in 2 divided doses x 10 days
Keflex *Cap:* 250, 333, 500, 750 mg; *Oral susp:* 125, 250 mg/5 ml (100, 200 ml) (strawberry)
▷ *clindamycin* (B)(G) 150-300 mg q 6 hours x 10 days
Pediatric: 8-16 mg/kg/day in 3-4 divided doses x 10 days
Cleocin *Cap:* 75 (tartrazine), 150 (tartrazine), 300 mg
Cleocin Pediatric Granules *Oral susp:* 75 mg/5 ml (100 ml) (cherry)
▷ *dicloxacillin* (B)(G) 500 mg q 6 hours x 10 days
Pediatric: 12.5-25 mg/kg/day in 4 divided doses x 10 days; *see page 632 for dose by weight*
Dynapen *Cap:* 125, 250, 500 mg; *Oral susp:* 62.5 mg/5 ml (80, 100, 200 ml)
▷ *erythromycin base* (B)(G) 500 mg q 6 hours x 10 days
Pediatric: <45 kg: 30-50 mg in 2-4 doses x 10 days; ≥45 kg: same as adult
Ery-Tab *Tab:* 250, 333, 500 mg ent-coat
PCE *Tab:* 333, 500 mg
Comment: *erythromycin* may increase INR with concomitant *warfarin*, as well as increase serum level of *digoxin, benzodiazepines*, and *statins*.
▷ *erythromycin ethylsuccinate* (B)(G) 400 mg q 6 hours x 10 days
Pediatric: 30-50 mg/kg/day in 4 divided doses q 6 hours x 10 days; may double dose with severe infection; max 100 mg/kg/day; *see page 635 for dose by weight*
EryPed *Oral susp:* 200 mg/5 ml (100, 200 ml) (fruit); 400 mg/5 ml (60, 100, 200 ml) (banana); *Oral drops:* 200, 400 mg/5 ml (50 ml) (fruit); *Chew tab:* 200 mg wafer (fruit)
E.E.S. *Oral susp:* 200, 400 mg/5 ml (100 ml) (fruit)
E.E.S. Granules *Oral susp:* 200 mg/5 ml (100, 200 ml) (cherry)
E.E.S. 400 Tablets *Tab:* 400 mg
Comment: *erythromycin* may increase INR with concomitant *warfarin*, as well as increase serum level of *digoxin, benzodiazepines*, and *statins*.

PEDICULOSIS HUMANUS CAPITIS (HEAD LICE)/ PEDICULOSIS PHTHIRUS (PUBIC LICE)

▷ *ivermectin* (C) thoroughly wet hair; leave on for 10 minutes; then rinse off with water; do not re-treat
Pediatric: <6 months, <33 lbs: not recommended; ≥6 months, ≥33 lbs: same as adult
Sklice *Lotn:* 0.5% (4 oz, 117 gm, laminate tube)

▷ *lindane* (C)(G) apply, leave on for 4 minutes, then thoroughly wash off
Pediatric: <2 years: not recommended; ≥2 years: same as adult
Kwell Shampoo *Shampoo:* 1% (60 ml)
▷ *malathion* (B)(G) thoroughly wet hair; allow to dry naturally; shampoo and rinse after 8-12 hours; use a fine tooth comb to remove lice and nits; if lice persist after 7-9 days, may repeat treatment
Pediatric: same as adult
Ovide (OTC) *Lotn:* 59% (2 oz)
▷ *permethrin* (B)(G) apply to washed and towel-dried hair; allow to remain on for 10 minutes, then rinse off; repeat after 7 days if needed
Pediatric: <2 months: not recommended; ≥2 months: same as adult
Nix (OTC) *Crm rinse:* 1% (2 oz w. comb)
▷ *pyrethrins with piperonyl butoxide* (C)(G) apply and leave on for 10 minutes, then wash off
A-200 *Shampoo:* pyr 0.33%+pip but 3%
Rid Mousse *Shampoo:* pyr 0.33%+pip but 4%
Rid Shampoo *Shampoo:* pyr 0.33%+pip but 3%

Comment: To remove nits, soak hair in equal parts white vinegar and water for 15-20 minutes.

 PELVIC INFLAMMATORY DISEASE (PID)

Comment: The following treatment regimens are published in the **2015 CDC Sexually Transmitted Diseases Treatment Guidelines.** Treatment regimens are presented by generic drug name first, followed by information about brands and dose forms. Treat all sexual partners. Because of the high risk for maternal morbidity and preterm delivery, pregnant women who have suspected PID should be hospitalized and treated with parenteral antibiotics. HIV-infected women with PID respond equally well to standard parenteral and antibiotic regimens as HIV-negative women.

OUTPATIENT REGIMENS
Regimen 1

▷ *ceftriaxone* 250 mg IM in a single dose plus *doxycycline*
▷ *doxycycline* 100 mg bid x 14 days with or without *metronidazole*
▷ *metronidazole* 500 mg PO bid x 14 days

Regimen 2

▷ *cefoxitin* 2 gm IM in a single dose plus *probebecid*
▷ *probenecid* 1 gm PO in a single dose administered concurrently plus *doxycycline* 100 mg bid x 14 days with or without *metronidazole*
▷ *metronidazole* 500 mg PO bid x 14 days

Regimen 3

▷ Other parenteral third-generation cephalosporin (e.g., *ceftizoxime* or *cefotaxime*) in a single dose) plus *doxycycline*
▷ *doxycycline* 100 mg bid x 14 days with or without *metronidazole*
▷ *metronidazole* 500 mg PO bid x 14 days

DRUG BRANDS AND DOSE FORMS

▷ *cefoxitin* (B)(G)
Mefoxin *Vial:* 1, 2 g
▷ *ceftriaxone* (B)(G)
Rocephin Vials 250, 500 mg; 1, 2 gm

▷ *doxycycline* (D)(G)
        Acticlate *Tab:* 75, 150**mg
        Adoxa *Tab:* 50, 75, 100, 150 mg ent-coat
        Doryx *Tab:* 50, 75, 100, 150, 200 mg del-rel
        Doxteric *Tab:* 50 mg del-rel
        Monodox *Cap:* 50, 75, 100 mg
        Oracea *Cap:* 40 mg del-rel
        Vibramycin *Tab:* 100 mg; *Cap:* 50, 100 mg; *Syr:* 50 mg/5 ml (raspberry-apple)
        (sulfites); *Oral susp:* 25 mg/5 ml (raspberry)
        Vibra-Tab *Tab:* 100 mg film-coat

Comment: *doxycycline* is contraindicated <8 years-of-age, in pregnancy, and lactation (discolors developing tooth enamel). A side effect may be photosensitivity (photophobia). Do not take with antacids, calcium supplements, milk or other dairy, or within 2 hours of taking another drug.

▷ *metronidazole* (not for use in 1st; B in 2nd, 3rd)
        Flagyl *Tab:* 250*, 500*mg
        Flagyl 375 *Cap:* 375 mg
        Flagyl ER *Tab:* 750 mg ext-rel

Comment: Alcohol is contraindicated during treatment with oral *metronidazole* and for 72 hours after therapy due to a possible *disulfiram*-like reaction (nausea, vomiting, flushing, headache).

▷ *probenecid* (B)(G)
        Benemid *Tab:* 500*mg; *Cap:* 500 mg

 PEPTIC ULCER DISEASE (PUD)

Helicobacter pylori **Eradication Regimens** *see page* 203
Antacids *see* GERD *page* 169

H2 ANTAGONISTS

▷ *cimetidine* (B)(G)
    Pediatric: <16 years: not recommended; ≥16 years: same as adult
        Tagamet 800 mg bid or 400 mg qid; max 2.4 gm/day
          Tab: 300, 400*, 800*mg
        Tagamet HB (OTC) *Prophylaxis:* 1 tab ac; *Treatment:* 1 tab bid
          Tab: 200 mg
        Tagamet HB Oral Suspension (OTC) *Prophylaxis:* 1 tsp ac; *Treatment:* 1 tsp bid
          Oral susp: 200 mg/20 ml (12 oz)
        Tagamet Liquid *Liq:* 300 mg/5 ml (mint-peach) (alcohol 2.8%)
▷ *famotidine* (B)(G) 20 mg bid or 40 mg q HS; *max 6 weeks*
    Pediatric: 0.5 mg/kg/day q HS or in 2 divided doses; max 40 mg/day
        Pepcid *Tab:* 20, 40 mg; *Oral susp:* 40 mg/5 ml (50 ml)
        Pepcid AC (OTC) 1 tab ac; max 2 doses/day
          Tab/Rapid dissolv tab: 10 mg
        Pepcid Complete (OTC) 1 tab ac; max 2 doses/day
          Tab: fam 10 mg+$CaCO_2$ 800 mg+mag *hydrox* 165 mg
        Pepcid RPD
          Tab: 20, 40 mg rapid-dissolv
▷ *nizatidine* (B)(G) 150 mg bid; max 12 weeks
    Pediatric: <12 years: not recommended; ≥12 years: same as adult
        Axid *Cap:* 150, 300 mg
        Axid AR (OTC) 1 tab ac; max 150 mg/day
          Tab: 75 mg

▷ *ranitidine* (B)(G)
Pediatric: <1 month: not recommended; 1 month-16 years: 2-4 mg/kg/day in 2 divided doses; max 300 mg/day; *Duodenal/Gastric Ulcer:* 2-4 mg/kg/day divided bid; max 300 mg/day; *Erosive Esophagitis:* 5-10 mg/kg/day divided bid; max 300 mg/day; >16 years: same as adult

    Zantac 150 mg bid <u>or</u> 300 mg q HS
      Tab: 150, 300 mg
    Zantac 75 (OTC) 1 tab ac
      Tab: 75 mg
    Zantac EFFERdose dissolve 25 mg tab in 5 ml water; dissolve 150 mg tab in 6-8 oz water
      Efferdose: 25, 150 mg effervescent (phenylalanine)
    Zantac Syrup *Syr:* 15 mg/ml (peppermint) (alcohol 7.5%)
▷ *ranitidine bismuth citrate* (C) 400 mg bid
Pediatric: <12 years: not recommended; ≥12 years: same as adult
    Tritec *Tab:* 400 mg

PROTON PUMP INHIBITORS (PPIs)

Comment: If hepatic impairment, <u>or</u> if patient is Asian, consider reducing the PPI dosage. Research has demonstrated associations between PPI use and fractures of the hip, wrist, and spine, hypomagnesemia, kidney injuries and chronic kidney disease, possible cardiovascular drug interactions, and infections (e.g., Clostridium difficile and pneumonia). Reducing the acidity of the stomach allows bacteria to thrive and spread to other organs like the lungs and intestines. This risk is increased with high dose and chronic use and greatest in the elderly. The most recent class-wide FDA warning cites reports of cutaneous and systemic lupus erythematosis (CLS/SLE) associates with PPIs in patients with both new onset and exacerbation of existing autoimmune disease. PPI treatment should be discontinued and the patient should be referred to a specialist. (http://www.fda.gov/Drugs/DrugSafety/InformationbyDrugClass/ucm213259.htm)

▷ *dexlansoprazole* (B)(G) 30-60 mg daily for up to 4 weeks
Pediatric: <18 years: not recommended; ≥18 years: same as adult
    Dexilant *Cap:* 30, 60 mg ent-coat del-rel granules; may open and sprinkle on applesauce; do not crush <u>or</u> chew granules
    Dexilant SoluTab *Tab:* 30 mg del-rel orally-disint
▷ *esomeprazole* (B)(OTC)(G) 20-40 mg daily; max 8 weeks; take 1 hour before food; swallow whole <u>or</u> mix granules with food <u>or</u> juice and take immediately; do not crush <u>or</u> chew granules
Pediatric: <1 year: not recommended; 1-11 years: <20 kg: 10 mg; ≥20 kg: 10-20 mg once daily; 12-17 years: 20-40 mg once daily; max 8 weeks; >17 years: same as adult
    Nexium *Cap:* 20, 40 mg ent-coat del-rel pellets
    Nexium for Oral Suspension *Oral susp:* 10, 20, 40 mg ent-coat del-rel granules/pkt (30 pkt/carton); mix in 2 tbsp water and drink immediately
▷ *lansoprazole* (B)(OTC)(G) 15-30 mg daily for up to 8 weeks; may repeat course; take before eating
Pediatric: <1 year: not recommended; 1-11, <30 kg: 15 mg once daily; ≥12 years: same as adult
    Prevacid *Cap:* 15, 30 mg ent-coat del-rel granules; swallow whole <u>or</u> mix granules with food <u>or</u> juice and take immediately; do not crush <u>or</u> chew granules; follow with water
    Prevacid for Oral Suspension *Oral susp:* 15, 30 mg ent-coat del-rel granules/pkt (30 pkt/carton); mix in 2 tbsp water and drink immediately; (strawberry)
    Prevacid SoluTab *ODT:* 15, 30 mg (strawberry) (phenylalanine)
    Prevacid 24HR 15 mg ent-coat del-rel granules; swallow whole <u>or</u> mix granules with food <u>or</u> juice and take immediately; do not crush <u>or</u> chew granules; follow with water

▷ *omeprazole* (C)(OTC)(G) 20-40 mg daily; take before eating; swallow whole or mix granules with applesauce and take immediately; do not crush or chew; follow with water
Pediatric: <1 year: not recommended; 5-<10 kg: 5 mg daily; 10-<20 kg: 10 mg daily; ≥20 kg: same as adult
  Prilosec *Cap:* 10, 20, 40 mg ent-coat del-rel granules
  Prilosec OTC *Tab:* 20 mg del-rel (regular, wild berry)
▷ *pantoprazole* (B)(G) initially 40 mg bid
Pediatric: <12 years: not recommended; ≥12 years: same as adult
  Protonix *Tab:* 40 mg ent-coat del-rel
  Protonix for Oral Suspension *Oral susp:* 40 mg ent-coat del-rel granules/pkt; mix in 1 tsp apple juice for 5 seconds or sprinkle on 1 tsp apple sauce, and swallow immediately; do not mix in water or any other liquid or food; take approximately 30 minutes prior to a meal; 30 pkt/carton
▷ *rabeprazole* (B)(OTC)(G) initially 20 mg daily; then titrate; may take 100 mg daily in divided doses or 60 mg bid
Pediatric: <12 years: not recommended; ≥12 years: 20 mg once daily; max 8 weeks
  AcipHex *Tab:* 20 mg ent-coat del-rel
  AcipHex Sprinkle *Cap:* 5, 10 mg del-rel

OTHER AGENTS

▷ *glycopyrrolate* (B)(G) initially 1-2 mg bid-tid; *Maintenance:* 1 mg bid; max 8 mg/day
Pediatric: <12 years: not recommended; ≥12 years: same as adult
  Robinul *Tab:* 1 mg (dye-free)
  Robinul Forte *Tab:* 2 mg (dye-free)
Comment: *glycopyrrolate* is an anticholinergic adjunct to PUD treatment.
▷ *mepenzolate* (B)(G) 25-50 mg divided qid, with meals and at HS
  Cantil *Tab:* 25 mg
▷ *sucralfate* (B)(G) Active ulcer: 1 gm qid; *Maintenance:* 1 gm bid
  Carafate *Tab:* 1*g; *Oral susp:* 1 gm/10 ml (14 oz)

PROPHYLAXIS

▷ *misoprostol* (X) 200 mg qid with food for prevention of NSAID-induced gastric ulcers
  Cytotec *Tab:* 100, 200 mg
Comment: *misoprostol* is a prostaglandin E1 analog indicated for the prevention of NSAID-induced gastric ulcers. Females of childbearing potential should have a negative serum pregnancy test within 2 weeks before starting and first dose on the 2nd or 3rd day of next the menstrual period. A contraceptive method should be maintained during therapy. Risks to pregnant females include: spontaneous abortion, premature birth, fetal anomalies, and uterine rupture.

 PERIPHERAL NEURITIS, DIABETIC NEUROPATHIC PAIN, PERIPHERAL NEUROPATHIC PAIN

▷ **Acetaminophen for IV Infusion** *see Pain page 344*
▷ **Ibuprophen for IV Infusion** *see Pain page 344*
▷ *acetaminophen* (B)(G) *see Fever page 165*

▷ *aspirin* (D)(G) *see Fever page 166*
Comment: *aspirin*-containing medications are contraindicated with history of allergic-type reaction to *aspirin*, children and adolescents with *Varicella* or other viral illness, and 3rd trimester of pregnancy.

ALPHA-2 DELTA LIGAND

➤ *pregabalin (GABA analog)* (C)(V) initially 150 mg daily divided bid-tid; may titrate within one week; max 600 mg divided bid-tid; discontinue over one week
Pediatric: <18 years: not recommended; ≥18 years: same as adult
  Lyrica *Cap:* 25, 50, 75, 100, 150, 200, 225, 300 mg; *Oral soln:* 20 mg/ml

SEROTONIN-NOREPINEPHRINE REUPTAKE INHIBITOR (SNRI)

➤ *duloxetine* (C) swallow whole; 30-60 mg once daily; may increase by 30 mg at 1 week intervals; usual target 60 mg daily; max 120 mg/day
Pediatric: <12 years: not recommended; ≥12 years: same as adult
  Cymbalta *Cap:* 20, 30, 60 mg ent-coat pellets
  Comment: **Cymbalta** is indicated for chronic pain syndromes (e.g., arthritis, fibromyalgia, lowback pain).

TOPICAL AND TRANSDERMAL NSAIDs

➤ *capsaicin* (B)(G) apply tid-qid prn to intact skin
Pediatric: <2 years: not recommended; ≥2 years: apply sparingly tid-qid prn
  Axsain *Crm:* 0.075% (1, 2 oz)
  Capsin *Lotn:* 0.025, 0.075% (59 ml)
  Capzasin-P (OTC) *Crm:* 0.025% (1.5 oz); *Lotn:* 0.025% (2 oz)
  Dolorac *Crm:* 0.025% (28 gm)
  Double Cap (OTC) *Crm:* 0.05% (2 oz)
  R-Gel *Gel:* 0.025% (15, 30 gm)
  Zostrix (OTC) *Crm:* 0.025% (0.7, 1.5, 3 oz)
  Zostrix HP (OTC) *Emol crm:* 0.075% (1, 2 oz)
➤ *capsaicin* 8% patch (B) apply up to 4 patches for one 60-minute application to clean dry skin; may prep area with topical anesthetic; wear nonlatex gloves; patches may be cut to size/shape; treatment may be repeated every 3 months; remove with cleansing gel after treatment
Pediatric: <18 years: not recommended
  Qutenza *Patch:* 8% 1640 mcg/cm (179 mg) (1 or 2 patches, each w. 1-50 gm tube cleansing gel/carton)
➤ *diclofenac epolamine transdermal patch* (C) apply one patch to affected area bid; remove during bathing; avoid non intact skin
Pediatric: <12 years: not recommended; ≥12 years: same as adult
  Flector Patch *Patch:* 180 mg/patch (30/carton)
➤ *capsaicin* (B)(G) apply tid to qid prn to intact skin
Pediatric: <2 years: not recommended; ≥2 years: same as adult
  Axsain *Crm:* 0.075% (1, 2 oz)
  Capsin *Lotn:* 0.025, 0.075% (59 ml)
  Capzasin-P (OTC) *Crm:* 0.025% (1.5 oz); *Lotn:* 0.025% (2 oz)
  Dolorac *Crm:* 0.025% (28 gm)
  Double Cap (OTC) *Crm:* 0.05% (2 oz)
  R-Gel *Gel:* 0.025% (15, 30 gm)
  Zostrix (OTC) *Crm:* 0.025% (0.7, 1.5, 3 oz)
  Zostrix HP (OTC) *Emol crm:* 0.075% (1, 2 oz)
➤ *capsaicin* 8% patch (B) apply up to 4 patches for one 60-minute application to clean dry skin; may prep area with topical anesthetic; wear non-latex gloves; patches may be cut to size/shape; treatment may be repeated every 3 months; remove with cleansing gel after treatment
Pediatric: <18 years: not recommended; ≥18 years: same as adult
  Qutenza *Patch:* 8% 1640 mcg/cm (179 mg) (1 or 2 patches w. 1-50 gm tube cleansing gel/carton)

▷ *lidocaine* 5% patch **(B)(G)** apply up to 3 patches at one time for up to 12 hours/24-hour period (12 hours on/12 hours off); patches may be cut into smaller sizes before removal of the release liner; do not re-use
Pediatric: <12 years: not recommended; ≥12 years: same as adult
  Lidoderm *Patch:* 5% (10x14 cm, 30/carton)

ORAL ANALGESICS

▷ *tramadol* **(C)(IV)(G)**
Comment: *tramadol* is known to be excreted in breast milk. The FDA and the European Medicines Agency (EMA) are investigating the safety of using *tramadol*-containing medications to treat pain in children 12-18 years because of the potential for serious side effects, including slowed or difficult breathing.
  Rybix ODT initially 100 mg once daily; may increase by 100 mg every 5 days; max 300 mg/day; *CrCl <30 mL/min or severe hepatic impairment:* not recommended; *Cirrhosis:* max 50 mg q 12 hours
  Pediatric: <12 years: contraindicated; 12-<18: use extreme caution; not recommended for children and adolescents with obesity, asthma, obstructive sleep apnea, or other chronic breathing problem, or for post-tonsillectomy/adenoidectomy pain; ≥18 years: same as adult
    ODT: 50 mg (mint) (phenylalanine)
  Ryzolt initially 100 mg once daily; may increase by 100 mg every; 5 days; max 300 mg/day; *CrCl <30 mL/min or severe hepatic impairment:* not recommended
  Pediatric: <18 years: not recommended; ≥18 years: same as adult
    Tab: 100, 200, 300 mg ext-rel
  Ultram 50-100 mg q 4-6 hours prn; max 400 mg/day; *CrCl <30 mL/min:* max 100 mg q 12 hours; *Cirrhosis:* max 50 mg q 12 hours
  Pediatric: <18 years: not recommended; ≥18 years: same as adult
    Tab: 50 mg
  Ultram ER initially 100 mg once daily; may increase by 100 mg every 5 days; max 300 mg/day; *CrCl <30 mL/min or severe hepatic impairment:* not recommended
  Pediatric: <18 years: not recommended; ≥18 years: same as adult
    Tab: 100, 200, 300 mg ext-rel
Comment: *tramadol* is known to be excreted in breast milk. The FDA and the European Medicines Agency (EMA) are investigating the safety of using *tramadol*-containing medications to treat pain in children 12-18 years because of the potential for serious side effects, including slowed or difficult breathing.
▷ *tramadol+acetaminophen* **(C)(IV)(G)** 2 tabs q 4-6 hours; max 8 tabs/day; 5 days; *CrCl <30 mL/min:* max 2 tabs q 12 hours; max 4 tabs/day x 5 days
  Pediatric: <18 years: not recommended; ≥18 years: same as adult
    Ultracet *Tab:* tram 37.5+acet 325 mg
Comment: *tramadol* is known to be excreted in breast milk. The FDA and the European Medicines Agency (EMA) are investigating the safety of using *tramadol*-containing medications to treat pain in children 12-18 years because of the potential for serious side effects, including slowed or difficult breathing.

MU-OPIOID AGONIST+NOREPINEPHRINE REUPTAKE INHIBITOR COMBINATION

▷ *tapentadol* **(C)**
  Pediatric: <18 years: not recommended; ≥18 years: same as adult
    Nucynta 50-100 mg q 4-6 hours prn; max 700 mg/day on the first day; 600 mg/day on subsequent days
    Tab: 50, 75, 100 mg
    Nucynta ER *Opioid-naïve:* initially 50 mg q 12 hours, then titrate to optimal dose within therapeutic range; usual therapeutic range 100-250 mg q 12 hours;

doses >500 mg not recommended; *Converting from Nucynta:* divide total **Nucynta** daily dose into 2 **Nucynta ER** doses and administer q 12 hours; converting from *oxycodone CR* and other opioids, see mfr recommendations

    Tab: 50, 100, 150, 200, 250 mg ext-rel

 ## PERIPHERAL VASCULAR DISEASE (PVD, ARTERIAL INSUFFICIENCY, INTERMITTENT CLAUDICATION)

ANTIPLATELET THERAPY

➤ *aspirin* (D)(OTC) usually 81 mg once daily; range 75-325 mg once daily

    Ecotrin *Tab/Cap:* 81, 325, 500 mg ent-coat

Comment: *aspirin*-containing medications are contraindicated with history of allergic-type reaction to *aspirin*, children and adolescents with *Varicella* or other viral illness, and 3rd trimester of pregnancy.

➤ *cilostazol* (C) 100 mg bid 1/2 hour before or 2 hours after breakfast or dinner; may reduce to 50 mg bid if used with CYP 3A4 (e.g., azole antifungals, macrolides, *diltiazem, fluvoxamine, fluoxetine, nefazodone, sertraline*) or CYP 2C19 (e.g., *omeprazole*) inhibitors

    Tab: 50, 100 mg

Comment: *cilostazol* may be used with *aspirin*. Cautious use with other antiplatelet agents and anticoagulants.

➤ *clopidogrel* (B) 75 mg daily

    Plavix *Tab:* 75 mg

➤ *dipyridamole* (B)(G) 25-100 mg tid-qid

    Persantine *Tab:* 25, 50, 75 mg

Comment: *dipyridamole* does not potentiate *warfarin* and may be taken concomitantly. Do not administer *dipyridamole* concomitantly with *aspirin*.

➤ *pentoxifylline* (C) 400 mg tid with food

    PentoPak *Tab:* 400 mg ext-rel

    Trental *Tab:* 400 mg sust-rel

➤ *ticlopidine* (B) 250 mg bid with food

    Ticlid *Tab:* 250 mg

Comment: Monitor for neutropenia; resolves after discontinuation.

➤ *warfarin* (X) adjust dose to maintain INR in recommended range; *see Anticoagulation Therapy page 589*

    Coumadin *Tab:* 1*, 2*, 2.5*, 5*, 7.5*, 10* mg

    Coumadin for Injection *Vial:* 2 mg/ml (5 mg) pwdr for reconstitution

Comment: Treatment for over-anticoagulation with *warfarin* is *vitamin K*.

 ## PERLECHE (ANGULAR STOMATITIS)

Comment: Perleche is a form of intertrigo. This localized tissue inflammation and maceration is characterized by constant exposure to saliva, which normally contains bacteria, yeast, and other organisms, in the natural anatomical furrow at the corners of the mouth. Perleche is often misdiagnosed as yeast infection, but almost never responds to anti-yeast agents. Patients with severe vitamin deficiencies (e.g., chronic alcoholism, malnutrition) are often at increased risk. Sensitivities or allergies to toothpaste may be contributing irritants.

Treatment: apply a small amount of a combination of 2.5% *hydrocortisone* cream and *miconazole* cream (which kills yeast, fungi, and many bacteria) to the affected area twice a day. Once the area is clear, recurrence can be prevented with local application of petroleum jelly.

PERTUSSIS (WHOOPING COUGH)

Prophylaxis *see* **Childhood Immunizations** *page* 546

POST-EXPOSURE PROPHYLAXIS AND TREATMENT

Comment: Antibiotics do not alter the course of illness, but they do prevent transmission. Infected persons should be isolated until after the fifth day of antibiotic treatment.

▷ *azithromycin* **(B)(G)** 500 mg x 1 dose on day 1, then 250 mg daily on days 2-5 or 500 mg daily x 3 days
Pediatric: 12 mg/kg/day x 5 days; max 500 mg/day; *see page* 621 *for dose by weight*
   Zithromax *Tab:* 250, 500, 600 mg; *Oral susp:* 100 mg/5 ml (15 ml); 200 mg/5 ml (15, 22.5, 30 ml) (cherry); *Pkt:* 1 gm for reconstitution (cherry-banana)
   Zithromax Tri-pak *Tab:* 3 x 500 mg tabs/pck
   Zithromax Z-pak *Tab:* 6 x 250 mg tabs/pck
   Zmax *Oral susp:* 2 gm ext-rel for reconstitution (cherry-banana) (148 mg Na⁺)
   Comment: *azithromycin* is the drug of choice for infants <1 month-of-age.
▷ *clarithromycin* **(C)(G)** 250 mg bid or 500 mg ext-rel daily x 10 days
Pediatric: <6 months: not recommended; ≥6 months: 7.5 mg/kg divided bid x 10 days; *see page* 630 *for dose by weight*
   Biaxin *Tab:* 250, 500 mg
   Biaxin Oral Suspension *Oral susp:* 125, 250 mg/5 ml (50, 100 ml) (fruit-punch)
   Biaxin XL *Tab:* 500 mg ext-rel
▷ *erythromycin base* **(B)(G)** 1 gm/day divided qid x 14 days
Pediatric: 40 mg/kg/day in divided doses x 14 days
   Ery-Tab *Tab:* 250, 333, 500 mg ent-coat
   PCE *Tab:* 333, 500 mg
▷ *erythromycin ethylsuccinate* **(B)(G)** 1 gm/day in 4 divided doses x 14 days
Pediatric: 40-50 mg/kg/day in 4 divided doses x 7 days; may double dose with severe infection; max 100 mg/kg/day; *see page* 635 *for dose by weight*
   EryPed *Oral susp:* 200 mg/5 ml (100, 200 ml) (fruit); 400 mg/5 ml (60, 100, 200 ml) (banana); Oral drops: 200, 400 mg/5 ml (50 ml) (fruit); *Chew tab:* 200 mg wafer (fruit)
   E.E.S. *Oral susp:* 200, 400 mg/5 ml (100 ml) (fruit)
   E.E.S. Granules *Oral susp:* 200 mg/5 ml (100, 200 ml) (cherry)
   E.E.S. 400 Tablets *Tab:* 400 mg
Comment: *erythromycin* may increase INR with concomitant *warfarin*, as well as increase serum level of *digoxin, benzodiazepines*, and *statins*.
▷ *trimethoprim+sulfamethoxazole (TMP-SMX)* **(C)(G)**
Pediatric: <2 months: not recommended; ≥2 months: 40 mg/kg/day of *sulfamethox-azole* in 2 doses bid x 10 days; *see page* 648 *for dose by weight*
   Bactrim, Septra 2 tabs bid x 10 days
      Tab: trim 80 mg+*sulfa* 400 mg*
   Bactrim DS, Septra DS 1 tab bid x 10 days
      Tab: trim 160 mg+*sulfa* 800 mg
   Bactrim Pediatric Suspension, Septra Pediatric Suspension
      Oral susp: trim 40 mg+*sulfa* 200 mg per 5 ml (100 ml) (cherry) (alcohol 0.3%)

 PHARYNGITIS: GONOCOCCAL

Comment: Treat all sexual contacts. Empiric therapy requires concomitant treatment for *Chlamydia*. Post-treatment culture recommended with PMHx history rheumatic fever.

PRIMARY THERAPY

▷ *azithromycin* (B)(G) 1 gm x 1 dose
　Pediatric: 12 mg/kg/day x 5 days; max 500 mg/day; *see page 621 for dose by weight*
　　Zithromax *Tab:* 250, 500, 600 mg; *Oral susp:* 100 mg/5 ml (15 ml); 200 mg/5 ml
　　(15, 22.5, 30 ml) (cherry); *Pkt:* 1 gm for reconstitution (cherry-banana)
　　Zithromax Tri-pak *Tab:* 3 x 500 mg tabs/pck
　　Zithromax Z-pak *Tab:* 6 x 250 mg tabs/pck
　　Zmax *Oral susp:* 2 gm ext-rel for reconstitution (cherry-banana) (148 mg Na$^+$)
　Comment: Per the CDC 2015 STD Treatment Guidelines, *azithromycin* should be
　used with *ceftriaxone* 250 mg.
▷ *ceftriaxone* (B)(G) 250 mg IM x 1 dose
　Pediatric: <45 kg: 125 mg IM x 1 dose; ≥45 kg: same as adult
　　Rocephin *Vial:* 250, 500 mg; 1, 2 gm

PHARYNGITIS: STREPTOCOCCAL

Comment: Acute rheumatic fever is a rare but serious autoimmune disease that may
occur following a group A *streptococcal* throat infection. It causes inflammatory lesions
in connective tissue, especially that of the heart, kidneys, joints, blood vessels, and
subcutaneous tissue. Prior to the broad availability of penicillin, rheumatic fever was a
leading cause of death in children and one of the leading causes of acquired heart disease
in adults. Strep throat is highly responsive to the penicillins and cephalosporins.

▷ *amoxicillin* (B)(G) 500-875 mg bid or 250-500 mg tid x 10 days
　Pediatric: <40 kg (88 lb): 20-40 mg/kg/day in 3 divided doses x 10 days or 25-45 mg/kg/
　day in 2 divided doses x 10 days; ≥40 kg: same as adult; *see page 616 for dose by weight*
　　Amoxil *Cap:* 250, 500 mg; *Tab:* 875*mg; *Chew tab:* 125, 200, 250, 400 mg
　　(cherry-banana-peppermint) (phenylalanine); *Oral susp:* 125, 250 mg/5 ml (80,
　　100, 150 ml) (strawberry); 200, 400 mg/5 ml (50, 75, 100 ml) (bubble gum); *Oral
　　drops:* 50 mg/ml (30 ml) (bubble gum)
　　Moxatag *Tab:* 775 mg ext-rel
　　Trimox *Tab:* 125, 250 mg; *Cap:* 250, 500 mg; *Oral susp:* 125, 250 mg/5 ml (80, 100,
　　150 ml) (raspberry-strawberry)
▷ *amoxicillin+clavulanate* (B)(G)
　　Augmentin 500 mg tid or 875 mg bid x 7-10 days
　　Pediatric: 40-45 mg/kg/day divided tid x 10 days or 90 mg/kg/day divided bid x
　　10 days *see pages 618-619 for dose by weight*
　　　Tab: 250, 500, 875 mg; *Chew tab:* 125, 250 mg (lemon-lime); 200, 400 mg
　　　(cherry-banana) (phenylalanine); *Oral susp:* 125 mg/5 ml (banana), 250 mg/5
　　　ml (75, 100, 150 ml) (orange); 200, 400 mg/5 ml (50, 75, 100 ml) (orange)
　　　(phenylalanine)
　　Augmentin ES-600 not recommended for adults
　　Pediatric: <3 months: not recommended; ≥3 months, <40 kg: 90 mg/kg/day in 2
　　divided doses x 7-10 days; ≥40 kg: not recommended
　　　Oral susp: 42.9 mg/5 ml (50, 75, 100, 125, 150, 200 ml) (strawberry cream)
　　　(phenylalanine)
　　Augmentin XR 2 tabs q 12 hours x 7-10 days
　　Pediatric: <16 years: use other forms; ≥16 years: same as adult
　　　Tab: 1000*mg ext-rel
▷ *azithromycin* (B)(G) 500 mg x 1 dose on day 1, then 250 mg daily on days 2-5 or 500
　mg daily x 3 days
　Pediatric: 12 mg/kg/day x 5 days; max 500 mg/day; *see page 621 for dose by weight*
　　Zithromax *Tab:* 250, 500, 600 mg; *Oral susp:* 100 mg/5 ml (15 ml); 200 mg/5 ml
　　(15, 22.5, 30 ml) (cherry); *Pkt:* 1 gm for reconstitution (cherry-banana)

Zithromax Tri-pak *Tab:* 3 x 500 mg tabs/pck
Zithromax Z-pak *Tab:* 6 x 250 mg tabs/pck
Zmax *Oral susp:* 2 gm ext-rel for reconstitution (cherry-banana) (148 mg Na⁺)

▷ *cefaclor* (B)(G) 250 mg tid or 375 mg bid x 5 days
Pediatric: <1 month: not recommended; 20-40 mg/kg bid or q 12 hours x 10 days; max 1 gm/day; *see page 622 for dose by weight*
Tab: 500 mg; *Cap:* 250, 500 mg; *Susp:* 125 mg/5 ml (75, 150 ml) (strawberry); 187 mg/5 ml (50, 100 ml) (strawberry); 250 mg/5 ml (75, 150 ml) (strawberry); 375 mg/5 ml (50, 100 ml) (strawberry)
Cefaclor Extended Release
Pediatric: <16 years: ext-rel not recommended; ≥16 years: same as adult
Tab: 375, 500 mg ext-rel

▷ *cefadroxil* (B) 1 gm in 1-2 doses x 10 days
Pediatric: 30 mg/kg/day in 2 divided doses x 10 days; *see page 623 for dose by weight*
Duricef *Cap:* 500 mg; *Tab:* 1 gm; *Oral susp:* 250 mg/5 ml (100 ml); 500 mg/5 ml (75, 100 ml) (orange-pineapple)

▷ *cefdinir* (B) 300 mg bid x 10 days
Pediatric: <6 months: not recommended; 6 months-12 years: 14 mg/kg/day in 1-2 doses x 10 days; *see page 624 for dose by weight;* >12 years: same as adult
Omnicef *Cap:* 300 mg; *Oral susp:* 125 mg/5 ml (60, 100 ml) (strawberry)

▷ *cefditoren pivoxil* (B) 200 mg bid x 10 days
Pediatric: <12 years: not recommended; ≥12 years: same as adult
Spectracef *Tab:* 200 mg
Comment: Spectracef is contraindicated with milk protein allergy or carnitine deficiency.

▷ *cefixime* (B)(G) 400 mg daily x 5 days
Pediatric: <6 months: not recommended; 6 months-12 years, <50 kg: 8 mg/kg/day in 1-2 divided doses x 10 days; *see page 625 for dose by weight;* >12 years, ≥50 kg: same as adult
Suprax *Tab:* 400 mg; *Cap:* 400 mg; *Oral susp:* 100, 200, 500 mg/5 ml (50, 75, 100 ml) (strawberry)

▷ *cefpodoxime proxetil* (B) 100 mg bid x 5-7 days
Pediatric: <2 months: not recommended; 2 months-12 years: 10 mg/kg/day in 2 divided doses x 5-7 days; *see page 626 for dose by weight;* >12 years: same as adult
Vantin *Tab:* 100, 200 mg; *Oral susp:* 50, 100 mg/5 ml (50, 75, 100 ml) (lemon creme)

▷ *cefprozil* (B) 500 mg daily x 10 days
Pediatric: <2 years: not recommended; 2-12 years: 7.5 mg/kg divided bid x 10 days; *see page 627 for dose by weight;* >12 years: same as adult
Cefzil *Tab:* 250, 500 mg; *Oral susp:* 125, 250 mg/5 ml (50, 75, 100 ml) (bubble gum) (phenylalanine)

▷ *ceftibuten* (B) 400 mg daily x 5 days
Pediatric: 9 mg/kg daily x 5 days; *see page 628 for dose by weight*
Cedax *Cap:* 400 mg; *Oral susp:* 90 mg/5 ml (30, 60, 90, 120 ml); 180 mg/5 ml (30, 60, 120 ml) (cherry)

▷ *cephalexin* (B)(G) 500 mg bid x 10 days
Pediatric: 25-50 mg/kg/day in 2 divided doses x 10 days; *see page 629 for dose by weight*
Keflex *Cap:* 250, 333, 500, 750 mg; *Oral susp:* 125, 250 mg/5 ml (100, 200 ml) (strawberry)

▷ *clarithromycin* (C)(G) 250 mg bid or 500 mg ext-rel daily x 10 days
Pediatric: <6 months: not recommended; ≥6 months: 7.5 mg/kg divided bid x 10 days; *see page 630 for dose by weight*
Biaxin *Tab:* 250, 500 mg

       Biaxin Oral Suspension *Oral susp:* 125, 250 mg/5 ml (50, 100 ml) (fruit-punch)
       Biaxin XL *Tab:* 500 mg ext-rel
➤ *dirithromycin* **(C)(G)** 500 mg daily x 10 days
    Pediatric: <12 years: not recommended; ≥12 years: same as adult
       Dynabac *Tab:* 250 mg
➤ *erythromycin base* **(B)(G)** 500 mg qid x 10 days
    Pediatric: <45 kg: 30-50 mg divided bid-qid x 10 days; ≥45 kg: same as adult
       Ery-Tab *Tab:* 250, 333, 500 mg ent-coat
       PCE *Tab:* 333, 500 mg

Comment: *erythromycin* may increase INR with concomitant *warfarin*, as well as increase serum level of *digoxin, benzodiazepines*, and *statins*.

➤ *erythromycin estolate* **(B)(G)** 250-500 mg qid x 10 days
    Pediatric: 20-50 mg/kg divided q 6 hours x 10 days; *see page 634 for dose by weight*
       Ilosone *Pulvule:* 250 mg; *Tab:* 500 mg; *Liq:* 125, 250 mg/5 ml (100 ml)

Comment: *erythromycin* may increase INR with concomitant *warfarin*, as well as increase serum level of *digoxin, benzodiazepines*, and *statins*.

➤ *erythromycin ethylsuccinate* **(B)(G)** 400 mg qid or 800 mg bid x 10 days
    Pediatric: 30-50 mg/kg/day in 4 divided doses x 7 days; may double dose with severe infection; max 100 mg/kg/day; *see page 635 for dose by weight*
       EryPed *Oral susp:* 200 mg/5 ml (100, 200 ml) (fruit); 400 mg/5 ml (60, 100, 200 ml) (banana); *Oral drops:* 200, 400 mg/5 ml (50 ml) (fruit); *Chew tab:* 200 mg wafer (fruit)
       E.E.S. *Oral susp:* 200, 400 mg/5 ml (100 ml) (fruit)
       E.E.S. Granules *Oral susp:* 200 mg/5 ml (100, 200 ml) (cherry)
       E.E.S. 400 Tablets *Tab:* 400 mg

Comment: *erythromycin* may increase INR with concomitant *warfarin*, as well as increase serum level of *digoxin, benzodiazepines*, and *statins*.

➤ *loracarbef* **(B)** 200 mg bid x 5 days
    Pediatric: 15 mg/kg/day in 2 divided doses x 5 days; *see page 642 for dose by weight*
       Lorabid *Pulvule:* 200, 400 mg; *Oral susp:* 100 mg/5 ml (50, 100 ml); 200 mg/5 ml (50, 75, 100 ml) (strawberry bubble gum)
➤ *penicillin g (benzathine)* **(B)(G)** 1.2 million units IM x 1 dose
    Pediatric: <60 lb: 300,000-600,000 units IM x 1 dose; ≥60 lb: 900,000 units x 1 dose
       Bicillin L-A *Cartridge-needle unit:* 600,000 units (1 ml); 1.2 million units (2 ml)
➤ *penicillin g (benzathine and procaine)* **(B)(G)** 2.4 million units IM x 1 dose
    Pediatric: <30 lb: 600,000 units IM x 1 dose; 30-60 lb: 900,000-1.2 million units IM x 1 dose; >60 lb: same as adult
       Bicillin C-R *Cartridge-needle unit:* 600,000 units (1 ml); 1.2 million units; (2 ml); 2.4 million units (4 ml)
➤ *penicillin v potassium* **(B)(G)** 500 mg bid or 250 mg qid x 10 days
    Pediatric: <12 years: 25-50 mg/kg day in 4 divided doses x 10 days; *see page 644 for dose by weight;* >12 years: same as adult
       Pen-Vee K *Tab:* 250, 500 mg; *Oral soln:* 125 mg/5 ml (100, 200 ml); 250 mg/5 ml (100, 150, 200 ml)
       Veetids *Tab:* 250, 500 mg; *Oral soln:* 125, 250 mg/5 ml (100, 200 ml)

PHEOCHROMOCYTOMA

ALPHA-BLOCKER

➤ *phenoxybenzamine* **(C)** initially 10 mg bid; increase every other day as needed; usually 20-40 mg bid-tid
       Dibenzyline *Cap:* 10 mg

PINWORM (*ENTEROBIUS VERMICULARIS*)

Comment: Treatment of all family members is recommended.

ANTHELMINTICS

Comment: Oral bioavailability of anthelmintics is enhanced when administered with a fatty meal (estimated fat content 40 gm). Treatment of all family members is recommended. Some clinicians recommend all household contacts of infected patients receive treatment, especially when multiple or repeated symptomatic infections occur, since such contacts commonly also are infected; retreatment after 14 to 21 days may be needed.

▷ *albendazole* (C) 400 mg x 1 dose; may repeat in 2-3 weeks if needed; take with a meal
  Pediatric: <20 kg: 200 mg as a single dose; ≥20 kg: same as adult
    Albenza *Tab:* 200 mg

▷ *mebendazole* (C) chew, swallow, or mix with food; 100 mg x 1 dose; may repeat in 3 weeks if needed; take with a meal
  Pediatric: <2 years: not recommended; ≥2 years: same as adult
    Emverm *Chew tab:* 100 mg
    Vermox (G) *Chew tab:* 100 mg

▷ *pyrantel pamoate* (C) 11 mg/kg x 1 dose; max 1 gm/dose; may repeat in 2-3 weeks if needed; take with a meal
  Pediatric: 25-37 lb: 1/2 tsp x 1 dose; 38-62 lb: 1 tsp x 1 dose; 63-87 lb: 1 tsp x 1 dose; 88-112 lb: 2 tsp x 1 dose; 113-137 lb: 2 tsp x 1 dose; 138-162 lb: 3 tsp x 1 dose; 163-187 lb: 3 tsp x 1 dose; >187 lb: 4 tsp x 1 dose
    Pin-X (OTC); *Cap:* 180 mg; *Liq:* 50 mg/ml (30 ml); 144 mg/ml (30 ml); *Oral susp:* 50 mg/ml (30 ml)

▷ *thiabendazole* (C) 50 mg/kg x 1 dose after a meal; max 3 gm; may repeat in 2-3 weeks if needed; take with a meal
  Pediatric: same as adult
    Mintezol *Chew tab:* 500*mg (orange); *Oral susp:* 500 mg/5 ml (120 ml) (orange)
    Comment: *thiabendazole* is not for prophylaxis and should not be used as first-line therapy for pinworms. May impair mental alertness. May not be available in the US.

 PITYRIASIS ALBA

Topical Corticosteroids *see page* 566

Comment: Pityriasis alba is a chronic skin disorder seen in children with a genetic predisposition to atopic disease. Treatment is directed toward controlling roughness and pruritus. There is no known treatment for the associated skin pigment changes. Pityriasis alba resolves spontaneously and permanently in the 2nd or 3rd decade of life.

COAL TAR PREPARATIONS

▷ *coal tar* (C)
  Pediatric: same as adult
    Scytera (OTC) apply qd-qid; use lowest effective dose
      Foam: 2%
    T/Gel Shampoo Extra Strength (OTC) use every other day; max 4 x/week; massage into affected area for 5 minutes; rinse; repeat
      Shampoo: 1%
    T/Gel Shampoo Original Formula (OTC) use every other day; max 7 x/week; massage into affected area for 5 minutes; rinse; repeat
      Shampoo: 0.5%

T/Gel Shampoo Stubborn Itch Control (OTC) use every other day; max 7 x/ week; massage into affected area for 5 minutes; rinse; repeat
    Shampoo: 0.5%

EMOLLIENTS AND OTHER MOISTURIZING AGENTS

see **Dermatitis: Atopic** *page* 122

 PITYRIASIS ROSEA

Topical Corticosteroids *see page* 566
Antihistamines *see* **Drugs for the Management of Allergy, Cough, and Cold Symptoms** *see page* 598

 PLAGUE (*YERSINIA PESTIS*)

Comment: *Yersinia pestis* is transmitted via the bite of a flea from an infected rodent <u>or</u> the bite, lick, <u>or</u> scratch of an infected cat. Untreated bubonic plague may progress to secondary pneumonic plague, which may be transmitted via contaminated respiratory droplet spread.

▷ *streptomycin* (C)(G) 15 mg/kg IM bid x 10 days
    Pediatric: same as adult
    Amp: 1 gm/2.5 ml <u>or</u> 400 mg/ml (2.5 ml)
    Comment: For patients with renal impairment, reduce dose of *streptomycin* to 20 mg/ kg/day if mild and 8 mg/kg/day q 3 days if advanced). For patients who are pregnant <u>or</u> who have hearing impairment, shorten the course of treatment to 3 days after fever has resolved.

▷ *moxifloxacin* (C)(G) 400 mg daily x 10 days
    Pediatric: <18 years: not recommended; ≥18 years: same as adult
    Avelox *Tab:* 400 mg; IV soln: 400 mg/250 mg (latex-free, preservative-free)

▷ *tetracycline* (D)(G) 500 mg qid <u>or</u> 25-50 mg/kg/day divided q 6 hours x 10 days
    Pediatric: <8 years: not recommended; ≥8 years: same as adult

Comment: *tetracycline* is contraindicated <8 years-of-age, in pregnancy, and lactation (discolors developing tooth enamel). A side effect may be photosensitivity (photophobia). Do not give with antacids, calcium supplements, milk or other dairy, or within two hours of taking another drug.

 PNEUMONIA: CHLAMYDIAL

RECOMMENDED REGIMEN

▷ *erythromycin base* (B)(G) 500 mg qid hours x 10-14 days
    Pediatric: <45 kg: 50 mg in 4 divided doses x 10-14 days; ≥45 kg: same as adult
    Ery-Tab *Tab:* 250, 333, 500 mg ent-coat
    PCE *Tab:* 333, 500 mg

Comment: *erythromycin* may increase INR with concomitant *warfarin*, as well as increase serum level of *digoxin, benzodiazepines*, and *statins*.

▷ *erythromycin ethylsuccinate* (B)(G) 400 mg qid x 10-14 days
    Pediatric: <45 kg: 50 mg/kg/day in 4 divided doses x 10-14 days; ≥45 kg: same as adult; *see page* 635 *for dose by weight*
    EryPed *Oral susp:* 200 mg/5 ml (100, 200 ml) (fruit); 400 mg/5 ml (60, 100, 200 ml) (banana); *Oral drops:* 200, 400 mg/5 ml (50 ml) (fruit); *Chew tab:* 200 mg wafer (fruit)

E.E.S. *Oral susp:* 200, 400 mg/5 ml (100 ml) (fruit)
E.E.S. Granules *Oral susp:* 200 mg/5 ml (100, 200 ml) (cherry)
E.E.S. 400 Tablets *Tab:* 400 mg

Comment: *erythromycin* may increase INR with concomitant *warfarin*, as well as increase serum level of *digoxin, benzodiazepines*, and *statins*.

ALTERNATE REGIMENS

▷ *azithromycin* (B)(G) 500 mg once daily x 10 days
Pediatric: 20 mg/kg per dose once daily x 3 days; max 500 mg/day; *see page* 621 *for dose by weight*
Zithromax *Tab:* 250, 500, 600 mg; *Oral susp:* 100 mg/5 ml (15 ml); 200 mg/5 ml (15, 22.5, 30 ml) (cherry); *Pkt:* 1 gm for reconstitution (cherry-banana)
Zithromax Tri-pak *Tab:* 3 x 500 mg tabs/pck
Zithromax Z-pak *Tab:* 6 x 250 mg tabs/pck
Zmax *Oral susp:* 2 gm ext-rel for reconstitution (cherry-banana) (148 mg Na$^+$)
▷ *levofloxacin* (C) *Uncomplicated:* 500 mg daily x 7 days; *Complicated:* 750 mg daily x 7 days
Pediatric: <18 years: not recommended; ≥18 years: same as adult
Levaquin *Tab:* 250, 500, 750 mg; *Oral soln:* 25 mg/ml (480 ml) (benzyl alcohol); *Inj conc:* 25 mg/ml for IV infusion after dilution (20, 30 ml single-use vial) (preservative-free); *Premix soln:* 5 mg/ml for IV infusion (50, 100, 150 ml) (preservative-free)

Comment: *levofloxacin* is contraindicated <18 years-of-age, and during pregnancy and lactation. Risk of tendonitis or tendon rupture.

PNEUMONIA: COMMUNITY ACQUIRED (CAP) AND COMMUNITY ACQUIRED BACTERIAL PNEUMONIA (CABP)

Comment: Over 70% of patients with uncomplicated community-acquired pneumonia (CAP) received prescriptions for antibiotics that exceeded national duration recommendations, according to a retrospective study that included 22,128 patients from 18 to 64 years-of-age with private insurance and 130,746 patients aged >65 years with Medicare, who were hospitalized with uncomplicated CAP. Length of antibiotic therapy (LOT) during hospital stay was estimated using the MarketScan Hospital Drug Database and outpatient LOT was determined using prescriptions filled at discharge. The researchers defined excessive duration as a LOT of more than 3 days.

REFERENCE

Yi, S. H., Hatfield, K. M., Baggs, J., Hicks, L. A., Srinivasan, A., Reddy, S., & Jernigan, J. A. (2017). Duration of Antibiotic Use Among Adults With Uncomplicated Community-Acquired Pneumonia Requiring Hospitalization in the United States. *Clinical Infectious Diseases.* doi:10.1093/cid/cix986

ANTI-INFFECTIVES

▷ *amoxicillin* (B)(G) 500-875 mg bid <u>or</u> 250-500 mg tid x 3-10 days
Pediatric: <40 kg (88 lb): 20-40 mg/kg/day in 3 divided doses x 3-10 days <u>or</u> 25-45 mg/kg/day in 2 divided doses x 3-10 days; ≥40 kg: same as adult
Amoxil *Cap:* 250, 500 mg; *Tab:* 875 mg; *Chew tab:* 125, 200, 250, 400 mg (cherry-banana-peppermint) (phenylalanine); *Oral susp:* 125, 250 mg/5 ml (80, 100, 150 ml) (strawberry); 200, 400 mg/5 ml (50, 75, 100 ml) (bubble gum); *Oral drops:* 50 mg/ml (30 ml) (bubble gum)
Moxatag *Tab:* 775 mg ext-rel
Trimox *Tab:* 125, 250 mg; *Cap:* 250, 500 mg; *Oral susp:* 125, 250 mg/5 ml (80, 100, 150 ml) (raspberry-strawberry)

➢ *amoxicillin+clavulanate* **(B)(G)** 500 mg tid <u>or</u> 875 mg bid x 3-10 days
    Augmentin 500 mg tid <u>or</u> 875 mg bid x 3-10 days
    Pediatric: 40-45 mg/kg/day divided tid x 10 days <u>or</u> 90 mg/kg/day divided bid x
    10 days *see pages 612-613 for dose by weight*
        Tab: 250, 500, 875 mg; *Chew tab:* 125, 250 mg (lemon-lime); 200, 400 mg
        (cherry-banana) (phenylalanine); *Oral susp:* 125 mg/5 ml (banana), 250 mg/5
        ml (75, 100, 150 ml) (orange); 200, 400 mg/5 ml (50, 75, 100 ml) (orange)
        (phenylalanine)
    Augmentin ES-600 not recommended for adults
    Pediatric: <3 months: not recommended; ≥3 months, <40 kg: 90 mg/kg/day in 2
    divided doses x 3-10 days; ≥40 kg: not recommended
        Oral susp: 42.9 mg/5 ml (50, 75, 100, 125, 150, 200 ml) (strawberry cream)
        (phenylalanine)
    Augmentin XR 2 tabs q 12 hours x 3-10 days
    Pediatric: <16 years: use other forms; ≥16 years: same as adult
        Tab: 1000*mg ext-rel

➢ *azithromycin* **(B)(G)** *Day 1,* 500 mg as a single dose <u>and</u> *Days 2-5,* 250 mg once daily
    <u>or</u> 500 mg once daily x 3 days
    Pediatric: <6 months: not recommended; ≥6 months: 10 mg/kg x 1 dose on day 1;
    then 5 mg/kg/day on days 2-5; max 500 mg/day; *see page 615 for dose by weight*
        Zithromax *Tab:* 250, 500, 600 mg; *Oral susp:* 100 mg/5 ml (15 ml); 200 mg/5 ml
        (15, 22.5, 30 ml) (cherry); *Pkt:* 1 gm for reconstitution (cherry-banana)
        Zithromax Tri-pak *Tab:* 3 x 500 mg tabs/pck
        Zithromax Z-pak *Tab:* 6 x 250 mg tabs/pck
        Zmax *Oral susp:* 2 gm ext-rel for reconstitution (cherry-banana) (148 mg Na⁺)

➢ *cefaclor* **(B)(G)** 250 mg tid <u>or</u> 375 mg bid 3-10 days
    Pediatric: <1 month: not recommended; 1 month-12 years: 20-40 mg/kg divided bid
    <u>or</u> q 12 hours x 3-10 days; max 1 gm/day; *see page 616 for dose by weight;* >12 years:
    same as adult
        Tab: 500 mg; *Cap:* 250, 500 mg; *Susp:* 125 mg/5 ml (75, 150 ml) (strawberry);
        187 mg/5 ml (50, 100 ml) (strawberry); 250 mg/5 ml (75, 150 ml) (strawber-
        ry); 375 mg/5 ml (50, 100 ml) (strawberry)
    Cefaclor Extended Release 375-500 mg bid x 3-10 days
    Pediatric: <16 years: ext-rel not recommended; ≥16 years: same as adult
        Tab: 375, 500 mg ext-rel

➢ *cefdinir* **(B)** 300 mg bid <u>or</u> 600 mg daily x 3-10 days
    Pediatric: <6 months: not recommended; 6 months-12 years: 14 mg/kg/day in a single
    <u>or</u> 2 divided doses x 3-10 days; *see page 618 for dose by weight;* >12 years: same as
    adult
        Omnicef *Cap:* 300 mg; *Oral susp:* 125 mg/5 ml (60, 100 ml) (strawberry)

➢ *cefpodoxime proxetil* **(B)** 200 mg bid x 3-10 days
    Pediatric: 2 months-12 years: 10 mg/kg/day in 2 divided doses x 3-5 days; *see page*
    620 for dose by weight; >12 years: same as adult
        Vantin *Tab:* 100, 200 mg; *Oral susp:* 50, 100 mg/5 ml (50, 75, 100 ml) (lemon
        creme)

➢ *ceftaroline fosamil* **(B)** administer by IV infusion after reconstitution every 12 hours x
    3-10 days; *CrCl ≥50 mL/min:* 600 mg; *CrCl >30-<50 mL/min:* 400 mg; *CrCl: >15-<30*
    mL/min: 300 mg; ES RD: 200 mg
    Pediatric: <18 years: not recommended; ≥18 years: same as adult
        Teflaro *Vial:* 400, 600 mg

➢ *ceftriaxone* **(B)(G)** 1-2 gm IM daily; x 1-3 days
    Pediatric: 50-75 mg/kg IM in 2 divided doses; max 2 gm/day x 1-3 days
        Rocephin *Vial:* 250, 500 mg; 1, 2 gm

➤ *clarithromycin* (C)(G) 500 mg bid <u>or</u> 500 mg ext-rel daily x 3-10 days
  Pediatric: <6 months: not recommended; ≥6 months: 7.5 mg/kg bid x 3-10 days
    Biaxin *Tab:* 250, 500 mg
    Biaxin Oral Suspension *Oral susp:* 125, 250 mg/5 ml (50, 100 ml) (fruit-punch)
    Biaxin XL *Tab:* 500 mg ext-rel
➤ *dirithromycin* (C)(G) 500 mg daily x 3-10 days
  Pediatric: <12 years: not recommended; ≥12 years: same as adult
    Dynabac *Tab:* 250 mg
➤ *doxycycline* (D)(G) 100 mg bid x 3-10 days
  Pediatric: <8 years: not recommended; ≥8 years, ≤100 lb: 2 mg/lb on first day in 2 divided doses, followed by 1 mg/lb/day in 1-2 divided doses; ≥8 years, >100 lb: same as adult; *see page 627 for dose by weight*
    Acticlate *Tab:* 75, 150**mg
    Adoxa *Tab:* 50, 75, 100, 150 mg ent-coat
    Doryx *Tab:* 50, 75, 100, 150, 200 mg del-rel
    Doxteric *Tab:* 50 mg del-rel
    Monodox *Cap:* 50, 75, 100 mg
    Oracea *Cap:* 40 mg del-rel
    Vibramycin Tab: 100 mg; *Cap:* 50, 100 mg; *Syr:* 50 mg/5 ml (raspberry-apple) (sulfites); *Oral susp:* 25 mg/5 ml (raspberry)
    Vibra-Tab *Tab:* 100 mg film-coat
Comment: *doxycycline* is contraindicated <8 years-of-age, in pregnancy, and lactation (discolors developing tooth enamel). A side effect may be photosensitivity (photophobia). Do not take with antacids, calcium supplements, milk <u>or</u> other dairy, <u>or</u> within 2 hours of taking another drug.
➤ *ertapenem* (B) 1 gm daily; *CrCl <30 mL/min:* 500 mg daily x 3-10 days; may switch to an oral antibiotic after 3 days if warranted; *IV infusion:* administer over 30 minutes; *IM injection:* reconstitute with lidocaine only
    Invanz *Vial:* 1 gm pwdr for reconstitution
➤ *erythromycin base* (B)(G) 500 mg q 6 hours x 14-21 days; <45 kg: 30-50 mg in 2-4 doses x 3-10 days; ≥45 kg: same as adult
    Ery-Tab *Tab:* 250, 333, 500 mg ent-coat
    PCE *Tab:* 333, 500 mg
Comment: **erythromycin** may increase INR with concomitant *warfarin*, as well as increase serum level of *digoxin*, *benzodiazepines*, and *statins*.
➤ *erythromycin estolate* (B) 500 mg q 6 hours x 3-10 days
    Ilosone *Pulvule:* 250 mg; *Tab:* 500 mg; *Liq:* 125, 250 mg/5 ml (100 ml)
Comment: **erythromycin** may increase INR with concomitant *warfarin*, as well as increase serum level of *digoxin*, *benzodiazepines*, and *statins*.
➤ *gemifloxacin* (C)(G) 320 mg daily x 3-10 days
  Pediatric: <18 years: not recommended; ≥18 years: same as adult
    Factive *Tab:* 320*mg
➤ *levofloxacin* (C) *250 mg* once daily x 3-10 days
  Pediatric: <18 years: not recommended; ≥18 years: same as adult
    Levaquin *Tab:* 250, 500, 750 mg; *Oral soln:* 25 mg/ml (480 ml) (benzyl alcohol); *Inj conc:* 25 mg/ml for IV infusion after dilution (20, 30 ml single-use vial) (preservative-free); *Premix soln:* 5 mg/ml for IV infusion (50, 100, 150 ml) (preservative-free)
➤ *linezolid* (C)(G) 400-600 mg q 12 hours x 10-14 days
  Pediatric: <5 years: 10 mg/kg q 8 hours x 10-14 days; 5-11 years: 10 mg/kg q 12 hours x 10-14 days; >11 years: same as adult
    Zyvox *Tab:* 400, 600 mg; *Oral susp:* 100 mg/5 ml (150 ml) (orange) (phenylalanine)

Comment: *linezolid* is indicated to treat susceptible vancomycin-resistant *E. faecium* infections.

➤ *loracarbef* (B) 400 mg bid x 3-10 days
  Pediatric: <12 years: 15 mg/kg/day in 2 divided doses x 7 days; *see page 612 for dose by weight table;* ≥12 years: 200 mg bid x 7 days
    Lorabid *Pulvule:* 200, 400 mg; *Oral susp:* 100 mg/5 ml (50, 100 ml); 200 mg/5 ml (50, 75, 100 ml) (strawberry bubble gum)

➤ *moxifloxacin* (C)(G) 400 mg daily x 3-10 days
  Pediatric: <18 years: not recommended; ≥18 years: same as adult
    Avelox *Tab:* 400 mg; IV soln: 400 mg/250 mg (latex-free, preservative-free)

➤ *ofloxacin* (C)(G) 400 mg bid x 3-10 days
  Pediatric: <18 years: not recommended; ≥18 years: same as adult
    Floxin *Tab:* 200, 300, 400 mg

➤ *penicillin v potassium* (B) 250-500 mg q 6 hours x 3-10 days
  Pediatric: <12 years: 25-75 mg/kg day divided q 6-8 hours x 5-7 days; *see page 614 for dose by weight table;* ≥12 years: same as adult
    Pen-VK *Tab:* 250, 500 mg; *Oral soln:* 125 mg/5 ml (100, 200 ml); 250 mg/5 ml (100, 150, 200 ml)

➤ *tedizolid phosphate* (B) administer 200 mg once daily x 6 days, via PO or IV infusion over 1 hour
    Sivextro *Tab:* 200 mg (6/blister pck)
Comment: Sivextro is indicated for the treatment of community acquired bacterial pneumonia (CABP)

➤ *telithromycin* (C) 2 x 400 mg tabs in a single dose once daily x 3-5 days
  Pediatric: <8 years: not recommended; ≥8 years: same as adult
    Ketek *Tab:* 300, 400 mg
Comment: *telithromycin* is contraindicated with PMHx hepatitis or jaundice associated with macrolide use.

➤ *tigecycline* (D)(G) 100 mg once; then 50 mg q 12 hours x 3-5 days; *Severe hepatic impairment (Child-Pugh Class C):* 100 mg once; then 25 mg q 12 hours x 3-5 days
  Pediatric: <18 years: not recommended; ≥18 years: same as adult
    Tygacil *Vial:* 50 mg pwdr for reconstitution and IV infusion (preservative-free)
Comment: Tygacil is indicated only for the treatment of adults (≥18 years-of-age) with community acquired bacterial pneumonia (CABP). *tigecycline* is contraindicated in pregnancy, and lactation (discolors developing tooth enamel). A side effect may be photo-sensitivity (photophobia). Do not give with antacids, calcium supplements, milk or other dairy, or within two hours of taking another drug.

➤ *trimethoprim+sulfamethoxazole* (TMP-SMX) (C)(G)
  Pediatric: <2 months: not recommended; ≥2 months: 40 mg/kg/day of *sulfamethoxazole* in 2 doses bid x 3-10 days; *see page 642 for dose by weight*
    Bactrim, Septra 2 tabs bid x 3-10 days
      Tab: trim 80 mg+*sulfa* 400 mg*
    Bactrim DS, Septra DS 1 tab bid x 3-10 days
      Tab: trim 160 mg+*sulfa* 800 mg*
    Bactrim Pediatric Suspension, Septra Pediatric Suspension 160/800 bid x 3-10 days
      Oral susp: trim 40 mg+*sulfa* 200 mg per 5 ml (100 ml) (cherry) (alcohol 0.3%)

PNEUMONIA: LEGIONELLA

ANTI-INFECTIVES

➤ *ciprofloxacin* (C) 500 mg bid x 14-21 days
  Pediatric: <18 years: not recommended; ≥18 years: same as adult

Cipro (G) *Tab:* 250, 500, 750 mg; *Oral susp:* 250, 500 mg/5 ml (100 ml) (strawberry)
Cipro XR *Tab:* 500, 1000 mg ext-rel
ProQuin XR *Tab:* 500 mg ext-rel
▷ *clarithromycin* (C)(G) 500 mg bid or 500 mg ext-rel daily x 14-21 days
Biaxin *Tab:* 250, 500 mg
Biaxin Oral Suspension *Oral susp:* 125, 250 mg/5 ml (50, 100 ml) (fruit-punch)
Biaxin XL *Tab:* 500 mg ext-rel
▷ *dirithromycin* (C)(G) 500 mg once daily x 14-21 days
Dynabac *Tab:* 250 mg
▷ *erythromycin base* (B)(G) 500 mg qid x 14-21 days
Pediatric: <45 kg: 30-50 mg in 2-4 divided doses x 14-21 days; ≥45 kg: same as adult
Ery-Tab *Tab:* 250, 333, 500 mg ent-coat
PCE *Tab:* 333, 500 mg

Comment: *erythromycin* may increase INR with concomitant *warfarin*, as well as
increase serum level of *digoxin, benzodiazepines*, and *statins*.

▷ *erythromycin estolate* (B)(G) 1-2 gm daily in divided doses x 14-21 days
Pediatric: 30-50 mg/kg/day in divided doses x 14-21 days; *see page* 634 *for dose by weight*
Ilosone *Pulvule:* 250 mg; *Tab:* 500 mg; *Liq:* 125, 250 mg/5 ml (100 ml)

Comment: *erythromycin* may increase INR with concomitant *warfarin*, as well as
increase serum level of *digoxin, benzodiazepines*, and *statins*.

▷ *trimethoprim+sulfamethoxazole (TMP-SMX)* (C)(G)
Pediatric: <2 months: not recommended; ≥2 months: 40 mg/kg/day of *sulfamethox-azole* in 2 doses bid x 10 days
Bactrim, Septra 2 tabs bid x 10 days
Tab: trim 80 mg+*sulfa* 400 mg*
Bactrim DS, Septra DS 1 tab bid x 10 days
Tab: trim 160 mg+*sulfa* 800 mg*
Bactrim Pediatric Suspension, Septra Pediatric Suspension
Oral susp: trim 40 mg+*sulfa* 200 mg per 5 ml (100 ml) (cherry) (alcohol 0.3%)

◯ PNEUMONIA: MYCOPLASMA

ANTI-INFECTIVES

▷ *azithromycin* (B)(G) 500 mg x 1 dose on day 1, then 250 mg daily on days 2-5 or 500
mg daily x 3 days or Zmax 2 gm in a single dose
Pediatric: 12 mg/kg/day x 5 days; max 500 mg/day; *see page* 621 *for dose by weight*
Zithromax *Tab:* 250, 500, 600 mg; *Oral susp:* 100 mg/5 ml (15 ml); 200 mg/5 ml
(15, 22.5, 30 ml) (cherry); *Pkt:* 1 gm for reconstitution (cherry-banana)
Zithromax Tri-pak *Tab:* 3 x 500 mg tabs/pck
Zithromax Z-pak *Tab:* 6 x 250 mg tabs/pck
Zmax *Oral susp:* 2 gm ext-rel for reconstitution (cherry-banana) (148 mg Na⁺)
▷ *clarithromycin* (C)(G) 500 mg bid or 500 mg ext-rel daily x 14-21 days
Pediatric: <6 months: not recommended; ≥6 months: 7.5 mg/kg bid x 7 days; *see page*
630 *for dose by weight*
Biaxin *Tab:* 250, 500 mg
Biaxin Oral Suspension *Oral susp:* 125, 250 mg/5 ml (50, 100 ml) (fruit-punch)
Biaxin XL *Tab:* 500 mg ext-rel
▷ *erythromycin base* (B)(G) 500 mg q 6 hours x 14-21 days
Pediatric: <45 kg: 30-50 mg in 2-4 doses x 14-21 days; ≥45 kg: same as adult
Ery-Tab *Tab:* 250, 333, 500 mg ent-coat
PCE *Tab:* 333, 500 mg

Comment: *erythromycin* may increase INR with concomitant *warfarin*, as well as
increase serum level of *digoxin, benzodiazepines*, and *statins*.

▷ *erythromycin ethylsuccinate* **(B)(G)** 400 mg qid x 14-21 days
Pediatric: 30-50 mg/kg/day in 4 divided doses x 14-21 days; may double dose with severe infection; max 100 mg/kg/day; *see page 635 for dose by weight*

EryPed *Oral susp:* 200 mg/5 ml (100, 200 ml) (fruit); 400 mg/5 ml (60, 100, 200 ml) (banana); *Oral drops:* 200, 400 mg/5 ml (50 ml) (fruit); *Chew tab:* 200 mg wafer (fruit)

E.E.S. *Oral susp:* 200, 400 mg/5 ml (100 ml) (fruit)

E.E.S. Granules *Oral susp:* 200 mg/5 ml (100, 200 ml) (cherry)

E.E.S. 400 Tablets *Tab:* 400 mg

Comment: *erythromycin* may increase INR with concomitant **warfarin**, as well as increase serum level of **digoxin, benzodiazepines**, and **statins**.

▷ *tetracycline* **(D)(G)** 500 mg qid
Pediatric: <8 years: not recommended; ≥8 years, <100 lb: 25-50 mg/kg/day in 2-4 divided doses; ≥8 years, ≥100 lb: same as adult; *see page 646 for dose by weight*

Achromycin V *Cap:* 250, 500 mg

Sumycin *Tab:* 250, 500 mg; *Cap:* 250, 500 mg; *Oral susp:* 125 mg/5 ml (100, 200 ml) (fruit) (sulfites)

PNEUMONIA: PNEUMOCOCCAL

TREATMENT

see CAP/CABP *page 378*

PROPHYLAXIS

▷ *pneumococcal* vaccine **(C)** 0.5 ml IM or SC in deltoid x 1 dose

Pneumovax

Pediatric: <2 years: not recommended; ≥2 years: same as adult
Vial: 25 mcg/0.5 ml (single-dose, 10/pck; multi-dose, 2.5 ml, 10/pck)

Pnu-Imune 23

Pediatric: <2 years: not recommended; ≥2 years: same as adult
Vial: 25 mcg/0.5 ml (0.5 ml single-dose, 5/pck; 2.5 ml)

Prevnar 13 for adults ≥50 years of age

Pediatric: total 4 doses: 2, 4, 6, and 12-15 months-of-age; may start at 6 weeks of age; administer first 3 doses 4-8 weeks apart and the 4th dose at least 2 months after the 3rd dose

Vial: 25 mcg/0.5 ml (single-dose, 10/pck); *Prefilled syringe:* (single-dose, 10/pck; 2.5 ml, multi-dose)

Comment: Pneumococcal vaccine contains 23 polysaccharide isolates representing approximately 85-90% of common U.S. isolates. Administer the pneumococcal vaccine in the anterolateral aspect of the thigh for infants and the deltoid for toddlers, children, and adults.

PNEUMONIA (*PNEUMOCYSTIS JIROVECI*)

▷ *atovaquone* **(C)** take with food; Treatment: 750 mg once daily x 21 days; Prophylaxis: 1500 mg once daily
Pediatric: see mfr pkg insert

Mepron *Susp:* 750 mg/5 ml (citrus)

▷ *trimethoprim+sulfamethoxazole (TMP-SMX)* **(C)(G)** Prophylaxis: 1 tab 3 x/week; Treatment: 1 tab daily x 3 weeks; *Septra* can be given if intolerable to *Bactrim*
Pediatric: <2 months: not recommended; ≥2 months: 40 mg/kg/day of *sulfamethoxazole* in 2 doses bid x 10 days

Bactrim, Septra 2 tabs bid x 10 days
Tab: trim 80 mg+sulfa 400 mg*
Bactrim DS, Septra DS 1 tab bid x 10 days
Tab: trim 160 mg+sulfa 800 mg*
Bactrim Pediatric Suspension, Septra Pediatric Suspension
Oral susp: trim 40 mg+sulfa 200 mg per 5 ml (100 ml) (cherry) (alcohol 0.3%)

 POLIOMYELITIS

PROPHYLAXIS

▷ *trivalent poliovirus vaccine, inactivated (type 1, 2, and 3)* (C)
Pediatric: <6 weeks: not recommended; ≥6 weeks: one dose at 2, 4, 6-18 months and
4-6 years of age
Ipol 0.5 ml SC or IM in deltoid area

 POLYCYSTIC OVARIAN SYNDROME (PCOS, STEIN-LEVENTHAL DISEASE)

See **Contraceptives** *page* 548
See **Type 2 Diabetes Mellitus** *page* 486

 POLYMYALGIA RHEUMATICA

Oral Corticosteroids *see page* 569
Calcium and Vitamin D Supplementation see **Hypocalcemia** *page* 255

Comment: Initial treatment is low-dose prednisone at 12-25 mg/day. May attempt a
very slow tapering regimen after 2-4 weeks. If relapse occurs, increase the daily dose of
corticosteroid to the previous effective dose. Most people with polymyalgia rheumatica
need to continue corticosteroid treatment for at least a year. Approximately 30-60%
of people will have at least one relapse during corticosteroid tapering. Joint guidelines
from the American Academy of Rheumatology (AAR) and the European League
Against Rheumatism (ELAR) suggest using concomitant *methotrexate* (MTX) along
with corticosteroids in some patients. It may be useful early in the course of treatment
or later, if the patient relapses or does not respond to corticosteroids. The American
Academy of Rheumatology (AAR) recommends the following daily doses for anyone
on a chronic oral corticosteroid regimen: Calcium 1,200-1,500 mg/day and vitamin D
800-1,000 IU/day.

▷ *methotrexate* (X) 7.5 mg x 1 dose per week or 2.5 mg x 3 at 12 hour intervals once a
week; max 20 mg/week; therapeutic response begins in 3-6 weeks; administer methotrexate injection SC only into the abdomen or thigh
Pediatric: <2 years: not recommended; ≥2 years: 10 mg/m² once weekly; max
20 mg/m²
Rasuvo *Autoinjector:* 7.5 mg/0.15 ml, 10 mg/0.20 ml, 12.5 mg/0.25 ml, 15 mg/0.30
ml, 17.5 mg/0.35 ml, 20 mg/0.40 ml, 22.5 mg/0.45 ml, 25 mg/0.50 ml, 27.5 mg/0.55
ml, 30 mg/0.60 ml (solution concentration for SC injection is 50 mg/ml)
Rheumatrex *Tab:* 2.5*mg (5, 7.5, 10, 12.5, 15 mg/week, 4/card unit dose pack)
TrexallR *Tab:* 5*, 7.5*, 10*, 15*mg (5, 7.5, 10, 12.5, 15 mg/week, 4/card unit dose
pack)
Comment: *methotrexate* (MTX) is contraindicated with immunodeficiency, blood
dyscrasias, alcoholism, and chronic liver disease.

POLYPS, NASAL

LONG-ACTING CORTICOSTEROID SINUS IMPLANT

▷ *mometasone furoate* the **Sinuva Sinus Implant** must be inserted by a physician trained in otolaryngology; the implant is loaded into a sterile delivery system supplied with the implant and placed in the ethmoid sinus under endoscopic visualization; the implant is left in the sinus to gradually release the corticosteroid over 90 days; the implant is removed at Day 90 <u>or</u> earlier at the physician's discretion using standard surgical instruments; repeat administration has not been studied.

Pediatric: <18 years: not established: ≥18 years: same as adult

Sinuva Sinus Implant *Sinus implant:* 1350 mcg w. sterile delivery system

Comment: **Sinuva** is a corticosteroid-eluting sinus implant indicated for the treatment of recurrent nasal polyp disease in patients who have ethmoid sinus surgery. Monitor nasal mucosa adjacent to the **Sinuva Sinus Implant** for any signs of bleeding (epistaxis), irritation, infection, <u>or</u> perforation. Avoid use in patients with nasal ulcers <u>or</u> trauma. Monitor patients with a change in vision <u>or</u> with a history of increased intraocular pressure, glaucoma, <u>and/or</u> cataracts closely. Potential worsening of existing tuberculosis; fungal, bacterial, viral, parasitic infection, <u>or</u> ocular herpes simplex. More serious <u>or</u> even fatal course of chickenpox <u>or</u> measles in susceptible patients. If corticosteroid effects such as hypercorticism and adrenal suppression appear in patients, consider sinus implant removal. To report suspected adverse reactions, contact Intersect ENT at 1-866 531-6004 <u>or</u> FDA at 1-800-FDA-1088 <u>or</u> www.fda.gov/medwatch

NASAL SPRAY CORTICOSTEROIDS

▷ *beclomethasone dipropionate* (C)

Beconase 1 spray in each nostril bid-qid

Pediatric: <6 years: not recommended; 6-12 years: 1 spray in each nostril tid; >12 years: same as adult

Nasal spray: 42 mcg/actuation (6.7 gm, 80 sprays; 16.8 gm, 200 sprays)

Beconase AQ 1-2 sprays in each nostril bid

Pediatric: <6: not recommended; ≥6 years: same as adult

Nasal spray: 42 mcg/actuation (25 gm, 180 sprays)

Beconase Inhalation Aerosol 1-2 sprays in each nostril bid to qid

Pediatric: <6: not recommended; 6-12 years: 1 spray in each nostril tid; >12 years: same as adult

Nasal spray: 42 mcg/actuation (6.7 gm, 80 sprays; 16.8 gm, 200 sprays)

Vancenase AQ 1-2 sprays in each nostril bid

Pediatric: <6 years: not recommended; ≥6 years: same as adult

Nasal spray: 84 mcg/actuation (25 gm, 200 sprays)

Vancenase AQ DS 1-2 sprays in each nostril once daily

Pediatric: <6 years: not recommended; ≥6 years: same as adult

Nasal spray: 84, 168 mcg/actuation (19 gm, 120 sprays)

Vancenase Pockethaler 1 spray in each nostril bid or qid

Pediatric: <6: not recommended; ≥6 years: 1 spray in each nostril tid

Pockethaler: 42 mcg/actuation (7 gm, 200 sprays)

QNASL Nasal Aerosol 2 sprays, 80 mcg/spray, in each nostril once daily

Pediatric: <12 years: 2 sprays, 40 mcg/spray, in each nostril once daily; ≥12 years: same as adult

Nasal spray: 40 mcg/actuation (4.9 gm, 60 sprays); 80 mcg/actuation (8.7 gm, 120 sprays)

▷ *budesonide* (C)

Rhinocort initially 2 sprays in each nostril bid in the AM and PM, <u>or</u> 4 sprays in each nostril in the AM; max 4 sprays each nostril/day; use lowest effective dose

Pediatric: <6 years: not recommended; ≥6 years: same as adult
Nasal spray: 32 mcg/actuation (7 gm, 200 sprays)
Rhinocort Aqua Nasal Spray initially 1 spray in each nostril once daily; max 4 sprays in each nostril once daily
Pediatric: <6 years: not recommended; ≥6-12 years: initially 1 spray in each nostril once daily; max 2 sprays in each nostril once daily
Nasal spray: 32 mcg/actuation (10 ml, 60 sprays)

▷ *ciclesonide* (C)
Pediatric: <6 years: not recommended; ≥6 years: same as adult
Omnaris 2 sprays in each nostril once daily
Nasal spray: 50 mcg/actuation (12.5 gm, 120 sprays)
Zetonna 1-2 sprays in each nostril once daily
Nasal spray: 37 mcg/actuation (6.1 gm, 60 sprays) (HFA)

▷ *dexamethasone* (C) 2 sprays in each nostril bid-tid; max 12 sprays/day; maintain at lowest effective dose
Pediatric: <6 years: not recommended; ≥6-12 years: 1-2 sprays in each nostril bid; max 8 sprays/day; maintain at lowest effective dose; >12 years: same as adult
Dexacort Turbinaire *Nasal spray:* 84 mcg/actuation (12.6 gm, 170 sprays)

▷ *fluticasone furoate* (C) 2 sprays in each nostril once daily; may reduce to 1 spray each nostril once daily
Pediatric: <2 years: not recommended; ≥2-11 years: 1 spray in each nostril once daily; ≥12 years: same as adult
Veramyst *Nasal spray:* 27.5 mcg/actuation (10 gm, 120 sprays) (alcohol-free)

▷ *fluticasone propionate* (C)
Flonase (OTC)(G) initially 2 sprays in each nostril once daily <u>or</u> 1 spray bid; maintenance 1 spray once daily
Pediatric: <4 years: not recommended; ≥4 years: initially 1 spray in each nostril once daily; may increase to 2 sprays in each nostril once daily; maintenance 1 spray in each nostril once daily; max 2 sprays in each nostril/day
Nasal spray: 50 mcg/actuation (16 gm, 120 sprays)
Xhance 1 spray per nostril bid (total daily dose 372 mcg); 2 sprays per nostril bid may also be effective in some patients (total daily dose 744 mcg)
Pediatric: <12 years: not established; ≥12 years: same as adult
Nasal spray: 93 mcg/actuation (16 ml, 120 metered sprays)
Comment: Available data from published literature on the use of inhaled <u>or</u> intranasal *fluticasone propionate* in pregnant women have not reported a clear association with adverse developmental outcomes. There are no available data on the presence of *fluticasone propionate* in human milk <u>or</u> effects on the breastfed child. The safety and efficacy of **Xhance** in pediatric patients have not been established.

▷ *flunisolide* (C) 2 sprays in each nostril bid; may increase to 2 sprays in each nostril tid; max 8 sprays/nostril/day
Pediatric: <6 years: not recommended; 6-14 years: initially 1 spray in each nostril tid <u>or</u> 2 sprays in each nostril bid; max 4 sprays/nostril/day; >14 years: same as adult
Nasalide *Nasal spray:* 25 mcg/actuation (25 ml, 200 sprays)
Nasarel *Nasal spray:* 25 mcg/actuation (25 ml, 200 sprays)

▷ *mometasone furoate* (C)(G) 2 sprays in each nostril once daily
Pediatric: <2 years: not recommended; 2-11 years: 1 spray in each nostril once daily; max 2 sprays in each nostril once daily; >11 years: same as adult
Nasonex *Nasal spray:* 50 mcg/actuation (17 gm, 120 sprays)

▷ *olopatadine* (C) 2 sprays in each nostril bid
Pediatric: <6 years: not recommended; 6-11 years: 1 spray each nostril bid; >11 years: same as adult

Patanase *Nasal spray:* 0.6%; 665 mcg/actuation (30.5 gm, 240 sprays) (benzalkonium chloride)

▷ **triamcinolone acetonide** (C)(G) initially 2 sprays in each nostril once daily; max 4 sprays in each nostril once daily <u>or</u> 2 sprays in each nostril bid <u>or</u> 1 spray in each nostril qid; maintain at lowest effective dose

Pediatric: <6 years: not recommended; ≥6 years: 1 spray in each nostril once daily; max 2 sprays in each nostril once daily

Nasacort Allergy 24HR (OTC) *Nasal spray:* 55 mcg/actuation (10 gm, 120 sprays)
Tri-Nasal *Nasal spray:* 50 mcg/actuation (15 ml, 120 sprays)

◯ POSTHERPETIC NEURALGIA

Acetaminophen for IV Infusion see *Pain page 344*
Oral Analgesics see *Pain page 338*

GAMMA AMINOBUTYRIC ACID ANALOG

▷ **gabapentin** (C) *CrCl 30-60 mL/min:* 600-1800 mg; *CrCl <30 mL/min* <u>or</u> *on hemodialysis:* not recommended; avoid abrupt cessation of **gabapentin** and **gabapentin enacarbil**. To discontinue, withdraw gradually over 1 week <u>or</u> longer.

Gralise initially 300 mg on Day 1; then 600 mg on Day 2; then 900 mg on Days 3-6; then 1200 mg on Days 7-10; then 1500 mg on Days 11-14; titrate up to 1800 mg on Day 15; take entire dose once daily with the evening meal; do not crush, split, <u>or</u> chew

Pediatric: <18 years: not recommended; ≥18 years: same as adult
Tab: 300, 600 mg

Neurontin (G) 300 mg daily x 1 day, then 300 mg bid x 1 day, then 300 mg tid continuously; max 1,800 mg/day in 3 divided doses; taper over 7 days
Pediatric: <3 years: not recommended; 3-12 years: initially 10-15 mg/kg/day in 3 divided doses; max 12 hours between doses; titrate over 3 days; 3-4 years: titrate to 40 mg/kg/day; 5-12 years: titrate to 25-35 mg/kg/day; max 50 mg/kg/day
Tab: 600*, 800*mg; *Cap:* 100, 300, 400 mg; *Oral soln:* 250 mg/5 ml (480 ml) (strawberry-anise)

▷ **gabapentin enacarbil** (C) avoid abrupt cessation of **gabapentin enacarbil;** to discontinue, withdraw gradually over 1 week or longer; 600 mg once daily at about 5:00 PM; if dose not taken at recommended time, next dose should be taken the following day; swallow whole; take with food; *CrCl 30-59 mL/min:* 600 mg on Day 1, Day 3, and every day thereafter; *CrCl <30 mL/min:* <u>or</u> on hemodialysis: not recommended
Pediatric: <18 years: not recommended; ≥18 years: same as adult
Horizant *Tab:* 600 ext-rel

Tricyclic Antidepressants (TCAs)

Comment: Co-administration of SSRIs and TCAs requires extreme caution.

▷ **amitriptyline** (C)(G) initially 75 mg/day in divided doses of 50-100 mg/day q HS; max 300 mg/day
Pediatric: <12 years: not recommended; ≥12 years: same as adult
Tab: 10, 25, 50, 75, 100, 150 mg

▷ **amoxapine** (C) initially 50 mg bid-tid; after 1 week may increase to 100 mg bid-tid; usual effective dose 200-300 mg/day; if total dose exceeds 300 mg/day, give in divided doses (max 400 mg/day); may give as a single bedtime dose (max 300 mg q HS)
Pediatric: <12 years: not recommended; ≥12 years: same as adult
Tab: 25, 50, 100, 150 mg

▷ **desipramine** (C)(G) 100-200 mg/day in single <u>or</u> divided doses; max 300 mg/day
Pediatric: <12 years: not recommended; ≥12 years: same as adult
 Norpramin *Tab:* 10, 25, 50, 75, 100, 150 mg
▷ **doxepin** (C)(G) 75 mg/day; max 150 mg/day
Pediatric: <12 years: not recommended; ≥12 years: same as adult
 Cap: 10, 25, 50, 75, 100, 150 mg; *Oral conc:* 10 mg/ml (4 oz w. dropper)
▷ **imipramine** (C)(G)
Pediatric: <12 years: not recommended; ≥12 years: same as adult
 Tofranil initially 75 mg daily (max 200 mg); adolescents initially 30-40 mg daily
 (max 100 mg/day); if maintenance dose exceeds 75 mg daily, may switch to **Tofra-
nil PM** for divided <u>or</u> bedtime dose
  Tab: 10, 25, 50 mg
 Tofranil PM initially 75 mg daily 1 hour before HS; max 200 mg
  Cap: 75, 100, 125, 150 mg
 Tofranil Injection 50 mg IM; lower dose for adolescents; switch to oral form as
 soon as possible
  Amp: 25 mg/2 ml (2 ml)
▷ **nortriptyline** (D)(G) initially 25 mg tid-qid; max 150 mg/day
Pediatric: <12 years: not recommended; ≥12 years: same as adult
 Pamelor *Cap:* 10, 25, 50, 75 mg; *Oral soln:* 10 mg/5 ml (16 oz)
▷ **protriptyline** (C) initially 5 mg tid; usual dose 15-40 mg/day in 3-4 divided doses;
max 60 mg/day
Pediatric: <12 years: not recommended; ≥12 years: same as adult
 Vivactil *Tab:* 5, 10 mg
▷ **trimipramine** (C) initially 75 mg/day in divided doses; max 200 mg/day
Pediatric: <12 years: not recommended; ≥12 years: same as adult
 Surmontil *Cap:* 25, 50, 100 mg

ALPHA-2 DELTA LIGAND

▷ **pregabalin** (GABA analog) (C)(V) initially 150 mg daily divided bid-tid and
may titrate within one week; max 600 mg divided bid-tid; discontinue over one week
Pediatric: <18 years: not recommended; ≥18 years: same as adult
 Lyrica *Cap:* 25, 50, 75, 100, 150, 200, 225, 300 mg; *Oral soln:* 20 mg/ml

TOPICAL AND TRANSDERMAL ANALGESICS

▷ **capsaicin** (B)(G) apply tid-qid prn to intact skin; avoid mucus membranes
Pediatric: <2 years: not recommended; ≥2 years: same as adult
 Double Cap (OTC) *Crm:* 0.05% (2 oz)
 Qutenza *Patch:* 8% (1-2, both with 50 gm tube of cleansing gel)
 Zostrix (OTC) *Crm:* 0.025% (0.7, 1.5, 3 oz)
 Zostrix HP (OTC) *Emol crm:* 0.075% (1, 2 oz)
Comment: Provides some relief by 1-2 weeks; optimal benefit may take 4-6 weeks.
▷ **diclofenac epolamine** (C) apply one patch to affected area bid; remove during bathing;
avoid non-intact skin; do not re-use
Pediatric: <12 years: not recommended; ≥12 years: same as adult
 Flector Patch *Patch:* 180 mg/patch (30/carton)
Comment: *diclofenac* is contraindicated with *aspirin* allergy and 3rd trimester of
pregnancy.
▷ **doxepin** (B) cream apply to affected area qid at intervals of at least 3-4 hours; max 8
days
Pediatric: <12 years: not recommended; ≥12 years: same as adult
 Prudoxin *Crm:* 5% (45 gm)
 Zonalon *Crm:* 5% (30, 45 gm)

▷ *tacrolimus* (C) apply to affected area bid; continue for 1 week after clearing
 Pediatric: <2 years: not recommended; 2-15 years: use 0.03% strength
  Protopic *Oint:* 0.03, 0.1% (30, 60 gm)

TOPICAL AND TRANSDERMAL ANESTHETICS

▷ *lidocaine* cream (B) apply to affected area bid prn
 Pediatric: <12 years: not recommended; ≥12 years: same as adult
  LidaMantle *Crm:* 3% (1, 2 oz)
  Lidoderm *Crm:* 3% (85 gm)
▷ *lidocaine* lotion (B) apply to affected area bid prn
 Pediatric: <12 years: not recommended; ≥12 years: same as adult
  LidaMantle *Lotn:* 3% (177 ml)
▷ *lidocaine* 5% patch (B)(G) apply up to 3 patches at one time for up to 12 hours/24-hour period (12 hours on/12 hours off); patches may be cut into smaller sizes before removal of the release liner; do not re-use
 Pediatric: <12 years: not recommended; ≥12 years: same as adult
  Lidoderm *Patch:* 5% (10x14 cm; 30/carton)
▷ *lidocaine+dexamethasone* (B)
 Pediatric: <12 years: not recommended; ≥12 years: same as adult
  Decadron Phosphate with Xylocaine *Lotn:* dexa 4 mg+lido 10 mg per ml (5 ml)
▷ *lidocaine+hydrocortisone* (B)(G) apply to affected area bid prn
 Pediatric: <12 years: not recommended; ≥12 years: same as adult
  LidaMantle HC *Crm:* lido 3%+hydro 0.5% (1, 3 oz); *Lotn:* (177 ml)

ORAL ANALGESICS

▷ *acetaminophen* (B)(G) *see Fever page* 165
▷ *aspirin* (D)(G) *see Fever page* 166
 Comment: *aspirin*-containing medications are contraindicated with history of allergic-type reaction to *aspirin*, children and adolescents with *Varicella* or other viral illness, and 3rd trimester of pregnancy.
▷ *tramadol* (C)(IV)(G)
Comment: *tramadol* is known to be excreted in breast milk. The FDA and the European Medicines Agency (EMA) are investigating the safety of using *tramadol*-containing medications to treat pain in children 12-18 years because of the potential for serious side effects, including slowed or difficult breathing.
  Rybix ODT initially 100 mg once daily; may increase by 100 mg every 5 days; max 300 mg/day; *CrCl <30 mL/min or severe hepatic impairment:* not recommended; *Cirrhosis:* max 50 mg q 12 hours
  Pediatric: <18 years: not recommended; ≥18 years: same as adult
   ODT: 50 mg (mint) (phenylalanine)
  Ryzolt initially 100 mg once daily; may increase by 100 mg every 5 days; max 300 mg/day; *CrCl <30 mL/min or severe hepatic impairment:* not recommended
  Pediatric: <18 years: not recommended; ≥18 years: same as adult
   Tab: 100, 200, 300 mg ext-rel
  Ultram 50-100 mg q 4-6 hours prn; max 400 mg/day; *CrCl <30 mL/min:* max 100 mg q 12 hours; *Cirrhosis:* max 50 mg q 12 hours
  Pediatric: <18 years: not recommended; ≥18 years: same as adult
   Tab: 50*mg
  Ultram ER initially 100 mg once daily; may increase by 100 mg every 5 days; max 300 mg/day; *CrCl <30 mL/min:* or *severe hepatic impairment:* not recommended
  Pediatric: <18 years: not recommended; ≥18 years: same as adult
   Tab: 100, 200, 300 mg ext-rel

▷ *tramadol+acetaminophen* (C)(IV)(G) 2 tabs q 4-6 hours; max 8 tabs/day; 5 days;
CrCl <30 mL/min: max 2 tabs q 12 hours; max 4 tabs/day x 5 days
Pediatric: <18 years: not recommended; ≥18 years: same as adult
   Ultracet *Tab: tram* 37.5+*acet* 325 mg

Comment: *tramadol* is known to be excreted in breast milk. The FDA and the
European Medicines Agency (EMA) are investigating the safety of using *tramadol*-
containing medications to treat pain in children 12-18 years because of the potential
for serious side effects, including slowed <u>or</u> difficult breathing.

TRICYCLIC ANTIDEPRESSANTS (TCAs)

Comment: Co-administration of TCAs with SSRIs requires extreme caution.
▷ *amitriptyline* (C)(G) titrate to achieve pain relief; max 300 mg/day
Pediatric: <12 years: not recommended; ≥12 years: same as adult
   Tab: 10, 25, 50, 75, 100, 150 mg
▷ *amoxapine* (C) titrate to achieve pain relief; if total dose exceeds 300 mg/day, give in
divided doses; max 400 mg/day
Pediatric: <12 years: not recommended; ≥12 years: same as adult
   Tab: 25, 50, 100, 150 mg
▷ *desipramine* (C)(G) titrate to achieve pain relief; max 300 mg/day
Pediatric: <12 years: not recommended; ≥12 years: same as adult
   Norpramin *Tab:* 10, 25, 50, 75, 100, 150 mg
▷ *doxepin* (C)(G) titrate to achieve pain relief; max 150 mg/day
Pediatric: <12 years: not recommended; ≥12 years: same as adult
   Cap: 10, 25, 50, 75, 100, 150 mg; *Oral conc:* 10 mg/ml (4 oz w. dropper)
▷ *imipramine* (C)(G)
Pediatric: <12 years: not recommended; ≥12 years: same as adult
   Tofranil titrate to achieve pain relief; max 200 mg/day; adolescents max 100 mg/day;
   if maintenance dose exceeds 75 mg/day, may switch to **Tofranil PM** at bedtime
      Tab: 10, 25, 50 mg
   Tofranil PM titrate to achieve pain relief; initially 75 mg at HS; max 200 mg at HS
      Cap: 75, 100, 125, 150 mg
   Tofranil Injection 50 mg IM; lower dose for adolescents; switch to oral form as
   soon as possible
      Amp: 25 mg/2 ml (2 ml)
▷ *nortriptyline* (D)(G) titrate to achieve pain relief; initially 10-25 mg tid-qid; max 150
mg/day; lower doses for elderly and adolescents
Pediatric: <12 years: not recommended; ≥12 years: same as adult
   Pamelor titrate to achieve pain relief; max 150 mg/day
      Cap: 10, 25, 50, 75 mg; *Oral soln:* 10 mg/5 ml (16 oz)
▷ *protriptyline* (C) titrate to achieve pain relief; initially 5 mg tid; max 60 mg/day
Pediatric: <12 years: not recommended; ≥12 years: same as adult
   Vivactil *Tab:* 5, 10 mg
▷ *trimipramine* (C) titrate to achieve pain relief; max 200 mg/day
Pediatric: <12 years: not recommended; ≥12 years: same as adult
   Surmontil *Cap:* 25, 50, 100 mg

◯ POST-TRAUMATIC STRESS DISORDER (PTSD)

Comment: No one pharmacological agent has emerged as the best treatment for PTSD.
A combination of pharmacological agents (e.g., antidepressants, non-adrenergic agents,
antipsychosis drugs) may comprise an individualized treatment plan to successfully
manage core symptoms of PTSD as well as associated anxiety, depression, sleep
disturbances, and co-occurring psychiatric disorders.

SELECTIVE SEROTONIN REUPTAKE INHIBITORS (SSRIs)

Comment: The FDA has approved two SSRIs for the treatment of PTSD: *paroxetine* and *sertraline*. However, the safety and efficacy of other SSRIs (*fluoxetine, citalopram, escitalopram, fluvoxamine*) have been tested in clinical practice. Co-administration of SSRIs with TCAs requires extreme caution. Concomitant use of MAOIs and SSRIs is absolutely contraindicated. Avoid St. John's wort and other serotonergic agents. A potentially fatal adverse event is *serotonin syndrome*, caused by serotonin excess. Milder symptoms require HCP intervention to avert severe symptoms which can be rapidly fatal without urgent/emergent medical care. Symptoms include restlessness, agitation, confusion, hallucinations, tachycardia, hypertension, dilated pupils, muscle twitching, muscle rigidity, loss of muscle coordination, diaphoresis, diarrhea, headache, shivering, piloerection, hyperpyrexia, cardiac arrhythmias, seizures, loss of consciousness, coma, death. Abrupt withdrawal or interruption of treatment with an antidepressant medication is sometimes associated with an *Antidepressant Discontinuation Syndrome* which may be mediated by gradually tapering the drug over a period of two weeks or longer, depending on the dose strength and length of treatment. Common symptoms of the *serotonin discontinuation Syndrome* include flu-like symptoms (nausea, vomiting, diarrhea, headaches, sweating), sleep disturbances (insomnia, nightmares, constant sleepiness), mood disturbances (dysphoria, anxiety, agitation), cognitive disturbances (mental confusion, hyperarousal), sensory and movement disturbances (imbalance, tremors, vertigo, dizziness, electric-shock-like sensations in the brain, often described by sufferers as "brain zaps."

➤ *paroxetine maleate* (D)(G)
Pediatric: <12 years: not recommended; ≥12 years: same as adult
　Paxil initially 20 mg daily in AM; may increase by 10 mg/day at weekly intervals as needed; max 60 mg/day
　　Tab: 10*, 20*, 30, 40 mg
　Paxil CR initially 25 mg daily in AM; may increase by 12.5 mg at weekly intervals as needed; max 62.5 mg/day
　　Tab: 12.5, 25, 37.5 mg cont-rel ent-coat
　Paxil Suspension initially 20 mg daily in AM; may increase by 10 mg/day at weekly intervals as needed; max 60 mg/day
　　Oral susp: 10 mg/5 ml (250 ml; orange)
➤ *paroxetine mesylate* (D)(G) initially 7.5 mg daily in AM; may increase by 10 mg/day at weekly intervals as needed; max 60 mg/day
Pediatric: <12 years: not recommended; ≥12 years: same as adult
　Brisdelle *Cap:* 7.5 mg
➤ *sertraline* (C) initially 50 mg daily; increase at 1 week intervals if needed; max 200 mg daily
Pediatric: <6 years: not recommended; 6-12 years: initially 25 mg daily; max 200 mg/day; 13-17 years: initially 50 mg daily; max 200 mg/day; ≥17 years: same as adult
　Zoloft *Tab:* 15*, 50*, 100*mg; *Oral conc:* 20 mg per ml (60 ml [dilute just before administering in 4 oz water, ginger ale, lemon-lime soda, lemonade, or orange juice]) (alcohol 12%)

ATYPICAL ANTIPSYCHOSIS DRUGS

➤ *olanzapine* (C)(G) initially 2.5-5 mg once daily at HS; increase by 5 mg every week to 20 mg at HS; usual maintenance 10-20 mg/day
　Zyprexa *Tab:* 2.5, 5, 7.5, 10, 15, 20 mg
　Zyprexa Zydis *ODT:* 5, 10, 15, 20 mg (phenylalanine)
➤ *quetiapine* (C)(G) initially 25 mg bid; increase total daily dose by 50 mg, as needed and tolerated, to max 300-600 mg/day
　Seroquel *Tab:* 25, 100, 200, 300 mg
　Seroquel XR *Tab:* 50, 150, 200, 300, 400 mg ext-rel

▷ *risperidone* (C)(G) initially 0.5-1 mg bid; titrate to 3 mg bid by the end of the first week; usual maintenance 4-6 mg/day
    Risperdal *Tab:* 0.25, 0.5, 1, 2, 3, 4 mg; *Soln:* 1 mg/ml (30 ml w. pipette); *Consta (Inj):* 25, 37.5, 50 mg
    Risperdal M-Tabs *M-tab:* 0.5, 1, 2, 3, 4 mg orally-disint (phenylalanine)

NON-ADRENERGIC AGENTS
ALPHA-1 ANTAGONISTS

Comment: *prazosin* is useful in reducing combat-trauma nightmares, normalizing dreams for combat veterans, and mediating other sleep disturbances.

▷ *prazosin* (C)(G) first dose at HS, 1 mg bid-tid; increase dose slowly; usual range 6-15 mg/day in divided doses; max 20-40 mg/day
Pediatric: <12 years: not recommended; ≥12 years: same as adult
    Minipress *Cap:* 1, 2, 5 mg

CENTRAL ALPHA-2 AGONISTS

Comment: *clonidine* is useful to reduce nightmares, hypervigilance, startle reactions, and outbursts of rage.

▷ *clonidine* (C)
Pediatric: <12 years: not recommended; ≥12 years: same as adult
    Catapres initially 0.1 mg bid; usual range 0.2-0.6 mg/day in divided doses; max 2.4 mg/day *Tab:* 0.1*, 0.2*, 0.3*mg
    Catapres-TTS initially 0.1 mg patch weekly; increase after 1-2 weeks if needed; max 0.6 mg/day
        Patch: 0.1, 0.2 mg/day (12/carton); 0.3 mg/day (4/carton)
    Kapvay (G) initially 0.1 mg bid; usual range 0.2-0.6 mg/day in divided doses; max 2.4 mg/day *Tab:* 0.1, 0.2 mg
    Nexiclon XR initially 0.18 mg (2 ml) suspension or 0.17 mg tab once daily; usual max 0.52 mg (6 ml suspension) once daily
        Tab: 0.17, 0.26 mg ext-rel; *Oral susp:* 0.09 mg/ml ext-rel (4 oz)

BETA-ADRENERGIC BLOCKER (NON-CARDIOSELECTIVE)

Comment: *propranolol* is useful to mediate hyperarousal. For other non-cardioselective beta-adrenergic blockers, *see* **Hypertension**, *page* 260

▷ *propranolol* (C)(G) 40-240 mg daily
Pediatric: <12 years: not recommended; ≥12 years: same as adult
    Inderal *Tab:* 10*, 20*, 40*, 60*, 80*mg
    Inderal LA initially 80 mg daily in a single dose; increase q 3-7 days; usual range 120-160 mg/day; max 320 mg/day in a single dose

SEROTONIN-NOREPINEPHRINE REUPTAKE INHIBITORS (SNRIs)

▷ *desvenlafaxine* (C)(G) swallow whole; initially 50 mg once daily; max 120 mg/day
Pediatric: <12 years: not recommended; ≥12 years: same as adult
    Pristiq *Tab:* 50, 100 mg ext-rel
▷ *duloxetine* (C)(G) swallow whole; initially 30 mg once daily x 1 week; then increase to 60 mg once daily; max 120 mg/day
Pediatric: <12 years: not recommended; ≥12 years: same as adult
    Cymbalta *Cap:* 20, 30, 40, 60 mg del-rel
▷ *venlafaxine* (C)(G)
    Effexor initially 75 mg/day in 2-3 divided doses; may increase at 4-day intervals in 75 mg increments to 150 mg/day; max 225 mg/day
Pediatric: <18 years: not recommended; ≥18 years: same as adult

Tab: 37.5, 75, 150, 225 mg
Effexor XR initially 75 mg q AM; may start at 37.5 mg daily x 4-7 days, then increase by increments of up to 75 mg/day at intervals of at least 4 days; usual max 375 mg/day
Pediatric: <18 years: not recommended; ≥18 years: same as adult
Tab/Cap: 37.5, 75, 150 mg ext-rel

5HT2/3 RECEPTOR BLOCKERS

▷ *mirtazapine* (C) initially 15 mg q HS; increase at intervals of 1-2 weeks; 1-2 weeks; usual range 15-60 mg/day; max 60 mg/day
Pediatric: <12 years: not recommended; ≥12 years: same as adult
Remeron *Tab:* 15*, 30*, 45*mg
Remeron SolTab *ODT:* 15, 30, 45 mg (orange) (phenylalanine)

SERTONIN+ACETYLCHOLINE+NOREPINEPHRINE+DOPAMINE BLOCKER

▷ *trazodone* (C)(G) initially 150 mg/day in divided doses with food; increase by 50 mg/day q 3-4 days; max 400 mg/day in divided doses <u>or</u> 50-400 mg at HS
Pediatric: <18 years: not recommended; ≥18 years: same as adult
Oleptro *Tab:* 50, 100*, 150*, 200, 250, 300 mg

TRICYCLIC ANTIDEPRESSANTS (TCAs)

▷ *amitriptyline* (C)(G) 10-20 mg at HS
Pediatric: <12 years: not recommended; ≥12 years: same as adult
Tab: 10, 25, 50, 75, 100, 150 mg
▷ *doxepin* (C)(G) 10-200 mg at HS
Pediatric: <12 years: not recommended; ≥12 years: same as adult
Cap: 10, 25, 50, 75, 100, 150 mg; *Oral conc:* 10 mg/ml (4 oz w. dropper)
▷ *imipramine* (C)(G) 10-200 mg q HS
Tofranil 100-300 mg at HS <u>or</u> divided bid <u>or</u> tid
Pediatric: <6 years: not recommended; 6-12 years: initially 25 mg; >12 years: 50 mg max 2.5 mg/kg/day
Tab: 10, 25, 50 mg
Tofranil PM initially 75 mg daily 1 hour before HS; max 200 mg
Pediatric: <12 years: not recommended; ≥12 years: same as adult
Cap: 75, 100, 125, 150 mg
Tofranil Injection 50 mg IM; lower dose for adolescents; switch to oral form as soon as possible
Amp: 25 mg/2 ml (2 ml)
▷ *nortriptyline* (D)(G) 10-150 mg q HS
Pediatric: <12 years: not recommended; ≥12 years: same as adult
Pamelor *Cap:* 10, 25, 50, 75 mg; *Oral soln:* 10 mg/5 ml

MONOAMINE OXIDASE INHIBITORS (MAOIs)

Comment: Many drug and food interactions with this class of drugs, use cautiously. MAOIs should be reserved for refractory depression that has not responded to other classes of antidepressants. Concomitant use of MAOIs and SSRIs is contraindicated. See mfr pkg insert for drug and food interactions. MAOIs have been used to reduce recurrent recollections of the trauma, nightmares, flashbacks, numbing, sleep disturbances, and social withdrawal in PTSD.

▷ *phenelzine* (C)(G) initially 15 mg tid; max 90 mg/day
Pediatric: <16 years: not recommended; ≥16 years: same as adult
Nardil *Tab:* 15 mg

▷ **selegiline** (C) initially 10 mg tid; max 60 mg/day
  Pediatric: <12 years: not recommended; ≥12 years: same as adult
    Emsam *Transdermal patch:* 6 mg/24 hrs, 9 mg/24 hrs, 12 mg/24 hrs
Comment: At the **Emsam** transdermal patch 6 mg/24 hrs dose, the dietary restrictions commonly required when using nonselective MAOIs are not necessary.

 PRECOCIOUS PUBERTY, CENTRAL (CPP)

Comment: GnRH-dependent CPP is defined by pubertal development occurring before the age of 8 years in girls and 9 years in boys. It is characterized by early pubertal changes such as breast development and start of menses in girls and increased testicular and penile growth in boys, appearance of pubic hair, as well as acceleration of growth velocity and bone maturation and tall stature during childhood, which often results in reduced adult height due to premature fusion of the growth plates.

GONADOTROPIN RELEASING HORMONE (GnRH) AGONIST

▷ **triptorelin** (X)
  Pediatric: <2 years: not recommended; ≥2 years: administer as a single 22.5 mg IM injection once every 24 weeks; must be administered under the supervision of a physician; monitor response with LH levels after a GnRH <u>or</u> GnRH agonist stimulation test, basal LH, <u>or</u> serum concentration of sex steroid levels beginning 1 to 2 months following initiation of therapy, during therapy as necessary to confirm maintenance of efficacy, and with each subsequent dose; measure height every 3-6 months and monitor bone age periodically; see mfr pkg insert for reconstitution and administration instructions
  Triptodur Single-use kit: 1 single-dose vial of **triptorelin** 22.5 mg w. Flip-Off seal containing sterile lyophilized white to slightly yellow powder cake, 1 sterile, glass syringe prefilled with 2 ml of sterile water for injection, 2 sterile 21 gauge, 1½" needles (thin-wall) with safety cover
  Comment: **Triptodur** is contraindicated in females who are pregnant since expected hormonal changes that occur with **triptorelin** treatment increase the risk for pregnancy loss. Available data with **triptorelin** use in pregnant females are insufficient to determine a drug-associated risk of adverse developmental outcomes. Based on mechanism of action in humans and findings of increased pregnancy loss in animal studies, **triptorelin** may cause fetal harm when administered to pregnant females. Advise pregnant females of the potential risk to a fetus. The estimated background risk of major birth defects and miscarriage is unknown. There are no data on the presence of **triptorelin** in human milk <u>or</u> the effects of the drug on the breastfed infant. The developmental and health benefits of breastfeeding should be considered along with the mother's clinical need for **triptorelin** and any potential adverse effects on the breastfed child from **triptorelin** <u>or</u> from the underlying maternal condition. During the early phase of therapy, gonadotropins and sex steroids rise above baseline because of the initial stimulatory effect of the drug. Therefore, a transient increase in clinical signs and symptoms of puberty, including vaginal bleeding, may be observed during the first weeks of therapy. Post-marketing reports with this class of drugs include symptoms of emotional lability, such as crying, irritability, impatience, anger, and aggression. Monitor for development <u>or</u> worsening of psychiatric symptoms during treatment with **Triptodur.** Post-marketing reports of convulsions have been observed in patients receiving GnRH agonists, including **triptorelin.** These included patients with a history of seizures, epilepsy, cerebrovascular disorders, central nervous system anomalies <u>or</u> tumors, and patients on concomitant medications that have been associated with convulsions such as bupropion and SSRIs. Convulsions have also been reported in patients in the absence of any of the conditions mentioned above.

PREGNANCY

see **Appendix Z: Prescription Prenatal Vitamins** *page* 594

Comment: Prenatal vitamins should have at least 400 mcg of folic acid content. Take one dose once daily. It is recommended that prenatal vitamins be started at least 3 months prior to conception to improve preconception nutritional status, and continued throughout pregnancy and the postnatal period, in lactating and nonlactating women, and throughout the childbearing years.

NAUSEA/VOMITING

▷ *doxyalamine succinate+pyridoxine* (A)(G) do not crush or chew; take on an empty stomach with water; initially 2 tabs at HS on day 1; may increase to 1 tab AM and 2 tabs at HS day 2; may increase to 1 tab AM, 1 tab mid-afternoon, 2 tabs at HS; max 4 tabs/day

Diclegis *Tab: doxyl* 10 mg+*pyri* 10 mg del-rel

Comment: Diclegis is the only FDA-approved drug for the treatment of morning sickness. It has not been studied in women with hyperemesis gravidarum.

▷ *ondansetron* (C)(G) 4-8 mg bid prn or 8 mg q 8 hours prn

Zofran *Tab:* 4, 8, 24 mg

Zofran Injection *Vial:* 2 mg/ml (2 ml single-dose); 2 mg/ml (20 ml multi-dose) for IV or IM administration

Zofran ODT *ODT:* 4, 8 mg (strawberry) (phenylalanine)

Zofran Oral Solution *Oral soln:* 4 mg/5 ml (50 ml) (strawberry)

Zuplenz Oral Soluble Film: 4, 8 mg orally-disint (10/carton) (peppermint)

▷ *promethazine* (C)(G) 12.5-50 mg PO/IM/rectally q 4-6 hours prn

Phenergan *Tab:* 12.5*, 25*, 50 mg; *Plain syr:* 6.25 mg/5 ml; *Fortis syr:* 25 mg/5 ml; *Rectal supp:* 12.5, 25, 50 mg; *Amp:* 25, 50 mg/ml (1 ml)

 PREMENSTRUAL DYSPHORIC DISORDER (PMDD)

NSAIDs *see page* 562
Opioid Analgesics *see* **Pain** *page* 345
Oral Contraceptives *see page* 548

ORAL ESTROGEN+PROGESTERONE COMBINATIONS

Comment: **Rajani** (a generic form of **Beyaz**) and **Yaz**; also available in generic Forms (**Gianvi, Ocella, Syeda, Vestura, Yasmin, Zarah**) have an FDA indication for treatment of PMDD in females who choose to use an OCP. Contraindicated with renal and adrenal insufficiency. Monitor K+ level during the first cycle if the patient is at risk for hyperkalemia for any reason. If the patient is taking a drug that increase serum potassium (e.g., ACEIs, ARBS, NSAIDs, K+ sparing diuretics), the patient is at risk for hyperkalemia.

▷ *ethinyl estradiol+drospirenone* (X)(G) Pre-menarchal: not indicated; Post-menarchal: 1 tab once daily x 28 days; repeat cycle; start on first Sunday after menses begins or on first day of next menses

Yaz *Tab: ethin estra* 20 mcg+*drospir* 3 mg

▷ *ethinyl+estradiol+drospirenone+levomefolate calcium* (X)(G) Pre-menarchal: not indicated; Post-menarchal: 1 tab once daily x 28 days; repeat cycle; start on first Sunday after menses begins or on first day of next menses preceded by a negative pregnancy test

Beyaz *Tab: ethin estra* 20 mcg+*drospir* 3 mg+*levo* 0.451 mg
Rajani *Tab: ethin estra* 20 mcg+*drospir* 3 mg+*levo* 0.451 mg

DIURETICS

▷ *spironolactone* (D)(G) initially 50-100 mg once daily <u>or</u> in divided doses; titrate at 2-week intervals
Pediatric: <12 years: not recommended; ≥12 years: same as adult
    Aldactone *Tab:* 25, 50*, 100*mg

ANTIDEPRESSANTS

▷ *fluoxetine* (C)(G)
    Prozac initially 20 mg daily; may increase after 1 week; doses >20 mg/day should be divided into AM and noon doses; max 80 mg/day
    Pediatric: <8 years: not recommended; 8-17 years: initially 10 <u>or</u> 20 mg/day; start lower weight children at 10 mg/day; if starting at 10 mg/day, may increase after 1 week to 20 mg/day; ≥17 years: same as adult
        Tab: 10*mg; *Cap:* 10, 20, 40 mg; *Oral soln:* 20 mg/5 ml (4 oz) (mint)
    Prozac Weekly following daily *fluoxetine* therapy at 20 mg/day for 13 weeks, may initiate **Prozac Weekly** 7 days after the last 20 mg *fluoxetine* dose
    Pediatric: <12 years: not recommended; ≥12 years: same as adult
        Cap: 90 mg ent-coat del-rel pellets
    Sarafem administer daily <u>or</u> 14 days before expected menses and through first full day of menses; initially 20 mg/day; max 80 mg/day
    Pediatric: <8 years: not recommended; 8-17 years: initially 10 or 20 mg/day; start lower weight children at 10 mg/day; if starting at 10 mg/day, may increase after 1 week to 20 mg/day
        Tab: 10, 15, 20 mg; *Cap:* 20 mg
▷ *paroxetine maleate* (D)(G)
    Pediatric: <12 years: not recommended; ≥12 years: same as adult
    Paxil initially 20 mg daily in AM; may increase by 10 mg/day at weekly intervals as needed; max 60 mg/day
        Tab: 10*, 20*, 30, 40 mg
    Paxil CR initially 25 mg daily in AM; may increase by 12.5 mg at weekly intervals as needed; max 62.5 mg/day; may start 14 days before and continue through day one of menses
        Tab: 12.5, 25, 37.5 mg cont-rel ent-coat
    Paxil Suspension initially 20 mg daily in AM; may increase by 10 mg/day at weekly intervals as needed; max 60 mg/day
        Oral susp: 10 mg/5 ml (250 ml) (orange)
▷ *paroxetine mesylate* (D)(G) initially 7.5 mg daily in AM; may increase by 10 mg/day at weekly intervals as needed; max 60 mg/day
    Pediatric: <12 years: not recommended; ≥12 years: same as adult
    Brisdelle *Cap:* 7.5 mg
▷ *sertraline* (C)
    For 2 weeks prior to onset of menses: initially 50 mg daily x 3; then increase to 100 mg daily for remainder of the cycle; *For full cycle:* initially 50 mg daily; then may increase by 50 mg/day each cycle to max 150 mg/day
    Pediatric: <12 years: not recommended; ≥12 years: same as adult
    Zoloft *Tab:* 25*, 50*, 100*mg; *Oral conc:* 20 mg per ml (60 ml) (alcohol 12%); dilute just before administering in 4 oz water, ginger ale, lemon-lime soda, lemonade, <u>or</u> orange juice
▷ *nortriptyline* (D)(G) initially 25 mg tid-qid; max 150 mg/day
    Pediatric: <12 years: not recommended; ≥12 years: same as adult
    Pamelor *Cap:* 10, 25, 50, 75 mg; *Oral soln:* 10 mg/5 ml

CALCIUM SUPPLEMENTS

▷ *calcium* **(C)** 1200 mg/day
see **Osteoporosis** *page* 331

 PRIMARY IMMUNODEFICIENCY IN ADULTS

▷ *recombinant human hyaluronidase (human normal immunoglobulin)* **(C)**
HyQvia see mfr pkg insert for dose by weight and dose schedule table
Vial: 10%; 2.5 gm/200 u, 5 gm/400 u, 10 gm/800 u, 20 gm/1600 u, 30 gm/2400
u (2 single-use/dual-vial unit (preservative-free)
Comment: HyQvia is an immune globulin with a recombinant human
hyaluronidase indicated for the treatment of primary immunodeficiency (PI) in
adults. This includes, but is not limited to, common variable immunodeficiency
(CVID), X-linked agammaglobulinemia, congenital agammaglobulinemia, Wiskott-
Aldrich syndrome, and severe combined immunodeficiencies. **HyQvia** contains
IgG antibodies, collected from human plasma donated by healthy people. **HyQvia**
is a dual vial unit with one vial of immune globulin infusion 10% (Human) and one
vial of recombinant human hyaluronidase. The hyaluronidase part of **HyQvia** helps
more of the immune globulin get absorbed into the body. HyQvia is a ready-for-
use sterile, liquid preparation of highly purified, concentrated, broad spectrum
IgG antibodies. The distribution of the IgG subclasses is similar to that of normal
plasma. Contains 100 mg/ml protein. **HyQvia** is collected only at FDA approved
blood establishments and is tested by FDA licensed serological tests for Hepatitis B
Surface Antigen (HBsAg), and for antibodies to Human Immunodeficiency Virus
(HIV-1/HIV-2) and Hepatitis C Virus (HCV) in accordance with U.S. regulatory
requirements. As an additional safety measure, mini-pools of the plasma are tested
for the presence of HIV-1 and HCV by FDA licensed Nucleic Acid Testing (NAT).
Protect from light. Use within 3 months after removal to room temperature but
within the expiration date on the carton and vial labels. Do not return vials to the
refrigerator after being stored at room temperature.

PROCTITIS: ACUTE (PROCTOCOLITIS, ENTERITIS)

Comment: The following regimen for the treatment of proctitis, proctocolitis, and
enteritis is published in the **2015 CDC Sexually Transmitted Diseases Treatment
Guidelines**.

RECOMMENDED REGIMEN

▷ *ceftriaxone* **(B)(G)** 250 mg IM in a single dose
Rocephin *Vial:* 250, 500 mg; 1, 2 gm
plus
▷ *doxycycline* 100 mg bid x 7 days
Acticlate *Tab:* 75, 150**mg
Adoxa *Tab:* 50, 75, 100, 150 mg ent-coat
Doryx *Tab:* 50, 75, 100, 150, 200 mg del-rel
Doxteric *Tab:* 50 mg del-rel
Monodox *Cap:* 50, 75, 100 mg
Oracea *Cap:* 40 mg del-rel
Vibramycin *Tab:* 100 mg; *Cap:* 50, 100 mg; *Syr:* 50 mg/5 ml (raspberry-apple)
(sulfites); *Oral susp:* 25 mg/5 ml (raspberry)
Vibra-Tab *Tab:* 100 mg film-coat

PROSTATITIS: ACUTE

ANTI-INFECTIVES

▷ *ciprofloxacin* (C) 500 mg bid x 4-6 weeks
  Pediatric: <18 years: not recommended; ≥18 years: same as adult
    Cipro (G) *Tab:* 250, 500, 750 mg; *Oral susp:* 250, 500 mg/5 ml (100 ml)
    (strawberry)
    Cipro XR *Tab:* 500, 1000 mg ext-rel
    ProQuin XR *Tab:* 500 mg ext-rel

Comment: *ciprofloxacin* is contraindicated <18 years-of-age, and during pregnancy and lactation. Risk of tendonitis or tendon rupture.

▷ *norfloxacin* (C) 400 mg bid x 28 days
  Pediatric: <18 years: not recommended; ≥18 years: same as adult
    Noroxin *Tab:* 400 mg

Comment: *norfloxacin* is contraindicated <18 years-of-age, and during pregnancy and lactation. Risk of tendonitis or tendon rupture.

▷ *ofloxacin* (C)(G) 300 mg x bid x 6 weeks
  Pediatric: <18 years: not recommended; ≥18 years: same as adult
    Floxin *Tab:* 200, 300, 400 mg

Comment: *ofloxacin* is contraindicated <18 years-of-age, and during pregnancy and lactation. Risk of tendonitis or tendon rupture.

▷ *trimethoprim+sulfamethoxazole (TMP-SMX)* (C)(G)
  Pediatric: <12 years: not recommended; ≥12 years: same as adult
    Bactrim, Septra 2 tabs bid x 10 days
      Tab: trim 80 mg+*sulfa* 400 mg*
    Bactrim DS, Septra DS 1 tab bid x 10 days
      Tab: trim 160 mg+*sulfa* 800 mg*
    Bactrim Pediatric Suspension, Septra Pediatric Suspension
      Oral susp: trim 40 mg+*sulfa* 200 mg per 5 ml (100 ml) (cherry) (alcohol 0.3%)

 PROSTATITIS: CHRONIC

ANTI-INFECTIVES

▷ *carbenicillin* (B) 2 tabs qid x 4-12 weeks
    Geocillin *Tab:* 382 mg

▷ *ciprofloxacin* (C) 500 mg bid x 3 or more months
  Pediatric: <18 years: not recommended; ≥18 years: same as adult
    Cipro (G) *Tab:* 250, 500, 750 mg; *Oral susp:* 250, 500 mg/5 ml (100 ml) (strawberry)
    Cipro XR *Tab:* 500, 1000 mg ext-rel
    ProQuin XR *Tab:* 500 mg ext-rel

Comment: *ciprofloxacin* is contraindicated <18 years-of-age, and during pregnancy and lactation. Risk of tendonitis or tendon rupture.

▷ *norfloxacin* (C) 400 mg bid x 4-12 weeks
  Pediatric: <18 years: not recommended; ≥18 years: same as adult
    Noroxin *Tab:* 400 mg

Comment: *norfloxacin* contraindicated <18 years-of-age, and during pregnancy and lactation. Risk of tendonitis or tendon rupture.

▷ *ofloxacin* (C)(G) 300 mg bid x 4-12 weeks
  Pediatric: <18 years: not recommended; ≥18 years: same as adult
    Floxin *Tab:* 200, 300, 400 mg

Comment: *ofloxacin* is contraindicated <18 years-of-age, and during pregnancy and lactation. Risk of tendonitis or tendon rupture.

▷ *trimethoprim+sulfamethoxazole* (C)(G)
  Pediatric: <18 years: See Appendix ___ for dose by weight; ≥18 years: same as adult
    Bactrim, Septra 2 tabs bid x 10 days
      Tab: trim 80 mg+*sulfa* 400 mg*
    Bactrim DS, Septra DS 1 tab bid x 10 days
      Tab: trim 160 mg+*sulfa* 800 mg
    Bactrim Pediatric Suspension, Septra Pediatric Suspension 20 ml bid x 10 days
      Oral susp: trim 40 mg+*sulfa* 200 mg per 5 ml (100 ml) (cherry) (alcohol
      0.3%)

SUPPRESSION THERAPY

▷ *trimethoprim+sulfamethoxazole (TMP-SMX)* (C)(G)
  Pediatric: <18 years: not recommended; ≥18 years: same as adult
    Bactrim, Septra 2 tabs bid x 10 days
      Tab: trim 80 mg+*sulfa* 400 mg*
    Bactrim DS, Septra DS 1 tab bid x 10 days
      Tab: trim 160 mg+*sulfa* 800 mg*
    Bactrim Pediatric Suspension, Septra Pediatric Suspension 20 ml bid x 10 days
      Oral susp: trim 40 mg+*sulfa* 200 mg per 5 ml (100 ml) (cherry) (alcohol 0.3%)

 PRURITUS

Topical Corticosteroids *see page* 566
Parenteral Corticosteroids *see page* 570
Oral Corticosteroids *see page* 569
OTC Antihistamines
OTC Eucerin Products
OTC Lac-Hydrin Products
OTC Lubriderm Products
OTC Aveeno Products

TOPICAL OIL

▷ *fluocinolone acetonide* 0.01% topical oil (C)
  Pediatric: <6 years: not recommended; ≥6 years: apply sparingly bid for up to 4 weeks
    Derma-Smoothe/FS Topical Oil apply sparingly tid
      Topical oil: 0.01% (4 oz) (peanut oil)

TOPICAL/TRANSDERMAL ANALGESICS

▷ *capsaicin* (B)(G) apply tid-qid prn to intact skin
  Pediatric: <2 years: not recommended; ≥2 years: same as adult
    Axsain *Crm:* 0.075% (1, 2 oz)
    Capsin (OTC) *Lotn:* 0.025, 0, 075% (59 ml)
    Capzasin-P (OTC) *Crm:* 0.025% (1.5 oz); Lotn: 0.025% (2 oz)
    Capzasin-HP (OTC) *Crm:* 0.075% (1.5 oz); Lotn: 0.075% (2 oz)
    Dolorac *Crm:* 0.025% (28 gm)
    Double Cap (OTC) *Crm:* 0.05% (2 oz)
    Qutenza (B) *Patch:* 8% (1-2, both with 50 gm tube of cleansing gel)
    R-Gel *Gel:* 0.025% (15, 30 gm)
    Zostrix (OTC) *Crm:* 0.025% (0.7, 1.5, 3 oz)
    Zostrix HP (OTC) *Emol crm:* 0.075% (1, 2 oz)
  Comment: Provides some relief by 1-2 weeks; optimal benefit may take 4-6 weeks.
▷ *doxepin* (B) cream apply to affected area qid at intervals of at least 3-4 hours; max 8 days
  Pediatric: <12 years: not recommended; ≥12 years: same as adult

      Prudoxin *Crm:* 5% (45 gm)
      Zonalon *Crm:* 5% (30, 45 gm)
▷ *pimecrolimus* 1% cream (C) <2 years: not recommended; ≥2 years: apply to affected area bid; do not apply an occlusive dressing
      Elidel *Crm:* 1% (30, 60, 100 gm)
Comment: *pimecrolimus* is indicated for short-term and intermittent long-term use. Discontinue use when resolution occurs. Contraindicated if the patient is immunosuppressed. Change to the 0.1% preparation or if secondary bacterial infection is present.
▷ *tacrolimus* (C) apply to affected area bid; continue for 1 week after clearing
    Pediatric: <2 years: not recommended; 2-15 years: use 0.03% strength; apply to affected area bid; continue for 1 week after clearing
      Protopic *Oint:* 0.03, 0.1% (30, 60 gm)

 PSEUDOBULBAR AFFECT (PBA) DISORDER

Comment: Pseudobulbar affect (PBA), emotional lability, labile affect, or emotional incontinence refers by to a neurologic disorder characterized by involuntary crying or uncontrollable episodes of crying and/or laughing, or other emotional outbursts. PBA occurs secondary to a neurologic disease or brain injury such as traumatic brain injury (TBI), stroke, Parkinson's disease, multiple sclerosis, amyotrophic lateral sclerosis (ALS, Lou Gehrig disease).
▷ *dextromethorphan+quinidine* (C)(G) 1 cap once daily x 7 days; then starting on day 8, 1 cap bid
    Pediatric: <12 years: not recommended; ≥12 years: same as adult
      Nuedexta *Cap:* dextro 20 mg+quini 10 mg
Comment: *dextromethorphan hydrobromide* is an uncompetitive NMDA receptor antagonist and sigma-1 agonist. *quinidine sulfate* is a CYP450 2D6 inhibitor. **Nuedexta** is contraindicated with an MAOI or within 14 days of stopping an MAOI, with prolonged QT interval, congenital long QT syndrome, history suggestive of torsades de pointes, or heart failure, complete atrioventricular (AV) block without implanted pacemaker or patients at high risk of complete AV block, and concomitant drugs that both prolong QT interval and are metabolized by CYP2D6 (e.g., *thioridazine* or *pimozide*). Discontinue **Nuedexta** if the following occurs: hepatitis or thrombocytopenia or any other hypersensitivity reaction. Monitor ECG in patients with left ventricular hypertrophy (LVH) or left ventricular dysfunction (LVD). *desipramine* exposure increases **Nuedexta** 8-fold; reduce *desipramine* dose and adjust based on clinical response. Use of **Nuedexta** with selective serotonin reuptake inhibitors (SSRIs) or tricyclic antidepressants (TCAs) increases the risk of serotonin syndrome. *paroxetine* exposure increases **Nuedexta** 2-fold; therefore, reduce **paroxetine** dose and adjust based on clinical response (*digoxin* exposure may increase *digoxin* substrate plasma concentration. **Nuedexta** is not recommended in pregnancy or breastfeeding. Safety and effectiveness of **Nuedexta** in children have not been established. To report suspected adverse reactions, contact Avanir Pharmaceuticals at 1-866-388-5041 or FDA at 1-800-FDA-1088 or www.fda.gov/medwatch

 PSEUDOGOUT

Injectable Acetaminophen *see Pain page* 344
NSAIDs *see page* 562
Opioid Analgesics *see Pain page* 345
Topical and Transdermal NSAIDs *see Pain page* 334

Parenteral Corticosteroids *see page* 570
Oral Corticosteroids *see page* 569
Topical Analgesic and Anesthetic Agents *see page* 560

 PSEUDOMEMBRANOUS COLITIS

Comment: Staphylococcal enterocolitis and antibiotic-associated pseudomembranous colitis caused by *C. difficile*.

ANTI-INFECTIVES

▷ *vancomycin* (B, caps; C, susp)(G) 500 mg to 2 gm in 3-4 doses x 7-10 days; max 2 gm/day
  Pediatric: 40 mg/kg/day in 3-4 doses x 7-10 days; max 2 gm/day
▷ *metronidazole* (not for use in 1st; B in 2nd, 3rd)(G) 500 mg tid x 14 days
    Flagyl *Tab:* 250*, 500*mg
    Flagyl 375 *Cap:* 375 mg
    Flagyl ER *Tab:* 750 mg ext-rel

 PSITTACOSIS

ANTI-INFECTIVES

▷ *tetracycline* (D)(G) 250 mg qid <u>or</u> 500 mg tid x 7-14 days
  Pediatric: <8 years: not recommended; ≥8 years, <100 lb: 25-50 mg/kg/day in 4 doses x 7-14 days; ≥8 years, ≥100 lb: same as adult
    Achromycin V *Cap:* 250, 500 mg
    Sumycin *Tab:* 250, 500 mg; *Cap:* 250, 500 mg; *Oral susp:* 125 mg/5 ml (100, 200 ml) (fruit) (sulfites)
  Comment: *tetracycline* is contraindicated <8 years-of-age, in pregnancy, and lactation (discolors developing tooth enamel). A side effect may be photo-sensitivity (photophobia). Do not give with antacids or calcium supplements within two hours of another drug.

 PSORIASIS, PLAQUE PSORIASIS

Emollients *see Dermatitis: Atopic page* 122
Topical Corticosteroids *see page* 566

VITAMIN D-3 DERIVATIVES

▷ *calcipotriene* (C)
  Pediatric: <12 years: not recommended; ≥12 years: same as adult
    Dovonex apply bid to lesions and gently rub in completely
      Crm: 0.005% (30, 120 gm)

VITAMIN D-3 DERIVATIVE+CORTICOSTEROID COMBINATIONS

▷ *calcipotriene+betamethasone dipropionate* (C)(G)
  Pediatric: <18 years: not recommended; ≥18 years: same as adult
    Enstilar apply to affected area and gently rub in once daily x up to 4 weeks; limit treatment area to 30% of body surface area; do not occlude; do not use on face, axillae, groin, <u>or</u> atrophic skin; max 100 gm/week
      Foam: calci 0.005%+*beta* 0.064% (60 gm spray can)

Taclonex apply to affected area and gently rub in once daily as needed, up to 4 weeks

Taclonex Ointment apply bid to lesions and gently rub in completely; limit treatment area to 30% of body surface area; do not occlude; do not use on face, axillae, groin, _or_ atrophic skin; max 100 gm/week

Oint: calci 0.005%+_beta_ 0.064% (60, 100 gm)

Taclonex Scalp Topical Suspension apply to affected area and gently rub in once daily x 2 weeks _or_ until cleared; max 8 weeks; limit treatment area to 30% of body surface area; do not occlude; do not use on face, axillae, groin, _or_ atrophic skin; max 100 gm/week

Bottle: (30, 60 gm; 120 gm [2 x 60 gm])

▷ _Calcitriol_ (C)

Pediatric: <18 years: not recommended; ≥18 years: same as adult

Vectical apply bid to lesions and gently rub in completely; max weekly dose should not exceed 200 gm

Oint: 3 mcg/gm (100 gm)

IMMUNOSUPPRESSANTS

▷ _alefacept_ (B) 7.5 mg IV bolus _or_ 15 mg IM once weekly x 12 weeks; may re-treat x 12 weeks

Pediatric: <12 years: not recommended; ≥12 years: same as adult

Amevive _IV dose pack:_ 7.5 mg single-use (w. 10 ml sterile water diluents [use 0.6 ml]; 1, 4/pck); _IM dose pack:_ 15 mg single-use (w. 10 ml sterile water diluent [use 0.6 ml]; 1, 4/pck

Comment: CD4+ and T-lymphocyte count should be checked prior to initiating treatment with _alefacept_ and then monitored. Treatment should be withheld if CD4+ T-lymphocyte counts are below 250 cells/mcl.

▷ _cyclosporine_ (C) 1.25 mg/kg bid; may increase after 4 weeks by 0.5 mg/kg/day; then adjust at 2-week intervals; max 4 mg/kg/day; administer with meals

Pediatric: <18 years: not recommended; ≥18 years: same as adult

Neoral _Cap:_ 25, 100 mg (alcohol)

Neoral Oral Solution _Oral soln:_ 100 mg/ml (50 ml) may dilute in room temperature apple juice _or_ orange juice (alcohol)

ANTIMITOTICS

▷ _anthralin_ (C) apply once daily

Pediatric: <12 years: not recommended; ≥12 years: same as adult

Zithranol-RR _Crm:_ 1.2% (15, 45 gm)

RETINOIDS

▷ _acitretin_ (X)(G) 25-50 mg once daily with main meal

Pediatric: <12 years: not recommended; ≥12 years: same as adult

Soriatane _Cap:_ 10, 25 mg

▷ _tazarotene_ (X)(G) apply once daily at HS

Pediatric: <12 years: not recommended; ≥12 years: same as adult

Avage Cream _Crm:_ 0.1% (30 gm)

Tazorac Cream _Crm:_ 0.05, 0.1% (15, 30, 60 gm)

Tazorac Gel _Gel:_ 0.05, 0.1% (30, 100 gm)

COAL TAR PREPARATIONS

▷ _coal tar_ (C)(G)

Pediatric: same as adult

Scytera (OTC) apply qd-qid; use lowest effective dose
> *Foam:* 2%

T/Gel Shampoo Extra Strength (OTC) use every other day; max 4 x/week; massage into affected areas for 5 minutes; rinse; repeat *Shampoo:* 1%

T/Gel Shampoo Original Formula (OTC) use every other day; max 7 x/week; massage into affected areas for 5 minutes; rinse; repeat *Shampoo:* 0.5%

T/Gel Shampoo Stubborn Itch Control (OTC) use every other day; max 7 x/week; massage into affected areas for 5 minutes; rinse; repeat *Shampoo:* 0.5%

INTERLEUKIN-17A ANTAGONIST

▷ *brodalumab* (B) inject SC into the upper arm, abdomen, or thigh; rotate sites; administer 210 mg SC (as two separate 150 mg SC injections) at weeks 0, 1, and 2; then 210 mg every 2 weeks
Pediatric: <18 years: not recommended; ≥18 years: same as adult
> **Siliq** *Prefilled pen:* 210 mg/1.5 ml solution, single-use (2/carton) (preservative-free)

Comment: **Siliq** is currently indicated for plaque psoriasis only. **Siliq** is contraindicated with Crohn's disease. *Black Box Warning (BBW):* Suicidal ideation and behavior, including completed suicides, have occurred in patients treated with **Siliq**. Prior to prescribing, weigh potential risks and benefits in patients with a history of depression and/or suicidal ideation or behavior. Patients with new or worsening suicidal thoughts and behavior should be referred to a mental health professional, as appropriate. Advise patients and caregivers to seek medical attention for manifestations of suicidal ideation or behavior, new onset or worsening depression, anxiety, or other mood changes. Avoid using live vaccines concurrently with **Siliq** therapy. There are no human data on **Siliq** use in pregnant women to inform a drug associated risk. Human IgG antibodies are known to cross the placental barrier; therefore, **Siliq** may be transmitted from the mother to the developing fetus. There are no data on the presence of *brodalumab* in human milk or effects on the breastfed infant. **Siliq** is available only through the re-stricted **Siliq** REMS Program.

▷ *secukinumab* (B) inject SC into the upper arm, abdomen, or thigh; rotate sites; administer 300 mg SC (as two separate 150 mg SC injections) at weeks 0, 1, 2, 3, and 4; then 300 mg every 4 weeks; for some patients, 150 mg/dose may be sufficient
Pediatric: <18 years: not recommended; ≥18 years: same as adult
> **Cosentyx** *Vial:* 150 mg/ml pwdr for SC inj after reconstitution single-use (preservative-free)

Comment: **Cosentyx** may be used as monotherapy or in combination with *methotrexate* (MTX). Avoid using live vaccines concurrently with **Siliq** therapy. For professional preparation and administration only.

INTERLEUKIN-12+INTERLEUKIN-23 ANTAGONIST

▷ *ustekinumab* (B) inject SC; rotate sites; <100 kg: 45 mg once; then 4 weeks later; then every 12 weeks; ≥100 kg: 90 mg once; then 4 weeks later; then every 12 weeks
Pediatric: <18 years: not recommended; ≥18 years: same as adult
> **Stelara** *Vial:* 45 mg/0.5 ml single-use (preservative-free)
> Comment: **Stelara** may be used as monotherapy or in combination with *methotrexate* (MTX).

TUMOR NECROSIS FACTOR (TNF) BLOCKERS

▷ *adalimumab* (B) initially 80 mg SC once followed by 40 mg once every other week starting one week after initial dose; inject into thigh or abdomen; rotate sites
Pediatric: <18 years: not recommended; ≥18 years: same as adult

> **Humira** *Prefilled syringe:* 20 mg/0.4 ml; 40 mg/0.8 ml single-dose (2/pck; 2, 6/ starter pck) (preservative-free)

▷ **adalimumab-adbm (B)** initially 80 SC; then, 40 mg SC every other week starting one week after initial dose; inject into thigh or abdomen; rotate sites
Pediatric: <18 years: not recommended; ≥18 years: same as adult

> **Cyltezo** *Prefilled syringe:* 40 mg/0.8 ml single-dose (preservative-free)

Comment: **Cyltezo** is biosimilar to **Humira** (*adalimumab*).

▷ **etanercept (B)** inject SC into thigh, abdomen, <u>or</u> upper arm; rotate sites; initially 50 mg twice weekly (3-4 days apart) for 3 months; then 50 mg/week maintenance <u>or</u> 25 mg <u>or</u> 50 mg per week for 3 months; then 50 mg/week maintenance
Pediatric: <4 years: not recommended; 4-17 years: Chronic moderate-to-severe plaque psoriasis; >17 years: same as adult

> **Enbrel** *Vial:* 25 mg pwdr for SC injection after reconstitution (4/carton w. supplies) (preservative-free, diluent contains benzyl alcohol); *Prefilled syringe:* 25, 50 mg/ml (preservative-free); *SureClick autoinjector:* 50 mg/ml (preservative-free)

▷ **golimumab (B)** administer SC <u>or</u> IV infusion (in combination with *methotrexate [MTX]*)
Pediatric: <18 years: not recommended; ≥18 years: same as adult

> **Simponi** 50 mg SC once monthly; rotate sites
> *Prefilled syringe, SmartJect autoinjector:* 50 mg/0.5 ml, single-use (preservative-free)
> **Simponi Aria** 2 mg/kg IV infusion week 0 and week 4; then every 8 weeks thereafter
> *Vial:* 50 mg/4 ml, single-use, soln for IV infusion after dilution (latex-free, preservative-free)

▷ **infliximab** *(tumor necrosis factor-alpha blocker)* must be refrigerated at 2°C to 8°C (36°F to 46°F); administer dose intravenously over a period of not less than 2 hours; do not use beyond the expiration date as this product contains no preservative; administer in conjunction with *methotrexate*, infuse 3 mg/kg at 0, 2 and 6 weeks; then every 8 weeks; some patients may benefit from increasing the dose up to 10 mg/kg <u>or</u> treatment as often as every 4 weeks
Pediatric: <6 years: not studied; ≥6-17 years: 3 mg/kg at 0, 2 and 6 weeks, then every 8 weeks; ≥18 years: same as adult

> **Remicade** *Vial:* 100 mg for reconstitution to 10 ml administration volume, single-dose (preservative-free)

Comment: **Remicade** is indicated to reduce signs and symptoms, and induce and maintain clinical remission, in adults and children ≥6 years-of-age with moderately to severely active disease who have had an inadequate response to conventional therapy <u>and</u> reduce the number of draining enterocutaneous and rectovaginal fistulas, and maintain fistula closure, in adults with fistulizing disease. Common adverse effects associated with **Remicade** included abdominal pain, headache, pharyngitis, sinusitis, and upper respiratory infections. In addition, **Remicade** might increase the risk for serious infections, including tuberculosis, bacterial sepsis, and invasive fungal infections. Available data from published literature on the use of *infliximab* products during pregnancy have not reported a clear association with *infliximab* products and adverse pregnancy outcomes. *infliximab* products cross the placenta and infants exposed *in utero* should not be administered live vaccines for at least 6 months after birth. Otherwise, the infant may be at increased risk of infection, including disseminated infection which can become fatal. Available information is insufficient to inform the amount of *infliximab* products present in human milk <u>or</u> effects on the breastfed infant. To report suspected adverse reactions, contact Merck Sharp & Dohme Corp., a subsidiary of Merck & Co. at 1-877-888-4231 <u>or</u> FDA at 1-800-FDA1088 <u>or</u> www.fda.gov/medwatch

▷ **infliximab-abda** *(tumor necrosis factor-alpha blocker)* **(B)**

Renflexis: see **infliximab** (Remicade) above for full prescribing information

Comment: **Renflexis** is a biosimilar to **Remicade** for the treatment of immune-disorders including Crohn's disease, ulcerative colitis, rheumatoid arthritis, ankylosing spondylitis, psoriatic arthritis and plaque psoriasis. **Renflexis** was approved under the FDA category for biosimilars and demonstrated no clinically meaningful differences for use, dosing regimens, strengths, dosage forms, and routes of administration from the FDA-approved biological product **Remicade**.

▷ **infliximab-dyyb** *(tumor necrosis factor-alpha blocker)* **(B)**

Inflectra: see **infliximab** (Remicade) above for full prescribing information

Comment: **Inflectra** is a biosimilar to **Remicade** for the treatment of immune-disorders including Crohn's disease, ulcerative colitis, rheumatoid arthritis, ankylosing spondylitis, psoriatic arthritis and plaque psoriasis. **Inflectra** was approved under the FDA category for biosimilars and demonstrated no clinically meaningful differences for use, dosing regimens, strengths, dosage forms, and routes of administration from the FDA-approved biological product **Remicade**.

Renflexis *see infliximab* (Remicade) above for full prescribing information

Comment: **Inflectra** is a biosimilar to **Remicade** for the treatment of immune-disorders including Crohn's disease, ulcerative colitis, rheumatoid arthritis, ankylosing spondylitis, psoriatic arthritis and plaque psoriasis. **Inflectra** was approved under the FDA category for biosimilars and demonstrated no clinically meaningful differences for use, dosing regimens, strengths, dosage forms, and routes of administration from the FDA-approved biological product **Remicade**.

▷ **infliximab-qbtx** *(tumor necrosis factor-alpha blocker)* **(B)**

Ifixi: see **infliximab** (Remicade) above for full prescribing information

Comment: **Ifixi** is a biosimilar to **Remicade** for the treatment of immune disorders including Crohn's disease, ulcerative colitis, rheumatoid arthritis, ankylosing spondylitis, psoriatic arthritis and plaque psoriasis. **Ifixi** was approved under the FDA category for biosimilars and demonstrated no clinically meaningful differences for use, dosing regimens, strengths, dosage forms, and routes of administration from the FDA-approved biological product **Remicade**.

MOISTURIZING AGENTS

Aquaphor Healing Ointment (OTC) *Oint:* (1.75, 3.5, 14 oz) (alcohol)

Eucerin Daily Sun Defense (OTC) *Lotn:* 6 oz (fragrance-free)

Comment: **Eucerin Daily Sun Defense** is a moisturizer with SPF 15.

Eucerin Facial Lotion (OTC) *Lotn:* 4 oz

Eucerin Light Lotion (OTC) *Lotn:* 8 oz

Eucerin Lotion (OTC) *Lotn:* 8, 16 oz

Eucerin Original Creme (OTC) *Crm:* 2, 4, 16 oz (alcohol)

Eucerin Plus Creme *Crm:* 4 oz

Eucerin Plus Lotion (OTC) *Lotn:* 6, 12 oz

Eucerin Protective Lotion (OTC) *Lotn:* 4 oz (alcohol)

Comment: **Eucerin Protective Lotion** is a moisturizer with SPF 25.

Lac-Hydrin Cream (OTC) *Crm:* 280, 385 gm

Lac-Hydrin Lotion (OTC) *Lotn:* 225, 400 gm

Lubriderm Dry Skin Scented (OTC) *Lotn:* 6, 10, 16, 32 oz

Lubriderm Dry Skin Unscented (OTC) *Lotn:* 3.3, 6, 10, 16 oz (fragrance-free)

Lubriderm Sensitive Skin Lotion (OTC) *Lotn:* 3.3, 6, 10, 16 oz (lanolin-free)

Lubriderm Dry Skin (OTC) *Lotn (scented):* 2.5, 6, 10, 16 oz;
Lotn (fragrance-free): 1, 2.5, 6, 10, 16 oz

Lubriderm Bath 1-2 capfuls in bath <u>or</u> rub onto wet skin as needed; then rinse (8 oz)

PSORIATIC ARTHRITIS

Injectable Acetaminophen *see Pain page* 344
NSAIDs *see page* 562
Opioid Analgesics *see Pain page* 345
Topical and Transdermal NSAIDs *see Pain page* 344
Parenteral Corticosteroids *see page* 570
Oral Corticosteroids *see page* 569
Topical Analgesic and Anesthetic Agents *see page* 560

TOPICAL/TRANSDERMAL ANALGESICS

▷ *capsaicin* **(B)(G)** apply tid-qid prn to intact skin
  Pediatric: <2 years: not recommended; ≥2 years: same as adult
    Axsain *Crm:* 0.075% (1, 2 oz)
    Capsin *Lotn:* 0.025, 0.075% (59 ml)
    Capzasin-P (OTC) *Crm:* 0.025% (1.5 oz); *Lotn:* 0.025% (2 oz)
    Dolorac *Crm:* 0.025% (28 gm)
    Double Cap (OTC) *Crm:* 0.05% (2 oz)
    Qutenza (B) *Patch:* 8% (1-2, both with 50 gm tube of cleansing gel)
    R-Gel *Gel:* 0.025% (15, 30 gm)
    Zostrix (OTC) *Crm:* 0.025% (0.7, 1.5, 3 oz)
    Zostrix HP (OTC) *Emol crm:* 0.075% (1, 2 oz)
Comment: Provides some relief by 1-2 weeks; optimal benefit may take 4-6 weeks.
▷ *diclofenac sodium* **(C; D ≥30 wks)** apply qid prn to intact skin
  Pediatric: <12 years: not recommended; ≥12 years: same as adult
    Pennsaid 1.5% in 10 drop increments, dispense and rub into front, side, and back
    of knee: usually; 40 drops (40 mg) qid
      Topical soln: 1.5% (150 ml)
    Pennsaid 2% apply 2 pump actuations (40 mg) and rub into front, side, and back
    of knee bid
      Topical soln: 2% (20 mg/pump actuation, 112 gm)
Comment: **Pennsaid** is indicated for the treatment of pain associated with osteoarthritis
of the knee.
    Pennsaid 2% apply 2 pump actuations (40 mg) and rub into front, side, and back
    of knee bid
    Solaraze Gel *Gel:* 3% (50 gm) (benzyl alcohol)
Comment: Contraindicated with *aspirin* allergy. As with other NSAIDs, **Solaraze Gel**
should be avoided in late pregnancy (≥30 weeks) because it may cause premature closure
of the ductus arteriosus.
    Voltaren Gel (G) *Gel:* 1% (100 gm)
Comment: Contraindicated with *aspirin* allergy. As with other NSAIDs, **Voltaren Gel**
should be avoided in late pregnancy (≥30 weeks) because it may cause premature closure
of the ductus arteriosus.
▷ *trolamine salicylate* apply tid-qid
    Mobisyl *Crm:* 10%
Comment: Provides some relief by 1-2 weeks; optimal benefit may take 4-6 weeks.

ORAL SALICYLATE

▷ *indomethacin* **(C)** initially 25 mg bid-tid, increase as needed at weekly intervals by
25-50 mg/day; max 200 mg/day
Pediatric: <14 years: usually not recommended; >2 years, if risk warranted: 1-2 mg/
kg/day in divided doses; max 3-4 mg/kg/day <u>or</u> 150-200 mg/day, whichever is less;
<14 years: ER cap not recommended

Cap: 25, 50 mg; *Susp;* 25 mg/5 ml (pineapple-coconut, mint) (alcohol 1%);
Supp: 50 mg; *ER Cap:* 75 mg ext-rel

Comment: *indomethacin* is indicated only for acute painful flares. Administer with food and/or antacids. Use lowest effective dose for shortest duration.

ORAL NSAIDs

See more **Oral NSAIDs** page 562

➤ *diclofenac sodium* (C)
> **Voltaren** 50 mg bid-qid or 75 mg bid or 25 mg qid with an additional 25 mg at HS if necessary
> *Tab:* 25, 50, 75 mg ent-coat
> **Voltaren XR** 100 mg once daily; rarely, 100 mg bid may be used
> *Tab:* 100 mg ext-rel

NSAID+PPI

➤ *esomeprazole+naproxen* (C)(G) 1 tab bid; use lowest effective dose for the shortest duration swallow whole; take at least 30 minutes before a meal
> *Pediatric:* <18 years: not recommended; ≥18 years: same as adult
> **Vimovo** *Tab:* nap 375 mg+eso 20 mg ext-rel; nap 500 mg+eso 20 mg ext-rel

Comment: **Vimovo** is indicated to improve signs/symptoms, and risk of gastric ulcer in patients at risk of developing NSAID-associated gastric ulcer.

COX-2 INHIBITORS

Comment: Cox-2 inhibitors are contraindicated with history of asthma, urticaria, and allergic-type reactions to *aspirin*, other NSAIDs, and sulfonamides, 3rd trimester of pregnancy, and coronary artery bypass graft (CABG) surgery.

➤ *celecoxib* (C)(G) 50-400 mg once daily-bid; max 800 mg/day
> *Pediatric:* <18 years: not recommended; ≥18 years: same as adult
> **Celebrex** *Cap:* 50, 100, 200, 400 mg

➤ *meloxicam* (C)(G)
> *Pediatric:* <18 years: not recommended; ≥18 years: same as adult
> **Mobic** <2 years, <60 kg: not recommended; ≥2, ≥60 kg: 0.125 mg/kg; max 7.5 mg once daily; ≥18 years: initially 7.5 mg once daily; max 15 mg once daily; *Hemodialysis:* max 7.5 mg/day
> *Tab:* 7.5, 15 mg; *Oral susp:* 7.5 mg/5 ml (100 ml) (raspberry)
> **Vivlodex** <18 years: not established; ≥18 years: initially 5 mg qd; may increase to max 10 mg/day; *Hemodialysis:* max 5 mg/day
> *Cap:* 5, 10 mg

PHOSPHODIESTERASE 4 (PDE4) INHIBITOR

➤ *apremilast* (C) swallow whole; initial titration over 5 days; maintenance 30 mg bid; *Day 1:* 10 mg in AM; *Day 2:* 10 mg AM and 10 mg PM; *Day 3:* 10 mg AM and 20 mg PM; *Day 4:* 20 mg AM and 20 mg PM; *Day 5:* 20 mg AM and 30 mg PM; *Day 6 and ongoing:* 30 mg AM and 30 mg PM
> *Pediatric:* <12 years: not recommended; ≥12 years: same as adult
> **Otezla** *Tab:* 10, 20, 30 mg; *2-Week Starter Pack*

Comment: Register pregnant patients exposed to by calling 877-311-8972.

INTERLEUKIN-12 AND INTERLEUKIN-23 ANTAGONIST

➤ *ustekinumab* (B) inject SC; rotate sites; <100 kg: 45 mg once; then 4 weeks later; then every 12 weeks; ≥100 kg: 90 mg once; then 4 weeks later; then every 12 weeks

Pediatric: <18 years: not recommended; ≥18 years: same as adult
> **Stelara** *Vial:* 45 mg/0.5 ml single-use (preservative-free)
Comment: Stelara may be used as monotherapy <u>or</u> in combination with ***methotrexate*** (MTX).

TUMOR NECROSIS FACTOR (TNF) BLOCKERS

▷ ***adalimumab*** **(B)** 40 mg SC once every other week; may increase to once weekly without ***methotrexate*** (MTX); administer in abdomen <u>or</u> thigh; rotate sites; 2-17 years, supervise first dose
Pediatric: <2 years, <10 kg: not recommended; 10-<15 kg: 10 mg every other week; 15-<30 kg: 20 mg every other week; 30 kg: 40 mg every other week
> **Humira** *Prefilled syringe:* 20 mg/0.4 ml; 40 mg/0.8 ml single-dose (2/pck; 2, 6/ starter pck) (preservative-free)
> **Comment: Humira** may use with ***methotrexate*** (MTX), DMARDS, corticoids, salicylates, NSAIDs, <u>or</u> analgesics.
▷ ***adalimumab-adbm*** **(B)** initially 80 SC; then, 40 mg SC every other week starting one week after initial dose; inject into thigh or abdomen; rotate sites
Pediatric: <18 years: not recommended; ≥18 years: same as adult
> **Cyltezo** *Prefilled syringe:* 40 mg/0.8 ml single-dose (preservative-free)
Comment: Cyltezo is biosimilar to **Humira** (***adalimumab***).
▷ ***etanercept*** **(B)** 25 mg SC twice weekly (72-96 hours apart) <u>or</u> 50 mg SC weekly; rotate sites
Pediatric: <4 years: not recommended; 4-17 years: 0.4 mg/kg SC twice weekly, 72-96 hours apart (max 25 mg/dose) <u>or</u> 0.8 mg/kg SC weekly (max 50 mg/dose); >17 years: same as adult
> **Enbrel** *Vial:* 25 mg pwdr for SC injection after reconstitution (4/carton w. supplies) (preservative-free; diluent contains benzyl alcohol); *Prefilled syringe:* 25, 50 mg/ml (preservative-free); *SureClick Autoinjector:* 50 mg/ml (preservative-free)
Comment: *etanercept* reduces pain, morning stiffness, and swelling. May be administered in combination with ***methotrexate***. Live vaccines should not be administered concurrently. Do not administer with active infection.
▷ ***golimumab*** **(B)** administer SC <u>or</u> IV infusion (in combination with ***methotrexate*** *[MTX]*)
Pediatric: <18 years: not recommended; ≥18 years: same as adult
> **Simponi** 50 mg SC once monthly; rotate sites
>> *Prefilled syringe, SmartJect autoinjector:* 50 mg/0.5 ml, single-use (preservative-free)
> **Simponi Aria** 2 mg/kg IV infusion week 0 and week 4; then every 8 weeks thereafter
>> *Vial:* 50 mg/4 ml, single-use, soln for IV infusion after dilution (latex-free, preservative-free)
Comment: Corticosteroids, nonbiologic DMARDs, <u>and/or</u> NSAIDs may be continued during treatment with ***golimumab***.
▷ ***infliximab*** *(tumor necrosis factor-alpha blocker)* must be refrigerated at 2°C to 8°C (36°F to 46°F); administer dose intravenously over a period of not less than 2 hours; do not use beyond the expiration date as this product contains no preservative; 5 mg/kg at 0, 2 and 6 weeks, then every 8 weeks; some adult patients who initially respond to treatment may benefit from increasing the dose to 10 mg/kg if response is lost later
Pediatric: <6 years: not studied; ≥6-17 years: mg/kg at 0, 2 and 6 weeks, then every 8 weeks; ≥18 years: same as adult
> **Remicade** *Vial:* 100 mg for reconstitution to 10 ml administration volume, single-dose (preservative-free)

Comment: **Remicade** is indicated to reduce signs and symptoms, and induce and maintain clinical remission, in adults and children ≥6 years-of-age with moderately to severely active disease who have had an inadequate response to conventional therapy and reduce the number of draining enterocutaneous and rectovaginal fistulas, and maintain fistula closure, in adults with fistulizing disease. Common adverse effects associated with **Remicade** included abdominal pain, headache, pharyngitis, sinusitis, and upper respiratory infections. In addition, **Remicade** might increase the risk for serious infections, including tuberculosis, bacterial sepsis, and invasive fungal infections. Available data from published literature on the use of *infliximab* products during pregnancy have not reported a clear association with *infliximab* products and adverse pregnancy outcomes. *infliximab* products cross the placenta and infants exposed *in utero* should not be administered live vaccines for at least 6 months after birth. Otherwise, the infant may be at increased risk of infection, including disseminated infection which can become fatal. Available information is insufficient to inform the amount of *infliximab* products present in human milk or effects on the breastfed infant. To report suspected adverse reactions, contact Merck Sharp & Dohme Corp., a subsidiary of Merck & Co. at 1-877-888-4231 or FDA at 1-800-FDA1088 or www.fda.gov/medwatch

▷ *infliximab-abda (tumor necrosis factor-alpha blocker)* (B)
   Renflexis: see *infliximab* (**Remicade**) above for full prescribing information
Comment: **Renflexis** is a biosimilar to **Remicade** for the treatment of immune-disorders including Crohn's disease, ulcerative colitis, rheumatoid arthritis, ankylosing spondylitis, psoriatic arthritis and plaque psoriasis. **Renflexis** was approved under the FDA category for biosimilars and demonstrated no clinically meaningful differences for use, dosing regimens, strengths, dosage forms, and routes of administration from the FDA-approved biological product **Remicade**.

▷ *infliximab-dyyb (tumor necrosis factor-alpha blocker)* (B)
   Inflectra: see *infliximab* (**Remicade**) above for full prescribing information
Comment: **Inflectra** is a biosimilar to **Remicade** for the treatment of immune-disorders including Crohn's disease, ulcerative colitis, rheumatoid arthritis, ankylosing spondylitis, psoriatic arthritis and plaque psoriasis. **Inflectra** was approved under the FDA category for biosimilars and demonstrated no clinically meaningful differences for use, dosing regimens, strengths, dosage forms, and routes of administration from the FDA-approved biological product **Remicade**.

▷ *infliximab-qbtx (tumor necrosis factor-alpha blocker)* (B)
   Ifixi: see *infliximab* (**Remicade**) above for full prescribing information
Comment: **Ifixi** is a biosimilar to **Remicade** for the treatment of immune disorders including Crohn's disease, ulcerative colitis, rheumatoid arthritis, ankylosing spondylitis, psoriatic arthritis and plaque psoriasis. **Ifixi** was approved under the FDA category for biosimilars and demonstrated no clinically meaningful differences for use, dosing regimens, strengths, dosage forms, and routes of administration from the FDA-approved biological product **Remicade**.

Selective Costimulation Modulator

▷ *abatacept* (C) administer as an IV infusion over 30 minutes at weeks 0, 2, and 4; then every 4 weeks thereafter; <60 kg, administer 500 mg/dose; 60-100 kg, administer 750 mg/dose; >100 kg, administer 1 gm/dose
   Pediatric: <6 years: not recommended; 6-17 years: administer as an IV infusion over 30 minutes at weeks 0, 2, and 4; then every 4 weeks thereafter; <75 kg, administer 10 mg/kg; same as adult (max 1 gm); >17 years: same as adult
      Orencia *Vial:* 250 mg pwdr for IV infusion after reconstitution (silicone-free) (preservative-free); *Prefilled syringe:* 125 mg/ml soln for SC injection (preservative-free); *ClickJect Autoinjector:* 125 mg/ml soln for SC injection

PULMONARY ARTERIAL HYPERTENSION (PAH) (WHO GROUP I)

ENDOTHELIAL RECEPTOR ANTAGONIST (ERA)

➤ *bosentan* (G) initiate at 62.5 mg orally twice daily; for patients weighing greater than 40 kg, increase to 125 mg orally twice daily after 4 weeks
Pediatric: <3 years: not established; 3-12: initiate at 62.5 mg orally twice daily; for patients weighing > 40 kg, increase to 125 mg orally twice daily after 4 weeks; >12 years: same as adult

      Tracleer *Tab:* 62.5, 125 mg film-coat; *Tab for oral suspension:* 32 mg

Comment: *bosentan* is an endothelin receptor antagonist (ERA) indicated for the treatment of pulmonary arterial hypertension (PAH) (WHO Group 1). **Tracleer** is the first ERA indicated for the treatment of PAH in patients aged 3 years and older with idiopathic or congenital PAH to improve pulmonary vascular resistance (PVR), which is expected to result in an improvement in exercise ability. The most common adverse events associated with **Tracleer** in clinical trials include respiratory tract infections, headache, edema, chest pain, syncope, flushing, hypotension, sinusitis, arthralgia, abnormal serum aminotransferases, palpitations, and anemia. Monitor hemoglobin levels after 1 and 3 months of treatment, then every 3 months thereafter. If signs of pulmonary edema occur, consider the diagnosis of associated pulmonary veno-occlusive disease (PVOD) and consider discontinuing **Tracleer**. Measure liver aminotransferases prior to initiation of treatment and then monthly. Reduce the dose and closely monitor patients developing aminotransferase elevations >3 x ULN. Co-administration of **Tracleer** with drugs metabolized by CYP2C9 and CYP3A can increase exposure to **Tracleer** and/or the co-administered drug. **Tracleer** use decreases contraceptive exposure and reduces effectiveness. There are no data on the presence of *bosentan* in human milk or the effects on the breastfed infant. However, because of the potential for serious adverse reactions, such as fluid retention and hepatotoxicity in breastfed infants, advise women not to breastfeed during treatment with **Tracleer** and pregnancy is contraindicated while taking **Tracleer**. To prevent pregnancy, females of reproductive potential must use two reliable forms of contraception during treatment and for one month after stopping **Tracleer** Due to the risks of hepatotoxicity and birth defects, **Tracleer** includes a boxed warning and is only available through the restricted **Tracleer** Risk Evaluation and Mitigation Strategy REMS Program, a restricted distribution program. Patients, prescribers, and pharmacies must enroll in the program to receive and administer **Tracleer**: http://www.tracleerrems.com/prescribers.aspx. To report adverse side effects, pregnancy, or other complications contact Actelion at 1-866-228-3546 or call 1-800-FDA-1088 or visit www.fda.gov/medwatch

PROSTACYCLIN RECEPTOR AGONIST

➤ *selexipag* (X) initially 200 mcg bid; increase by 200 mcg bid to highest tolerated dose up to 1600 mcg bid; *Moderate hepatic impairment (Child-Pugh Class B):* initially 200 mcg once daily; increase by 200 mcg once daily at weekly intervals as tolerated; swallow whole; may take with food to improve tolerability
Pediatric: <12 years: not recommended; ≥12 years: same as adult

    Uptravi
        Tab: 200, 400, 600, 800, 1000, 1200, 1400, 1600 mcg; *Titration pck:* 140 x 200 mcg + 60 x 800 mcg)

    Comment: Discontinue **Uptravi** if pulmonary veno-occlusive disease is confirmed or severe hepatic impairment (Child-Pugh Class C). May be potentiated by concomitant strong CYP2C8 inhibitors (e.g., gemfibrozil); *Nursing mothers:* not recommended. Discontinue breastfeeding or discontinue the drug.

GUANYLATE CYCLASE STIMULATOR

Endothelin Receptor Antagonist, Selective for the Endothelin Type-A (ETA) Receptor

➢ *ambrisentan* (X)(G) initiate treatment at 5 mg once daily, with <u>or</u> without *tadalafil* 20 mg once daily; at 4-week intervals, either the dose of **Letairis** <u>or</u> *tadalafil* can be increased, as needed and tolerated, to **Letairis** 10 mg <u>or</u> *tadalafil* 40 mg; do not split, crush, <u>or</u> chew

Pediatric: <12 years: not recommended; ≥12 years: same as adult

Letairis *Tab:* 5, 10 mg *film-coat*

Comment: In patients with PAH, plasma ET-1 concentrations are increased as much as 10-fold and correlate with increased mean right atrial pressure and disease severity. ET-1 and ET-1 mRNA concentrations are increased as much as 9-fold in the lung tissue of patients with PAH, primarily in the endothelium of pulmonary arteries. These findings suggest that ET-1 may play a critical role in the pathogenesis and progression of PAH. When taken with *tadalafil*, **Letairis** is indicated to reduce the risk of disease progression and hospitalization, to reduce the risk of hospitalization due to worsening PAH, and to improve exercise tolerance. **Letairis** is contraindicated in idiopathic pulmonary fibrosis (IPF). Exclude pregnancy before the initiation of treatment with **Letairis**. Females of reproductive potential must use acceptable methods of contraception during treatment with **Letairis** and for one month after treatment. Obtain monthly pregnancy tests during treatment and 1 month after discontinuation of treatment. Females can only receive **Letairis** through the **Letairis** Risk Evaluation and Mitigation Strategy (REMS) Program, a restricted distribution program, because of the risk of embryo-fetal toxicity: www.Letairisrems.com <u>or</u> 1-866-664-5327.

➢ *riociguat* (X) initially 0.5-1 mg tid; titrate every 2 weeks as tolerated (SBP ≥95 and absence of hypotensive symptoms) to highest tolerated dose; max 2.5 mg tid

Pediatric: <12 years: not recommended; ≥12 years: same as adult

Adempas *Tab:* 0.5, 1, 1.5, 2, 2.5 mg

Comment: If **Adempas** is interrupted for ≥3 days, re-titrate. Consider titrating to dosage higher than 2.5 mg tid, if tolerated, in patients who smoke. Consider a starting dose of 0.5 mg tid when initiating **Adempas** in patients receiving strong cytochrome P450 (CYP) and P-glycoprotein/breast cancer resistance protein (P-gp/BCRP) inhibitors such as azole antimycotics (e.g., *ketoconazole, itraconazole*) <u>or</u> HIV protease inhibitors (e.g., *ritonavir*). Monitor for signs and symptoms of hypotension with strong CYP and P-gp/BCRP inhibitors. Obtain pregnancy tests prior to initiation and monthly during treatment. **Adempas** has consistently shown to have teratogenic effects when administered to animals. Females can only receive **Adempas** through the Adempas Risk Evaluation and Mitigation Strategy (REMS) Program, a restricted distribution program: **www.AdempasREMS.com** <u>or</u> 855-4 ADEMPAS. It is not known if **Adempas** is present in human milk; however, *riociguat* <u>or</u> its metabolites were present in the milk of rats. Because of the potential for serious adverse reactions in nursing infants from *riociguat*, discontinue nursing <u>or</u> **Adempas**. In placebo-controlled clinical trials, serious bleeding has occurred (including hemoptysis, hematemesis, vaginal hemorrhage, catheter site hemorrhage, subdural hematoma, and intra-abdominal hemorrhage. Safety and efficacy have not been demonstrated in patients with creatinine clearance <15 mL/min <u>or</u> on dialysis <u>or</u> severe hepatic impairment (Child-Pugh Class C).

Endothelin Receptor Antagonist, Selective for the Endothelin Type-A (ETA) Receptor

PHOSPHODIESTERASE TYPE 5 (PDE5) INHIBITORS, CGMP-SPECIFIC DRUGS

➢ *sildenafil citrate* (B)(G) *Orally:* initially 5 <u>or</u> 20 mg tid, 4-6 hours apart; max 20 mg tid; *IV bolus:* 2.5 mg <u>or</u> 10 mg bolus injection tid, 4-6 hours apart; max 10 mg tid; the dose does not need to be adjusted for body weight

Pediatric: <12 years: not recommended; ≥12 years: same as adult

> **Revatio** *Tab:* 20 mg film-coat; *Oral susp:* 10 mg/ml pwdr for reconstitution (1.12 gm, 112 ml) (grape) (sorbitol); *Vial:* 10 mg/12.5 ml (0.8 mg/ml)

Comment: A 10 mg IV dose is predicted to provide pharmacological effect equivalent to the 20 mg oral dose. **Revatio** is contraindicated with concomitant nitrate drugs including *nitroglycerin, isosorbide dinitrate,* isosorbide mononitrate, and some recreational drugs such as "poppers." Taking **Revatio** with a nitrate can cause a sudden and serious decrease in blood pressure. **Revatio** is contraindicated with concomitant guanylate cyclase stimulator drugs such as *riociguat* (Adempas). Avoid the use of grapefruit products while taking **Revatio**. Stop **Revatio** and get emergency medical help if sudden vision loss. **Revatio** is contraindicated with other phosphodiesterase type 5 (PDE5) Inhibitors, cGMP-specific drugs such as *avanafil* (Stendra), *tadalafil* (Cialis) or *vardenafil* (Levitra). Caution with history of recent MI, stroke, life-threatening arrhythmia, hypotension, hypertension, cardiac failure, unstable angina, retinitis pigmentosa, CYP3A4 inhibitors (e.g., *cimetidine,* the azoles, *erythromycin,* protease inhibitors (e.g., *ritonavir*), CYP3A4 inducers (e.g., *rifampin, carbamazepine, phenytoin, phenobarbital*), alcohol, antihypertensive agents. Side effects include headache, flushing, nasal congestion, rhinitis, dyspepsia, and diarrhea. Use **Revatio** with caution in patients with anatomical deformation of the penis (e.g., angulation, cavernosal fibrosis, or Peyronie's disease) or in patients who have conditions, which may predispose them to priapism (e.g., sickle cell anemia, multiple myeloma, or leukemia). In the event of an erection that persists longer than 4 hours, the patient should seek immediate medical assistance. If priapism (painful erection greater than 6 hours in duration) is not treated immediately, penile tissue damage and permanent loss of potency could result.

> *tadalafil* (B)(G) 40 mg once daily; *CrCl 31-80 mL/min:* initially 20 mg once daily; increase to 40 mg once daily if tolerated; *CrCl <30 mL/min:* not recommended; *Mild or moderate hepatic cirrhosis (Child-Pugh Class A or B):* initially 20 mg once daily. *Severe hepatic cirrhosis (Child-Pugh Class C):* not recommended; *use with* **ritonavir**; *Receiving* **ritonavir** *for at least 1 week:* initiate *tadalafil* at 20 mg once daily; may increase to 40 mg once daily if tolerated; *Already on* **tadalafil***:* stop *tadalafil* at least 24 hours prior to initiating *ritonavir;* resume *tadalafil* at 20 mg once daily after at least 1 week; may increase to 40 mg once daily if tolerated
> *Pediatric:* <12 years: not recommended; ≥12 years: same as adult
>> **Adcirca** *Tab:* 20 mg
>> Comment: Contraindicated with concomitant organic nitrates and guanylate cyclase stimulators (e.g., *riociguat*).

> *treprostinil* (B) swallow whole; take with food
>> **Orenitram** *Tab:* 0.125, 0.25, 1, 2.5 mg ext-rel
>> Comment: **Orenitram** is indicated to improve exercise capacity. It is contraindicated with severe hepatic impairment (Child-Pugh Class C). **Orenitram** inhibits platelet aggregation and increases the risk of bleeding. Concomitant administration of **Orenitram** with diuretics, antihypertensive agents or other vasodilators increases the risk of symptomatic hypotension.

 PYELONEPHRITIS: ACUTE

URINARY TRACT ANALGESIA

> *phenazopyridine* (B)(G) 95-200 mg q 6 hours prn; max 2 days
> *Pediatric:* <12 years: not recommended; ≥12 years: same as adult
>> **AZO Standard, Prodium, Uristat (OTC)** *Tab:* 95 mg
>> **AZO Standard Maximum Strength (OTC)** *Tab:* 97.5 mg
>> **Pyridium, Urogesic** *Tab:* 100, 200 mg
>> **Urogesic** *Tab:* 100, 200 mg

OUTPATIENT ANTI-INFECTIVE TREATMENT

Comment: Acute pyelonephritis can be treated with a single IM antibiotic administration followed by a PO antibiotic regimen and close follow up. Example: **Rocephin** 1 gm IM followed by **Bactrim DS**, *cephalexin*, *ciprofloxacin*, *levofloxacin*, or *loracarbef*.

➤ *cephalexin* (B)(G) 1-4 gm/day in 4 divided doses x 10-14 days
   Pediatric: 25-50 mg/kg/day in 4 divided doses x 10-14 days; *see page 629 for dose by weight*
      Keflex *Cap:* 250, 333, 500, 750 mg; *Oral susp:* 125, 250 mg/5 ml (100, 200 ml) (strawberry)
➤ *ciprofloxacin* (C) 500 mg bid or 1000 mg XR once daily x 3-14 days
   Pediatric: <18 years: not recommended; ≥18 years: same as adult
      Cipro (G) *Tab:* 250, 500, 750 mg; *Oral susp:* 250, 500 mg/5 ml (100 ml) (strawberry)
      Cipro XR *Tab:* 500, 1000 mg ext-rel
      ProQuin XR *Tab:* 500 mg ext-rel
➤ *levofloxacin* (C) *Uncomplicated:* 500 mg once daily x 10 days; *Complicated:* 750 mg once daily x 10 days
   Pediatric: <18 years: not recommended; ≥18 years: same as adult
      Levaquin *Tab:* 250, 500, 750 mg; *Oral soln:* 25 mg/ml (480 ml) (benzyl alcohol); *Inj conc:* 25 mg/ml for IV infusion after dilution for IV infusion (50, 100, 150 ml) (preservative-free)
➤ *loracarbef* (B) 400 mg bid x 14 days
   Pediatric: 15 mg/kg/day in 2 divided doses x 14 days; *see page 642 for dose by weight*
      Lorabid *Pulvule:* 200, 400 mg; *Oral susp:* 100 mg/5 ml (50, 100 ml); 200 mg/5 ml (50, 75, 100 ml) (strawberry bubble gum)
➤ *trimethoprim+sulfamethoxazole (TMP-SMX)* (D)(G) bid x 10 days
   Pediatric: <2 months: not recommended; ≥2 months: 40 mg/kg/day of *sulfamethoxazole* in 2 divided doses x 10 days; *see page 648 for dose by weight*
      Bactrim, Septra 2 tabs bid x 10 days
         Tab: trim 80 mg+*sulfa* 400 mg*
      Bactrim DS, Septra DS 1 tab bid x 10 days
         Tab: trim 160 mg+*sulfa* 800 mg*
      Bactrim Pediatric Suspension, Septra Pediatric Suspension
         Oral susp: trim 40 mg+*sulfa* 200 mg per 5 ml (100 ml) (cherry) (alcohol 0.3%)

 RABIES

PRE-EXPOSURE PROPHYLAXIS

Comment: Postpone pre-exposure prophylaxis during acute febrile illness or infection. Have *epinephrine* 1:1000 readily available.
➤ *rabies immune globulin, human (HRIG)* (C) 3 injections of 1 ml IM each on day 0, 7, and either day 21 or 28; booster doses 1 ml IM every 2 years
   Pediatric: same as adult (except for infants administer in the vastus lateralis muscle)
      Imovax *Vial:* 2.5 u/ml (1 ml, single-dose)

POST-EXPOSURE PROPHYLAXIS (PEP)

Comment: Have *epinephrine* 1:1000 readily available.
➤ *rabies immune globulin, human (HRIG)* (C) 20 IU/kg infiltrated into wound area as much as feasible, then remaining dose administered IM at site remote from vaccine administration
   Pediatric: same as adult
      BayRab, KedRAB, Imogam Rabies *Vial:* 150 IU/ml (2, 10 ml)

Comment: Administer *immune globulin, human (HRIG)* concurrently with a full course of rabies vaccine.

▷ *rabies vaccine, human diploid cell* (C) *Not previously immunized:* administer first dose 1 ml in the deltoid as soon as possible after exposure; then repeat on days 3, 7, 14, 28 <u>or</u> 30, and 90; administer 1st dose with rabies immune globulin; *Previously immunized:* only 2 doses are administered, immediately after exposure and again 3 days later; no rabies immune globulin is needed

Pediatric: same as adult (except for infants administer in vastus lateralis muscle)

Imovax, RabAvert *Vial:* 2.5 IU/ml (2.5 IU of freeze-dried vaccine w. diluent)

TETANUS PROPHYLAXIS VACCINE

see Tetanus page 460 for patients not previously immunized

 RESPIRATORY SYNCYTIAL VIRUS (RSV)

PROPHYLAXIS

▷ *palivizumab* 15 mg/kg IM administered monthly throughout the RSV season
Synagis *Vial:* 100 mg/ml

TREATMENT

See Bronchiolitis page 58

 RESTLESS LEGS SYNDROME (RLS)

GAMMA AMINOBUTYRIC ACID ANALOGS

▷ *gabapentin* (C)(G) 100 mg once daily x 1 day; then 100 mg bid x 1 day; then 100 mg tid thereafter; max 900 mg tid

Gralise (C) initially 300 mg on Day 1; then 600 mg on Day 2; then 900 mg on Days 3-6; then 1200 mg on Days 7-10; then 1500 mg on Days 11-14; titrate up to 1800 mg on Day 15; take entire dose once daily with the evening meal; do not crush, split, <u>or</u> chew

Pediatric: <12 years: not recommended; ≥12 years: same as adult

Tab: 300, 600 mg

Neurontin (G) 100 mg daily x 1 day, then 100 mg bid x 1 day, then 100 mg tid continuously; max 900 mg tid

Pediatric: <3 years: not recommended; 3-12 years: initially 10-15 mg/kg/day in 3 divided doses; max 12 hours between doses; titrate over 3 days; 3-4 years: titrate to 40 mg/kg/day; 5-12 years: titrate to 25-35 mg/kg/day; max 50 mg/kg/day;

▷ *gabapentin enacarbil* (C) 600 mg once daily at about 5:00 PM; if dose not taken at recommended time, next dose should be taken the following day; swallow whole; take with food; *CrCl 30-59 mL/min:* 600 mg on Day 1, Day 3, and every day thereafter; *CrCl <30 mL/min* <u>or</u> on hemodialysis: not recommended

Pediatric: <12 years: not recommended; ≥12 years: same as adult

Horizant *Tab:* 600 ext-rel

Comment: Avoid abrupt cessation of *gabapentin* and *gabapentin enacarbil*. To discontinue, withdraw gradually over 1 week <u>or</u> longer.

DOPAMINE RECEPTOR AGONISTS

▷ *pramipexole dihydrochloride* (C)(G) initially 0.125 mg once daily 2-3 hours before bedtime; may double dose every 4-7 days; max 0.75 mg/day

Pediatric: <12 years: not recommended; ≥12 years: same as adult

Mirapex *Tab:* 0.125, 0.25*, 0.5*, 0.75*, 1*, 1.5*mg

▷ *ropinirole* (C) take once daily 1-3 hours prior to bedtime; initially 0.25 mg on days 1 and 2; then 0.5 mg on days 3-7; increase by 0.5 mg/day at 1 week intervals to 3 mg; max 4 mg/day
Pediatric: <12 years: not recommended; ≥12 years: same as adult
Requip *Tab:* 0.25, 0.5, 1, 2, 3, 4, 5 mg

▷ *rotigotine* transdermal patch (C) apply to clean, dry, intact skin on abdomen, thigh, hip, flank, shoulder, or upper arm; initially 1 mg/24 Hrs patch once daily; may increase weekly by 1 mg/24 Hrs if needed; max 3 mg/24 Hrs once daily; rotate sites and allow 14 days before reusing site; if hairy, shave site at least 3 days before application to site; avoid abrupt cessation; reduce by 1 mg/24 Hrs every other day
Pediatric: <12 years: not recommended; ≥12 years: same as adult
Neupro *Trans patch:* 1 mg/24 Hrs, 2 mg/24 Hrs, 3 mg/24 Hrs, 4 mg/24 Hrs, 6 mg/24 Hrs, 8 mg/24 Hrs (30/carton) (sulfites)

RETINITIS: CYTOMEGALOVIRUS (CMV)

Comment: *cidofovir* and *valganciclovir* are nucleoside analogs and prodrugs of *ganciclovir* indicated for the treatment of AIDS-related *cytomegalovirus* (CMV) retinitis and prevention of CMV disease in adult kidney, heart, and kidney-pancreas transplant patients at high risk, and for prevention of CMV disease in pediatric kidney and heart transplant patients at high risk.

▷ *cidofovir* (C) administer via IV infusion over 1 hour; pre-treat with oral *probenecid* (2 gm, 3 hours prior to starting the *cidofovir* infusion and 1 gm, 2 and 8 hours after the infusion is ended) and 1 liter of IV NaCl should be infused immediately before each dose of *cidofovir* (a 2nd liter of NaCl should also be infused either during or after each dose of *cidofovir* if a fluid load is tolerable); *Induction:* 5 mg/kg once weekly for 2 consecutive weeks; *Maintenance:* 5 mg/kg once every 2 weeks; reduce to 3 mg/kg if serum creatinine (sCr) increases 0.3-0.4 mg/dL above baseline; discontinue if sCr increases to >0.5 mg/dL above baseline or if >3+ proteinuria develops
Pediatric: <12 years: not recommended; ≥12 years: same as adult
Vistide *Vial:* 75 mg/ml (5 ml) (preservative-free)

Comment: *cidofovir* is a nucleoside analog indicated for treatment of AIDS-related *cytomegalovirus* (CMV) retinitis.

▷ *valganciclovir* (C)(G) take with food; *Induction:* 900 mg bid x 21 days; *Maintenance:* 900 mg daily; *CrCl <60 mL/min:* reduce dose (see mfr pkg insert; hemodialysis or *CrCl <10 mL/min* not recommended (use *ganciclovir*)
Pediatric: <4 months: not recommended; 4 months-16 years: see mfr pkg insert for dosing calculation equation
Valcyte *Tab:* 450 mg (preservative-free); *Oral pwdr for reconstitution:* 50 mg/ml (tutti-frutti)

RHEUMATOID ARTHRITIS (RA)

Injectable Acetaminophen *see Pain page* 344
NSAIDs *see page* 562
Opioid Analgesics *see Pain page* 345
Topical and Transdermal NSAIDs *see Pain page* 344
Parenteral Corticosteroids *see page* 570
Oral Corticosteroids *see page* 569
Topical Analgesic and Anesthetic Agents *see page* 526

TOPICAL/TRANSDERMAL ANALGESICS

▷ *capsaicin* cream (B)(G) apply tid-qid prn to intact skin
Pediatric: <2 years: not recommended; ≥2 years: same as adult

Axsain *Crm:* 0.075% (1, 2 oz)
Capsin *Lotn:* 0.025, 0.075% (59 ml)
Capzasin-P (OTC) *Crm:* 0.025% (1.5 oz); *Lotn:* 0.025% (2 oz)
Dolorac *Crm:* 0.025% (28 gm)
Double Cap (OTC) *Crm:* 0.05% (2 oz)
Qutenza (B) *Patch:* 8% (1-2, both with 50 gm tube of cleansing gel)
R-Gel *Gel:* 0.025% (15, 30 gm)
Zostrix (OTC) *Crm:* 0.025% (0.7, 1.5, 3 oz)
Zostrix HP (OTC) *Emol crm:* 0.075% (1, 2 oz)

▷ *trolamine salicylate*
Mobisyl apply tid-qid
Crm: 10%

Comment: Provides some relief by 1-2 weeks; optimal benefit may take 4-6 weeks.

ORAL SALICYLATE

▷ *indomethacin* (C) initially 25 mg bid-tid, increase as needed at weekly intervals by 25-50 mg/day; max 200 mg/day
Pediatric: <14 years: usually not recommended; >2 years, if risk warranted: 1-2 mg/kg/day in divided doses; max 3-4 mg/kg/day (or 150-200 mg/day, whichever is less; <14 years: ER cap not recommended
Cap: 25, 50 mg; *Susp:* 25 mg/5 ml (pineapple-coconut, mint) (alcohol 1%); *Supp:* 50 mg; *ER Cap:* 75 mg ext-rel

Comment: *indomethacin* is indicated only for acute painful flares. Administer with food and/or antacids. Use lowest effective dose for shortest duration.

ORAL NSAID

See more **Oral NSAIDs** *page* 562

▷ *diclofenac sodium* (C)(G)
Voltaren 50 mg bid-qid or 75 mg bid or 25 mg qid with an additional 25 mg at HS if necessary
Pediatric: <12 not recommended; ≥12 years: same as adult
Tab: 25, 50, 75 mg ent-coat
Voltaren XR 100 mg once daily; rarely, 100 mg bid may be used
Pediatric: <18 not recommended; ≥18 years: same as adult
Tab: 100 mg ext-rel

ORAL NSAID+PPI

▷ *esomeprazole+naproxen* (C)(G) 1 tab bid; use lowest effective dose for the shortest duration swallow whole; take at least 30 minutes before a meal
Pediatric: <18 not recommended; ≥18 years: same as adult
Vimovo *Tab:* nap 375 mg+eso 20 mg ext-rel; nap 500 mg+eso 20 mg ext-rel
Comment: **Vimovo** is indicated to improve signs/symptoms, and risk of gastric ulcer in patients at risk of developing NSAID-associated gastric ulcer.

COX-2 INHIBITORS

Comment: Cox-2 inhibitors are contraindicated with history of asthma, urticaria, and allergic-type reactions to *aspirin*, other NSAIDs, and sulfonamides, 3rd trimester of pregnancy, and coronary artery bypass graft (CABG) surgery.
▷ *celecoxib* (C)(G) 50-400 mg once daily-bid; max 800 mg/day
Pediatric: <18 years: not recommended; ≥18 years: same as adult
Celebrex *Cap:* 50, 100, 200, 400 mg

➤ *meloxicam* (C)(G)

    Mobic <2 years, <60 kg: not recommended; ≥2, ≥60 kg: 0.125 mg/kg; max 7.5 mg once daily; ≥18 years: initially 7.5 mg once daily; max 15 mg once daily; *Hemodialysis:* max 7.5 mg/day

        Tab: 7.5, 15 mg; *Oral susp:* 7.5 mg/5 ml (100 ml) (raspberry)

    Vivlodex <18 years: not established; ≥18 years: initially 5 mg qd; may increase to max 10 mg/day; Hemodialysis: max 5 mg/day

        Cap: 5, 10 mg

JANUS KINASE (JAK) INHIBITOR

➤ *tofacitinib* (C) 5 mg twice daily; reduce to 5 mg once daily for moderate-to-severe renal impairment or moderate hepatic impairment, concomitant potent CYP3A4 inhibitors, or drugs that result in both CYP3A4 and potent CYP2C19 inhibition
    Pediatric: <12 years: not recommended; ≥12 years: same as adult
    Xeljanz *Tab:* 5 mg
    Xeljanz XR *Tab:* 11 mg ext-rel

Comment: Xeljanz is indicated for moderate-to-severe RA as monotherapy in patients who have inadequate response or intolerance to *methotrexate* (MTX) and/or in combination with other non-biologic DMARDs.

DISEASE MODIFYING ANTI-RHEUMATIC DRUGS (DMARDs)

Comment: DMARDs are first-line treatment options for RA. DMARDs include penicillamine, gold salts (*auranofin, aurothio-glucose*), immunosuppressants, and *hydroxychloroquine*. The DMARDs reduce ESR, reduce RF, and favorably affect the outcome of RA. Immunosuppressants may require 6 weeks to affect benefits and 6 months for full improvement.

➤ *auranofin (gold salt)* (C) 3 mg bid or 6 mg once daily; if inadequate response after 6 months, increase to 3 mg tid
    Pediatric: <12 years: not recommended; ≥12 years: same as adult
    Ridaura *Vial:* 100 mg/20 ml

➤ *azathioprine* (D) 1 mg/kg/day in a single or divided doses; may increase by 0.5 mg/kg/day q 4 weeks; max 2.5 mg/kg/day; minimum trial to ascertain effectiveness is 12 weeks
    Pediatric: <12 years: not recommended; ≥12 years: same as adult
    Azasan *Tab* 75*, 100*mg
    Imuran *Tab* 50*mg

➤ *cyclosporine (immunosuppressant)* (C) 1.25 mg/kg bid; may increase after 4 weeks by 0.5 mg/kg/day; then adjust at 2 week intervals; max 4 mg/kg/day; administer with meals
    Pediatric: <12 years: not recommended; ≥12 years: same as adult
    Neoral *Cap:* 25, 100 mg (alcohol)
    Neoral Oral Solution *Oral soln:* 100 mg/ml (50 ml) may dilute in room temperature apple juice or orange juice (alcohol)
    Comment: Neoral is indicated for RA unresponsive to *methotrexate (MTX)*.

➤ *hydroxychloroquine* (C) 400-600 mg/day
    Pediatric: <12 years: not recommended; ≥12 years: same as adult
    Plaquenil *Tab:* 200 mg

Comment: May require several weeks to achieve beneficial effects. If no improvement in 6 months, discontinue.

➤ *leflunomide* (X)(G) initially 100 mg once daily x 3 days; maintenance dose 20 mg once daily; max 20 mg daily
    Pediatric: <18 years: not recommended; ≥18 years: same as adult
    Arava *Tab:* 10, 20, 100 mg

Comment: **Arava** is contraindicated with breastfeeding.

▷ *methotrexate (MTX)* (X) 7.5 mg x 1 dose per week or 2.5 mg x 3 at 12 hour intervals once a week; max 20 mg/week; therapeutic response begins in 3-6 weeks; administer **methotrexate** injection SC only into the abdomen or thigh

Pediatric: <2 years: not recommended; ≥2 years: 10 mg/m² once weekly; max 20 mg/m²

Rasuvo *Autoinjector:* 7.5 mg/0.15 ml, 10 mg/0.20 ml, 12.5 mg/0.25 ml, 15 mg/0.30 ml, 17.5 mg/0.35 ml, 20 mg/0.40 ml, 22.5 mg/0.45 ml, 25 mg/0.50 ml, 27.5 mg/0.55 ml, 30 mg/0.60 ml (solution concentration for SC injection is 50 mg/ml)

Rheumatrex *Tab:* 2.5*mg (5, 7.5, 10, 12.5, 15 mg/week, 4/card unit-of-use dose pack)

Trexall *Tab:* 5*, 7.5*, 10*, 15*mg (5, 7.5, 10, 12.5, 15 mg/week, 4/card unit-of-use dose pack)

Comment: *methotrexate (MTX)* is contraindicated with immunodeficiency, blood dyscrasias, alcoholism, and chronic liver disease.

▷ *penicillamine* (D) 125-250 mg once daily initially; may increase by 125-250 mg/day q 1-3 months; max 1.5 gm/day

Pediatric: <12 years: not recommended; ≥12 years: same as adult

Cuprimine *Cap:* 125, 250 mg

Depen *Tab:* 250 mg

▷ *sulfasalazine* (C; D in 2nd, 3rd)(G) initially 0.5 gm once daily bid; gradually increase every 4 days; usual maintenance 2-3 gm/day in equally divided doses at regular intervals; max 4 gm/day

Pediatric: <6 years: not recommended; 6-16 years: initially 1/4 to 1/3 of maintenance dose; increase weekly; maintenance 30-50 mg/kg/day in 2 divided doses at regular intervals; max 2 gm/day; >16 years: same as adult

Azulfidine *Tab:* 500 mg

Azulfidine EN *Tab:* 500 mg ent-coat

TUMOR NECROSIS FACTOR (TNF) BLOCKERS

▷ *adalimumab* (B) 40 mg SC once every other week; may increase to once weekly without *methotrexate* (MTX); administer in abdomen or thigh; rotate sites; 2-17 years, supervise first dose

Pediatric: <2 years, <10 kg: not recommended; 10-<15 kg: 10 mg every other week; 15-<30 kg: 20 mg every other week; ≥30 kg: 40 mg every other week

Humira *Prefilled syringe:* 20 mg/0.4 ml; 40 mg/0.8 ml single-dose (2/pck; 2, 6/starter pck) (preservative-free)

Comment: **Humira** may use with *methotrexate* (MTX), DMARDs, corticosteroids, salicylates, NSAIDs, or analgesics.

▷ *adalimumab-adbm* (B) initially 80 SC; then, 40 mg SC every other week starting one week after initial dose; inject into thigh or abdomen; rotate sites

Pediatric: <18 years: not recommended; ≥18 years: same as adult

Cyltezo *Prefilled syringe:* 40 mg/0.8 ml single-dose (preservative-free)

Comment: **Cyltezo** is biosimilar to **Humira** (*adalimumab*).

▷ *certolizumab pegol* (B) 400 mg SC on day 1, at week 2, and at week 4; then 200 mg every other week; rotate sites

Pediatric: <12 years: not recommended; ≥12 years: same as adult

Cimzia *Vial:* 200 mg single-dose w. supplies (2/pck, 2, 6/starter pck); *Prefilled syringe:* 200 mg single-dose w. supplies (2/pck, 2, 6/starter pck) (preservative-free)

▷ *etanercept* (B) 25 mg SC twice weekly, 72-96 hours apart or 50 mg SC weekly; rotate sites

Pediatric: <4 years: not recommended; 4-17 years: 0.4 mg/kg SC twice weekly, 72-96 hours apart (max 25 mg/dose) or 0.8 mg/kg SC weekly (max 50 mg/dose)

Enbrel *Vial:* 25 mg pwdr for SC injection after reconstitution (4/carton w. supplies) (preservative-free; diluent contains benzyl alcohol); *Prefilled syringe:* 50 mg/ml (preservative-free); *SureClick autoinjector:* 50 mg/ml (preservative-free)

Comment: *etanercept* reduces pain, morning stiffness, and swelling. May be administered in combination with ***methotrexate***. Live vaccines should not be administered concurrently. Do not administer with active infection.

▷ ***golimumab*** (B) administer SC <u>or</u> IV infusion (in combination with ***methotrexate*** [MTX])

Pediatric: <12 years: not recommended; ≥12 years: same as adult

Simponi 50 mg SC once monthly; rotate sites

Prefilled syringe, SmartJect autoinjector: 50 mg/0.5 ml, single-use (preservative-free)

Simponi Aria 2 mg/kg IV infusion week 0 and week 4; then every 8 weeks thereafter

Vial: 50 mg/4 ml, single-use, soln for IV infusion after dilution (latex-free, preservative-free)

Comment: corticosteroids, non-biologic DMARDs, <u>and/or</u> NSAIDs may be continued during treatment with ***golimumab***.

▷ ***infliximab*** *(tumor necrosis factor-alpha blocker)* must be refrigerated at 2°C to 8°C (36°F to 46°F); administer dose intravenously over a period of not less than 2 hours; do not use beyond the expiration date as this product contains no preservative; 5 mg/kg at 0, 2 and 6 weeks, then every 8 weeks.

Pediatric: <6 years: not studied; ≥6-17 years: mg/kg at 0, 2 and 6 weeks, then every 8 weeks; ≥18 years: same as adult

Remicade *Vial:* 100 mg for reconstitution to 10 ml administration volume, single-dose (preservative-free)

Comment: Use ***infliximab*** concomitantly with ***methotrexate*** when there has been insufficient response to ***methotrexate*** alone. **Remicade** is indicated to reduce signs and symptoms, and induce and maintain clinical remission, in adults and children ≥6 years-of-age with moderately to severely active disease who have had an inadequate response to conventional therapy <u>and</u> reduce the number of draining enterocutaneous and rectovaginal fistulas, and maintain fistula closure, in adults with fistulizing disease. Common adverse effects associated with **Remicade** included abdominal pain, headache, pharyngitis, sinusitis, and upper respiratory infections. In addition, **Remicade** might increase the risk for serious infections, including tuberculosis, bacterial sepsis, and invasive fungal infections. Available data from published literature on the use of ***infliximab*** products during pregnancy have not reported a clear association with ***infliximab*** products and adverse pregnancy outcomes. ***infliximab*** products cross the placenta and infants exposed *in utero* should not be administered live vaccines for at least 6 months after birth. Otherwise, the infant may be at increased risk of infection, including disseminated infection which can become fatal. Available information is insufficient to inform the amount of ***infliximab*** products present in human milk <u>or</u> effects on the breastfed infant. To report suspected adverse reactions, contact Merck Sharp & Dohme Corp., a subsidiary of Merck & Co. at 1-877-888-4231 <u>or</u> FDA at 1-800-FDA1088 <u>or</u> www.fda.gov/medwatch

▷ ***infliximab-abda*** *(tumor necrosis factor-alpha blocker)* (B)

Renflexis: see ***infliximab*** (**Remicade**) above for full prescribing information

Comment: **Renflexis** is a biosimilar to **Remicade** for the treatment of immune-disorders including Crohn's disease, ulcerative colitis, rheumatoid arthritis, ankylosing spondylitis, psoriatic arthritis and plaque psoriasis. **Renflexis** was approved under the FDA category for biosimilars and demonstrated no clinically meaningful differences for use, dosing regimens, strengths, dosage forms, and routes of administration from the FDA-approved biological product **Remicade**.

▷ *infliximab-dyyb (tumor necrosis factor-alpha blocker)* (B)
  Inflectra: see *infliximab* (Remicade) above for full prescribing information
Comment: Inflectra is a biosimilar to Remicade for the treatment of immune-disorders including Crohn's disease, ulcerative colitis, rheumatoid arthritis, ankylosing spondylitis, psoriatic arthritis and plaque psoriasis. Inflectra was approved under the FDA category for biosimilars and demonstrated no clinically meaningful differences for use, dosing regimens, strengths, dosage forms, and routes of administration from the FDA-approved biological product Remicade.

▷ *infliximab-qbtx (tumor necrosis factor-alpha blocker)* (B)
  Ifixi: see *infliximab* (Remicade) above for full prescribing information
Comment: Ifixi is a biosimilar to Remicade for the treatment of immune disorders including Crohn's disease, ulcerative colitis, rheumatoid arthritis, ankylosing spondylitis, psoriatic arthritis and plaque psoriasis. Ifixi was approved under the FDA category for biosimilars and demonstrated no clinically meaningful differences for use, dosing regimens, strengths, dosage forms, and routes of administration from the FDA-approved biological product Remicade.

Interleukin-1 Receptor Antagonist

▷ *anakinra (interleukin-1 receptor antagonist)* (B) 100 mg SC once daily; discard any unused portion
  Pediatric: <12 years: not recommended; ≥12 years: same as adult
    Kineret *Prefilled syringe:* 100 mg/single-dose syringe (7, 28/pck) (preservative-free)

Interleukin-6 Receptor Antagonists

▷ *sarilumab* 200 mg SC every 2 weeks on the same day; if necessary, the dosage can be reduced 150 mg every 2 weeks to manage potential laboratory abnormalities, such as neutropenia, thrombocytopenia, and liver enzyme elevations; SC injections may be self-administered
  Pediatric: <18 years: not recommended; ≥18 years: same as adult
    Kevzara *Prefilled syringe:* 150, 200 mg (1.4 ml, single-use)
Comment: *sarilumab* is a human monoclonal antibody that binds to the interleukin-6 receptor (IL-6R), and has been shown to inhibit IL-6R mediated signaling. IL-6 is a cytokine in the body that, in excess and over time, can contribute to the inflammation associated with RA. Kevzara received FDA approval in May, 2017 for use in patients with active moderate-to-severe rheumatoid arthritis (RA) in adults who have had an inadequate response or intolerance to one or more disease modifying antirheumatic drugs (DMARDs). Kevzara may be used as monotherapy or in combination with *methotrexate* or other conventional DMARDs. Monitor patient for dose related laboratory changes including elevated LFTs, neutropenia, and thrombocytopenia. Kevzara should not be initiated in patients with an absolute neutrophil count (ANC) <2000/mm³, platelet count <150,000/mm³, or liver transaminases above 1.5 times the upper limit of normal (ULN). Registration in the Pregnancy Exposure Registry (1-877-311-8972) is encouraged for monitoring pregnancy outcomes in women exposed to Kevzara during pregnancy. Negative side effects of Kevzara should be reported to the FDA at www.fda.gov/medwatch or call 1-800-FDA-1088 or call Sanofi-Aventis at 1-800-633-1610. The limited available data with Kevzara in pregnant women are not sufficient to determine whether there is a drug-associated risk for major birth defects and miscarriage. Monoclonal antibodies, such as *sarilumab*, are actively transported across the placenta during the third trimester of pregnancy and may affect immune response in the infant exposed *in utero*. It is not known whether *sarilumab* passes into breast milk; therefore, breastfeeding is not recommended while using Kevzara.

▷ *tocilizumab* (B) *IV Infusion:* administer over 1 hour; do not administer as bolus <u>or</u> IV push; *Adults, PJIA, and SJIA, ≥30 kg:* dilute to 100 mL in 0.9% <u>or</u> 0.45% NaCl. *PJIA and SJIA, <30 kg:* dilute to 50 mL in 0.9% <u>or</u> 0.45% NaCl.

    Adults: IV Infusion: Whether used in combination with DMARDs <u>or</u> as monotherapy, the recommended IV infusion starting dose is 4 mg/kg IV every 4 weeks followed by an increase to 8 mg/kg IV every 4 weeks based on clinical response; Max 800 mg per infusion in RA patients; *SC Administration: ≥100 kg:* 162 mg SC once weekly on the same day; *<100 kg:* 162 mg SC every other week on the same day followed by an increase according to clinical response; SC injections may be self-administered

    Pediatric: <2 years: not recommended; ≥2 years: weight-based dosing according to diagnosis: *PJIA: ≥30 kg:* 8 mg/kg SC every 4 weeks; *<30 kg:* 10 mg/kg SC every 4 weeks; *SJIA: ≥30 kg:* 8 mg/kg SC every 2 weeks; *<30 kg:* 12 mg/kg SC every 2 weeks

        Actemra *Vial:* 80 mg/4 ml, 200 mg/10 ml, 400 mg/20 ml, single-use, for IV infusion after dilution; *Prefilled syringe:* 162 mg (0.9 ml, single-dose)

Comment: *tocilizumab* is an interleukin-6 receptor-α inhibitor indicated for use in moderate-to-severe rheumatoid arthritis (RA) that has not responded to conventional therapy, and also for some subtypes of juvenile idiopathic arthritis (JIA). **Actemra** may be used alone <u>or</u> in combination with **methotrexate** and in RA, other DMARDs may be used. Monitor patient for dose related laboratory changes including elevated LFTs, neutropenia, and thrombocytopenia. **Actemra** should not be initiated in patients with an absolute neutrophil count (ANC) below 2000 per mm^3, platelet count below 100,000 per mm^3, <u>or</u> who have ALT <u>or</u> AST above 1.5 times the upper limit of normal (ULN). Registration in the Pregnancy Exposure Registry (1-877-311-8972) is encouraged for monitoring pregnancy outcomes in women exposed to **Actemra** during pregnancy. The limited available data with **Actemra** in pregnant women are not sufficient to determine whether there is a drug-associated risk for major birth defects and miscarriage. Monoclonal antibodies, such as *tocilizumab*, are actively transported across the placenta during the third trimester of pregnancy and may affect immune response in the infant exposed *in utero*. It is not known whether *tocilizumab* passes into breast milk; therefore, breastfeeding is not recommended while using **Actemra**.

Selective Co-stimulation Modulator

▷ *abatacept* (C) administer as an IV infusion over 30 minutes at weeks 0, 2, and 4; then every 4 weeks thereafter; <60 kg, administer 500 mg/dose; 60-100 kg, administer 750 mg/dose; >100 kg, administer 1 gm/dose

    Pediatric: <6 years: not recommended; 6-17 years: administer as an IV infusion over 30 minutes at weeks 0, 2, and 4; then every 4 weeks thereafter; <75 kg, administer 10 mg/kg; same as adult (max 1 gm)

        Orencia *Vial:* 250 mg pwdr for IV infusion after reconstitution (silicone-free) (preservative-free); *Prefilled syringe:* 125 mg/ml soln for SC injection (preservative-free); *ClickJect Autoinjector:* 125 mg/ml soln for SC injection

CD20 ANTIBODY

▷ *rituximab* (C) administer corticosteroid 30 minutes prior to each infusion; concomitant **methotrexate** therapy, administer a 1000 mg IV infusion at 0 and 2 weeks; then every 24 weeks <u>or</u> based on response, but not sooner than every 16 weeks.

    Pediatric: <6 years: not recommended; ≥6 years: same as adult

        Rituxan *Vial:* 10 mg/ml (10, 50 ml) (preservative-free)

INTRA-ARTICULAR INJECTION

▷ *sodium hyaluronate* 20 mg as intra-articular injection weekly x 5 weeks
   Pediatric: <12 years: not recommended; ≥12 years: same as adult
      Hyalgan *Prefilled syringe:* 20 mg/2 ml
Comment: Remove joint effusion and inject with *lidocaine* if possible before injecting
Hyalgan.

 RHINITIS/SINUSITIS: ALLERGIC

Drugs for the Management of Allergy, Cough, and Cold Symptoms *see page* 598
Parenteral Corticosteroids *see page* 570
Oral Corticosteroids *see page* 569

Comment: The Joint Task Force on Practice Parameters, which comprises
representatives of the American Academy of Allergy, Asthma and Immunology
(AAAAI) and the American College of Allergy, Asthma and Immunology (ACAAI),
has provided guidance to healthcare providers on the initial pharmacologic treatment
of seasonal allergic rhinitis in patients aged ≥12 years. For initial treatment of seasonal
allergic rhinitis in persons aged ≥12 years: routinely prescribe monotherapy with an
intranasal corticosteroid rather than an intranasal corticosteroid in combination with an
oral antihistamine. For initial treatment of seasonal allergic rhinitis in persons aged ≥15
years: recommend an intranasal corticosteroid over a leukotriene. For initial treatment
of seasonal allergic rhinitis in persons aged ≥15 years: recommend an intranasal
corticosteroid over a leukotriene receptor antagonist. For initial treatment of moderate
to severe seasonal allergic rhinitis in persons aged ≥12 years: recommend a combination
of an intranasal corticosteroid and an intranasal antihistamine.

REFERENCE
Wallace, D. V., Dykewicz, M. S., Oppenheimer, J., Portnoy, J. M., & Lang, D. M. (2017). Pharmacologic
   treatment of seasonal allergic rhinitis: Synopsis of guidance from the 2017 joint task force on practice
   parameters. *Annals of Internal Medicine, 167*(12), 876. doi:10.7326/m17-2203

SECOND GENERATION ANTIHISTAMINES

Comment: The following drugs are second generation antihistamines. As such
they minimally sedating, much less so than the first generation antihistamines. All
antihistamines are excreted into breast milk.
▷ *cetirizine* (C)(OTC)(G) initially 5-10 mg once daily; 5 mg once daily; ≥65 years: use
  with caution
   Pediatric: <6 years: not recommended; ≥6 years: same as adult
      Children's Zyrtec Chewable *Chew tab:* 5, 10 mg (grape)
      Children's Zyrtec Allergy Syrup *Syr:* 1 mg/ml (4 oz) (grape, bubble gum) (sug-
      ar-free, dye-free)
      Zyrtec *Tab:* 10 mg
      Zyrtec Hives Relief *Tab:* 10 mg
      Zyrtec Liquid Gels *Liq gel:* 10 mg
▷ *desloratadine* (C)
      Clarinex 1/2-1 tab once daily
      Pediatric: <6 years: not recommended; ≥6 years: same as adult
        Tab: 5 mg
      Clarinex RediTabs 5 mg once daily
      Pediatric: <6 years: not recommended; 6-12 years: 2.5 mg once daily; ≥12 years:
      same as adult
        ODT: 2.5, 5 mg (tutti-frutti) (phenylalanine)

Clarinex Syrup 5 mg (10 ml) once daily
Pediatric: <6 months: not recommended; 6-11 months: 1 mg (2 ml) once daily;
1-5 years: 1.25 mg (2.5 ml) once daily; 6-11 years: 2.5 mg (5 ml) once daily; ≥12
years: same as adult
   Syr: 0.5 mg per ml (4 oz) (tutti-frutti) (phenylalanine)
Desloratadine ODT 1 tab once daily
Pediatric: <6 years: not recommended; 6-11 years: 1/2 tab once daily; ≥12 years:
same as adult
   ODT: 5 mg

➤ *fexofenadine* (C)(OTC)(G) 60 mg once daily-bid <u>or</u> 180 mg once daily; *CrCl <90 mL/
min:* 60 mg once daily
Pediatric: <6 months: not recommended; 6 months-2 years: 15 mg bid; *CrCl ≤90 mL/
min:* 15 mg once daily; 2-11 years: 30 mg bid; *CrCl ≤90 mL/min:* 30 mg once daily;
≥12 years: same as adult
   Allegra *Tab:* 30, 60, 180 mg film-coat
   Allegra Allergy *Tab:* 60, 180 mg film-coat
   Allegra ODT *ODT:* 30 mg (phenylalanine)
   Allegra Oral Suspension *Oral susp:* 30 mg/5 ml (6 mg/ml) (4 oz)

➤ *levocetirizine* (B)(OTC) administer dose in the PM; *Seasonal Allergic Rhinitis:* <2
years: not recommended; may start at ≥2 years; *Chronic Idiopathic Urticaria (CIU),
Perennial Allergic Rhinitis:* <6 months: not recommended; may start at ≥ 6 months;
Dosing by Age: 6 months-5 years: max 1.25 mg once daily; 6-11 years: max 2.5 mg
once daily; ≥12 years: 2.5-5 mg once daily; *Renal Dysfunction <12 years:* contraindicated; *Renal Dysfunction ≥12 years:* CrCl 50-80 ml/min: 2.5 mg once daily; CrCl
30-50 mL/min: 2.5 mg every other day; CrCl: 10-30 mL/min: 2.5 mg twice weekly
(every 3-4 days); CrCl <10 mL/min, ESRD <u>or</u> hemodialysis: contraindicated
   Children's Xyzal Allergy 24HR *Oral Soln:* 0.5 mg/ml (150 ml)
   Xyzal Allergy 24HR *Tab:* 5*mg

➤ *loratadine* (C)(OTC)(G) 5 mg bid <u>or</u> 10 mg once daily; *Hepatic <u>or</u> Renal Insufficiency:*
see mfr pkg insert
Pediatric: <2 years: not recommended; 2-5 years: 5 mg once daily; ≥6 years: same as
adult
   Children's Claritin Chewables *Chew tab:* 5 mg (grape) (phenylalanine)
   Children's Claritin Syrup 1 mg/ml (4 oz) (fruit) (sugar-free, alcohol-free, dye-
free; sodium 6 mg/5 ml)
   Claritin *Tab:* 10 mg
   Claritin Hives Relief *Tab:* 10 mg
   Claritin Liqui-Gels *Liq gel:* 10 mg
   Claritin RediTabs 12 Hours *ODT:* 5 mg (mint)
   Claritin RediTabs 24 Hours *ODT:* 10 mg (mint)

FIRST GENERATION ANTIHISTAMINES

➤ *diphenhydramine* (B)(G) 25-50 mg q 6-8 hours; max 100 mg/day
Pediatric: <2 years: not recommended; 2-6 years: 6.25 mg q 4-6 hours; max 37.5 mg/
day; >6-12 years: 12.5-25 mg q 4-6 hours; max 150 mg/day; >12 years: same as adult
   Benadryl (OTC) *Chew tab:* 12.5 mg (grape) (phenylalanine); *Liq:* 12.5 mg/5 ml
(4, 8 oz); *Cap:* 25 mg; *Tab:* 25 mg; *Dye-free soft gel:* 25 mg; *Dye-free liq:* 12.5 mg/5
ml (4, 8 oz)

➤ *diphenhydramine injectable* (B)(G) 25-50 mg IM immediately; then q 6 hours prn
Pediatric: <12 years: *See mfr pkg insert:* 1.25 mg/kg up to 25 mg IM x 1 dose; then q 6
hours prn; ≥12 years: same as adult
   Benadryl Injectable *Vial:* 50 mg/ml (1 ml single-use); 50 mg/ml (10 ml
multidose); *Amp:* 10 mg/ml (1 ml); *Prefilled syringe:* 50 mg/ml (1 ml)

▷ *hydroxyzine* (C)(G) 50-100 mg/day divided qid prn
  Pediatric: <6 years: 50 mg/day divided qid prn; ≥6 years-12 years: 50 mg/day divided qid prn; >12 years: same as adult
    Atarax *Tab:* 10, 25, 50, 100 mg; *Syr:* 10 mg/5 ml (alcohol 0.5%)
    Vistaril *Cap:* 25, 50, 100 mg; *Oral susp:* 25 mg/5 ml (4 oz) (lemon)
Comment: *hydroxyzine* is contraindicated in early pregnancy and in patients with a prolonged QT interval. It is not known whether this drug is excreted in human milk; therefore, *hydroxyzine* should not be given to nursing mothers.

ALLERGEN EXTRACTS

Comment: Allergen extracts (**Grastek**, **Oralair**, **Ragwitek**) are not for immediate relief of allergic symptoms. Contraindicated with severe, unstable, and uncontrolled asthma, history of eosinophilic esophagitis, and severe local or systemic reaction. First dose under supervision HCP and observe ≥30 minutes. Subsequent doses may be taken at home.
▷ *short ragweed pollen allergen extract* (C) one SL tab once daily
  Pediatric: <18 years: not established; ≥18 years: same as adult
    Ragwitek *SL tab: Ambrosia artemisiifolia 12 amb a 1-unit* (30, 90/blister pck)
Comment: Initiate **Ragwitek** at least 12 weeks before onset of ragweed pollen season and continue throughout season.
▷ *sweet vernal, orchard, perennial rye, timothy, Kentucky blue grass mixed pollen allergen extract* (C) 300 IR once daily
  Pediatric: <10 years: not established; 10-17 years: Day 1: 100 IR; Day 2: 200 IR; Day 3 and thereafter: 300 IR once daily
    Oralair *SL tab:* 100, 300 IR (index of reactivity) (30/blister pck)
Comment: **Oralair** is indicated for grass pollen-induced allergic rhinitis with or without conjunctivitis confirmed by positive skin test. Initiate **Oralair** at least 4 months before onset of grass pollen season and continue throughout season.
▷ *Timothy grass pollen allergen extract* (C) one SL tab once daily
  Pediatric: <5 years: not established; ≥5 years: same as adult
    Grastek *SL tab:* 2800 bioequivalent allergy units (BAUS) (30/blister pck)
Comment: **Grastek** is indicated for grass pollen-induced allergic rhinitis with or without conjunctivitis confirmed by positive skin test. Initiate **Grastek** at least 12 weeks before onset of grass pollen season and continue throughout season.

NASAL DECONGESTANT

▷ *tetrahydrozoline* (C)
    Tyzine 2-4 drops or 3-4 sprays in each nostril q 3-8 hours prn
    Pediatric: <6 years: not recommended; ≥6 years: same as adult
      Nasal spray: 0.1% (15 ml); *Nasal drops:* 0.1% (30 ml)
    Tyzine Pediatric Nasal Drops 2-3 sprays or drops in each nostril q 3-6 hours prn
      Nasal drops: 0.05% (15 ml)

LEUKOTRIENE RECEPTOR ANTAGONISTS (LRAs)

Comment: For prophylaxis and chronic treatment only. Not for primary (rescue) treatment of acute asthma attack.
▷ *montelukast* (B)(G) 10 mg once daily in the PM; for EIB, take at least 2 hours before exercise; max 1 dose/day
  Pediatric: 12 months: not recommended; 12-23 months: one 4 mg granule pkt daily; 2-5 years: one 4 mg chew tab or granule pkt daily; 6-14 years: one 5 mg chew tab daily daily; ≥15 years: same as adult
    Singulair *Tab:* 10 mg

    Singulair Chewable *Chew tab:* 4, 5 mg (cherry, phenylalanine)

    Singulair Oral Granules: 4 mg/pkt; take within 15 minutes of opening pkt; may mix with applesauce, carrots, rice, <u>or</u> ice cream

▷ *zafirlukast* (B)(G) 20 mg bid, 1 hour ac <u>or</u> 2 hours pc

    Pediatric: <7 years: not recommended; 7-11 years: 10 mg bid 1 hour ac <u>or</u> 2 hours pc; >11 years: same as adult

        Accolate *Tab:* 10, 20 mg

▷ *zileuton* (C)(G)

    Pediatric: <12 years: not recommended; ≥12 years: same as adult

        Zyflo 1 tab qid (total 2400 mg/day)

        Tab: 600 mg

        Zyflo CR 2 tab bid (total 2400 mg/day)

        Tab: 600 mg ext-rel

NASAL CORTICOSTEROIDS

▷ *beclomethasone dipropionate* (C)

    Beconase 1 spray in each nostril bid-qid

    Pediatric: <6 years: not recommended; 6-12 years: 1 spray in each nostril tid; >12 years: same as adult

    Nasal spray: 42 mcg/actuation (6.7 gm, 80 sprays; 16.8 gm, 200 sprays)

    Beconase AQ 1-2 sprays in each nostril bid

    Pediatric: <6: not recommended; ≥6 years: same as adult

    Nasal spray: 42 mcg/actuation (25 gm, 180 sprays)

    Beconase Inhalation Aerosol 1-2 sprays in each nostril bid to qid

    Pediatric: <6: not recommended; 6-12 years: 1 spray in each nostril tid; >12 years: same as adult

    Nasal spray: 42 mcg/actuation (6.7 gm, 80 sprays; 16.8 gm, 200 sprays)

    Vancenase AQ 1-2 sprays in each nostril bid

    Pediatric: <6 years: not recommended; ≥6 years: same as adult

    Nasal spray: 84 mcg/actuation (25 gm, 200 sprays)

    Vancenase AQ DS 1-2 sprays in each nostril once daily

    Pediatric: <6 years: not recommended; ≥6 years: same as adult

    Nasal spray: 84, 168 mcg/actuation (19 gm, 120 sprays)

    Vancenase Pockethaler 1 spray in each nostril bid <u>or</u> qid

    Pediatric: <6: not recommended; ≥6 years: 1 spray in each nostril tid

    Pockethaler: 42 mcg/actuation (7 gm, 200 sprays)

    QNASL Nasal Aerosol 2 sprays, 80 mcg/spray, in each nostril once daily

    Pediatric: <12 years: 2 sprays, 40 mcg/spray, in each nostril once daily; ≥12 years: same as adult

    Nasal spray: 40 mcg/actuation (4.9 gm, 60 sprays); 80 mcg/actuation (8.7 gm, 120 sprays)

▷ *budesonide* (C)

    Rhinocort initially 2 sprays in each nostril bid in the AM and PM, <u>or</u> 4 sprays in each nostril in the AM; max 4 sprays each nostril/day; use lowest effective dose

    Pediatric: <6 years: not recommended; ≥6 years: same as adult

    Nasal spray: 32 mcg/actuation (7 gm, 200 sprays)

    Rhinocort Aqua Nasal Spray initially 1 spray in each nostril once daily; max 4 sprays in each nostril once daily

    Pediatric: <6 years: not recommended; ≥6-12 years: initially 1 spray in each nostril once daily; max 2 sprays in each nostril once daily

    Nasal spray: 32 mcg/actuation (10 ml, 60 sprays)

▷ *ciclesonide* (C)
  Pediatric: <6 years: not recommended; ≥6 years: same as adult
    Omnaris 2 sprays in each nostril once daily
      Nasal spray: 50 mcg/actuation (12.5 gm, 120 sprays)
    Zetonna 1-2 sprays in each nostril once daily
      Nasal spray: 37 mcg/actuation (6.1 gm, 60 sprays) (HFA)
▷ *dexamethasone* (C) 2 sprays in each nostril bid-tid; max 12 sprays/day; maintain at
  lowest effective dose
  Pediatric: <6 years: not recommended; ≥6-12 years: 1-2 sprays in each nostril bid;
  max 8 sprays/day; maintain at lowest effective dose; >12 years: same as adult
    Dexacort Turbinaire *Nasal spray:* 84 mcg/actuation (12.6 gm, 170 sprays)
▷ *fluticasone furoate* (C) 2 sprays in each nostril once daily; may reduce to 1 spray each
  nostril once daily
  Pediatric: <2 years: not recommended; ≥2-11 years: 1 spray in each nostril once daily;
  ≥12 years: same as adult
    Veramyst *Nasal spray:* 27.5 mcg/actuation (10 gm, 120 sprays) (alcohol-free)
▷ *fluticasone propionate* (C)(OTC)(G) initially 2 sprays in each nostril once daily <u>or</u> 1
  spray bid; maintenance 1 spray once daily
  Pediatric: <4 years: not recommended; ≥4 years: initially 1 spray in each nostril once
  daily; may increase to 2 sprays in each nostril once daily; maintenance 1 spray in each
  nostril once daily; max 2 sprays in each nostril/day
    Flonase *Nasal spray:* 50 mcg/actuation (16 gm, 120 sprays)
▷ *flunisolide* (C) 2 sprays in each nostril bid; may increase to 2 sprays in each nostril
  tid; max 8 sprays/nostril/day
  Pediatric: <6 years: not recommended; 6-14 years: initially 1 spray in each nostril tid
  <u>or</u> 2 sprays in each nostril bid; max 4 sprays/nostril/day; >14 years: same as adult
    Nasalide *Nasal spray:* 25 mcg/actuation (25 ml, 200 sprays)
    Nasarel *Nasal spray:* 25 mcg/actuation (25 ml, 200 sprays)
▷ *mometasone furoate* (C)(G) 2 sprays in each nostril once daily
  Pediatric: <2 years: not recommended; 2-11 years: 1 spray in each nostril once daily;
  max 2 sprays in each nostril once daily; >11 years: same as adult
    Nasonex *Nasal spray:* 50 mcg/actuation (17 gm, 120 sprays)
▷ *olopatadine* (C) 2 sprays in each nostril bid
  Pediatric: <6 years: not recommended; 6-11 years: 1 spray each nostril bid; >11 years:
  same as adult
    Patanase *Nasal spray:* 0.6%; 665 mcg/actuation (30.5 gm, 240 sprays) (benzalko-
    nium chloride)
▷ *triamcinolone acetonide* (C)(G) initially 2 sprays in each nostril once daily; max 4
  sprays in each nostril once daily <u>or</u> 2 sprays in each nostril bid <u>or</u> 1 spray in each
  nostril qid; maintain at lowest effective dose
  Pediatric: <6 years: not recommended; ≥6 years: 1 spray in each nostril once daily;
  max 2 sprays in each nostril once daily
    Nasacort Allergy 24HR (OTC) *Nasal spray:* 55 mcg/actuation (10 gm, 120 sprays)
    Tri-Nasal *Nasal spray:* 50 mcg/actuation (15 ml, 120 sprays)

NASAL MAST CELL STABILIZERS

▷ *cromolyn sodium* (B)(OTC) 1 spray in each nostril tid-qid; max 6 sprays in each
  nostril/day
  Pediatric: <2 years: not recommended; ≥2 years: same as adult
    Children's NasalCrom, NasalCrom *Nasal spray:* 5.2 mg/spray (13 ml, 100 sprays;
    26 ml, 200 sprays)
  Comment: Begin 1-2 weeks before exposure to known allergen. May take 2-4 weeks
  to achieve maximum effect.

NASAL ANTIHISTAMINES

▷ *azelastine* (C)

Astelin Ready Spray 2 sprays in each nostril bid
Pediatric: <5 years: not recommended; ≥5-12 years: 1 spray in each nostril once daily bid; >12 years: same as adult
Nasal spray: 137 mcg/actuation (30 ml, 200 sprays) (benzalkonium chloride)
Astepro 0.15% Nasal Spray 1 or 2 sprays each nostril once daily bid
Pediatric: <12 years: not recommended; ≥12 years: same as adult
Nasal spray: 205.5 mcg/actuation (17 ml, 106 sprays; 30 ml, 200 sprays) (benzalkonium chloride)

NASAL ANTIHISTAMINE+CORTICOSTEROID COMBINATION

▷ *azelastine/fluticasone* (C)(G) 1 spray in each nostril bid
Pediatric: <6 years: not recommended; ≥6 years: same as adult
Dymista *Nasal spray:* azel 137 mcg/*flutic* 50 mcg per actuation (23 gm, 120 sprays) (benzalkonium chloride)

NASAL ANTICHOLINERGICS

▷ *ipratropium bromide* (B)(G)

Atrovent Nasal Spray 0.03% 2 sprays in each nostril bid-tid
Pediatric: <6 years: not recommended; ≥6 years: same as adult
Nasal spray: 21 mcg/actuation (30 ml, 345 sprays)
Atrovent Nasal Spray 0.06% 2 sprays in each nostril tid-qid; max 5-7 days
Pediatric: <5 years: not recommended; ≥5-11 years: 2 sprays in each nostril tid; >11 years: same as adult
Nasal spray: 42 mcg/actuation (15 ml, 165 sprays)

Comment: Avoid use with narrow-angle glaucoma, prostate hyperplasia, and bladder neck obstruction.

◯ RHINITIS MEDICAMENTOSA

Comment: The nasal/oral regimen selected should be instituted with concurrent weaning from the nasal decongestant.

Nasal Corticosteroids *see Rhinitis, Sinusitis: Allergic page 425*
Oral Corticosteroids *see page 562*
Parenteral Corticosteroids *see page 570*
OTC Decongestants
OTC Antihistamine+Decongestant Combinations

NASAL ANTICHOLINERGICS

▷ *ipratropium bromide* (B)(G)

Atrovent Nasal Spray 0.03% stop nasal decongestant; 2 sprays in each nostril bid-tid with progressive weaning as tolerated
Pediatric: <6 years: not recommended; ≥6 years: same as adult
Nasal spray: 21 mcg/actuation (30 ml, 345 sprays)
Atrovent Nasal Spray 0.06% stop nasal decongestant; 2 sprays in each nostril tid-qid with progressive weaning as tolerated
Pediatric: <5 years: not recommended; ≥5-11 years: 2 sprays in each nostril tid; ≥11 years: same as adult
Nasal spray: 42 mcg/actuation (15 ml, 165 sprays)

Comment: Avoid use with narrow-angle glaucoma, prostate hyperplasia, and bladder neck obstruction

NASAL ANTIHISTAMINE

▷ *azelastine* (C) 2 sprays in each nostril bid
  Pediatric: <5 years: not recommended; ≥5-12 years: 1 spray in each nostril bid
    Astelin Ready Spray *Nasal spray:* 137 mcg/actuation (30 ml, 200 sprays)

FIRST GENERATION ANTIHISTAMINES

▷ *diphenhydramine* (B)(G) 25-50 mg q 6-8 hours; max 100 mg/day
  Pediatric: <2 years: not recommended; 2-6 years: 6.25 mg q 4-6 hours; max 37.5 mg/day; >6-12 years: 12.5-25 mg q 4-6 hours; max 150 mg/day; >12 years: same as adult
    Benadryl (OTC) *Chew tab:* 12.5 mg (grape) (phenylalanine); *Liq:* 12.5 mg/5 ml (4, 8 oz); *Cap:* 25 mg; *Tab:* 25 mg; *Dye-free soft gel:* 25 mg; *Dye-free liq:* 12.5 mg/5 ml (4, 8 oz)
▷ *diphenhydramine* injectable (B)(G) 25-50 mg IM immediately; then q 6 hours prn
  Pediatric: <12 years: *See mfr pkg insert:* 1.25 mg/kg up to 25 mg IM x 1 dose; then q 6 hours prn; ≥12 years:
    Benadryl Injectable *Vial:* 50 mg/ml (1 ml single-use); 50 mg/ml (10 ml multi-dose); *Amp:* 10 mg/ml (1 ml); *Prefilled syringe:* 50 mg/ml (1 ml)
▷ *hydroxyzine* (C)(G) 25 mg tid prn; max 600 mg/day
  Pediatric: <6 years: 50 mg/day divided qid prn; ≥6 years: 50-100 mg/day divided qid prn; max 600 mg/day
    Atarax *Tab:* 10, 25, 50, 100 mg; *Syr:* 10 mg/5 ml (alcohol 0.5%)
    Vistaril *Cap:* 25, 50, 100 mg; *Oral susp:* 25 mg/5 ml (4 oz) (lemon)

SECOND GENERATION ANTIHISTAMINES

Comment: Second generation antihistamines are sedating, but much less so than the first generation antihistamines. All antihistamines are excreted into breast milk.
▷ *cetirizine* (C)(OTC)(G) <6 years: not recommended; ≥6-<65 years: initially 5-10 mg once daily; ≥65 years: 5 mg once daily
    Children's Zyrtec Chewable *Chew tab:* 5, 10 mg (grape)
    Children's Zyrtec Allergy Syrup *Syr:* 1 mg/ml (4 oz) (grape, bubble gum) (sugar-free, dye-free)
    Zyrtec *Tab:* 10 mg
    Zyrtec Hives Relief *Tab:* 10 mg
    Zyrtec Liquid Gels *Liq gel:* 10 mg
▷ *desloratadine* (C)
    Clarinex <6 years: not recommended; ≥6 years: 1/2-1 tab once daily
      Tab: 5 mg
    Clarinex RediTabs <6 years: not recommended; 6-12 years: 2.5 mg once daily; ≥12 years: 5 mg once daily
      ODT: 2.5, 5 mg (tutti-frutti) (phenylalanine)
    Clarinex Syrup <6 months: not recommended; 6-11 months: 1 mg (2 ml) once daily; 1-5 years: 1.25 mg (2.5 ml) once daily; 6-11 years: 2.5 mg (5 ml) once daily; ≥12 years: 5 mg (10 ml) once daily
      Tab: 0.5 mg per ml (4 oz) (tutti-frutti) (phenylalanine)
    Desloratadine ODT
▷ *fexofenadine* (C)(OTC)(G) 6 months-2 years: 15 mg bid; *CrCl ≤90 mL/min:* 15 mg once daily; 2-11 years: 30 mg bid; *CrCl ≤90 mL/min:* 30 mg once daily ≥12 years and older: ≥12 years: 60 mg once daily-bid or 180 mg once daily; *CrCl <90 mL/min:* 60 mg once daily **Allegra** *Tab:* 30, 60, 180 mg film-coat
    Allegra Allergy *Tab:* 60, 180 mg film-coat
    Allegra ODT *ODT:* 30 mg (phenylalanine)
    Allegra Oral Suspension *Oral susp:* 30 mg/5 ml (6 mg/ml) (4 oz)

▷ *levocetirizine* (B)(OTC) administer dose in the PM; *Seasonal Allergic Rhinitis:* <2 years: not recommended; may start at ≥2 years; *Chronic Idiopathic Urticaria (CIU), Perennial Allergic Rhinitis:* <6 months: not recommended; may start at ≥ 6 months; *Dosing by Age:* 6 months-5 years: max 1.25 mg once daily; 6-11 years: max 2.5 mg once daily; ≥12 years: 2.5-5 mg once daily; *Renal Dysfunction <12 years:* contraindicated; *Renal Dysfunction ≥12 years:* CrCl 50-80 ml/min: 2.5 mg once daily; CrCl 30-50 mL/min: 2.5 mg every other day; CrCl: 10-30 mL/min: 2.5 mg twice weekly (every 3-4 days); CrCl <10 mL/min, ESRD or hemodialysis: contraindicated [alpha corrected]

Children's Xyzal Allergy 24HR *Oral Soln:* 0.5 mg/ml (150 ml)
Xyzal Allergy 24HR *Tab:* 5*mg

▷ *loratadine* (C)(OTC)(G) 5 mg bid or 10 mg once daily; *Hepatic or Renal Insufficiency:* see mfr pkg insert
Pediatric: <2 years: not recommended; 2-5 years: 5 mg once daily; ≥6 years: same as adult

Children's Claritin Chewables *Chew tab:* 5 mg (grape) (phenylalanine)
Children's Claritin Syrup 1 mg/ml (4 oz) (fruit) (sugar-free, alcohol-free, dye-free, sodium 6 mg/5 ml)
Claritin *Tab:* 10 mg
Claritin Hives Relief *Tab:* 10 mg
Claritin Liqui-Gels *Liq gel:* 10 mg
Claritin RediTabs 12 Hours *ODT:* 5 mg (mint)
Claritin RediTabs 24 Hours *ODT:* 10 mg (mint)

⬤ RHINITIS: VASOMOTOR

NASAL ANTICHOLINERGICS

Comment: Avoid use with narrow-angle glaucoma, prostate hyperplasia, and bladder neck obstruction

▷ *ipratropium bromide* (B)(G)
Atrovent Nasal Spray 0.03% stop nasal decongestant; 2 sprays in each nostril bid-tid with progressive weaning as tolerated
Pediatric: <6 years: not recommended; ≥6 years: same as adult
Nasal spray: 21 mcg/actuation (30 ml, 345 sprays)
Atrovent Nasal Spray 0.06% stop nasal decongestant; 2 sprays in each nostril tid-qid with progressive weaning as tolerated
Pediatric: <5 years: not recommended; ≥5-11 years: 2 sprays in each nostril tid; >11 years: same as adult
Nasal spray: 42 mcg/actuation (15 ml, 165 sprays)

⬤ ROSEOLA INFANTUM (EXANTHEM SUBITUM)

Antipyretics *see Fever page* 165

Comment: Roseola infantum (also known as exanthem subitum, sixth disease, pseudorubella, exanthem criticum, and three-day fever) is a generally mild clinical syndrome, commonly occurring in children <3 years-of-age, characterized by sudden onset of high fever (may exceed 40°C [104°F]) that lasts 3 days and resolves abruptly, and is followed by development of a rash lasting ≤3 days. Roseola usually is caused by human herpesvirus 6 (HHV-6). Treatment is antipyretics (aspirin is contraindicated) and adequate hydration. Monitor for febrile seizures. As with the common cold, roseola spreads from person to person through contact with an infected person's respiratory secretions or saliva. The disease can occur at any time of year.

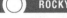 **ROCKY MOUNTAIN SPOTTED FEVER (*RICKETTSIA RICKETTSII*)**

ANTI-INFECTIVES

▷ *doxycycline* (D)(G) 200 mg on first day; then 100 mg bid x 7-10 days
  Pediatric: <8 years: not recommended; ≥8 years, <100 lb: 2-2.5 mg/kg q 12 hours x
  7-10 days; ≥8 years, ≥100 lb: same as adult

  Acticlate *Tab:* 75, 150**mg
  Adoxa *Tab:* 50, 75, 100, 150 mg ent-coat
  Doryx *Tab:* 50, 75, 100, 150, 200 mg del-rel
  Doxteric *Tab:* 50 mg del-rel
  Monodox *Cap:* 50, 75, 100 mg
  Oracea *Cap:* 40 mg del-rel
  Vibramycin *Tab:* 100 mg; *Cap:* 50, 100 mg; *Syr:* 50 mg/5 ml (raspberry-apple)
    (sulfites); *Oral susp:* 25 mg/5 ml (raspberry)
  Vibra-Tab *Tab:* 100 mg film-coat

Comment: *doxycycline* contraindicated <8 years-of-age, in pregnancy, and
lactation (discolors developing tooth enamel). A side effect may be photosensitivity
(photophobia). Do not take with antacids, calcium supplements, milk or other dairy, or
within 2 hours of taking another drug.

▷ *tetracycline* (D)(G) 500 mg q 6 hours x 7-10 days
  Pediatric: <8 years: not recommended; ≥8 years, <100 lb: 10 mg/kg/day q 6 hours x
  7-10 days; ≥8 years, ≥100 lb: same as adult

  Achromycin V *Cap:* 250, 500 mg
  Sumycin *Tab:* 250, 500 mg; *Cap:* 250, 500 mg; *Oral susp:* 125 mg/5 ml (100, 200
    ml) (fruit) (sulfites)

Comment: *tetracycline* is contraindicated <8 years-of-age, in pregnancy, and
lactation (discolors developing tooth enamel). A side effect may be photosensitivity
(photophobia). Do not give with antacids, calcium supplements, milk or other dairy, or
within two hours of taking another drug.

 ROTAVIRUS GASTROENTERITIS

PROPHYLAXIS

Comment: RotaTeq targets the most common strains of rotavirus (G1, G2, G3, G4),
which are responsible for more than 90% of rotavirus disease in the United States.

▷ *rotavirus vaccine, live* not recommended for adults
  Pediatric: <6 weeks or >32 weeks: not recommended; >6 weeks and <32 weeks: administer 1st dose at 6-12 weeks of age; administer 2nd and 3rd doses at 4-10-week intervals for
  a total of 3 doses; if an incomplete dose is administered, do not administer a replacement
  dose, but continue with the remaining doses in the recommended series

  RotaTeq *Oral susp:* 2 ml single-use tube (fetal bovine serum [trace], preservative-
    free, thimerosal-free)

 ROUNDWORM (*ASCARIASIS*)

ANTHELMINTICS

Comment: Oral bioavailability of anthelmintics is enhanced when administered with a
fatty meal (estimated fat content 40 gm).

▷ *albendazole* (C) take with a meal; swallow, chew, crush, or mix with food; 400 mg
  once daily x 7 days

Pediatric: <2 years: 200 mg once daily x 3 days; may repeat in 3 weeks if needed; 2-12 years: 400 mg once daily x 3 days; may repeat in 3 weeks if needed; >12 years: same as adult

    Albenza *Tab:* 200 mg

▷ *mebendazole* **(C)** take with a meal; swallow, chew, crush, or mix with food; 100 mg bid x 3 days; may repeat in 3 weeks if needed
Pediatric: <2 years: not recommended; ≥2 years: same as adult

    Emverm *Chew tab:* 100 mg

    Vermox (G) *Chew tab:* 100 mg

▷ *pyrantel pamoate* **(C)** take with a meal; may open capsule and sprinkle or mix with food; treat x 3 days; may repeat in 2-3 weeks if needed; 11 mg/kg once daily x 3 days; max 1 gm/dose
Pediatric: 25-37 lb: 1/2 tsp x 1 dose; 38-62 lb: 1 tsp x 1 dose; 63-87 lb: 1 tsp x 1 dose; 88-112 lb: 2 tsp x 1 dose; 113-137 lb: 2 tsp x 1 dose; 138-162 lb: 3 tsp x 1 dose; 163-187 lb: 3 tsp x 1 dose; >187 lb: 4 tsp x 1 dose

    Antiminth (OTC) *Cap:* 180 mg; *Liq:* 50 mg/ml (30 ml); 144 mg/ml (30 ml); *Oral susp:* 50 mg/ml (60 ml)

    Pin-X (OTC) *Cap:* 180 mg; *Liq:* 50 mg/ml (30 ml); 144 mg/ml (30 ml); *Oral susp:* 50 mg/ml (30 ml)

▷ *thiabendazole* **(C)** 25 mg/kg bid x 7 days; max 1.5 gm/dose; max 3000 mg/day; take with a meal
Pediatric: same as adult

    Mintezol *Chew tab:* 500*mg (orange); *Oral susp:* 500 mg/5 ml (120 ml) (orange)

Comment: *thiabendazole* is not for prophylaxis. May impair mental alertness. May not be available in the US.

 RUBELLA (GERMAN MEASLES)

Antipyretics *see* **Fever** *page* 165
See **Childhood Immunizations** *page* 546

Comment: Rubella is highly contagious and highly teratogenic. Quarantine is mandatory to prevent a community outbreak. Herd immunity is the best prevention.

PROPHYLAXIS VACCINE

Comment: <12 months: not recommended; ≥12 months: 25 mcg SC; if vaccinated <12 months, re-vaccinate at 12 months; administer in the upper posterior arm.

▷ *rubella virus, live, attenuated+neomycin* vaccine **(C)**
Pediatric: <12 months: not recommended (if vaccinated <12 months, revaccinate at 12 months); ≥12 months: 25 mcg SC

    Meruvax II 25 mcg SC

▷ *measles, mumps, rubella, live, attenuated, neomycin vaccine* **(C)**

    MMR II 25 mcg SC (preservative-free)

Comment: Contraindications: hypersensitivity to *neomycin* or eggs, primary or acquired immune deficiency, immunosuppressant therapy, bone marrow or lymphatic malignancy, and pregnancy (within 3 months following vaccination).

    see **Childhood Immunizations** *page* 546

TREATMENT

▷ *immune globulin* (Ig) 0.25 ml/kg IM (0.5 mg/kg in immunocompromised children)

RUBEOLA (RED MEASLES)

Antipyretics *see* **Fever** *page 165*
See **Childhood Immunizations** *page 546*

PROPHYLAXIS VACCINE

▷ *measles, mumps, rubella, live, attenuated, neomycin vaccine* (C)
   MMR II 25 mcg SC (preservative-free)
Comment: Contraindications: hypersensitivity to *neomycin* or eggs, primary or
acquired immune deficiency, immunosuppressant therapy, bone marrow or lymphatic
malignancy, and pregnancy (within 3 months following vaccination).

TREATMENT

▷ *immune globulin* (Ig) 0.25 ml/kg IM (0.5 mg/kg in immunocompromised children)

 SALMONELLOSIS

ANTI-INFECTIVES

▷ *ciprofloxacin* (C) 500 mg bid x 3-5 days
   Pediatric: <18 years: not recommended; ≥18 years: same as adult
      Cipro (G) *Tab:* 250, 500, 750 mg; *Oral susp:* 250, 500 mg/5 ml (100 ml) (strawberry)
      Cipro XR *Tab:* 500, 1000 mg ext-rel
      ProQuin XR *Tab:* 500 mg ext-rel
Comment: *ciprofloxacin* is contraindicated <18 years-of-age, and during pregnancy and
lactation. Risk of tendonitis or tendon rupture.
▷ *trimethoprim+sulfamethoxazole (TMP-SMX)* (D)(G)
   Pediatric: <2 months: not recommended; ≥2 months: 40 mg/kg/day of *sulfamethoxazole* in 2 divided doses bid x 10 days; *see page 648 for dose by weight*
      Bactrim, Septra 2 tabs bid x 10 days
         Tab: trim 80 mg+*sulfa* 400 mg*
      Bactrim DS, Septra DS 1 tab bid x 10 days
         Tab: trim 160 mg+*sulfa* 800 mg*
      Bactrim Pediatric Suspension, Septra Pediatric Suspension
         Oral susp: trim 40 mg+*sulfa* 200 mg per 5 ml (100 ml) (cherry) (alcohol 0.3%)

 SCABIES (*SARCOPTES SCABIEI*)

Comment: This section presents treatment regimens for scabies infestation published
in the **2015 CDC Sexually Transmitted Diseases Treatment Guidelines**, as well as other
available treatments.

RECOMMENDED REGIMEN

▷ *permethrin* (B)(G) massage into skin from head to soles of feet; leave on x 8-14 hours,
   then rinse off
   Pediatric: <2 months: not recommended; ≥2 months: same as adult
      Acticin, Elimite *Crm:* 5% (60 gm)

ALTERNATIVE REGIMEN

▷ *lindane* (B)(G) 1 oz of lotion or 30 gm of cream apply to all skin surfaces from neck
   down to the soles of the feet; leave on x 8 hours, then wash off thoroughly; may repeat
   if needed in 14 days

Pediatric: <2 months: not recommended; ≥2 months: same as adult
Kwell *Lotn:* 1% (60, 473 ml); *Crm:* 1% (60 gm); *Shampoo:* 1% (60, 473 ml)

OTHER TOPICAL TREATMENTS

▷ *crotamiton* (C) massage into skin from chin down; repeat in 24 hours
Pediatric: <12 years: not recommended; ≥12 years: same as adult
Eurax *Lotn:* 10% (60 gm); *Crm:* 10% (60 gm)

SCARLET FEVER (SCARLATINA)

Comment: Microorganism responsible for scarlet fever is Group A beta-hemolytic
Streptococcus (GABHS). Strep cultures and screens will be positive.

▷ *azithromycin* (B)(G) 500 mg x 1 dose on day 1, then 250 mg once daily on days 2-5 <u>or</u>
500 mg once daily x 3 days
Pediatric: 12 mg/kg/day x 5 days; max 500 mg/day; *see page 621 for dose by weight*
Zithromax *Tab:* 250, 500, 600 mg; *Oral susp:* 100 mg/5 ml (15 ml); 200 mg/5 ml
(15, 22.5, 30 ml) (cherry); *Pkt:* 1 gm for reconstitution (cherry-banana)
Zithromax Tri-pak *Tab:* 3 x 500 mg tabs/pck
Zithromax Z-pak *Tab:* 6 x 250 mg tabs/pck
Zmax *Oral susp:* 2 gm ext-rel for reconstitution (cherry-banana) (148 mg Na$^+$)

▷ *cefadroxil* (B)
Pediatric: 15-30 mg/kg/day in 2 divided doses x 10 days; *see page 623 for dose by weight*
Duricef *Cap:* 500 mg; *Tab:* 1 gm; *Oral susp:* 250 mg/5 ml (100 ml); 500 mg/5 ml
(75, 100 ml) (orange-pineapple)

▷ *cephalexin* (B)(G)
Pediatric: 25-50 mg/kg/day in 2 divided doses x 10 days; *see page 629 for dose by weight*
Keflex *Cap:* 250, 333, 500, 750 mg; *Oral susp:* 125, 250 mg/5 ml (100, 200 ml)
(strawberry)

▷ *clarithromycin* (C)(G) 250 mg bid <u>or</u> 500 mg ext-rel once daily x 10 days
Pediatric: <6 months: not recommended; ≥6 months: 7.5 mg/kg bid x 10 days; *see page 630 for dose by weight*
Biaxin *Tab:* 250, 500 mg
Biaxin Oral Suspension *Oral susp:* 125, 250 mg/5 ml (50, 100 ml) (fruit punch)
Biaxin XL *Tab:* 500 mg ext-rel

▷ *clindamycin* (B)(G) 150-300 mg q 6 hours x 10 days
Pediatric: 8-16 mg/kg/day in 3-4 divided doses x 10 days
Cleocin *Cap:* 75 (tartrazine), 150 (tartrazine), 300 mg
Cleocin Pediatric Granules *Oral susp:* 75 mg/5 ml (100 ml) (cherry)

▷ *erythromycin estolate* (B)(G) 250 mg q 6 hours x 10 days
Pediatric: 20-50 mg/kg q 6 hours x 10 days; *see page 634 for dose by weight*
Ilosone *Pulvule:* 250 mg; *Tab:* 500 mg; *Liq:* 125, 250 mg/5 ml (100 ml)

Comment: *erythromycin* may increase INR with concomitant *warfarin*, as well as
increase serum level of *digoxin, benzodiazepines,* and *statins.*

▷ *erythromycin ethylsuccinate* (B)(G) 400 mg qid <u>or</u> 800 mg bid x 10 days
Pediatric: 30-50 mg/kg/day in 4 divided doses x 10 days; may double dose with severe
infection; max 100 mg/kg/day; *see page 635 for dose by weight*
EryPed *Oral susp:* 200 mg/5 ml (100, 200 ml) (fruit); 400 mg/5 ml (60, 100,
200 ml) (banana); *Oral drops:* 200, 400 mg/5 ml (50 ml) (fruit); *Chew tab:* 200 mg
wafer (fruit)

E.E.S. *Oral susp:* 200, 400 mg/5 ml (100 ml) (fruit)
E.E.S. Granules *Oral susp:* 200 mg/5 ml (100, 200 ml) (cherry)
E.E.S. 400 Tablets *Tab:* 400 mg
Comment: *erythromycin* may increase INR with concomitant *warfarin*, as well as increase serum level of *digoxin, benzodiazepines*, and *statins*.

➤ *penicillin g (benzathine and procaine)* (B)(G) 2.4 million units IM x 1 dose
Pediatric: <30 lb: 600,000 units IM x 1 dose; 30-60 lb: 900,000-1.2 million units IM x 1 dose
Bicillin C-R Cartridge-needle unit: 600,000 units (1 ml); 1.2 million units; (2 ml); 2.4 million units (4 ml)

➤ *penicillin v potassium* (B) 250 mg tid x 10 days
Pediatric: 25-50 mg/kg day in 4 divided doses x 10 days; ≥12 years: same as adult; *see page 644 for dose by weight*
Pen-Vee K *Tab:* 250, 500 mg; *Oral soln:* 125 mg/5 ml (100, 200 ml); 250 mg/5 ml (100, 150, 200 ml)

 SCHISTOSOMIASIS

TREMATODICIDE

Comment: *praziquantel* is a trematodicide indicated for the treatment of infections due to all species of genus *Schistosoma* (e.g., *Schistosoma mekongi, Schistosoma japonicum, Schistosoma mansoni*, and *Schistosoma hematobium)* and infections due to liver flukes (i.e., *Clonorchis sinensis, Opisthorchis viverrini). praziquantel* induces a rapid contraction of schistosomes by a specific effect on the permeability of the cell membrane. The drug further causes vacuolization and disintegration of the schistosome tegument.

➤ *praziquantel* (B) 20 mg/kg tid as a one-day treatment; take the 3 doses at intervals of not less than 4 hours and not more than 6 hours; swallow whole with water during meals; holding the tablets in the mouth leaves a bitter taste which can trigger gagging or vomiting.
Pediatric: <4 years: not established; ≥4 years: same as adult
Biltricide *Tab:* 600 mg film-coat
Comment: Concomitant administration with strong Cytochrome P450 (P450) inducers, such as *rifampin*, is contraindicated since therapeutically effective blood levels of *praziquantel* may not be achieved. In patients receiving *rifampin* who need immediate treatment for schistosomiasis, alternative agents for schistosomiasis should be considered. However, if treatment with *praziquantel* is necessary, *rifampin* should be discontinued 4 weeks before administration of *praziquantel*. Treatment with *rifampin* can then be restarted one day after completion of *praziquantel* treatment. Concomitant administration of other P450 inducers (e.g., antiepileptic drugs such as *phenytoin, phenobarbital, carbamazepine*) and *dexamethasone*, may also reduce plasma levels of *praziquantel*. Concomitant administration of P450 inhibitors (e.g., *cimetidine, ketoconazole, itraconazole, erythromycin*) may increase plasma levels of *praziquantel*. Patients should be warned not to drive a car or operate machinery on the day of Biltricide treatment and the following day. There are no adequate or well-controlled studies in pregnant women. This drug should be used during pregnancy only if clearly needed. *praziquantel* appears in the milk of nursing women at a concentration of about 1/4 that of maternal serum. It is not known whether a pharmacological effect is likely to occur in children. Women should not nurse on the day of Biltricide treatment and during the subsequent 72 hours.

SCHIZOPHRENIA AND SCHIZOPHRENIA WITH CO-MORBID PERSONALITY DISORDER

Other Antipsychosis Drugs *see* **Appendix Q: Antipsychosis Drugs** *pages* 581
Tardive Dyskinesia *see page* 456

Comment: A team of researchers examined the effects of antipsychotics on mortality risk in schizophrenia patients. They studied data on 29,823 patients with schizophrenia in Sweden, aged 16 to 64 years and found mortality among patients with schizophrenia was 40% lower when they used antipsychotics as compared to when they did not. Long-acting injection (LAI) use was associated with an approximately 33% lower risk of death compared with the oral use of the same medication. The lowest mortality was observed with use of once-monthly *paliperidone* LAI, oral aripiprazole, and risperidone LAI.

REFERENCE

Taipale, H., Mittendorfer-Rutz, E., Alexanderson, K., Majak, M., Mehtälä, J., Hoti, F., ... Tiihonen, J. (2017). Antipsychotics and mortality in a nationwide cohort of 29,823 patients with schizophrenia. *Schizophrenia Research.* doi:10.1016/j.schres.2017.12.010

➢ *aripiprazole lauroxil* (C) administer by IM injection in the deltoid (441 mg dose only) or gluteal (441 mg, 662 mg, 882 mg or 1064 mg) muscle by a qualified healthcare professional; initiate at a dose of 441 mg, 662 mg or 882 mg administered monthly, or 882 mg every 6 weeks, or 1064 mg every 2 months
Pediatric: <18 years: not recommended; ≥18 years: same as adult
  Aristada *Prefilled syringe:* 441, 662, 882, 1064 mg single-use, ext-rel susp
Comment: **Aristada** is an atypical antipsychotic available in 4 doses with 3 dosing duration options for flexible dosing. For patients naïve to *aripiprazole*, establish tolerability with oral *aripiprazole* prior to initiating treatment with **Aristada**. **Aristada** can be initiated at any of the 4 doses at the appropriate dosing duration option. In conjunction with the first injection, administer treatment with oral *aripiprazole* for 21 consecutive days for all 4 dose sizes. The most common adverse event associated with **Aristada** is akathisia. Patients are also at increased risk for developing neuroleptic malignant syndrome, tardive dyskinesia, pathological gambling or other compulsive behaviors, orthostatic hypotension, hyperglycemic, dyslipidemia, and weight gain. Hypersensitive reactions can occur and range from pruritus or urticaria to anaphylaxis. Stroke, transient ischemic attacks, and falls have been reported in elderly patients with dementia-related psychosis who were treated with *apriprazole*. **Aristada** is not for treatment of people who have lost touch with reality (psychosis) due to confusion and memory loss (dementia). May cause extrapyramidal and/or withdrawal symptoms in neonates exposed in utero in the third trimester of pregnancy. **aripiprazole** is present in human breast milk; however, there are insufficient data to assess the amount in human milk or the effects on the breast-fed infant. The development and health benefits of breastfeeding should be considered along with the mother's clinical need for **Aristada** and any potential adverse effects on the breastfed infant from **Aristada** or from the underlying maternal condition. For more information or to report suspected ASEs, contact the National Pregnancy Registry for Atypical Antipsychotics at 1-866-961-2388 or visit http://womensmentalhealth.org/clinical-and-research-programs/pregnancyregistry/. Limited published data on aripiprazole use in pregnant women are not sufficient to inform any drug-associated risks for birth defects or miscarriage. To report suspected adverse reactions, contact Alkermes at 1-866-274-7823 or FDA at 1-800-FDA-1088 or www.fda.gov/medwatch

SEIZURE DISORDER

Status Epilepticus *see Status Epilepticus page* 448
Anticonvulsant Drugs *see page* 584

 SEXUAL ASSAULT (STD/STI/VD EXPOSURE)

Comment: The following treatment regimens for victims of sexual assault are published in the **2015 CDC Sexually Transmitted Diseases Treatment Guidelines**.

RECOMMENDED PROPHYLAXIS REGIMEN

▷ *ceftriaxone* 250 mg IM in a single dose plus *metronidazole* 2 gm in a single dose plus *azithromycin* 1 gm in a single dose

ALTERNATE PROPHYLAXIS REGIMENS

Regimen 1

▷ *ceftriaxone* 250 mg IM in a single dose plus *metronidazole* 2 gm in a single dose plus *doxycycline* 100 mg bid x 7 days

Regimen 2

▷ *cefixime* 400 mg in a single dose plus *metronidazole* 2 gm in a single dose plus *azithromycin* 1 gm in a single dose

Regimen 3

▷ *cefixime* 400 mg in a single dose plus *metronidazole* 2 gm in a single dose plus *doxycycline* 100 mg bid x 7 days

Regimen 4

▷ *azithromycin* (B) 1 gm as a single dose plus *metronidazole* 2 gm in a single dose

DRUG BRANDS AND DOSE FORMS

▷ *azithromycin* (B)(G)
>   **Zithromax** *Tab:* 250, 500, 600 mg; *Oral susp:* 100 mg/5 ml (15 ml); 200 mg/5 ml (15, 22.5, 30 ml) (cherry); *Pkt:* 1 gm for reconstitution (cherry-banana)
>   **Zithromax Tri-pak** *Tab:* 3 x 500 mg tabs/pck
>   **Zithromax Z-pak** *Tab:* 6 x 250 mg tabs/pck
>   **Zmax** *Oral susp:* 2 gm ext-rel for reconstitution (cherry-banana) (148 mg Na⁺)

▷ *cefixime* (B)(G)
>   **Suprax** *Tab:* 400 mg; *Cap:* 400 mg; *Oral susp:* 100, 200, 500 mg/5 ml (50, 75, 100 ml) (strawberry)

▷ *ceftriaxone* (B)(G)
>   **Rocephin** *Vial:* 250, 500 mg; 1, 2 gm

▷ *doxycycline* (D)(G)
>   **Acticlate** *Tab:* 75, 150**mg
>   **Adoxa** *Tab:* 50, 75, 100, 150 mg ent-coat
>   **Doryx** *Tab:* 50, 75, 100, 150, 200 mg del-rel
>   **Doxteric** *Tab:* 50 mg del-rel
>   **Monodox** *Cap:* 50, 75, 100 mg
>   **Oracea** *Cap:* 40 mg del-rel
>   **Vibramycin** *Tab:* 100 mg; *Cap:* 50, 100 mg; *Syr:* 50 mg/5 ml (raspberry-apple) (sulfites); *Oral susp:* 25 mg/5 ml (raspberry)
>   **Vibra-Tab** *Tab:* 100 mg film-coat

Comment: *doxycycline* is contraindicated <8 years-of-age, in pregnancy, and lactation (discolors developing tooth enamel). A side effect may be photosensitivity (photophobia). Do not take with antacids, calcium supplements, milk or other dairy, or within 2 hours of taking another drug.

▷ *metronidazole* (not for use in 1st; B in 2nd, 3rd)(G)

    Flagyl *Tab:* 250*, 500*mg

    Flagyl 375 *Cap:* 375 mg

    Flagyl ER *Tab:* 750 mg ext-rel

Comment: Alcohol is contraindicated during treatment with oral *metronidazole* and for 72 hours after therapy due to a possible *disulfiram*-like reaction (nausea, vomiting, flushing, headache).

 SHIGELLOSIS (GENUS *SHIGELLA*)

ANTI-INFECTIVES

▷ *azithromycin* (B)(G) 500 mg x 1 dose on day 1, then 250 mg once daily on days 2-5 or 500 mg once daily x 3 days or **Zmax** 2 gm in a single dose

    Pediatric: <6 months: not recommended; ≥6 months: 10 mg/kg x 1 dose on day 1; then 5 mg/kg/day on days 2-5; max 500 mg/day; *see page 621 for dose by weight*

    Zithromax *Tab:* 250, 500, 600 mg; *Oral susp:* 100 mg/5 ml (15 ml); 200 mg/5 ml (15, 22.5, 30 ml) (cherry); *Pkt:* 1 gm for reconstitution (cherry-banana)

    Zithromax Tri-pak *Tab:* 3 x 500 mg tabs/pck

    Zithromax Z-pak *Tab:* 6 x 250 mg tabs/pck

    Zmax *Oral susp:* 2 gm ext-rel for reconstitution (cherry-banana) (148 mg Na⁺)

▷ *ciprofloxacin* (C) 500 mg bid x 3 days

    Pediatric: <18 years: not recommended; ≥18 years: same as adult

    Cipro (G) *Tab:* 250, 500, 750 mg; *Oral susp:* 250, 500 mg/5 ml (100 ml) (strawberry)

    Cipro XR *Tab:* 500, 1000 mg ext-rel

    ProQuin XR *Tab:* 500 mg ext-rel

▷ *ofloxacin* (C)(G) 400 mg bid x 3 days

    Pediatric: <18 years: not recommended; ≥18 years: same as adult

    Floxin *Tab:* 200, 300, 400 mg

▷ *tetracycline* (D)(G) 250-500 mg qid x 5 days

    Pediatric: <8 years: not recommended; ≥8 years, <100 lb: 25-50 mg/kg/day in 4 divided doses x 5 days; ≥8 years, ≥100 lb: same as adult; *see page 646 for dose by weight*

    Achromycin V *Cap:* 250, 500 mg

    Sumycin *Tab:* 250, 500 mg; *Cap:* 250, 500 mg; *Oral susp:* 125 mg/5 ml (100, 200 ml) (fruit) (sulfites)

▷ *trimethoprim+sulfamethoxazole* (TMP-SMX) (D)(G)

    Bactrim, Septra 2 tabs bid x 10 days

        Tab: trim 80 mg+*sulfa* 400 mg*

    Bactrim DS, Septra DS 1 tab bid x 10 days

        Tab: trim 160 mg+*sulfa* 800 mg*

    Bactrim Pediatric Suspension, Septra Pediatric Suspension 20 ml bid x 10 days

        Oral susp: trim 40 mg+*sulfa* 200 mg per 5 ml (100 ml) (cherry) (alcohol 0.3%)

 SHOCK: SEPTIC, DISTRIBUTIVE

Comment: Septic shock is the most common form of distributive shock and is characterized by considerable mortality (treated, around 30%; untreated, probably >80%). In the United States, septic shock is the leading cause of non-cardiac death in

intensive care units. **Giapreza (angiotensin** II) *received accelerated review and FDA approval December 2017* to increase blood pressure, when added to conventional interventions used to raise blood pressure, to prevent/treat dangerously low hypotension resulting from septic and other distributive shock states. There is a potential for venous and arterial thrombotic and thromboembolic events in patients who receive **Giapreza**. Therefore, use concurrent venous thromboembolism (VTE) prophylaxis. **Giapreza** is available March 2018.

ANGIOTENSIN II

▷ *angiotensin II* dilute in 0.9% NaCl; must be administered as an IV infusion; initial infusion rate 20 ng/kg/min; titrate as frequently as every 5 minutes by increments of up to 15 ng/kg/min as needed; during the first 3 hours, max 80 ng/kg/min; max maintenance dose 40 ng/kg/min; diluted solution may be stored at room temperature or refrigerated; discard after 24 hours.
Dilution/Concentration:
Giapreza 1 ml (2.5 mg/ml) in 500 ml 0.9%NaCl = 5,000 ng/ml
     1 ml (2.5.mg/ml in 250 ml 0.9%NaCl = 10,000 ng/ml
     2 ml (5 mg/ml) in 500 ml 0.9%NaCl = 10,000 ng/ml
   Giapreza Vial: 2.5 mg in ml, 5 mg/2 ml (2.5 mg/ml)
Comment: The safety and efficacy of **Giapreza** in pediatric patients have not been established. It is not known whether **Giapreza** is present in human milk and no data are available on the effects of angiotensin II on the breastfed child. The published data on angiotensin II use in pregnant women are not sufficient to determine a drug-associated risk of adverse developmental outcomes. However, Delaying treatment in pregnant women with hypotension associated with septic or other distributive shock is likely to increase the risk of shock-associated maternal and fetal morbidity and mortality.

 SICKLE CELL DISEASE (SCD)

▷ *hydroxyurea*
Comment: *hydroxyurea* has an FDA-approved "orphan drug" designation for the treatment of sickle cell disease SCD). It is an antimetabolite indicated to reduce the frequency of painful crises and to reduce the need for blood transfusions in patients with sickle cell anemia SCA) with recurrent moderate to severe painful crises. *Blac Box Warning (BBW): hydroxyurea* may cause severe myelosuppression. Do not administer if bone marrow function is markedly depressed. Monitor blood counts at baseline and every 2 weeks throughout treatment. Blood counts within an acceptable range are defined as: *neutrophils* ≥ 2,500 cells/mm3, *platelets* ≥95,000 cells/mm3, *Hgb* ≥5.3 gm/ dL, *reticulocytes* ≥95,000 cells/mm3 if the Hgb <9 gm/dL. Discontinue *hydroxyurea* until hematologic recovery if blood counts are considered toxic. Treatment may be resumed after reducing the *hydroxyurea* dose by 2.5 mg/kg/day from the dose associated with hematological toxicity. *CrCl <60 mL/min:* reduce dose by 50%. *hydroxyurea* is carcinogenic. Advise sun protection and monitor patients for malignancies. Avoid live vaccines when using *hydroyurea*. Discontinue *hydroxyurea* if vasculitic toxicity occurs. Risks with concomitant use of antiretroviral drugs: pancreatitis, hepatotoxicity, and neuropathy. Monitor for signs and symptoms in patients with HIV infection using antiretroviral drugs. If patients with HIV infection are treated with *hydroxyurea*, and in particular, in combination with *didanosine* and/or *stavudine*, close monitoring for signs and symptoms of pancreatitis is recommended. Permanently discontinue *hydroxyurea* in patients who develop signs and symptoms of pancreatitis. *hydroxyurea* can cause fetal harm (embryotoxic and teratogenic effects in animal studies). Advise patients regarding potential risk to a fetus and use of effective contraception during and after

treatment with **hydroxyurea** for at least 6 months after therapy is ended. Advise females to immediately report pregnancy. *Hydroxyurea* may damage spermatozoa and testicular tissue, resulting in possible genetic abnormalities. Azoospermia or oligospermia, sometimes reversible, has been observed in men. Inform male patients about the possibility of sperm conservation before the initiation of *hydroxyurea* therapy. Males with female sexual partners of reproductive potential should use effective contraception during and after treatment for at least 1 year. *hydroxyurea* is excreted in human milk. Discontinue breastfeeding during treatment. To report suspected adverse reactions, contact Bristol-Myers Squibb at 1-800-721-5072 or FDA at 1-800-FDA-1088 or www. fda.gov/medwatch

Droxia use actual or ideal body weight (whichever is less) for dosing; initially 15 mg/kg once daily; if the blood counts are within an acceptable range, increase the dose by 5 mg/kg/day every 12 weeks to the highest dose that does not produce toxic blood counts over 24 consecutive weeks (dosage should not exceed 35 mg/kg/day)

Pediatric: <18 years: not established: ≥18 years: same as adult

    Cap: 200, 300, 400 mg

Hydrea (see **Droxia** for prescribing information)

    Tab: 500 mg

Siklos use actual or ideal body weight (whichever is less) for dosing. *initially* 20 mg/kg once daily; may be increased by 5 mg/kg/day every 8 weeks, or sooner if a severe painful crisis occurs, until a maximum toleraeded dose or 35 mg/kg/day is reached; reduce the dose of **Siklos** by 50% (10 mg) in patients with CrCl <60 mL/min or with ESRD

Pediatric: <2 years: not recommended; ≥2 years: same as adult

    Tab: 100 mg; 1,000***mg

Comment: Safety and effectiveness of **Siklos** have been established in pediatric patients aged 2-18 years with sickle cell anemia (SSA) with recurrent moderate to severe painful crises and is the only *hydroxyurea* approved for use in children. Use of **Siklos** in these age groups is supported by evidence from a non-interventional cohort study, the European Sickle Cell Disease prospective Cohort study, ESCORT-HU, in which 405 pediatric patients ages 2 to <18 were treated with **Siklos**: n=274 children (2-11 years) and n=108 adolescents 12-16 years). Pediatric patients aged 2-16 years had a higher risk of neutropenia than patients >16 years. Continuous follow-up of the growth of treated children is recommended.

AMINO ACID

▷ *L-glutamine powder* take 5-15 gm orally, twice daily, based on body weight; <30 kg, <66 lb (1 pkt bid), 30-65 kg, 66-143 lb (2 pkts bid), >65 kg, >143 lb (3 pkts bid); mix each dose in 8 oz. (240 ml) of cold or room temperature beverage or 4-6 oz of food before ingestion

Pediatric: <5 years: not established; ≥5 years: same as adult

    Endari *Oral Powder:* 5 gm/paper-foil-plastic laminate pkt (60 pkts/carton)

Comment: **Endari** is an amino acid indicated to reduce the acute complications of sickle cell disease. Common adverse reactions include constipation, nausea, abdominal pain, headache, cough, pain in extremity, back pain, chest pain There are no available data on **Endari** use in pregnancy to inform a drug-associated risk of major birth defects and miscarriage. There are no data on the presence of **Endari** in human milk or effects on the breastfed infant. The developmental and health benefits from breastfeeding should be considered along with the mother's clinical need for **Endari** and any potential adverse effects on the breastfed child from **Endari** or from the underlying maternal condition. To report suspected adverse reactions, contact Emmaus Medical at 1-877-420-6493 or FDA at 1-800-FDA-1088 or www.fda.gov/medwatch

CHIMERIC (MURINE/HUMAN) MONOCLONAL ANTIBODY

▷ *basiliximab* (B)
Pediatric: <6 months: not recommended; 6 months-12 years: 14 mg/kg/day in a single or 2 divided doses x 10 days; 12 years: same as adult; see page 618 for dose by weight

Simulect *Vial:* 10, 20 mg (6 ml) for reconstitution and IV infusion (pre-serva-tive-free 10 mg vial: contains 10 mg *basiliximab*, 3.61 mg monobasic potassium phosphate, 0.50 mg disodium hydrogen phosphate (anhydrous), 0.80 mg sodium chloride, 10 mg sucrose, 40 mg mannitol, 20 mg glycine, to be reconstituted in 2.5 mL of Sterile Water for Injection, USP *20 mg vial; contains* 20 mg *basiliximab*, 7.21 mg monobasic potassium phosphate, 0.99 mg disodium hydrogen phosphate (anhydrous), 1.61 mg sodium chloride, 20 mg sucrose, 80 mg mannitol and 40 mg glycine, to be reconstituted in 5 mL of Sterile Water for Injection, US

Comment: **Simulect** is indicated for the prophylaxis of acute organ rejection in patients receiving renal transplantation when used as part of an immunosuppressive regimen that includes *cyclosporine* (modified) and corticosteroids. The efficacy of **Simulect** for the prophylaxis of acute rejection in recipients of other solid organ allografts has not been demonstrated. No dose adjustment is necessary when Simulect is added to triple immunosuppression regimens including *cyclosporine*, corticosteroids, and either *azathioprine* or *mycophenolate mofetil*. It is not known whether **Simulect** is excreted in human milk. A decision should be made to discontinue nursing <u>or</u> to discontinue the drug, taking into account the importance of the drug to the mother.

 SINUSITIS AND RHINOSINUSITIS: ACUTE BACTERIAL (ABRS)

ANTI-INFECTIVES

▷ *amoxicillin* (B)(G) 500-875 mg bid <u>or</u> 250-500 mg tid x 10 days
Pediatric: <40 kg (88 lb): 20-40 mg/kg/day in 3 divided doses x 10 days or 25-45 mg/kg/day in 2 divided doses x 10 days; see page 616 for dose by weight

Amoxil *Cap:* 250, 500 mg; *Tab:* 875*mg; *Chew tab:* 125, 200, 250, 400 mg (cherry-banana-peppermint) (phenylalanine); *Oral susp:* 125, 250 mg/5 ml (80, 100, 150 ml) (strawberry); 200, 400 mg/5 ml (50, 75, 100 ml) (bubble gum); *Oral drops:* 50 mg/ml (30 ml) (bubble gum)
Moxatag *Tab:* 775 mg ext-rel
Trimox *Tab:* 125, 250 mg; *Cap:* 250, 500 mg; *Oral susp:* 125, 250 mg/5 ml (80, 100, 150 ml) (raspberry-strawberry)

▷ *amoxicillin+clavulanate* (B)(G)
Augmentin 500 mg tid or 875 mg bid x 10 days
Pediatric: 40-45 mg/kg/day divided tid x 10 days or 90 mg/kg/day divided bid x 10 days see pages 618-619 for dose by weight
Tab: 250, 500, 875 mg; *Chew tab:* 125, 250 mg (lemon-lime); 200, 400 mg (cherry-banana) (phenylalanine); *Oral susp:* 125 mg/5 ml (banana), 250 mg/5 ml (75, 100, 150 ml) (orange); 200, 400 mg/5 ml (50, 75, 100 ml) (orange) (phenylalanine)
Augmentin ES-600 not recommended for adults
Pediatric: <3 months: not recommended; ≥3 months, <40 kg: 90 mg/kg/day in 2 divided doses x 10 days; ≥40 kg: not recommended
Oral susp: 42.9 mg/5 ml (50, 75, 100, 125, 150, 200 ml) (strawberry cream) (phenylalanine)
Augmentin XR 2 tabs q 12 hours x 10 days
Pediatric: <16 years: use other forms; ≥16 years: same as adult
Tab: 1000*mg ext-rel

▷ *cefaclor* (B)(G) 250-500 mg q 8 hours x 10 days; max 2 gm/day
Pediatric: <1 month: not recommended; 20-40 mg/kg bid or q 12 hours x 10 days;
max 1 gm/day; *see page 622 for dose by weight*
Tab: 500 mg; *Cap:* 250, 500 mg; *Susp:* 125 mg/5 ml (75, 150 ml) (strawberry); 187
mg/5 ml (50, 100 ml) (strawberry); 250 mg/5 ml (75, 150 ml) (strawberry); 375 mg/5
ml (50, 100 ml) (strawberry)
Pediatric: <16 years: ext-rel not recommended; ≥16 years: same as adult
Cefaclor Extended Release *Tab:* 375, 500 mg ext-rel
▷ *cefdinir* (B) 300 mg bid or 600 mg once daily x 10 days
Pediatric: <6 months: not recommended; 6 months-12 years: 14 mg/kg/day in a single
or 2 divided doses x 10 days; 12 years: same as adult; *see page 624 for dose by weight*
Omnicef *Cap:* 300 mg; *Oral susp:* 125 mg/5 ml (60, 100 ml) (strawberry)
▷ *cefixime* (B)(G) 400 mg once daily x 10 days
Pediatric: <6 months: not recommended; 6 months-12 years, <50 kg: 8 mg/kg/day in
1-2 divided doses x 10 days; *see page 625 for dose by weight;* >12 years, >50 kg: same
as adult
Suprax *Tab:* 400 mg; *Cap:* 400 mg; *Oral susp:* 100, 200, 500 mg/5 ml (50, 75, 100
ml) (strawberry)
▷ *cefpodoxime proxetil* 200 mg bid x 10 days
Pediatric: <2 months: not recommended; 2 months-12 years: 10 mg/kg/day (max 400
mg/dose) or 5 mg/kg/day bid (max 200 mg/dose) x 10 days; *see page 626 for dose by
weight*
Vantin *Tab:* 100, 200 mg; *Oral susp:* 50, 100 mg/5 ml (50, 75, 100 mg) (lemon
creme)
▷ *cefprozil* (B) 250-500 mg bid x 10 days
Pediatric: <6 months: not recommended; 6 months-12 years: *Mild:* 7.5 mg/kg bid x 10
days; *Moderate/Severe:* 15 mg/kg q 12 hours x 10 days; *see page 627 for dose by weight;*
>12 years: same as adult
Cefzil *Tab:* 250, 500 mg; *Oral susp:* 125, 250 mg/5 ml (50, 75, 100 ml) (bubble
gum) (phenylalanine)
▷ *ceftibuten* (B) 400 mg once daily x 10 days
Pediatric: <12 years: 9 mg/kg once daily x 10 days; max 400 mg/day; *see page 628 for
dose by weight;* ≥12 years: 400 mg once daily x 10 days
Cedax *Cap:* 400 mg; Oral susp: 90 mg/5 ml (30, 60, 90, 120 ml); 180
Cedax *Cap:* 400 mg; *Oral susp:* 90 mg/5 ml (30, 60, 90, 120 ml); 180 mg/5 ml (30,
60, 120 ml) (cherry)
▷ *ciprofloxacin* (C) 500 mg bid x 10 days
Pediatric: <18 years: not recommended; ≥18 years: same as adult
Cipro (G) *Tab:* 250, 500, 750 mg; *Oral susp:* 250, 500 mg/5 ml (100 ml) (strawberry)
Cipro XR *Tab:* 500, 1000 mg ext-rel
ProQuin XR *Tab:* 500 mg ext-rel
Comment: ciprofloxacin is contraindicated <18 years-of-age, and during pregnancy and
lactation. Risk of tendonitis or tendon rupture.
▷ *clarithromycin* (C)(G) 500 mg bid or 1000 mg ext-rel once daily x 10 days
Pediatric: <6 months: not recommended; ≥6 months: 7.5 mg/kg bid x 10 days; *see
page 630 for dose by weight*
Biaxin *Tab:* 250, 500 mg
Biaxin Oral Suspension *Oral susp:* 125, 250 mg/5 ml (50, 100 ml) (fruit punch)
Biaxin XL *Tab:* 500 mg ext-rel
▷ *levofloxacin* (C) *Uncomplicated:* 500 mg once daily x 10-14 days; *Complicated:* 750 mg
once daily x 10-14 days
Pediatric: <18 years: not recommended; ≥18 years: same as adult

Levaquin *Tab:* 250, 500, 750 mg; *Oral soln:* 25 mg/ml (480 ml) (benzyl alcohol); *Inj conc:* 25 mg/ml for IV infusion after dilution (20, 30 ml single-use vial) (preservative-free); *Premix soln:* 5 mg/ml for IV infusion (50, 100, 150 ml) (preservative-free)

Comment: *levofloxacin* is contraindicated <18 years-of-age, and during pregnancy and lactation. Risk of tendonitis or tendon rupture.

▷ *loracarbef* (B) 400 mg bid x 10 days
  Pediatric: 15 mg/kg/day in 2 divided doses x 10 days; *see page 642 for dose by weight*
    Lorabid *Pulvule:* 200, 400 mg; *Oral susp:* 100 mg/5 ml (50, 100 ml);
    200 mg/5 ml (50, 75, 100 ml) (strawberry bubble gum)

▷ *moxifloxacin* (C)(G) 400 mg once daily x 10 days
  Pediatric: <18 years: not recommended; ≥18 years: same as adult
    Avelox *Tab:* 400 mg

Comment: *moxifloxacin* is contraindicated <18 years-of-age, and during pregnancy and lactation. Risk of tendonitis or tendon rupture.

▷ *trimethoprim+sulfamethoxazole* (TMP-SMX) (D)(G)
  Pediatric: <2 months: not recommended; ≥2 months: 40 mg/kg/day of
  sulfamethoxazole in 2 divided doses bid x 10 days; *see page 648 for dose by weight*
    Bactrim, Septra 2 tabs bid x 10 days
      Tab: trim 80 mg+*sulfa* 400 mg*
    Bactrim DS, Septra DS 1 tab bid x 10 days
      Tab: trim 160 mg+*sulfa* 800 mg*
    Bactrim Pediatric Suspension, Septra Pediatric Suspension
      Oral susp: trim 40 mg+*sulfa* 200 mg per 5 ml (100 ml) (cherry) (alcohol 0.3%)

SJÖGREN-LARSSON-SYNDROME (SLS)

Comment: Sjögren-Larsson-Syndrome is a chronic autoimmune disorder that causes the white blood cells to attack the moisture-producing glands. Sjögren's syndrome can occur in association with other autoimmune diseases, including systemic lupus erythematosus, rheumatoid arthritis, scleroderma, systemic sclerosis, cryoglobulinemia, or polyarteritis nodosa. The disease can affect the eyes, mouth, parotid gland, pancreas, gastrointestinal system, blood vessels, lungs, kidneys, skin, and nervous system. Erythrocyte sedimentation rate (ESR) is elevated in 80% of patients. Rheumatoid factor is present in 52% of primary cases and 98% of secondary-type cases. A mild normochromic normocytic anemia is present in 50% of patients, and leukopenia occurs in up to 42% of patients. Creatinine clearance is diminished in up to 50% of patients. Anti-nuclear antibody (ANA) is positive in 70% of patients. SS-A and SS-B are marker antibodies for Sjögren's syndrome—70% of patients are positive for SS-A and 40% are positive for SS-B.

CHOLINERGIC (MUSCARINIC) AGONIST COMBINATION

▷ *cevimeline* (C)(G) 30 mg tid
    Evoxac *Cap:* 30 mg
    Comment: *cevimeline* is contraindicated in acute iritis, narrow angle glaucoma, and uncontrolled asthma.

▷ *pilocarpine* (C)(G) 5 mg qid or 7.5 mg tid
    Salagen *Tab:* 5, 7.5 mg

ORAL ENZYME RINSE

▷ *xylitol+solazyme+selectobac* swish 5 ml for 30 seconds bid-tid
    Orazyme Dry Mouth Rinse *Oral soln:* 1.5, 16 oz

SKIN: CALLUSED

KERATOLYTICS

▶ *salicylic acid* (C)(OTC) apply lotion, cream or gel to affected area once daily-bid; apply patch to affected area and leave on x 48 hours with max 5 applications/14 days
  Pediatric: <12 years: not recommended; ≥12 years: same as adult
▶ *urea* (C)
  Pediatric: <12 years: not recommended; ≥12 years: same as adult
  Carmol 40 apply to affected area with applicator stick provided once daily-tid; smooth over until cream is absorbed; protect surrounding tissue; may cover with adhesive bandage or gauze secured with adhesive tape
  Crm/Gel: 40% (30 gm)
  Keratol 40 apply to affected area with applicator stick provided once daily-tid; smooth over until cream is absorbed; protect surrounding tissue; may cover with adhesive bandage or gauze secured with adhesive tape
  Crm: 40% (1, 3, 7 oz); *Gel:* 40% (15 ml); *Lotn:* 40% (8 oz)
  Comment: The moisturizing effect of **Carmol 40** and **Keratol 40** is enhanced by applying while the skin is still moist (after washing or bathing).

 SKIN INFECTION: BACTERIAL (CARBUNCLE, FOLLICULITIS, FURUNCLE)

Comment: Abscesses usually require surgical incision and drainage.

ANTIBACTERIAL SKIN CLEANSERS

▶ *hexachlorophene* (C) dispense 5 ml into wet hand, work up into lather; then apply to area to be cleansed; rinse thoroughly
  pHisoHex *Liq clnsr:* 5, 16 oz

TOPICAL ANTI-INFECTIVES

▶ *mupirocin* (B)(G) apply to lesions bid
  Pediatric: same as adult
  Bactroban *Oint:* 2% (22 gm); *Crm:* 2% (15, 30 gm)
  Centany *Oint:* 2% (15, 30 gm)
▶ *polymyxin b+neomycin* (C) oint apply once daily-tid
  Neosporin (OTC) *Oint:* 15 gm

ORAL ANTI-INFECTIVES

▶ *amoxicillin* (B)(G) 500-875 mg bid or 250-500 mg tid x 10 days
  Pediatric: <40 kg (88 lb): 20-40 mg/kg/day in 3 divided doses x 10 days or
  25-45 mg/kg/day in 2 divided doses x 10 days; *see page 616 for dose by weight*
  Amoxil *Cap:* 250, 500 mg; *Tab:* 875*mg; *Chew tab:* 125, 200, 250, 400 mg (cherry-banana-peppermint) (phenylalanine); *Oral susp:* 125, 250 mg/5 ml (80, 100, 150 ml) (strawberry); 200, 400 mg/5 ml (50, 75, 100 ml) (bubble gum); *Oral drops:* 50 mg/ml (30 ml) (bubble gum)
  Moxatag *Tab:* 775 mg ext-rel
  Trimox *Tab:* 125, 250 mg; *Cap:* 250, 500 mg; *Oral susp:* 125, 250 mg/5 ml (80, 100, 150 ml) (raspberry-strawberry)
▶ *azithromycin* (B)(G) 500 mg x 1 dose on day 1, then 250 mg once daily on days 2-5 or 500 mg once daily x 3 days or **Zmax** 2 gm in a single dose
  Pediatric: 12 mg/kg/day x 5 days; max 500 mg/day; *see page 621 for dose by weight*

    Zithromax *Tab:* 250, 500, 600 mg; *Oral susp:* 100 mg/5 ml (15 ml); 200 mg/5 ml (15, 22.5, 30 ml) (cherry); *Pkt:* 1 gm for reconstitution (cherry-banana)

    Zithromax Tri-pak *Tab:* 3 x 500 mg tabs/pck

    Zithromax Z-pak *Tab:* 6 x 250 mg tabs/pck

    Zmax *Oral susp:* 2 gm ext-rel for reconstitution (cherry-banana) (148 mg Na⁺)

▷ *cefaclor* (B)(G) 250-500 mg q 8 hours x 10 days; max 2 gm/day
Pediatric: <1 month: not recommended; 20-40 mg/kg bid <u>or</u> q 12 hours x 10 days; max 1 gm/day; *see page 622 for dose by weight*
    Tab: 500 mg; *Cap:* 250, 500 mg; *Susp:* 125 mg/5 ml (75, 150 ml) (strawberry); 187 mg/5 ml (50, 100 ml) (strawberry); 250 mg/5 ml (75, 150 ml) (strawberry); 375 mg/5 ml (50, 100 ml) (strawberry)

    Cefaclor Extended Release
        Pediatric: <16 years: ext-rel not recommended; ≥16 years: same as adult
        Tab: 375, 500 mg ext-rel

▷ *cefadroxil* (B) 1-2 gm in a single <u>or</u> 2 divided doses x 10 days
Pediatric: 15-30 mg/kg/day in 2 divided doses x 10 days; *see page 623 for dose by weight*
    Duricef *Cap:* 500 mg; *Tab:* 1 gm; *Oral susp:* 250 mg/5 ml (100 ml); 500 mg/5 ml (75, 100 ml) (orange-pineapple)

▷ *cefdinir* (B) 300 mg bid x 10 days
Pediatric: <6 months: not recommended; 6 months-12 years: 14 mg/kg/day in 1-2 divided doses x 10 days; *see page 624 for dose by weight*
    Omnicef *Cap:* 300 mg; *Oral susp:* 125 mg/5 ml (60, 100 ml) (strawberry)

▷ *cefditoren pivoxil* (B) 200 mg bid x 10 days
Pediatric: <12 years: not recommended; ≥12 years: same as adult
    Spectracef *Tab:* 200 mg

Comment: Contraindicated with milk protein allergy <u>or</u> carnitine deficiency.

▷ *cefpodoxime proxetil* (B) 400 mg bid x 7-14 days
Pediatric: <2 months: not recommended; 2 months-12 years: 10 mg/kg/day (max 400 mg/dose) <u>or</u> 5 mg/kg/day bid (max 200 mg/dose) x 7-14 days; *see page 626 for dose by weight*
    Vantin *Tab:* 100, 200 mg; *Oral susp:* 50, 100 mg/5 ml (50, 75, 100 mg) (lemon creme)

▷ *cefprozil* (B) 250-500 mg bid <u>or</u> 500 mg once daily x 10 days
Pediatric: 2-12 years: 7.5 mg/kg bid x 10 days; >12 years: same as adult; *see page 627 for dose by weight*
    Cefzil *Tab:* 250, 500 mg; *Oral susp:* 125, 250 mg/5 ml (50, 75, 100 ml) (bubble gum) (phenylalanine)

▷ *ceftriaxone* (B)(G) 1-2 gm IM once daily; max 4 gm/day
Pediatric: 50-75 mg/kg IM in 1-2 divided doses; max 2 gm/day
    Rocephin *Vial:* 250, 500 mg; 1, 2 gm

▷ *cephalexin* (B)(G) 500 mg bid x 10 days
Pediatric: 25-50 mg/kg/day in 4 divided doses x 10 days; *see page 629 for dose by weight*
    Keflex *Cap:* 250, 333, 500, 750 mg; *Oral susp:* 125, 250 mg/5 ml (100, 200 ml) (strawberry)

▷ *clarithromycin* (C)(G) 250-500 mg bid <u>or</u> 500-1000 mg ext-rel once daily x 7-14 days
Pediatric: <6 months: not recommended; ≥6 months: 7.5 mg/kg bid x 7-14 days; *see page 630 for dose by weight*
    Biaxin *Tab:* 250, 500 mg
    Biaxin Oral Suspension *Oral susp:* 125, 250 mg/5 ml (50, 100 ml) (fruit punch)
    Biaxin XL *Tab:* 500 mg ext-rel

▷ *dicloxacillin* (B) 500 mg qid x 10 days
Pediatric: 12.5-25 mg/kg/day in 4 divided doses x 10 days; *see page 632 for dose by weight*
    Dynapen *Cap:* 125, 250, 500 mg; *Oral susp:* 62.5 mg/5 ml (80, 100, 200 ml)

➤ *dirithromycin* (C)(G) 500 mg once daily x 5-7 days
  Pediatric: <12 years: not recommended; ≥12 years: same as adult
      Dynabac *Tab:* 250 mg
➤ *doxycycline* (D)(G) 100 mg bid x 9 days
  Pediatric: <8 years: not recommended; ≥8 years, <100 lb: 1 mg/lb in a single dose
  once daily x 9 days; *see page 633 for dose by weight;* >8 years, ≥100 lb: same as adult
      Acticlate *Tab:* 75, 150**mg
      Adoxa *Tab:* 50, 75, 100, 150 mg ent-coat
      Doryx *Tab:* 50, 75, 100, 150, 200 mg del-rel
      Doxteric *Tab:* 50 mg del-rel
      Monodox *Cap:* 50, 75, 100 mg
      Oracea *Cap:* 40 mg del-rel
      Vibramycin *Tab:* 100 mg; *Cap:* 50, 100 mg; *Syr:* 50 mg/5 ml (raspberry-apple)
      (sulfites); *Oral susp:* 25 mg/5 ml (raspberry)
      Vibra-Tab *Tab:* 100 mg film-coat
Comment: *doxycycline* is contraindicated <8 years-of-age, in pregnancy, and
lactation (discolors developing tooth enamel). A side effect may be photosensitivity
(photophobia). Do not take with antacids, calcium supplements, milk or other dairy, or
within 2 hours of taking another drug.
➤ *erythromycin base* (B)(G) 250-500 mg tid x 10 days
  Pediatric: 30-50 mg/kg/day in 2-4 divided doses x 10 days
      Ery-Tab *Tab:* 250, 333, 500 mg ent-coat
      PCE *Tab:* 333, 500 mg
Comment: *erythromycin* may increase INR with concomitant *warfarin*, as well as
increase serum level of *digoxin, benzodiazepines,* and *statins.*
➤ *erythromycin estolate* (B)(G) 250-500 mg q 6 hours x 10 days
  Pediatric: 20-50 mg/kg q 6 hours x 10 days; *see page 634 for dose by weight*
      Ilosone *Pulvule:* 250 mg; *Tab:* 500 mg; *Liq:* 125, 250 mg/5 ml (100 ml)
Comment: *erythromycin* may increase INR with concomitant *warfarin*, as well as
increase serum level of *digoxin, benzodiazepines,* and *statins.*
➤ *erythromycin ethylsuccinate* (B)(G) 400 mg qid x 10 days
  Pediatric: 30-50 mg/kg/day in 4 divided doses x 10 days; may double dose with severe
  infection; max 100 mg/kg/day; *see page 635 for dose by weight*
      EryPed *Oral susp:* 200 mg/5 ml (100, 200 ml) (fruit); 400 mg/5 ml (60, 100, 200
      ml) (banana); *Oral drops:* 200, 400 mg/5 ml (50 ml) (fruit); *Chew tab:* 200 mg
      wafer (fruit)
      E.E.S. *Oral susp:* 200, 400 mg/5 ml (100 ml) (fruit)
      E.E.S. Granules *Oral susp:* 200 mg/5 ml (100, 200 ml) (cherry)
      E.E.S. 400 Tablets *Tab:* 400 mg
Comment: *erythromycin* may increase INR with concomitant *warfarin*, as well as
increase serum level of *digoxin, benzodiazepines,* and *statins.*
➤ *gemifloxacin* (C)(G) 320 mg once daily x 5-7 days
  Pediatric: <18 years: not recommended; ≥18 years: same as adult
      Factive *Tab:* 320*mg
Comment: *gemifloxacin* is contraindicated <18 years-of-age, and during pregnancy and
lactation. Risk of tendonitis or tendon rupture.
➤ *levofloxacin* (C) *Uncomplicated:* 500 mg once daily x 7-10 days; *Complicated:* 750 mg
  once daily x 7-10 days
  Pediatric: <18 years: not recommended; ≥18 years: same as adult
      Levaquin *Tab:* 250, 500, 750 mg; *Oral soln:* 25 mg/ml (480 ml) (benzyl alcohol);
      Inj conc: 25 mg/ml for IV infusion after dilution (20, 30 ml single-use vial) (pre-
      servative-free); *Premix soln:* 5 mg/ml for IV infusion (50, 100, 150 ml) (preserva-
      tive-free)

Comment: *levofloxacin* is contraindicated <18 years-of-age, and during pregnancy and lactation. Risk of tendonitis or tendon rupture.

▷ *linezolid* (C)(G) 400-600 mg q 12 hours x 10-14 days
   Pediatric: <5 years: 10 mg/kg q 8 hours x 10-14 days; 5-11 years: 10 mg/kg q 12 hours x 10-14 days; >11 years: same as adult
      Zyvox *Tab:* 400, 600 mg; *Oral susp:* 100 mg/5 ml (150 ml) (orange) (phenylalanine)
   Comment: *linezolid* is indicated to treat susceptible vancomycin-resistant *E. faecium* infections.

▷ *loracarbef* (B) 200 mg bid x 7 days
   Pediatric: 15 mg/kg/day in 2 divided doses x 7 days; *see page* 642 *for dose by weight*
      Lorabid *Pulvule:* 200, 400 mg; *Oral susp:* 100 mg/5 ml (50, 100 ml); 200 mg/5 ml (50, 75, 100 ml) (strawberry bubble gum)

▷ *minocycline* (D)(G) 200 mg on first day; then 100 mg q 12 hours x 9 more days
   Pediatric: <8 years: not recommended; ≥8 years, <100 lb: 2 mg/lb on first day in 2 divided doses, followed by 1 mg/lb q 12 hours x 9 more days; ≥8 years, ≥100 lb: same as adult
      Dynacin *Cap:* 50, 100 mg
      Minocin *Cap:* 50, 75, 100 mg; *Oral susp:* 50 mg/5 ml (60 ml) (custard) (sulfites, alcohol 5%)

Comment: *minocycline* is contraindicated <8 years-of-age, in pregnancy, and lactation (discolors developing tooth enamel). A side effect may be photosensitivity (photophobia). Do not give with antacids, calcium supplements, milk or other dairy, or within two hours of taking another drug.

▷ *moxifloxacin* (C)(G) 400 mg once daily x 10 days
   Pediatric: <18 years: not recommended; ≥18 years: same as adult
      Avelox *Tab:* 400 mg

Comment: *moxifloxacin* is contraindicated <18 years-of-age, and during pregnancy and lactation. Risk of tendonitis or tendon rupture.

▷ *ofloxacin* (C)(G) 400 mg bid x 10 days
   Pediatric: <18 years: not recommended; ≥18 years: same as adult
      Floxin *Tab:* 200, 300, 400 mg

Comment: *ofloxacin* is contraindicated <18 years-of-age, and during pregnancy and lactation. Risk of tendonitis or tendon rupture.

▷ *tetracycline* (D)(G) 500 mg qid x 10 days
   Pediatric: <8 years: not recommended; ≥8 years, <100 lb: 25-50 mg/kg/day in 4 divided doses x 10 days; ≥8 years, ≥100 lb: same as adult; *see page* 646 *for dose by weight*
      Achromycin V *Cap:* 250, 500 mg
      Sumycin *Tab:* 250, 500 mg; *Cap:* 250, 500 mg; *Oral susp:* 125 mg/5 ml (100, 200 ml) (fruit) (sulfites)

⬤ SLEEP APNEA: OBSTRUCTIVE (HYPOPNEA SYNDROME)

ANTI-NARCOLEPTIC AGENTS

▷ *armodafinil* (C)(IV)(G) *OSAHS:* 150-250 mg once daily in the AM; *SWSD:* 150 mg 1 hour before starting shift; reduce dose with severe hepatic impairment
   Pediatric: <17 years: not recommended; ≥17 years: same as adult
      Nuvigil *Tab:* 50, 150, 200, 250 mg

▷ *modafinil* (C)(IV) 100-200 mg q AM; max 400 mg/day
   Pediatric: <16 years: not recommended; ≥16 years: same as adult
      Provigil *Tab:* 100, 200*mg

Comment: *modafinil* promotes wakefulness in patients with excessive sleepiness due to obstructive sleep apnea/hypopnea syndrome.

SLEEPINESS: EXCESSIVE SHIFT WORK SLEEP DISORDER (SWSD)

ANTI-NARCOLEPTIC AGENT

▷ *armodafinil* (C)(IV)(G) *OSAHS:* 150-250 mg once daily in the AM; *SWSD:* 150 mg 1 hour before starting shift; reduce dose with severe hepatic impairment
  Pediatric: <17 years: not recommended; ≥17 years: same as adult
    Nuvigil *Tab:* 50, 150, 200, 250 mg
▷ *modafinil* (C)(IV) 100-200 mg q AM; max 400 mg/day
  Pediatric: <16 years: not recommended; ≥16 years: same as adult
    Provigil *Tab:* 100, 200*mg

Comment: Provigil promotes wakefulness in patients with narcolepsy, shift work sleep disorder, and excessive sleepiness due to obstructive sleep apnea/hypopnea syndrome.

 SMALLPOX (*VARIOLA MAJOR*)

PROPHYLAXIS

▷ *vaccina virus* **vaccine** *(dried, calf lymph type)* (C)
  Pediatric: <12 months: not recommended; 12 months-18 years, non-emergency: not recommended
    DRYvax
      Kit: vial dried smallpox vaccine (1), 0.25 ml diluent in syringe (1), vented needle (1), 100 individually wrapped bifurcated needles (5 needles/strip, 20 strips) (polymyxin b sulfate+dihydrostreptomycin+sulfate, chlortetracycline HCL+neomycin sulfate+glycerin+phenol)

Comment: DRYvax is a dried live vaccine with approximately 100 million *Infectious vaccina* viruses (pock-forming units [pfu] per ml). Contact with immunosuppressed individuals should be avoided until the scab has separated from the skin (2 to 3 weeks) and/or a protective occlusive dressing covers the inoculation site. Scarification only. Do not inject IV, IM, or SC. Revaccination is recommended every 10 years.

 SPINAL MUSCULAR ATROPHY (SMA)

Comment: Spinal muscular atrophy (SMA) is a group of inherited disorders characterized by motor neuron loss in the spinal cord and lower brainstem, muscle weakness, and atrophy. Survival motor neuron (SMN) protein is essential for the maintenance of motor neurons. Because of a defect in, or loss of, the SMN1 gene, patients with SMA do not produce enough SMN protein. It is the most common genetic cause of death in infants, but can affect people at any age. **Spinraza (*nusinersen*)** is the first FDA-approved drug to treat SMA.

SURVIVAL MOTOR NEURON-2 (SMN2)-DIRECTED ANTISENSE OLIGONUCLEOTIDE

▷ *nusinersen* 12 mg per intrathecal administration; initially four loading doses: the first 3 loading doses administered at 14-day intervals; the 4th loading dose administered 30 days after the 3rd loading dose; the maintenance dose is administered every 4 months after the 4th loading dose; prior to administration, 5 ml cerebral spinal fluid (CSF) should be removed; the intrathecal bolus injection should be administered over 1-3 minutes using a spinal anesthetic needle.
  Pediatric: same as adult
    Spinraza *Vial:* 12 mg/5 ml (2.4 mg/ml) single-dose, solution for intrathecal administration (preservative-free)

Comment: At baseline and prior to each dose, obtain a platelet count and coagulation laboratory testing (there is increased risk for thrombocytopenia and coagulation abnormalities) and quantitative spot urine protein testing (to monitor for renal toxicity). Store **Spinraza** in a refrigerator between 2°C to 8°C (36°F to 46°F) in the original carton to protect from light. Do not freeze. Prior to administration, unopened vials of **Spinraza** can be removed from and returned to the refrigerator, if necessary. If removed from the original carton, the total combined time out of refrigeration should not exceed 30 hours at a temperature that does not exceed 25°C (77°F). **Spinraza** has no labeled contraindications. **Spinraza** has not been studied in pregnant or lactating females, or in patients with renal or hepatic impairment.

 SPRAIN

Comment: RICE: Rest; Ice; Compression; Elevation.

Injectable Acetaminophen *see Pain page* 344
NSAIDs *see page* 562
Opioid Analgesics *see Pain page* 345
Topical and Transdermal NSAIDs *see Pain page* 344
Parenteral Corticosteroids *see page* 570
Oral Corticosteroids *see page* 569
Topical Analgesic & Anesthetic Agents *see page* 560

 STATUS ASTHMATICUS

Inhaled Beta-2 Agonists (Bronchodilators) *see Asthma page* 30
Oral Beta-2 Agonists (Bronchodilators) *see Asthma page* 37
Inhaled Anticholinergics *see Asthma page* 32
Inhaled Anticholinergic+Beta-2 Agonist Combination *see Asthma page* 30
Methylxanthines *see Asthma page* 30
Parenteral Corticosteroids *see page* 570
Oral Corticosteroids *see page* 569

EPINEPHRINE

➢ *epinephrine* (C)(G) 0.3-0.5 mg (0.3-0.5 ml of a 1:1000 soln) SC q 20-30 minutes as needed up to 3 doses
Pediatric: <2 years: 0.05-0.1 ml; 2-6 years: 0.1 ml; 6-12 years: 0.2 ml; All: q 20-30 minutes as needed up to 3 doses; >12 years: same as adult

ANAPHYLAXIS EMERGENCY TREATMENT KITS

➢ *epinephrine* (C) 0.3 ml IM <u>or</u> SC in thigh; may repeat if needed
Pediatric: 0.01 mg/kg SC <u>or</u> IM in thigh; may repeat if needed; <15 kg: not recommended; 15-30 kg: 0.15 mg; >30 kg: same as adult
  AdrenaClick *Auto-injector:* 0.15, 0.3 mg (1 mg/ml; 2/carton) (sulfites)
  Auvi-Q *Auto-injector:* 0.15, 0.3 mg (1 mg/ml; 2/carton w. 1 non active training device) (sulfites)
  EpiPen *Autoinjector 0.3 mg* (epi 1:1000, 0.3 ml (2/carton) (sulfites)
  EpiPen Jr *Autoinjector 0.15 mg* (epi 1:2000, 0.3 ml (2/carton) (sulfites)
  Twinject *Autoinjector: 0.15, 0.3 mg* (epi 1:1000, 2/carton) (sulfites)
➢ *epinephrine+chlorpheniramine* (C) epinephrine 0.3 ml SC <u>or</u> IM <u>plus</u> 4 tabs *chlorpheniramine* by mouth

Pediatric: infants-2 years: 0.05-0.1 ml SC or IM; 2-6 years: 0.15 ml SC or IM plus 1 tab *chlor;* 6-12 years: 0.2 ml SC or IM plus 2 tabs *chlor;* >12 years: same as adult

    Ana-Kit: 0.3 ml syringes of *epi* 1:1000 (2/carton) for self-injection plus *chlor* 2 mg chewable tabs x 4

STATUS EPILEPTICUS

Anticonvulsant Drugs *see page 584*

▷ *diazepam* injectable (D)(IV) initially 5-10 mg IV in large vein; may repeat q 10-15 minutes; max 30 mg; may repeat in 2-4 hours if needed; do not dilute; may give IM if IV not accessible

Pediatric: 1 month-5 years: 0.2-0.5 mg IV q 2-5 minutes; max 5 mg; >5 years: 1 mg IV q 2-5 minutes; max 10 mg; may repeat in 2-4 hours if needed

    Diastat *Rectal gel delivery system:* 2.5 mg

    Diastat AcuDial *Rectal gel delivery system:* 10, 20 mg

    Valium Injectable *Vial:* 5 mg/ml (10 ml); *Amp:* 5 mg/ml (2 ml); *Prefilled syringe:* 5 mg/ml (5 ml)

    Valium Intensol Oral Solution *Conc oral soln:* 5 mg/ml (30 ml w. dropper) (alcohol 19%)

    Valium Oral Solution *Oral soln:* 5 mg/5 ml (500 ml) (wintergreen-spice)

▷ *lorazepam* injectable (D)(IV) 4 mg IV over 2 minutes (dilute first); may repeat in 10-15 minutes; may give IM if needed (undiluted)

Pediatric: <18 years: not recommended; ≥18 years: same as adult

    Ativan Injectable *Vial:* 2 mg/ml (1, 10 ml); *Tubex:* 2 mg/ml (0.5 ml); *Cartridge:* 2, 4 mg/ml (1 ml)

▷ *phenytoin (injectable)* (D)(G) 10-15 mg/kg IV, not to exceed 50 mg/minute; follow with 100 mg orally or IV q 6-8 hours; do not dilute in IV fluid

Pediatric: 15-20 mg/kg IV, not to exceed 1-2 mg/kg/minute

    Dilantin *Vial:* 50 mg/ml (2, 5 ml); *Amp:* 50 mg/ml (2 ml)

Comment: Monitor *phenytoin* serum levels. Therapeutic serum level: 10-20 gm/ml. Side effects include gingival hyperplasia.

STYE (HORDEOLUM)

OPHTHALMIC ANTI-INFECTIVES

▷ *erythromycin* ophthalmic ointment (B) 1 cm up to 6 x/day

Pediatric: same as adult

    Ilotycin Ophthalmic Ointment *Ophth oint:* 5 mg/gm (1/8 oz)

▷ *erythromycin* ophthalmic solution (B) initially 1-2 drops q 1-2 hours; may then increase dose interval

Pediatric: same as adult

    Isopto Cetamide Ophthalmic Solution *Ophth soln:* 15% (15 ml)

▷ *gentamicin* ophthalmic ointment (C) 1 cm bid-tid

Pediatric: same as adult

    Garamycin Ophthalmic Ointment *Ophth oint:* 3 mg/gm (3.5 gm)

    Genoptic Ophthalmic Ointment *Ophth oint:* 3 mg/gm (3.5 gm)

    Gentacidin Ophthalmic Ointment *Ophth oint:* 3 mg/gm (3.5 gm)

▷ *polymyxin b+bacitracin* ophthalmic ointment (C) apply 1/2 inch q 3-4 hours

Pediatric: same as adult

    Polysporin *Ophth oint:* *poly* b 10,000 U+*bac* 500 units per gm (3.75 gm)

▷ *polymyxin b+bacitracin+neomycin* ophthalmic ointment (C)(G) apply 1/2 inch q 3-4 hours

Pediatric: same as adult
> **Neosporin Ophthalmic Ointment** *Ophth oint: poly* b 10,000 U+*bac* 400
> U+*neo* 3.5 mg/gm (3.75 gm)

▷ *polymyxin b+neomycin+gramicidin* ophthalmic solution (C) 1-2 drops 2-3 times q
1 hour; then 1-2 drops bid-qid x 7-10 days
Pediatric: same as adult
> **Neosporin Ophthalmic Solution**
> *Ophth soln: poly* b 10,000 U+*neo* 1.75 mg/gm 0.025 mg/ml (10 ml)

▷ *sodium sulfacetamide* ophthalmic solution and ointment (C)
> **Bleph-10 Ophthalmic Solution** 2 drops q 4 hour x 7-14 days
> *Pediatric:* <2 years: not recommended; ≥2 years: 1-2 drops q 2-3 hours during the
> day
> *Ophth soln:* 10% (2.5, 5, 15 ml; benzalkonium chloride)
> **Bleph-10 Ophthalmic Ointment** apply 1/2 inch qid and HS
> *Pediatric:* <2 years: not recommended; ≥2 years: apply 1/4-1/3 inch qid and HS
> *Ophth oint:* 10% (3.5 gm) (phenylmercuric acetate)

SUNBURN

▷ *prednisone* (C)(G) 10 mg qid x 4-6 days if severe and extensive
▷ *silver sulfadiazine* (C)(G) apply topically to burn once daily-bid
Pediatric: <12 years: not recommended; ≥12 years: same as adult
> **Silvadene** *Crm:* 1% (20, 50, 85, 400, 1000 gm jar; 20 gm tube)

Comment: *silver sulfadiazine* is contradicted in sulfa allergy, late pregnancy, within the
first 2 months after birth, premature infants.

SYPHILIS (*TREPONEMA PALLIDUM*)

Comment: The following treatment regimens for *T. pallidum* are published in the **2015
CDC Sexually Transmitted Diseases Treatment Guidelines.** Treat all sexual contacts.
Consider testing for other STDs. *Penicillin g*, administered parenterally, is the preferred
drug for treating all stages of syphilis. The preparation used (i.e., benzathine, aqueous
procaine, or aqueous crystalline), the dosage, and the length of treatment depend on the
stage and clinical manifestations of the disease. Combinations of *benzathine penicillin,
procaine penicillin,* and oral *penicillin* preparations are not appropriate (e.g., **Bicillin
C-R**). All women should be screened serologically for syphilis early in pregnancy. There
are no proven alternatives to *penicillin* for the treatment of syphilis during pregnancy.
Pregnant patients who are allergic to penicillin should be desensitized and treated
with *penicillin*. Sexual transmission of *T. pallidum* is thought to occur only when
mucocutaneous syphilis at any stage should be evaluated clinically and serologically and
treated with a recommended regimen according to CDC guidelines.

PRIMARY, SECONDARY, AND EARLY LATENT (<1 YEAR) SYPHILIS
Regimen 1
▷ *penicillin g (benzathine)* 2.4 million units IM in a single dose

LATE LATENT, LATENT SYPHILIS OF UNKNOWN DURATION, AND TERTIARY SYPHILIS
Regimen 1
▷ *penicillin g (benzathine)* 7.2 million units total administered in 3 divided doses of 2.4
million units each IM at 1 week intervals

REGIMEN: ADULT, NEUROSYPHILIS
Regimen 1
▷ *aqueous crystalline penicillin g* 18-24 million units per day, administered as 3-4 million units IV every 4 hours <u>or</u> continuous IV infusion, for 10-14 days

ALTERNATIVE REGIMEN: ADULT, NEUROSYPHILIS
Regimen 1
▷ *penicillin g (procaine)* 2.4 million units IM once daily x 10-14 days <u>plus</u> *probenecid* 500 mg qid x 10-14 days

PRIMARY AND SECONDARY SYPHILIS IN HIV-INFECTED PERSONS
Regimen 1
▷ *penicillin g (benzathine)* 2.4 million units IM in a single dose

LATENT SYPHILIS AMONG HIV-INFECTED PERSONS
Comment: Treatment is the same as for HIV-negative persons.

CONGENITAL SYPHILIS
Regimen 1
▷ *aqueous crystalline penicillin g* 100,000-150,000 units/kg/day, administered as 50,000 units IV every 12 hours during the first 7 days of life and every 8 hours thereafter for a total of 10 days

ALTERNATE REGIMEN
Regimen 1
▷ *penicillin g (benzathine)* 50,000 units/kg IM in a single dose

Regimen 2
▷ *penicillin g (procaine)* 50,000 units/kg/dose IM, administered in a single daily dose x 10 days

OLDER INFANTS AND CHILDREN
Regimen 1
▷ *aqueous crystalline penicillin g* 200,000-300,000 units/kg/day, administered as 50,000 units IV every 12 hours during the first 7 days of life and every 4-6 hours thereafter for a total of 10 days

DRUG BRANDS AND DOSE FORMS
▷ *aqueous crystalline penicillin g* (B)(G)
▷ *penicillin g (benzathine)* (B)(G)
  Bicillin L-A *Cartridge-needle unit:* 600,000 million units (1 ml); 1.2 million units (2 ml); 2.4 million units (4 ml)
▷ *penicillin g (procaine)* (B)(G)
  Bicillin C-R Cartridge-needle unit: 600,000 units (1 ml); 1.2 million units; (2 ml); 2.4 million units (4 ml)
▷ *probenecid* (B)(G)
  Benemid *Tab:* 500*mg; *Cap:* 500 mg

SYSTEMIC LUPUS ERYTHEMATOSIS (SLE)

NSAIDs *see page* 562
Oral Corticosteroids *see page* 569

Comment: All SLE patients should routinely be given *hydroxychloroquine* HCQ and supplemental vitamin D as low levels of vitamin D are associated with higher rates of ESRD; supplemental vitamin D reduces urine protein (the best predictor of future renal failure). Vitamin D insufficiency and deficiency are more common in patients with SLE than in the general population. Vitamin D supplementation may decrease disease activity and improve fatigue. In addition, supplementation may improve endothelial function, which may reduce cardiovascular disease. A disease-modifying anti-rheumatic drug (DMARD) should be added when a patient's prednisone dose cannot be tapered and also when hemolysis is present and hemoglobin is abnormally low in the setting of mild-to-moderate hematological involvement. Other DMARDs, such as *methotrexate (MTX)*, *azathioprine*, *mycophenolate mofetil* (MMF), *cyclosporine* (CYC), and other calcineurin-inhibitors should be considered in cases of arthritis, cutaneous disease, serositis, vasculitis, or cytopaenias if HCQ is insufficient. For refractory cases, *belimumab* (Benlysta) or *rituximab* (Rituxan), may be considered. The recommended dose of *rituximab*, if required, is either 750 mg/m² (to a maximum of 1 gm per day) at day 1 and day 15, or 375 mg/m² once a week for 4 doses. In patients with SLE without major organ manifestations, glucocorticoids and antimalarial agents may be beneficial. NSAIDs may be used for short periods in patients at low risk for complications from these drugs. Consider immunosuppressive agents (e.g., *azathioprine*, MMF, MTX) in refractory cases or when steroid doses cannot be reduced to levels for long-term use.

REFERENCES

Gordon, C., Amissah-Arthur, M.-B., Gayed, M., Brown, S., Bruce, I. N., . . . D'Cruz, D. (2017). The British Society for Rheumatology guideline for the management of systemic lupus erythematosus in adults. *Rheumatology*. doi:10.1093/rheumatology/kex286

Groot, N., de Graeff, N., Avcin, T., Bader-Meunier, B., Brogan, P., Dolezalova, P., . . . Beresford, M. W. (2017). European evidence-based recommendations for diagnosis and treatment of childhood-onset systemic lupus erythematosus: the SHARE initiative. *Annals of the Rheumatic Diseases, 76*(11), 1788–1796. doi:10.1136/annrheumdis-2016-210960

Leach, MZ. (November 7, 2017). First UK guidelines for adults with lupus. *Rheumatology Network*. Retrieved November 13, 2017 http://www.rheumatologynetwork.com/article/first-uk-guidelines-adults-lupus

CD20 ANTIBODY

▷ *rituximab* (C) administer corticosteroid 30 minutes prior to each infusion; concomitant *methotrexate* therapy, administer a 1000 mg IV infusion at 0 and 2 weeks; then every 24 weeks or based on response, but not sooner than every 16 weeks.
   Pediatric: <6 years: not recommended; >6 years: same as adult
      Rituxan *Vial:* 10 mg/ml (10, 50 ml) (preservative-free)

B-LYMPHOCYTE STIMULATOR (BLyS)-SPECIFIC INHIBITOR

▷ *belimumab*
      SC administration: 200 mg SC once weekly. May be self-administered by the patient in the home setting.
Comment: *Benlysta* was initially approved as an intravenous formulation administered in a hospital or clinic setting as a weight-dosed IV infusion every four weeks. Patients can now self-administer **Benlysta** as a once weekly SC injection after being trained by a health care provider.

IV infusion: 10 mg/kg at 2-week intervals for the first 3 doses and at 4-week intervals thereafter; reconstitute, dilute, and administer as an intravenous infusion over a period of 1 hour. Consider administering premedication for prophylaxis against infusion reactions and hypersensitivity reactions. Must be administered in a hospital <u>or</u> clinic setting by a qualified healthcare provider
Pediatric: <18 years: not established; ≥18 years: same as adult

> **Benlysta Prefilled syringe:** 200 mg/ml (1 ml) single-dose (4/carton);
> *Autoinjector:* 200 mg (1 ml) single-dose (4/carton); *Vial:* 120 mg/5 ml, 400
> mg/ 20 ml, single-dose, pwdr for reconstitution and IV infusion (4/carton)

Comment: **Benlysta** is indicated for the treatment of patients >18 years-of-age with active, autoantibody-positive, systemic lupus erythematosus who are receiving standard therapy. Common adverse reactions include nausea, diarrhea, pyrexia, nasopharyngitis, bronchitis, insomnia, pain in extremity, depression, migraine, and pharyngitis. The efficacy of **Benlysta** has not been evaluated in patients with severe active lupus nephritis <u>or</u> severe active central nervous system lupus. **Benlysta** has not been studied in combination with other biologics <u>or</u> intravenous *cyclophosphamide.* Therefore, use of Benlysta is not recommended in these situations. Limited data on use of **Benlysta** in pregnancy women, from observational studies, published case reports, and post-marketing surveillance, is insufficient to determine whether there is a drug-associated risk for major birth defects <u>or</u> miscarriage. Monoclonal antibodies, such as *belimumab,* are actively transported across the placenta during the third trimester of pregnancy and may affect immune response in the in utero-exposed infant. Monoclonal antibodies are increasingly transported across the placenta as pregnancy progresses, with the largest amount transferred during the third trimester. No information is available on the presence of *belimumab* in human milk <u>or</u> the effects of the drug on the breastfed infant. As there are risks to the mother and fetus associated with SLE, risks and benefits should be considered prior to administering live <u>or</u> live-attenuated vaccines to infants exposed to **Benlasta** in utero. Monitor the infant of a treated mother for B-cell reduction and other immune dysfunction. There is a pregnancy exposure registry that monitors pregnancy outcomes in females exposed to **Benlysta** during pregnancy. Healthcare professionals are encouraged to register patients by calling 1-877-681-6296. To report suspected adverse reactions, contact GlaxoSmithKline at 1-877-423-6597 <u>or</u> FDA at 1-800-FDA-1088 <u>or</u> www.fda. gov/medwatch

DISEASE MODIFYING ANTI-RHEUMATIC DRUGS (DMARDs)

Comment: DMARDs include *penicillamine*, gold salts (*auranofin, aurothioglucose*), immunosuppressants, and *hydroxychloroquine*. The DMARDs reduce ESR, reduce RF, and favorably affect SLE symptoms. Immunosuppressants may require 6 weeks to affect benefits and 6 months for full improvement.

➢ *auranofin (gold salt)* **(C)** 3 mg bid <u>or</u> 6 mg once daily; if inadequate response after 6 months, increase to 3 mg tid
Pediatric: <12 years: not recommended; ≥12 years: same as adult
Ridaura *Vial:* 100 mg/20 ml

➢ *azathioprine* **(D)** 1 mg/kg/day in a single <u>or</u> divided doses; may increase by 0.5 mg/ kg/day q 4 weeks; max 2.5 mg/kg/day; minimum trial to ascertain effectiveness is 12 weeks
Pediatric: <12 years: not recommended; ≥12 years: same as adult
Azasan *Tab* 75*, 100*mg
Imuran *Tab* 50*mg

➢ *cyclosporine (immunosuppressant)* **(C)** 1.25 mg/kg bid; may increase after 4 weeks by 0.5 mg/kg/day; then adjust at 2 week intervals; max 4 mg/kg/day; administer with meals

Pediatric: <12 years: not recommended; ≥12 years: same as adult
    Neoral *Cap:* 25, 100 mg (alcohol)
    Neoral Oral Solution *Oral soln:* 100 mg/ml (50 ml) may dilute in room temperature apple juice <u>or</u> orange juice (alcohol)

Comment: **Neoral** is indicated for RA unresponsive to **methotrexate** (MTX).

▷ *leflunomide* **(X)(G)** initially 100 mg once daily x 3 days; maintenance dose 20 mg once daily; max 20 mg daily
Pediatric: <18 years: not recommended; ≥18 years: same as adult
    Arava *Tab:* 10, 20, 100 mg

Comment: **Arava** is contraindicated with breastfeeding.

▷ *methotrexate* **(X)** 7.5 mg x 1 dose per week <u>or</u> 2.5 mg x 3 at 12 hour intervals once a week; max 20 mg/week; therapeutic response begins in 3-6 weeks; administer *methotrexate* injection SC only into the abdomen <u>or</u> thigh
Pediatric: <2 years: not recommended; ≥2 years: 10 mg/m^2 once weekly; max 20 mg/m^2
    Rasuvo *Autoinjector:* 7.5 mg/0.15 ml, 10 mg/0.20 ml, 12.5 mg/0.25 ml, 15 mg/0.30 ml, 17.5 mg/0.35 ml, 20 mg/0.40 ml, 22.5 mg/0.45 ml, 25 mg/0.50 ml, 27.5 mg/0.55 ml, 30 mg/0.60 ml (solution concentration for SC injection is 50 mg/ml)
    Rheumatrex *Tab:* 2.5*mg (5, 7.5, 10, 12.5, 15 mg/week, 4/card unit-of-use dose pack)
    Trexall *Tab:* 5*, 7.5*, 10*, 15*mg (5, 7.5, 10, 12.5, 15 mg/week, 4/card unit-of-use dose pack)

Comment: *methotrexate* (MTX) is contraindicated with immunodeficiency, blood dyscrasias, alcoholism, and chronic liver disease.

▷ *penicillamine* **(D)** 125-250 mg once daily initially; may increase by 125-250 mg/day q 1-3 months; max 1.5 mg/day
Pediatric: <12 years: not recommended; ≥12 years: same as adult
    Cuprimine *Cap:* 125, 250 mg
    Depen *Tab:* 250 mg

▷ *sulfasalazine* **(C; D in 2nd, 3rd)(G)** initially 0.5 gm once daily bid; gradually increase every 4 days; usual maintenance 2-3 gm/day in equally divided doses at regular intervals; max 4 gm/day
Pediatric: <6 years: not recommended; 6-16 years: initially 1/4 to 1/3 of maintenance dose; increase weekly; maintenance 30-50 mg/kg/day in 2 divided doses at regular intervals; max 2 gm/day
    Azulfidine *Tab:* 500 mg
    Azulfidine EN *Tab:* 500 mg ent-coat

ANTIMALARIALS

▷ *atovaquone* **(C)(G)** take as a single dose with food <u>or</u> a milky drink at the same time each day; repeat dose if vomited within 1 hour; *Prophylaxis:* 1,500 mg once daily; *Treatment:* 750 mg bid x 21 days
Pediatric: <13 years: not established; ≥13 years: same as adult
    Mepron *Susp:* 750 mg/5 ml

▷ *atovaquone+proguanil* **(C)(G)** >40 kg: take as a single dose with food <u>or</u> a milky drink at the same time each day; repeat dose if vomited within 1 hour; *Prophylaxis:* 1 tab daily starting 1-2 days before entering endemic area, during stay, and for 7 days after return; *Treatment (acute, uncomplicated):* 4 tabs daily x 3 days
Pediatric: <5 kg: not recommended; 5-40 kg:
Prophylaxis: daily dose starting 1-2 days before entering endemic area, during stay, and for 7 days after return; 5-20 kg: 1 ped tab; 21-30 kg: 2 ped tabs; 31-40 kg: 3 ped tabs; ≥40 kg: same as adult; *Treatment (acute, uncomplicated):* daily dose x 3 days; 5-8 kg: 2 ped tabs; 9-10 kg: 3 ped tabs; 11-20 kg: 1 adult tab; 21-30 kg: 2 adult tabs; 31-40 kg: 3 adult tabs; >40 kg: same as adult

> Malarone *Tab: atov* 250 mg+*prog* 100 mg
> Malarone Pediatric *Tab: atov* 62.5 mg+*prog* 25 mg

Comment: *atovaquone* is antagonized by *tetracycline* and *metoclopramide*. Concomitant *rifampin* is not recommended (may elevate LFTs).

➤ *chloroquine* (C)(G) *Prophylaxis:* 500 mg once weekly (on the same day of each week); start 2 weeks prior to exposure, continue while in the endemic area, and continue 4 weeks after departure; *Treatment:* initially 1 gm; then 500 mg 6 hours, 24 hours, and 48 hours after initial dose or initially 200-250 mg IM; may repeat in 6 hours; max 1 gm in first 24 hours; continue to 1.875 gm in 3 days
Pediatric: Suppression: 8.35 mg/kg (max 500 mg) weekly (on the same day of each week); *Treatment:* initially 16.7 mg/kg (max 1 gm); then 8.35 mg/kg (max 500 mg) 6 hours, 24 hours, and 48 hours after initial dose, or initially 6.25 mg/kg IM; may repeat in 6 hours; max 12.5 mg/kg/day
Pediatric:
> Aralen *Tab:* 500 mg; *Amp:* 50 mg/ml (5 ml)

Comment: There are no adequate and well-controlled studies evaluating the safety and efficacy of *chloroquine* in pregnant women. Usage of *chloroquine* during pregnancy should be avoided except in the suppression or treatment of malaria when the benefit outweighs the potential risk to the fetus. Because of the potential for serious adverse reactions in nursing infants from chloroquine, a decision should be made whether to discontinue nursing or to discontinue the drug, taking into account the potential clinical benefit of the drug to the mother. Since this drug is known to concentrate in the liver, it should be used with caution in patients with hepatic disease or alcoholism or in conjunctionwith known hepatotoxic drugs.

➤ *hydroxychloroquine* (C)(G) 400-600 mg/day
Pediatric: <12 years: not recommended; ≥12 years: same as adult
> Plaquenil *Tab:* 200 mg

Comment: May require several weeks to achieve beneficial effects. If no improvement in 6 months, discontinue.

➤ *mefloquine* (C) *Prophylaxis:* 250 mg once weekly (on the same day of each week); start 1 week prior to exposure, continue while in the endemic area, and continue for 4 weeks after departure; *Treatment:* 1,250 mg as a single dose
Pediatric: <6 months: not recommended; *Prophylaxis:* ≥6 months: 3-5 mg/kg (max 250 mg) weekly (on the same day of each week); start 1 week prior to exposure, continue while in the endemic area, and continue for 4 weeks after departure; *Treatment:* ≥6 months: 25-50 mg/kg as a single dose; max 250 mg
> Lariam *Tab:* 250*mg

Comment: *mefloquine* is contraindicated with active or recent history of depression, generalized anxiety disorder, psychosis, schizophrenia or any other psychiatric disorder or history of convulsions.

➤ *quinine sulfate* (C)(G) 1 tab or cap every 8 hours x 7 days
Pediatric: <16 years: not recommended; ≥16 years: same as adult
> *Tab:* 260 mg; *Cap:* 260, 300, 325 mg
> Qualaquin *Cap:* 324 mg

Comment: *Qualaquin* is indicated in the treatment of uncomplicated *P. falciparum* malaria (including chloroquine-resistant strains).

 TAPEWORM (CESTODE)

ANTHELMINTICS

Comment: Oral bioavailability of anthelmintics is enhanced when administered with a fatty meal (estimated fat content 40 gm).

▷ *albendazole* **(C)(G)** take with a meal; may crush and mix with food; 400 mg bid x 7 days; may repeat in 3 weeks if needed
Pediatric: <2 years: 200 mg once daily x 3 days; may repeat in 3 weeks; ≥2-12 years: 400 mg once daily x 3 days; may repeat in 3 weeks; ≥12 years: same as adult
    Albenza *Tab:* 200 mg

Comment: *albendazole* is a broad-spectrum benzimidazole carbamate anthelmintic.

▷ *nitazoxanide* **(B)** take with a meal; may crush and mix with food; 500 mg q 12 hours x 3 days
Pediatric: <12 months: not recommended; ≥12 months: treat q 12 hours x 3 days; <11 years: [susp] 12-47 months: 5 ml; 4-11 years: 10 ml; ≥11 years: [tab/susp] 500 mg
    Alinia *Tab:* 500 mg; *Oral susp:* 100 mg/5 ml (60 ml)

▷ *praziquantel* **(B)(G)** take with a meal; may crush and mix with food; 5-10 mg/kg as a single dose
Pediatric: <4 years: not established; ≥4 years: same as adult
    Biltricide *Tab:* 600 mg film-coat (scored for half or quarter dose)

Comment: Therapeutically effective levels of **Biltricide** may not be achieved when administered concomitantly with strong P450 inducers, such as *rifampin.* Females should not breastfeed on the day of **Biltricide** treatment and during the subsequent 72 hours. Use caution with hepatosplenic patients who have moderate to severe liver impairment (Child-Pugh Class B and C).

 TARDIVE DYSKINESIA

Comment: Tardive dyskinesia is a treatable, albeit irreversible, neurological disorder characterized by repetitive involuntary movements, usually of the jaw, lips and tongue, such as grimacing, sticking out the tongue and smacking the lips. Some affected people also experience involuntary movement of the extremities or difficulty breathing. This condition is most often an adverse side effect associated with the older "typical" antipsychotic drugs. Risk is decreased with the newer "atypical" antipsychotic drugs. The first and only FDA-approved treatment for this disorder is *valbenazine* (**Ingrezza**), a vesicular monoamine transporter 2 (VMAT2) inhibitor.

REFERENCE
Davis, M. C., Miller, B. J., Kalsi, J. K., Birkner, T., & Mathis, M. V. (May 10, 2017). Efficient trial design—FDA approval of valbenazine for tardive dyskinesia. *The New England Journal of Medicine, 376*(26), 2503–2506.

VESICULAR MONOAMINE TRANSPORTER 2 (VMAT2) INHIBITOR

▷ *valbenazine* initially 40 mg once daily; after one week, increase to the recommended 80 mg once daily; take with or without food; recommended dose for patients with moderate or severe hepatic impairment is 40 mg once daily; consider dose reduction based on tolerability in known CYP2D6 poor metabolizers; concomitant use of strong CYP3A4 inducers is not recommended; avoid concomitant use of MAOIs
Pediatric: <18 years: not established; ≥18 years: same as adult
    Ingrezza *Cap:* 40 mg

Comment: Safety and effectiveness of **Ingrezza** have not been established in pediatric patients. No dose adjustment is required for elderly patients. The limited available data on **Ingrezza** use in pregnant women are insufficient to inform a drug-associated risk. There is no information regarding the presence of **Ingrezza** or its metabolites in human milk, the effects on the breastfed infant, or the effects on milk production. However, women are advised not to breastfeed during treatment and for 5 days after the final dose. To report suspected adverse reactions, contact Neurocrine Biosciences, Inc. at 877-641-3461 or FDA at 1-800-FDA-1088 or www.fda.gov/medwatch.

TEMPOROMANDIBULAR JOINT (TMJ) DISORDER

Injectable Acetaminophen *see* **Pain** *page* 344
NSAIDs *see page* 562
Opioid Analgesics *see* **Pain** *page* 345
Topical and Transdermal NSAIDs *see* **Pain** *page* 344
Parenteral Corticosteroids *see page* 570
Oral Corticosteroids *see page* 569
Topical Analgesic and Anesthetic Agents *see page* 560

SKELETAL MUSCLE RELAXANTS

➤ *baclofen* (C)(G) 5 mg tid; titrate up by 5 mg every 3 days to 20 mg tid; max 80 mg/day
   Pediatric: <12 years: not recommended; ≥12 years: same as adult
      Lioresal *Tab:* 10*, 20*mg
Comment: *baclofen* is indicated for muscle spasm pain and chronic spasticity associated with multiple sclerosis and spinal cord injury or disease. Potential for seizures or hallucinations on abrupt withdrawal.
➤ *carisoprodol* (C)(G) 1 tab tid or qid
   Pediatric: <12 years: not recommended; ≥12 years: same as adult
      Soma *Tab:* 350 mg
➤ *chlorzoxazone* (G) 1 caplet qid; max 750 mg qid
   Pediatric: <12 years: not recommended; ≥12 years: same as adult
      Parafon Forte DSC *Cplt:* 500*mg
➤ *cyclobenzaprine* (B)(G) 10 mg tid; usual range 20-40 mg/day in divided doses; max 60 mg/day x 2-3 weeks or 15 mg ext-rel once daily; max 30 mg ext-rel/day x 2-3 weeks
   Pediatric: <15 years: not recommended; ≥15 years: same as adult
      Amrix *Cap:* 15, 30 mg ext-rel
      Fexmid *Tab:* 7.5 mg
      Flexeril *Tab:* 5, 10 mg
➤ *dantrolene* (C) 25md daily x 7 days; then 25 mg tid x 7 days; then 50 mg tid x 7 days; max 100 mg qid
   Pediatric: 0.5 mg/kg daily x 7 days; then 0.5 mg/kg tid x 7 days; then 1 mg/kg tid x 7 days; then 2 mg/kg tid; max 100 mg qid
      Dantrium *Tab:* 25, 50, 100 mg
Comment: *dantrolene* is indicated for chronic spasticity associated with multiple sclerosis and spinal cord injury or disease.
➤ *diazepam* (C)(IV) 2-10 mg bid-qid; may increase gradually
   Pediatric: <6 months: not recommended; ≥6 months: initially 1-2.5 mg bid-qid; may increase gradually
      Diastat *Rectal gel delivery system:* 2.5 mg
      Diastat AcuDial *Rectal gel delivery system:* 10, 20 mg
      Valium *Tab:* 2, 5, 10 mg
      Valium Intensol Oral Solution *Conc oral soln:* 5 mg/ml (30 ml w. dropper) (alcohol 19%)
      Valium Oral Solution *Oral soln:* 5 mg/5 ml (500 ml) (wintergreen spice)
➤ *metaxalone* (B) 1 tab tid-qid
   Pediatric: <12 years: not recommended; ≥12 years: same as adult
      Skelaxin *Tab:* 800*mg
➤ *methocarbamol* (C)(G) initially 1.5 gm qid x 2-3 days; maintenance, 750 mg every 4 hours or 1.5 gm 3 x daily; max 8 gm/day
   Pediatric: <16 years: not recommended; ≥16 years: same as adult
      Robaxin *Tab:* 500 mg
      Robaxin 750 *Tab:* 750 mg

Robaxin Injection 10 ml IM <u>or</u> IV; max 30 ml/day; max 3 days; max 5 ml/ gluteal injection q 8 hours; max IV rate 3 ml/min
Vial: 100 mg/ml (10 ml)
▷ *nabumetone* (C)
Pediatric: <12 years: not recommended; ≥12 years: same as adult
Relafen *Tab:* 500, 750 mg
Relafen 500 *Tab:* 500 mg
▷ *orphenadrine citrate* (C)(G) 1 tab bid
Pediatric: <12 years: not recommended; ≥12 years: same as adult
Norflex *Tab:* 100 mg sust-rel
▷ *tizanidine* (C) 1-4 mg q 6-8 hours; max 36 mg/day
Pediatric: <12 years: not recommended; ≥12 years: same as adult
Zanaflex *Tab:* 2*, 4**mg; *Cap:* 2, 4, 6 mg

SKELETAL MUSCLE RELAXANT+NSAID COMBINATIONS

Comment: *aspirin*-containing medications are contraindicated with history of allergic-type reaction to *aspirin*, children and adolescents with *Varicella* <u>or</u> other viral illness, and 3rd trimester of pregnancy.
▷ *carisoprodol+aspirin* (C)(III)(G) 1-2 tabs qid
Pediatric: <12 years: not recommended; ≥12 years: same as adult
Soma Compound *Tab: caris* 200 mg+*asp* 325 mg (sulfites)
▷ *meprobamate+aspirin* (D)(IV) 1-2 tabs tid <u>or</u> qid
Pediatric: <12 years: not recommended; ≥12 years: same as adult
Equagesic *Tab: mepro* 200 mg+*asp* 325*mg

SKELETAL MUSCLE RELAXANT+NSAID+CAFFEINE COMBINATIONS

Comment: *aspirin*-containing medications are contraindicated with history of allergic-type reaction to *aspirin*, children and adolescents with *Varicella* <u>or</u> other viral illness, and 3rd trimester of pregnancy.
▷ *orphenadrine+aspirin+caffeine* (D)(G)
Pediatric: <12 years: not recommended; ≥12 years: same as adult
Norgesic 1-2 tabs tid-qid
Tab: orphen 25 mg+*asp* 385 mg+*caf* 30 mg
Norgesic Forte 1 tab tid <u>or</u> qid; max 4 tabs/day
Tab: orphen 50 mg+*asp* 770 mg+*caf* 60*mg

SKELETAL MUSCLE RELAXANT+NSAID+CODEINE COMBINATIONS

▷ *carisoprodol+aspirin+codeine* (D)(III)(G) 1-2 tabs qid prn
Pediatric: <18 years: not recommended; ≥18 years: not recommended
Soma Compound w. Codeine *Tab: caris* 200 mg+*asp* 325 mg+*cod* 16 mg
(sulfites)
Comment: *Codeine* is known to be excreted in breast milk. <12 years: not recommended; 12-<18: use extreme caution; not recommended for children and adolescents with asthma <u>or</u> other chronic breathing problem. The FDA and the European Medicines Agency (EMA) are investigating the safety of using *codeine* containing medications to treat pain, cough and colds, in children 12-<18 years because of the potential for serious side effects, including slowed <u>or</u> difficult breathing. *aspirin*-containing medications are contraindicated with history of allergic-type reaction to *aspirin*, children and adolescents with *Varicella* <u>or</u> other viral illness, and 3rd trimester of pregnancy.

TESTOSTERONE DEFICIENCY, HYPOTESTOSTERONEMIA, HYPOGONADISM

Comment: *testosterone* is contraindicated in male breast cancer and prostate cancer. *testosterone* replacement therapy is indicated in males with primary hypogonadism (congenital or acquired due to cryptorchidism, bilateral torsion, orchitis, vanishing testis syndrome, or orchidectomy), or hypogonadotropic hypogonadism (congenital or acquired), and delayed puberty not secondary to a pathological disorder (x-ray of the hand and wrist to determine bone age should be obtained every 6 months to assess the effect of treatment on the epiphyseal centers).

ORAL ANDROGENS

▷ *fluoxymesterone* (X)(III) *Hypogonadism:* <12 years: use by specialist only; Puberty: 5-20 mg once daily; *Delayed puberty:* use low dose and limit duration to 4-6 months
  Halotestin *Tab:* 2*, 5*, 10*mg (tartrazine)
▷ *methyltestosterone* (X)(III) usually 10-50 mg once daily; for delayed puberty, use low dose and limit duration to 4-6 months
  Android *Cap:* 10 mg
  Methitest *Tab:* 10*mg
  Testred *Cap:* 10 mg
▷ *testosterone* (X)(III) 30 mg q 12 hours to gum region, just above the incisor tooth on either side of the mouth; hold system in place for 30 seconds; rotate sites with each application
  Striant *Buccal tab:* 30 mg (6 blister pks; 10 buccal systems/blister pck)
  Comment: Serum total *testosterone* concentrations may be checked 4 to 12 weeks after initiating treatment with **Striant**. To capture the maximum serum concentration, an early morning sample (just prior to applying the AM dose) is recommended.

TOPICAL ANDROGENS

Comment: Wash hands after application. Allow solution to dry before it touches clothing. Do not wash site for at least 2 hours after application. Pregnant and nursing women, and children, must avoid skin contact with application sites on men. If there is contact, wash the area as soon as possible with soap and water.
▷ *testosterone* (X)(III)(G)
  Pediatric: <18 years: not recommended; ≥18 years: same as adult
  AndroGel 1% (G) initially apply 25 mg once daily in the AM to clean, dry, intact skin of the shoulders, upper arms, and/or abdomen; do not apply to scrotum; may increase to 75 mg/day and then to 100 mg/day if needed
    Gel: 25 mg/2.5 gm pkt (30 pkts/carton); 50 mg/5 gm pkt (30 pkts/carton)
  AndroGel 1.62% (G) initially apply 25 mg once daily in the AM to clean, dry, intact skin of the shoulders and upper arms intact skin of the upper arms; do not apply to abdomen or genitals; may adjust dose between 1 and 4 pump actuations based on the pre-dose morning serum testosterone concentration at approximately 14 and 28 days after starting treatment or adjusting dose
    Gel: 20.25 mg/1.25 gm pkt; 40.5 mg/2.5 gm pkt; *20.25* mg/1.25 gm pump actuation (60 metered dose actuations)
  Axiron apply to clean dry intact skin of the axillae; do not apply to the scrotum, penis, abdomen, shoulders, or upper arms; initially apply 60 mg (30 mg/axilla) once daily in the AM; adjust dose based on serum testosterone concentration 2 to 8 hours after applying and at least 14 days after starting therapy or following dose adjustment; may increase dose in 30 mg increments if serum

testosterone <300 ng/dL up to 120 mg; reduce dose to 30 mg if levels >1050 ng/dL; discontinue if serum testosterone remains at >1050 ng/dL; to apply a 120 mg dose, apply 30 mg to each axilla and allow to dry, then repeat

Soln: 30 mg/1.5 ml pump actuation (60 metered dose actuations) (alcohol, latex-free)

Fortesta (G) initially 40 mg of testosterone (4 pump actuations) applied to the thighs once daily in the AM; may adjust between 10 mg minimum and 70 mg maximum

Gel: 10 mg/0.5 gm pump actuation (120 metered dose actuations) (ethanol)

Comment: The **Fortesta** dose should be based on the serum *testosterone* concentration 2 hours after applying **Fortesta** and at approximately 14 days and 35 days after starting treatment or following dose adjustment. Dose adjustment criteria: ≤500 ng/dL, increase daily dose by 10 mg; 500-≤1250 ng/dL, no change; 1250-≤2500 ng/dL, decrease daily dose by 10 mg; ≥2500 ng/dL, decrease daily dose by 20 mg.

Testim (G) initially apply 5 gm once daily in the AM to clean, dry, intact skin of the shoulders and/or upper arms; do not apply to the genitals or abdomen; may increase to 10 gm after 2 weeks

Gel: 1%, clear, hydroalcoholic (5 mg/5 gm pkt, 30 pkts/carton)

Vogelxo Gel (G) 1% initially apply 5 gm once daily in the AM to clean, dry, intact skin of the shoulders, upper arms, and/or abdomen; do not apply to scrotum; may increase to 7.5 gm/day and then to 10 gm/day if needed

Gel: 50 mg/5 gm pkt (30 pkts/carton); 50 mg/5 gm tube (30 tubes/carton); *Pump:* 12.5 mg/1.25 gm pump actuation, 60 metered dose actuations)

INTRANASAL ANDROGENS

▷ *testosterone (nasal gel)* **(X)(III)** initially one pump actuation each nostril (33 mg) 3 x/ day, at least 6-8 hours apart, at the same times each day max: 6 pump actuation/day
Pediatric: <18 years: not established; ≥18 years: same as adult
Natesto *Gel:* 5.5 mg/0.122 gm pump actuation (60 metered dose actuations)

TRANSDERMAL ANDROGEN PATCH

▷ *testosterone* **(X)(III)**
Androderm initially apply 4 mg nightly at approximately 10 PM to clean, dry area of the arm, back, or upper buttocks; leave on x 24 hours; may increase to 7.5 mg or decrease to 2.5 mg based on confirmed AM serum testosterone concentrations
Pediatric: <15 years: not recommended; ≥15 years: same as adult
Transdermal patch: 2, 4 mg/24 Hr

 TETANUS (*CLOSTRIDIUM TETANI*)

PROPHYLAXIS

see **Childhood Immunizations** *page* 546

POSTEXPOSURE PROPHYLAXIS IN PREVIOUSLY NONIMMUNIZED PERSONS

▷ *tetanus immune globulin, human* **(C)** 250 mg deep IM in a single dose
Pediatric: >7 years: same as adult
BayTET, Hyper-TET
Vial: 250 units single-dose; *Prefilled syringe:* 250 units
▷ *tetanus toxoid vaccine* **(C)** 0.5 ml IM x 3 dose series
Vial: 5 Lf units/0.5 ml (0.5, 5 ml); *Prefilled syringe:* 5 Lf units/0.5 ml (0.5 ml)

Comment: Dose of **BayTET/HyperTET** S/D is calculated as 4 units/kg. However, it may be advisable to administer the entire contents of the syringe of **BayTET/HyperTET** S/D (250 units) regardless of the child's size, since theoretically the same amount of toxin will be produced in the child's body by the infecting tetanus organism as it will in an adult's body. At the same time but in a different extremity and with a different syringe, administer Diphtheria and Tetanus Toxoids and Pertussis Vaccine Adsorbed (DTP) or Diphtheria and Tetanus Toxoids Adsorbed (For Pediatric Use) (DT), if pertussis vaccine is contraindicated, should be administered per mfr pkg insert. Tetanus immune globulin may interact with live viral vaccines such as measles, mumps, rubella, and polio. It is also unknown if **BayTET/HyperTET** can cause fetal harm when administered to a pregnant woman or can affect reproduction capacity. The single injection of tetanus toxoid only initiates the series for producing active immunity in the recipient. Impress upon the patient the need for further toxoid injections in 1 month and 1 year, otherwise the active immunization series is incomplete. If a contraindication to using tetanus toxoid-containing preparations exists for a person who has not completed a primary series of tetanus toxoid immunization, and that person has a wound that is neither clean nor minor, only passive immunization should be given using tetanus immune globulin.

 THREADWORM (*STRONGYLOIDES STERCORALIS*)

ANTHELMINTICS

Comment: Oral bioavailability of anthelmintics is enhanced when administered with a fatty meal (estimated fat content 40 gm).

▷ *albendazole* (C) take with a meal; may crush and mix with food; may repeat in 3 weeks if needed; 400 mg bid x 7 days
Pediatric: <2 years: 200 mg bid x 7 days; 2-12 years: 400 mg once daily x 7 days; >12 years: same as adult
　　Albenza *Tab:* 200 mg

Comment: *albendazole* is a broad-spectrum benzimidazole carbamate anthelmintic.

▷ *ivermectin* (C) take with water; chew or crush and mix with food; may repeat in 3 months if needed; 200 mcg/kg as a single dose
Pediatric: <15 kg: not recommended; ≥15 kg: same as adult
　　Stromectol *Tab:* 3, 6*mg

▷ *mebendazole* (C)(G) take with a meal; chew or crush and mix with food; may repeat in 3 weeks if needed; 100 mg bid x 3 days
Pediatric: <2 years: not recommended; ≥2 years: same as adult
　　Emverm *Chew tab:* 100 mg
　　Vermox *Chew tab:* 100 mg

▷ *praziquantel* (B)(G) take with a meal; may crush and mix with food; 5-10 mg/kg as a single dose
Pediatric: <4 years: not established; ≥4 years: same as adult
　　Biltricide *Tab:* 600**mg film-coat (cross-scored for half or quarter dose)

Comment: Therapeutically effective levels of **Biltricide** may not be achieved when administered concomitantly with strong P450 inducers, such as rifampin. Females should not breastfeed on the day of **Biltricide** treatment and during the subsequent 72 hours. Use caution with hepatosplenic patients who have moderate to severe liver impairment (Child-Pugh Class B and C).

▷ *pyrantel pamoate* (C) take with a meal; may open capsule and sprinkle or mix with food; treat x 3 days; may repeat in 2-3 weeks if needed; treat x 3 days; 11 mg/kg/dose; max 1 gm/dose; <25 lb: not recommended; 25-37 lb: 1/2 tsp/dose; 38-62 lb: 1 tsp/dose; 63-87 lb: 1 tsp/dose; 88-112 lb: 2 tsp/dose; 113-137 lb: 2 tsp/dose; 138-162 lb: 3 tsp/dose; 163-187 lb: 3 tsp/dose; >187 lb: 4 tsp/dose

> **Antiminth** *Cap:* 180 mg; *Liq:* 50 mg/ml (30 ml); 144 mg/ml (30 ml); *Oral susp:* 50 mg/ml (60 ml)
> **Pin-X** *Cap:* 180 mg; *Liq:* 50 mg/ml (30 ml); 144 mg/ml (30 ml); *Oral susp:* 50 mg/ml (30 ml)

▷ *nitazoxanide* (B) take with a meal; may crush and mix with food; <12 months: not recommended; ≥12 months: treat q 12 hours x 3 days; <11 years: [use suspension]; 1-3 years: 5 ml; 4-11 years: 10 ml; >11 years: [use tab or suspension] 500 mg
   Alinia *Tab:* 500 mg; *Oral susp:* 100 mg/5 ml (60 ml)

▷ *thiabendazole* (C) take with a meal; may crush and mix with food; treat x 7 days; <30 lb: consult mfr pkg insert; ≥30 lb: 25 mg/kg/dose bid with meals; 30-50 lb: 250 mg bid with meals; >50 lb: 10 mg/lb/dose bid with meals; max 1.5 gm/dose; max 3 gm/day
   Mintezol *Chew tab:* 500*mg (orange); *Oral susp:* 500 mg/5 ml (120 ml) (orange)

Comment: *thiabendazole* is not for prophylaxis. May impair mental alertness. May not be available in the US.

TINEA CAPITIS

Comment: Tinea capitis must be treated with a systemic anti-fungal.

FOR SEVERE KERION PRURITUS

▷ *prednisone* (C) 1 mg/kg/day for 7-14 days
   see **Oral Corticosteroids** page 569

SYSTEMIC ANTI-FUNGALS

▷ *griseofulvin, microsize* (C)(G) 500 mg once daily x 4-6 weeks or longer; max 1 gm/day
Pediatric: <30 lb: 5 mg/lb/day; 30-50 lb: 125-250 mg/day; >50 lb: 250-500 mg/day; 5 mg/lb/day x 4-6 weeks or longer; see page 640 for dose by weight
   Grifulvin V *Tab:* 250, 500 mg; *Oral susp:* 125 mg/5 ml (120 ml) (alcohol 0.02%)

▷ *griseofulvin, ultramicrosize* (C)(G) 375 mg/day in a single or divided doses x 4-6 weeks or longer
Pediatric: <2 years: not recommended; ≥2 years: 3.3 mg/lb/day in a single or divided doses x 4-6 weeks or longer
   Gris-PEG *Tab:* 125, 250 mg

Comment: *griseofulvin* should be taken with fatty foods (e.g., milk, ice cream). Liver enzymes should be monitored.

▷ *ketoconazole* (C)(G) initially 200 mg once daily; max 400 mg/day x 4 weeks
Pediatric: <2 years: not recommended; ≥2 years: 3.3-6.6 mg/kg once daily x 4 weeks
   Nizoral *Tab:* 200 mg

Comment: Caution with *ketoconazole* due to concerns about potential for hepatotoxicity.

TINEA CORPORIS

TOPICAL ANTI-FUNGALS

▷ *butenafine* (C)(G) apply bid x 1 week or once daily x 4 weeks
Pediatric: <12 years: not recommended; ≥12 years: same as adult
   Lotrimin Ultra (OTC) *Crm:* 1% (12, 24 gm)
   Mentax *Crm:* 1% (15, 30 gm)

Comment: *butenafine* is a benzylamine, not an azole. Fungicidal activity continues for at least 5 weeks after last application.

▷ *ciclopirox* (B)
  Loprox Cream apply bid; max 4 weeks
    Pediatric: <10 years: not recommended; ≥10 years: same as adult
      Crm: 0.77% (15, 30, 90 gm)
  Loprox Lotion apply bid; max 4 weeks
    Pediatric: <10 years: not recommended; ≥10 years: same as adult
      Lotn: 0.77% (30, 60 ml)
  Loprox Gel apply bid; max 4 weeks
    Pediatric: <16 years: not recommended; ≥16 years: same as adult
      Gel: 0.77% (30, 45 gm)
▷ *clotrimazole* (B)(G) apply to affected area bid x 7 days
  Pediatric: same as adult
    Lotrimin *Crm:* 1% (15, 30, 45 gm)
    Lotrimin AF (OTC) *Crm:* 1% (12 gm); *Lotn:* 1% (10 ml); *Soln:* 1% (10 ml)
▷ *econazole* (C) apply once daily x 14 days
  Pediatric: same as adult
    Spectazole *Crm:* 1% (15, 30, 85 gm)
▷ *ketoconazole* (C) apply once daily x 14 days
  Pediatric: <12 years: not recommended; ≥12 years: same as adult
    Nizoral Cream *Crm:* 2% (15, 30, 60 gm)
▷ *luliconazole* (C) apply to affected area and 1 inch into the immediate surrounding
  area(s) once daily
  Pediatric: <18 years: not recommended; ≥18 years: same as adult
    Luzu Cream 1% *Crm:* 1% (30, 60 gm)
▷ *miconazole* 2% (C) apply once daily-bid x 2 weeks
  Pediatric: same as adult
    Lotrimin AF Spray Liquid (OTC) *Spray liq:* 2% (113 gm) (alcohol 17%)
    Lotrimin AF Spray Powder (OTC) *Spray pwdr:* 2% (90 gm) (alcohol 10%)
    Monistat-Derm *Crm:* 2% (1, 3 oz); *Spray liq:* 2% (3.5 oz); *Spray pwdr:* 2%
    (3 oz)
▷ *naftifine* (B)(G)
  Pediatric: <12 years: not recommended; ≥12 years: same as adult
    Naftin Cream apply once daily x 14 days
      Crm: 1% (15, 30, 60 gm)
    Naftin Gel apply bid x 14 days
      Gel: 1% (20, 40, 60 gm)
▷ *oxiconazole nitrate* (B)(G) apply once daily-bid x 2 weeks
  Pediatric: same as adult
    Oxistat *Crm:* 1% (15, 30, 60 gm); *Lotn:* 1% (30 ml)
▷ *sulconazole* (C) apply once daily-bid x 3 weeks
  Pediatric: <12 years: not recommended; ≥12 years: same as adult
    Exelderm *Crm:* 1% (15, 30, 60 gm); *Lotn:* 1% (30 mg)
▷ *terbinafine* (B)(G)
  Pediatric: <12 years: not recommended; ≥12 years: same as adult
    Lamisil Cream (OTC) apply to affected and surrounding area once daily-bid x 1-4
    weeks until significantly improved
      Crm: 1% (15, 30 gm)
    Lamisil AT Cream (OTC) apply to affected and surrounding area once daily-bid x
    1-4 weeks until significantly improved
      Crm: **1% (15, 30 gm)**
    Lamisil Solution (OTC) apply to affected and surrounding area once daily x 1 week
      Soln: 1% (30 ml spray bottle)

TOPICAL ANTIFUNGAL+STEROID COMBINATION

▷ *clotrimazole+betamethasone* (C)(G) apply bid x 2 weeks; max 4 weeks
   Pediatric: <12 years: not recommended; ≥12 years: same as adult
      Lotrisone *Crm: clotrim* 1 mg+*beta* 0.5 mg (15, 45 gm); *Lotn: clotrim* 1 mg+*beta*
      0.5 mg (30 ml)

SYSTEMIC ANTIFUNGALS

▷ *griseofulvin, microsize* (C)(G) 500 mg/day x 2-4 weeks; max 1 gm/day
   Pediatric: <30 lb: 5 mg/lb/day; 30-50 lb: 125-250 mg/day; >50 lb: 250-500 mg/day; *see
   page* 640 *for dose by weight*
      Grifulvin V *Tab:* 250, 500 mg; *Oral susp:* 125 mg/5 ml (120 ml) (alcohol 0.02%)
▷ *griseofulvin, ultramicrosize* (C)(G) 375 mg/day in a single or divided doses x 2-4
   weeks
   Pediatric: <2 years: not recommended; ≥2 years: 3.3 mg/lb/day in a single or divided
   doses
      Gris-PEG *Tab:* 125, 250

Comment: *griseofulvin* should be taken with fatty foods (e.g., milk, ice cream). Liver
enzymes should be monitored.
▷ *ketoconazole* (C) initially 200 mg once daily; max 400 mg/day x 4 weeks
   Pediatric: <2 years: not recommended; ≥2 years: 3.3-6.6 mg/kg/day x 4 weeks
      Nizoral *Tab:* 200 mg

Comment: Caution with *ketoconazole* due to concerns about potential for hepatotoxicity.

 TINEA CRURIS (JOCK ITCH)

TOPICAL ANTIFUNGALS

▷ *butenafine* (B)(G) apply bid x 1 week or once daily x 4 weeks
   Pediatric: <12 years: not recommended; ≥12 years: same as adult
      Lotrimin Ultra (C)(OTC) *Crm:* 1% (12, 24 gm)
      Mentax *Crm:* 1% (15, 30 gm)
   Comment: *butenafine* is a benzylamine, not an azole. Fungicidal activity continues for
   at least 5 weeks after last application.
▷ *ciclopirox* (B)
      Loprox Cream apply bid; max 4 weeks
         Pediatric: <10 years: not recommended; ≥10 years: same as adult
         Crm: 0.77% (15, 30, 90 gm)
      Loprox Lotion apply bid; max 4 weeks
         Pediatric: <10 years: not recommended; ≥10 years: same as adult
         Lotn: 0.77% (30, 60 ml)
      Loprox Gel apply bid; max 4 weeks
         Pediatric: <16 years: not recommended; ≥16 years: same as adult
         Gel: 0.77% (30, 45 gm)
▷ *clotrimazole* (B)(G) apply to affected area bid x 7 days
   Pediatric: same as adult
      Lotrimin *Crm:* 1% (15, 30, 45 gm)
      Lotrimin AF (OTC) *Crm:* 1% (12 gm); *Lotn:* 1% (10 ml); *Soln:* 1% (10 ml)
▷ *econazole* (C) apply once daily x 2 weeks
   Pediatric: same as adult
      Spectazole *Crm:* 1% (15, 30, 85 gm)
▷ *ketoconazole* (C)(G) apply bid x 4 weeks
   Pediatric: <12 years: not recommended; ≥12 years: same as adult
      Nizoral Cream *Crm:* 2% (15, 30, 60 gm)

▷ *luliconazole* (C) apply to affected area and 1 inch into the immediate surrounding area(s) once daily
   Pediatric: <18 years: not recommended; ≥18 years: same as adult
      Luzu Cream 1% *Crm:* 1% (30, 60 gm)
▷ *miconazole 2%* (C)(G) apply once daily-bid x 2 weeks
   Pediatric: same as adult
      Lotrimin AF Spray Liquid (OTC) *Spray liq:* 2% (113 gm) (alcohol 17%)
      Lotrimin AF Spray Powder (OTC) *Spray pwdr:* 2% (90 gm) (alcohol 10%)
      Monistat-Derm *Crm:* 2% (1, 3 oz); *Spray liq:* 2% (3.5 oz); *Spray pwdr:* 2% (3 oz)
▷ *naftifine* (B)(G)
   Pediatric: <12 years: not recommended; ≥12 years: same as adult
      Naftin Cream apply once daily x 2 weeks
         Crm: 1% (15, 30, 60 gm)
      Naftin Gel apply bid x 2 weeks
         Gel: 1% (20, 40, 60 gm)
▷ *oxiconazole nitrate* (B)(G) apply once daily-bid x 2 weeks
   Pediatric: same as adult
      Oxistat *Crm:* 1% (15, 30, 60 gm); *Lotn:* 1% (30 ml)
▷ *sulconazole* (C) apply once daily-bid x 3 weeks
   Pediatric: <12 years: not recommended; ≥12 years: same as adult
      Exelderm *Crm:* 1% (15, 30, 60 gm); *Lotn:* 1% (30 mg)
▷ *terbinafine* (B)(G)
   Pediatric: <12 years: not recommended; ≥12 years: same as adult
      Lamisil Cream (OTC) apply bid x 1-4 weeks
         Crm: 1% (15, 30 gm)
      Lamisil AT Cream (OTC) apply to affected and surrounding area once daily-bid x 1-4 weeks until significantly improved
         Crm: 1% (15, 30 gm)
      Lamisil Solution (OTC) apply to affected and surrounding area once daily x 1 week
         Soln: 1% (30 ml spray bottle)
▷ *tolnaftate* (C)(OTC)(G) apply sparingly bid x 2-4 weeks
   Pediatric: <2 years: not recommended; ≥2 years: same as adult
      Tinactin *Crm:* 1% (15, 30 gm); *Pwdr:* 1% (45, 90 gm); *Soln:* 1% (10 ml); *Aerosol liq:* 1% (4 oz); *Aerosol pwdr:* 1% (3.5, 5 oz)
▷ *undecylenic acid* apply bid x 4 weeks
   Pediatric: same as adult
      Desenex (OTC) *Pwdr:* 25% (1.5, 3 oz); *Spray pwdr:* 25% (2.7 oz); *Oint:* 25% (0.5, 1 oz)

TOPICAL ANTIFUNGAL+ANTI-INFLAMMATORY AGENTS

▷ *clotrimazole+betamethasone* (C)(G) apply bid x 4 weeks; max 4 weeks
   Pediatric: <12 years: not recommended; ≥12 years: same as adult
   Crm: clotrim 10 mg+*beta* 0.5 mg (15, 45 gm); *Lotn: clotrim* 10 mg+*beta* 0.5 mg (30 ml)

SYSTEMIC ANTIFUNGALS

▷ *griseofulvin, microsize* (C)(G) 1 gm once daily x 2 weeks
   Pediatric: <30 lb: 5 mg/lb/day; 30-50 lb: 125-250 mg/day; >50 lb: 250-500 mg/day; 5 mg/lb/day x 4-6 weeks <u>or</u> longer; *see page* 640 *for dose by weight*
      Grifulvin V *Tab:* 250, 500 mg; *Oral susp:* 125 mg/5 ml (120 ml) (alcohol 0.02%)
▷ *griseofulvin, ultramicrosize* (C) 375 mg/day in a single <u>or</u> divided doses x 2 weeks
   Pediatric: <2 years: not recommended; ≥2 years: 3.3 mg/lb/day in a single <u>or</u> divided doses
      Gris-PEG *Tab:* 125, 250 mg
Comment: *griseofulvin* should be taken with fatty foods (e.g., milk, ice cream). Liver enzymes should be monitored.

▷ **ketoconazole** (C) initially 200 mg once daily; max 400 mg once daily x 4 weeks
  Pediatric: <2 years: not recommended; ≥2 years: 3.3-6.6 mg/kg/day
    Nizoral *Tab:* 200 mg
Comment: Caution with **ketoconazole** due to concerns about potential for hepatotoxicity.

◯ TINEA PEDIS (ATHLETE'S FOOT)

TOPICAL ANTIFUNGALS

▷ **butenafine** (B)(G) apply bid x 1 week or once daily x 4 weeks
  Pediatric: <12 years: not recommended; ≥12 years: same as adult
    Lotrimin Ultra (C)(OTC) *Crm:* 1% (12, 24 gm)
    Mentax *Crm:* 1% (15, 30 gm)
Comment: **butenafine** is a benzylamine, not an azole. Fungicidal activity continues for at least 5 weeks after last application.
▷ **Burrows solution** wet dressings
▷ **ciclopirox** (B)
    Loprox Cream apply bid; max 4 weeks
      Pediatric: <10 years: not recommended; ≥10 years: same as adult
      Crm: 0.77% (15, 30, 90 gm)
    Loprox Lotion apply bid; max 4 weeks
      Pediatric: <10 years: not recommended; ≥10 years: same as adult
      Lotn: 0.77% (30, 60 ml)
    Loprox Gel apply bid; max 4 weeks
      Pediatric: <16 years: not recommended; ≥16 years: same as adult
      Gel: 0.77% (30, 45 gm)
▷ **clotrimazole** (C)(G) apply bid to affected area x 4 weeks
  Pediatric: same as adult
    Desenex *Crm:* 1% (0.5 oz)
    Lotrimin *Crm:* 1% (15, 30, 45, 90 gm); *Lotn:* 1% (30 ml); *Soln:* 1% (10, 30 ml)
    Lotrimin AF (OTC) *Crm:* 1% (15, 30, 45, 90 gm); *Lotn:* 1% (20 ml); *Soln:* 1% (20 ml)
▷ **econazole** (C) apply once daily x 4 weeks
  Pediatric: same as adult
    Spectazole *Crm:* 1% (15, 30, 85 gm)
▷ **ketoconazole** (C) apply once daily x 6 weeks
  Pediatric: <12 years: not recommended; ≥12 years: same as adult
    Nizoral Cream *Crm:* 2% (15, 30, 60 gm)
▷ **luliconazole** (C) apply to affected area and 1 inch into the immediate surrounding area(s) once daily
  Pediatric: <18 years: not recommended; ≥18 years: same as adult
    Luzu Cream 1% *Crm:* 1% (30, 60 gm)
▷ **miconazole 2%** (C)(G) apply bid x 4 weeks
  Pediatric: same as adult
    Lotrimin AF Spray Liquid (OTC) *Spray liq:* 2% (113 gm) (alcohol 17%)
    Lotrimin AF Spray Powder (OTC) *Spray pwdr:* 2% (90 gm; alcohol 10%)
    Monistat-Derm *Crm:* 2% (1, 3 oz); *Spray liq:* 2% (3.5 oz); *Spray pwdr:* 2% (3 oz)
▷ **naftifine** (B)(G)
  Pediatric: <12 years: not recommended; ≥12 years: same as adult
    Naftin Cream apply once daily x 4 weeks
      Crm: 1% (15, 30, 60 gm)
    Naftin Gel apply bid x 4 weeks
      Gel: 1% (20, 40, 60 gm)

> *oxiconazole nitrate* (B)(G) apply once daily-bid x 4 weeks
  Pediatric: same as adult
      Oxistat *Crm:* 1% (15, 30, 60 gm); *Lotn:* 1% (30 ml)
> *sertaconazole* (C) apply once daily-bid x 4 weeks
  Pediatric: <12 years: not recommended; ≥12 years: same as adult
      Ertaczo *Crm:* 2% (15, 30 gm)
> *sulconazole* (C) apply once daily-bid x 4 weeks
  Pediatric: <12 years: not recommended; ≥12 years: same as adult
      Exelderm *Crm:* 1% (15, 30, 60 gm); *Lotn:* 1% (30 mg)
> *terbinafine* (B)(G)
  Pediatric: <12 years: not recommended; ≥12 years: same as adult
      Lamisil Cream (OTC) apply bid x 1-4 weeks
        Crm: 1% (15, 30 gm)
      Lamisil AT Cream (OTC) apply to affected and surrounding area once daily-bid x
        1-4 weeks until significantly improved
        Crm: 1% (15, 30 gm)
      Lamisil Solution (OTC) apply to affected and surrounding area bid x 1 week
        Soln: 1% (30 ml spray bottle)
> *tolnaftate* (C)(OTC)(G) apply sparingly bid x 2-4 weeks
  Pediatric: <2 years: not recommended; ≥2 years: same as adult
      Tinactin *Crm:* 1% (15, 30 gm); *Pwdr:* 1% (45, 90 gm); *Soln:* 1% (10 ml); *Aerosol
      liq:* 1% (4 oz); *Aerosol pwdr:* 1% (3.5, 5 oz)

TOPICAL ANTIFUNGAL+ANTI-INFLAMMATORY COMBINATION

> *clotrimazole+betamethasone* (C)(G) apply bid x 4 weeks; max 4 weeks
  Pediatric: <12 years: not recommended; ≥12 years: same as adult
      Lotrisone *Crm:* clotrim 1 mg+beta 0.5 mg (15, 45 gm); *Lotn:* clotrim 1 mg+beta
      0.5 mg (30 ml)

SYSTEMIC ANTIFUNGALS

> *griseofulvin, microsize* (C)(G) 1 gm once daily x 4-8 weeks
  Pediatric: <30 lb: 5 mg/lb/day; 30-50 lb: 125-250 mg/day; >50 lb: 250-500 mg/day; 5
  mg/lb/day x 4-6 weeks or longer; *see page* 640 *for dose by weight*
      Grifulvin V *Tab:* 250, 500 mg; *Oral susp:* 125 mg/5 ml (120 ml) (alcohol 0.02%)
> *griseofulvin, ultramicrosize* (C) 750 mg/day in a single or divided doses x 4-6 weeks
  Pediatric: <2 years: not recommended; ≥2 years: 3.3 mg/lb/day in a single or divided
  doses
      Gris-PEG *Tab:* 125, 250
Comment: *griseofulvin* should be taken with fatty foods (e.g., milk, ice cream). Liver
enzymes should be monitored.
> *ketoconazole* (C) initially 200 mg once daily; max 400 mg/day x 4 weeks
  Pediatric: <2 years: not recommended; ≥2 years: 3.3-6.6 mg/kg once daily x 4 weeks
      Nizoral *Tab:* 200 mg
Comment: Caution with *ketoconazole* due to concerns about potential for hepatotoxicity.

◯ TINEA VERSICOLOR

Comment: Resolution may take 3-6 months.

TOPICAL ANTIFUNGALS

> *butenafine* (G) apply once daily x 2 weeks
  Pediatric: <12 years: not recommended; ≥12 years: same as adult

      Lotrimin Ultra (C)(OTC) *Crm:* 1% (12, 24 gm)

      Mentax (B) *Crm:* 1% (15, 30 gm)

    Comment: *butenafine* is a benzylamine, not an azole. Fungicidal activity continues for at least 5 weeks after last application.

▷ *ciclopirox* (B)

      Loprox Cream apply bid; max 4 weeks

     Pediatric: <10 years: not recommended; ≥10 years: same as adult

        Crm: 0.77% (15, 30, 90 gm)

      Loprox Lotion apply bid; max 4 weeks

     Pediatric: <10 years: not recommended; ≥10 years: same as adult

        Lotn: 0.77% (30, 60 ml)

      Loprox Gel apply bid; max 4 weeks

     Pediatric: <16 years: not recommended; ≥16 years: same as adult

        Gel: 0.77% (30, 45 gm)

▷ *clotrimazole* (B)(G) apply bid x 7 days

    Pediatric: same as adult

      Lotrimin *Crm:* 1% (15, 30, 45 gm)

      Lotrimin AF (OTC) *Crm:* 1% (12 gm); *Lotn:* 1% (10 ml); *Soln:* 1% (10 ml)

▷ *econazole* (C) apply once daily x 2 weeks

    Pediatric: same as adult

      Spectazole *Crm:* 1% (15, 30, 85 gm)

▷ *miconazole* 2% (C)(G) apply once daily x 2 weeks

    Pediatric: same as adult

      Lotrimin AF Spray Liquid (OTC) *Spray liq:* 2% (113 gm) (alcohol 17%)

      Lotrimin AF Spray Powder (OTC) *Spray pwdr:* 2% (90 gm) alcohol 10%)

      Monistat-Derm *Crm:* 2% (1, 3 oz); *Spray liq:* 2% (3.5 oz); *Spray pwdr:* 2% (3 oz)

▷ *ketoconazole* (C)(G)

    Pediatric: <12 years: not recommended; ≥12 years: same as adult

      Nizoral Cream apply once daily x 2 weeks

        Crm: 2% (15, 30, 60 gm)

      Nizoral Shampoo lather into area and leave on 5 minutes x 1 application

        Shampoo: 2% (4 oz)

▷ *oxiconazole nitrate* (B)(G) apply once daily x 2 weeks

    Pediatric: same as adult

      Oxistat *Crm:* 1% (15, 30, 60 gm); *Lotn:* 1% (30 ml)

▷ *selenium sulfide* shampoo (C)(G) apply after shower, allow to dry, leave on overnight; then scrub off vigorously in AM; repeat in 1 week and again q 3 months until resolution occurs

    Pediatric: same as adult

      Selsun Blue *Shampoo:* 1% (120, 210, 240, 330 ml); 2.5% (120 ml)

▷ *sulconazole* (C) apply once daily-bid x 3 weeks

    Pediatric: <12 years: not recommended; ≥12 years: same as adult

      Exelderm *Crm:* 1% (15, 30, 60 gm); *Lotn:* 1% (30 mg)

▷ *terbinafine* (B) apply bid to affected and surrounding area x 1 week

    Pediatric: <12 years: not recommended; ≥12 years: same as adult

      Lamisil Solution (OTC) *Soln:* 1% (30 ml spray bottle)

ORAL ANTI-FUNGALS

▷ *ketoconazole* (C) initially 200 mg once daily; max 400 mg/day x 4 weeks

    Pediatric: <2 years: not recommended; ≥2 years: 3.3-6.6 mg/kg once daily x 4 weeks

      Nizoral *Tab:* 200 mg

TOBACCO DEPENDENCE, TOBACCO CESSATION, NICOTINE WITHDRAWAL SYNDROME

Comment: According to findings from the Population Assessment of Tobacco and Health (PATH) Study (respondents=10, 384, mean age=14.3), any use of e-cigarettes, hookah, non-cigarette combustible tobacco, or smokeless tobacco was independently associated with traditional cigarette smoking 1 year later and use of more than 1 of these products increases the odds of progressing to traditional cigarette use.

REFERENCE

Watkins, S. L., Glantz, S. A., & Chaffee, B. W. (2018). Association of Noncigarette Tobacco Product Use With Future Cigarette Smoking Among Youth in the Population Assessment of Tobacco and Health (PATH) Study, 2013-2015. *JAMA Pediatrics, 172*(2), 181. doi:10.1001/jamapediatrics.2017.4173

NON-NICOTINE PRODUCTS

Alpha4-Beta4 Nicotinic Acetylcholine Receptor Partial Agonist

▷ *varenicline* (C) set target quit date; begin therapy 1 week prior to target quit date; take after eating with a full glass of water; initially 0.5 mg once daily for 3 days; then 0.5 mg bid x 4 days; then 1 mg bid; treat x 12 weeks; may continue treatment for 12 more weeks
   Pediatric: <18 years: not recommended; ≥18 years: same as adult
      Chantix *Tab:* 0.5, 1 mg; *Starting Month Pak:* 0.5 mg x 11 tabs + 1 mg x 42 tabs; *Continuing Month Pak:* 1 mg x 56 tabs

Comment: Caution with **Chantix** due to potential risk for anxiety or suicidal ideation.

AMINOKETONES

▷ *bupropion HBr* (C)(G)
   Pediatric: Safety and effectiveness in the pediatric population have not been established. When considering the use of **Aplenzin** in a child or adolescent, balance the potential risks with the clinical need
      Aplenzin initially 100 mg bid for at least 3 days; may increase to 375 or 400 mg/day after several weeks; then after at least 3 more days, 450 mg in 4 divided doses; max 450 mg/day, 174 mg/single dose
         Tab: 174, 348, 522 mg
▷ *bupropion HCl* (C)(G)
   Pediatric: Safety and effectiveness in the pediatric population have not been established. When considering the use of **Forfivo XL** in a child or adolescent, balance the potential risks with the clinical need
      Forfivo XL do not use for initial treatment; use immediate-release *bupropion* forms for initial titration; switch to **Forfivo XL** 450 mg once daily when total dose/day reaches 450 mg; may switch to **Forfivo XL** when total dose/day reaches 300 mg for 2 weeks and patient needs 450 mg/day to reach therapeutic target; swallow whole, do not crush or chew
         Tab: 450 mg ext-rel
      Wellbutrin initially 100 mg bid for at least 3 days; may increase to 375 or 400 mg/day after several weeks; then after at least 3 more days, 450 mg in 4 divided doses; max 450 mg/day, 150 mg/single dose
         Tab: 75, 100 mg
      Wellbutrin SR initially 150 mg in AM for at least 3 days; may increase to 150 mg bid if well tolerated; usual dose 300 mg/day; max 400 mg/day
         Tab: 100, 150 mg sust-rel

Wellbutrin XL initially 150 mg in AM for at least 3 days; increase to 150 mg bid if well tolerated; usual dose 300 mg/day; max 400 mg/day

Tab: 150, 300 mg sust-rel

Zyban 150 mg once daily x 3 days; then 150 mg bid x 7-12 weeks; max 300 mg/day

Tab: 150 mg sust-rel

Comment: Contraindications to *bupropion* include seizure disorder, eating disorder, concurrent MAOI and alcohol use. Smoking should be discontinued after the 7th day of therapy with *bupropion*. Avoid bedtime dose.

TRANSDERMAL NICOTINE SYSTEMS (D)

Habitrol (OTC) initially one 21 mg/24 hr patch/day x 4-6 weeks; then one 14 mg/24 hr patch/day x 2-4 weeks; then one 7 mg/24 hr patch/day x 2-4 weeks; then discontinue

Pediatric: <12 years: not recommended; ≥12 years: same as adult

Transdermal patch: 7, 14, 21 mg/24 hr

Nicoderm CQ (OTC) initially one 21 mg/24 hr patch/day x 6 weeks, then one 14 mg/24 hr patch/day x 2 weeks; then one 7 mg/24 hr patch/day x 2 weeks

Pediatric: <12 years: not recommended; ≥12 years: same as adult

Transdermal patch: 7, 14, 21 mg/24 hr

Comment: Nicoderm CQ is available as a clear patch.

Nicotrol Step-down Patch (OTC) 1 patch/day x 6 weeks

Pediatric: <12 years: not recommended; ≥12 years: same as adult

Transdermal patch: 5, 10, 15 mg/16 hr (7/pck)

Nicotrol Transdermal (OTC) 1 patch/day x 6 weeks

Pediatric: <12 years: not recommended; ≥12 years: same as adult

Transdermal patch: 15 mg/16 hour (7/pck)

Prostep initially one 22 mg/24 hr patch/day x 4-8 weeks; then discontinue <u>or</u> one 11 mg/24 hr patch/day x 2-4 additional weeks

Pediatric: <12 years: not recommended; ≥12 years: same as adult

Transdermal patch: 11, 22 mg/24 hr (7/pck)

NICOTINE GUM

▷ *nicotine polacrilex* (D) chew one piece of gum slowly and intermittently over 30 minutes q 1-2 hours x 6 weeks; then q 2-4 hours x 3 weeks; then q 4-8 hours x 3 weeks; max 24 pieces/day; 2 mg if smoked <25 cigarettes/day; 4 mg if smoked >24 cigarettes/day

Pediatric: <12 years: not recommended; ≥12 years: same as adult

Nicorette (OTC) *Gum squares:* 2, 4 mg (108 piece starter kit and 48 piece refill) (orange, mint, <u>or</u> original, sugar-free)

NICOTINE LOZENGE

▷ *nicotine polacrilex* (X)(OTC)(G) dissolve over 20-30 minutes; minimize swallowing; do not eat <u>or</u> drink for 15 min before and during use; Use 2 mg lozenge if first cigarette smoked >30 minutes after waking; Use 4 mg lozenge if first cigarette smoked within 30 min of waking; 1 lozenge q 1-2 hours (at least 9/day) x 6 weeks; then q 2-4 hours x 3 weeks; then q 4-8 hours x 3 weeks; then stop; max 5 lozenges/6 hours and 20 lozenges/day

Pediatric: <18 years: not recommended; ≥18 years: same as adult

Commit Lozenge *Loz:* 2, 4 mg (72/pck) (phenylalanine)

Nicorette Mini Lozenge (G) *Loz:* 2, 4 mg (72/pck) (mint; phenylalanine)

NICOTINE INHALATION PRODUCTS

▷ *nicotine* 0.5 mg aqueous nasal spray (D)

Pediatric: <12 years: not recommended; ≥12 years: same as adult

Nicotrol NS 1-2 doses/hour nasally; max 5 doses/hour <u>or</u> 40 doses/day; usual max 3 months
Nasal spray: 0.5 mg/spray; 10 mg/ml (10 ml, 200 doses)

▷ *nicotine* 10 mg inhalation system (D)
Pediatric: <12 years: not recommended; ≥12 years: same as adult
Nicotrol Inhaler individualize therapy; at least 6 cartridges/day x 3-6 weeks; max 16 cartridges/day x first 12 weeks; then reduce gradually over 12 more weeks
Inhaler: 10 mg/cartridge, 4 mg delivered (42 cartridge/pck) (menthol)

Comment: Nicotrol Inhaler is a smoking replacement; to be used with decreasing frequency. Smoking should be discontinued before starting therapy. Side effects include cough, nausea, mouth, <u>or</u> throat irritation. This system delivers nicotine, but no tars <u>or</u> carcinogens. Each cartridge lasts about 20 minutes with frequent continuous puffing and provides nicotine equivalent to 2 cigarettes.

 TONSILLITIS: ACUTE

ANTI-INFECTIVES

▷ *amoxicillin* (B)(G) 500-875 mg bid <u>or</u> 250-500 mg tid x 10 days
Pediatric: <40 kg (88 lb): 20-40 mg/kg/day in 3 divided doses x 10 days <u>or</u> 25-45 mg/kg/day in 2 divided doses x 10 days; *see page 616 for dose by weight*
Amoxil *Cap:* 250, 500 mg; *Tab:* 875*mg; *Chew tab:* 125, 200, 250, 400 mg (cherry-banana-peppermint) (phenylalanine); *Oral susp:* 125, 250 mg/5 ml (80, 100, 150 ml) (strawberry); 200, 400 mg/5 ml (50, 75, 100 ml) (bubble gum); *Oral drops:* 50 mg/ml (30 ml) (bubble gum)
Moxatag *Tab:* 775 mg ext-rel
Trimox *Tab:* 125, 250 mg; *Cap:* 250, 500 mg; *Oral susp:* 125, 250 mg/5 ml (80, 100, 150 ml) (raspberry-strawberry)

▷ *azithromycin* (B)(G) 500 mg x 1 dose on day 1, then 250 mg once daily on days 2-5 <u>or</u> 500 mg once daily x 3 days <u>or</u> Zmax 2 gm in a single dose
Pediatric: 12 mg/kg/day x 5 days; max 500 mg/day; *see page 621 for dose by weight*
Zithromax *Tab:* 250, 500, 600 mg; *Oral susp:* 100 mg/5 ml (15 ml); 200 mg/5 ml (15, 22.5, 30 ml) (cherry); *Pkt:* 1 gm for reconstitution (cherry-banana)
Zithromax Tri-pak *Tab:* 3 x 500 mg tabs/pck
Zithromax Z-pak *Tab:* 6 x 250 mg tabs/pck
Zmax *Oral susp:* 2 gm ext-rel for reconstitution (cherry-banana) (148 mg Na$^+$)

▷ *cefaclor* (B)(G) 250-500 mg q 8 hours x 10 days; max 2 gm/day
Pediatric: <1 month: not recommended; 20-40 mg/kg bid <u>or</u> q 12 hours x 10 days; max 1 gm/day; *see page 622 for dose by weight*
Tab: 500 mg; *Cap:* 250, 500 mg; *Susp:* 125 mg/5 ml (75, 150 ml) (strawberry); 187 mg/5 ml (50, 100 ml) (strawberry); 250 mg/5 ml (75, 150 ml) (strawberry); 375 mg/5 ml (50, 100 ml) (strawberry)
Cefaclor Extended Release *Tab:* 375, 500 mg ext-rel
Pediatric: <16 years: ext-rel not recommended; ≥16 years; same as adult

▷ *cefadroxil* (B) 1 gm once daily <u>or</u> divided bid x 10 days
Pediatric: 30 mg/kg/day in 2 divided doses x 10 days; *see page 623 for dose by weight*
Duricef *Cap:* 500 mg; *Tab:* 1 gm; *Oral susp:* 250 mg/5 ml (100 ml); 500 mg/5 ml (75, 100 ml) (orange-pineapple)

▷ *cefdinir* (B) 300 mg bid x 5-10 days <u>or</u> 600 mg once daily x 10 days
Pediatric: <6 months: not recommended; 6 months-12 years: 14 mg/kg/day in a single <u>or</u> 2 divided doses x 10 days; >12 years: same as adult; *see page 624 for dose by weight*
Omnicef *Cap:* 300 mg; *Oral susp:* 125 mg/5 ml (60, 100 ml) (strawberry)

➤ *cefditoren pivoxil* (B) 200 mg bid x 10 days
  Pediatric: <12 years: not recommended; ≥12 years: same as adult
    Spectracef *Tab:* 200 mg
Comment: Contraindicated with milk protein allergy <u>or</u> carnitine deficiency.
➤ *ceftibuten* (B) 200 mg once daily x 10 days
  Pediatric: 9 mg/kg once daily x 10 days; max 400 mg/day; *see page 628 for dose by weight*
    Cedax *Cap:* 400 mg; *Oral susp:* 90 mg/5 ml (30, 60, 90, 120 ml); 180 mg/5 ml (30, 60, 120 ml) (cherry)
➤ *cefixime* (B)(G) 400 mg once daily x 10 days
  Pediatric: <6 months: not recommended; 6 months-12 years, <50 kg: 8 mg/kg/day in a single <u>or</u> 2 divided doses x 10 days; *see page 625 for dose by weight;* >12 years, >50 kg: same as adult
    Suprax *Tab:* 400 mg; *Cap:* 400 mg; *Oral susp:* 100, 200, 500 mg/5 ml (50, 75, 100 ml) (strawberry)
➤ *cefpodoxime proxetil* (B) 200 mg bid x 5-7 days
  Pediatric: <2 months: not recommended; 2 months-12 years: 10 mg/kg/day (max 400 mg/dose) <u>or</u> 5 mg/kg/day bid (max 200 mg/dose) x 5-7 days; *see page 626 for dose by weight*
    Vantin *Tab:* 100, 200 mg; *Oral susp:* 50, 100 mg/5 ml (50, 75, 100 mg) (lemon creme)
➤ *cefprozil* (B) 500 mg once daily x 10 days
  Pediatric: 2-12 years: 7.5 mg/kg bid x 10 days; >12 years: same as adult; *see page 627 for dose by weight*
    Cefzil *Tab:* 250, 500 mg; *Oral susp:* 125, 250 mg/5 ml (50, 75, 100 ml) (bubble gum) (phenylalanine)
➤ *cephalexin* (B)(G) 250 mg tid x 10 days
  Pediatric: 25-50 mg/kg/day in 4 divided doses x 10 days; *see page 629 for dose by weight*
    Keflex *Cap:* 250, 333, 500, 750 mg; *Oral susp:* 125, 250 mg/5 ml (100, 200 ml) (strawberry)
➤ *clarithromycin* (C)(G) 250 mg bid <u>or</u> 500 mg ext-rel once daily 10 days
  Pediatric: <6 months: not recommended; ≥6 months: 7.5 mg/kg bid x 10 days; *see page 630 for dose by weight*
    Biaxin *Tab:* 250, 500 mg
    Biaxin Oral Suspension *Oral susp:* 125, 250 mg/5 ml (50, 100 ml) (fruit punch)
    Biaxin XL *Tab:* 500 mg ext-rel
➤ *dirithromycin* (C)(G) 500 mg once daily x 10 days
  Pediatric: <12 years: not recommended; ≥12 years: same as adult
    Dynabac *Tab:* 250 mg
➤ *erythromycin base* (B)(G) 300-400 mg tid x 10 days
  Pediatric: 30-50 mg/kg/day in 2-4 divided doses x 10 days
    Ery-Tab *Tab:* 250, 333, 500 mg ent-coat
    PCE *Tab:* 333, 500 mg
Comment: *erythromycin* may increase INR with concomitant *warfarin*, as well as increase serum level of *digoxin, benzodiazepines,* and *statins.*
➤ *erythromycin ethylsuccinate* (B)(G) 400 mg qid x 7 days
  Pediatric: 30-50 mg/kg/day in 4 divided doses x 7 days; may double dose with severe infection; max 100 mg/kg/day; *see page 635 for dose by weight*
    EryPed *Oral susp:* 200 mg/5 ml (100, 200 ml) (fruit); 400 mg/5 ml (60, 100, 200 ml) (banana); *Oral drops:* 200, 400 mg/5 ml (50 ml) (fruit); *Chew tab:* 200 mg wafer (fruit)
    E.E.S. *Oral susp:* 200, 400 mg/5 ml (100 ml) (fruit)

E.E.S. Granules *Oral susp:* 200 mg/5 ml (100, 200 ml) (cherry)
E.E.S. 400 Tablets *Tab:* 400 mg

Comment: *erythromycin* may increase INR with concomitant *warfarin*, as well as increase serum level of *digoxin, benzodiazepines*, and *statins*.

▷ *loracarbef* (B) 200 mg bid x 10 days
  Pediatric: 15 mg/kg/day in 2 divided doses x 10 days; *see page 642 for dose by weight*
    Lorabid *Pulvule:* 200, 400 mg; *Oral susp:* 100 mg/5 ml (50, 100 ml); 200 mg/5 ml (50, 75, 100 ml) (strawberry bubble gum)

▷ *penicillin v potassium* (B)(G) 250 mg tid x 10 days
  Pediatric: 25-50 mg/kg day in 4 divided doses x 10 days; ≥12 years: same as adult; *see page 644 for dose by weight*
    Pen-Vee K *Tab:* 250, 500 mg; *Oral soln:* 125 mg/5 ml (100, 200 ml); 250 mg/5 ml (100, 150, 200 ml)

 TRICHINOSIS (*TRICHINELLA SPIRALIS*)

Comment: Trichinosis is caused by eating raw <u>or</u> undercooked pork <u>or</u> wild game infected with the larvae of a parasitic worm, *Trichinella spiralis*. The initial symptoms are abdominal discomfort, nausea, vomiting, diarrhea, fatigue, and fever beginning one to two days following ingestion. These parasites then invade other organs (e.g., muscles) causing muscle aches, itching, fever, chills, and joint pains that begins about two to eight weeks after ingestion. The treatment is oral anthelmintics which may cause abdominal pain, diarrhea, and (rarely) hypersensitivity reactions, convulsions, neutropenia, agranulocytosis, and hepatitis.

ANTHELMINTICS

Comment: Oral bioavailability of anthelmintics is enhanced when administered with a fatty meal (estimated fat content 40 gm).

▷ *albendazole* (C) take with a meal; may crush and mix with food; may repeat in 3 weeks if needed; 400 mg as once daily x 7 days
  Pediatric: <2 years: 200 mg once daily x 3 days; may repeat in 3 weeks; 2-12 years: 400 mg once daily x 3 days; may repeat in 3 weeks; >12 years: same as adult
    Albenza *Tab:* 200 mg

Comment: *albendazole* is a broad-spectrum benzimidazole carbamate anthelmintic.

▷ *ivermectin* (C) take with water; chew or crush and mix with food; may repeat in 3 months if needed; 200 mcg/kg as a single dose
  Pediatric: <15 kg: not recommended; ≥15 kg: same as adult
    Stromectol *Tab:* 3, 6*mg

▷ *mebendazole* (C)(G) take with a meal; chew or crush and mix with food; may repeat in 3 weeks if needed; <2 years: not recommended; ≥2 years: 100 mg bid x 3 days
  Pediatric: <2 years: not recommended; ≥2 years: same as adult
    Emverm *Chew tab:* 100 mg
    Vermox (G) *Chew tab:* 100 mg

▷ *pyrantel pamoate* (C) take with a meal; may open capsule and sprinkle or mix with food; treat x 3 days; may repeat in 2-3 weeks if needed; treat x 3 days; 11 mg/kg/dose; max 1 gm/dose; <25 lb: not recommended; 25-37 lb: 1/2 tsp/dose; 38-62 lb: 1 tsp/dose; 63-87 lb: 1 tsp/dose; 88-112 lb: 2 tsp/dose; 113-137 lb: 2 tsp/dose; 138-162 lb: 3 tsp/dose; 163-187 lb: 3 tsp/dose; >187 lb: 4 tsp/dose
    Antiminth *Cap:* 180 mg; *Liq:* 50 mg/ml (30 ml); 144 mg/ml (30 ml); *Oral susp:* 50 mg/ml (60 ml)
    Pin-X (OTC) *Cap:* 180 mg; *Liq:* 50 mg/ml (30 ml); 144 mg/ml (30 ml); *Oral susp:* 50 mg/ml (30 ml)

▷ *thiabendazole* (C) take with a meal; may crush and mix with food; treat x 7 days; 25 mg/kg bid x 7 days; max 1.5 gm/dose; take with a meal
Pediatric: same as adult; <30 lb: consult mfr pkg insert; ≥30 lb: 25 mg/kg in 2 divided doses/day with meals; 30-50 lbs: 250 mg bid with meals; >50 lb: 10 mg/lb/dose bid with meals; max 3 gm/day

Mintezol *Chew tab:* 500*mg (orange); *Oral susp:* 500 mg/5 ml (120 ml) (orange)
Comment: *thiabendazole* is not for prophylaxis. May impair mental alertness. May not be available in the US.

 TRICHOMONIASIS (*TRICHOMONAS VAGINALIS*)

Comment: The following treatment regimens for *Trichomoniasis* are published in the **2015 CDC Sexually Transmitted Diseases Treatment Guidelines**. Treat all sexual contacts. A multi-dose treatment regimen should be considered in HIV-positive women.

RECOMMENDED REGIMENS (NON-PREGNANT)
Regimen 1
▷ *metronidazole* 2 gm once in a single dose

Regimen 2
▷ *tinidazole* 2 gm once in a single dose

RECOMMENDED ALTERNATE REGIMEN
Regimen 1
▷ *metronidazole* 500 mg bid x 7 days

DRUG BRANDS AND DOSE FORMS
▷ *metronidazole* (not for use in 1st; B in 2nd, 3rd)(G)
    Flagyl *Tab:* 250*, 500*mg
    Flagyl 375 *Cap:* 375 mg
    Flagyl ER *Tab:* 750 mg ext-rel
▷ *tinidazole* (not for use in 1st; B in 2nd, 3rd)
    Tindamax *Tab:* 250*, 500*mg

RECOMMENDED REGIMENS: PREGNANCY/LACTATION

Comment: All pregnant women should be considered for treatment. Women can be treated with 2 gm *metronidazole* in a single dose at any stage of pregnancy. Lactating women who are administered *metronidazole* should be instructed to interrupt breastfeeding for 12-24 hours after receiving the 2 gm dose of *metronidazole*.

 TRICHOTILLOMANIA

Comment: Trichotillomania is on the obsessive-compulsive spectrum within the larger DS-5 category, Anxiety Disorders, and depression is frequently a co-morbid disorder. Hence, medications used to treat OCD can be helpful in treating trichotillomania. Recommended psychotropic agents include *clomipramine* (**Anafranil**) and *fluvoxamine* (**Luvox**). Other medications that research suggests may have some benefit include the SSRIs *fluoxetine* (**Prozac**), *sertraline* (**Zoloft**), *paroxetine* (**Paxil**), the mood stabilizer *lithium carbonate* (**Lithobid, Eskalith**), the OTC supplement **N-acetylcysteine**, an amino acid that influences neurotransmitters related to mood, **olanzapine** (**Zyprexa**), an atypical anti-psychotic, and *valproate* (**Depakote**), an anticonvulsant.

TRICYCLIC ANTIDEPRESSANT (TCA) COMBINATIONS

▷ *clomipramine* (C)(G) initially 25 mg daily in divided doses; gradually increase to 100 mg during first 2 weeks; max 250 mg/day; total maintenance dose may be given at HS
  Pediatric: <10 years: not recommended; ≥10 years: initially 25 mg daily in divided doses; gradually increase; max 3 mg/kg or 100 mg, whichever is smaller
    Anafranil *Cap:* 25, 50, 75 mg

SELECTIVE SEROTONIN REUPTAKE INHIBITORS (SSRIs)

▷ *fluoxetine* (C)(G)
    Prozac initially 20 mg daily; may increase after 1 week; doses >20 mg/day should be divided into AM and noon doses; max 80 mg/day
    Pediatric: <8 years: not recommended; 8-17 years: initially 10 mg/day; may increase after 1 week to 20 mg/day; range 20-60 mg/day; range for lower weight children, 20-30 mg/day
        Cap: 10, 20, 40 mg; *Tab:* 30*, 60*mg; *Oral soln:* 20 mg/5 ml (4 oz) (mint)
    Prozac Weekly following daily fluoxetine therapy at 20 mg/day for 13 weeks, may initiate **Prozac Weekly** 7 days after the last 20 mg fluoxetine dose
    Pediatric: <12 years: not recommended; ≥12 years: same as adult
        Cap: 90 mg ent-coat del-rel pellets
▷ *fluvoxamine* (C)(G)
Comment: fluvoxamine has a specific FDA indication for OCD.
    Luvox initially 50 mg q HS; adjust in 50 mg increments at 4-7 day intervals; range 100-300 mg/day; over 100 mg/day, divide into 2 doses giving the larger dose at HS
    Pediatric: <8 years: not recommended; 8-17 years: initially 25 mg q HS; adjust in 25 mg increments q 4-7 days; usual range 50-200 mg/day; over 50 mg/day, divide into 2 doses giving the larger dose at HS; >17 years: same as adult
        Tab: 25, 50*, 100*mg
    Luvox CR initially 100 mg once daily at HS; may increase by 50 mg increments at 1 week intervals; max 300 mg/day; swallow whole
    Pediatric: <18 years: not recommended; ≥18 years: same as adult
        Cap: 100, 150 mg ext-rel
▷ *paroxetine maleate* (D)(G)
    Pediatric: <12 years: not recommended; ≥12 years: same as adult
    Paxil initially 20 mg daily in AM; may increase by 10 mg/day at weekly intervals as needed; max 60 mg/day
        Tab: 10*, 20*, 30, 40 mg
    Paxil CR initially 25 mg daily in AM; may increase by 12.5 mg at weekly intervals as needed; max 62.5 mg/day
        Tab: 12.5, 25, 37.5 mg cont-rel ent-coat
    Paxil Suspension initially 20 mg daily in AM; may increase by 10 mg/day at weekly intervals as needed; max 60 mg/day
        Oral susp: 10 mg/5 ml (250 ml) (orange)
▷ *paroxetine mesylate* (D)(G) <12 years: not recommended; ≥12 years: initially 7.5 mg daily in AM; may increase by 10 mg/day at weekly intervals as needed; max 60 mg/day
    Brisdelle *Cap:* 7.5 mg
▷ *sertraline* (C)(G) initially 50 mg daily; increase at 1 week intervals if needed; max 200 mg daily; dilute oral concentrate immediately prior to administration in 4 oz water, ginger ale, lemon-lime soda, lemonade, or orange juice
    Pediatric: <6 years: not recommended; 6-12 years: initially 25 mg daily; max 200 mg/day; 13-17 years: initially 50 mg daily; max 200 mg/day; >17 years: same as adult
        Zoloft *Tab:* 25*, 50*, 100*mg; *Oral conc:* 20 mg per ml (60 ml) (alcohol 12%)

Lithium Salts Mood Stabilizer

▷ **lithium carbonate** (D)(G) swallow whole; *Usual maintenance:* 900-1200 mg/day in 2-3 divided doses
Pediatric: <12 years: not recommended; ≥12 years: same as adult
    Lithobid *Tab:* 300 mg slow-rel

Comment: Signs and symptoms of **lithium** toxicity can occur below 2 mEq/L and include blurred vision, tinnitus, weakness, dizziness, nausea, abdominal pains, vomiting, diarrhea to (severe) hand tremors, ataxia, muscle twitches, nystagmus, seizures, slurred speech, decreased level of consciousness, coma, death.

Valproate Mood Stabilizer

▷ **divalproex sodium** (D)(G) take once daily; swallow ext-rel form whole; initially 25 mg/kg/day in divided doses; max 60 mg/kg/day; *Elderly:* reduce initial dose and titrate slowly
Pediatric: <12 years: not recommended; ≥12 years: same as adult
    Depakene *Cap:* 250 mg; *Syr:* 250 mg/5 ml (16 oz)
    Depakote *Tab:* 125, 250 mg
    Depakote ER *Tab:* 250, 500 mg ext-rel
    Depakote Sprinkle *Cap:* 125 mg

ANTIPSYCHOTIC

▷ **olanzapine** (C) initially 2.5-10 mg daily; increase to 10 mg/day within a few days; then by 5 mg/day at weekly intervals; max 20 mg/day
    Zyprexa *Tab:* 2.5, 5, 7.5, 10 mg
    Zyprexa Zydis *ODT:* 5, 10, 15, 20 mg (phenylalanine)

◯ TRIGEMINAL NEURALGIA (TIC DOULOUREUX)

ANTICONVULSANTS

▷ **baclofen** (C)(G) initially 5-10 mg tid with food; usual dose 10-80 mg/day
Pediatric: <12 years: not recommended; ≥12 years: same as adult
    Lioresal *Tab:* 10*, 20*mg

Comment: Potential for seizures <u>or</u> hallucinations on abrupt withdrawal of **baclofen**.

▷ **carbamazepine** (C)
    Carbatrol initially 200 mg bid; may increase weekly as needed by 200 mg/day; usual maintenance 800 mg-1.2 gm/day
    Pediatric: <12 years: max <35 mg/kg/day; use ext-rel form above 400 mg/day; 12-15 years: max 1 gm/day in 2 divided doses; >15 years: usual maintenance 1.2 gm/day in 2 divided doses
        Cap: 200, 300 mg ext-rel
    Tegretol (G) initially 100 mg bid <u>or</u> 1/2 tsp susp qid; may increase dose by 100 mg q 12 hours <u>or</u> by 1/2 tsp susp q 6 hours; usual maintenance 400-800 mg/day; max 1200 mg/day
    Pediatric: <6 years: initially 10-20 mg/kg/day in 2 divided doses; increase weekly as needed in 3-4 divided doses; max 35 mg/kg/day in 3-4 divided doses; ≥6 years: initially 100 mg bid; increase weekly as needed by 100 mg/day in 3-4 divided doses; max 1 gm/day in 3-4 divided doses
        Tab: 200*mg; *Chew tab:* 100*mg; *Oral susp:* 100 mg/5 ml (450 ml) (citrus-vanilla)
    Tegretol XR (G) initially 200 mg bid; may increase weekly by 200 mg/day in 2 divided doses

> *Pediatric:* <6 years: use other forms; ≥6 years: initially 100 mg bid; may increase weekly by 100 mg/day in 2 divided doses; max 1 gm/day
>> *Tab:* 100, 200, 400 mg ext-rel

▷ *clonazepam* (D)(IV)(G) initially 0.25 mg bid; increase to 1 mg/day after 3 days
Pediatric: <10 years, <30 kg: initially 0.1-0.3 mg/kg/day; may increase up to 0.05 mg/kg/day bid-tid; usual maintenance 0.1-0.2 mg/kg/day tid
>> **Klonopin** *Tab:* 0.5*, 1, 2 mg
>> **Klonopin Wafers** dissolve in mouth with <u>or</u> without water
>>> *Wafer:* 0.125, 0.25, 0.5, 1, 2 mg orally-disint

▷ *divalproex sodium* (D) initially 250 mg bid; gradually increase to max 1000 mg/day if needed
Pediatric: <10 years: not recommended; ≥10 years: same as adult
>> **Depakene** *Cap:* 250 mg; *Syr:* 250 mg/5 ml
>> **Depakote** *Tab:* 125, 250 mg
>> **Depakote ER** *Tab:* 250, 500 mg ext-rel
>> **Depakote Sprinkle** *Cap:* 125 mg

▷ *phenytoin* (D) 400 mg/day in divided doses
>> **Dilantin** *Cap:* 30, 100 mg; *Oral susp:* 125 mg/5 ml (8 oz); *Infatab:* 50 mg

Comment: Monitor *phenytoin* serum levels. Therapeutic serum level: 10-20 gm/ml. Side effects include gingival hyperplasia.

▷ *valproic acid* (D) initially 15 mg/kg/day; may increase weekly by 5-10 mg/kg/day; max 60 mg/kg/day <u>or</u> 250 mg/day
>> **Depakene** *Cap:* 250 mg; *Syr:* 250 mg/5 ml

TRICYCLIC ANTIDEPRESSANTS (TCAs)

Comment: Co-administration of TCAs with SSRIs requires extreme caution.

▷ *amitriptyline* (C)(G) titrate to achieve pain relief; max 300 mg/day
Pediatric: <12 years: not recommended; ≥12 years: same as adult
>> *Tab:* 10, 25, 50, 75, 100, 150 mg

▷ *amoxapine* (C) titrate to achieve pain relief; if total dose exceeds 300 mg/day, give in divided doses; max 400 mg/day
Pediatric: <12 years: not recommended; ≥12 years: same as adult
>> *Tab:* 25, 50, 100, 150 mg

▷ *desipramine* (C)(G) titrate to achieve pain relief; max 300 mg/day
Pediatric: <12 years: not recommended; ≥12 years: same as adult
>> **Norpramin** *Tab:* 10, 25, 50, 75, 100, 150 mg

▷ *doxepin* (C)(G) titrate to achieve pain relief; max 150 mg/day
Pediatric: <12 years: not recommended; ≥12 years: same as adult
>> *Cap:* 10, 25, 50, 75, 100, 150 mg; *Oral conc:* 10 mg/ml (4 oz w. dropper)

▷ *imipramine* (C)(G)
Pediatric: <12 years: not recommended; ≥12 years: same as adult
>> **Tofranil** titrate to achieve pain relief; max 200 mg/day; adolescents max 100 mg/day; if maintenance dose exceeds 75 mg/day, may switch to **Tofranil PM** at bedtime
>>> *Tab:* 10, 25, 50 mg
>> **Tofranil PM** titrate to achieve pain relief; initially 75 mg at HS; max 200 mg at HS
>>> *Cap:* 75, 100, 125, 150 mg
>> **Tofranil Injection** 50 mg IM; lower dose for adolescents; switch to oral form as soon as possible
>>> *Amp:* 25 mg/2 ml (2 ml)

▷ *nortriptyline* (D)(G) titrate to achieve pain relief; initially 10-25 mg tid-qid; max 150 mg/day; lower doses for elderly and adolescents
Pediatric: <12 years: not recommended; ≥12 years: same as adult

　　　Pamelor titrate to achieve pain relief; max 150 mg/day
　　　　Cap: 10, 25, 50, 75 mg; *Oral soln:* 10 mg/5 ml (16 oz)
▷ *protriptyline* (C) titrate to achieve pain relief; initially 5 mg tid; max 60 mg/day
　　Pediatric: <12 years: not recommended; ≥12 years: same as adult
　　　Vivactil *Tab:* 5, 10 mg
▷ *trimipramine* (C) titrate to achieve pain relief; max 200 mg/day
　　Pediatric: <12 years: not recommended; ≥12 years: same as adult
　　　Surmontil *Cap:* 25, 50, 100 mg

TUBERCULOSIS (TB): PULMONARY (*MYCOBACTERIUM TUBERCULOSIS*)

SCREENING

▷ *purified protein derivative (PPD)* (C) 0.1 ml intradermally; examine inoculation site for induration at 48 to 72 hours.
　Pediatric: same as adult
　　Aplisol, Tubersol *Soln:* 5 US units/0.1 ml (1, 5 ml)

PROPHYLAXIS VACCINE

The only tuberculosis vaccine uses attenuation of the related organism *Mycobacterium bovis* by culture in bile-containing media to create the *Bacillus Calmette-Guerin* (BCG) vaccination strain. It was first used experimentally in 1921 by Albert Calmette and Camille Guerin and is currently in widespread use outside of the United States. It is not available in the US. The BCG vaccine protects newborns against tuberculosis-related meningitis and other systemic tuberculosis infections, but it has limited protection against active pulmonary disease. Once vaccinated, the patient will be PPD positive.

ANTI-TUBERCULAR AGENTS

Comment: Avoid *streptomycin* in pregnancy. *pyridoxine* (*vitamin B6*) 25 mg once daily x 6 months should be administered concomitantly with *INH* for prevention of side effects. *rifapentine* produces red-orange discoloration of body tissues and body fluids and may stain contact lenses.
▷ *bedaquiline* (B)(G)
　　Sirturo *Tab:* 100 mg
Comment: *bedaquiline* is a diarylquinoline antimycobacterial ATP synthase for the treatment of pulmonary multi-drug resistant TB (MDR-TB).
▷ *ethambutol (EMB)* (B)(G)
　　Myambutol *Tab:* 100, 400*mg
▷ *isoniazid (INH)* (C) *Tab:* 300*mg
▷ *pyrazinamide (PZA)* (C) *Tab:* 500*mg
▷ *rifampin (RIF)* (C)(G)
　　Rifadin, Rimactane *Cap:* 150, 300 mg
▷ *rifapentine* (C)
　　Priftin *Tab:* 150 mg (24, 32 pck)
Comment: The 32-count packs of **Priftin** are intended for patients with active tuberculosis infection (TB). The 24-count packs are are intended for patients with latent tuberculosis infection (LTBI) who are at high risk for progression to tuberculosis disease. **Priftin** for active TB is indicated for patients ≥12 years-of-age. **Priftin** for LTBI is indicated for patients ≥2 years-of-age.
▷ *rilpivirine* (C) *Tab:* 25 mg
　　Rifabutin *Cap:* 150 mg
▷ *streptomycin (SM)* (C)(G) *Amp:* 1 gm/2.5 ml <u>or</u> 400 mg/ml (2.5 ml)

COMBINATION AGENTS

▷ *rifampin+isoniazid* (C)
    Rifamate *Cap: rif* 300 mg+*iso* 150 mg
▷ *rifampin+isoniazid+pyrazinamide* (C)
    Rifater *Tab: rif* 120 mg+*iso* 50 mg+*pyr* 300 mg

PROPHYLAXIS AFTER EXPOSURE TO TUBERCULOSIS, WITH NEGATIVE PPD

▷ *isoniazid* (C) 300 mg once daily in a single dose x at least 6 months
    Pediatric: 10-20 mg/kg/day x 9 months

PROPHYLAXIS AFTER EXPOSURE, WITH NEW PPD CONVERSION

▷ *isoniazid* (C) 300 mg once daily in a single dose x 12 months
    Pediatric: 10-20 mg/kg/day x 9 months
    Tab: 100, 300*mg; *Syr:* 50 mg/5 ml; *Inj:* 100 mg/ml
▷ *rifampin* (C) 600 mg once daily + *isoniazid* (C) 300 mg once daily x 4 months
    Pediatric: *rifampin* (C) 10-20 mg/kg + *isoniazid* (C) 10-20 mg/kg once daily x 4 months
▷ *rifapentine* (C) 600 mg once weekly + *isoniazid* (C) 300 mg once weekly x 12 weeks
    Pediatric: ≤12 years: Treat x 12 weeks; 10-14 kg: *rifapentine* (C) 300 mg once weekly
    + *isoniazid* (C) 25 mg/kg (max 900 mg) once weekly; 14.1-25 kg: *rifapentine* (C) 450
    mg once weekly + *isoniazid* (C) 25 mg/kg (max 900 mg) once weekly; 25.1-32 kg:
    rifapentine (C) 600 mg once weekly + *isoniazid* (C) 25 mg/kg (max 900 mg) once
    weekly; 32.1-50 kg: *rifapentine* (C) 750 mg once weekly + *isoniazid* (C) 25 mg/kg
    (max 900 mg) once weekly; >50 kg: *rifapentine* (C) 900 mg once weekly + *isoniazid*
    (C) 25 mg/kg (max 900 mg) once weekly; >12 years: same as adult

TREATMENT REGIMENS (≥12 YEARS)

Regimen 1

▷ *rifampin* (C) 600 mg + *isoniazid* (C) 300 mg + *pyrazinamide* (C) 2 gm + *ethambutol*
    (C) 15-25 mg/kg <u>or</u> *streptomycin* (C) 1 gm once daily x 8 weeks; then *isoniazid* (C)
    300 mg + *rifampin* (C) 600 mg once daily x 16 weeks <u>or</u> *isoniazid* 900 mg + *rifampin*
    (C) 600 mg 2-3 x/week x 16 weeks

Regimen 2

▷ *rifampin* 600 mg + *isoniazid* 300 mg + *pyrazinamide* 2 gm + *ethambutol* 15-25 mg/
    kg <u>or</u> *streptomycin* 1 gm once daily x 2 weeks; then *rifampin* 600 mg + *isoniazid* 900
    mg + *pyrazinamide* 4 gm + *ethambutol* 50 mg/kg <u>or</u> *streptomycin* 1.5 gm 2 x/week x
    6 weeks; then *isoniazid* 300 mg + *rifampin* 600 mg once daily x 16 weeks <u>or</u> 2 x/week
    x 16 weeks *rifampin* 600 mg once daily x 16 weeks <u>or</u> 2 x/week x 16 weeks

Regimen 3

▷ *rifampin* 600 mg + *isoniazid* 900 mg + *pyrazinamide* 3 gm + *ethambutol* 25-30 mg/
    kg <u>or</u> *streptomycin* 1.5 gm 3 x/week x 6 months

Regimen 4 (for smear and culture negative for pulmonary TB in adult)

▷ Options 1, 2, <u>or</u> 3 x 8 weeks; then *isoniazid* 300 mg + *rifampin* 600 mg once daily x 16
    weeks; then *rifampin* 600 mg + *isoniazid* 300 mg + *pyrazinamide* 2 gm + *ethambutol*
    15-25 mg/kg <u>or</u> *streptomycin* 1 gm once daily x 8 weeks <u>or</u> 2-3 x/week x 8 weeks

Regimen 5 (for smear and culture negative for pulmonary TB in adult)

▷ *rifapentine* 600 mg twice weekly x 2 months (at least 72 hours between doses) +
    once daily *isoniazid* 300 mg, *ethambutol* 15-25 mg/kg + *pyrazinamide* 2 gm; then
    rifapentine 600 mg once weekly x 4 months + once daily *isoniazid* 300 mg + another
    appropriate anti-tuberculosis agent for susceptible organisms

Regimen 6 (when pyrazinamide is contraindicated)

▷ *rifampin* 600 mg + *isoniazid* 300 mg + *ethambutol* 15-25 mg/kg + *streptomycin* 1 gm once daily x 4-8 weeks; then *isoniazid* 300 mg + *rifampin* 600 mg once daily x 24 weeks or 2 x/week x 24 weeks

PEDIATRIC TREATMENT REGIMENS (<12 YEARS)

Regimen 1

▷ *rifampin* 10-20 mg/kg + *isoniazid* 10-20 mg/kg + *pyrazinamide* 15-20 mg/kg + *ethambutol* 15-25 mg/kg or *streptomycin* 20-40 mg/kg once daily x 8 weeks; then *isoniazid* 10-20 mg/kg + *rifampin* 10-20 mg/kg once daily x 16 weeks or *isoniazid* 20-40 mg/kg + *rifampin* 10-20 mg/kg 2-3 x/week x 16 weeks

Regimen 2

▷ *rifampin* 10-20 mg/kg + *isoniazid* 10-20 mg/kg + *pyrazinamide* 15-30 mg/kg + *ethambutol* 15-25 mg/kg or *streptomycin* 20-40 mg/kg once daily x 2 weeks; then *rifampin* 10-20 mg/kg + *isoniazid* 20-40 mg/kg + *pyrazinamide* 50-70 mg/kg + *ethambutol* 50 mg/kg or *streptomycin* 25-30 mg/kg 2 x/week x 6 weeks; then *isoniazid* 10-20 mg/kg + *rifampin* 10-20 mg/kg once daily x 16 weeks or *rifampin* 10-20 mg/kg + *isoniazid* 20-40 mg/kg 2 x/week x 16 weeks

Regimen 3

▷ *rifampin* 10-20 mg/kg + *isoniazid* 20-40 mg/kg + *pyrazinamide* 50-70 mg/kg + *ethambutol* 25-30 mg/kg or *streptomycin* 25-30 mg/kg 3 x/week x 6 months

Regimen 4 (when pyrazinamide is contraindicated)

▷ *rifampin* 10-20 mg/kg + *isoniazid* 10-20 mg/kg + *ethambutol* 15-25 mg/kg + *streptomycin* 20-40 mg/kg once daily x 4-8 weeks; then *isoniazid* 10-20 mg/kg + *rifampin* 10-20 mg/kg once daily x 24 weeks or *rifampin* 10-20 mg/kg + *isoniazid* 20-40 mg/kg 2 x/week x 24 weeks

POLYPEPTIDE ANTIBIOTIC ISOLATED FROM STREPTOMYCES CAPREOLUS

Comment: *capreomycin sulfate* is a complex of 4 microbiologically active components which have been characterized in part; however, complete structural determination of all the components has not been established. **Capastat Sulfate**, which is to be used concomitantly with other appropriate anti-tuberculosis agents, is indicated in pulmonary infections caused by *capreomycin*-susceptible strains of *M. tuberculosis* when the primary agents (i.e., *isoniazid*, *rifampin*, *ethambutol*, *aminosalicylic acid*, and *streptomycin*) have been ineffective or cannot be used because of toxicity or the presence of resistant tubercle bacilli.

▷ *capreomycin sulfate* (C)(G) may be administered deep IM in a large muscle mass after reconstitution with 2 ml 0.9%NS or sterile water or via IV infusion over 60 minutes after reconstitution and dilution in 100 ml 0.9%NS; usual dose is 1 gm daily (not to exceed 20 mg/kg/day) via IM or IV infusion for 60 to 120 days; see mfr pkg insert for dosage table based on kg body weight and toute of administration
Pediatric: <18 years: not recommended; ≥18 years: same as adult

  Capastat *Vial:* 1 gm pwdr for reconstitution with 2 ml 0.9%NS or sterile water
Comment: Black Box Warning (BBW): The use of *capreomycin sulfate* in patients with renal insufficiency or preexisting auditory impairment must be undertaken with great caution, and the risk of additional cranial nerve VIII impairment or renal injury should be weighed against the benefits to be derived from therapy. Since other parenteral antituberculosis agents (e.g., *streptomycin*, *viomycin*) also have similar

and sometimes irreversible toxic effects, particularly on cranial nerve VIII and renal function, simultaneous administration of these agents with **Capastat Sulfate** is not recommended. Use with non-antituberculosis drugs (e.g., *polymyxin A sulfate, colistin sulfate, amikacin, gentamicin, tobramycin, vancomycin, kanamycin*, and *neomycin*) having ototoxic or nephrotoxic potential should be undertaken only with great caution. Audiometric measurements and assessment of vestibular function should be performed prior to initiation of therapy with **Capastat Sulfate** and at regular intervals during treatment. Renal injury, with tubular necrosis, elevation of the blood urea nitrogen (BUN) or serum creatinine, and abnormal urinary sediment, has been noted. Slight elevation of the BUN and serum creatinine (sCr) has been observed in a significant number of patients receiving prolonged therapy. The appearance of casts, red cells, and white cells in the urine has been noted in a high percentage of these cases. The safety of the use of **Capastat Sulfate** in pregnancy has not been determined. Safety and effectiveness in pediatric patients have not been established. It is not known whether this drug is excreted in human milk.

 TYPE 1 DIABETES MELLITUS

Comment: Target glycosylated hemoglobin (HbA1c) is <7%. Addition of daily ACE-I and/or ARB therapy is strongly recommended for renal protection. Insulin may be indicated in the management of Type 2 diabetes with or without concomitant oral anti-diabetic agents.

TREATMENT FOR ACUTE HYPOGLYCEMIA

➤ *glucagon (recombinant)* (B) administer SC, IM, or IV; if patient does not respond in 15 minutes, may administer a single dose or 2 divided doses; <20 kg: 0.5 mg or 20-30 mg/kg; ≥20 kg: 1 mg
Pediatric: same as adult

INHALED INSULIN
Rapid-Acting Inhalation Powder Insulin

➤ *insulin human (inhaled)* (C) one inhaler may be used for up to 15 days, then discard; dose at meal times as follows: *Insulin naïve:* initially 4 units at each meal; adjust according to blood glucose monitoring
Conversion from SC to inhaled mealtime insulin:
SC 1-4 units: inhal 4 units
SC 5-8 units: inhal 8 units
SC 9-12 units: inhal 12 units
SC 13-16 units: inhal 16 units
SC 17-20 units: inhal 20 units
SC 21-24 units: inhal 24 units
Pediatric: <18 years: not established; ≥18 years: same as adult
    Afrezza Inhalation Powder administer at the beginning of the meal; *Mealtime insulin naïve:* initially 4 units at each meal; *Using SC prandial insulin:* convert dose to **Afrezza** using a conversion table (see mfr pkg insert); *Using SC pre-mixed:* divide 1/2 of total daily injected pre-mixed insulin equally among 3 meals of the day; administer 1/2 total injected pre-mixed dose as once daily injected basal insulin dose
      Inhal: 4, 8, 12 unit single-inhalation color-coded cartridges (30, 60, 90/pkg w. 2 disposable inhalers)

Comment: **Afrezza** is not a substitute for long-acting insulin. **Afrezza** must be used in combination with long-acting insulin in patients with T1DM. **Afrezza** is not recommended for the treatment of diabetic ketoacidosis. **Afrezza** is contraindicated with chronic lung disease because of the risk of acute bronchospasm. The use of **Afrezza** is not recommended in patients who smoke or who have recently stopped smoking. Each card contains 5 blister strips with 3 cartridges each (total 15 cartridges). The doses are color-coded. **Afrezza** is contraindicated with chronic respiratory disease (e.g., asthma, COPD) and patients prone to episodes of hypoglycemia.

INJECTABLE INSULINS

Rapid-Acting Insulins

▷ *insulin aspart (recombinant)* **(B)** onset <15 minutes; peak 1-3 hours; duration 3-5 hours; administer 5-10 minutes prior to a meal; SC or infusion pump or IV infusion
Pediatric: <3 years: not recommended; ≥3 years: same as adult
   NovoLog *Vial:* 100 U/ml (10 ml); *PenFill cartridge:* 100 U/ml (3 ml, 5/pck) (zinc, m-cresol)

▷ *insulin glulisine (rDNA origin)* **(C)** onset <15 minutes; peak 1 hour; duration 2-4 hours; administer up to 15 minutes before, or within 20 minutes after starting a meal; use with an intermediate or long-acting insulin; SC only; may administer via insulin pump; do not dilute or mix with other insulin in pump
Pediatric: <4 years: not recommended; ≥4 years: same as adult
   Apidra *Vial:* 100 U/ml (10 ml); *Cartridge:* 100 U/ml (3 ml, 5/pck; m-cresol)

▷ *insulin lispro (recombinant)* **(B)** onset <15 minutes; peak 1 hour; duration 3.5-4.5 hours; administer up to 15 minutes before, or immediately after, a meal; SC or IV infusion pump only
Pediatric: <3 years: not recommended; ≥3 years: same as adult
   Admelog *Vial:* 100 U/ml (10 ml) (zinc, m-cresol); *Prefilled disposable SoloStar pen (disposable):* 100 U/ml (3 ml) (5/pck) (zinc, m-cresol)
   Humalog *Vial:* 100 U/ml (10 ml); *Prefilled disposable KwikPen:* 100 U/ml (3 ml, 5/pck) (zinc, m-cresol); *HumaPen Memoir* and *HumaPen Luxura HD* inj device for *Humulog cartridges* (100 U/ml, 3 ml 5/pck) (zinc, m-cresol)

▷ *insulin regular* **(B)**
   Humulin R U-100 *(human, recombinant)* **(OTC)** onset 30 minutes; peak 2-4 hours; duration up to 6-8 hours; SC or IV or IM
      Vial: 100 U/ml (10 ml)
   Humulin R U-500 *(human, recombinant)* onset 30 minutes; peak 1.75-4 hours; duration up to 24 hours; SC only; for in-hospital use only
      Vial: 500 U/ml (20 ml); *KwikPen:* 3 ml (2, 5/carton)

Comment: **Humulin R U-500** formulation is 5 times more concentrated than standard U-100 concentration, indicated for adults and children who require ≥200 units of insulin/day, allowing patients to inject 80% less liquid to receive the desired dose. Recommend using U-500 syringe (BD, Eli Lilly). The U-500 syringe (0.5 ml, 6 mm x 31 gauge) is marked in 5 unit increments and allows for dosing up to 250 units.

   Iletin II Regular *(pork)* **(OTC)** onset 30 minutes; peak 2-4 hours; duration 6-8 hours; SC, IV or IM
      Vial: 100 U/ml (10 ml)
   Novolin R *(human)* **(OTC)** onset 30 minutes; peak 2.5-5 hours; duration 8 hours; SC, IV, or IM
      Vial: 100 U/ml (10 ml); *PenFill cartridge:* 100 U/ml (1.5 ml, 5/pck); *Prefilled syringe:* 100 U/ml (1.5 ml, 5/pck)

▷ *pramlintide* *(amylin analog/amylinomimetic)* **(C)** administer immediately before major meals (≥250 kcal or ≥30 gm carbohydrates); initially 15 mcg; titrate in 15 mcg increments for 3 days if no significant nausea occurs; if nausea occurs at 45 or 60 mcg, reduce to 30 mcg; if not tolerated, consider discontinuing therapy; *Maintenance:* 60 mcg (30 mcg *only* if 60 mcg not tolerated)
   Symlin *Vial:* 0.6 mg/ml (5 ml) (m-cresol, mannitol)

Comment: **Symlin** is indicated as adjunct to mealtime insulin with or without a sulfo-nylurea and/or *metformin* when blood glucose control is suboptimal despite optimal insulin therapy. Do not mix with insulin. When initiating **Symlin**, reduce preprandial short/rapid-acting insulin dose by 50% and monitor pre- and post-prandial and bedtime blood glucose. Do not use in patients with poor compliance, HgbA1c is >9%, recurrent hypoglycemia requiring assistance in the previous 6 months, or if taking a prokinetic drug. With Type 2 DM, initial therapy is 60 mcg/dose and max is 120 mcg/dose.

RAPID-ACTING+INTERMEDIATE-ACTING INSULIN

Insulin Aspart Protamine Suspension+Insulin Aspart Combinations

▷ *insulin aspart protamine suspension 70%/insulin aspart 30% (recombinant)* (B)(G) onset 15 min; peak 2.4 hours; duration up to 24 hours; SC only
Pediatric: not recommended
NovoLog Mix 70/30 (OTC) *Vial:* 100 U/ml (10 ml)
NovoLog Mix 70/30 FlexPen (OTC) *Prefilled disposable pen:* 100 U/ml (3 ml, 5/pck); *PenFill cartridge:* 100 U/ml (3 ml, 5/pck)

LONG-ACTING INSULINS

▷ *insulin detemir (human)* (B) administer SC once daily with evening meal or at HS as a basal insulin; may administer twice daily (AM/PM); administer in the deltoid, abdomen, or thigh; onset 1-2 hours; peak 6-8 hours; duration 24 hours; switching from another basal insulin, dose should be the same on a unit-to-unit basis; may need more *insulin detemir* when switching from **NPH**; *Type 1:* starting dose 1/3 of total daily insulin requirements; rapid-acting or short-acting, pre-meal insulin should be used to satisfy the remainder of daily insulin requirements; *Type 2 (inadequately controlled on oral antidiabetic agents):* initially 10 units or 0.1-0.2 units/kg, once daily in the evening or divided twice daily (AM/PM); do not add-mix or dilute *insulin detemir* with other insulins.
Pediatric: <2 years: not recommended; ≥2 years: same as adult
Levemir *Vial:* 100 U/ml (10 ml); *FlexPen:* 100 U/ml (3 ml, 5/pck; (zinc, m-cresol)
▷ *insulin glargine (recombinant)* (C)
Basaglar administer SC once daily, at the same time each day, as a basal insulin in the deltoid, abdomen, or thigh; onset 1-1.5 hours, no pronounced peak, duration 20-24 hours; *T1DM (adults and children >6 years-of-age):* initially 1/3 of total daily insulin dose; administer the remainder of the total dose as short- or rapid-acting pre-prandial insulin; *T2DM (adults only):* initially 2 units/kilogram or up to 10 units once daily; *Switching from once daily insulin glargine 300 units/ml (i.e., Toujeo) to 100 units/ml:* initially 80% of the insulin glargine 300 units/ml; *Switching from twice daily NPH:* initially 80% of the total daily NPH dose; do not add-mix or dilute *insulin glargine* with other insulins.
Pediatric: <6 years: not established; ≥6 years: individualize and adjust as needed
Prefilled KwikPen (disposable), 100 U/ml (3 ml) (5/carton) (m-cresol)
Lantus administer SC once daily at the same time each day as a basal insulin; onset 1-1.5 hours, no pronounced peak, duration 20-24 hours; initial average starting dose 10 units for insulin-naïve patients; *Switching from once daily NPH or Ultralente insulin:* initial dose of *insulin glargine* should be on a unit-for-unit basis; *Switching from twice daily NPH insulin:* start at 20% lower than the total daily **NPH** dose
Pediatric: <6 years: not recommended; ≥6 years: same as adult
Vial: 100 U/ml (10 ml); *Cartridge:* 100 U/ml (3 ml, for use in the *OptiPen One Insulin Delivery Device*) (5/carton) (m-cresol); *SoloStar pen (disposable):* 100 U/ml (3 ml) (5/carton)
Toujeo administer SC once daily at the same time each day as a basal insulin; in the upper arm, abdomen, or thigh; onset of action 6 hours; duration 20-24 hours;

T2DM, insulin naïve: initially 0.2 units/kg; titrate every 3-4 days; *T1DM, insulin naïve:* initially 1/3-1/2 total daily insulin dose; remainder as short-acting insulin divided between each meal; *Switch from once daily long- or intermediate-acting insulin:* on a unit-for-unit basis; *Switching from **Lantus:*** a higher daily dose is expected; *Switching from twice daily **NPH:*** reduce initial dose by 20% of total daily NPH dose
> *Pediatric:* <18 years: not established; ≥18 years: same as adult
>> *Soln for SC injection:* 300 units/ml prefilled disposable SoloStar Pen (1.5 ml, 3-5/carton)

▷ **insulin isophane suspension (NPH)** (B)
> *Pediatric:* <18 years: not recommended; ≥18 years: same as adult
>> **Humulin N** *(human, recombinant)* **(OTC)** onset 1-2 hours; peak 6-12 hours; duration 18-24 hours; SC only
>>> *Vial:* 100 U/ml (10 ml); *Prefilled disposable pen:* 100 U/ml (3 ml, 5/pck)
>> **Novolin N** *(recombinant)* **(OTC)** onset 1.5 hours; peak 4-12 hours; duration 24 hours; SC only
>>> *Vial:* 100 U/ml (10 ml); *PenFill cartridge:* 1.5 ml (5/pck); *KwikPens:* 1.5 ml (5/pck)
>> **Iletin II NPH** *(pork)* **(OTC)** onset 1-2 hours; peak 6-12 hours; duration 18-26 hours; SC only
>>> *Vial:* 100 U/ml (10 ml)

▷ **insulin zinc suspension** *(lente)* (B)
> *Pediatric:* <18 years: not recommended; ≥18 years: same as adult
>> **Humulin L** *(human)* **(OTC)** onset 1-3 hours; peak 6-12 hours; duration 18-24 hours; SC only
>>> *Vial:* 100 U/ml (10 ml)
>> **Iletin II Lente** *(pork)* **(OTC)** onset 1-3 hours; peak 6-12 hours; duration 18-26 hours; SC only
>>> *Vial:* 100 U/ml (10 ml)
>> **Novolin L** *(human)* **(OTC)** onset 2.5 hours; peak 7-15 hours; duration 22 hours; SC only
>>> *Vial:* 100 U/ml (10 ml)

Ultra Long-Acting Insulin

▷ **insulin degludec (insulin analog)** (C) administer by SC injection once daily at any time of day, with or without food, into the upper arm, abdomen, or thigh; titrate every 3-4 days; *Insulin naïve with type 1 diabetes:* initially 1/3-1/2 of total daily insulin dose, usually 0.2-0.4 units/kg; administer the remainder of the total dose as short-acting insulin divided between each daily meal; *Insulin naive with type 2 diabetes:* initially 10 units once daily; adjust dose of concomitant oral antidiabetic agent; *Already on insulin (type 1 or type 2):* initiate at same unit dose as total daily long- or intermediate-acting insulin unit dose
> *Pediatric:* <1 year: not established; ≥1 year: same as adult
>> **Tresiba FlexTouch** *Pen:* 100 U/ml (3 ml, 5 pens/carton), 200 U/ml (3 ml, 3 pens/carton) (zinc, m-cresol)

Comment: Tresiba U-200 FlexTouch is the only long-acting insulin in a 160-unit pen allowing up to 160 units in a single injection. The U-200 dose counter always shows the desired dose (i.e., no conversion from U/100 to U-200 is required)

▷ **insulin extended zinc suspension** *(Ultralente) (human)* (B) onset 4-6 hours; peak 8-20 hours; duration 24-48 hours; SC only
> *Pediatric:* <18 years: not recommended; ≥18 years: same as adult
>> **Humulin U (OTC)** *Vial:* 100 U/ml (10 ml)

Insulin Lispro Protamine+Insulin Lispro Combinations

▷ *insulin lispro protamine75%+insulin lispro 25% (B)*
　　Pediatric: <18 years: not recommended; ≥18 years: same as adult
　　　Humalog Mix 75/25 *(human)* onset 15 minutes; peak 30 minutes to 1 hour; duration 24 hours; SC only
　　　　Vial: 100 U/ml (10 ml); *Prefilled disposable KwikPen:* 100 U/ml (3 ml, 5/pck) (zinc, m-cresol); *HumaPen Memoir* and *HumaPen Luxura* HD inj device for *Humalog cartridges* (100 U/ml, 3 ml, 5/pck) (zinc, m-cresol)
▷ *insulin lispro protamine 50%+insulin lispro 50% (B)*
　　Pediatric: <18 years: not recommended; ≥18 years: same as adult
　　　Humalog Mix 50/50 *(recombinant)* **(B)** onset 15 minutes; peak 2.3 hours; range 1-5 hours; SC only
　　　　Vial: 100 U/ml (10 ml); *Prefilled disposable KwikPen:* 100 U/ml (3 ml, 5/pck) (zinc, m-cresol); *HumaPen Memoir* and *HumaPen LUXURA* HD inj device for *Humalog cartridges* (100 U/ml, 3 ml, 5/pck) (zinc, m-cresol)

Insulin Isophane Suspension (NPH)+Insulin Regular Combinations

▷ *NPH 70%+regular 30% (B)*
　　Pediatric: <18 years: not recommended; ≥18 years
　　　Humulin 70/30 *(human, recombinant)* **(OTC)** onset 30 minutes; peak 2-12 hours; duration up to 24 hours; SC only
　　　　Vial: 100 U/ml (10 ml)
　　　Novolin 70/30 *(recombinant)* **(OTC)** onset 30 minutes; peak 2-12 hours; duration up to 24 hours; SC only
　　　　Vial: 100 U/ml (10 ml)
▷ *NPH 50%+regular 50% (B)*
　　Pediatric: <18 years: not recommended; ≥18 years: same as adult
　　　Humulin 50/50 *(human)* **(OTC)** onset 30 minutes; peak 3-5 hours; duration up to 24 hours; SC only
　　　　Vial: 100 U/ml (10 ml)

Insulin Lispro Protamine+Insulin Lispro Combinations

▷ *insulin lispro protamine 75%+insulin lispro 25% (B)*
　　Pediatric: <18 years: not recommended; ≥18 years: same as adult
　　　Humalog Mix 75/25 *(recombinant)* onset 15 minutes; peak 30-90 minutes; duration 24 hours; SC only
　　　　Vial: 100 U/ml (10 ml); *Prefilled disposable KwikPen:* 100 U/ml (3 ml, 5/pck) (zinc, m-cresol); *HumaPen Memoir* and *HumaPen LUXURA* HD inj device for *Humalog cartridges* (100 U/ml, 3 ml 5/pck) (zinc, m-cresol)
▷ *insulin lispro protamine 50%+insulin lispro 50% (B)*
　　Pediatric: <18 years: not recommended; ≥18 years: same as adult
　　　Humalog Mix 50/50 *(recombinant)* onset 15 minutes; peak 1 hour; duration up to 16 hours; SC only
　　　　Vial: 100 U/ml (10 ml); *Prefilled disposable KwikPen:* 100 U/ml (3 ml, 5/pck) (zinc, m-cresol); *HumaPen Memoir* and *HumaPen LUXURA* HD inj device for *Humalog cartridges* (100 U/ml, 3 ml 5/pck) (zinc, m-cresol); U/ml (3 ml, 5/pck) (zinc, m-cresol); *HumaPen Memoir* and *HumaPen LUXURA* HD inj device for *Humalog cartridges* (100 U/ml, 3 ml 5/pck) (zinc, m-cresol); (100 U/ml, 3 ml 5/pck (zinc, m-cresol)

Basal Insulin+GLP-1 RA Combinations

▷ *insulin degludec (insulin analog)+liraglutide* **(C)** for treatment of type 2 diabetes only in adults inadequately controlled on <50 units of basal insulin daily or ≤1.8 mg of

liraglutide daily; administer by SC injection once daily, with or without food, into the upper arm, abdomen, or thigh; titrate every 3-4 days
Pediatric: <18 years: not recommended; ≥18 years: same as adult
Xultophy Prefilled pen: 100/3.6 U/ml (3 ml, 5 pens/carton)

▷ *insulin glargine (insulin analog)+lixisenatide* (C) for treatment of type 2 diabetes only in adults inadequately controlled on <60 units of basal insulin daily or *lixisenatide*; administer by SC injection once daily, with or without food, into the upper arm, abdomen, or thigh; titrate every 3-4 days
Pediatric: <18 years: not recommended; ≥18 years: same as adult
Soliqua Prefilled pen: 100/33 U/ml (3 ml, 5 pens/carton) covering 15-60 mg *insulin glargine* 100 units/ml and 15-20 mcg of *lixisenatide (m-cresol)*

TYPE 2 DIABETES MELLITUS

Comment: Normal fasting glucose is <100 mg/dL. Impaired glucose tolerance is a risk factor for type 2 diabetes and a marker for cardiovascular disease risk; it occurs early in the natural history of these two diseases. Impaired fasting glucose is >100 mg/dL and <125 mg/dL. Impaired glucose tolerance is OGTT, 2 hour post-load 75 gm glucose >140 mg/dL and <200 mg/dL. Target pre-prandial glucose is 80 mg/dL to 120 mg/dL. Target bedtime glucose is 100 mg/dL to 140 mg/dL. Target glycosylated hemoglobin (HbA1c) is <7.0%. Additional medications to be considered for initiation at onset of T2DM, particularly in the presence of hypertension, include an angiotensin-converting enzyme inhibitor (ACEI), angiotensin II receptor blocker (ARB), thiazide-like diuretic, or a calcium channel blocker (CCB). Consider diabetes screening at age 25 years for persons in high-risk groups (non-Caucasian, positive family history for DM, obesity). Hypertension and hyperlipidemia are common comorbid conditions. Macrovascular complications include cerebral vascular disease, coronary artery disease, and peripheral vascular disease. Microvascular complications include retinopathy, nephropathy, neuropathy, and cardiomyopathy. Oral hypoglycemics are contraindicated in pregnancy.

REFERENCE
American Diabetes Association. Standards of Medical Care in Diabetes—2017. *Diabetes Care.* 2017: 40(suppl 1), S1–S135

Insulins *see Type 1 Diabetes Mellitus page* 481

TREATMENT FOR ACUTE HYPOGLYCEMIA

▷ *glucagon (recombinant)* (B) administer SC, IM, or IV; if patient does not respond in 15 minutes, may administer a single or 2 divided doses
Adults and Children: <20 kg: 0.5 mg or 20-30 mg/kg; ≥20 kg: 1 mg

SULFONYLUREAS

Comment: Sulfonylureas are secretagogues (i.e., stimulate pancreatic insulin secretion); therefore, the patient taking a sulfonylurea should be alerted to the risk for hypoglycemia. Action is dependent on functioning beta cells in the pancreatic islets.

First Generation Sulfonylureas

▷ *chlorpropamide* (C)(G) initially 250 mg/day with breakfast; max 750 mg
Pediatric: <12 years: not recommended; ≥12 years: same as adult
Diabinese *Tab:* 100*, 250*mg

▷ *tolazamide* (C)(G) initially 100-250 mg/day with breakfast; increase by 100-250 mg/day at weekly intervals; maintenance 100 mg 1 gm/day; max 1 gm/day
Pediatric: <12 years: not recommended; ≥12 years: same as adult
Tolinase *Tab:* 100, 250, 500 mg
▷ *tolbutamide* (C) initially 1-2 gm in divided doses; max 2 gm/day
Pediatric: <12 years: not recommended; ≥12 years: same as adult
Tab: 500 mg

Second Generation Sulfonylureas

▷ *glimepiride* (C) initially 1-2 mg once daily with breakfast; after reaching dose of 2 mg, increase by 2 mg at 1-2 week intervals as needed; usual maintenance 1-4 mg once daily; max 8 mg/day
Pediatric: <12 years: not recommended; ≥12 years: same as adult
Amaryl *Tab:* 1*, 2*, 4*mg
▷ *glipizide* (C)(G)
Pediatric: <12 years: not recommended; ≥12 years: same as adult
Glucotrol initially 5 mg before breakfast; increase by 2.5-5 mg every few days if needed; max 15 mg/day; max 40 mg/day in divided doses
Tab: 5*, 10*mg
Glucotrol XL initially 5 mg with breakfast; usual range 5-10 mg/day; max 20 mg/day
Tab: 2.5, 5, 10 mg ext-rel
▷ *glyburide* (C)(G) initially 2.5-5 mg/day with breakfast; increase by 2.5 mg at weekly intervals; maintenance 1.25-20 mg/day in a single or 2 divided doses; max 20 mg/day
Pediatric: <12 years: not recommended; ≥12 years: same as adult
DiaBeta, Micronase *Tab:* 1.25*, 2.5*, 5*mg
▷ *glyburide, micronized* (B)
Pediatric: <12 years: not recommended; ≥12 years: same as adult
Glynase PresTab initially 1.5-3 mg/day with breakfast; increase by 1.5 mg at weekly intervals if needed; usual maintenance 0.75-12 mg/day in single or divided doses; max 12 mg/day
Tab: 1.5*, 3*, 6*mg

ALPHA-GLUCOSIDASE INHIBITORS

Comment: Alpha-glucosidase inhibitors block the enzyme that breaks down carbohydrates in the small intestine, delaying digestion and absorption of complex carbohydrates, and lowering peak post-prandial glycemic concentrations. Use as monotherapy or in combination with a sulfonylurea. Contraindicated in inflammatory bowel disease, colon ulceration, and intestinal obstruction. Side effects include flatulence, diarrhea, and abdominal pain.
▷ *acarbose* (B) initially 25 mg tid ac, increase at 4-8 week intervals; or initially 25 mg once daily, increase gradually to 25 mg tid; usual range 50-100 mg tid; max 100 mg tid
Pediatric: <12 years: not recommended; ≥12 years: same as adult
Precose *Tab:* 25, 50, 100 mg
▷ *miglitol* (B) initially 25 mg tid at the start of each main meal, titrated to 50 mg tid at the start of each main meal; max 100 mg tid
Pediatric: <12 years: not recommended; ≥12 years: same as adult
Glyset *Tab:* 25, 50, 100 mg

BIGUANIDE

Comment: The biguanides decrease gluconeogenesis by the liver in the presence of insulin. Action is dependent on the presence of circulating insulin. Lower hepatic glucose production leads to lower overnight, fasting, and pre-prandial plasma glucose levels. Common side effects include GI distress, nausea, vomiting, bloating, and flatulence which usually eventually resolve. May be used as monotherapy (in adults only) or with a sulfonylurea or insulin. The only biguanide is *metformin*.

▷ *metformin* (B)(G) take with meals

Comment: *metformin* is contraindicated with renal impairment, metabolic acidosis, ketoacidosis. *Metformin* is contraindicated in patients with decreased tissue perfusion or hemodynamic instability, alcohol abuse, advanced liver disease, acute unstable acute congestive heart failure, or any condition that may lead to lactic acidosis. Suspend *metformin*, prior to, and for 48 hours after, surgery or receiving IV iodinated contrast agents. *Metformin* is associates with weight loss. Clinicians should consider adding either a sulfonylurea, a thiazolidindione (TZD), an SGLT-2 inhibitor, or a DPP-4 inhibitor to metformin to improve glycemic control when a second oral therapy is considered.

Pediatric: <17 years: not recommended; ≥17 years: same as adult
Tab: 500, 1000 mg ext-rel

    Glucophage initially 500 mg bid; may increase by 500 mg/day at 1 week intervals; max 1 gm bid or 2.5 gm in 3 divided doses; or initially 850 mg once daily in AM; may increase by 850 mg/day in divided doses at 2 week intervals; max 2000 mg/day; take with meals
Pediatric: <10 years: not recommended; ≥10-16 years: use only as monotherapy; >16 years: same as adult dose same as adult
    Tab: 500, 850, 1000*mg

    Glucophage XR initially 500 mg by mouth every evening; may increase by 500 mg/day at 1 week intervals; max 2 gm/day
Pediatric: <10 years: not recommended; ≥10-16 years: use immediate release form; >16 years: same as adult
    Tab: 500, 750 mg ext-rel

    Glumetza ER (G) initially 1000 mg once daily; may increase by 500 mg/day at week intervals; max 2 gm/day
Pediatric: <18 years: not recommended; ≥18 years: same as adult
    Tab: 500, 1000 mg ext-rel

    Riomet XR initially 500 mg once daily; may increase by 500 mg/day at 1 week intervals; max 2 gm/day in divided doses; take with meals
Pediatric: <10 years: not recommended; ≥10 years: monotherapy only
    Oral soln: 500 mg/ml (4 oz; cherry)

MEGLITINIDES

Comment: Meglitinides are secretagogues (i.e., stimulate pancreatic insulin secretion) in response to a meal. Action is dependent on functioning beta cells in the pancreatic islets. Use as monotherapy or in combination with *metformin*.

▷ *nateglinide* (C) 60-120 mg tid ac 1-30 minutes prior to start of the meal
Pediatric: <12 years: not recommended; ≥12 years: same as adult
    Starlix *Tab:* 60, 120 mg

▷ *repaglinide* (C)(G) initially 0.5 mg with 2-4 meals/day; take 30 minutes ac; titrate by doubling dose at intervals of at least 1 week; range 0.5-4 mg with 2-4 meals/day; max 16 mg/day
Pediatric: <12 years: not recommended; ≥12 years: same as adult
    Prandin *Tab:* 0.5, 1, 2 mg

THIAZOLIDINEDIONES (TZDs)

Comment: The TZDs decrease hepatic gluconeogenesis and reduce insulin resistance (i.e., increase glucose uptake and utilization by the muscles). Liver function tests are indicated before initiating these drugs. Do not start if ALT more than 3 times greater than normal. Recheck ALT monthly for the first six months of therapy; then every two months for the remainder of the first year and periodically thereafter. Liver function tests should be obtained at the first symptoms suggestive of hepatic dysfunction (nausea, vomiting, fatigue, dark urine, anorexia, abdominal pain).

➢ *pioglitazone* (C)(G) initially 15-30 mg once daily; max 45 mg/day as a monotherapy; usual max 30 mg/day in combination with *metformin*, insulin, <u>or</u> a sulfonylurea
Pediatric: <18 years: not recommended; ≥18 years: same as adult
    Actos *Tab:* 15, 30, 45 mg

➢ *rosiglitazone* (C)(G) initially 4 mg/day in a single <u>or</u> 2 divided doses; may increase after 8-12 weeks; max 8 mg/day as a monotherapy <u>or</u> combination therapy with *metformin* <u>or</u> a sulfonylurea; not for use with *insulin*
Pediatric: <18 years: not recommended; ≥18 years: same as adult
    Avandia *Tab:* 2, 4, 8 mg

DIPEPTIDYL PEPTIDASE-4 (DPP-4) INHIBITOR+THIAZOLIDINEDIONE COMBINATION

Comment: The FDA has reported that *alogliptin*-containing drugs may increase the risk of heart failure, especially in patients who already have cardiovascular <u>or</u> renal disease. The drug **Oseni** (*alogliptin+pioglitazone*) is in this risk group.

➢ *alogliptin+pioglitazone* (C) take 1 dose once daily with first meal of the day; max: *rosiglitazone* 8 mg and max *glimepiride* per day; same precautions as *alogliptin* and *pioglitazone*
Pediatric: <18 years: not recommended; ≥18 years: same as adult
    Oseni
        Tab: **Oseni 12.5/15** *alo* 12.5 mg+*pio* 15 mg;
            Oseni 12.5/30 *alo* 12.5 mg+*pio* 30 mg
            Oseni 12.5/45 *alo* 12.5 mg+*pio* 45 mg
            Oseni 25/15 *alo* 25+*pio* 15 mg
            Oseni 25/30 *alo* 25+*pio* 30 mg
            Oseni 25/45 *alo* 25 mg+*pio* 45 mg

SECOND GENERATION SULFONYLUREA+BIGUANIDE COMBINATIONS

Comment: *Metaglip* and *Glucovance* are combination secretagogues (sulfonylureas) and insulin sensitizers (biguanides). *Sulfonylurea:* Action is dependent on functioning beta cells in the pancreatic islets; patient should be alerted to the risk for hypoglycemia. Common side effects of the biguanide include GI distress, nausea, vomiting, bloating, and flatulence which usually eventually resolve. Take with food. *metformin* is contraindicated with renal impairment, metabolic acidosis, ketoacidosis. Suspend *metformin*, prior to, and for 48 hours after, surgery <u>or</u> receiving IV iodinated contrast agents.

➢ *glipizide+metformin* (C) take with meals; *Primary therapy:* 2.5/250 once daily <u>or</u> if FBS is 280-320 mg/dL, may start at 2.5/250 bid; may increase by 1 tab/day every 2 weeks; max 10/2000 per day in 2 divided doses; *Second Line Therapy:* 2.5/500 <u>or</u> 5/500 bid; may increase by up to 5/500 every 2 weeks; max: 20/2000 per day; Same precautions as *glipizide* and *metformin*
Pediatric: <12 years: not recommended; ≥12 years: same as adult
    Metaglip
        Tab: **Metaglip 2.5/250** *glip* 2.5 mg+*met* 250 mg
            Metaglip 2.5/500 *glip* 2.5 mg+*met* 500 mg
            Metaglip 5/500 *glip* 5 mg+*met* 500 mg

➢ *glyburide+metformin* (B) take with meals; *Primary therapy (initial therapy if HgbA1c <9.0%):* initially 1.25/250 once daily; max *glyburide* 20 mg and *metformin* 2000

mg per day; *Primary therapy (initial therapy if HbA1c >9.0% or FBS >200):* initially 1.25/250 bid; max *glyburide* 20 mg and *metformin* 2000 mg per day; *Second line therapy (initial therapy if HbA1c >7.0%):* initially 2.5/500 or 5/500 bid; max *glyburide* 20 mg and *metformin* 2000 mg per day; *Previously treated with a sulfonylurea and metformin:* dose to approximate total daily doses of *glyburide* and *metformin* already being taken; max: *glyburide* 20 mg and *metformin* 2000 mg per day; Same precautions as *glyburide* and *metformin*
Pediatric: <12 years: not recommended; ≥12 years: same as adult
    Glucovance
      Tab: Glucovance **1.25/250** *glyb* 1.25 mg+*met* 250 mg
           Glucovance **2.5/500** *glyb* 2.5 mg+*met* 500 mg
           Glucovance **5/500** *glyb* 5 mg+*met* 500 mg
Comment: *metformin* is contraindicated with renal impairment, metabolic acidosis, ketoacidosis. Suspend *metformin*, prior to, and for 48 hours after, surgery or receiving IV iodinated contrast agents.

THIAZOLIDINEDIONE (TZD)+BIGUANIDE COMBINATION

▷ *pioglitazone+metformin* (C) take in divided doses with meals; *Previously on metformin alone:* initially 15 mg/500 mg or 15 mg/850 mg once or twice daily; *Previously on pioglitazone alone:* initially 15 mg/500 mg bid; *Previously on pioglitazone and metformin:* switch on a mg/mg basis; may increase after 8-12 weeks; max: *pioglitazone* 45 mg and *metformin* 2000 mg per day; Same precautions as *pioglitazone* and *metformin*
Pediatric: <12 years: not recommended; ≥12 years: same as adult
    Actoplus Met, Actoplis Met R (G)
      Tab: Actoplus Met **15/500** *pio* 15 mg+*met* 500 mg
           Actoplus Met **15/850** *pio* 15 mg+*met* 850 mg
           Actoplus Met XR **15/1000** *pio* 15 mg+*met* 1000 mg
           Actoplus Met XR **30/1000** *pio* 30 mg+*met* 1000 mg
Comment: *metformin* is contraindicated with renal impairment, metabolic acidosis, ketoacidosis. Suspend *metformin*, prior to, and for 48 hours after, surgery or receiving IV iodinated contrast agents.
▷ *rosiglitazone+metformin* (C)(G) take in divided doses with meals; *Previously on metformin alone:* add *rosiglitazone* 4 mg/day; may increase after 8-12 weeks; *Previously on rosiglitazone alone:* add *metformin* 1000 mg/day; may increase after 1-2 weeks; *Previously on rosiglitazone and metformin:* switch on a mg/mg basis; may increase *rosiglitazone* by 4 mg and/or *metformin* by 500 mg per day; max: *rosiglitazone* 8 mg and *metformin* 2000 mg per day; Same precautions as *rosiglitazone* and *metformin*
Pediatric: <12 years: not recommended; ≥12 years: same as adult
    Avandamet
      Tab: Avandamet **2/500** *rosi* 2 mg+*met* 500 mg
           Avandamet **2/1000** *rosi* 2 mg+*met* 1000 mg
           Avandamet **4/500** *rosi* 4 mg+*met* 500 mg
           Avandamet **4/1000** *rosi* 4 mg+*met* 1000 mg
Comment: *rosiglitazone* has been withdrawn from retail pharmacies. In order to enroll and receive *rosiglitazone*, healthcare providers and patients must enroll in the *Avandia-Rosiglitazone Medicines Access Program.* The program limits the use of *rosiglitazone* to patients already being treated successfully, and those whose blood sugar cannot be controlled with other antidiabetic medicines. *metformin* is contraindicated with renal impairment, metabolic acidosis, ketoacidosis. Suspend *metformin*, prior to, and for 48 hours after, surgery or receiving IV iodinated contrast agents.

THIAZOLIDINEDIONE (TZD)+SULFONYLUREA COMBINATIONS

➤ *pioglitazone+glimepiride* (C)(G) take 1 dose daily with first meal of the day; *Previously on sulfonylurea alone:* initially 30 mg/2 mg; *Previously on pioglitazone and glimepiride:* switch on a mg/mg basis; max: *pioglitazone* 30 mg and *glimepiride* 4 mg per day; Same precautions as *pioglitazone* and *glimepiride*
Pediatric: <18 years: not recommended; ≥18 years: same as adult
> Duetact
> > *Tab:* **Duetact 30/2** *pio* 30 mg+*glim* 2 mg
> > **Duetact 304** *pio* 30 mg+*glim* 4 mg

➤ *rosiglitazone+glimepiride* (C) take 1 dose daily with first meal of the day; max: *rosiglitazone* 8 mg and *glimepiride* 4 mg per day; Same precautions as *rosiglitazone* and *glimepiride*
Pediatric: <18 years: not recommended; ≥18 years: same as adult
> Avandaryl
> > *Tab:* **Avandaryl 4/1** *rosi* 4 mg+*glim* 1 mg
> > **Avandaryl 4/2** *rosi* 4 mg+*glim* 2 mg
> > **Avandaryl 4/4** *rosi* 4 mg+*glim* 4 mg
> > **Avandaryl 8/2** *rosi* 8 mg+*glim* 2 mg
> > **Avandaryl 8/4** *rosi* 8 mg+*glim* 4 mg

GLUCAGON-LIKE PEPTIDE-1 (GLP-1) RECEPTOR AGONISTS

Comment: GLP-1 receptor agonists act as an agonist at the GLP-1 receptors. They have a longer half-life than the native protein allowing them to be dosed once daily. They increase intracellular cAMP resulting in *insulin* release in the presence of increased serum concentration, decrease *glucagon* secretion, and delay gastric emptying, thus, reducing fasting, pre-meal, and post-prandial glucose throughout the day. GLP-1 receptor agonists are not a substitute for *insulin*, not for treatment of DKA, and not for post-prandial administration.

➤ *dulaglutide* (C) administer by SC injection into the upper arm, abdomen, or thigh once weekly on the same day and the same time of day, with or without food; initially 0.75 mg SC once weekly; may increase to 1.5 mg SC once weekly
Pediatric: <18 years: not established; ≥18 years: same as adult
> Trulicity *Prefilled pen/syringe:* 0.75, 1.5 mg/0.5 ml single-dose disposable autoinjector (4/pck)

➤ *exenatide* (C) administer by SC injection into the upper arm, abdomen, or thigh
Pediatric: <12 years: not recommended; ≥12 years: same as adult
> Bydureon inject immediately after mixing; administer 2 mg SC once weekly; administer on the same day, at any time of day; with or without meals; if switching from **Byetta**, discontinue **Byetta** and instead administer Bydureon and continue the same once weekly administration schedule with ydureon
> > *Vial:* 2 mg w. 0.65 ml diluent, single-dose; *Prefilled pen:* 2 mg w. 0.65 ml diluent, single-dose
> Bydureon BCise administer 2 mg by subcutaneous injection once weekly; at any time of day; with or without meals; if switching from **Byetta** to **Bydureon**, disconcontinue **Byetta** and start **Bydureon BBCise** SC once weekly on the same day of the week
> > *Autoinjector:* 2 mg (0.85 ml) single-dose
> Byetta inject within 60 minutes before AM and PM meals, or before the 2 main meals of the day, approx ≥6 hours apart; initially 5 mcg/dose; may increase to 10 mcg/dose after one month
> > *Prefilled pen:* 250 mcg/ml (5, 10 mcg/dose; 60 doses, needles not included) (m-cresol, mannitol)

▷ *liraglutide* (C) administer by SC injection into the upper arm, abdomen, or thigh once daily; initially 0.6 mg/day for 1 week; then 1.2 mg/day; may increase to 1.8 mg/day
Pediatric: <18 years: not recommended; ≥18 years: same as adult
  Victoza *Prefilled pen:* 6 mg/ml (3 ml; needles not included)

▷ *lixisenatide* (C) administer SC in the upper arm, abdomen, or thigh once daily; initially 10 mcg SC x 14 days; maintenance: 20 mcg beginning on day 15; administer within one hour of the first meal of the day and the same meal of the day
Pediatric: <18 years: not established; ≥18 years: same as adult
  Adlyxin Soln for SC inj; *Starter Pen:* 50 mcg/ml (14 doses of 10 mcg; 3 ml); *Maintenance Pen:* 100 mcg/ml (14 doses of 20 mcg); *Starter Pack:* 1 prefilled starter pen and 1 prefilled maintenance pen; *Maintenance Pack:* 2 prefilled maintenance pens

Comment: **Adlyxin** is indicated as an adjunct to diet and exercise for T2DM. Not indicated for treatment of T1DM. Do not use with **Victoza, Saxenda,** other GLP-1 receptor agonists, or insulin. Contraindicated with gastroparesis and GFR <15 mL/min. Poorly controlled diabetes in pregnancy increases the maternal risk for diabetic ketoacidosis, pre-eclampsia, spontaneous abortions, preterm delivery, stillbirth and delivery complications. Poorly controlled diabetes increases the fetal risk for major birth defects, still birth, and macrosomia related morbidity. **Adlyxin** should be used during pregnancy only if the potential benefit justifies the potential risk to the fetus. Estimated background risk of major birth defects and miscarriage in clinically recognized pregnancies is 2-4% and 15-20%, respectively.

▷ *semaglutide* administer SC in the upper arm, abdomen, or thigh once weekly at any time of day, with or without meals; initially 0.25 mg once weekly; after 4 weeks, increase the dose to 0.5 mg once weekly; if after at least 4 weeks additional glycemic control is needed, increase to 1 mg once weekly (usual main-maintenance dose); if a dose is missed, administer within 5 days of the missed dose
Pediatric: <18 years: not recommended; ≥18 years: same as adult
  Ozempic *Prefilled pen:* 2 mg/1.5 ml (1.34 mg/ml) single-patient-use; 0.25, 0.5, 1 mg/injection

Comment: *semaglutide* is contraindicated with personal or family history of medullary thyroid carcinoma or with multiple endocrine neoplasia syndrome type 2. **Ozempic** has not been studied in patients with a history of pancreatitis. Consider another antidiabetic therapy. **Ozempic** is not recommended in females or males with reproductive potential. Discontinue in women at least 2 months before a planned pregnancy due to the long washout period for *semaglutide*. Not recommended as first-line therapy for patients inadequately controlled on diet and exercise. There are no data on the presence of *semaglutide* in human milk or the effects on the breastfed infant.

BASAL INSULIN+GLP-1 RA COMBINATIONS

▷ *insulin degludec (insulin analog)+liraglutide* (C) for treatment of type 2 diabetes only when inadequately controlled on <50 units of basal *insulin* daily or ≤1.8 mg of *liraglutide* daily; administer by SC injection once daily, with or without food, into the upper arm, abdomen, or thigh; titrate every 3-4 days
Pediatric: <18 years: not recommended: ≥18 years: same as adult
  Xultophy *Prefilled pen:* 100/3.6 U/ml (3 ml, 5 pens/carton)

▷ *insulin glargine (insulin analog)+lixisenatide* (C) for treatment of type 2 diabetes only when inadequately controlled on <60 units of basal *insulin* daily or *lixisenatide*; administer by SC injection once daily, with or without food, into the upper arm, abdomen, or thigh; titrate every 3-4 days
Pediatric: <18 years: not recommended: ≥18 years: same as adult
  Soliqua *Prefilled pen:* 100/33 U/ml (3 ml, 5 pens/carton) covering 15-60 mg *insulin glargine* 100 units/ml and 15-20 mcg of *lixisenatide (m-cresol)*

SODIUM-GLUCOSE CO-TRANSPORTER 2 (SGLT2) INHIBITORS

Comment: SGLT2 inhibitors block the SGLT2 protein involved in 90% of glucose reabsorption in the proximal renal tubule, resulting in increased renal glucose excretion (typically >2000 mg/dL), and lower blood glucose levels (low risk of hypoglycemia), modest weight loss, and mild reduction in blood pressure (probably due to sodium loss). These agents probably also increase insulin sensitivity, decrease gluconeogenesis, and improve *insulin* release from pancreatic beta cells. SGLT2 inhibitors are contraindicated in T1DM, and are decreased <u>or</u> contraindicated with decreased GFR, increased SCr, renal failure, ESRD, renal dialysis, metabolic acidosis, <u>or</u> diabetic ketoacidosis. The most common ASEs are increased urination, UTI, and female genital mycotic infection (due to the glycosuria). These effects may be managed with adequate oral hydration and post-voiding genital hygiene. OTC **Vagisil** wet wipes are recommended to completely remove any post-voiding glucose film, and, thus, reduce potential risk of UTI and vaginal candidiasis, and reverse initial signs/symptoms of candida vaginalis. The SGLT2 inhibitors are not recommended in nursing women. There is potential for a hypersensitivity reaction to include angioedema and anaphylaxis. Caution with SGLT2 use due to reports of increased risk of treatment-emergent bone fractures.

▷ *canagliflozin* (C) take one tab before the first meal of the day; initially 100 mg; may titrate up to max 300 mg once daily; *GFR <45 mL/min:* do not initiate
  Pediatric: <18 years: not established; ≥18 years: same as adult
    Invokana *Tab:* 100, 300 mg
Comment: **Invokana** is contraindicated with GFR <45 *mL/min;* If GFR 45-≤60 *mL/min,* max 100 mg once daily <u>or</u> consider other antihyperglycemic

▷ *dapagliflozin* (C) take one tab before the first meal of the day; initially 5 mg; may increase to max 10 mg once daily
  Pediatric: <18 years: not established; ≥18 years: same as adult
    Farxiga *Tab:* 5, 10 mg
Comment: **Farxiga** is contraindicated with GFR <60 mL/min.

▷ *empagliflozin* (C) take one tab before the first meal of the day; initially 10 mg; may increase to max 25 mg once daily
  Pediatric: <18 years: not established; ≥18 years: same as adult
    Jardiance *Tab:* 10, 25 mg
Comment: **Jardiance** is contraindicated with GFR <45 mL/min.

▷ *ertugliflozin* (C) take one tab before the first meal of the day; initially 5 mg; may increase to max 15 mg once daily
  Pediatric: <18 years: not established; ≥18 years: same as adult
    Steglatro *Tab:* 5, 15 mg

SODIUM-GLUCOSE CO-TRANSPORTER 2 (SGLT2) INHIBITOR+BIGUANIDE COMBINATIONS

Comment: Caution with **SGLT2** use due to reports of increased risk of treatment-emergent bone fractures. *metformin* is contraindicated with renal impairment, metabolic acidosis, ketoacidosis. Suspend *metformin*, prior to, and for 48 hours after, surgery <u>or</u> receiving IV iodinated contrast agents.

▷ *canagliflozin+metformin* (C) take 1 dose twice daily with meals; max daily dose 300/2000; *GFR 45-≤60 mL/min: canagliflozin* max 100 mg once daily <u>or</u> consider other antihyperglycemic; *GFR <45 mL/min:* do not initiate
  Pediatric: <18 years: not established; ≥18 years: same as adult
    Invokamet
      Tab: Invokamet 50/500 *cana* 50 mg+*met* 500 mg
        Invokamet 50/1000 *cana* 50 mg+*met* 1000 mg

        Invokamet 150/500 *cana* 150 mg+*met* 500 mg
        Invokamet 150/1000 *cana* 150 mg+*met* 1000 mg

▷ *dapagliflozin+metformin* (C) swallow whole; do not crush or chew; take once daily first meal of the day; max daily dose 10/2000
  Pediatric: <18 years: not established; ≥18 years: same as adult
      Xigduo XR
        Tab: **Xigduo XR 5/500** *dapa* 5 mg+*met* 500 mg ext-rel
             Xigduo XR 5/1000 *dapa* 5 mg+*met* 1000 mg ext-rel
             Xigduo XR 10/500 *dapa* 10 mg+*met* 500 mg ext-rel
             Xigduo XR 10/1000 *dapa* 10 mg+*met* 1000 mg ext-rel

      Comment: **Xigduo** is contraindicated with GFR <60 mL/min, SCr >1.5 (men) or SCr >1.4 (women)

▷ *empagliflozin+metformin* (C) take 1 dose twice daily with meals; max daily dose 25/2000
  Pediatric: <18 years: not established; ≥18 years: same as adult
      Synjardy
        Tab: **Synjardy 5/500** *empa* 5 mg+*met* 500 mg
             Synjardy 5/1000 *empa* 5 mg+*met* 1000 mg
             Synjardy 12.5/500 *empa* 12.5 mg+*met* 500 mg
             Synjardy 12.5/1000 *empa* 12.5 mg+*met* 1000 mg
      Synjardy XR
        Tab: **Synjardy XR 5/1000** *empa* 5 mg+*met* 1000 mg
             Synjardy XR 12.5/1000 *empa* 12.5 mg+*met* 1000 mg
             Synjardy XR 10/1000 *empa* 10 mg+*met* 1000 mg
             Synjardy XR 25/1000 *empa* 25 mg+*met* 1000 mg

      Comment: **Synjardy** is contraindicated with GFR <45 mL/min, SCr >1.5 (men), or SCr >1.4 (women).

▷ *ertugliflozin+metformin* (C) take 1 dose twice daily with meals; max daily dose 15/2000
  Pediatric: <18 years: not established; ≥18 years: same as adult
      Segluormet
      Tab: **Segluormet 2.5/500** *ertu* 2.5 mg+*met* 500 mg
           Segluormet 2.5/1000 *ertu* 2.5 mg+*met* 1000 mg
           Segluormet 7.5/500 *ertu* 7.5 mg+*met* 500 mg
           Segluormet 7.5/1000 *ertu* 7.5 mg+*met* 1000 mg

SODIUM-GLUCOSE CO-TRANSPORTER 2 (SGLT2) INHIBITOR+DIPEPTIDYL PEPTIDASE-4 (DPP-4) INHIBITOR COMBINATIONS

Comment: Caution with **SGLT2** use due to reports of increased risk of treatment-emergent bone fractures and increased risk for UTI and Candida vaginalis secondary to drug-associated glycosuria.

▷ *dapagliflozin+saxagliptin* (C) initially 5/10 once daily, at any time of day, with or without food; if a dose is missed and it is ≥12 hours until the next dose, the dose should be taken; if a dose is missed and it is <12 hours until the next dose, the missed dose should be skipped and the next dose taken at the usual time.
  Pediatric: <18 years: not recommended: ≥18 years: same as adult
      Qtern *Tab:* dapa 10 mg+saxa 5 mg film-coat

Comment: **Qtern** should not be used during pregnancy. If pregnancy is detected, treatment with **Qtern** should be discontinued. It is unknown whether **Qtern** and/or its metabolites are excreted in human milk. Do not use with CrCl <60 mL/min or eGFR <60 mL/min/1.73 m² or ESRD or severe hepatic impairment or history of pancreatitis.

▷ *empagliflozin+linagliptin* (C) initially 10/5 once daily with the first meal of the day; max daily dose 25/5

Pediatric: <18 years: not established; ≥18 years: same as adult
Glyxambi
> *Tab:* **Glyxambi 10/5** *empa* 10 mg+*lina* 5 mg
> **Glyxambi 25/5** *empa* 25 mg+*lina* 5 mg

Comment: **Glyxambi** is contraindicated with GFR <45 mL/min.

▷ *ertugliflozin+sitagliptin* (C) initially 5/100 once daily with the first meal of the day; max daily dose 15/100
Pediatric: <18 years: not established; ≥18 years: same as adult
Steglujan
> *Tab:* **Steglujan 5/100** ertu 5 mg+glip 100 mg
> **Steglujan 15/100** ertu 15 mg+glip 100 mg

Comment: Steglujan is contraindicated with GFR <45 mL/min.

DIPEPTIDYL PEPTIDASE-4 (DPP-4) INHIBITOR

Comment: DPP-4 is an enzyme that degrades incretin hormones glucagon-like peptide-1 (GLP-1) and glucose-dependent insulinotropic polypeptide (GIP). Thus, DPP-4 inhibitors increase the concentration of active incretin hormones, stimulating the release of *insulin* in a glucose-dependent manner and decreasing the levels of circulating *glucagon*. The FDA has reported that *saxagliptin*- and *alogliptin*-containing drugs may increase the risk of heart failure, especially in patients who already have cardiovascular or renal disease. Drugs in this risk group include **Nesina** (*alogliptin*) and **Onglyza** (*saxagliptin*)

▷ *alogliptin* (B) take twice daily with meals; max 25 mg day
Pediatric: <18 years: not recommended; ≥18 years: same as adult
Nesina *Tab:* 6.25, 12.5, 25 mg

▷ *linagliptin* (B) 5 mg once daily
Pediatric: <18 years: not recommended; ≥18 years: same as adult
Tradjenta *Tab:* 5 mg

▷ *saxagliptin* (B) 2.5-5 mg once daily
Pediatric: <18 years: not recommended; ≥18 years: same as adult
Onglyza *Tab:* 2.5, 5 mg

▷ *sitagliptin* (B) as monotherapy or as combination therapy with metformin or a TZD
Pediatric: <18 years: not recommended; ≥18 years: same as adult
Januvia 25-100 mg once daily
> *Tab:* 25, 50, 100 mg

DIPEPTIDYL PEPTIDASE-4 (DPP-4) INHIBITOR+BIGUANIDE COMBINATIONS

Comment: DPP-4 inhibitor+*metformin* combinations are contraindicated with renal impairment (men: SCr ≥1.5 mg/dL; women: SCr ≥1.4 mg/dL) or abnormal CrCl, metabolic acidosis, ketoacidosis, or history of angioedema. Suspend *metformin*, prior to, and for 48 hours after, surgery or receiving IV iodinated contrast agents. Avoid in the elderly, malnourished, dehydrated, or with clinical or lab evidence of hepatic disease. For other DPP-4 and/or *metformin* precautions, see mfr pkg insert. The FDA has reported that *saxagliptin*- and *alogliptin*-containing drugs may increase the risk of heart failure, especially in patients who already have cardiovascular or renal disease. These drugs include: **Onglyza** (*saxagliptin*), **Kombiglyze XR** (*saxagliptin+metformin*), **Nesina** (*alogliptin*), **Kazano** (*alogliptin+metformin*), and **Oseni** (*alogliptin+pioglitazone*).

▷ *alogliptin+metformin* (B) take twice daily with meals; max *alogliptin* 25 mg/day, max *metformin* 2000 mg/day
Pediatric: <18 years: not recommended; ≥18 years: same as adult
Kazano
> *Tab:* **Kazano 12.5/500** *algo* 12.5 mg+*met* 500 mg
> **Kazano 2.5/1000** *algo* 12.5 mg+*met* 1000 mg

▷ *linagliptin+metformin* (B)
   Pediatric: <18 years: not recommended; ≥18 years: same as adult
      Jentadueto take twice daily with meals; max *linagliptin* 5 mg/day, max *metformin* 2000 mg/day
         Tab: **Jentadueto 2.5/500** *lina* 2.5 mg+*met* 500 mg film-coat
              Jentadueto 2.5/850 *lina* 2.5 mg+*met* 850 mg film-coat
              Jentadueto 2.5/1000 *lina* 2.5 mg+*met* 1000 mg film-coat
      Jentadueto XR *Currently not treated with metformin*: initiate **Jentadueto XR 5/1000** once daily; *Already treated with metformin*: initiate **Jentadueto XR** 5 mg *linagliptin* total daily dose and a similar total daily dose of *metformin* once daily; *Already treated with linagliptin and metformin* <u>or</u> *Jentadueto*: switch to **Jentadueto XR** containing 5 mg of *linagliptin* total daily dose and a similar total daily dose of *metformin* once daily; max *linagliptin 5 mg* <u>and</u> *metformin 2,000 mg*; take as a single dose once daily; take with food; do not crush <u>or</u> chew *eGFR <30 mL/min*: contraindicated; *eGFR 30-45 mL/min*: not recommended
         Tab: **Jentadueto 2.5/1000** *lina* 2.5 mg+*met* 1,000 mg film-coat ext-rel
              Jentadueto 5/1000 *lina* 5 mg+*met* 1,000 mg film-coat ext-rel
▷ *saxagliptin+metformin* (B) take once daily with meals; max *saxagliptin* 5 mg/day, max *metformin* 2,000 mg/day; do not crush <u>or</u> chew
   Pediatric: <18 years: not recommended; ≥18 years: same as adult
      Kombiglyze XR
         Tab: **Kombiglyze XR 5/500** *saxa* 5 mg+*met* 500 mg
              Kombiglyze XR 2.5/1000 *saxa* 2.5 mg+*met* 1,000 mg
              Kombiglyze XR 5/1000 *saxa* 5 mg+*met* 1,000 mg
Comment: The FDA has reported that *saxagliptin*-containing drugs may increase the risk of heart failure, especially in patients who already have cardiovascular <u>or</u> renal disease. The drug Kombiglyze XR (*saxagliptin+metformin*) is in this risk group. *metformin* is contraindicated with renal impairment, metabolic acidosis, ketoacidosis. Suspend *metformin*, prior to, and for 48 hours after, surgery <u>or</u> receiving IV iodinated contrast agents.
▷ *sitagliptin+metformin* (B) take twice daily with meals; max *sitagliptin* 100 mg/day, max *metformin* 2000 mg/day
   Pediatric: <18 years: not recommended; ≥18 years: same as adult
      Janumet
         Tab: **Janumet 50/500** *sita* 50 mg+*met* 500 mg
              Janumet 50/1000 *sita* 50 mg+*met* 1,000 mg
      Janumet XR
         Tab: **Janumet XR 50/500** *sita* 50 mg+*met* 500 mg ext-rel
              Janumet XR 50/1000 *sita* 50 mg+*met* 1,000 mg ext-rel
              Janumet XR 100/1000 *sita* 100 mg+*met* 1,000 mg ext-rel
Comment: *metformin* is contraindicated with renal impairment, metabolic acidosis, ketoacidosis. Suspend *metformin*, prior to, and for 48 hours after, surgery <u>or</u> receiving IV iodinated contrast agents.

MEGLITINIDE+BIGUANIDE COMBINATION

▷ *repaglinide+metformin* (C)(G) take in 2-3 divided doses within 30 minutes before food; max 4/1000 per meal and 10/2000 per day
   Pediatric: <18 years: not recommended; ≥18 years: same as adult
      Prandimet
         Tab: **Prandimet 1/500** *repa* 1 mg+*met* 500 mg
              Prandimet 2/500 *repa* 2 mg+*met* 500 mg
Comment: *metformin* is contraindicated with renal impairment, metabolic acidosis, ketoacidosis. Suspend *metformin*, prior to, and for 48 hours after, surgery <u>or</u> receiving IV iodinated contrast agents.

DIPEPTIDYL PEPTIDASE-4 (DPP-4) INHIBITOR+HMG-COA REDUCTASE INHIBITOR COMBINATION

➤ *sitagliptin+simvastatin* (B) take once daily in the PM; swallow whole; adjust dose if needed after 4 weeks; *Concomitant* **verapamil** or **diltiazem**: max 100/10 once daily; *Concomitant* **amiodarone, amlodipine,** or **ranolazine**: max 100/20 once daily; *Homogenous familial hypercholesterolemia*: max 100/40 once daily; *Chinese patients taking lipid-modifying doses (>1 gm/day niacin) of* **niacin**-*containing products*: caution with 100/40 dose; increase risk of myopathy
  Pediatric: <18 years: not recommended; ≥18 years: same as adult
    Juvisync
      Tab: Juvisync 100/10 *sita* 100 mg+*simva* 10 mg
        Juvisync 100/20 *sita* 100 mg+*simva* 20 mg
        Juvisync 100/40 *sita* 100 mg+*simva* 40 mg

DOPAMINE RECEPTOR AGONIST

➤ *bromocriptine mesylate* (B) take with food in the morning within 2 hours of waking; initially 0.8 mg once daily; may increase by 0.8 mg/week; max 4.8 mg/week; *Severe psychotic disorders*: not recommended
  Pediatric: <12 years: not recommended; ≥12 years: same as adult
    Cycloset *Tab*: 0.8 mg
    Comment: **Cycloset** is an adjunct to diet and exercise to improve glycemic control. Contraindicated with syncopal migraines, nursing mothers, and other ergot-related drugs.

Bile Acid Sequestrant

➤ *colesevelam* (B) *Monotherapy*: 3 tabs bid or 6 tabs once daily or one **1.875 gm pkt bid** or one 3.75 gm pkt once daily
  Pediatric: <12 years: not recommended; ≥12 years: same as adult
    WelChol *Tab*: 625 mg; *Pwdr for oral susp*: 1.875 gm pwdr pkts (60/carton); 3.75 gm pwdr pkts (30/carton) (citrus) (phenylalanine)
  Comment: *colesevelam* (WelChol) is indicated as an adjunctive therapy to improve glycemic control in adults with type 2 diabetes. It can be added to *metformin*, sulfonylureas, or *insulin* alone or in combination with other antidiabetic agents

◯ TYPHOID FEVER (*SALMONELLA TYPHI*)

PRE-EXPOSURE PROPHYLAXIS

➤ *typhoid* vaccine, oral, live, attenuated strain
    Vivotif Berna 1 cap every other day, 1 hour before a meal, with a lukewarm (not > body temperature) or cold drink for a total of 4 doses; do not crush or chew; complete therapy at least 1 week prior to expected exposure; re-immunization recommended every 5 years if repeated exposure
      Pediatric: <6 years: not recommended; ≥6 years: same as adult
      Cap: ent-coat
➤ *typhoid Vi polysaccharide* vaccine (C)
    Pediatric: <2 years: not recommended; ≥2 years: same as adult
    Typhim Vi 0.5 ml IM in deltoid; re-immunization recommended every 2 years if repeated exposure
      Vial: 20, 50 dose; *Prefilled syringe*: 0.5 ml
  Comment: Febrile illness may require delaying administration of the vaccine; have *epinephrine* 1:1000 readily available.

TREATMENT

➤ **azithromycin (B)(G)** 8-10 mg/kg/day; *Mild Illness:* treat x 7 days; *Severe Illness:* treat x 14 days
Pediatric: 8-10 mg/kg/day; max 500 mg/day; *Mild Illness:* treat x 7 days; *Severe Illness:* treat x 14 days; *see page 621 for dose by weight*
    Zithromax *Tab:* 250, 500, 600 mg; *Oral susp:* 100 mg/5 ml (15 ml); 200 mg/5 ml (15, 22.5, 30 ml) (cherry); *Pkt:* 1 gm for reconstitution (cherry-banana)
    Zithromax Tri-pak *Tab:* 3 x 500 mg tabs/pck
    Zithromax Z-pak *Tab:* 6 x 250 mg tabs/pck
    Zmax *Oral susp:* 2 gm ext-rel for reconstitution (cherry-banana) (148 mg Na$^+$)
➤ **cefixime (B)(G)** *Mild Illness:* 15-20 mg/kg/day x 7-14 days; *Severe Illness:* 20 mg/kg/day x 10-14 days
Pediatric: <6 months: not recommended; 6 months-12 years, <50 kg: *Mild Illness:* 15-20 mg/kg/day x 7-14 days; *Severe Illness:* 20 mg/kg/day x 10-14 >50 kg: same as adult; *see page 625 for dose by weight*
    Suprax *Tab:* 400 mg; *Cap:* 400 mg; *Oral susp:* 100, 200, 500 mg/5 ml (50, 75, 100 ml) (strawberry)
➤ **ciprofloxacin (C)** 15 mg/kg/day; *Mild Illness:* treat x 5-7 days; *Severe Illness:* treat x 10-14 days
Pediatric: <18 years: not recommended; ≥18 years: same as adult
    Cipro (G) *Tab:* 250, 500, 750 mg; *Oral susp:* 250, 500 mg/5 ml (100 ml) (strawberry)
    Cipro XR *Tab:* 500, 1000 mg ext-rel
    ProQuin XR *Tab:* 500 mg ext-rel
Comment: *ciprofloxacin* is contraindicated <18-years-of-age, and during pregnancy and lactation. Risk of tendonitis or tendon rupture.
➤ **ofloxacin (C)** 15 mg/kg/day; *Mild Illness:* treat x 5-7 days; *Severe Illness:* treat x 10-14 days
Pediatric: <18 years: not recommended; ≥18 years: same as adult
    Floxin *Tab:* 200, 300, 400 mg
Comment: *ofloxacin* is contraindicated <18-years-of-age, and during pregnancy and lactation. Risk of tendonitis or tendon rupture.
➤ **cefotaxime** 80 mg/kg/day IM/IV x 10-14 days; max 2 gm/day
Pediatrics: 80 mg/kg/day IM/IV x 10-14 days; max 2 gm/day
    Claforan *Vial:* 500 mg; 1, 2 gm
➤ **ceftriaxone (B)(G)** 75 mg/kg/day IM/IV x 10-14 days; max 2 gm/day
Pediatrics: 75 mg/kg/day IM/IV x 10-14 days; max 2 gm/day
    Rocephin *Vial:* 250, 500 mg; 1, 2 gm
➤ **trimethoprim+sulfamethoxazole (TMP-SMX) (D)(G)** 8-40 mg/kg/day x 14 days
Pediatric: <2 months: not recommended; ≥2 months: 8-40 mg/kg/day of *sulfamethoxazole* in 2 divided doses bid x 10 days; *see page 648 for dose by weight*
    Bactrim, Septra 2 tabs bid x 10 days
    Tab: trim 80 mg+*sulfa* 400 mg*
    Bactrim DS, Septra DS 1 tab bid x 10 days
    Tab: trim 160 mg+*sulfa* 800 mg*
    Bactrim Pediatric Suspension, Septra Pediatric Suspension 20 ml bid x 10 days
    Oral susp: trim 40 mg+*sulfa* 200 mg per 5 ml (100 ml) (cherry) (alcohol 0.3%)

ULCER: DIABETIC, NEUROPATHIC (LOWER EXTREMITY); VENOUS INSUFFICIENCY (LOWER EXTREMITY)

NUTRITIONAL SUPPLEMENT

➤ **L-methylfolate calcium (as metafolin)+pyridoxyl 5-phosphate+methylcobalamin** take 1 cap daily

Pediatric: <12 years: not recommended; ≥12 years: same as adult

    Metanx *Cap:* metafo 3 mg+*pyrid* 35 mg+*methyl* 2 mg (gluten-free, yeast-free, lactose-free)

Comment: **Metanx** is indicated as adjunct treatment of endothelial dysfunction <u>and/or</u> hyperhomocysteinemia in patients who have lower extremity ulceration.

DEBRIDING+CAPILLARY STIMULANT AGENT

▷ *trypsin+balsam peru+castor oil* apply at least twice daily; may cover with a wet bandage

    Granulex *Aerosol liq:* tryp 0.12 mg+*bal peru* 87 mg+*cast* 788 mg per 0.82 ml

GROWTH FACTOR

▷ *becaplermin* (C) apply once daily with a cotton swab <u>or</u> tongue depressor; then cover with saline moistened gauze dressing; rinse after 12 hours; then re-cover with a clean saline dressing

    Regranex *Gel:* 0.01% (2, 7.5, 15 gm) (parabens)

Comment: Store in refrigerator; do not freeze. Not for use in wounds that close by primary intention.

 ULCER: PRESSURE, DECUBITUS

DEBRIDING/CAPILLARY STIMULANT AGENT

    Granulex (*trypsin* 0.1 mg+*balsam peru* 72.5 mg+*castor oil* 650 mg per 0.82 ml) apply at least twice daily; may cover with a wet bandage
    Aerosol liq: (2, 4 oz)

GROWTH FACTOR

▷ *becaplermin* (C) apply once daily with a cotton swab <u>or</u> tongue depressor; then cover with saline moistened gauze dressing; rinse after 12 hours; then recover with a clean saline dressing

    Regranex *Gel:* 0.01% (2, 7.5, 15 gm) (parabens)

Comment: Store in refrigerator; do not freeze. Not for use in wounds that close by primary intention.

 ULCERATIVE COLITIS (UC)

Comment: Standard treatment regimen is anti-infective, anti-spasmodic, and bowel rest; progressing to clear liquids; then to high fiber.

Parenteral Corticosteroids *see page* 570

Oral Corticosteroids *see page* 569

▷ *budesonide micronized* (C)(G) 9 mg once daily in the AM for up to 8 weeks; may repeat an 8-week course; *Maintenance of remission:* 6 mg once daily for up to 3 months; taper other systemic steroids when transferring to *budesonide*

Pediatric: <12 years: not recommended; ≥12 years: same as adult

    Entocort EC *Cap:* 3 mg ent-coat granules
    Uceris *Tab:* 9 mg ext-rel

RECTAL CORTICOSTEROIDS

▷ *hydrocortisone* rectal (C)

Pediatric: <12 years: not recommended; ≥12 years: same as adult

    Anusol-HC Suppositories 1 supp rectally 3 x/day <u>or</u> 2 supp rectally 2 x/day for 2 weeks; max 8 weeks

    Rectal supp: 25 mg (12, 24/pck)

Cortenema 1 enema q HS x 21 days <u>or</u> until symptoms controlled
Enema: 100 mg/60 ml (1, 7/pck)
Cortifoam 1 applicator full once daily-bid x 2-3 weeks and every 2nd day thereafter until symptoms are controlled
Aerosol: 80 mg/applicator (14 application/container)
Proctocort 1 supp rectally in AM and PM x 2 weeks; for more severe cases, may increase to 1 supp rectally 3 times daily <u>or</u> 2 supp rectally twice daily; max 4-8 weeks
Rectal supp: 30 mg (12, 24/pck)

Comment: Use *hydrocortisone* foam as adjunctive therapy in the distal portion of the rectum when *hydrocortisone* enemas cannot be retained.

RECTAL CORTICOSTEROID+ANESTHETIC

Hydrocortisone+Pramoxine

Proctofoam HC apply to anal/rectal area 3-4 times daily; max 4-8 weeks
Rectal foam: hydrocort 1%+*pram* 1% (10 gm w. applicator)

SALICYLATES

Comment: symptoms of salicylate toxicity include hematemesis, tachypnea, hyperpnea, tinnitus, deafness, lethargy, seizures, confu-sion, or dyspnea. Severe intoxication may lead to electrolyte and blood pH imbalance and potentially to other organ (e.g., renal and liver) involvement. There is no specific antidote for mesalamine overdose; however, conventional therapy for salicylate toxicity may be beneficial in the event of acute overdosage. This includes preven-tion of further gastrointestinal tract absorption by emesis and, if necessary, by gastric lavage. Fluid and electrolyte imbalance should be corrected by the administration of appropriate intravenous ther-apy. Adequate renal function should be maintained.

▷ *balsalazide disodium* (B)

Comment: *balsalazide* 6.75 gm provides 2.4 gm of *mesalazine* to the colon.

Colazal 3 x 750 mg caps/day (6.75 gm/day), with <u>or</u> without food, x 8 weeks; may require treatment for up to 12 weeks; swallow whole <u>or</u> may be opened and sprinkled on applesauce, then chewed <u>or</u> swallowed immediately
Pediatric: <5 years: not recommended; 5-17 years: 1 x 750 mg cap 3 x/day (2.25 gm/day), with <u>or</u> without food for up to 8 weeks <u>or</u> 3 x 750 mg caps/day (6.75 gm/day), with <u>or</u> without food, x 8 weeks; swallow whole <u>or</u> may be opened and sprinkled on applesauce, then chewed <u>or</u> swallowed immediately
Cap: 750 mg

Comment: **Colazal** is a locally-acting aminosalicylate indicated for the treatment of mildly to moderately active ulcerative colitis in patients ≥5 years. Safety and effectiveness of **Colazal** >8 weeks in children (5-17 years) and >12 weeks in patients ≥18 years has not been established.

Giazo is a locally-acting aminosalicylate indicated for the treatment of mildly to moderately active ulcerative colitis <u>only</u> in male patients ≥18 years; take 3 x 1.1 gm tabs bid (6.6 gm/day) for up to 8 weeks
Pediatric: <18 years: not recommended; >18 years: same as adult
Tab: 1.1 gm (sodium 126 mg/tab) film-coat

Comment: Effectiveness of **Giazo** in female patients has not been demonstrated in clinical trials. Safety and effectiveness of **Giazo** > 8 weeks has not been established.

▷ *mesalamine* (B)

Apriso *Maintenance: of Remission* 4 x 0.375 gm caps (1.5 gm/day) once daily in the morning, for maintenance of remission with <u>or</u> without food; do not co-administer with antacids
Pediatric: <18 years: not recommended; ≥18 years: same as adult
Cap: 0.375 gm ext-rel (phenylalanine 0.56 mg/cap)

Comment: **Apriso** is a locally-acting aminosalicylate indicated for the maintenance of remission of ulcerative colitis in adults.

Asacol HD (G) Induction of Remission: 2 x 800 mg tab (1600 mg) tid x 6 weeks; *Maintenance of Remission:* 1.6 gm/day in divided doses; take on an empty stomach, at least 1 hour before or 2 hours after a meal; swallow whole; do not crush, break, or chew
Pediatric: <18 years: not recommended; ≥18 years: same as adult
Tab: 800 mg del-rel

Comment: **Asacol HD** is an aminosalicylate indicated for the treatment of moderately active ulcerative colitis in adults. Do not substitute one **Asacol HD 800** tablet for two **mesalamine** delayed-release 400 mg oral products

Canasa 1 x 1,000 mg suppository administered rectally once daily at bedtime for 3 to 6 weeks.
Pediatric: <18 years: not recommended; ≥18 years: same as adult
Rectal supp: 1 gm del-rel (30, 42/pck)

Comment: **Canasa** is an aminosalicylate indicated in adults for the treatment of mildly to moderately active ulcerative proctitis. Safety and effectiveness of **Canasa** beyond 6 weeks have not been established.

Delzicol Treatment: 2 x 400 mg caps (800 mg/day) 3 x/day x 6 weeks; *Maintenance:* 4 x 400 mg caps (1.6 gm/day) in 2-4 divided doses once daily; swallow whole; take with or without food; do not crush or chew
Pediatric: ≥5-17 years: twice daily dosing for 6 weeks; see mfr pkg **insert** for weight-based dosing table; **≥18 years: same as adult**
Cap: 400 mg del-rel

Comment: 2 x 400 mg **Dezlicol** caps have not been shown to be interchangeable or substitutable with one *mesalamine* delayed-release 80 mg tablet. Evaluate renal function prior to initiation of **Dezlicol**.

Lialda (G) Induction of Remission: 2-4 x 1.2 gm tabs (2.4-4.8 gm) once daily for up to 8 weeks; *Maintenance: of Remission:* 2 x 1.2 gm tabs (2.4 gm) once daily; swallow whole; do not crush or chew
Pediatric: <18 years: not recommended; ≥18 years: same as adult
Tab: 1.2 gm del-rel

Comment: **Lialda** is a locally-acting 5-aminosalicylic acid (5-ASA) indicated for the induction of remission in adults with active, mild to moderate ulcerative colitis and for the maintenance of remission of ulcerative colitis. Safety and effectiveness of **Lialda** in pediatric patients have not been established.

Pentasa Induction of Remission: 1 gm qid for up to 8 weeks
Pediatric: <18 years: not recommended; ≥18 years: same as adult
Cap: 250, 500 mg ext-rel

Comment: **Pentasa** is an aminosalicylate anti-inflammatory agent indicated for the induction of remission and for the treatment of patients with mildly to moderately active ulcerative colitis.

Rowasa Suppository 1 supp rectally bid x 3-6 weeks; retain for 1-3 hours or longer
Pediatric: <18 years: not recommended; ≥18 years: same as adult
Rectal supp: 500 mg (12, 24/pck)

Rowasa Rectal Suspension 4 gm (60 ml) rectally by enema q HS; retain for 8 hours x 3-6 weeks (sulfite-free)
Pediatric: <18 years: not recommended; ≥18 years: same as adult
Enema: 4 gm/60 ml (7, 14, 28/pck; kit, 7, 14, 28/pck w. wipes)

Comment: *RowasaRectal Suspension Enema* is indicated for the treatment of active mild to moderate distal ulcerative colitis, proctosigmoiditis, and proctitis.

▶ **olsalazine (C) Maintenance of Remission:** 1 gm/day in 2 divided doses; take with food
Pediatric: <18 years: not recommended; ≥18 years: same as adult
Dipentum *Cap:* 250 mg

Comment: *osalazine* is the sodium salt of a salicylate, disodium 3,3'-azobis (6-hydroxybenzoate) a compound that is effectively bioconverted to 5-amino-salicylic acid (5-ASA), which has anti-inflammatory activity in ulcerative colitis. The conversion of *olsalazine* to *mesalamine* (5-ASA) in the colon is similar to that of *sulfasalazine*, which is converted into *sulfapyridine* and *mesalamine*. *olsalazine* is indicated for the maintenance of remission of ulcerative colitis in patients who are intolerant of *sulfasalazine*.

▷ *sulfasalazine* (B; D in 2nd, 3rd)(G) Induction of Remission: 3-4 gm/day in evenly divided doses with dosage intervals not exceeding eight hours; in some cases, it is advisable to initiate therapy with a smaller dosage, e.g., 1-2 gm/day, to reduce possible gastrointestinal intolerance. If daily doses exceeding 4 gm are required to achieve desired effects, the increased risk of toxicity should be kept in mind; **Maintenance of Remission: 4 gm/day in divided doses**
Pediatric: <2 years: not recommended; 2-16 years: initially 40-60 mg/kg/day in 3 to 6 divided doses; max 30 mg/kg/day in 4 divided doses; max 2 gm/day in divided doses; >16 years: same as adult
  Azulfidine *Tab:* 500*mg
  Azulfidine EN-Tabs *Tab:* 500 mg ent-coat

TUMOR NECROSIS FACTOR (TNF) BLOCKER

▷ *adalimumab* (B) initially 180 mg SC (as 4 injections in 1 day or divided over 2 days) on week 0; then 80 mg at week 2; start 40 mg every other week maintenance at week 4; only continue if evidence of clinical remission by 8 weeks; administer in abdomen or thigh; rotate sites
Pediatric: <18 years: not recommended; ≥18 years: same as adult
  Humira *Prefilled syringe:* 20 mg/0.4 ml; 40 mg/0.8 ml single-dose (2/pck; 2, 6/ starter pck) (preservative-free)
▷ *adalimumab-adbm* (B) *First dose (Day 1):* 160 mg SC (4 x 40 mg injections in one day or 2 x 40 mg injections per day for two consecutive days); *Second dose two weeks later (Day 15):* 80 mg SC; *Two weeks later (Day 29):* begin a maintenance dose of 40 mg SC every other week (only continue in patients who have shown evidence of clinical remission by eight weeks (Day 57) of therapy.
Pediatric: <18 years: not recommended; ≥18 years: same as adult
  Cyltezo *Prefilled syringe:* 40 mg/0.8 ml single-dose (preservative-free)
Comment: Cyltezo is biosimilar to Humira (*adalimumab*).
▷ *infliximab* (*tumor necrosis factor-alpha blocker*) must be refrigerated at 2°C to 8°C (36°F to 46°F); administer dose via IV infusion over a period of not less than 2 hours; do not use beyond the expiration date as this product contains no preservative; 5 mg/ kg at 0, 2 and 6 weeks, then every 8 weeks.
Pediatric: <6 years: not studied; ≥6-17 years: mg/kg at 0, 2 and 6 weeks, then every 8 weeks; ≥18 years: same as adult
  Remicade *Vial:* 100 mg for reconstitution to 10 ml administration volume, single-dose (preservative-free)
Comment: **Remicade** is indicated to reduce signs and symptoms, and induce and maintain clinical remission, in adults and children ≥6 years-of-age with moderately to severely active disease who have had an inadequate response to conventional therapy and reduce the number of draining enterocutaneous and rectovaginal fistulas, and maintain fistula closure, in adults with fistulizing disease. Common adverse effects associated with **Remicade** included abdominal pain, headache, pharyngitis, sinusitis, and upper respiratory infections. In addition, **Remicade** might increase the risk for serious infections, including tuberculosis, bacterial sepsis, and invasive fungal infections. Available data from published literature on the use of *infliximab* products during pregnancy have not reported a clear association with *infliximab* products

and adverse pregnancy outcomes. *infliximab* products cross the placenta and infants exposed *in utero* should not be administered live vaccines for at least 6 months after birth. Otherwise, the infant may be at increased risk of infection, including disseminated infection which can become fatal. Available information is insufficient to inform the amount of *infliximab* products present in human milk or effects on the breast-fed infant. To report suspected adverse reactions, contact Merck Sharp & Dohme Corp., a subsidiary of Merck & Co. at 1-877-888-4231 or FDA at 1-800-FDA1088 or www.fda.gov/medwatch.

▷ *infliximab-abda (tumor necrosis factor-alpha blocker)* (B)
  Renflexis: see *infliximab* (Remicade) above for full prescribing information
Comment: Renflexis is a biosimilar to Remicade for the treatment of immune-disorders including Crohn's disease, ulcerative colitis, rheumatoid arthritis, ankylosing spondylitis, psoriatic arthritis and plaque psoriasis. Renflexis was approved under the FDA category for biosimilars and demonstrated no clinically meaningful differences for use, dosing regimens, strengths, dosage forms, and routes of administration from the FDA-approved biological product Remicade.

▷ *infliximab-dyyb (tumor necrosis factor-alpha blocker)* (B)
  Inflectra: see *infliximab* (Remicade) above for full prescribing information
Comment: Inflectra is a biosimilar to Remicade for the treatment of immune-disorders including Crohn's disease, ulcerative colitis, rheumatoid arthritis, ankylosing spondylitis, psoriatic arthritis and plaque psoriasis. Inflectra was approved under the FDA category for biosimilars and demonstrated no clinically meaningful differences for use, dosing regimens, strengths, dosage forms, and routes of administration from the FDA-approved biological product Remicade.

▷ *infliximab-qbtx (tumor necrosis factor-alpha blocker)* (B)
  Ifixi: see *infliximab* (Remicade) above for full prescribing information
Comment: Ifixi is a biosimilar to Remicade for the treatment of immune disorders including Crohn's disease, ulcerative colitis, rheumatoid arthritis, ankylosing spondylitis, psoriatic arthritis and plaque psoriasis. Ifixi was approved under the FDA category for biosimilars and demonstrated no clinically meaningful differences for use, dosing regimens, strengths, dosage forms, and routes of administration from the FDA-approved biological product Remicade.

INTEGRIN RECEPTOR ANTAGONIST

▷ *vedolizumab* (B) administer by IV infusion over 30 minutes; 300 mg at weeks 0, 2, 6; then once every 8 weeks
  Pediatric: <12 years: not established; ≥12 years: same as adult
    Entyvio *Vial:* 300 mg (20 ml) single-dose, pwdr for IV infusion after reconstitution (preservative-free)
Comment: To report suspected adverse reactions, contact Takeda Pharmaceuticals at 1-877-TAKEDA-7 (1-877-825-3327) or FDA at 1800-FDA-1088 or www.fda.gov/medwatch

ANTI-DIARRHEAL AGENTS

▷ *difenoxin+atropine* (C) 2 tabs; then 1 tab after each loose stool or 1 tab q 3-4 hours; max 8 tabs/day x 2 days
    Motofen *Tab: dif* 1 mg+*atro* 0.025 mg
▷ *diphenoxylate+atropine* (C)(G) 2 tabs or 10 ml qid
    Lomotil *Tab: diphen* 2.5 mg+*atro* 0.025 mg; *Liq: diphen* 2.5 mg+*atro* 0.025 mg/5 ml (2 oz w. dropper)
▷ *loperamide* (B)(G)
    Imodium (OTC) 4 mg initially; then 2 mg after each loose stool; max 16 mg/day
      Cap: 2 mg

Imodium A-D (OTC) 4 mg initially; then 2 mg after each loose stool; usual max 8 mg/day x 2 days

Cplt: 2 mg; *Liq:* 1 mg/5 ml (2, 4 oz)

▷ **loperamide+simethicone (B)(G)**

Imodium Advanced (OTC) 2 tabs chewed after first loose stool; then 1 after the next loose stool; max 4 tabs/day

Chew tab: loper 2 mg+simeth 125 mg

 URETHRITIS: NONGONOCOCCAL (NGU)

Comment: The following treatment regimens for NGU are published in the **2015 CDC Sexually Transmitted Diseases Treatment Guidelines.** Treatment regimens are for adults only; consult a specialist for treatment of patients less than 18 years-of-age. Treatment regimens are presented by generic drug name first, followed by information about brands and dose forms. All persons who have confirmed or suspected urethritis should be tested for gonorrhea and chlamydia. Men treated for NGU should be instructed to abstain from sexual intercourse for 7 days after a single dose regimen or until completion of a 7-day regimen.

RECOMMENDED REGIMEN: UNCOMPLICATED NGU

▷ *azithromycin* 1 gm in a single dose or 100 mg orally bid x 7 days

plus

▷ *doxycycline* 100 mg bid x 7 days

PERSISTENT-RECURRENT NGU

Men Initially Treated With Azithromycin+Doxycycline

▷ *azithromycin* 1 gm PO in a single dose

Men Who Fail a Regimen of Azithromycin

▷ *moxifloxacin* 400 mg PO once daily x 7 days

Heterosexual Men Who Live in Areas Where *T. Vaginalis* is Highly Prevalent

▷ *metronidazole* 2 gm PO in a single dose

or

▷ *tinidazole* 2 gm PO in a single dose

ALTERNATIVE REGIMENS

▷ *erythromycin base* 500 mg PO qid x 7 days

or

▷ *erythromycin ethylsuccinate* 800 mg PO qid x 7 days

or

▷ *levofloxacin* 500 mg once daily x 7 days

or

▷ *ofloxacin* 300 mg PO bid x 7 days

DRUG BRANDS AND DOSE FORMS

▷ *azithromycin* (B)(G)

Zithromax *Tab:* 250, 500, 600 mg; *Oral susp:* 100 mg/5 ml (15 ml); 200 mg/5 ml (15, 22.5, 30 ml) (cherry); *Pkt:* 1 gm for reconstitution (cherry-banana)

      Zithromax Tri-pak *Tab:* 3 x 500 mg tabs/pck

      Zithromax Z-pak *Tab:* 6 x 250 mg tabs/pck

      Zmax *Oral susp:* 2 gm ext-rel for reconstitution (cherry-banana) (148 mg Na$^+$)

▷ *doxycycline* (D)(G)

      Acticlate *Tab:* 75, 150**mg

      Adoxa *Tab:* 50, 75, 100, 150 mg ent-coat

      Doryx *Tab:* 50, 75, 100, 150, 200 mg del-rel

      Doxteric *Tab:* 50 mg del-rel

      Monodox *Cap:* 50, 75, 100 mg

      Oracea *Cap:* 40 mg del-rel

      Vibramycin *Tab:* 100 mg; *Cap:* 50, 100 mg; *Syr:* 50 mg/5 ml (raspberry-apple) (sulfites); *Oral susp:* 25 mg/5 ml (raspberry)

      Vibra-Tab *Tab:* 100 mg film-coat

▷ *erythromycin base* (B)

      Ery-Tab *Tab:* 250, 333, 500 mg ent-coat

      PCE *Tab:* 333, 500 mg

Comment: *erythromycin* may increase INR with concomitant *warfarin*, as well as increase serum level of *digoxin, benzodiazepines,* and *statins.*

▷ *erythromycin ethylsuccinate* (B)(G)

      EryPed *Oral susp:* 200 mg/5 ml (100, 200 ml) (fruit); 400 mg/5 ml (60, 100, 200 ml) (banana); *Oral drops:* 200, 400 mg/5 ml (50 ml) (fruit); *Chew tab:* 200 mg wafer (fruit)

      E.E.S. *Oral susp:* 200, 400 mg/5 ml (100 ml) (fruit)

      E.E.S. Granules *Oral susp:* 200 mg/5 ml (100, 200 ml) (cherry)

      E.E.S. 400 Tablets *Tab:* 400 mg

Comment: *erythromycin* may increase INR with concomitant *warfarin*, as well as increase serum level of *digoxin, benzodiazepines,* and *statins.*

▷ *levofloxacin* (C)

      Levaquin *Tab:* 250, 500, 750 mg; *Oral soln:* 25 mg/ml (480 ml) (benzyl alcohol); *Inj conc:* 25 mg/ml for IV infusion after dilution (20, 30 ml single-use vial) (preservative-free); *Premix soln:* 5 mg/ml for IV infusion (50, 100, 150 ml) (preservative-free)

▷ *metronidazole* (not for use in 1st; B in 2nd, 3rd)(G)

      Flagyl *Tab:* 250*, 500*mg

      Flagyl 375 *Cap:* 375 mg

      Flagyl ER *Tab:* 750 mg ext-rel

▷ *moxifloxacin* (C)(G)

      Avelox *Tab:* 400 mg

Comment: *moxifloxacin* is contraindicated <18 years-of-age, and during pregnancy and lactation. Risk of tendonitis or tendon rupture.

▷ *ofloxacin* (C)(G)

      Floxin *Tab:* 200, 300, 400 mg

Comment: *ofloxacin* is contraindicated <18 years-of-age, and during pregnancy and lactation. Risk of tendonitis or tendon rupture.

▷ *tinidazole* (not for use in 1st; B in 2nd, 3rd)

      Tindamax *Tab:* 250*, 500*mg

URINARY RETENTION: UNOBSTRUCTIVE

▷ *bethanechol* (C) 10-30 mg tid

      Urecholine *Tab:* 5, 10, 25, 50 mg

Comment: Contraindicated in presence of urinary obstruction. *atropine* 0.4 mg administered SC reverses *bethanechol* toxicity.

URINARY TRACT INFECTION (UTI, CYSTITIS: ACUTE)

URINARY TRACT ANALGESIA

Comment: Except when contraindicated, *ibuprofen* <u>or</u> other inflammatory agent of choice is a recommended adjunct <u>or</u> monotherapy in the treatment of UTI dysuria, frequency, and urgency which is due to inflammation and associated smooth muscle spasms/colic.

OTC **AZO Standard**
OTC **AZO Standard Maximum Strength**
OTC **Prodium**
OTC Uristat

ANTISPASMODIC AGENT

▷ *flavoxate* (B)(G) 100-200 mg tid-qid
   Pediatric: <12 years: not recommended; >12 years: same as adult
      Urispas *Tab:* 100 mg
Comment: *flavoxate* hydrochloride tablets are indicated for symptomatic relief of dysuria, urgency, nocturia, suprapubic pain, frequency and incontinence as may occur in cystitis, prostatitis, urethritis, urethrocystitis/urethrotrigonitis. *flavoxate* is not indicated for definitive treatment, but is compatible with drugs used for the treatment of UTI. *flavoxate* is contraindicated in patients who have any of the following obstructive conditions: pyloric <u>or</u> duodenal obstruction, obstructive intestinal lesions, ileus, achalasia, GI hemorrhage, and obstructive uropathies of the lower urinary tract. Used with caution with glaucoma. It is not known whether *flavoxate* is excreted in human milk.

URINARY TRACT ANALGESIC-ANTISPASMODIC AGENTS

▷ *hyoscyamine* (C)(G)
      Anaspaz 1-2 tabs q 4 hours prn; max 12 tabs/day
         Tab: 0.125*mg
      Pediatric: <2 years: not recommended; 2-12 years: 0.0625-0.125 mg q 4 hours prn; max 0.75 mg/day; >12 years: same as adult
      Levbid 1-2 tabs q 12 hours prn; max 4 tabs/day
      Pediatric: <12 years: not recommended; ≥12 years: same as adult
         Tab: 0.375*mg ext-rel
      Levsin 1-2 tabs q 4 hours prn; max 12 tabs/day
      Pediatric: <6 years: not recommended; 6-12 years: 1 tab q 4 hours prn; ≥12 years: same as adult
         Tab: 0.125*mg
      Levsin Drops Use SL <u>or</u> PO forms
      Pediatric: 3.4 kg: 4 drops q 4 hours prn; max 24 drops/day; 5 kg: 5 drops q 4 hours prn; max 30 drops/day; 7 kg: 6 drops q 4 hours prn; max 36 drops/day; 10 kg: 8 drops q 4 hours prn; max 40 drops/day
         Oral drops: 0.125 mg/ml (15 ml) (orange) (alcohol 5%)
      Levsin Elixir 5 ml q 4 hours prn ←fix raised font left
      Pediatric: <10 kg: use drops; 10-19 kg: 1.25 ml q 4 hours prn; 20-39 kg: 2.5 ml q 4 hours prn; 40-49 kg: 3.75 ml q 4 hours prn; >50 kg:
         Elix: 0.125 mg/5 ml (16 oz) (orange) (alcohol 20%)
      Levsinex SL 1-2 tabs q 4 hours; max 12 tabs/day
      Pediatric: <2 years: not recommended; 2-12 years: 1 tab q 4 hours; max 6 tabs/day; >12 years: same as adult
         Tab: 0.125 mg sublingual

Levsinex Timecaps 1-2 caps q 12 hours; may adjust to 1 cap q 8 hours
Pediatric: <2 years: not recommended; 2-12 years: 1 cap q 12 hours; max 2 caps/day; >12 years: same as adult
> *Cap:* 0.375 mg time-rel

NuLev dissolve 1-2 tabs on tongue, with <u>or</u> without water, q 4 hours prn; max 12 tabs/day
Pediatric: <2 years: not recommended; 2-12 years: dissolve 1 tab on tongue, with <u>or</u> without water, q 4 hours prn; max 6 tabs/day; >12 years:
> *ODT:* 0.125 mg (mint) (phenylalanine)

➤ *methenamine+phenyl salicylate+methylene blue+benzoic acid+atropine sulfate+hyoscyamine* (C)(G) 2 tabs qid prn
Pediatric: <6 years: not recommended; ≥6 years: same as adult
Urised *Tab:* meth 40.8 mg+phenyl salic 18.1 mg+meth blue 5.4 mg+benz acid 4.5 mg+atro sulf 0.03 mg+hyoscy 0.03 mg

Comment: Urised imparts a blue-green color to urine which may stain fabrics.

➤ *methenamine+phenyl salicylate+methylene blue+sod phosphate monobasic+hyoscyamine* (C) 1 cap qid prn
Pediatric: <6 years: not recommended; ≥6 years: same as adult
Uribel *Cap:* meth 118 mg+phenyl salic 36 mg+meth blue 10 mg+sod phos mono 40.8 mg+hyoscy 0.12 mg

➤ *methenamine+phenyl salicylate+methylene blue+sod biphosphate+hyoscyamine* (C) 1 tab qid prn
Pediatric: <6 years: not recommended; ≥6 years: same as adult
Urelle *Cap:* meth 81 mg+phenyl salic 32.4 mg+meth blue 10.8 mg+sod biphos 40.8 mg+hyoscy 0.12 mg

➤ *phenazopyridine* (B)(G) 100-200 mg q 6 hours prn; max 2 days
Pediatric: <12 years: not recommended; ≥12 years: same as adult
AZO Standard, Prodium, Uristat (OTC) *Tab:* 95 mg
AZO Standard Maximum Strength (OTC) *Tab:* 97.5 mg
Pyridium, Urogesic *Tab:* 100, 200 mg

Comment: *phenazopyridine* imparts an orange-red color to urine which may stain fabrics.

ANTI-INFECTIVES

➤ *acetyl sulfisoxazole* (C)(G)
Gantrisin initially 2-4 gm in a single <u>or</u> divided doses; then, 4-8 gm/day in 4-6 divided doses x 3-10 days
Pediatric: <12 years: not recommended; ≥12 years: same as adult
> *Tab:* 500 mg

Gantrisin initially 2-4 gm in a single <u>or</u> divided doses; then, 4-8 gm/day in 4-6 divided doses x 3-10 days
Pediatric: <2 months: not recommended; 2 months-12 years: initial dose 75 mg/kg/ day; then 150 mg/kg/day in 4-6 divided doses x 3-10 days; max 6 gm/day; >12 years: same as adult
> *Oral susp:* 500 mg/5 ml (4, 16 oz); *Syr:* 500 mg/5 ml (16 oz)

➤ *amoxicillin* (B)(G) 500-875 mg bid <u>or</u> 250-500 mg tid x 3-10 days
Pediatric: <40 kg (88 lb): 20-40 mg/kg/day in 3 divided doses x 10 days <u>or</u> 25-45 mg/kg/day in 2 divided doses 3-10 days; *see page 586 for dose by weight table;* ≥40 kg: same as adult
Amoxil *Cap:* 250, 500 mg; *Tab:* 875*mg; *Chew tab:* 125, 200, 250, 400 mg (cherry-banana-peppermint) (phenylalanine); *Oral susp:* 125, 250 mg/5 ml (80, 100, 150 ml) (strawberry); 200, 400 mg/5 ml (50, 75, 100 ml) (bubble gum); *Oral drops:* 50 mg/ml (30 ml) (bubble gum)
Moxatag *Tab:* 775 mg ext-rel

Trimox *Tab:* 125, 250 mg; *Cap:* 250, 500 mg; *Oral susp:* 125, 250 mg/5 ml (80, 100, 150 ml) (raspberry-strawberry)

▷ *amoxicillin+clavulanate* (B)(G)

Augmentin 500 mg tid <u>or</u> 875 mg bid x 3-10 days

Pediatric: <40 kg: 40-45 mg/kg/day divided tid x 3-10 days <u>or</u> 90 mg/kg/day divided bid x 10 days; *see page 588 for dose by weight table;* ≥40 kg: same as adult

Tab: 250, 500, 875 mg; *Chew tab:* 125, 250 mg (lemon-lime); 200, 400 mg (cherry-banana) (phenylalanine); *Oral susp:* 125 mg/5 ml (banana), 250 mg/5 ml (75, 100, 150 ml) (orange); 200, 400 mg/5 ml (50, 75, 100 ml) (orange) (phenylalanine)

Augmentin ES-600 <3 months: not recommended; ≥3 months, <40 kg: 90 mg/kg/day divided q 12 hours x 3-10 days; *see page 589 for dose by weight table;* ≥40 kg: not recommended

Oral susp: 600 mg/5 ml (50, 75, 100, 125, 150, 200 ml) (strawberry cream) (phenylalanine)

Augmentin XR <16 years: use other forms; ≥16 years: 2 tabs q 12 hours x 3-10 days

Tab: 1000*mg ext-rel

▷ *ampicillin* (B) 500 mg qid x 3-10 days

Pediatric: <12 years: 50-100 mg/kg/day in 4 divided doses x 3-10 days; *see page 586 for dose by weight table;* ≥12 years: same as adult

Omnipen, Principen *Cap:* 250, 500 mg; *Oral susp:* 125, 250 mg/5 ml (100, 150, 200 ml) (fruit)

▷ *carbenicillin* (B) 1-2 tabs qid x 3-10 days

Pediatric: <12 years: not recommended; ≥12 years: same as adult

Geocillin *Tab:* 382 mg

Tab: 375, 500 mg ext-rel

▷ *cefaclor* (B)(G) 250-500 mg q 8 hours x 3-10 days; max 2 gm/day

Pediatric: <1 month: not recommended; 1 month-12 years: 20-40 mg/kg divided bid x 10 days; *see page 592 for dose by weight table;* max 1 gm/day; >12 years: same as adult

Tab: 500 mg; *Cap:* 250, 500 mg; *Susp:* 125 mg/5 ml (75, 150 ml) (strawberry); 187 mg/5 ml (50, 100 ml) (strawberry); 250 mg/5 ml (75, 150 ml) (strawberry); 375 mg/5 ml (50, 100 ml) (strawberry)

Cefaclor Extended Release 500 mg bid x 3-10 days (clinically equivalent to 250 mg immed-rel caps tid); swallow whole; take with meals

Pediatric: <16 years: not recommended; ≥16 years: same as adult

Tab: 375, 500 mg ext-rel

▷ *cefadroxil* (B) 1-2 gm in a single <u>or</u> 2 divided doses x 3-10 days

Pediatric: <12 years: 30 mg/kg/day in 2 divided doses x 3-10 days; *see page 593 for dose by weight table;* ≥12 years: same as adult

Duricef *Cap:* 500 mg; *Tab:* 1 gm; *Oral susp:* 250 mg/5 ml (100 ml); 500 mg/5 ml (75, 100 ml) (orange-pineapple)

▷ *cefixime* (B)(G) 400 mg once daily x 5 days

Pediatric: <6 months: not recommended; 6 months-12 years, <50 kg: 8 mg/kg/day in 1-2 divided doses x 5 days; *see page 595 for dose by weight table;* >12 years, >50 kg: same as adult

Suprax *Tab:* 400 mg; *Cap:* 400 mg; *Oral susp:* 100, 200, 500 mg/5 ml (50, 75, 100 ml) (strawberry)

▷ *cefpodoxime proxetil* (B) 100 mg bid x 3-10 days

Pediatric: <2 months: not recommended; 2 months-12 years: 10 mg/kg/day (max 400 mg/dose) <u>or</u> 5 mg/kg/day bid (max 200 mg/dose) x 3-10 days: *see page 596 for dose by weight table;* ≥12 years: same as adult

Vantin *Tab:* 100, 200 mg; *Oral susp:* 50, 100 mg/5 ml (50, 75, 100 mg) (lemon creme)

▷ *cephalexin* (B)(G) 500 mg bid x 3-10 days
Pediatric: <12 years: 25-50 mg/kg/day in 4 divided doses x 3-10 days; *see page* 599 *for dose by weight table;* ≥12 years:
  Keflex *Cap:* 250, 333, 500, 750 mg; *Oral susp:* 125, 250 mg/5 ml (100, 200 ml) (strawberry)

▷ *ciprofloxacin* (C) 500 mg bid or 1000 mg XR once daily x 3-7 days
Pediatric: <18 years: not recommended; ≥18 years: same as adult
  Cipro (G) *Tab:* 250, 500, 750 mg; *Oral susp:* 250, 500 mg/5 ml (100 ml) (strawberry)
  Cipro XR *Tab:* 500, 1000 mg ext-rel
  ProQuin XR *Tab:* 500 mg ext-rel
Comment: *ciprofloxacin* is contraindicated <18 years-of-age, and during pregnancy and lactation. Risk of tendonitis or tendon rupture.

▷ *doxycycline* (D)(G) 100 mg bid x 3-10 days
Pediatric: <8 years: not recommended; ≥8 years, <100 lb: 2 mg/lb on first day in 2 divided doses, followed by 1 mg/lb/day in a single or 2 divided doses x 3-10 days; ≥8 years, ≥100 lb: same as adult
  Acticlate *Tab:* 75, 150**mg
  Adoxa *Tab:* 50, 75, 100, 150 mg ent-coat
  Doryx *Tab:* 50, 75, 100, 150, 200 mg del-rel
  Doxteric *Tab:* 50 mg del-rel
  Monodox *Cap:* 50, 75, 100 mg
  Oracea *Cap:* 40 mg del-rel
  Vibramycin *Tab:* 100 mg; *Cap:* 50, 100 mg; *Syr:* 50 mg/5 ml (raspberry-apple) (sulfites); *Oral susp:* 25 mg/5 ml (raspberry)
  Vibra-Tab *Tab:* 100 mg film-coat
Comment: *doxycycline* is contraindicated <8 years-of-age, in pregnancy, and lactation (discolors developing tooth enamel). A side effect may be photosensitivity (photophobia). Do not take with antacids, calcium supplements, milk or other dairy, or within 2 hours of taking another drug.

▷ *enoxacin* (C) 200 mg q 12 hours x 3-10 days
Pediatric: <18 years: not recommended; ≥18 years: same as adult
  Penetrex *Tab:* 200, 400 mg
Comment: *enoxacin* is contraindicated <18 years-of-age, and during pregnancy and lactation. Risk of tendonitis or tendon rupture.

▷ *fosfomycin* (B) take as a single dose on an empty stomach; dissolve 1 sachet pkt in 3-4 oz cold water and drink immediately
Pediatric: <12 years: not established; ≥12 years: same as adult
  Monurol *Single-dose sachet pkts:* 3 gm (mandarin orange) (saccharin, sucrose)
Comment: *fosfomycin tromethamine* is a single-dose synthetic, broad spectrum, bactericidal antibiotic for treatment of uncomplicated UTI. Repeat dosing does not improve clinical efficacy. Safety and effectiveness in children ≥12 years have not been established in adequate and well-controlled studies.

▷ *levofloxacin* (C) 250 mg once daily x 3-7 days
Pediatric: <18 years: not recommended; ≥18 years: same as adult
  Levaquin *Tab:* 250, 500, 750 mg; *Oral soln:* 25 mg/ml (480 ml) (benzyl alcohol); *Inj conc:* 25 mg/ml for IV infusion after dilution (20, 30 ml single-use vial) (preservative-free); *Premix soln:* 5 mg/ml for IV infusion (50, 100, 150 ml) (preservative-free)
Comment: *levofloxacin* is contraindicated <18 years-of-age, and during pregnancy and lactation. Risk of tendonitis or tendon rupture.

▷ *lomefloxacin* (C) 400 mg once daily x 3-7 days
Pediatric: <18 years: not recommended; ≥18 years: same as adult
  Maxaquin *Tab:* 400 mg

Comment: *lomefloxacin* is contraindicated <18 years-of-age, and during pregnancy and lactation. Risk of tendonitis or tendon rupture.

▷ *minocycline* (D)(G) 100 mg q 12 hours x 3-10 days
Pediatric: <8 years: not recommended; ≥8 years, <100 lb: 1-2 mg/lb in 2 divided doses x 3-10 days; ≥8 years, ≥100 lb: same as adult
    Dynacin *Cap:* 50, 100 mg
    Minocin *Cap:* 50, 75, 100 mg; *Oral susp:* 50 mg/5 ml (60 ml) (custard) (sulfites, alcohol 5%)

Comment: *minocycline* is contraindicated <8 years-of-age, in pregnancy, and lactation (discolors developing tooth enamel). A side effect may be photo-sensitivity (photophobia). Do not give with antacids, calcium supplements, milk or other dairy, or within two hours of taking another drug.

▷ *nalidixic acid* (B) 1 gm qid x 3-10 days
Pediatric: <3 months: not recommended; ≥3 months-<12 years: 25 mg/lb/day in 4 divided doses x 3-10 days; ≥12 years: same as adult
    NegGram *Tab:* 250, 500 mg; 1 gm; *Cap:* 250, 500 mg; *Oral susp:* 250 mg/5 ml

▷ *nitrofurantoin* (B)(G)
    Furadantin 50-100 mg qid x 3-10 days
Pediatric: <1 month: not recommended; ≥1 month-12 years: 5-7 mg/kg/ day in 4 divided doses x 3-10 days; *see page* 613 *for dose by weight table;* >12 years: same as adult
        Oral susp: 25 mg/5 ml (60 ml)
    Macrobid 100 mg q 12 hours x 3-10 days
Pediatric: <12 years: not recommended; ≥12 years: same as adult
        Cap: 100 mg
    Macrodantin 50-100 mg qid x 3-10 days
Pediatric: <12 years: not recommended; ≥12 years: same as adult
        Cap: 25, 50, 100 mg

▷ *norfloxacin* (C) 400 mg once daily x 3-7 days
Pediatric: <18 years: not recommended; ≥18 years: same as adult
    Noroxin *Tab:* 400 mg

Comment: *norfloxacin* is contraindicated <18 years-of-age, and during pregnancy and lactation. Risk of tendonitis or tendon rupture.

▷ *ofloxacin* (C)(G) 200 mg q 12 hours x 3-7 days
Pediatric: <18 years: not recommended; ≥18 years: same as adult
    Floxin *Tab:* 200, 300, 400 mg
    Floxin UroPak *Tab:* 200 mg (6/pck)

Comment: *ofloxacin* is contraindicated <18 years-of-age, and during pregnancy and lactation. Risk of tendonitis or tendon rupture.

▷ *trimethoprim* (C)(G)
    Primsol 100 mg q 12 hours or 200 mg once daily x 10 days
Pediatric: <6 months: not recommended; ≥6 months-12 years: 10 mg/kg/ day in 2 divided doses x 10 days; >12 years: same as adult
        Oral soln: 50 mg/5 ml (bubble gum) (dye-free, alcohol-free)
    Proloprim 100 mg q 12 hours or 200 mg once daily x 10 days
Pediatric: <12 years: not recommended; ≥12 years: same as adult
        Tab: 100, 200 mg
    Trimpex 100 mg q 12 hours or 200 mg once daily x 10 days
Pediatric: <12 years: not recommended; ≥12 years: same as adult
        Tab: 100 mg

▷ *trimethoprim+sulfamethoxazole* (TMP-SMX) (D)(G)
    Bactrim, Septra 2 tabs bid x 3-10 days
Pediatric: <12 years: not recommended; ≥12 years: same as adult
        Tab: trim 80 mg+sulfa 400 mg*

Bactrim DS, Septra DS 1 tab bid x 3-10 days
Pediatric: <12 years: not recommended; ≥12 years: same as adult
  Tab: trim 160 mg+sulfa 800 mg*
Bactrim Pediatric Suspension, Septra Pediatric Suspension use tabs
Pediatric: <2 months: not recommended; ≥2 months-12 years: 40 mg/kg/day of *sulfamethoxazole* in 2 doses bid; >12 years: use tabs
  Oral susp: trim 40 mg+sulfa 200 mg per 5 ml (100 ml) (cherry) (alcohol 0.3%)

PARENTERAL THERAPY FOR COMPLICATED cUTI

▷ *ertapenem* (B) 1 gm once daily; *CrCl <30 mL/min:* 500 mg once daily; treat x 10-14 days; may switch to an oral antibiotic after 3 days if warranted; *IV infusion:* administer over 30 minutes; *IM injection:* reconstitute
Pediatric: <18 years: not recommended; ≥18 years same as adult
  Invanz *Vial:* 1 gm pwdr for reconstitution

▷ *meropenem+vaborbactam* administer 4 gm (*meropenem* 2 gm and *vaborbactam* 2 gm) every 8 hours by IV infusion; administer over 3 hours; treat for up to 14 days; monitor urine cultures and eGFR; *eGFR 30-49 mL/min:* 2 gm (*meropenem* 1 gm and *vaborbactam* 1 gm) every 8 hours; *eGFR 15-29 mL/min:* 2 gm (*meropenem* 1 gm and *vaborbactam* 1 gm) every 12 hours; *eGFR <15 mL/min:* 1 gm (*meropenem* 0.5 gm and *vaborbactam* 0.5 gm) every 12 hours; *ESRD:* administer 1 gm (*meropenem* 0.5 gm and *vaborbactam* 0.5 gm) every 12 hours <u>after</u> dialysis
Pediatric: <18 years: not recommended; ≥18 years same as adult
  Vabomere *Vial:* mero 1 gm+vabor 1 gm pwdr for reconstitution and dilution
Comment: **Vabomere** (formerly **Carbavance**) is a carbapenem *(meropenem)* and beta-lactamase inhibitor *(vaborbactam)* combination indicated for the treatment of complicated urinary tract infections (cTIs). Administer **abomere** with caution with history of hyper-sensitivity to penicillin, cephalosporin, other betalactams <u>or</u> other allergens. Discontinue immediately if allergic reaction occurs. Vabomere is not recommended with concomitant *valproic acid* <u>or</u> *divalproex sodium*. Discontinue **Vabomere** if *C. difficile*-associated diarrhea is suspected <u>or</u> confirmed. Monitor, and reevaluate risk/ benefit if signs of neuromotor impairment (e.g., seizures, focal tremors, myoclonus, delirium, paresthesias), renal impairment, thrombocytopenia, <u>and/or</u> superinfection.

LONG-TERM PROPHYLACTIC-SUPPRESSION THERAPY

▷ *methenamine hippurate* (C) 1 gm once daily
Pediatric: <6 years: 0.25 gm/30 lb once daily; 6-12 years: 25-50 mg/kg/day once daily <u>or</u> 0.5-1 gm once daily; >12 years:
  Hiprex *Tab:* 1 gm; *Oral susp:* 500 mg/5 ml (480 ml)
  Urex *Tab:* 1 gm; *Oral susp:* 500 mg/5 ml (480 ml)
▷ *nitrofurantoin* (B)(G)
  Furadantin 50-100 mg as a single dose at bedtime
  Pediatric: <1 month: not recommended; ≥1 month-12 years: 1 mg/kg as a single dose at bedtime; >12 years: same as adult
    Oral susp: 25 mg/5 ml (60 ml)
  Macrobid 50-100 mg as a single dose at bedtime
  Pediatric: <12 years: not recommended; ≥12 years: same as adult
    Cap: 100 mg
  Macrodantin 50-100 mg as a single dose at bedtime
  Pediatric: <12 years: not recommended; ≥12 years: same as adult
    Cap: 25, 50, 100 mg
  Furadantin 50-100 mg as a single dose at bedtime
  Pediatric: <12 years: not recommended; ≥12 years: same as adult
    Oral susp: 25 mg/5 ml (60 ml)

Macrobid 100 mg as a single dose at bedtime
Pediatric: <12 years: not recommended; ≥12 years: same as adult
  Cap: 100 mg
Macrodantin 50-100 mg as a single dose at bedtime
Pediatric: <12 years: not recommended; ≥12 years: same as adult
  Cap: 25, 50, 100 mg

 UROLITHIASIS (RENAL CALCULI, KIDNEY STONES)

Acetaminophen for IV Infusion *see Pain page* 344
NSAIDs *see page* 562
Opioid Analgesics *see Pain page* 345

PREVENTION OF CALCIUM STONES

▷ *chlorothiazide* (B)(G) 50 mg bid
  Pediatric: <6 months: up to 15 mg/lb/day in 2 divided doses; ≥6 months-12 years: 10 mg/lb/day in 2 divided doses; max 375 mg/day; >12 years: Same as adult
    Diuril *Tab:* 250*, 500*mg; *Oral susp:* 250 mg/5 ml (237 ml)
▷ *hydrochlorothiazide* (B)(G) 50 mg bid
  Pediatric: <12 years: not recommended; ≥12 years: same as adult
    Esidrix *Tab:* 25, 50 mg
    Microzide *Cap:* 12.5 mg

PREVENTION OF CYSTINE STONES

▷ *penicillamine* (D) 1-4 gm/day
  Pediatric: <12 years: not recommended; ≥12 years: same as adult
    Cuprimine *Cap:* 125, 250 mg
    Depen *Titratable tab:* 250 mg
▷ *potassium citrate* (C)(G) 30 mEq qid
  Pediatric: <12 years: not recommended; ≥12 years: same as adult
    Urocit-K *Tab:* 5, 10, 15 mEq ext-rel

Comment: *potassium citrate* is contraindicated in hyperkalemia. Encourage patients to limit salt intake and maintain liberal hydration (urine volume should be at least 2 liters/day). Target urine pH is 6.0-7.0 and urine citrate at least 320 mg/day and close to the normal mean of 640 mg/day. Take with food.

PREVENTION OF URIC ACID STONES

▷ *allopurinol* (C)(G) 200-300 mg in 1-3 doses; max 800 mg/day; max single dose 300 mg
  Pediatric: <6 years: max 150 mg/day; 6-10 years: max 400 mg/day; max single dose 300 mg; >10 years: same as adult
    Zyloprim *Tab:* 100*, 300*mg
▷ *potassium citrate* (C)(G) 30 mEq qid
    Urocit-K *Tab:* 5, 10, 15 mEq ext-rel

Comment: *potassium citrate* is contraindicated in hyperkalemia. Encourage patients to limit salt intake and maintain liberal hydration (urine volume should be at least 2 liters/day). Target urine pH is 6.0-7.0 and urine citrate at least 320 mg/day and close to the normal mean of 640 mg/day. Take with food.

ALPHA-1A BLOCKERS

Comment: Alpha-1A blockers facilitate stone passage.

▷ *alfuzosin* (B)(G) 10 mg once daily taken immediately after the same meal each day
  UroXatral *Tab*: 10 mg ext-rel
▷ *tamsulosin* (B)(G) initially 0.4 mg once daily; may increase to 0.8 mg once daily after 2-4 weeks if needed
  Pediatric: ≤18 years: with radiopaque lower ureteral stones of 10-12 mm or smaller have received the following doses: *tamsulosin* 0.2 mg PO at bedtime (≤4 years) and 0.4 mg PO at bedtime (>4 years); administer x 28 days or until definite stone passage (i.e., evidence of stone on urine straining); >18 years:
  Flomax *Cap*: 0.4 mg

Comment: *tamsulosin* 0.4 mg may be taken with **Avodart** 0.5 mg once daily as combination therapy. *tamsulosin* is taken with standard analgesia (e.g., ibuprofen); mild somnolence is common. If pain is controlled with oral analgesia, clear liquids are tolerated, and there is no evidence of infection, monitor closely for spontaneous passage for 3 to 4 weeks prior to definitive therapy, since most data demonstrate safe lower uretal stone expulsion in the first 10 days of conservative medical management.

ANTISPASMODIC AGENT

▷ *flavoxate* (B)(G) 100-200 mg tid-qid
  Pediatric: <12 years: not recommended; >12 years: same as adult
  Urispas Tab: 100 mg

Comment: *flavoxate* hydrochloride tablets are indicated for symptomatic relief of dysuria, urgency, nocturia, suprapubic pain, frequency and incontinence as may occur in cystitis, prostatitis, urethritis, urethrocystitis/urethrotrigonitis. *flavoxate* is not indicated for definitive treatment, but is compatible with drugs used for the treatment of UTI. flavoxate is contraindicated in patients who have any of the following obstructive conditions: pyloric or duodenal obstruction, obstructive intestinal lesions, ileus, achalasia, GI hemorrhage, and obstructive uropathies of the lower urinary tract. Used with caution with glaucoma. It is not known whether *flavoxate* is excreted in human milk.

ACETAMINOPHEN FOR IV INFUSION

▷ *acetaminophen* injectable (B) administer by IV infusion over 15 minutes; 1,000 mg q 6 hours prn or 650 mg q 4 hours prn; max 4,000 mg/day
  Pediatric: <2 years: not recommended; 2-13 years <50 kg: 15 mg/kg q 6 hours prn or 2.5 mg/kg q 4 hours prn; max 750 mg/single dose; max 75 mg/kg per day; >13 years: same as adult
  Ofirmev *Vial*: 10 mg/ml (100 ml) (preservative-free)

Comment: The **Ofirmev** vial is intended for single-use. If any portion is withdrawn from the vial, use within 6 hours. Discard the unused portion. For pediatric patients, withdraw the intended dose and administer via syringe pump. Do not admix **Ofirmev** with any other drugs. **Ofirmev** is physically incompatible with *diazepam* and *chlorpromazine hydrochloride*.

IBUPROFEN FOR IV INFUSION

▷ *ibuprofen* (B) dilute dose in 0.9% NS, D5W, or Lactated Ringers (LR) solution; administer by IV infusion over at least 10 minutes; do not administer via IV bolus or IM; 400-800 mg q 6 hours prn; maximum 3,200 mg/day
  Pediatric: <6 months; not recommended; 6 months-<12 years: 10 mg/kg q 4-6 hours prn; max 400 mg/dose; max 40 mg/kg or 2,400 mg/24 hours, whichever is less; 12-17 years: max 400 mg q 4-6 hours prn; max 2,400 mg/24 hours
  Caldolor *Vial*: 800 mg/8 ml single-dose

Comment: Prepare **Caldolor** solution for IV administration as follows: 100 mg dose: dilute 1 ml of **Caldolor** in at least 100 ml of diluent (IVF); 200 mg dose: dilute 2 ml of **Caldolor** in at least 100 ml of diluent; 400 mg dose: dilute 4 ml of **Caldolor** in at least 100 ml of diluent; 800 mg dose: dilute 8 ml of **Caldolor** in at least 200 ml of diluent. **Caldolor** is also indicated for management of fever. For adults with fever, 400 mg via IV infusion, followed by 400 mg q 4-6 hours or 100-200 mg q 4 hours prn.

MU OPIOID ANALGESICS

▷ *tramadol* (C)(IV)(G)

Comment: *tramadol* is known to be excreted in breast milk. The FDA and the European Medicines Agency (EMA) are investigating the safety of using *tramadol*-containing medications to treat pain in children 12-18 years because of the potential for serious side effects, including slowed or difficult breathing.

 Rybix ODT initially 100 mg once daily; may increase by 100 mg every 5 days; max 300 mg/day; *CrCl <30 mL/min or severe hepatic impairment*: not recommended; *Cirrhosis*: max 50 mg q 12 hours

 Pediatric: <12 years: contraindicated; 12-<18: use extreme caution; not recommended for children and adolescents with obesity, asthma, obstructive sleep apnea, or other chronic breathing problem, or for post-tonsillectomy/adenoidectomy pain; ≥18 years: same as adult

  ODT: 50 mg (mint) (phenylalanine)

 Ryzolt initially 100 mg once daily; may increase by 100 mg every 5 days; max 300 mg/day; CrCl <30 mL/min or severe hepatic impairment: not recommended

 Pediatric: <12 years: contraindicated; 12-<18: use extreme caution; not recommmended for children and adolescents with obesity, asthma, obstructive sleep apnea, or other chronic breathing problem, or for post-tonsillectomy/adenoidectomy pain; ≥18 years: same as adult

  Tab: 100, 200, 300 mg ext-rel

 Ultram 50-100 mg q 4-6 hours prn; max 400 mg/day; *CrCl <30 mL/min*, max 100 mg q 12 hours; cirrhosis, max 50 mg q 12 hours

 Pediatric: <12 years: contraindicated; 12-<18: use extreme caution; not recommended for children and adolescents with obesity, asthma, obstructive sleep apnea, or other chronic breathing problem, or for post-tonsillectomy/ adenoidectomy pain; ≥18 years: same as adult

  Tab: 50*mg

 Ultram ER initially 100 mg once daily; may increase by 100 mg every 5 days; max 300 mg/day; *CrCl <30 mL/min or severe hepatic impairment*: not recommended

 Pediatric: <12 years: contraindicated; 12-<18: use extreme caution; not recommended for children and adolescents with obesity, asthma, obstructive sleep apnea, or other chronic breathing problem, or for post-tonsillectomy/adenoidectomy pain; ≥18 years: same as adult

  Tab: 100, 200, 300 mg ext-rel

▷ *tramadol+acetaminophen* (C)(IV)(G) 2 tabs q 4-6 hours; max 8 tabs/day x 5 days; *CrCl <30 mL/min*: max 2 tabs q 12 hours; max 4 tabs/day x 5 days

 Pediatric: <12 years: contraindicated; 12-<18: use extreme caution; not recommended for children and adolescents with obesity, asthma, obstructive sleep apnea, or other chronic breathing problem, or for post-tonsillectomy/adenoidectomy pain; same as adult

 Ultracet *Tab*: tram 37.5+acet 325 mg

Comment: *tramadol* is known to be excreted in breast milk. The FDA and the European Medicines Agency (EMA) are investigating the safety of using **tramadol**-containing medications to treat pain in children 12-18 years because of the potential for serious side effects, including slowed or difficult breathing.

INTRANASAL (TRANSMUCOSAL) OPIOID ANALGESICS

▷ *butorphanol tartrate* nasal spray (C)(IV) initially 1 spray (1 mg) in one nostril and may repeat after 60-90 minutes in opposite nostril if needed or 1 spray in each nostril and may repeat q 3-4 hours prn

Pediatric: <18 years: not recommended; ≥18 years: same as adult
>   **Butorphanol Nasal Spray** *Nasal spray:* 1 mg/actuation (10 mg/ml, 2.5 ml)
>   **Stadol Nasal Spray** *Nasal spray:* 1 mg/actuation (10 mg/ml, 2.5 ml)
▷ *fentanyl* nasal spray **(C)(II)** initially 1 spray (100 mcg) in one nostril and may repeat after 2 hours; when adequate analgesia is achieved, use that dose for subsequent breakthrough episodes; *Titration steps:* 100 mcg using 1 x 100 mcg spray; 200 mcg using 2 x 100 mcg spray (1 spray in each nostril); 400 mcg using 1 x 400 mcg spray; 800 mcg using 2 x 400 mcg (1 spray in each nostril); max 800 mcg; limit to ≤4 doses per day
   Pediatric: <18 years: not recommended; ≥18 years: same as adult
>   **Lazanda Nasal Spray** *Nasal spray:* 100, 400 mcg/100 mcl (8 sprays/bottle)
Comment: **Lazanda Nasal Spray** is available by restricted distribution program. Call 855-841-4234 or visit https://www.fda.gov/downloads/drugs/drugsafety/ postmarketdrugsafetyinformationforpatientsandproviders/ucm261983.pdf to enroll. **Lazanda Nasal Spray** is indicated for the management of breakthrough pain in cancer patients who are already receiving and who are tolerant to opioid therapy for their underlying persistent cancer pain. Patients considered opioid tolerant are those who are taking at least 60 mg of oral morphine/day, 25 mcg of transdermal *fentanyl*/hour, 30 mg oral *oxycodone*/day, 8 mg oral *hydromorphone*/day, 25 mg oral *oxymorphone*/ day, or an equianalgesic dose of another opioid for a week or longer. Patients must remain on around-the-clock opioids when using **Lazanda Nasal Spray**. As such, it is contraindicated in the management of acute or post-op pain, including headache/ migraine, or dental pain.

Comment: The Transmucosal Immediate Release **Fentanyl** (TIRF) Risk Evaluation and Mitigation Strategy (REMS) program is an FDA-required program designed to ensure informed risk-benefit decisions before initiating treatment, and while patients are treated to ensure appropriate use of TIRF medicines. The purpose of the TIRF REMS Access program is to mitigate the risk of misuse, abuse, addiction, overdose and serious complications due to medication errors with the use of TIRF medicines. You must enroll in the TIRF REMS Access program to prescribe, dispense, or distribute TIRF medicines. To register, call the TIRF REMS Access program at 1-866-822-1483 or register online at https://www.tirfremsaccess.com/TirfUI/rems/home.action.

 URTICARIA: MILD-TO-ACUTE HIVES AND CHRONIC SPONTANEOUS/ IDIOPATHIC URTICARIA (CSU/CIU)

Topical Corticosteroids *see page* 566
Oral Corticosteroids *see page* 569
Parenteral Corticosteroids *see page* 563

MILD-TO-MODERATE URTICARIA (HIVES, ANGIOEDEMA)
Second Generation Oral Antihistamines
Comment: The following drugs are second generation antihistamines. As such they minimally sedating, much less so than the first generation antihistamines. All antihistamines are excreted into breast milk.
▷ *cetirizine* **(C)(OTC)(G)** initially 5-10 mg once daily; 5 mg once daily; ≥65 years: use with caution
   Pediatric: <6 years: not recommended; ≥6 years: same as adult
>   **Children's Zyrtec Chewable** *Chew tab:* 5, 10 mg (grape)
>   **Children's Zyrtec Allergy Syrup** *Syr:* 1 mg/ml (4 oz) (grape, bubble gum) (sugar-free, dye-free)
>   **Zyrtec** *Tab:* 10 mg

    Zyrtec Hives Relief *Tab:* 10 mg
    Zyrtec Liquid Gels *Liq gel:* 10 mg
➤ *desloratadine* (C)
    Clarinex 1/2-1 tab once daily
    Pediatric: <6 years: not recommended; ≥6 years: same as adult
      Tab: 5 mg
    Clarinex RediTabs 5 mg once daily
    Pediatric: <6 years: not recommended; 6-12 years: 2.5 mg once daily; ≥12 years:
    same as adult
      ODT: 2.5, 5 mg (tutti-frutti) (phenylalanine)
    Clarinex Syrup 5 mg (10 ml) once daily
    Pediatric: <6 months: not recommended; 6-11 months: 1 mg (2 ml) once daily;
    1-5 years: 1.25 mg (2.5 ml) once daily; 6-11 years: 2.5 mg (5 ml) once daily; ≥12
    years: same as adult
      Syr: 0.5 mg per ml (4 oz) (tutti-frutti) (phenylalanine)
    Desloratadine ODT 1 tab once daily
    Pediatric: <6 years: not recommended; 6-11 years: 1/2 tab once daily; ≥12 years:
    same as adult
      ODT: 5 mg
➤ *fexofenadine* (C)(OTC)(G) 60 mg once daily-bid <u>or</u> 180 mg once daily; *CrCl <90 mL/ min:* 60 mg once daily
    Pediatric: <6 months: not recommended; 6 months-2 years: 15 mg bid; *CrCl ≤90 mL/ min:* 15 mg once daily; 2-11 years: 30 mg bid; *CrCl ≤90 mL/min:* 30 mg once daily;
    ≥12 years: same as adult
    Allegra *Tab:* 30, 60, 180 mg film-coat
    Allegra Allergy *Tab:* 60, 180 mg film-coat
    Allegra ODT *ODT:* 30 mg (phenylalanine)
    Allegra Oral Suspension *Oral susp:* 30 mg/5 ml (6 mg/ml) (4 oz)
➤ *levocetirizine* (B)(OTC) administer dose in the PM; *Seasonal Allergic Rhinitis:* <2 years: not recommended; may start at ≥2 years; *Chronic Idiopathic Urticaria (CIU), Perennial Allergic Rhinitis:* <6 months: not recommended; may start at ≥ 6 months; *Dosing by Age:* 6 months-5 years: max 1.25 mg once daily; 6-11 years: max 2.5 mg once daily; ≥12 years: 2.5-5 mg once daily; *Renal Dysfunction <12 years:* contrain-dicated; *Renal Dysfunction ≥12 years:* CrCl 50-80 ml/min: 2.5 mg once daily; CrCl 30-50 mL/min: 2.5 mg every other day; CrCl: 10-30 mL/min: 2.5 mg twice weekly (every 3-4 days); CrCl <10 mL/min, ESRD <u>or</u> hemodialysis: contraindicated
    Children's Xyzal Allergy 24HR *Oral Soln:* 0.5 mg/ml (150 ml)
    Xyzal Allergy 24HR *Tab:* 5*mg
➤ *loratadine* (C)(OTC)(G) 5 mg bid <u>or</u> 10 mg once daily; *Hepatic <u>or</u> Renal Insufficiency:* see mfr pkg insert
    Pediatric: <2 years: not recommended; 2-5 years: 5 mg once daily; ≥6 years: same as adult
    Children's Claritin Chewables *Chew tab:* 5 mg (grape) (phenylalanine)
    Children's Claritin Syrup 1 mg/ml (4 oz) (fruit) (sugar-free, alcohol-free, dye-free; sodium 6 mg/5 ml)
    Claritin *Tab:* 10 mg
    Claritin Hives Relief *Tab:* 10 mg
    Claritin Liqui-Gels *Liq gel:* 10 mg
    Claritin RediTabs 12 Hours *ODT:* 5 mg (mint)
    Claritin RediTabs 24 Hours *ODT:* 10 mg (mint)

First Generation Oral Antihistamines

➤ *diphenhydramine* (B)(G) 25-50 mg q 6-8 hours; max 100 mg/day
    Pediatric: <2 years: not recommended; 2-6 years: 6.25 mg q 4-6 hours; max 37.5 mg/day; >6-12 years: 12.5-25 mg q 4-6 hours; max 150 mg/day; >12 years: same as adult

Benadryl (OTC) *Chew tab:* 12.5 mg (grape) (phenylalanine); *Liq:* 12.5 mg/ 5 ml (4, 8 oz); *Cap:* 25 mg; *Tab:* 25 mg; *Dye-free soft gel:* 25 mg; *Dye-free liq:* 12.5 mg/5 ml (4, 8 oz)

▷ *hydroxyzine* (C)(G) 50 mg/day divided qid prn; 50-100 mg/day divided qid prn
  Pediatric: <6 years: 50 mg/day divided qid prn; ≥6 years: same as adult
  Atarax *Tab:* 10, 25, 50, 100 mg; *Syr:* 10 mg/5 ml (alcohol 0.5%)
  Vistaril *Cap:* 25, 50, 100 mg; *Oral susp:* 25 mg/5 ml (4 oz) (lemon)

Comment: *hydroxyzine* is contraindicated in early pregnancy and in patients with a prolonged QT interval. It is not known whether this drug is excreted in human milk; therefore, *hydroxyzine* should not be given to nursing mothers.

SEVERE URTICARIA
Parenteral Antihistamine

▷ *diphenhydramine* injectable (B)(G) 25-50 mg IM immediately; then q 6 hours prn
  Pediatric: <12 years: *See mfr pkg insert:* 1.25 mg/kg up to 25 mg IM x 1 dose; then q 6 hours prn; ≥12 years: same as adult
  Benadryl Injectable *Vial:* 50 mg/ml (1 ml single-use); 50 mg/ml (10 ml multi-dose); *Amp:* 10 mg/ml (1 ml); *Prefilled syringe:* 50 mg/ml (1 ml)

Parenteral Epinephrine

▷ *epinephrine* (C) 1:1000 0.01 ml/kg SC; max 0.3 ml
  Pediatric: 0.01 mg/kg SC

CHRONIC SPONTANEOUS/IDIOPATHIC URTICARIA
IgE Blocker (IgG1k Monoclonal Antibody)

Comment: Xolair *(omalizumab)* is a humanized monoclonal antibody that specifically binds to free immunoglobulin E in the blood and on the surface of selected B lymphocytes, but not on the surface of mast cells, antigen-presenting dendritic cells, or basophils. In the US *omalizumab* is approved for adults at 150 mg or 300 mg subcutaneously administered every 4 weeks for the treatment of CSU not responsive to high-dose antihistamines. In three published, pivotal, phase 3 randomized trials, the clinical response rate to **omalizumab** at 300 mg every 4 weeks, as defined by a weekly 7-day Urticaria Activity Score (UAS7) ≤6 at 12 weeks, was 52% in ASTERIA I, 66% in ASTERIA II, and 52% in GLACIAL. Good control of disease activity was defined as a UAS7 score of ≤6 on the 0- to 42-point UAS7, which correlates well with minimal or no patient symptoms

REFERENCE
Finlay, A. Y., Kaplan, A. P., Beck, L. A., Antonova, E. N., Balp, M.-M., Zazzali, J., … Maurer, M. (2017). Omalizumab substantially improves dermatology-related quality of life in patients with chronic spontaneous urticaria. *Journal of the European Academy of Dermatology and Venereology, 31*(10), 1715–1721. doi:10.1111/jdv.14384

Comment: A multicenter open-label study of 286 patients with CSU, conducted by the Catalan and Balearic Chronic Urticaria Network (XUrCB) at 15 hospitals, found about two-thirds of patients with CSU treated with the approved dose of *omalizumab* achieved good disease control. Three-quarters of the non-responders achieved good disease control upon up-dosing to 450 or 600 mg (twice the approved dose) every 4 weeks, without increase in adverse events.

REFERENCE
https://www.mdedge.com/familypracticenews/article/155732/urticaria/updosing-omalizumab-chronic-urticaria-pays

▷ *omalizumab* (B) 150-375 mg SC every 2-4 weeks based on body weight and pre-treatment serum total IgE level; max 150 mg/injection site
  Pediatric: <12 years: not recommended; ≥12 years: 30-90 kg + IgE >30-100 IU/ml 150 mg q 4 weeks; 90-150 kg + IgE >30-100 IU/ml or 30-90 kg + IgE >100-200 IU/ml or 30-60 kg + IgE >200-300 IU/ml 300 mg q 4 hours; >90-150 kg + IgE >100-200 IU/ml or >60-90 kg + IgE >200-300 IU/ml or 30-70 kg + IgE >300-400 IU/ml 225 mg q 2 weeks; >90-150 kg + IgE >200-300 IU/ml or >70-90 kg + IgE >300-400 IU/ml or 30-70 kg + IgE >400-500 IU/ml or 30-60 kg + IgE >500-600 IU/ml or 30-60 kg + IgE >600-700 IU/ml 375 mg q 2 weeks
    Xolair *Vial:* 150 mg pwdr for SC injection after reconstitution (preservative-free)

⬤ UTERINE FIBROIDS

See **Progesterone-only Contraceptives** *page* 559

▷ *medroxyprogesterone acetate* (X) 10 mg daily
    Provera *Tab:* 2.5, 5, 10 mg
▷ *Oral contraceptives* (X) with 35 mcg estrogen equivalent

SELECTIVE PROGESTERONE RECEPTOR MODULATOR

▷ *ulipristal acetate (UPA)* (X)(G) 5-10 mg once daily
Comment: Ulipristal acetate is currently approved in the United States as an emergency contraceptive (a single 30 mg dose), but is marketed for treating symptomatic fibroids in Canada and Europe. It is not yet available in a dose form appropriate for treatment of uterine fibroids (i.e., 5, 10 mg). The drug reduced dysfunctional uterine bleeding in about 90% of patients in the European trials. Women with uterine fibroids taking UPA experienced significant improvement of quality of life, compared with those taking placebo according to researchers' reported outcomes of VENUS II, a phase 3, prospective, randomized, double-blind, double-dummy, placebo-controlled study. Its design incorporated both parallel and crossover elements: Some patients who were on placebo crossed over to one of two doses of UPA after a washout period, and some patients on each active arm crossed over to placebo. The women (n=432) were between 18 and 50 years and premenopausal. At 13 weeks, uterine bleeding was controlled in 91% of the women receiving 5 mg of *ulipristal acetate*, 92% of those receiving 10 mg of *ulipristal* acetate, and 19% of those receiving placebo (P<0.001). Of women taking 5 mg of UPA, 91% achieved control (40.5%-42% became amenorrheic); of those taking 10 mg, 92% achieved control (54.8%-57.3% became amenorrheic) (controlled in 92%). These results compared to amenorrhea rates of 0%-8% (controlled in 19%) for women on placebo (*p*< .0001 for all values).
    Ella *Tab:* 30 mg
    Logilia *Tab:* 30 mg

REFERENCE
Donnez, J., Tatarchuk, T. F., Bouchard, P., Puscasiu, L., Zakharenko, N. F., Ivanova, T., . . . Loumaye, E. (2012). Ulipristal acetate versus placebo for fibroid treatment before surgery. *New England Journal of Medicine, 366*(5), 409–420. doi:10.1056/nejmoa1103182

⬤ VAGINAL IRRITATION: EXTERNAL

OTC Replens Vaginal Moisturizer
OTC Vagisil Intimate Moisturizer
Comment: Vagisil has no effect on condom integrity.

VERTIGO

▷ *meclizine* (B)(G) 25-100 mg/day in divided doses
Pediatric: <12 years: not established; ≥12 years: same as adult
    Antivert *Tab:* 12.5, 25, 50*mg
    Bonine (OTC) *Cap:* 15, 25, 30 mg; *Tab:* 12.5, 25, 50 mg; *Chew tab/Film-coat tab:* 25 mg
    Dramamine II (OTC) *Tab:* 25*mg
    Zentrip *Strip:* 25 mg orally-disint
▷ *methscopolamine bromide* (B) 1 tab q 6 hours prn
Pediatric: <12 years: not recommended; ≥12 years: same as adult
    Pamine *Tab:* 2.5 mg
    Pamine Forte *Tab:* 5 mg
▷ *scopolamine* (C) 0.4-0.8 mg tab (may repeat in 8 hours) or 1 x 1.5 mg transdermal patch behind ear (effective x 3 days; may replace every 4th day)
Pediatric: <12 years: not recommended; ≥12 years: same as adult
    Scopace *Tab:* 0.4 mg
    Transderm Scop *Transdermal patch:* 1.5 mg (4/carton)

VITILIGO

RE-PIGMENTATION AGENTS

▷ *methoxsalen* (C) Apply to well-defined area of vitiligo; then expose area to source of UVA (ultraviolet A) <u>or</u> sunlight; initial exposure no more than 1/2 predicted minimal erythemal dose; repeat weekly
Pediatric: <12 years: not recommended; ≥12 years: same as adult
    Oxsoralen *Lotn:* 1% (30 ml)
Comment: *methoxsalen* may only be applied by a health care provider. Do not dispense to patient.
▷ *trioxsalen* (C) 10 mg daily, taken 2-4 hours before ultraviolet light exposure; max 14 days and 28 tabs
Pediatric: <12 years: not recommended; ≥12 years: same as adult
    Trisoralen *Tab:* 5 mg

DEPIGMENTING AGENTS

▷ *hydroquinone* (C)(G) apply sparingly to affected area and rub in bid
    Lustra *Crm:* 4% (1, 2 oz) (sulfites)
    Lustra AF *Crm:* 4% (1, 2 oz) (sunscreen, sulfites)
▷ *monobenzone* (C) apply sparingly to affected area and rub in bid-tid; depigmentation occurs in 1-4 months
Pediatric: same as adult
    Benoquin *Crm:* 20% (1.25 oz)
▷ *tazarotene* (X)(G) apply daily at HS
Pediatric: <12 years: not recommended; ≥12 years: same as adult
    Avage Cream *Crm:* 0.1% (30 gm)
    Tazorac Cream *Crm:* 0.05, 0.1% (15, 30, 60 gm)
    Tazorac Gel *Gel:* 0.05, 0.1% (30, 100 gm)
▷ *tretinoin* (C) apply daily at HS
Pediatric: <12 years: not recommended; ≥12 years: same as adult
    Avita *Crm/Gel:* 0.025% (20, 45 gm)
    Renova *Crm:* 0.02% (40 gm); 0.05% (40, 60 gm)
    Retin-A Cream *Crm:* 0.025, 0.05, 0.1% (20, 45 gm)

Retin-A Gel *Gel:* 0.01, 0.025% (15, 45 gm) (alcohol 90%)
Retin-A Liquid *Liq:* 0.05% (28 ml) (alcohol 55%)
Retin-A Micro *Microspheres:* 0.04, 0.1% (20, 45 gm)

COMBINATION AGENTS

▷ *hydroquinone+fluocinolone+tretinoin* (C) apply sparingly to affected area and rub in daily at HS
Pediatric: <12 years: not recommended; ≥12 years: same as adult
    Tri-Luma *Crm: hydroquin* 4%+*fluo* 0.01%+*tretin* 0.05% (30 gm) (parabens, sulfites)
▷ *hydroquinone+padimate o+oxybenzone+octyl methoxycinnamate* (C) apply sparingly to affected area and rub in bid
Pediatric: <12 years: not recommended; ≥16 years: same as adult
    Glyquin *Crm:* 4% (1 oz jar)
▷ *hydroquinone+ethyl dihydroxypropyl PABA+dioxybenzone+oxybenzone* (C) apply sparingly to affected area and rub in bid; max 2 months
Pediatric: <12 years: not recommended; ≥12 years: same as adult
    Solaquin *Crm: hydroquin* 2%+*PABA* 5%+*dioxy* 3%+*oxy* 2% (1 oz) (sulfites)
▷ *hydroquinone+padimate+dioxybenzone+oxybenzone* (C) apply sparingly to affected area and rub in bid; max 2 months
Pediatric: <12 years: not recommended; ≥12 years: same as adult
    Solaquin Forte *Crm: hydroquin* 4%+*pad* 0.5%+*dioxy* 3%+*oxy* 2% (1oz)
    (sunscreen, sulfites)
▷ *hydroquinone+padimate+dioxybenzone* (C) apply sparingly to affected area and rub in bid; max 2 months
Pediatric: <12 years: not recommended; ≥12 years: same as adult
    Solaquin Forte Gel: *hydroquin* 4%+*pad* 0.5%+*dioxy* 3% (1 oz) (alcohol, sulfites)

◯ WART: COMMON (*VERRUCA VULGARIS*)

▷ *salicylic acid* (G)
Pediatric: same as adult
    Duo Film (OTC) apply daily-bid; max 12 weeks; *Liq:* 17% (1/2 oz w. applicator)
    Duo Film Patch for Kids (OTC) apply 1 patch q 48 hours; max 12 weeks
        Patch: 40% (18/pck)
    Occlusal HP (OTC) apply daily-bid; max 12 weeks
        Liq: 17% (10 ml w. applicator)
    Wart-Off (OTC) apply one drop at a time to sufficiently cover wart, let dry; repeat 1-2 times daily; max 12 weeks
        Liq: 17% (0.45 oz)
▷ *trichloroacetic acid* apply after wart is pared and repeat weekly
▷ Cryotherapy with liquid nitrogen <u>or</u> cryoprobe <u>or</u> cryospray; repeat applications every 1-2 weeks as needed to destroy lesion
    Histofreeze (see pkg insert for application freeze time

ORAL RETINOID

▷ *acitretin* (X)(G) 25-50 mg once daily with main meal
Pediatric: <18 years: not recommended; ≥18 years: same as adult
    Soriatane *Cap:* 10, 25 mg

REFERENCES

Can Oral Retinoids Have An Impact For Recalcitrant Warts? https://www.podiatrytoday.com/blogged/can-oral-retinoids-have-impact-recalcitrant-warts

Joshipura, D., Goldminz, A., Greb, J., & Gottlieb A. (2017). Acitretin for the treatment of recalcitrant plantar warts. *Dermatol Online Journal, 23*(3).

WART: PLANTAR (VERRUCA PLANTARIS)

▷ *salicylic acid* (G)
 Duo Plant Gel (OTC) apply daily bid; max 12 weeks
  Gel: 17% (1/2 oz)
 Mediplast cut to size of wart and apply; remove q 1-2 days, peel keratin, and reapply; repeat as long as needed
 Occlusal-HP (OTC) apply once daily-bid; max 12 weeks
  Liq: 17% (10 ml w. applicator)
 Wart-Off (OTC) apply one drop at a time to sufficiently cover wart, let dry; repeat 1-2 times daily; max 12 weeks
  Liq: 17% (0.45 oz)
▷ *trichloroacetic acid* apply after wart is pared and repeat weekly

ORAL RETINOID

▷ *acitretin* (**X**)(G) 25-50 mg once daily with main meal
 Pediatric: <12 years: not recommended; ≥12 years: same as adult
 Soriatane *Cap:* 10, 25 mg

REFERENCES

Can Oral Retinoids Have An Impact For Recalcitrant Warts? https://www.podiatrytoday.com/blogged/can-oral-retinoids-have-impact-recalcitrant-warts

Joshipura, D., Goldminz, A., Greb, J., & Gottlieb A. (2017). Acitretin for the treatment of recalcitrant plantar warts. *Dermatol Online Journal, 23*(3).

 WART: VENEREAL, HUMAN PAPILLOMAVIRUS (HPV), CONDYLOMA ACUMINATA

Comment: This section contains treatment regimens for genital warts published in the **2015 CDC Sexually Transmitted Diseases Treatment Guidelines** as well as other treatment options. Due to the increased risk of cervical cancer with HPV, Pap smears should be done q 3 months during active disease and then q 3-6 months for the next 2 years.

PATIENT-APPLIED AGENTS
Regimen 1

▷ *imiquimod* (C)
 Pediatric: <12 years: not recommended; ≥12 years: same as adult
 Aldara (G) rub into lesions before bedtime and remove with soap and water 6-10 hours later; treat 3 times per week; max 16 weeks
  Crm: 5% (12 single-use pkts/carton)
 Zyclara rub into lesions before bedtime and remove with soap and water 8 hours later; treat 3 times per week; max 1 packet per treatment; max 8 weeks
  Crm: 3.75% (28 single-use pkts/carton) (parabens)

Regimen 2

▷ *podofilox 0.5% cream* (C) apply bid (q 12 hours) x 3 days; then discontinue for 4 days; may repeat if needed; max 4 treatment cycles
 Condylox *Soln:* 0.5% (3.5 ml); *Gel:* 0.5% (3.5 gm)

Regimen 3

▷ *sinecatechins 15% ointment* (C) apply to each lesion tid for up to 16 weeks
 Veregen *Oint:* 15% (15, 30 gm)

PROVIDER-ADMINISTERED AGENTS

Regimen 1

▷ Cryotherapy with liquid nitrogen <u>or</u> cryoprobe; repeat applications every 1-2 weeks as needed

Regimen 2

▷ *trichloroacetic acid (TCA) 80-90%* (C) apply to warts; repeat weekly if needed
Comment: TCA is the preferred treatment during pregnancy. Immediate application of sodium bicarbonate paste following treatment decreases pain.

Regimen 3

▷ *podofilox 0.5% cream* (C) apply bid (q 12 hours) x 3 days; then discontinue for 4 days; may repeat if needed; max 4 treatment cycles
Condylox *Soln:* 0.5% (3.5 ml); *Gel:* 0.5% (3.5 gm)

Regimen 4

▷ *interferon alfa-n3* (C) 0.05 ml injected into base of wart twice weekly for up to 8 weeks; max 0.5 ml/session (20 warts/session)
Alferon N *Vial:* 5 million units/ml (1 ml)

Regimen 5

▷ *interferon alfa-2b* (C) 0.1 ml injected into base of wart three times weekly for up to 3 weeks; max 0.5 ml/session (5 warts/session)
Intron A *Vial:* 1 million units/0.1 ml (0.5, 1 ml)

Regimen 6

▷ Surgical removal either by tangential scissor excision, tangential shave excision, curettage, <u>or</u> electrosurgery

⬤ WEST NILE VIRUS

Comment: The principal route of human infection with West Nile virus is through the bite of an infected mosquito. Additional routes of infection have become a parent during the 2002 West Nile epidemic. It is important to note that these other methods of transmission represent a very small proportion of cases. Other methods of transmission include blood transfusion, organ transplantation, mother-to-child (ingestion of breast milk and transplacental) and occupational. Symptoms of mild disease will generally last a few days. Symptoms of severe disease may last several weeks, although neurological effects may be permanent. There is no specific treatment for West Nile virus infection; treatment is symptomatic and supportive. About 8 in 10 infected with West Nile virus do not develop any symptoms. About 1 in 5 develop a fever with other symptoms such as headache, body aches, joint pains, vomiting, diarrhea, <u>or</u> rash. Most people with this level of disease recover completely, but fatigue and weakness can last for weeks to months. About 1 in 150 people who are infected develop a severe illness affecting the central nervous system (encephalitis meningitis. Symptoms of severe illness include high fever, headache, neck stiffness, stupor, disorientation, coma, tremors, convulsions, muscle weakness, vision loss, numbness and paralysis. About 1 in 10 who develop severe illness affecting the central nervous system die. There is currently no preventive vaccine. However, the National Institutes of Health have announced that an experimental vaccine to protect against West Nile Virus has entered human trial. The developers say because the vaccine uses inactivated virus it should be suitable for a wide range of people. The trial tested the safety of the vaccine, called **HydroVax-001**, and its ability to produce an immune response in human subjects. The randomized, placebo-controlled, double-blind clinical trial was conducted by researchers at Duke University School of Medicine, Durham, NC, and enrolled 50 healthy volunteers, men and women 18-50 years-of-age. Participants were randomly assigned to one of the three groups. One group volunteers (n=20) received a low dose of the vaccine (1 mcg), another group (n=20) received a higher dose (4 mcg), and a third group (n=10) received a placebo. All participants received their doses via IM injection on day 1 and day 29 of the trial and are followed for 14 months. Results of the completed trial are pending.

REFERENCE
https://www.cdc.gov/westnile/symptoms/index.html

 WHIPWORM (TRICHURIASIS)

ANTHELMINTICS

▷ *albendazole* (C) 400 mg as a single dose; may repeat in 3 weeks; take with a meal
Pediatric: <2 years: 200 mg daily x 3 days; may repeat in 3 weeks; 2-12 years: 400 mg daily x 3 days; may repeat in 3 weeks; >12 years: same as adult
Albenza *Tab:* 200 mg

▷ *mebendazole* (C) chew, swallow, or mix with food; 100 mg bid x 3 days; may repeat in 3 weeks if needed; take with a meal
Pediatric: <2 years: not recommended; ≥2 years: same as adult
Emverm *Chew tab:* 100 mg
Vermox (G) *Chew tab:* 100 mg

▷ *pyrantel pamoate* (C) 11 mg/kg x 1 dose; max 1 gm/dose; take with a meal
Pediatric: 25-37 lb: 1/2 tsp x 1 dose; 38-62 lb: 1 tsp x 1 dose; 63-87 lb: 1 tsp x 1 dose; 88-112 lb: 2 tsp x 1 dose; 113-137 lb: 2 tsp x 1 dose; 138-162 lb: 3 tsp x 1 dose; 163-187 lb: 3 tsp x 1 dose; >187 lb: 4 tsp x 1 dose
Antiminth (OTC) *Cap:* 180 mg; *Liq:* 50 mg/ml (30 ml); 144 mg/ml (30 ml); *Oral susp:* 50 mg/ml (60 ml)
Pin-X (OTC) *Cap:* 180 mg; *Liq:* 50 mg/ml (30 ml); 144 mg/ml (30 ml); *Oral susp:* 50 mg/ml (30 ml)

▷ *thiabendazole* (C) 25 mg/kg bid x 7 days; max 1.5 gm/dose; take with a meal
Pediatric: same as adult; <30 lb: consult mfr pkg insert; >30 lb: 2 doses/day with meals; 30-50 lb: 250 mg bid with meals; >50 lb: 10 mg/lb/dose bid with meals; max 3 gm/day
Mintezol *Chew tab:* 500*mg (orange); *Oral susp:* 500 mg/5 ml (120 ml) (orange)

Comment: *thiabendazole* is not for prophylaxis. May impair mental alertness. May not be available in the US.

 WOUND: INFECTED, NONSURGICAL, MINOR

TETANUS PROPHYLAXIS VACCINE
Previously Immunized (within previous 5 years)

▷ *tetanus toxoid* vaccine (C) 0.5 ml IM x 1 dose
Vial: 5 Lf units/0.5 ml (0.5, 5 ml); *Prefilled syringe:* 5 Lf units/0.5 ml (0.5 ml)

Not Previously Immunized
see **Tetanus** *page 460*

TOPICAL ANTI-INFECTIVES

▷ *mupirocin* (B)(G) apply to lesions bid
  Pediatric: same as adult
    Bactroban *Oint:* 2% (22 gm); *Crm:* 2% (15, 30 gm)
    Centany *Oint:* 2% (15, 30 gm)

ORAL ANTI-INFECTIVES

▷ *azithromycin* (B)(G) 500 mg x 1 dose on day 1, then 250 mg daily on days 2-5 <u>or</u> 500 mg daily x 3 days <u>or</u> Zmax 2 gm in a single dose
  Pediatric: 10 mg/kg x 1 dose on day 1, then 5 mg/kg/day on days 2-5; max 500 mg/day; *see page 621 for dose by weight*
    Zithromax *Tab:* 250, 500, 600 mg; *Oral susp:* 100 mg/5 ml (15 ml); 200 mg/5 ml (15, 22.5, 30 ml) (cherry); *Pkt:* 1 gm for reconstitution (cherry-banana)
    Zithromax Tri-pak *Tab:* 3 x 500 mg tabs/pck
    Zithromax Z-pak *Tab:* 6 x 250 mg tabs/pck
    Zmax *Oral susp:* 2 gm ext-rel for reconstitution (cherry-banana) (148 mg Na$^+$)
▷ *amoxicillin+clavulanate* (B)(G)
    Augmentin 500 mg tid or 875 mg bid x 10 days
    Pediatric: 40-45 mg/kg/day divided tid x 10 days or 90 mg/kg/day divided bid x 10 days *see pages 618-619 for dose by weight*
      Tab: 250, 500, 875 mg; *Chew tab:* 125, 250 mg (lemon-lime); 200, 400 mg (cherry-banana) (phenylalanine); *Oral susp:* 125 mg/5 ml (banana), 250 mg/5 ml (75, 100, 150 ml) (orange); 200, 400 mg/5 ml (50, 75, 100 ml) (orange) (phenylalanine)
    Augmentin ES-600 not recommended for adults
    Pediatric: <3 months: not recommended; ≥3 months, <40 kg: 90 mg/kg/day in 2 divided doses x 10 days; ≥40 kg: not recommended
      Oral susp: 42.9 mg/5 ml (50, 75, 100, 125, 150, 200 ml) (strawberry cream) (phenylalanine)
    Augmentin XR 2 tabs q 12 hours x 10 days
    Pediatric: <16 years: use other forms; ≥16 years: same as adult
      Tab: 1000*mg ext-rel
▷ *cefaclor* (B)(G) 250-500 mg q 8 hours x 10 days; max 2 gm/day
  Pediatric: <1 month: not recommended; 20-40 mg/kg bid <u>or</u> q 12 hours x 10 days; max 1 gm/day; *see page 622 for dose by weight*
  Tab: 500 mg; *Cap:* 250, 500 mg; *Susp:* 125 mg/5 ml (75, 150 ml) (strawberry); 187 mg/5 ml (50, 100 ml) (strawberry); 250 mg/5 ml (75, 150 ml) (strawberry); 375 mg/5 ml (50, 100 ml) (strawberry)
    Cefaclor Extended Release *Tab:* 375, 500 mg ext-rel
    Pediatric: <16 years: ext-rel not recommended
▷ *cefadroxil* 1 gm/day in 1-2 divided doses x 10 days
  Pediatric: 15-30 mg/kg/day in 2 divided doses x 10 days; *see page 623 for dose by weight*
    Duricef *Cap:* 500 mg; *Tab:* 1 gm; *Oral susp:* 250 mg/5 ml (100 ml); 500 mg/5 ml (75, 100 ml) (orange-pineapple)
▷ *cefdinir* (B) 300 mg bid <u>or</u> 600 mg daily x 10 days
  Pediatric: <6 months: not recommended; 6 months-12 years: 14 mg/kg/day in 1-2 divided doses x 10 days; *see page 624 for dose by weight*
    Omnicef *Cap:* 300 mg; *Oral susp:* 125 mg/5 ml (60, 100 ml) (strawberry)
▷ *cefpodoxime proxetil* (B) 400 mg bid x 7-14 days
  Pediatric: <2 months: not recommended; 2 months-12 years: 10 mg/kg/day (max 400 mg/dose) <u>or</u> 5 mg/kg/day bid (max 200 mg/dose) x 7-14 days; *see page 626 for dose by weight*

      Vantin *Tab:* 100, 200 mg; *Oral susp:* 50, 100 mg/5 ml (50, 75, 100 mg; lemon creme)

      Pediatric: see page 626 for dose by weight

➤ *cefprozil* (B) 250-500 mg q 12 hours <u>or</u> 500 mg daily x 10 days

    Pediatric: <2 years: not recommended; 2-12 years: 7.5 mg/kg-15 mg/kg q 12 hours x 10 days; see page 627 for dose by weight; >12 years: same as adult

      Cefzil *Tab:* 250, 500 mg; *Oral susp:* 125, 250 mg/5 ml (50, 75, 100 ml) (bubble gum, phenylalanine)

➤ *cephalexin* (B)(G) 2 gm 1 hour before procedure

    Pediatric: 50 mg/kg/day in 4 divided doses x 10 days; see page 629 for dose by weight

      Keflex *Cap:* 250, 333, 500, 750 mg; *Oral susp:* 125, 250 mg/5 ml (100, 200 ml) (strawberry)

      Pediatric: see page 629 for dose by weight

➤ *clarithromycin* (C)(G) 500 mg <u>or</u> 500 mg ext-rel for 7-10 days

    Pediatric: see page 630 for dose by weight

      Biaxin *Tab:* 250, 500 mg

      Biaxin Oral Suspension *Oral susp:* 125, 250 mg/5 ml (50, 100 ml) (fruit-punch)

      Biaxin XL *Tab:* 500 mg ext-rel

➤ *dirithromycin* (C)(G) 500 mg daily x 7 days

    Pediatric: <12 years: not recommended

      Dynabac *Tab:* 250 mg

➤ *erythromycin base* (B)(G) 500 mg qid x 14 days

    Pediatric: 30-50 mg/kg/day in 2-4 divided doses x 10 days

      Ery-Tab *Tab:* 250, 333, 500 mg ent-coat

      PCE *Tab:* 333, 500 mg

Comment: *erythromycin* may increase INR with concomitant *warfarin*, as well as increase serum level of *digoxin, benzodiazepines*, and *statins*.

➤ *erythromycin ethylsuccinate* (B)(G) 400 mg qid x 7 days

    Pediatric: 30-50 mg/kg/day in 4 divided doses x 7 days; may double dose with severe infection; max 100 mg/kg/day; see page 635 for dose by weight

      EryPed *Oral susp:* 200 mg/5 ml (100, 200 ml) (fruit); 400 mg/5 ml (60, 100, 200 ml) (banana); *Oral drops:* 200, 400 mg/5 ml (50 ml) (fruit); *Chew tab:* 200 mg wafer (fruit)

      E.E.S. *Oral susp:* 200, 400 mg/5 ml (100 ml) (fruit)

      E.E.S. Granules *Oral susp:* 200 mg/5 ml (100, 200 ml) (cherry)

      E.E.S. 400 Tablets *Tab:* 400 mg

Comment: *erythromycin* may increase INR with concomitant *warfarin*, as well as increase serum level of *digoxin, benzodiazepines*, and *statins*.

➤ *gemifloxacin* (C)(G) 320 mg daily x 5-7 days

    Pediatric: <18 years: not recommended; ≥18 years: same as adult

      Factive *Tab:* 320*mg

➤ *levofloxacin* (C) *Uncomplicated:* 500 mg daily x 7 days; *Complicated:* 750 mg daily x 7 days

    Pediatric: <18 years: not recommended; ≥18 years: same as adult

      Levaquin *Tab:* 250, 500, 750 mg

Comment: *levofloxacin* is contraindicated <18 years-of-age, and during pregnancy and lactation. Risk of tendonitis or tendon rupture.

➤ *loracarbef* (B) 200-400 mg bid x 7 days

    Pediatric: 15 mg/kg/day in 2 divided doses x 7 days; see page 642 for dose by weight

      Lorabid *Pulvule:* 200, 400 mg; *Oral susp:* 100 mg/5 ml (50, 100 ml); 200 mg/5 ml (50, 75, 100 ml) (strawberry bubble gum)

▷ *ofloxacin* (C)(G) 400 mg bid x 10 days
  Pediatric: <18 years: not recommended; ≥18 years: same as adult
      Floxin *Tab:* 200, 300, 400 mg
Comment: *levofloxacin* is contraindicated <18 years-of-age, and during pregnancy and lactation. Risk of tendonitis or tendon rupture.

 WRINKLES: FACIAL

TOPICAL RETINOIDS

Comment: Wash the affected area with a soap-free cleanser; pat dry and wait 20 to 30 minutes; then apply topical retinoid sparingly to affected area. Use only once daily in the PM. Avoid eyes, ears, nostrils, and mouth.
▷ *adapalene* (C)(G)
  Pediatric: <12 years: not recommended; ≥12 years: same as adult
      Differin *Crm:* 0.1% (15, 45 gm); *Gel:* 0.1% (15, 45 gm); *Pad:* 0.1% (30/pck) (alcohol 30%)
      Differin Solution *Soln:* 0.1% (30 ml; alcohol 30%)
▷ *tazarotene* (X)(G) apply daily at HS
  Pediatric: <12 years: not recommended; ≥12 years: same as adult
      Avage Cream *Crm:* 0.1% (5, 30 gm)
      Tazorac Cream *Crm:* 0.05, 0.1% (15, 30, 60 gm)
      Tazorac Gel *Gel:* 0.05, 0.1% (30, 100 gm)
▷ *tretinoin* (C) apply daily at HS
  Pediatric: <12 years: not recommended; ≥12 years: same as adult
      Atralin Gel *Gel:* 0.05% (45 gm)
      Avita *Crm:* 0.025% (20, 45 gm); *Gel:* 0.025% (20, 45 gm)
      Renova *Crm:* 0.02% (40 gm); 0.05% (40, 60 gm)
      Retin-A Cream *Crm:* 0.025, 0.05, 0.1% (20, 45 gm)
      Retin-A Gel *Gel:* 0.01, 0.025% (15, 45 gm; alcohol 90%)
      Retin-A Liquid *Soln:* 0.05% (alcohol 55%)
      Retin-A Micro Gel *Gel:* 0.04, 0.08, 0.1% (20, 45 gm)
      Tretin-X Cream *Crm:* 0.075% (35 gm) (parabens-free, alcohol-free, propylene glycol-free)
      Retin-A Micro *Microspheres:* 0.04, 0.1% (20, 45 gm)
Comment: topical *treatinoin* is effective for mitigation of fine wrinkles, mottled hyperpigmentation, and tactile roughness of skin. No mitigating effect on deep wrinkles, skin yellowing, lentigines, telangiectasia, skin laxity, keratinocytic atypia, melanocytic atypia, or dermal elastosis. Avoid sun exposure. Cautious use of concomitant astringents, alcohol-based products, sulfur-containing products, salicylic acid-containing products, soap, and other topical agents.

 XEROSIS

MOISTURIZING AGENTS

      Aquaphor Healing Ointment (OTC) *Oint:* 1.75, 3.5, 14 oz (alcohol)
      Eucerin Daily Sun Defense (OTC) *Lotn:* 6 oz (fragrance-free)
Comment: **Eucerin Daily Sun Defense** is a moisturizer with SPF 15 sunscreen.
      Eucerin Facial Lotion (OTC) *Lotn:* 4 oz
      Eucerin Light Lotion (OTC) *Lotn:* 8 oz
      Eucerin Lotion (OTC) *Lotn:* 8, 16 oz

Eucerin Original Creme (OTC) *Crm:* 2, 4, 16 oz (alcohol)
Eucerin Plus Creme (OTC) *Crm:* 4 oz
Eucerin Plus Lotion (OTC) *Lotn:* 6, 12 oz
Eucerin Protective Lotion (OTC) *Lotn:* 4 oz (alcohol)

Comment: **Eucerin Protective** is a moisturizer with SPF 25 sunscreen.
Lac-Hydrin Cream (OTC) *Crm:* 280, 385 gm
Lac-Hydrin Lotion (OTC) *Lotn:* 225, 400 gm
Lubriderm Dry Skin Scented (OTC) *Lotn:* 6, 10, 16, 32 oz
Lubriderm Dry Skin Unscented (OTC) *Lotn:* 3.3, 6, 10, 16 oz (fragrance-free)
Lubriderm Sensitive Skin Lotion (OTC) *Lotn:* 3.3, 6, 10, 16 oz (lanolin-free)
Lubriderm Dry Skin (OTC) *Lotn:* 2.5, 6, 10, 16 oz (scented); 1, 2.5, 6, 10, 16 oz (fragrance-free)
Lubriderm Bath & Shower Oil (OTC) 1-2 capfuls in bath <u>or</u> rub onto wet skin as needed, then rinse; *Oil:* 8 oz
Moisturel *Crm:* 4, 16 oz; *Lotn:* 8, 12 oz; *Clnsr:* 8.75 oz

Topical Oil

▷ *fluocinolone acetonide* 0.01% topical oil **(C)**
Pediatric: <6 years: not recommended; ≥6 years: apply sparingly bid for up to 4 weeks
Derma-Smoothe/FS Topical Oil apply sparingly tid
Topical oil: 0.01% (4 oz; peanut oil)

 ZIKA VIRUS

Comment: The Zika virus is transmitted via the bite of an infected mosquito and is associated with severe teratogenicity: a unique and distinct pattern of birth defects, called congenital Zika syndrome, characterized by the following five features: (1) Severe microcephaly in which the skull has partially collapsed; (2) Decreased brain tissue with a specific pattern of brain damage, including subcortical calcifications; (3) Damage to the back of the eye, including macular scarring and focal pigmentary retinal mottling; (4) Congenital contractures, such as clubfoot and arthrogryposis; (5) Hypertonia restricting body movement. Congenital Zika virus infection has also been associated with other abnormalities, including but not limited to brain atrophy and asymmetry, abnormally formed <u>or</u> absent brain structures, hydrocephalus, and neuronal migration disorders. Other anomalies include excessive and redundant scalp skin. Reported neurologic findings include, hyperreflexia, irritability, tremors, seizures, brainstem dysfunction, and dysphagia. Reported eye abnormalities include, but are not limited to, focal pigmentary mottling and chorioretinal atrophy in the macula, optic nerve hypoplasia, cupping, and atrophy, other retinal lesions, iris colobomas, congenital glaucoma, microphthalmia, lens subluxation, cataracts, and intraocular calcifications. **A synthetic DNA-based preventive vaccine showed promising immune responses with no severe adverse reactions in humans,** an interim analysis of a phase I trial found. Following three doses of vaccine, 100% of patients produced binding antibodies, and 95% of patients produced binding antibodies following two doses of the vaccine, Examining immunogenicity, 41% of participants had detectable binding antibody responses 4 weeks after the first dose, the authors said, with a 74% antibody response at week 6 (2 weeks after the second dose). **The vaccine is not yet available to the public.** The FDA formally approved Roche's cobas Zika molecular test for use on whole donor blood and blood products and living organ donors; it's the first such approval granted.

REFERENCES

Paz-Bailey, gm et al. Zika virus persistence in body fluids, final report in body fluids-Final report. ASTMH 2017. Paper presented at the 66th Annual Meeting of the American Society of Tropical Medicine and Hygiene, November 5-9, Baltimore, MD

Rosenberg, E, et al. Prevalence and incidence of Zika virus infection among household contacts of Zika patients, Puerto Rico, 2016-2017. ASTMH 2017

Tebas, P., Roberts, C. C., Muthumani, K., Reuschel, E. L., Kudchodkar, S. B., Zaidi, F. I., . . . Maslow, J. N. (2017). Safety and immunogenicity of an anti–zika virus dna vaccine—preliminary report. *New England Journal of Medicine.* doi:10.1056/nejmoa1708120

ZOLLINGER-ELLISON SYNDROME

Comment: Zollinger-Ellison Syndrome is a condition in which a gastrin-secreting tumor or hyperplasia of the islet cells in the pancreas causes overproduction of gastric acid, resulting in recurrent peptic ulcers.

PROTON PUMP INHIBITORS (PPIs)

Comment: If hepatic impairment, or if patient is Asian, consider reducing the PPI dose.

▷ *dexlansoprazole* (B)(G) 30-60 mg daily for up to 4 weeks

Pediatric: <18 years: not recommended; ≥18 years: same as adult

Dexilant *Cap:* 30, 60 mg ent-coat del-rel granules; may open and sprinkle on applesauce; do not crush or chew granules

Dexilant SoluTab *Tab:* 30 mg del-rel orally-disint

▷ *esomeprazole* (B)(OTC)(G) 20-40 mg daily; max 8 weeks; take 1 hour before food; swallow whole or mix granules with food or juice and take immediately; do not crush or chew granules

Pediatric: <1 year: not recommended; 1-11 years, <20 kg: 10 mg; ≥20 kg: 10-20 mg once daily; 12-17 years: 20-40 mg once daily; max 8 weeks

Nexium *Cap:* 20, 40 mg ent-coat del-rel pellets

Nexium for Oral Suspension *Oral susp:* 10, 20, 40 mg ent-coat del-rel granules/pkt; mix in 2 tbsp water and drink immediately; 30 pkt/carton

▷ *esomeprazole+aspirin* (D) take one dose daily; max 8 weeks; take 1 hour before food

Yosprala

Tab: **Yosprala 40/81** *esom* 40 mg+*asp* 81 mg del-rel

Yosprala 40/325 *esom* 40 mg+*asp* 325 mg del-rel

Comment: *aspirin*-containing medications are contraindicated with history of allergic-type reaction to *aspirin*, children and adolescents with *Varicella* or other viral illness, and 3rd trimester of pregnancy.

▷ *lansoprazole* (B)(OTC)(G) 15-30 mg daily for up to 8 weeks; may repeat course; take before eating

Pediatric: <1 year: not recommended; 1-11 years, <30 kg: 15 mg once daily; >11 years: same as adult

Prevacid *Cap:* 15, 30 mg ent-coat del-rel granules; swallow whole or mix granules with food or juice and take immediately; do not crush or chew granules; follow with water

Prevacid for Oral Suspension *Oral susp:* 15, 30 mg ent-coat del-rel granules/pkt; mix in 2 tbsp water and drink immediately; 30 pkt/carton (strawberry)

Prevacid SoluTab *ODT:* 15, 30 mg (strawberry) (phenylalanine)

Prevacid 24HR *Oral granules:* 15 mg ent-coat del-rel granules; swallow whole or mix granules with food or juice and take immediately; do not crush or chew granules; follow with water

▷ *omeprazole* (C)(OTC)(G) 20-40 mg daily; take before eating; swallow whole <u>or</u> mix granules with applesauce and take immediately; do not crush <u>or</u> chew; follow with water

> **Prilosec** *Cap:* 10, 20, 40 mg ent-coat del-rel granules
> *Pediatric:* <18 years: not recommended; ≥18 years: same as adult
> **Prilosec** *Tab:* 20 mg del-rel (regular, wild berry)
> *Pediatric:* <1 year: not recommended; 5-<10 kg: 5 mg daily; 10-<20 kg: 10 mg daily; ≥20 kg: same as adult

▷ *pantoprazole* (B)(G) initially 40 mg bid
> *Pediatric:* <12 years: not recommended; ≥12 years: same as adult
> **Protonix** *Tab:* 40 mg ent-coat del-rel
> **Protonix for Oral Suspension** *Oral susp:* 40 mg ent-coat del-rel granules/pkt; mix in 1 tsp apple juice for 5 seconds <u>or</u> sprinkle on 1 tsp apple sauce, and swallow immediately; do not mix in water <u>or</u> any other liquid <u>or</u> food; take approximately 30 minutes prior to a meal; 30 pkt/carton any other liquid <u>or</u> food; take approximately 30 minutes prior to a meal; 30 pkt/carton

▷ *rabeprazole* (B)(OTC)(G) initially 20 mg daily; then titrate; may take 100 mg daily in divided doses <u>or</u> 60 mg bid
> *Pediatric:* <12 years: not recommended; ≥12 years: 20 mg once daily; max 8 weeks
> **AcipHex** *Tab:* 20 mg ent-coat del-rel

SECTION II

APPENDICES

APPENDIX A. U.S. FDA PREGNANCY CATEGORIES

Comment: For drugs FDA-approved *after June 30, 2015*, the 5-letter categories are no longer used and there is no replacement (categorical nomenclature) at this time. Rather, information regarding special populations, including pregnant and breastfeeding females, is addressed in a structured narrative format. Prescribers should refer to the drug's FDA labeling (https://www.fda.gov/Drugs/default.htm) or the manufacturer's package insert for this information. Prescription drugs submitted for FDA approval after June 30, 2015 use the new format immediately, while labeling for prescription drugs approved on or after June 30, 2015 are phased in gradually. Although drugs approved prior to June 29, 2015 are not subject to the FDA's **Pregnancy and Lactation Labeling Final Rule (PLLR)**, the *pregnancy letter category must be removed by June 29, 2018*. Labeling for over-the-counter (OTC) medicines will not change, as OTC drugs are not affected by the new FDA pregnancy labeling. For a more detailed explanation of the final rule **and** new narrative format, **visit** https://www.drugs.com/pregnancy-categories.html

Category	Description
A	Controlled studies in women have failed to demonstrate risk to the fetus in the first trimester of pregnancy and there is no evidence of risk in later trimesters.
B	Animal reproduction studies have not demonstrated risk to the fetus, but there are no controlled studies in pregnant women, or animal studies have demonstrated an adverse effect, but controlled studies in pregnant women have not documented risk to the fetus in the first trimester of pregnancy and there is no evidence of risk in later trimesters.
C	Risk to the fetus cannot be ruled out. Animal reproduction studies have demonstrated adverse effects on the fetus (i.e., teratogenic or embryocidal effects or other) but there are no controlled studies in pregnant women or controlled studies in women and animals are not available.
D	There is positive evidence of human fetal risk, but benefits from use by pregnant women may be acceptable despite the potential risk (e.g., if the drug is needed in a life-threatening situation or for a serious disease for which safer drugs cannot be used or are ineffective.
X	Studies in animals or humans have demonstrated fetal abnormalities or there is evidence of fetal risk based on human experience, or both, and the risk of using the drug in pregnant women clearly outweighs any possible benefit. The drug is contraindicated in women who are pregnant or who may become pregnant.

APPENDIX B. U.S. SCHEDULE OF CONTROLLED SUBSTANCES

Schedule	Description
I	High potential for abuse and of no currently accepted medical use. Not obtainable by prescription, but may be legally procured for research, study, or instructional use. (Examples: *heroin, LSD, marijuana, mescaline, peyote*)
II	High abuse potential and high liability for severe psychological or physical dependence potential. Prescription required and cannot be refilled. Prescription must be written in ink or typed and signed. A verbal prescription may be allowed in an emergency by the dispensing pharmacist, but must be followed by a written prescription within 72 hours. Includes opium derivatives, other opioids, and short-acting barbiturates.
III	Potential for abuse is less than that for drugs in schedules I and II. Moderate to low physical dependence and high psychological dependence potential. Prescription required. May be refilled up to 5 times in 6 months. Prescription may be verbal (telephone) or written. Includes certain stimulants and depressants not included in the above schedules, and preparations containing limited quantities of certain opioids.
IV	Lower potential for abuse than Schedule III drugs. Prescription required. May be refilled up to 5 times in 6 months. Prescription may be verbal (telephone) or written.
V	Abuse potential less than that for Schedule IV drugs. Preparations contain limited quantities of certain narcotic drugs. Generally intended for antitussive and anti-diarrheal purposes and may be distributed without a prescription provided that • such distribution is made only by a pharmacist; • not more than 240 ml or not more than 48 solid dosage units of any substance containing opium, nor more than 120 ml or not more than 24 solid dosage units of any other controlled substance may be distributed at retail to the same purchaser in any given 48-hour period without a valid prescription order; • the purchaser is at least 18 years old; • the pharmacist knows the purchaser or requests suitable identification; • the pharmacist keeps an official written record of: name and address of purchaser, name, and quantity of controlled substance purchased, date of sale, initials of dispensing pharmacist. This record is to be made available for inspection and copying by the U.S. officers authorized by the Attorney General; • other federal, state, or local law does not reuire a prescription order. Under jurisdiction of the Federal Controlled Substances Act. Refillable up to 5 times within 6 months.

APPENDIX C. BLOOD PRESSURE GUIDELINES¶

APPENDIX C.1. BLOOD PRESSURE CLASSIFICATIONS (≥18 YEARS)

Classification	SBP mmHg		DBP mmHg
Normal	<120	and	<80
Elevated BP	120-129	and	<80
Stage I Hypertension	130-139	or	80-89
Stage 2 Hypertension	≥140	or	≥90
Hypertensive Crisis	>180	and/or	>120

¶Adapted from Vogt, C. New AHA/ACC guidelines lower high BP threshold. *Consultant360.* November 14, 2017. Retrieved from https://www.consultant360.com/exclusives/new-ahaacc-guidelines-lower-high-bp-threshold

2017 ACC/AHA/AAPA/ABC/ACPM/AGS/APhA/ASH/ASPC/NMA/PCNA Guideline for the Prevention, Detection, Evaluation, and Management of High Blood Pressure in Adults: A report of the American College of Cardiology/American Heart Association Task Force on Clinical Practice Guidelines. Retrieved from http://hyper.ahajournals.org/content/hypertensionaha/early/2017/11/10/HYP.0000000000000065.full.pdf

APPENDIX C.2. BLOOD PRESSURE CLASSIFICATIONS (<18 YEARS)¶

Age Group	Significant		Severe	
	SBP	DBP	SBP	DBP
Newborn <7 days	>96		>106	
Newborn 8-30 days	>104		>110	
Infant 30 days-2 years	>112	>74	>118	>82
Children 3-5 years	>116	>76	>124	>84
Children 6-9 years	>122	>78	>130	>86
Children 10-12 years	>126	>82	>134	>90
Adolescents 13-15 years	>136	>86	>144	>92
Adolescents 16-18 years	>142	>92	>150	>98

¶Adapted from American Pharmacists Association. (2015). *Pediatric and neonatal dosage handbook: A universal resource for clinicians treating pediatric and neonatal patients* (22nd ed.). Hudson, Ohio: Lexicomp.

APPENDIX C.3. IDENTIFIABLE CAUSES OF HYPERTENSION (JNC-8)

• Obstructive sleep apnea • Chronic kidney disease • Primary aldosteronism • Renovascular disease	• *Prescription Drugs:* oral contraceptives, sympathomimetics, venlafaxine, bupropion, clozapine, buspirone, bromocriptine, carbamazepine, metoclopramide

(continued)

(continued)

• Excess sodium ingestion • Herbal supplements • Coarctation of the aorta • Pheochromocytoma • Thyroid disease • Parathyroid disease • Cushing's syndrome	• *Illicit, Over-the-Counter Drugs, and Herbal Products:* excess alcohol consumption, alcohol withdrawal, anabolic steroids, cocaine, cocaine withdrawal, phenylpropanolamine analogs, ephedra alkalois, ergot containing herbal products, St. John's wart, nicotine withdrawal

APPENDIX C.4. CVD RISK FACTORS (JNC-8)

• Hypertension • Obesity (BMI ≥30 kg/m^2) • Dyslipidemia • Diabetes mellitus • Cigarette smoking • Physical inactivity	• Microalbuminuria, GFR <60 mL/min • Age (men >55 yrs, women >65 yrs) • Family History of premature CVD (men <55 yrs, women <65 yrs)

APPENDIX C.5. DIAGNOSTIC WORKUP OF HYPERTENSION (JNC-8)

• Assess risk factors and comorbidities • Reveal identifiable causes of hypertension • Assess for presence of target organ damage • History and physical examination • Urinalysis, blood glucose, hematocrit, lipid panel, potassium, creatinine, calcium, (*optional* urine albumin/Cr ratio), EKG

APPENDIX C.6. RECOMMENDATIONS FOR MEASURING BLOOD PRESSURE (JNC-8)

• Blood pressure should be measured after the patient has emptied their bladder and has been seated for 5 minutes with back supported and legs resting on the ground (not crossed) • Arm used for measurement should rest on a table, at heart level. • Use a sphygmomanometer/stethoscope <u>or</u> automated electronic device (preferred) with the correct size arm cuff • Take two readings one to two minutes apart, and average the readings (preferred) • Measure blood pressure in both arms at initial valuation; use the higher reading for measurements thereafter • Confirm the diagnosis of HTN at a subsequent visit one to four weeks after the first • If blood pressure is very high (e.g., systolic 180 mmHg <u>or</u> higher), <u>or</u> timely follow-up unrealistic, treatment can be started after just one set of measurements

APPENDIX C.7. PATIENT-SPECIFIC FACTORS TO CONSIDER WHEN SELECTING DRUG TREATMENT FOR HYPERTENSION (JNC-8* AND ASH**)

JNC-8:

- Nonblack, including those with diabetes: thiazide, CCB, ACEI, or ARB
- African American, including those with diabetes: thiazide or CCB
- CKD; regimen should include an ACEI or ARB (including African Americans)
- Can initiate with two agents, especially if systolic >20 mmHg above goal or diastolic >10 mmHg above goal
- If goal not reached: stress adherence to medication and lifestyle, increase dose or add a second or third agent from one of the recommended classes
- Choose a drug outside of the classes recommended above only if these options have been exhausted. Consider specialist referral

ASH:

- **Nonblack <60 years of age:** *First-line:* ACEI or ARB; *Second-line (add-on):* CCB or thiazide; *Third-line:* CCB plus ACEI or ARB plus thiazide
- **Nonblack 60 years of age and older:** *First-line:* CCB or thiazide preferred, ACEI, or ARB; *Second-line (add-on):* CCB, thiazide, ACEI, or ARB (don't use ACEI plus ARB); *Third-line:* CCB plus ACEI or ARB plus thiazide
- **African American:** *First-line:* CCB or thiazide; *Second-line (add-on):* ACEI or ARB. *Third-line:* CCB plus ACEI or ARB plus thiazide

Comorbidities (ASH):

- **Diabetes:** *First-line:* ACEI or ARB (can start with CCB or thiazide in African Americans); *Second-line:* add CCB or thiazide (can add ACEI or ARB in African Americans); *Third-line:* CCB plus ACEI or ARB plus thiazide
- **CKD:** *First-line:* ARB or ACEI (ACEI for African Americans) *Second-line (add-on):* CCB or thiazide; *Third-line:* CCB plus ACEI or ARB plus thiazide
- **CAD:** *First-line:* BB plus ARB or ACEI; *Second-line (add-on):* CCB or thiazide; *Third-line:* BB plus ARB or ACEI plus CCB plus thiazide
- **Stroke history:** *First-line:* ACEI or ARB; *Second-line:* add CCB or thiazide; *Third-line:* CCB plus ACEI or ARB plus thiazide
- **Heart failure:** ACEI or ARB plus BB plus diuretic plus aldosterone antagonist. Amlodipine can be added for additional BP control (Start with ACEI, BB, diuretic. Can add BB even before ACE-I optimized. Use diuretic to manage fluid.)
- In patients 60 years of age or older who do not have diabetes or chronic kidney disease, the goal blood pressure level is now <150/90 mmHg
- In patients 18 to 59 years of age without major comorbidities, and in patients 60 years of age or older who have diabetes, chronic kidney disease, or both conditions, the new goal blood pressure level is <140/90 mmHg

APPENDIX C.8. BLOOD PRESSURE TREATMENT RECOMMENDATIONS (JNC-8)[¶]

- First-line and later-line treatments should now be limited to 4 classes of medications: thiazide-type diuretics, calcium channel blockers (CCBs), ACEIs, and ARBs
- Second- and third-line alternatives included higher doses or combinations of ACEIs, ARBs, thiazide-type diuretics, and CCBs

(continued)

(continued)

- Several medications are now designated as later-line alternatives, including the following:
  - Beta-blockers
  - Alpha-blockers
  - Alpha₁/beta-blockers (e.g., *carvedilol*)
  - Vasodilating beta-blockers (e.g., *nebivolol*)
  - Central alpha₂-adrenergic agonists (e.g, *clonidine*)
  - Direct vasodilators (e.g., *hydralazine*)
  - Loop diuretics (e.g., *furosemide*)
  - Aldosterone antagonists (e.g., *spironolactone*)
  - Peripherally acting adrenergic antagonists (e.g., *reserpine*)
- When initiating therapy, patients of African descent without chronic kidney disease should use CCBs and thiazides instead of ACEIs.
- Use of ACEIs and ARBs is recommended in all patients with chronic kidney disease regardless of ethnic background, either as first-line therapy <u>or</u> in addition to first-line therapy.
- ACEIs and ARBs should not be used in the same patient simultaneously.
- CCBs and thiazide-type diuretics should be used instead of ACEIs and ARBs in patients over the age of 75 with impaired kidney function due to the risk of hyperkalemia, increased creatinine, and further renal impairment.

[1]Adapted from: PL Detail-Document, Treatment of Hypertension: JNC 8 and More. *Pharmacist's Letter/Prescriber's Letter*, February 2014.

 APPENDIX D. TARGET LIPID RECOMMENDATIONS (ATP-IV)[1]

APPENDIX D.1. TARGET TC, TG, HDL-C, NON-HDL-C

Total cholesterol (TC)	<200 mg/dL
Triglyceride (TRG)	<150 mg/dL
High-density lipoprotein (HDL-C)	>40 mg/dL (male) >50 mg/dL (female)
Non-high-density lipoprotein (Non-HDL-C)	<130 mg/dL; 30 mg/dL above the LDL-C treatment target

[1]Adapted from the National Cholesterol Education Program Expert Panel on Detection, Evaluation, and Treatment of High Blood Cholesterol in Adults (Adult Treatment Panel IV, 2012)

APPENDIX D.2. TARGET LDL-C (ATP IV)[†]

Risk Assessment[††]	LDL Target	Initiate TLC[†††]	Initiate Drug Therapy
0-1	<160 mg/dL	≥160 mg/dL	≥190 mg/dL (optional at 160-189 mg/dL)
2 <u>or</u> more plus 10-year risk <10%	<130 mg/dL	≥130 mg/dL	≥160 mg/dL

(continued)

(*continued*)

Risk Assessment[††]	LDL Target	Initiate TLC[†††]	Initiate Drug Therapy
2 or more plus 10-year risk <20%	<130 mg/dL <100 mg/dL optional	≥130 mg/dL	≥130 mg/dL
CHD or CHD risk equivalents 10-year risk >20%	<100 mg/dL <70 mg/dL optional	≥100 mg/dL	≥100 mg/dL

[†]Treatment decisions based on LDL-C

Calculation: LDL-C = TC - [(TRG ÷ 5) + HDL-C]

[††]Risk factors include age (men ≥45 years and women ≥55 years)

[†††]Therapeutic lifestyle changes (e.g., exercise, weight loss, low fat diet)

APPENDIX D.3. NON-HDL-C CLASSIFICATIONS (ATP-IV)[¶]

Desirable	<130 mg/dL	Non-HDL-C is calculated as total cholesterol minus HDL-C. The addition of non-HDL-C to the Lipid Panel reflects the recognition of this calculated value as a predictive factor in cardiovascular disease based on the National Cholesterol Education III studies. The reference ranges for non-HDL-C are based on National Cholesterol Education III guidelines: Non-HDL-C is thought to be a better predictor of CVD than LDL-C; treatment goal for non-HDL-C is usually 30 mg/dL above the LDL-C treatment target. For example, if the LDL-C treatment goal is <70 mg/dL, the non-HDL-C treatment target would be <100 mg/dL.
Borderline high	139-159 mg/dL	
High	160-189 mg/dL	
Very high	≥190 mg/dL	

[¶]Adapted from the National Cholesterol Education Program Expert Panel on Detection, Evaluation, and Treatment of High Blood Cholesterol in Adults (Adult Treatment Panel IV, 2012).

APPENDIX E. EFFECTS OF SELECTED DRUGS ON INSULIN ACTIVITY

Hyper- and Hypoglycemic Drug Effects	
Drugs That May Cause Hyperglycemia	Drugs That May Cause Hypoglycemia
Calcium channel blockers	Alcohol
Thiazide diuretics	Beta-blockers
Corticosteroids	MAO inhibitors

(*continued*)

Hyper- and Hypoglycemic Drug Effects	
Drugs That May Cause Hyperglycemia	Drugs That May Cause Hypoglycemia
Nicotinic acid	Salicylates
Oral contraceptives	NSAIDs
Phenytoin	Warfarin
Sympathomimetics diazoxide	Phenylbutazone

APPENDIX F. GLYCOSYLATED HEMOGLOBIN (HBA1C) AND AVERAGE BLOOD GLUCOSE EQUIVALENT

HbA1c and Average Blood Glucose Equivalent			
HbA1c	GLU	HbA1c	GLU
4%	60 mg/dL	14%	360 mg/dL
5%	90 mg/dL	15%	390 mg/dL
6%	120 mg/dL	16%	420 mg/dL
7%	150 mg/dL	17%	450 mg/dL
8%	180 mg/dL	18%	480 mg/dL
9%	210 mg/dL	19%	510 mg/dL
10%	240 mg/dL	20%	540 mg/dL
11%	270 mg/dL	21%	570 mg/dL
12%	300 mg/dL	22%	600 mg/dL
13%	330 mg/dL	23%	630 mg/dL

APPENDIX G. ROUTINE IMMUNIZATION RECOMMENDATIONS[1]

APPENDIX G.1. ADMINISTRATION OF VACCINES

- Prior to 1 year-of-age, administer IM vaccinations in the vastus lateralis muscle
- After 1 year-of-age, administer vaccinations in the posterolateral upper arm
- Influenza vaccine should be administered annually for all ages ≥6 months
- Inactivated vaccines (e.g., pneumococcal, meningococcal, and inactivated influenza vaccines), are generally acceptable and live vaccines are generally avoided, in persons with immune deficiencies or immunocompromising conditions
- Additional information about routine vaccinations, unknown vaccination status, travel vaccinations, vaccinations in pregnancy, and other vaccines, is available at: www.cdc.gov/vaccines/hcp/acip-recs/index.html
www.cdc.gov/mmwr/preview/mmwrhtml rr6002a1/htm
wwwnc.cdc.gov/travel/destinations/list

(*continued*)

(continued)

www.cdc.gov/vaccines/adult/rec-vac/pregnant.html
www.cdc.gov/flu/protect/vaccine/vaccines/htm

- **DTaP** (*diphtheria-tetanus-toxoid, acellular pertussis*); minimum age 6 wks
- **DTaP** should not be administered at or after the 7th birthday
- The 4th dose of **DTaP** vaccine can be administered as early as age 12 months, provided that the interval between doses 3 and 4 is at least 6 months
- **DTaP** and **IPV** should be administered at or before school entry
- **HAV** (*hepatitis A vaccine*) is recommended for all children at 1 year (12-23 months) of age
- **HAV** 2-dose series should be administered at least 6 months apart
- **HBV** (*hepatitis B vaccine*) is a 3-dose series initiated at birth; administer 2nd dose at 1-2 months; administer the 3rd dose at age 6 months (not before ≥24 weeks)
- **HBV** should be offered to all children who have not received the full series
- Infants born to HVsAG-positive mothers should be tested for HBsAG and antibody to HBsAg after completion of the **HBV** series (at age 9-18 months)
- **Hib** (*hemophilus influenzae* type b conjugate vaccine) minimum age 6 months
- **Hib** is not recommended if age >5 years
- **HPV** (*human papillovirus vaccine*) vaccine should be administered anytime between 11 and 12 years-of-age
- **HPV** is a 3-series vaccine administered months 0, 1, 6; females may receive HPV/4 or HPV/2; males should receive HPV/2
- **HPV** if not previously received at 11 or 12 years-of-age, may be initiated at any time between 13 and 26 years-of-age
- **IIV** (*inactivated influenza vaccine*) can be administered >6 months (use age-appropriate formulation), pregnant women, and persons with hives-only allergy to eggs
- **IHD** (*influenza high dose*) (**Fluzone High Dose**) may be recommended to persons ≥65 years of age
- **IPV** (*inactivated poliovirus vaccine*) minimum age 4 weeks
- An all-**IPV** schedule is recommended to eliminate the risk of vaccine-associated paralytic polio (VAPP) associated with **OPV** (*oral poliovirus vaccine*)
- **LAIV** (*live attenuated influenza vaccine*) may be administered intranasally (**FluMist**)
- **Men** (*meningococcal vaccine*) should be administered to all children at the 11-12 year old visit as well as to unvaccinated adolescents 15 years-of-age (usually at high school entry)
- **Men** should be administered to all college freshmen living in dormitories\
- Use MPSV4 for children aged 2-10 years and MCV4 for older children, although MPSV4 is an acceptable alternative for prophylaxis in men
- **MMR** (*mumps-measles-rubella*) should be administered at age 12 months in high-risk areas; if indicated, tuberculin testing can be done at the same visit
- **MMR** should be administered at age 11-12 years unless 2 doses were given after the first birthday; the interval between doses should be at least 4 weeks
- **MMR** adults born <1957 are generally considered immune to measles and mumps; all adults born ≥1957 should have documentation of at least I dose of MMR vaccine unless there is a medical contraindication or laboratory evidence of immunity to each of the 3 disease components; documentation of provider-diagnosed disease is not acceptable evidence of immunity to any of the 3 disease components
- **PCV-13** (*pneumococcal vaccine*) does not replace 23-valent pneumococcal polysaccharide in children age ≥24 months
- **PCV-13** when PCV-13 and PCV-23 are indicated, administer PCV-13 first; do not administer PCV-13 and PCV-23 in the same visit

(continued)

(*continued*)

- **PCV-13** adults ≥65 years-of-age, who have <u>not</u> received PCV-13 <u>or</u> PCV-23, should receive PCV-13 followed by PCV-23 6-12 months later
- **PCV-23** (*pneumococcal vaccine 23 trivalent*) minimum age 6 weeks
- **PCV-23** adults ≥65 years of age, who have received **PCV-23**, but <u>not</u> received PCV-13, should receive. **PCV-13** at least I year later; adults ≥65 years of age, who have <u>not</u> received **PCV-23**, should receive
- **PCV-13** followed by **PCV-23** 6-12 months later
- **RIV** (*recombinant influenza vaccine*; **FluBlok**) may be administered to any adult >18 years-of-age, including pregnant women
- **RIV** does <u>not</u> contain any egg protein; can be administered to anyone with egg allergy at any severity
- Older infants and children previously vaccinated with **PCV** should receive 3 doses (if age 7-11 months), 2 doses (if age 12-23 months) <u>or</u> 1 dose (if age >24 months)
- **Rot** (*rotavirus vaccine*) is a live attenuated oral vaccine for infants age >6 weeks <u>or</u> <32 weeks *only*; administer the 1st dose at 6-12 weeks-of-age; administer 2nd and 3rd doses at 4-10-week intervals for a total of 3 doses
- **Rot** If an incomplete dose is administered, *do <u>not</u>* administer a replacement dose, but continue with the remaining doses in the recommended series
- **Td** (*tetanus-diphtheria vaccine*) should be repeated every 10 years throughout life (<u>or</u> if at-risk injury ≥5 years after previous dose)
- **Td** should <u>*not*</u> be administered until minimum age ≥7 years
- **TdaP** (*tetanus-diphtheria-acellular pertussis*) administer 1 dose to pregnant women during each pregnancy, preferably during 27-36 weeks gestation, regardless of interval since prior Td <u>or</u> TdaP
- **TdaP** persons ≥11 years of age who have <u>not</u> received **Tdap** vaccine <u>or</u> for whom vaccine status is unknown, should receive 1 dose of **TdaP** followed by a **Td** booster every 10 years
- **Var** should be administered to children at age 11-12 years who have <u>not</u> had chicken-pox <u>or</u> who report having had chickenpox but do <u>not</u> have laboratory documentation of immunity
- **Var** If <u>not</u> received between age 11 and 12 years, administer 2 doses at least 4 weeks apart anytime after 12 years-of-age <u>or</u> a 2nd dose if previously only received 1 dose
- **VarZ** (*herpes zoster vaccine*) should be administered in a single dose once at ≥60 years-of-age, whether <u>or</u> <u>not</u> the person reports a prior episode of active herpes zoster infection
- **VarZ** is contraindicated in pregnancy and immune deficiency
- DTaP and IPV can be initiated as early as 4 weeks in areas of high endemicity <u>or</u> outbreak.

¶Adapted from DHHS CDC 2015.

APPENDIX G.2. CONTRAINDICATIONS TO VACCINES¶

All vaccines	Previous anaphylactic reaction to the vaccine, moderate <u>or</u> severe illness with <u>or</u> without fever
Live or live attenuated (LAVs)	Immunocompromised, receiving immunosuppressive doses of corticosteroids

(*continued*)

(continued)

TDaP/DTaP, Td	Encephalopathy within 7 days of following previous dose
Hib	Previous anaphylactic reaction to the vaccine, moderate or severe illness with or without fever
HBV	Anaphylactic reaction to baker's yeast
HAV	Previous anaphylactic reaction to the vaccine Moderate or severe illness with or without fever
Influenza	Allergy to eggs (*except* **FluBlok** which does not contain any egg protein)
IPV	Anaphylactic reaction to neomycin or streptomycin
Pneumococcal	Hypersensitivity to diphtheria toxoid
MMR	Anaphylactic reaction to eggs or neomycin, pregnancy, immunocompromised (mumps, measles, rubella are LAVs)
Meningococcal	Encephalopathy within 7 days following previous dose
Rotavirus	<6 months or >32 months, (Rotavirus is an LAV)
HPV	Pregnancy (pregnancy testing is not required); however, if administered, defer the remaining dose(s) until completion or termination of pregnancy
Varicella	Pregnancy, immunocompromised (Varicella is an LAV)
Herpes zoster	Pregnancy (HZ is a live vaccine)

[¶] Adapted from DHHS CDC 2015.

APPENDIX G.3. ROUTE OF ADMINISTRATION AND DOSE OF VACCINES[¶]

Vaccine	Route	Dose
Single Vaccines		
Diphtheria-Tetanus-Pertussis (DTaP, Dtap, DT)	IM	0.5 ml
Haemophilus influenza type b (Hib)	IM	0.5 ml
Hepatitis A vaccine (HAV)	IM	0.5 ml: age <18 yrs 1.0 ml: age ≥19 yrs
Hepatitis B vaccine (HBV)	IM	0.5 ml: age <18 yrs 1.0 ml: age ≥19 yrs
Human Papillomavirus (HPV)	IM	0.5 ml
Influenza **(Fluzone Intradermal)**	ID	0.5 ml
Influenza, inactivated (IIV), recombinant (RIV)	IM	0.25 ml: age 6-35 months 0.5 ml: age ≥3 yrs

(continued)

(continued)

Vaccine	Route	Dose
Influenza, live attenuated (LAIV)	NS	0.2 ml; 0.1 ml in each nostril
Meningococcal conjugate	IM	0.5 ml
Meningococcal polysaccharide (MPSV)	SC	0.5 ml
Meningococcal sero group B (Men B)	IM	0.5 ml
Mumps-Measles-Rubella (MMR)	SC	0.5 ml
Pneumococcal conjugate (PCV)	IM	0.5 ml
Pneumococcal polysaccharide (PPSV)	IM/SC	0.5 ml
Polio, Inactivated (IPV)	IM/SC	0.5 ml
Rotavirus (**Rotarix**)	PO	1 ml
Rotavirus (**Rotateq**)	PO	2 ml
Tetanus (Td)	IM	0.5 ml
Varicella	SC	0.5 ml
Herpes Zoster	SC	0.65 ml: age ≥60 yrs
Combination Vaccines		
MMR-Var (**ProQuad**)	SC	0.5 ml: age ≤12 yrs
HBV-HAV (**Twinrix**)	IM	1 ml: >18 yrs
DTaP-HBV-IPV (**Pediarix**)	IM	0.5 ml
DTaP-IPV-Hib (**Pentacel**)	IM	0.5 ml
DTaP-IPV (**Kinrix, Quadracel**)	IM	0.5 ml
Hib-HBV (**Comvax**)	IM	0.5 ml
Hib-MenCY (**MenHibrix**)	IM	0.5 ml

¶ Adapted from DHHS CDC 2015

APPENDIX G.4. ADVERSE REACTIONS TO VACCINES¶

Vaccine	Signs and Symptoms	Treatment
Inactivated antigens: DTP, Dtap, DTaP, Td, IPV, influenza inactivated (IIV) recombinant (RIV) Live attenuated viruses: MMR, Meningococcal, rotavirus, varicella, herpes zoster	Local tenderness Erythema Swelling Low-grade fever Drowsiness Fretfulness Decreased appetite Prolonged crying Unusual cry	*acetaminophen* or *ibuprofen* for age and/or weight; *aspirin* and *aspirin*-containing products are contraindicated

¶ Adapted from DHHS CDC 2015.

APPENDIX G.5. MINIMUM INTERVALS BETWEEN VACCINE DOSES[1]

Type	#1 to #2	#2 to #3	#3 to #4	#4 to #5
HBV	4 weeks	5 months		
HAV	6 months			
DTaP	4 weeks	4 weeks	6 months	6 months
IPV	4 weeks	4 weeks	4 weeks	
MMR	4 weeks			
Var	4 weeks			
Rotavirus	4 weeks	4 weeks; do not administer >32 weeks of age		
PCV-13	4 weeks (if #1 at age <12 months and current age <24 months); 8 weeks (as last dose if #1 at age >12 months or current age 24-59 months); No more doses needed if healthy and #1 at age ≥24 months	4 weeks if age <12 months; 8 weeks (as last dose if age ≥12 months); No more doses needed if healthy and previous dose at age ≥24 months	8 weeks (as last dose; only necessary for age 12 months to 5 years who received 3 doses before age 12 months)	
Hib	4 weeks (if #1 at age <12 months); 8 weeks (as last dose if #1 at age 12-14 months); No more doses needed if healthy and #1 at age ≥15 months	4 weeks if age 12 months; 8 weeks (as last dose if age ≥12 months); No more doses needed if previous dose at age ≥15 months	8 weeks (as last dose; only necessary for age 12 months to 2 years who received 3 doses before age 12 months)	
HPV	4 weeks	20 weeks (24 weeks after #1		

[1] Adapted from DHHS CDC 2015

APPENDIX G.6. RECOMMENDED CHILDHOOD IMMUNIZATION SCHEDULE[1]

Type	Birth	1 month	2 months	4 months	6 months	6-18 months	12-15 months	15-18 months	4-6 years	11-12 years
HBV	✓	✓			✓					
DTaP			✓	✓	✓		✓		✓	
IPV			✓	✓		✓			✓	
Hib			✓	✓	✓		✓			
Rotavirus			✓	✓	✓					
MMR							✓		✓	
TDaP										✓
Varicella							✓		✓	
PVC-13			✓	✓	✓		✓			
HAV								✓		
Meningitis										✓
HPV										✓✓✓

[1]Adapted from DHHS CDC 2015.

✓ = immunization due.

✓✓✓ = HPV 3-dose series, months 0, 1, 6.

APPENDIX G.7. RECOMMENDED CHILDHOOD (BIRTH-12 YEARS) IMMUNIZATION CATCH-UP SCHEDULE[¶]

Vaccine	Minimum Interval Between Doses			
	#1 to #2	#2 to #3	#3 to #4	#4 to #5
HBV	4 weeks	8 weeks (16 weeks after #1)		
DTaP	4 weeks	4 weeks	6 months	6 months
IPV	4 weeks	4 weeks	4 weeks	
MMR	4 weeks			
Var	4 weeks			
Rotavirus	4 weeks	4 weeks; do not administer >32 weeks of age		
PCV	2 months	2 months	2 months	6-15 months
HPV	4 weeks	20 weeks (24 weeks after #1		

[¶]Adapted from DHHS CDC 2015

APPENDIX G.8. RECOMMENDED SCHEDULE FOR MISSED CHILDHOOD IMMUNIZATIONS (13-21 YEARS)[¶]

Type	19-21 yrs	22-26 yrs	27-49 yrs	50-59 yrs	60-65 yrs	≥65 yrs
Influenza	1 dose annually					
HBV	3 dose series: months 0, 1, 6					
Td/TdaP	Substitute Tdap for Td one time; then continue Td once every 10 years					
MMR*	Born >1957: 2 doses, 4 weeks apart					
Varicella*	Without evidence of immunity: 2 doses, 4 weeks apart					
Herpes zoster*					1 time dose	
PVC-13/ PVC-23					1 time dose	
HAV	Single Antigen, 2 doses: months 0, 6-12 (**Havrix**); 0, 6-18 (**Vaqta**)					
Meningitis	1 or more doses					

(*continued*)

(*continued*)

Type	19-21 yrs	22-26 yrs	27-49 yrs	50-59 yrs	60-65 yrs	≥65 yrs
HPV (female)*β	3 doses; months 0, 1, 6					
HPV (male)β	3 doses; months 0, 1, 6					

¶ Adapted from DHHS CDC 2015

* Contraindicated in pregnancy

β Only if not previously vaccinated between 11-12 years-of-age

◯ APPENDIX H. CONTRACEPTIVES

APPENDIX H.1. CONTRAINDICATIONS AND RECOMMENDATIONS

- All contraceptives are pregnancy category X
- No non-barrier contraceptives protect against STDs
- **Absolute Contraindication**:
  - HTN >35 years-of-age
  - DM >35 years-of-age
  - LDL-C >160 or TG >250
  - Known or suspected pregnancy
  - Known or suspected carcinoma of the breast
  - Known or suspected carcinoma of the endometrium
  - Known or suspected estrogen-dependent neoplasia
  - Undiagnosed abnormal genital bleeding
  - Cerebral vascular or coronary artery disease
  - Cholestatic jaundice of pregnancy or jaundice with prior use
  - Hepatic adenoma or carcinoma or benign liver tumor
  - Active or past history of thrombophlebitis or thromboembolic disorder
- **Relative Contraindications**
  - Lactation
  - Asthma
  - Ulcerative colitis
  - Migraine or vascular headache
  - Cardiac or renal dysfunction
  - Gestational diabetes, prediabetes, diabetes mellitus
  - Diastolic BP 90 mmHg or greater or hypertension by any other criteria
  - Psychic depression
  - Varicose veins
  - Smoker >35 years-of-age
  - Sickle-cell or sickle-hemoglobin C disease
  - Cholestatic jaundice during pregnancy, active gallbladder disease
  - Hepatitis or mononucleosis during the preceding year
  - First-order family history of fatal or nonfatal rheumatic CVD or diabetes prior to age 50 years

(*continued*)

(*continued*)

- Drug(s) with known interaction(s)
- Elective surgery or immobilization within 4 weeks
- Age >50 years
- **Recommendations**
  - Start the first pill on the first Sunday after menses begins. Thereafter, each new pill pack will be started on a Sunday.
  - Take each daily pill in the same 3-hour window (e.g., 9A-12N, 12N-3P; a 4-hour window prior to bedtime is not recommended).
  - If 1 pill is missed, take it as soon as possible and the next pill at the regular time.
  - If 2 pills are missed, take both pills as soon as possible and then two pills the following day. A barrier method should be used for the remainder of the pill pack.
  - If 3 pills are missed before 10th cycle day, resume taking OCs on a regular schedule and take precautions.
  - If 3 pills are missed after the 10th cycle day, discard the current pill pack and begin a new one 7 days after the last pill was taken.
  - If very low-dose OCs are used or if combination OCs are begun after the 5th day of the menstrual cycle, an additional method of birth control should be used for the first 7 days of OC use.
  - If nausea occurs as a side effect, select an OC with *lower **estrogen*** content.
  - If breakthrough bleeding occurs during the first half of the cycle, select an OC with *higher **progesterone*** content.
  - Symptoms of a serious nature include loss of vision, diplopia, unilateral numbness, weakness, or tingling, severe chest pain, severe pain in left arm or neck, severe leg pain, slurring of speech, and abdominal tenderness or mass.

APPENDIX H.2. 28-DAY ORAL CONTRACEPTIVES WITH ESTROGEN AND PROGES-TERONE CONTENT

Comment: **Beyaz, Loryna, Syeda, Safyral, Yasmin,** and **Yaz** are contraindicated with renal and adrenal insufficiency. Monitor k^+ level during the first cycle if the patient is at risk for hyperkalemia for any reason. If the patient is taking drugs that increase potassium (e.g., ACEIs, ARBS, NSAIDs, K^+ sparing diuretics), the patient is at risk for hyperkalemia.

Combined Oral Contraceptive	Estrogen (mcg)	Progesterone (mg)
Alesse-21, Alesse-28 (X)(G) *ethinyl estradiol+levonorgestrel*	20	0.1
Altavera (X) *ethinyl estradiol+levonorgestrel*	30	0.15
Apri (X)(G) *ethinyl estradiol+desogestrel*	30	0.15
Aranelle (X)(G) *ethinyl estradiol+norethindrone*	35	0.5 1 0.5
Aviane (X)(G) *ethinyl estradiol+levonorgestrel*	20	0.1

(*continued*)

(*continued*)

Combined Oral Contraceptive	Estrogen (mcg)	Progesterone (mg)
Balziva (X)(G) *ethinyl estradiol+norethindrone*	35	0.4
Beyaz (X)(G) *ethinyl estradiol+drospirenone* <u>plus</u> levomefolate calcium 0.451 mcg (28 tabs)	20	3
Blisovi 24Fe (X)(G) *ethinyl estradiol+norethindrone* plus *ferrous fumarate* 75 mg (4 tabs)	20	1
Brevicon-21, Brevicon-28 (X)(G) *ethinyl estradiol+norethindrone*	35	0.5
Camrese (X) *ethinyl estradiol+levonorgestrel*	30 10	0.15
Camrese Lo (X) *ethinyl estradiol+levonorgestrel*	20 10	0.1
Cesia (X)(G) *ethinyl estradiol+desogestrel*	25 25 25	0.1 0.125 0.15
Cryselle (X)(G) *ethinyl estradiol+norgestrel*	30	0.3
Cyclessa (X)(G) *ethinyl estradiol+desogestrel*	25 25 25	0.1 0.125 0.15
Demulen 1/35-21, Demulen 1/35-28 (X)(G) *ethinyl estradiol+ethynodiol diacetate*	35	1
Demulen 1/50-21, Demulen 1/50-28 (X)(G) *ethinyl estradiol+ethynodiol diacetate*	50	1
Desogen (X)(G) *ethinyl estradiol+desogestrel diacetate*	30	0.15
Enpresse (X)(G) *ethinyl estradiol+levonorgestrel*	30 40 30	0.05 0.075 0.125
Estrostep Fe (X) *ethinyl estradiol+norethindrone* plus *ferrous fumarate* 75 mg	20 30 35	1 1 1
Femcon Fe (X)(G) *ethinyl estradiol+norethindrone* <u>plus</u> *ferrous fumarate* 75 mg	35	0.4

(*continued*)

(*continued*)

Combined Oral Contraceptive	Estrogen (mcg)	Progesterone (mg)
Generess Fe Chew tab (X)(G) *ethinyl estradiol+norethindrone* <u>plus</u> *ferrous fumarate* 75 mg	25	0.8
Genora (X)(G) *ethinyl estradiol+norethindrone*	35 35 35	0.5 1 0.5
Gianvi (X)(G) *ethinyl estradiol+drospirenone*	20	3
Gildess 1.5/30 (X)(G) *ethinyl estradiol+norethindrone*	30	1.5
Introvale (X) *ethinyl estradiol+levonorgestrel*	30	0.15
Jenest-28 (X) *ethinyl estradiol+norethindrone*	35 35	0.5 1
Jolessa (X)(G) *ethinyl estradiol+levonorgestrel*	30	0.15
Junel 1/20 (X)(G) *ethinyl estradiol+norethindrone*	20	1
Junel 1.5/30 (X)(G) *ethinyl estradiol+norethindrone*	30	1.5
Junel Fe 1/20 (X)(G) *ethinyl estradiol+norethindrone* <u>plus</u> *ferrous fumarate* 75 mg	20	1
Junel Fe 1.5/30 (X)(G) *ethinyl estradiol+norethindrone* <u>plus</u> *ferrous fumarate* 75 mg	30	1.5
Kaitlib Fe Chew Tab (X)(G) *ethinyl estradiol+norethindrone* <u>plus</u> *ferrous fumarate* 75 mg	25	0.8
Kariva (X)(G) *ethinyl estradiol+desogestrel*	20 10	0.15 0.15
Kelnor 1/35 (X)(G) *ethinyl estradiol+ethynodiol diacetate*	35	1
Leena (X) *ethinyl estradiol+norethindrone*	35 35 35	0.5 1 0.5

(*continued*)

(continued)

Combined Oral Contraceptive	Estrogen (mcg)	Progesterone (mg)
Lessina 28 (X)(G) *ethinyl estradiol+levonorgestrel*	20	0.1
Levlen 21, Levlen 28 (X)(G) *ethinyl estradiol+levonorgestrel*	30	0.15
Levlite 28 (X)(G) *ethinyl estradiol+levonorgestrel*	20	0.1
Levora-21, Levora-28 (X)(G) *ethinyl estradiol+levonorgestrel*	30	0.15
Loestrin 21 1/20 (X)(G) *ethinyl estradiol+norethindrone*	20	1
Loestrin 21 1.5/30 (X)(G) *ethinyl estradiol+norethindrone*	30	1.5
Loestrin Fe 1/20 (X)(G) *ethinyl estradiol+norethindrone* <u>plus</u> *ferrous fumarate* 75 mg	20	1
Loestrin Fe 1.5/30 (X)(G) *ethinyl estradiol+norethindrone* <u>plus</u> *ferrous fumarate* 75 mg (4 tabs)	30	1.5
Loestrin 24 Fe (X)(G) *ethinyl estradiol+norethindrone* <u>plus</u> *ferrous fumarate* 75 mg (4 tabs)	20	1
Lo Loestrin Fe (X) *ethinyl estradiol+norethindrone* <u>plus</u> *ferrous fumarate* 75 mg (2 tabs)	10	1
Lomedia 24 Fe (X)(G) *ethinyl estradiol+norethindrone* <u>plus</u> *ferrous fumarate* 75 mg	20	1
Lo/Ovral-21, Lo/Ovral-28 (X)(G) *ethinyl estradiol+norgestrel*	30	0.3
Loryna (X) *ethinyl estradiol+drospirenone*	20	3
Low-Ogestrel-21, Low-Ogestrel-28 (X)(G) *ethinyl estradiol/norgestrel*	30	0.3
Lutera (X)(G) *ethinyl estradiol+levonorgestrel*	20	0.1

(continued)

(*continued*)

Combined Oral Contraceptive	Estrogen (mcg)	Progesterone (mg)
Lybrel (X) *ethinyl estradiol+levonorgestrel*	20	0.09
Mibelas 24 FE (X)(G) *ethinyl estradiol+norethindrone* <u>plus</u> *ferrous fumarate 75 mg*	20	1
Microgestin 1/20 (X)(G) *ethinyl estradiol+norethindrone*	20	1
Microgestin Fe 1/20 (X)(G) *ethinyl estradiol+norethindrone* <u>plus</u> *ferrous fumarate 75* mg	20	1
Microgestin 1.5/30 (X)(G) *ethinyl estradiol+norethindrone*	30	1.5
Microgestin Fe 1.5/30 (X)(G) *ethinyl estradiol+norethindrone* <u>plus</u> *ferrous fumarate 75 mg*	30	1.5
Mircette (X)(G) *ethinyl estradiol+desogestrel diacetate*	20 10	0.15
Minastrin 24 FE (X)(G) *ethinyl estradiol+norethindrone* <u>plus</u> *ferrous fumarate 75 mg*	20	1
Modicon 0.5/35-28 (X)(G) *ethinyl estradiol+norethindrone*	35	0.5
MonoNessa (X)(G) *ethinyl estradiol+norgestimate*	35	0.25
Natazia (X)(G) *estradiol valerate+dienogest*	30 20 20 10	— 2 3 —
Necon 0.5/35-21, Necon 0.5/35-28 (X)(G) *ethinyl estradiol+norethindrone*	35	0.5
Necon 1/35-21, Necon 1/35-28 (X)(G) *ethinyl estradiol+norethindrone*	35	0.5
Necon 10/11-21, Necon 10/11-28 (X)(G) *ethinyl estradiol+norethindrone*	35 35	0.5 1
Necon 1/50-21, Necon 1/50-28 (X)(G) *mestranol+norethindrone*	50	1

(*continued*)

(*continued*)

Combined Oral Contraceptive	Estrogen (mcg)	Progesterone (mg)
Nelova 0.5/35-21, Nelova 0.5/35-28 (X)(G) *ethinyl estradiol+norethindrone*	35	0.5
Nelova 1/35-21, Nelova 1/35-28 (X)(G) *ethinyl estradiol+norethindrone*	35	1
Nelova 10/11-21, Nelova 10/11-28 (X)(G) *ethinyl estradiol/norethindrone*	35 35	0.5 1
Nelova 1/50-21, Nelova 1/50-28 (X)(G) *mestranol+norethindrone*	50	1
Neocon 7/7/7 (X)(G) *ethinyl estradiol+norethindrone*	35 35 35	0.5 0.75 1
Nordette-21, Nordette-28 (X)(G) *ethinyl estradiol+levonorgestrel*	30	0.15
Norinyl 1/35-21, Norinyl 1/35-28 (X)(G) *ethinyl estradiol+norethindrone*	35	1
Norinyl 1/50-21, Norinyl 1/50-28 (X)(G) *mestranol+norethindrone*	50	1
Nortrel 0.5/35 (X)(G) *ethinyl estradiol/norethindrone*	35	0.5
Nortrel 1/35-21, Nortrel 1/35-28 (X)(G) *ethinyl estradiol+norethindrone*	35	1
Nortrel 7/7/7-28 (X)(G) *ethinyl estradiol+norethindrone*	35 35 35	0.5 0.75 1
Ocella (X)(G) *ethinyl estradiol+drospirenone*	30	3
Ortho-Cept 28 (X)(G) *ethinyl estradiol+desogestrel*	30	0.15
Ortho-Cyclen 28 (X)(G) *ethinyl estradiol+norgestimate*	35	0.25
Ortho-Novum 1/35-21, Ortho-Novum 1/35-28 (X)(G) *ethinyl estradiol+norethindrone*	35	1
Ortho-Novum 1/50-21, Ortho-Novum 1/50-28 (X)(G) *mestranol+norethindrone*	50	1

(*continued*)

(continued)

Combined Oral Contraceptive	Estrogen (mcg)	Progesterone (mg)
Ortho-Novum 7/7/7-28 (X)(G) *ethinyl estradiol+norethindrone*	35 35 35	0.5 0.75 1
Ortho-Novum 10/11-28 (X) *ethinyl estradiol+norethindrone*	35 35	0.5 1
Ortho Tri-Cyclen 21, Ortho Tri-Cyclen 28 (X)(G) *ethinyl estradiol+norgestimate*	35 35 35	0.18 0.215 0.25
Ortho Tri-Cyclen Lo (X)(G) *ethinyl estradiol+norgestimate*	25 25 25	0.18 0.215 0.25
Ovcon 35 Fe (X)(G) *ethinyl estradiol+norethindrone* plus *ferrous* *fumarate* 75 mg (4 tabs)	35	0.4
Ovcon 50-28, Ovcon 50-28 (X)(G) *ethinyl estradiol+norethindrone*	50	1
Ovral-21, Ovral-28 (X)(G) *ethinyl estradiol+norgestrel*	50	0.5
Portia (X)(G) *ethinyl estradiol+levonorgestrel*	30	0.15
Previfem (X) *ethinyl estradiol+norgestimate*	35	0.25
Quasense (X) *ethinyl estradiol+levonorgestrel*	30	0.15
Reclipsen (X)(G) *ethinyl estradiol+desogestrel* plus *ferrous fumarate* 75 mg (4 tabs)	30	0.15
Safyral (X)(G) *ethinyl estradiol+drospirenone* plus *levomefolate calcium* 0.451 mg	30	3
Sprintec 28 (X)(G) *ethinyl estradiol+norgestimate*	35	0.25
Syeda (X) *ethinyl estradiol+drospirenone*	30	3

(continued)

(continued)

Combined Oral Contraceptive	Estrogen (mcg)	Progesterone (mg)
Tarina Fe 1/20 (X)(G) *ethinyl estradiol+norethindrone* <u>plus</u> *ferrous fumarate* 75 mg (7 tabs)	20	1
Taytulla Fe 1/20 (X)(G) (Softgel caps) *ethinyl estradiol+norethindrone* <u>plus</u> *ferrous fumarate* 75 mg (4 Softgel caps)	20	1
Tilia Fe (X)(G) *ethinyl estradiol+norethindrone* <u>plus</u> *ferrous fumarate* 75 mg (7 tabs)	20 30 35	1 1 1
Tri-Legest 21 (X)(G) *ethinyl estradiol+norethindrone*	20 30 35	1 1 1
Tri-Legest Fe (X)(G) *ethinyl estradiol+norethindrone* <u>plus</u> *ferrous fumarate* 75 mg (7 tabs)	20 30 35	1 1 1
Tri-Levlen 21, Tri-Levlen 28 (X)(G) *ethinyl estradiol+levonorgestrel*	30 40 30	0.05 0.075 0.125
Tri-Lo-Estarylla (X)(G) *ethinyl estradiol+norgestimate*	25 25 25	0.18 0.215 0.25
Tri-Lo-Sprintec (X)(G) *ethinyl estradiol+norgestimate*	25 25 25	0.18 0.215 0.25
TriNessa (X)(G) *ethinyl estradiol+norgestimate*	35 35 35	0.18 0.215 0.25
Tri-Norinyl 21, Tri-Norinyl 28 (X)(G) *ethinyl estradiol+norethindrone*	35 35 35	0.5 1 0.5
Triphasil-21, Triphasil-28 (X)(G) *ethinyl estradiol+levonorgestrel*	30 40 30	0.050 0.075 0.125
Tri-Previfem (X)(G) *ethinyl estradiol+norgestimate*	35 35 35	0.18 0.215 0.25

(continued)

(*continued*)

Combined Oral Contraceptive	Estrogen (mcg)	Progesterone (mg)
Tri-Sprintec (X)(G)	35	0.18
ethinyl estradiol+norgestimate	35	0.215
	35	0.25
Trivora (X)(G)	30	0.05
ethinyl estradiol+levonorgestrel	40	0.075
	30	0.125
Velivet (X)(G)	25	0.1
ethinyl estradiol+desogestrel	25	0.125
	25	0.15
Yasmin (X)(G)	30	3
ethinyl estradiol+drospirenone		
Yaz (X)(G)	20	3
ethinyl estradiol+drospirenone		
Zovia 1/35E-28 (X)(G)	35	1
ethinyl estradiol+ethynodiol diacetate		
Zovia 1/50E-28 (X)(G)	50	1
ethinyl estradiol+ethynodiol diacetate		

APPENDIX H.3. EXTENDED-CYCLE ORAL CONTRACEPTIVES

91 Day
➤ *ethinyl estradiol+levonorgestrel* (X) 1 tab daily x 91 days; repeat (no tablet-free days)
    Ashlyna (G) *Tab: levonor* 15 mcg+*eth est* 30 mcg (84)+*eth est* 10 mcg (7)
    (91 tabs/pck)
    Jolessa (G) *Tab: levonor* 15 mcg+*eth est* 30 mcg (84)+inert tabs (7m91 tabs/pck)
    LoSeasonique *Tab: levonor* 0.1 mcg+*eth est* 20 mcg (84)+*eth est* 10 mcg (7)
    (91 tabs/pck)
    Quartette (G) *Tab: levonor* 15 mcg+*eth est* 30 mcg (84)+*eth est* 10 mcg (7)
    (91 tabs/pck)
    Quasense (G) *Tab: levonor* 15 mcg+*eth est* 30 mcg (84)+inert tabs (7)
    (91 tabs/pck)
    Seasonale (G) *Tab: levonor* 15 mcg+*eth est* 30 mcg (84)+inert tabs (7)
    (91 tabs/pck)
    Seasonique (G) *Tab: levonor* 15 mcg+*eth est* 30 mcg (84)+*eth est* 10 mcg (7)
    (91 tabs/pck)
365 Day
➤ *ethinyl estradiol+levonorgestrel* (X) 1 tab daily x 28 days; repeat (no tablet-free days)
    Lybrel *Tab: levonor* 0.09 mcg+*eth est* 20 mcg (28 tabs/pck)

APPENDIX H.4. PROGESTERONE-ONLY ORAL CONTRACEPTIVES ("MINI-PILL")

Brand	Progesterone	mcg
Comment: Take progestin-only pills at the same time each day (within a 3-hour time window). If a pill is missed, another method of contraception should be used for the remainder of the pill pack.		
Camila (X)(G)	*norethindrone*	35
Errin (X)(G)	*norethindrone*	35
Jolivette (X)(G)	*norethindrone*	35
Micronor (X)(G)	*norethindrone*	35
Nora-BE (X)(G)	*norethindrone*	35
Nor-QD (X)(G)	*norethindrone*	35
Ortho Micronor (X)(G)	*norethindrone*	35
Ovrette (X)(G)	*norgestrel*	7.5

APPENDIX H.5. INJECTABLE CONTRACEPTIVES

H.5.1: Injectable Progesterone

90 Days
Comment: Administer first dose within 5 days of onset of normal menses, within 5 days postpartum if not breastfeeding, or at 6 weeks postpartum if breastfeeding exclusively. Do not use for >2 years unless other methods are inadequate.

▷ *medroxyprogesterone* (X)(G)
    Depo-Provera 150 mg deep IM q 3 months
      Vial: 150 mg/ml (1 ml); *Prefilled syringe:* 150 mg/ml
    Depo-SubQ 104 mg SC q 3 months
      Prefilled syringe: 104 mg/ml (0.65 ml) (parabens)

APPENDIX H.6. TRANSDERMAL CONTRACEPTIVE

Ethinyl Estradiol+Norelgestromin
Comment: Apply the transdermal patch to the abdomen, buttock, upper-outer arm, or upper torso. *Do* not apply the transdermal patch to the breast. Rotate the site (however, may use the same anatomical area).

▷ *ethinyl estradiol+norelgestromin* (X)(G) apply one patch once weekly x 3 weeks; then 1 patch-free week; then repeat sequence
    Ortho Evra
      Transdermal patch: eth est 20 mcg+*norel* 150 mcg per day (1, 3/pck)

APPENDIX H.7. CONTRACEPTIVE VAGINAL RINGS

Ethinyl Estradiol+Etonogestrel

Comment: The vaginal ring should be inserted prior to, or on 5th day, of the menstrual cycle. Use of a backup method is recommended during the first week. When switching from oral contraceptives, the vaginal ring should be inserted anytime within 7 days after the last active tablet and no later than the day a new pill pack would have been started (no back up method is needed). If the ring is accidently expelled for less than 3 hours, it should be rinsed with cool to lukewarm water and reinserted promptly. If ring removal lasts for more than 3 hours, an additional contraceptive method should be used. If the ring is lost, a new ring should be inserted and the regimen continued without alteration.

▷ *etonogestrel+ethinyl estradiol* (X) insert 1 ring vaginally and leave in place for 3 weeks; then remove for 1 ring-free week; then repeat
    NuvaRing
        Vag ring: eth est 15 mcg/*eton* 120 mcg per day (1, 3/pck)

APPENDIX H.8. SUBDERMAL CONTRACEPTIVES

Comment: Implants must be inserted within 7 days of the onset of menses. A complete physical examination is required annually. Remove if pregnancy, thromboembolic disorder including thrombophlebitis, jaundice, visual disturbances. Not for use by patients with hypertension, diabetes, hyperlipidemia, impaired liver function, epilepsy, asthma, migraine, depression, cardiac or renal insufficiency, thromboembolic disorder including thrombophlebitis, pro-longed immobilization, or who are smokers.

▷ *etonogestrel* (X) implant rod subdermally in the upper inner non-dominant arm; remove and replace at the end of 3 years
    Implanon, Nexplanon
        Implantable rod: 68 mg implant for subdermal insertion (w. insertion device; latex-free)

▷ *levonorgestrel* (X) implant rods subdermally in the upper inner non-dominant arm; remove and replace at the end of 5 years
    Norplant
        Implantable rods: 6-36 mg implants (total 216 mg) for subdermal insertion (1 kit w. sterile supplies)

APPENDIX H.9. INTRAUTERINE CONTRACEPTIVES

Comment: Indicated in women who have had at least one child and who are in a stable, mutually monogamous relationship. Reexamine after menses within 3 months (recommend 4-6 weeks) to check placement.

▷ *levonorgestrel* (X)
    Kyleena *IUD:* 19.5 mg (replace at least every 5 years)
    Liletta *IUD:* 52 mg (replace at least every 3 years)
    Mirena *IUD:* 52 mg (replace at least every 5 years)
    Skyla *IUD:* 13.5 mg (replace at least every 3 years)

APPENDIX H.10. EMERGENCY CONTRACEPTION

> **Comment:** Emergency contraception must be started within 72 hours after unprotected intercourse following a negative urine hCG pregnancy test. If vomiting occurs within 1 hour of taking a dose, repeat the dose.

> ➤ *ethinyl estradiol+levonorgestrel* (X) 2 tabs as soon as possible after unprotected intercourse <u>or</u> contraceptive failure, then 2 more 12 hours after first dose
> *Premenarchal:* not applicable
> > **Preven** *Tab:* eth est 50 mcg+levonor 250 mcg (4/pck) <u>*plus*</u> *Pregnancy test:* 1 hCG home pregnancy test
> > **Yuzpe Regimen** *Tab:* eth est 50 mcg+levonor 250 mcg (4/pck)

> ➤ *levonorgestrel* (X)(OTC)(G) 1 tab as soon as possible, within 72 hours, after unprotected sex <u>or</u> suspected contraceptive failure
> *Premenarchal:* not applicable; <17 years (prescription required); ≥17 years (OTC)
> > **My Way** *Tab:* 1.5 mg (1/pck)
> > **Plan B One Step** *Tab:* 1.5 mg (1/pck)
> > **EContra EZ** *Tab:* 1.5 mg (1/pck)

> ➤ *ulipristal* (X)(G) take 1 tab as soon as possible within 120 hours (5 days) after unprotected intercourse <u>or</u> contraceptive failure; may repeat dose if vomiting occurs within 3 hours
> *Pediatric:* premenarchal: not applicable
> > **ella** *Tab:* 30 mg (1/pck)
> > **Logilia** *Tab:* 30 mg (1/pck)

APPENDIX I. ANESTHETIC AGENTS FOR LOCAL INFILTRATION AND DERMAL/MUCOSAL MEMBRANE APPLICATION

Agents and Indications	
Brand/*generic*	**Indication(s)**
AnaMantle HC *lidocaine 3%+hydrocortisone 0.5%*	Local anesthetic+steroid; for hemorrhoids, pruritus ani, anal fissure
Decadron Phosphate with Xylocaine *dexamethasone 4 mg+lidocaine 10 mg/ml (5 ml)*	Local anesthetic+steroid; infiltration by injection
Dyclone *dyclonine 0.5%, 0.1%*	Local anesthetic; infiltration by injection
Duranest (B) *etidocaine 1% (30 ml)* **Duranest (B) w. Epinephrine** *Inj: etido 1.5%+epi 1:200,000 (30 ml)* *Dental Cartridge: etido 1.5%+epi 1:200,000 (1.8 ml)*	Nerve block and local anesthetic; mouth, pharynx, larynx, trachea, esophagus, anogenital area, urethra Local anesthetic: dental procedures

(continued)

(continued)

Agents and Indications	
Brand/*generic*	**Indication(s)**
Ela-Max 4% Cream (B) *lidocaine 4%* **Ela-Max 5% Cream (B)** *lidocaine 5%*	Local dermal anesthetic and for anorectal irritation and pain
Emla Cream (B) (5, 30 gm) **Emla Anesthetic Disc (B)** (2 discs/box) *lidocaine 2.5%+prilocaine 2.5%*	Local dermal anesthetic; preparation for phlebotomy, PIV starts, injections
Flector Patch (C/D) (30/box) *diclofenac epolamine 180 mg*	Local dermal NSAID analgesic
Exparel (B) *Vial:* 13.3 mg/ml (20 ml) *bupivacaine liposome 1.3% susp for inj*	Surgical site injection for postop pain management
LidaMantle (B) cream (1, 2 oz) **LidaMantle (B)** lotion (177 ml) **Lidoderm** cream **(B)** (85 gm) *lidocaine 3%* **Lidoderm (B)(G)** adhesive patch (10 cm x14 cm; 30/box) *lidocaine 5%*	Local dermal anesthetic lotion, cream, and adhesive patch
Ophthaine (B) (15 ml) *proparacaine 0.5% ophthalmic solution*	Ophthalmic anesthetic for examination and removal of foreign body (eye)
Pliaglis Cream (B) (30 g) *lidocaine 7%+tetracaine 7%*	Local dermal anesthetic for superficial dermatological procedures
Qutenza (B) (1, 2 patches, each *with 50 g tube of cleansing gel*) *capsaicin 8% patch*	Local dermal NSAID analgesic for postherpetic neuralgia
Septocaine, Ultican (G) *articaine hcl+epinephrine 4%/1:200,000*	Local, infiltrate, or conductive anesthesia in both simple and complex dental procedures
Synera Topical Patch (B) (2, 10/pck) *lidocaine 70 mg+tetracaine 70 mg*	Local dermal anesthetic for venous access <u>or</u> skin lesion removal
Tetracaine Ophthalmic Solution (B) (15 ml) *proparacaine 0.5% ophthalmic solution*	Ophthalmic anesthetic for examination/ removal of foreign body (eye)
Xylocaine Jelly (B) (5, 10, 20, 30 ml) *lidocaine 2% aqueous*	For procedures of the urethra, painful urethritis, and endotracheal intubation

(continued)

(continued)

Agents and Indications	
Brand/*generic*	Indication(s)
Xylocaine Ointment (B) (3.5, 35 gm) *lidocaine 5% water miscible*	For procedures of the urethra, painful urethritis, and endotracheal intubation
Xylocaine Topical Solution (B) (100 ml) *lidocaine 2% solution* **Xylocaine Viscous (B)** (50 ml) *lidocaine 2% viscous solution*	Anesthetic for the nasal and oropharyngeal mucosa and the proximal portions of the GI tract
Zingo *lidocaine monohydrate 0.5 mg*	Hand-held, needle-free device, helium-powered delivery system that numbs site in 1-3 minutes delivers 0.5 mg sterile lidocaine HCL monohydrate sterile lidocaine HCL pwdr for intradermal injection for the management of venous access pain
Zostrix (B) (0.7, 1.5, 3 oz) *capsaicin 0.025% cream* **Zostrix HP (B)** (1, 2 oz) *capsaicin 0.075% emollient cream*	Local dermal NSAID analgesic

APPENDIX J. NSAIDs

Comment: NSAIDs should be taken with food to decrease gastric upset. Dosing of NSAIDs should be scheduled rather than PRN for maximal benefit. NSAIDs are contraindicated with sulfonamide *or* **aspirin** allergy, 3rd trimester pregnancy (causes premature closure of the ductus arteriosus), and coronary artery bypass graft (CABG) surgery. Concomitant use of **misoprostol** (**Cytotec**) with NSAIDs reduces gastric upset and potential for ulceration; however, **misoprostol** is pregnancy category X. Administration of **misoprostol** in pregnancy can cause spontaneous abortion, premature birth, birth defects, and uterine rupture (beyond the 8th week of pregnancy). NSAIDs and **warfarin** (**Coumadin**) are synergistic. With all patients, use the lowest effective dose for the shortest time necessary. NSAIDs should be taken with food to reduce the risk of gastrointestinal adverse side effects (GIASE).

> **Legend:** GI Adverse Side Effects:
>   (+) mild; (++) frequent; (+++) more frequent/severe

▷ *celecoxib* **(C/D)(G)(+)** 100 mg twice daily *or* 200 mg once daily *or* 200 mg twice daily *or* 400 mg once daily; <50 kg, start at lowest dose
Pediatric: <2 years: not recommended; ≥2 years, >10<25 kg: 50 mg twice daily; ≥25 kg: 100 mg once daily
    Celebrex *Cap:* 50, 100, 200, 400 mg

(continued)

(continued)

▷ *diclofenac potassium* (C/D)(G)(+++) 50 mg tid <u>or</u> qid <u>or</u> 25 mg tid <u>or</u> qid and may add 25 mg at HS
  Pediatric: <12 years: not recommended; ≥12 years: same as adult
    Cataflam *Tab:* 50 mg
    Zipsor *Gel cap:* 25 mg

▷ *diclofenac sodium* (D)(+++)
  Pediatric: <12 years: not recommended; ≥12 years: same as adult
    Dyloject administer 37.5 mg IV bolus over 15 seconds q 6 hours; max 150 mg/day
      Vial: 37.5 mg/ml (25/box)
    Pennsaid 1% in 10 drop increments, dispense and rub into front, side, and back of knee: usually 40 drops (40 mg) qid
      Topical soln: 1.5% (150 ml)
    Pennsaid 2% apply 2 pump actuations (40 mg) and rub into front, side, and back of knee bid
      Topical soln: 2% (20 mg/pump actuation; 112 g)
    Solaraze Gel apply to affected areas bid
      Gel: 3% (30 mg (100 g)
    Voltaren 50 mg bid <u>or</u> qid <u>or</u> 75 mg bid <u>or</u> 25 mg qid with an additional 25 mg at HS if necessary
      Tab: 25, 50, 75 mg ent-coat
    Voltaren XR 100 mg once daily; rarely, 100 mg bid may be used
      Tab: 100 mg ext-rel
    Zorvolex 35 mg tid
      Gelcap: 18, 35 mg ext-rel

▷ *diclofenac sodium+misoprostol* (X)(++)
  Pediatric: <12 years: not recommended; ≥12 years: same as adult
    Arthrotec *Tab:* 50, 75 mg

▷ *diflunisal* (C/D)(G)(+++) initially 1 gm as a single dose followed by 500 mg q 8-12 hours <u>or</u> 500 mg as a single dose followed by 250 mg q 8-12 hours
  Pediatric: <12 years: not recommended; ≥12 years: same as adult
    Dolobid *Tab:* 500*mg

▷ *etodolac* (C/D)(G)(+)
  Pediatric: <12 years: not recommended; ≥12 years: same as adult
    Lodine initially 600 mg to 1 gm/day in 2-3 divided doses; usual max 1 gm/day in divided doses; may increase to 1.2 g/day when needed
      Tab: 400, 500 mg; *Cap:* 200, 300 mg
    Lodine XL 400 mg to 1 gm once daily; max 1.2 gm/day
      Tab: 400, 500, 600 mg ext-rel

▷ *fenoprofen* (B/D)(++) 300-600 mg tid-qid; max 3.2 g/day
  Pediatric: <12 years: not recommended; ≥12 years: same as adult
    Nalfon *Tab:* 200 mg

▷ *flurbiprofen* (B/D)(G)(++) 200-300 mg/day in 2-4 divided doses; max single dose 100 mg; reduce dosage for renal impairment
  Pediatric: <12 years: not recommended; ≥12 years: same as adult
    Ansaid *Tab:* 50, 100 mg

(continued)

▷ **ibuprofen+famotidine** (B/D)(++) 1 tab 3 times daily; swallow whole; use lowest effective dose for the shortest duration
Pediatric: <12 years: not recommended; ≥12 years: same as adult
  Duexis *Tab:* ibu 800 mg/*fam* 26.6 mg

▷ **indomethacin** (B/D)(G)(+++) 75-100 mg daily in 3-4 divided doses; max 200 mg/day
Pediatric: <14 years: not recommended; ≥14 years: same as adult
  Indocin *Cap:* 25, 50 mg; *Rectal supp:* 50 mg; *Oral susp:* 25 mg/5 ml; *Vial:* 1 mg pwdr for reconstitution and IV infusion
  Indocin SR *Cap:* 75 mg ext-rel
  Tivorbex *Cap:* 20, 40 mg

▷ **ketoprofen** (C/D)(G)(++) 75 mg tid or 50 mg qid; max 300 mg/day
Pediatric: <18 years: not recommended; ≥18 years: same as adult
  Orudis *Cap:* 50, 75 mg
  Oruvail *Cap:* 100, 150, 200 mg ext-rel

▷ **ketorolac tromethamine** (C/D)(G)(+++)
Pediatric: <17 years: not recommended; ≥17 years: same as adult
  Sprix *17-64 years:* 1 spray each nostril (total dose 31,5 mg) every 6-8 hours prn; max 4 doses/24 hours (total daily dose 126 mg); ≥65 *years, renal impairment or <50 kg:* 1 spray in one nostril (total dose 15.75 mg) every 6-8 hours prn; max 4 doses/24 hours (63 mg); discard used bottle after 24 hours
    Nasal spray: 15.75 mg/100 mcl nasal spray (8 sprays, 1.7 g)
  Toradol 60 mg as a single IM dose; max 30 mg as a single IV dose; may administer 30 mg IV and 30 mg IM as a single dose; oral dosing is indicated *only* as continuation therapy to IM or IV dosing; oral formulation should *never* be administered as an initial dose; initiate oral dosing at 20 mg followed by 10 mg q 4-6 hours prn; max oral dosing 40 mg/day; >65 years, initiate oral dosing at 10 mg followed by 10 mg q 4-6 hours prn; max 40 mg/day; the combined duration of IV/IM/PO dosing is not to exceed 5 days
    Tab: 10 mg; *Inj* 15, 30, 60 mg/ml

▷ **magnesium choline trisalicylate** (C/D)(G)(+)
Pediatric: <12 years: not recommended; ≥12 years: same as adult
  Trilisate *Tab:* 500*, 750*mg; 1*gm; *Oral susp:* 5 mg/5 ml (cherry cordial)

▷ **meclofenamate sodium** (B/D)(G)(++) 50-100 mg q 4-6 hours or 300-400 mg/day in 3-4 equal doses; max 400 mg/day
Pediatric: <14 years: not recommended; ≥14 years: same as adult
  Meclofen *Cap:* 50, 100 mg

▷ **mefenamic acid** (C)(G)(++) 500 mg once; then, 250 mg q 6 hours
Pediatric: <14 years: not recommended; ≥14 years: same as adult
  Ponstel *Cap:* 250 mg

▷ **meloxicam** (C/D)(G)(+) 7.5 mg once daily; max 15 mg/day; hemodialysis max 7.5 mg/day
Pediatric: <2 years: not recommended; ≥2 years: 0.125 mg/kg; max 7.5 mg once daily
  Mobic *Tab:* 7.5, 15 mg; *Oral susp:* 7.5 mg/5 ml (100 ml) (raspberry)

(continued)

▷ *nabumetone* (C/D)(G)(+) 1-2 gm/day in a single dose or 2 divided doses; max 2 gm/day; <50 kg, max 1 gm/day
Pediatric: <12 years: not recommended; ≥12 years: same as adult
   Tab: 500, 750 mg

▷ *naproxen* (B)(G)(++) 275-550 mg twice daily or 275 mg every 6-8 hours; max 1.375 gm first day; then, max 1.1 gm/day; acute gout: 825 mg once, then 275 mg every 8 hours
Pediatric: <2 years: not recommended; ≥2 years: 5 mg/kg bid; max 15 mg/kg/day has been used; use suspension
   Naprosyn *Tab:* 250, 375, 500 mg
   Naprosyn Suspension *Oral susp:* 125 mg/5 ml

▷ *naproxen+esomeprazole (as magnesium trihydrate)* (C/D)(++)(G) one 375/20 or one 500/20 tab twice daily; take at least 30 minutes before meals; take lowest effective dose
Pediatric: <18 years: not recommended; ≥18 years: same as adult
   Vimovo 375/20 *Tab:* nap 375 mg+eso 20 mg
   Vimovo 500/20 *Tab:* nap 500 mg+eso 20 mg

▷ *oxaprozin* (C/D)(++) 1.2 gm once daily; max 1.8 gm or 26 mg/kg daily, whichever is less, in divided doses; low body weight, milder disease, or on dialysis: initially 600 mg once daily; max 1.2 gm daily
Pediatric: <6 years: not recommended; 6-16 years, 21-31 kg: 600 mg once daily; 32-54 kg: 900 mg once daily; ≥55 kg: 1.2 gm once daily
   Daypro *Tab:* 600*

▷ *piroxicam* (C/D)(G)(+++) 20 mg once daily
Pediatric: <12 years: not recommended; ≥12 years: same as adult
   Feldene *Cap:* 10, 20 mg
Comment: Because of the long half-life, steady state blood levels of *piroxicam* are not reached for 7-12 days. Therefore, expect a progressive response over several weeks.

▷ *salsalate* (C/D)(G)(+) 1.5 gm bid or 1 gm tid
Pediatric: <12 years: not recommended; ≥12 years: same as adult: 500*, 750*mg
   Cap: 500 mg

▷ *sulindac* (B/D)(G)(+++) 150-200 mg bid; max 400 mg/day; usually x 7-14 days
Pediatric: <14 years: not recommended; ≥14 years: same as adult
   Clinoril *Tab:* 150*, 200*mg

▷ *tolmetin* (C/D)(G)(+++) initially 400 mg tid; usual range 600 mg to 1.8 gm/day in divided doses; max 1,800 mg/day
Pediatric: <2 years: not recommended; ≥2 years: 20 mg/kg divided tid to qid; usual range 15-30 mg/kg/day divided tid to qid: max 30 mg/kg/day
   Tab: 200*mg

▷ *piroxicam* (C/D)(G)(+++) 20 mg once daily
Pediatric: not recommended
   Feldene *Cap:* 10, 20 mg

APPENDIX K. TOPICAL CORTICOSTEROIDS BY POTENCY

Comment: All topical, oral, and parenteral corticosteroids are pregnancy category C. Use with caution in infants and children. Steroids should be applied sparingly and for the shortest time necessary. Do not use in the diaper area. Do not use an occlusive dressing. Systemic absorption of topical corticosteroids can induce reversible hypothalamic-pituitary-adrenal (HPA) axis suppression with the potential for clinical glucocorticoid insufficiency.

Potency guide: Face: Low potency
Ears/Scalp margin: Intermediate potency
Eyelids: Hydrocortisone in ophthalmic ointment base 1%
Chest/Back: Intermediate potency
Skin folds: Low potency

Generic Name and Pregnancy Category	Brands, Formulation, and Dosing Frequency	Strength and Volume
Low Potency		
alclometasone dipropionate (C)	**Aclovate** Crm bid-tid	0.05% (15,45, 60 gm)
	Aclovate Oint bid-tid	0.05% (15,45, 60 gm)
fluocinolone acetonide (C)	**Synalar** Crm bid-qid	0.025% (15, 60 gm)
hydrocortisone base <u>or</u> *acetate* (C)(G)	**Anusol-HC** Crm bid-qid	2.5% (30 gm)
	Hytone Crm bid-qid	1% (1, 2 oz)
	Hytone Oint bid-qid	1% (1 oz)
	Hytone Lotn bid-qid	1% (2 oz)
	Hytone Crm bid-qid	2.5% (1, 2 oz)
	Hytone Oint bid-qid	2.5% (1 oz)
	Hytone Lotn bid-qid	2.5% (1 oz)
	U-cort Crm bid-qid	1% (7, 28, 35 gm)
triamcinolone acetonide (C)(G)	**Kenalog** Crm bid-qid	0.025% (15, 80 gm)
	Kenalog Lotn bid-qid	0.025% (60 ml)
	Kenalog Oint bid-qid	0.025% (15, 60, 80 gm)
Intermediate Potency		
betamethasone valerate (C)(G)	**Luxiq** Foam bid	0.12% (100 gm)
clocortolone pivalate (C)	**Cloderm** Crm bid	0.1% (30, 45, 75, 90 gm)
desonide (C)(G)	**Desonate** Gel/Formulation bid-tid	0.05% (15, 60 gm)
	DesOwen Crm bid-tid	0.05% (15, 60 gm)
	DesOwen Lotn bid-tid	0.05% (2, 4 fl oz)
	DesOwen Oint bid-tid	0.05% (15, 60 gm)
	Tridesilon Crm bid-qid	0.05% (15, 60 gm)
	Tridesilon Oint bid-qid	0.05% (15, 60 gm)
	Verdeso Foam	

(continued)

(*continued*)

Generic Name and Pregnancy Category	Brands, Formulation, and Dosing Frequency	Strength and Volume
desoximetasone (C)(G)	**Topicort-LP** Emol Crm bid	0.05% (15, 60 gm; 4 oz)
fluocinolone acetonide (C)(G)	**Capex** Shampoo **Derma-Smoothe/FS** Oil tid **Derma-Smoothe/FS** Shampoo **Synalar** Crm bid-qid **Synalar** Oint bid-qid	0.01% (4 oz) 0.01% (4 oz) 0.01% (4 oz) 0.025% (15, 30, 60 gm) 0.025% (15, 60 gm)
flurandrenolide (C)(G)	**Cordran-SP** Crm bid to tid **Cordran** Oint bid-tid **Cordran-SP** Crm bid-tid **Cordran** Lotn bid-tid **Cordran** Oint bid-tid	0.025% (30, 60 gm) 0.025% (30, 60 gm) 0.05% (15, 30, 60 gm) 0.05% (15, 60 ml) 0.05% (15, 30, 60 gm)
fluticasone propionate (C)(G)	**Cutivate** Oint bid **Cutivate** Crm qd-bid **Cutivate** Lotn qd-bid	0.005% (15, 30, 60 gm) 0.05% (15, 30, 60 gm) 0.05%
hydrocortisone probutate (C)	**Pandel** Crm qd-bid	0.1% (15, 45 gm)
hydrocortisone butyrate (C)(G)	**Locoid** Crm bid-tid **Locoid** Oint bid-tid **Locoid** Soln bid-tid	0.1% (15, 45 gm) 0.1% (15, 45 gm) 0.1% (30, 60 ml)
hydrocortisone valerate (C)(G)	**Westcort** Crm bid-tid **Westcort** Oint bid-tid	0.2% (15, 45, 60, 120 gm) 0.2% (15, 45, 60 gm)
mometasone furoate (C)	**Elocon** Crm qd **Elocon** Lotn qd **Elocon** Oint qd	0.1% (15, 45 gm) 0.1% (30, 60 ml) 0.1% (15, 45 gm)
prednicarbate	**Dermatop** Emol Crm bid **Dermatop** Oint bid	0.1% (15, 60 gm)
triamcinolone acetonide (C)(G)	**Kenalog** Crm bid-tid **Kenalog** Lotn bid-tid **Kenalog** Emul Spray bid-tid	0.1% (15, 60, 80 gm) 0.1% (60 ml) 0.2% (63, 100 gm)
High Potency		
amcinonide (C)(G)	Crm bid-tid Lotn bid Oint bid	0.1% (15, 30, 60 gm) 0.1% (20, 60 ml) 0.1% (15, 30, 60 gm)
Betamethasone dipropionate (C)	**Servivo Spray** Emul Spray bid	0.05% (60, 120 ml)

(*continued*)

(continued)

Generic Name and Pregnancy Category	Brands, Formulation, and Dosing Frequency	Strength and Volume
betamethasone dipropionate, augmented (C)	**Diprolene AF** Emol Crm qd-bid **Diprolene** Lotn qd-bid	0.05% (15, 50 gm) 0.05% (30, 60 ml)
desoximetasone (C)(G)	**Topicort** Gel bid **Topicort** Emol Crm bid **Topicort** Oint bid	0.05% (15, 60 gm) 0.25% (15, 60 gm) 0.25% (15, 60 gm)
diflorasone diacetate (C)	**Psorcon e** Emol Crm bid **Psorcon e** Emol Oint qd-tid	0.05% (15, 30, 60 gm) 0.05% (15, 30, 60 gm)
fluocinonide (C)	**Lidex** Crm bid-qid **Lidex** Gel bid-qid **Lidex** Oint bid-qid **Lidex** Soln bid-qid **Lidex-E** Emol Crm bid-qid	0.05% (15, 30, 60, 120 gm) 0.05% (15, 30, 60 gm) 0.05% (15, 30, 60, 120 gm) 0.05% (20, 60 ml) 0.05% (15, 30, 60 gm)
flurandrenolide (C)	**Cordan** Oint bid-tid **Cordan** Crm bid-tid	0.05% (15, 30, 60 gm) 0.025% (30, 60, 120 gm) 0.05% (15, 30, 60, 120 gm)
halcinonide (C)	**Halog** Crm bid-tid **Halog** Oint bid-tid **Halog** Soln bid-tid **Halog-E** Emol Crm qd-tid	0.1% (15, 30, 60, 240 gm) 0.1% (15, 30, 60, 120 gm) 0.1% (20, 60 ml) 0.1% (15, 30, 60 gm)
triamcinolone acetonide (C)(G)	**Kenalog** Crm bid-tid	0.5% (20 gm)
Super High Potency		
betamethasone dipropionate, augmented (C)(G)	**Diprolene** Oint qd-bid **Diprolene** Gel qd-bid	0.05% (15, 50 gm) 0.05% (15, 50 gm)
clobetasol propionate (C) (G)	**Clobex** Shampoo daily **Clobex** Spray bid **Cormax** Oint bid **Cormax** Scalp App **Olux** Foam **Olux E** Foam **Temovate** Crm bid **Temovate** Gel bid **Temovate** Oint bid **Temovate** Scalp App bid **Temovate-E** Emol Crm bid	0.05% (4 oz) 0.05% (2, 4.5 oz) 0.05% (15, 45 gm) 0.05% (15, 45 gm) 0.05% (50, 100 gm) 0.05% (50, 100 gm) 0.05% (15, 30, 45, 60 gm) 0.05% (15, 30, 60 gm) 0.05% (15, 30, 45, 60 gm) 0.05% (25, 50 ml) 0.05% (15, 30, 60 gm)

(continued)

(*continued*)

Generic Name and Pregnancy Category	Brands, Formulation, and Dosing Frequency	Strength and Volume
fluocinonide (C)(G)	**Vanos** Oint qd-tid	0.1% (30, 60, 120 gm)
flurandrenolide (C)	**Cordran** Tape q 12 hours	4 mcg/sq cm (roll of 3″x 80″)
halobetasol propionate (C)	**Ultravate** Crm qd-bid **Ultravate** Oint qd to bid	0.05% (15, 45 gm) 0.05% (15, 45 gm)

 APPENDIX L. ORAL CORTICOSTEROIDS

Comment: Systemic corticosteroids increase glucose intolerance, reduce the action of insulin and oral hypoglycemic agents, reduce adrenal cortex activity, decrease immunity, mask signs of infection, impair wound healing, suppress growth in children, and promote osteoporosis, fluid retention, and weight gain. Use systemic steroids with caution, using the lowest possible dose to affect clinical response, and withdraw (wean) gradually in tapering doses to avoid adrenal insufficiency. The American Academy of Rheumatology (AAR) recommends the following daily doses for anyone on a chronic systemic corticosteroid regimen: Calcium 1,200-1,500 mg/day and vitamin D 800-1,000 IU/day.

ORAL CORTICOSTEROIDS

▷ *betamethasone* (C)(G) initially 0.6-7.2 mg daily
    Pediatric: <12 years: not recommended; ≥12 years: same as adult
        Celestone *Tab:* 0.6 mg; *Syr:* 0.6 mg/5 ml (120 ml)

▷ *cortisone* (D)(G) initially 25-300 mg daily <u>or</u> every other day
    Pediatric: <12 years: not recommended; ≥12 years: same as adult
        Cortone Acetate *Tab:* 25 mg

▷ *dexamethasone* (C)(G) initially 0.75-9 mg/day
    Pediatric: <12 years: not recommended; ≥12 years: same as adult
        Decadron *Tab:* 0.5*, 0.75*, 4*mg; *Syr:* 0.5 mg/5 ml (100 ml)
        Decadron 5-12 Pak *Tabs:* 0.75*mg (12/pck)

▷ *hydrocortisone* (C)(G) 20-240 mg daily
    Pediatric: <12 years: 2-8 mg/day; ≥12 years: same as adult
        Cortef *Tab:* 5, 10, 20 mg; *Oral susp:* 10 mg/5 ml
        Hydrocortone *Tab:* 10 mg

▷ *methylprednisolone* (C)(G) 4-48 mg/day
    Pediatric: <12 years: not recommended; ≥12 years: same as adult
        Medrol *Tab:* 2*, 4*, 8*, 16*, 24*, 32*mg
        Medrol Dosepak *Dosepak:* 4*mg tabs (21/pck)

▷ *prednisolone* (C)(G) initially 5-60 mg/day in 1-2 doses x 3-5 days
    Pediatric: 0.14-2 mg/kg/day in 3-4 doses x 3-5 days
        Flo-Pred *Susp:* 5, 15 mg/5 ml
        Orapred *Soln:* 15 mg/5 ml (grape) (dye-free, alcohol 2%)

(*continued*)

(*continued*)

> Orapred ODT *Tab:* 10, 15, 30 mg orally disintegrating (grape)
> Pediapred *Soln:* 5 mg/5 ml (raspberry) (sugar-, alcohol-, dye-free)
> Prelone *Syr:* 15 mg/5 ml
> Comment: Flo-Pred does not require refrigeration <u>or</u> shaking prior to use.

▷ *prednisone* (C)(G) initially 5-60 mg/day in 1-2 doses x 3-5 days
  Pediatric: 0.14-2 mg/kg/day in 3-4 doses x 3-5 days
    Deltasone *Tab:* 2.5*, 5*, 10*, 20*, 50*mg

▷ *prednisone (delayed release)* (C)(G) initially 5-60 mg/day in 1-2 doses x 3-5 days
  Pediatric: 0.14-**2 mg**/kg/day in 3-4 doses x 3-5 days
    Rayos *Tab:* 1, 2, 5 mg del-rel

▷ *triamcinolone* (C)(G) initially 4-48 mg/day in 1-2 doses x 3-5 days
  Pediatric: 0.14-2 mg/kg/day in 3-4 doses x 3-5 days
    Aristocort *Tab:* 4*mg
    Aristocort Forte *Susp:* 40 mg/ml (benzoyl alcohol)
    Aristocort Aristopak *Tab:* 4*mg (16/pck)

APPENDIX M. PARENTERAL CORTICOSTEROIDS

Comment: Systemic glucocorticosteroids increase glucose intolerance, reduce the action of insulin and oral hypoglycemic agents, reduce adrenal cortex activity, decrease immunity, mask signs of infection, impair wound healing, suppress growth in children, and promote osteoporosis, fluid retention, and weight gain. Use systemic steroids with caution, using the lowest possible dose to affect clinical response, and withdraw (wean) gradually in tapering doses to avoid adrenal insufficiency. The American Academy of Rheumatology (AAR) recommends the following daily doses for anyone on a chronic systemic corticosteroid regimen: Calcium 1,200-1,500 mg/day and vitamin D 800-1,000 IU/day.

▷ *betamethasone* (C)(G)
    Celestone 0.5-9 mg IM/IV x 1 dose
      Vial: 3 mg/ml (10 ml)
    Celestone Soluspan 0.5-9 mg IM/IV x 1 dose; usual IM dose 6 mg
      Vial: 6 mg/ml (10 ml)

▷ *cortisone* (D)(G) 20-300 mg IM
  Pediatric: <12 years: not recommended; ≥12 years: same as adult
    Cortone Acetate *Vial:* 50 mg/ml (10 ml)

▷ *dexamethasone* (C)(G) initially 0.5-9 mg IM/IV daily
  Pediatric: <12 years: not recommended; ≥12 years: same as adult
    Decadron *Vial:* 4, 24 mg/ml for IM use (5 ml, sulfites)
    Dalalone D.P. *Vial:* 16 mg/ml (1, 5 ml)
    Decadron-LA *Vial:* 8 mg/ml (1, 5 ml)

▷ *hydrocortisone* (C)(G) initially 100-500 mg IM/IV daily
  Pediatric: 2-8 mg/kg loading dose (max 250 mg); then 8 mg/kg/day
    Hydrocortone *Vial:* 50 mg/ml (5 ml)
    Solu-Cortef *Vial:* 100 mg (2 ml); 250 mg (2 ml); 500 mg (4 ml); 1 gm (8 ml)

(*continued*)

(*continued*)

▷ *hydrocortisone phosphate* (C)(G) for IM, IV, and SC injection
  Pediatric: <12 years: not recommended; ≥12 years: same as adult
    Hydrocortone *Vial:* 50 mg/ml (2 ml)

▷ *methylprednisolone* (C)(G) 40-120 mg IM/week for 1-4 weeks
  Pediatric: <12 years: not recommended; ≥12 years: same as adult
    Depo-Medrol *Vial:* 20 mg/ml (5 ml); 40 mg/ml (5, 10 ml); 80 mg/ml (5 ml)

▷ *methylprednisolone sodium succinate* (C)(G) 10-40 mg IV initially; then, IM <u>or</u> IV
  Pediatric: 1-2 mg/kg loading dose; then 1.6 mg/kg/day in divided doses at least 6 hours apart
    Solu-Medrol *Vial:* 40 mg (1 ml), 125 mg (2 ml), 500 mg (4 ml); 1 g (8 ml); 2 g (8 ml)

▷ *triamcinolone* (C)(G) 40 mg IM/week
  Pediatric: <12 years: not recommended; ≥12 years: same as adult
    Aristocort *Vial:* 25 mg/ml (5 ml)
    Aristocort Forte *Vial:* 40 mg/ml (1, 5 ml) (*do* not *administer IV*)
    Aristospan *Vial:* 5 mg/ml (5 ml); 20 mg/ml (1, 5 ml)
    TAC-3 *Vial:* 3 mg/ml (5 ml) for intralesional and intradermal use

Injectable Corticosteroid/Anesthetic

▷ *dexamethasone/lidocaine* (C) 0.1-0.75 ml into painful area
    Decadron Phosphate with Xylocaine *Vial: dexa* 4 mg/*lido* 10 mg per ml (5 ml)

⬤ APPENDIX N. INHALATIONAL CORTICOSTEROIDS

Comment: Inhaled corticosteroids are indicated for the long-term control of asthma. Inhaled corticosteroids are not indicated for exercise induced asthma <u>or</u> for relief of acute symptoms (i.e., "rescue"). Low doses are indicated for mild persistent asthma, medium doses are indicated for moderate persistent asthma, and high doses are reserved for severe cases. Titrate to lowest effective dose. To reduce the potential for adverse effects with inhalers, the patient should use a spacer <u>or</u> holding chamber and rinse the mouth and spit after every inhalation treatment. Linear growth should be monitored in children. When inhaled doses exceed 1,000 mcg/day, consider supplements of calcium (1-1.5 gm/day), vitamin D (400 IU/day).

▷ *beclomethasone* (C)
    Beclovent 2 inhalations tid-qid <u>or</u> 4 inhalations bid; max 20 inhalations/day
    Pediatric: <6 years: not recommended; 6-12 years: 1-2 inhalations tid-qid <u>or</u> 4 inhalations bid; max 10 inhalations/day
      Inhaler: 42 mcg/actuation (6.7 g, 80 inh); 16.8 g (200 inh)
    Qvar *Previously using only bronchodilators:* initiate 40-80 mcg bid; max 320 mcg/day; *Previously using an inhaled corticosteroid:* initiate 40-160 mcg bid; max 320 mcg/day; Previously taking a systemic corticosteroid: attempt to wean off the systemic drug after approximately 1 week after initiating Qvar
    Pediatric: <12 years: not recommended; ≥12 years: same as adult
      Inhaler: 40, 80 mcg/actuation metered-dose aerosol w. dose counter (8.7 g, 120 inh) (CFC-free)

(*continued*)

Vanceril 2 inhalations tid to qid <u>or</u> 4 inhalations bid
Pediatric: <6 years: not recommended; 6-12 years: 1-2 inhalations tid to qid
  Inhaler: 42 mcg/actuation (16.8 g, 200 inh)
Vanceril Double Strength 2 inhalations bid
Pediatric: <6 years: not recommended; 6-12 years: 1-2 inhalations bid; >12 years: same as adult
  Inhaler: 84 mcg/actuation (12.2 g, 120 inh)

▷ *budesonide* (B)(G)
Pulmicort Respules use turbuhaler
Pediatric: <12 months: not recommended; ≥12 months to 8 years: *Previously using only bronchodilators:* initiate 0.5 mg/day once daily <u>or</u> in 2 divided doses; may start at 0.25 mg/day; *Previously using inhaled orticosteroids:* initiate 0.5 mg/day daily <u>or</u> in 2 divided doses; max 1 mg/day; *Previously using oral ortico-steroids:* initiate 1 mg/day daily <u>or</u> in 2 divided doses
  Inhal susp: 0.25 mg/2 ml (30/box)
Pulmicort Turbuhaler 1-2 inhalations bid; *Previously on oral corticosteroids:* 2-4 inhalations bid
Pediatric: <6 years: not recommended; 6-12 years: 1-2 inhalations bid; >12 years: same as adult
  Turbuhaler: 200 mcg/actuation (200 inh)

▷ *flunisolide* (C)(G)
AeroBid, AeroBid M initially 2 inhalations bid; max 8 inhalations/day
Pediatric: <6 years: not recommended; 6-15 years: 2 inhalations bid; ≥16 years: same as adult
  Inhaler: 250 mcg/actuation (7 gm, 100 inh)

▷ *fluticasone* (C)(G)
Flovent HFA initially 88 mcg bid; if previously using an inhaled corticosteroid, initially 88-220 mcg bid; if previously taking an oral corticosteroid, initially 880 mcg/day
Pediatric: use **Rotadisk**: initially 50-88 mcg inh bid; <4 years: not recommend-ed; 4-11 years: initially 50-88 mcg bid; >11 years: initially 100 mcg bid; if pre-viously using an inhaled corticosteroid, initially 100-200 mcg bid; *Previously taking an oral corticosteroid;* initially 1000 mcg bid
  Inhaler: 44 mcg/actuation (7.9 g, 60 inh; 13 g, 120 inh); 110 mcg/actuation (13 g, 120 inh); 220 mcg/actuation (13 g, 120 inh)
Rotadisk 50 mcg/actuation (60 blisters/disk); 100 mcg/actuation (60 blisters/disk); 250 mcg/actuation (60 blisters/disk)
Pediatric: <12 years: not recommended; ≥12 years: same as adult

▷ *mometasone furoate* (C) *Previously using a bronchodilator* <u>or</u> *inhaled corticosteroid:* 220 mcg q PM <u>or</u> bid; max 440 mcg q PM <u>or</u> 220 mcg bid; *Previously using an oral corticosteroid:* 440 mcg bid; max 880 mcg/day
Pediatric: <12 years: not recommended; ≥12 years: same as adult
Asmanex Twisthaler *Inhaler:* 220 mcg/actuation (6.7 gm, 80 inh); 16.8 gm (200 inh)

APPENDIX O. ANTIARRHYTHMIA DRUGS

Antiarrhythmics by Classification With Dose Forms		
Brand/Generic and Pregnancy Category	**Class and Indication(s)**	**Dose Form(s)**
Betapace *sotalol* (B)	*Class:* Class II and III Antiarrhythmic *Indications:* Documented life-threatening ventricular arrhythmias	*Tab:* 80*, 120*, 160*, 240*mg
Betapace AF *sotalol* (B)	*Class:* Class II and III Antiarrhythmic *Indications:* Maintenance of normal sinus rhythm in patients with highly symptomatic atrial fibrillation or atrial flutter who are currently in sinus rhythm	*Tab:* 80*, 120*, 160*mg
Calan *verapamil* (C)(G)	*Class:* Calcium Channel Blocker *Indications:* Control (with *digitalis*) of ventricular rate in patients with chronic atrial fibrillation or atrial flutter; prophylaxis of repetitive paroxysmal supraventricular tachycardia	*Tab:* 40, 80*, 120*mg
Cordarone *amiodarone* (D)(G)	*Class:* Class III Antiarrhythmic *Indications:* Documented life threatening recurrent refractory ventricular fibrillation or hemodynamically unstable ventricular tachycardia	*Tab:* 200*mg
Quinidex *quinidine sulfate* (C) (G)	*Class:* Class I Antiarrhythmic *Indications:* Atrial and ventricular arrhythmias	*Tab:* 300 mg ext-rel
Inderal *propranolol* (C)(G) **Inderal XL** *propranolol* ext-rel (C)(G) **InnoPran XL** *Propranolol ext-rel* (C)	*Class:* Beta-Blocker *Indications:* Atrial and ventricular arrhythmias; tachyarrhythmias due to *digitalis* intoxication; reduce mortality and risk of reinfarction in stabilized patients after myocardial infarction	*Tab:* 10*, 20*, 40*, 60*, 80* mg; *Cap:* 60, 80, 120, 160 mg sust-rel *Cap:* 80, 120 mg ext-rel
Mexitil *mexiletine* (C)	*Class:* Class IB Antiarrhythmic *Indications:* Documented life-threatening ventricular arrhythmias	*Cap:* 150, 200, 250 mg

(continued)

(*continued*)

Antiarrhythmics by Classification With Dose Forms		
Brand/Generic and Pregnancy Category	Class and Indication(s)	Dose Form(s)
Multaq *dronedarone* (C)	*Class:* IB Antiarrhythmic *Indications:* Paroxysmal or persistent atrial fibrillation or atrial flutter	*Tab:* 400 mg
Norpace *disopyramide* (C)	*Class:* Class I Antiarrhythmic *Indications:* Documented life threatening ventricular arrhythmias	*Cap:* 100, 150 mg
Procanbid *procainamide* (C)(G)	*Class:* Class IA Antiarrhythmic *Indications:* Life threatening ventricular arrhythmias	*Tab:* 500, 1000 mg ext-rel
Quinaglute *quinidine gluconate* (C)(G)	*Class:* Class I Antiarrhythmic *Indications:* Atrial and ventricular arrhythmias	*Tab:* 324 mg ext-rel
Rythmol *propafenone* (C)(G)	*Class:* Class IC Antiarrhythmic *Indications:* Documented lifethreatening ventricular arrhythmias; prolonged recurrence of paroxysmal atrial fibrillation and/or atrial flutter or paroxysmal supraventricular tachycardia associated with disabling symptoms in patients without structural heart disease	*Tab:* 150*, 225*, 300*mg *Cap:* 225, 325, 425 mg ext-rel
Sectral *acebutolol* (B)(G)	*Class:* Beta-Blocker *Indications:* Ventricular arrhythmias	*Cap:* 200, 400 mg
Sotylize *sotalol* (B)	*Class:* Class II and III Antiarrhythmic *Indications:* Documented life threatening ventricular arrhythmias, and highly symptomatic A-flutter/A-fib	*Oral soln:* 5 mg/ml
Tambocor *flecainide acetate* (C) (G)	*Class:* Class IC Antiarrhythmic *Indications:* Documented life threatening ventricular arrhythmias; paroxysmal atrial fibrillation and/or atrial flutter or paroxysmal supraventricular tachycardia in patients without structural heart disease	*Tab:* 50, 100*, 150* mg

(*continued*)

(continued)

Antiarrhythmics by Classification With Dose Forms		
Brand/Generic and Pregnancy Category	**Class and Indication(s)**	**Dose Form(s)**
Tenormin *atenolol* (C)(G)	*Class:* Beta-Blocker *Indications:* Reduce mortality and in stabilized patients after myocardial infarction	*Tab:* 25, 50, 100 mg *Inj:* 5 mg/ml (10 ml) for IV administration
timolol maleate (C) (G)	*Class:* Beta-Blocker *Indications:* Reduce mortality and in stabilized patients after myocardial infarction	*Tab:* 5, 10*, 20*mg
dofetilide (C)(G)	*Class:* Class III Antiarrhythmic *Indications:* Maintenance of normal sinus rhythm in patients with atrial fibrillation <u>or</u> atrial flutter of >1 week duration who were converted to normal sinus rhythm (only for highly symptomatic patients); conversion to normal sinus rhythm	*Cap:* 125, 250, 500 mcg
Tonocard *tocainide* (C)(G)	*Class:* Class I Antiarrhythmic *Indications:* Documented life-threatening ventricular arrhythmias	*Tab:* 400*, 600*mg
Toprol XL *metoprolol* (C)(G)	*Class:* Beta-Blocker *Indications:* Ischemic, hypertensive, <u>or</u> cardiomyopathic heart failure	*Tab:* 25*, 50*, 100*, 200*mg

APPENDIX P. ANTINEOPLASIA DRUGS

Comment: A new lab test offers potential for early detection of multiple cancer types with a single blood sample. Researchers studied 1,005 persons with non-metastatic, clinically-detected, stage 2 and 3 cancers of the ovary, liver, stomach, pancreas, esophagus, colorectum, lung, or breast. The blood test, CancerSEEK, accurately identified <u>cancer</u> cases 33-98% (M=70%) of the time in the study cohort, with accuracy reportedly 69-98% for the five <u>cancers</u> that currently have no widely used screening test: ovarian, pancreatic, stomach, <u>liver</u> and esophageal cancers. CancerSEEK combines tests that look for 16 genes and 10 proteins (mutations in cell-free DNA), linked to cancer. The researchers also tested blood samples from 812 healthy people, to see how often the test gave false-positive results, and were reported to be less than 1%. These findings represent a promising future for screening and early detection of cancer in asymptomatic persons. Optimally, cancers would be detected early enough that they could be cured by surgery alone, but even cancers that are not curable by surgery alone will respond better to systemic therapies when there is less advanced disease.

Anne Marie Lennon, MD, PhD, Johns Hopkins Kimmel Cancer Center, Baltimore and Len Lichtenfeld, MD, Deputy Chief Medical Officer, American Cancer Society, Atlanta. Online and print announcements, January 2018: PR Newswire, Science, U.S. News & World Report, Los Angeles Times, Forbes, The Guardian, Chicago Tribune

REFERENCE

Cohen, J. D., Li, L., Wang, Y., Thoburn, C., Afsari, B., Danilova, L., . . . Papadopoulos, N. (2018). Detection and localization of surgically resectable cancers with a multi-analyte blood test. *Science, 359*(6378), 926–930. doi:10.1126/science.aar3247

Antineoplastics with Classification and Dose Forms		
Brand, Generic and Pregnancy Category	**Class and Indications**	**Dose Form(s)**
Alecensa *alectinib*	Kinase Inhibitor	*Cap:* 150 mg
Aliqopa *copanlisib*	Kinase Inhibitor	*Vial:* 60 mg pwdr for injection, single dose
Alkeran *melphalan* (D)(G)	Alkylating Agent	*Tab:* 2*mg
Alunbrig *brigatinib*	Kinase Inhibitor	*Tab:* 30, 90 mg
Arimidex *anastrozole* (D)	Aromatase Inhibitor	*Tab:* 1 mg
Aromasin *exemestane* (D)	Aromatase Inactivator	*Tab:* 25 mg
Arranon *nelarabine* (D)	Nucleoside Analog	*Vial:* 250 mg for IV infusion
Bavencio *avelumab* (D)	Programmed Death Ligand-1 (PD-L1) Blocking Antibody	*Vial:* 200 mg/10 ml (20 mg/ml), single-dose
Bevyxxa *betrixiban*	Factor Xa (FXa) Inhibitor	*Cap:* 40, 80 mg
Blincyto *blinatumomab*	**Bispecific CD19-directed CD3 T-cell Engager**	*Vial:* 35 mcg pwdr for reconstitution, single-dose
bortizomib	Kinase Inhibitor	*Vial:* 3.5 mg pwdr for reconstitution, single-dose
Calquence *acalabrutinib*	Kinase Inhibitor	*Cap:* 100 mg

(continued)

(continued)

Antineoplastics with Classification and Dose Forms		
Brand, Generic and Pregnancy Category	**Class and Indications**	**Dose Form(s)**
Casodex *bicalutamide*	Antiandrogen	*Tab:* 50 mg
Clolar *clofarabine* (X)	Purine Nucleoside Metabolic Inhibitor	*Vial:* 20 mg/20 ml single-dose
Cytoxan *Cyclophosphamide* (D)	Alkylating Agent	*Tab:* 25, 50 mg
Daralex *daratumumab*	Human CD38-directed Monoclonal Antibody	*Vial:* 100 mg/5 ml, 400 mg/20 ml, single-dose
Eligard *leuprolide acetate* (X)	GnRH Analog	*Inj:* 7.5 mg ext-rel per monthly SC injection
Taxotere *docetaxel* (G)		*Vial:* 20 mg/2 ml (10 mg/ml) single-dose, 80 mg/8 ml (10 mg/ml), 160 mg/16 ml (10 mg/ml) multi-dose
Endari *l-glutamine*	Amino Acid	*Oral Pwdr:* 5 grams of L-glutamine pwdr per paper-foil-plastic laminate pkt
Eulexin *flutamide* (D)	Antiandrogen	*Cap:* 125 mg
Faslodex *fulvestrant* (D)(G)	Estrogen Receptor Antagonist	*Prefilled syringe for IM inj:* 50 mg/ml (2.5, 5 ml/syringe)
Femara *letrozole* (D)	Aromatase Inhibitor	*Tab:* 2.5 mg
Gleevec *imatinib mesylate* (D)	Signal Transduction Inhibitor	*Cap:* 100 mg
Hydrea *hydroxyurea* (D)(G)	Substituted Urea	*Cap:* 500 mg
Ibrance *palbociclib*	Kinase Inhibitor	*Cap:* 75, 100, 150 mg
Imbruvica *imbrutinib*	Kinase Inhibitor	*Tab:* 140 mg

(continued)

(continued)

Antineoplastics with Classification and Dose Forms		
Brand, Generic and Pregnancy Category	**Class and Indications**	**Dose Form(s)**
Imfinzi *durvalumab*	Programmed Death Ligand-1 (PD-L1) Blocking Antibody	*Vial:* 120 mg/2.4 ml (50 mg/ml, single-dose; 500 mg/10 ml (50 mg/ml, single-dose)
Inhifa *enasidenib*	Isocitrate Dehydrogenase-2 Inhibitor	*Tab:* 50, 100 mg
Iressa *gefitinib* (D)	Epidermal Growth Factor Receptor Tyrosine Kinase Inhibitor	*Tab:* 250 mg
Keytruda *pembrolizumab*	Programmed Death Receptor-1 (PD-1)-Blocking Antibody	*Vial:* 50 mg, single-dose for reconstitution; 100 mg/4 ml (25 mg/ml) single dose
Kisquali Femara Co-Pack *ribociclib+letrozole*	Cyclin-dependent Kinase Inhibitor+Aromatase Inhibitor	*Tab:* 600/2.5, 400/2.5, 200/2.5 mg
Kymriah *tisagenlecleucel*	CD19-directed Genetically Modified Autologous T cell Immunotherapy	*IV bag:* frozen suspension for IV infusion after thawing
Kyprolis, *carfilzomib*	Protease Inhibitor	*Vial:* 30, 60 mg, single-dose, pwdr for reconstitution
Lartruvo *olaratumab*	Platelet-derived Growth Factor Receptor Alpha (PDGFR-α) Blocking Antibody	*Vial:* 500 mg/50 ml (10 mg/ml, single-dose)
Lemvina *lenvatinib*	Kinase Inhibitor	*Cap:* 4, 10 mg
Leukeran *chlorambucil* (D)(G)	Alkylating Agent	*Tab:* 2 mg
Leupron *leuprolide* (X)	GnRH Analog	*Susp for IM inj:* 1 mg (daily); 7.5 mg depot (monthly); 22.5 mg depot (every 3 months); 30 mg depot (every 4 months)
Lynparza *olaparib*	Poly (ADP-ribose) Polymerase (PARP)-Inhibitor	*Tab:* 100, 150 mg

(continued)

(continued)

Antineoplastics with Classification and Dose Forms		
Brand, Generic and Pregnancy Category	Class and Indications	Dose Form(s)
Megace, Megace Oral Suspension, Megace ES, *megestrol acetate* (D) (G)	Progestin	*Tab:* 20*, 40*mg; *Susp:* 40 mg/ml; ES concentrate: 125 mg/ml, 625 mg/5 ml
Mekinist *trametinib*	Kinase Inhibitor	*Tab:* 0.5, 2 mg
Nerlynx *neratinib*	Kinase Inhibitor	*Tab:* 40 mg
Nexavar *sorafenib* (D)	Multikinase Inhibitor	*Tab:* 200 mg
Nilandron *nilutamide*	Nonsteroidal Orally Active Antiandrogen	*Tab:* 150 mg
Nolvadex *tamoxifen citrate* (D) (G)	Antiestrogen	*Tab:* 10, 20 mg
Opdivo *nivolumab*	Programmed Death Receptor-1 (PD-1)-Blocking Antibody	*Vial:* 40 mg/4 ml, 100 mg/10 ml (10 mg/ml, single dose)
Revlimid *lenalidomide*	Thalidomide Analogue	*Cap:* 2.5, 5, 10, 15, 20, 25 mg
Responsa *inotuzumab ozogamicin*	CD22-directed Antibody-Drug Conjugade (ADC)	*Vial:* 0.9 mg, single-dose, for reconstitution
Rituxan Hyclea *rituximab+ hyaluronidase*	Combination of **rituximab**, a CD20-directed Cytolytic Antibody and **hyaluronidase human**, an endoglycosidase	*Vial:* 1,400 mg **rituximab** and 23,400 Units **hyaluronidase human** per 11.7 ml (120 mg/2,000 Units per ml) single-dose; 1,600 mg **rituximab** and 26,800 Units **hyaluronidase human** per 13.4 ml (120 mg/2,000 Units per ml) single-dose
Rubraca *rucaparib*	Poly ADP-ribose Polymerase (PARP)-Inhibitor	*Tab:* 200, 300 mg

(continued)

(*continued*)

Antineoplastics with Classification and Dose Forms		
Brand, Generic and Pregnancy Category	Class and Indications	Dose Form(s)
Rydapt *midostaurin*	Kinase Inhibitor	*Tab:* 40 mg
Stivarga *regorafenib*	Kinase Inhibitor	*Tab:* 40 mg
Sutent *sunitinib malate*	Kinase Inhibitor	*Cap:* 12.5, 25, 37.5, 50 mg
Tagrisso *osimertinib*	Kinase Inhibitor	*Tab:* 40, 80 mg
Tarceva *erlotinib* (D)	Kinase Inhibitor	*Tab:* 25, 100, 150 mg
Tasigna *nilotinib*	Kinase Inhibitor	*Cap:* 150, 200 mg
Tecentriq *atezolizumab*	Programmed Death Ligand-1 (PD-L1) Blocking Antibody	*Vial:* 1,200 mg/20 ml (60 mg/ml, single-dose)
Treanda *bendamustine*	Alkylating Agent	*Vial:* 45 mg/0.5 ml, 180 mg/2 ml solution, single-dose; 25, 100 mg pwdr for reconstitution, single-dose
Vectibix *panitumumab*	Epidermal Growth Factor Receptor (EGFR) Antagonist	*Vial:* 100 mg/5 ml, 200 mg/10 ml, 400 mg/20 ml (20 mg/ml, single-use)
Velcade *bortezomib* (D)	Proteasome Inhibitor	*Vial:* 3.5 mg (pwdr for IV infusion after reconstitution)
Venclexta *venetoclax*	BCL-2 Inhibitor	*Tab:* 10, 50, 100 mg
Viadur (X) *leuprolide acetate*	GnRH Analog	*SC implant:* 65 mg depot (replace every 12 months)
Vyxeos *daunorubicin+ cytarabine*	***daunorubicin:*** Anthracycline Topoisomerase Inhibitor; ***cytarabine:*** Nucleoside Metabolic Inhibitor	*Vial:* daun 44 mg/cytar 100 mg (pwdr for IV injection after reconstitution)
Xeloda (D) *capecitabine*	***Fluoropyrimidine*** (prodrug of *5-fluorouracil*)	*Tab:* 150, 500 mg

(*continued*)

(*continued*)

Antineoplastics with Classification and Dose Forms		
Brand, Generic and Pregnancy Category	**Class and Indications**	**Dose Form(s)**
Yescarta *axicabtagene ciloleucel*	Chimeric Antigen Receptor T Cell (CAR T) Therapy	*Infusion bag:* (68 ml)
Zejula *niraparib*	Poly ADP-ribose Polymerase (PARP)-Inhibitor	*Cap:* 100 mg
Zoladex *goserelin acetate*	GnRH Analog	*SC implant:* 3.6 mg depot (28 days), 10.8 mg depot (3-month)
Zometa *zoledronic acid* (D)	Bisphosphonate	*Vial:* 4 mg pwdr for reconstitution for IV infusion, single-dose
Zykadia *ceritinib*	Kinase Inhibitor	*Cap:* 150 mg

 APPENDIX Q. ANTIPSYCHOSIS DRUGS

ANTIPSYCHOTICS WITH DOSE FORMS

Comment: Patients receiving an antipsychotic agent should be monitored closely for the following adverse side effects: neuroleptic malignant syndrome, extrapyramidal reactions, tardive dyskinesia, blood dyscrasias, anticholinergic effects, drowsiness, hypotension, photo-sensitivity, retinopathy, and lowered seizure threshold. Use lower doses for elderly or debilitated patients. Prescriptions should be written for the smallest practical amount. Foods and beverages containing alcohol are contraindicated for patients receiving any psychotropic drug. *Neuroleptic Malignant Syndrome* (NMS) and *Tardive Dyskinesia* (TD) are adverse side effects (ASEs) most often associated with the older antipsychotic drugs. Risk is decreased with the newer "atypical" antipsychotic drugs. However, these syndromes can develop, although much less commonly, after relatively brief treatment periods at low doses. Given these considerations, antipsychotic drugs should be prescribed in a manner that is most likely to minimize the occurrence. NMS, a potentially fatal symptom complex, is characterized by hyperpyrexia, muscle rigidity, altered mental status and evidence of autonomic instability (irregular pulse or blood pressure, tachycardia, diaphoresis, and cardiac dysrhythmia). Additional signs may include elevated creatine phosphor-kinase (CPK), myoglobinuria (rhabdomyolysis), and acute renal failure (ARF). TD is a syndrome consisting of potentially irreversible, involuntary, dyskinetic movements that can develop in patients with antipsychotic drugs. Characteristics include repetitive involuntary movements, usually of the jaw, lips and tongue, such as grimacing, sticking out the tongue and smacking the lips. Some affected people also experience involuntary movement of the extremities or difficulty breathing.

(*continued*)

The syndrome may remit, partially or completely, if antipsychotic treatment is withdrawn. If signs and symptoms of NMS and/or TD appear in a patient, management should include immediate discontinuation of antipsychotic drugs and other drugs not essential to concurrent therapy, intensive symptomatic treatment, medical monitoring, and treatment of any concomitant serious medical problems. The risk of developing NMS and/or TD, and the likelihood that either syndrome will become irreversible, is believed to increase as the duration of treatment and the total cumulative dose of antipsychotic drugs administered to the patient increase. The first and only FDA-approved treatment for TD is *valbenazine* (**Ingrezza**) (*see page* 456)

ANTIPSYCHOTICS WITH DOSE FORMS

▷ *aripiprazole* (C)(G)
> **Abilify** *Tab:* 2, 5, 10, 15, 20, 30 mg; *Oral soln:* 1 mg/ml (150 ml) (orange crèam; parabens)
> **Abilify Discmelt** *Tab:* 15 mg orally disintegrating (vanilla) (phenylalanine)
> **Abilify Maintena** *Vial:* 300, 400 mg ext-rel pwdr for IM injection after reconstitution; 300, 400 mg single-dose prefilled dual chamber syringes w. supplies
> **Aristada** *Prefilled syringe:* 441, 662, 882, 1064 mg, ext-rel susp for IM injection, single-dose w. safety needle

▷ *aripiprazole lauroxil* (C)
> **Aristada** Prefilled *syringe:* single-use, ext-rel injectable suspension: 441mg (1.6 ml), 662 mg (2.4 ml), 882 mg (3.2 ml), 1064 mg (3.9 ml)

▷ *asenapine* (C)
> **Saphris** *SL tab:* 2.5, 5, 10 mg

▷ *brexpizole* (C)
> **Rexulti** *Tab:* 0.25, 0.5, 1, 2, 3, 4 mg

▷ *bupropion* (C)
> **Forfivo XL** *Tab:* 450 mg ext-rel

▷ *cariprazine* (NE)
> **Vraylar** *Cap:* 1.5, 3, 4.5, 6 mg

▷ *chlorpromazine* (C)(G)
> **Thorazine** *Tab:* 10, 25, 50, 100, 200 mg; *Cap:* 30, 75, 150 mg sust-rel; *Syr:* 10 mg/5 ml (4 oz) (orange-custard); *Vial/Amp:* 25 mg/ml (1, 2 ml) (sulfites)

▷ *clozapine* (B)(G)
> **Clozapine ODT** (G) *ODT:* 150, 200 mg
> **Clozaril** (G) *Tab:* 25*, 100*mg; *ODT:* 150, 200 mg
> **FazaClo ODT** (G) *ODT:* 12.5, 25, 100, 150, 200 mg (phenylalanine)
> **Versacloz** *Oral susp:* 50 mg/ml (100 ml)

▷ *fluphenazine* (C)(G)
> **Prolixin** *Tab:* 1, 2.5, 5*, 10 mg (tartrazine); *Conc:* 5 mg/ml (4 oz w. calib dropper) (alcohol 14%); *Elix:* 5 mg/ml (2 oz w. calib dropper) (alcohol 14%); *Vial:* 25 mg/ml (10 ml)

▷ *fluphenazine decanoate* (C)(G)
> **Prolixin Decanoate** *Vial:* 25 mg/ml (5 ml) (benzyl alcohol)

(*continued*)

> ▷ *fluphenazine* (C)(G)
> **Prolixin Ethanate** *Vial:* 25 mg (5 ml) (benzyl alcohol)

> ▷ *fluphenazine decanoate* (C)(G)
> **Prolixin Decanoate** *Vial:* 25 mg/ml (5 ml) (benzyl alcohol)

> ▷ *haloperidol* (B)(G)
> **Haldol** *Tab:* 0.5*, 1*, 2*, 5*, 10*, 20*mg
> **Haldol Lactate** *Vial:* 5 mg for IM injection, single-dose
> **Haldol Decanoate** *Vial:* 50, 100 mg for IM injection, single-dose

> ▷ *iloperidone* (C)
> **Fanapt** *Tab:* 1, 2, 4, 6, 8, 10, 12 mg

> ▷ *loxapine* (C)
> **Adasuve** *Oral inhal pwdr:* 10 mg single-use disposable inhaler (5/box)

> ▷ *lurasidone* (B)
> **Latuda** *Tab:* 20, 40, 80 mg

> ▷ *olanzapine fumarate* (C)(G)
> **Zyprexa** *Tab:* 2.5, 5, 7.5, 10, 15, 20 mg
> **Zyprexa Zydis** *ODT:* 5, 10, 15, 20 mg (phenylalanine)

> ▷ *paliperidone palmitate* (C)(G)
> **Invega** *Tab:* 3, 6, 9 mg ext-rel
> **Invega Sustenna** *Prefilled syringe:* 39, 78, 117, 156, 234 mg ext-rel suspension w. needle
> **Invega Trinza** *Prefilled syringe:* 273, 410, 546, 819 mg ext-rel suspension

> ▷ *pimozide* (C)(G)
> **Orap** *Tab:* 1, 2 mg

> ▷ *prochlorperazine* (C)(G)
> **Compazine** *Tab:* 5, 10 mg; *Cap:* 10, 15 mg sus-rel; *Syr:* 5 mg/5 ml (4 oz) (fruit); *Supp:* 2.5, 5, 25 mg

> ▷ *quetiapine* (C)(G)
> **Seroquel** *Tab:* 25, 100, 200, 300 mg
> **Seroquel XR** *Tab:* 50, 150, 200, 300, 400 mg ext-rel

> ▷ *risperidone* (C)(G)
> **Risperdal** *Tab:* 0.25, 0.5, 1, 2, 3, 4 mg; *Soln:* 1 mg/ml (30 ml w. pipette); *Consta Inj:* 25, 37.5, 50 mg
> **Risperdal M-Tabs** *M-tab:* 0.5, 1, 2, 3, 4 mg orally-disint (phenylalanine)

> ▷ *thioridazine* (C)(G) *Tab:* 10, 25, 50, 100 mg

> ▷ *trifluoperazine* (C)(G)
> **Stelazine** *Tab:* 1, 2, 5, 10 mg; *Conc:* 10 mg/ml; (2 oz w. calib dropper (banana-vanilla) (sulfites); *Vial:* 2 mg/ml (10 ml)

> ▷ *ziprasidone* (C)(G)
> **Geodon** *Cap:* 20, 40, 60, 80 mg

APPENDIX R. ANTICONVULSANT DRUGS

ANTICONVULSANTS WITH DOSE FORMS

➤ *brivaracetam* (C)
    Briviact *Tab:* 10, 25, 50, 75, 100 mg; *Oral soln:* 10 mg/ml (300 ml); *Vial:* 50 mg/
      5 ml single-dose for IV inj

➤ *carbamazepine* (D)(G)
    Carbatrol *Cap:* 200, 300 mg ext-rel
    Carnexiv *Vial:* 200 mg/20 ml (10 mg/ml) single-dose for IV infusion
    Equetro *Cap:* 100, 200, 300 mg ext-rel
    Tegretol *Tab:* 100*, 200*mg; *Chew tab:* 100*mg
    Tegretol Suspension *Oral susp:* 100 mg/5 ml (450 ml) (citrus vanilla) (sorbitol)
    Tegretol-XR *Tab:* 100, 200, 400 mg ext-rel

➤ *clobazam* (C)(IV)
    Onfi *Tab:* 10*, 20*mg
    Onfi Oral Suspension *Oral susp:* 2.5 mg/ml (120 ml w. 2 dosing syringes) (berry)

➤ *clonazepam* (D)(IV)(G)
    Clonazepam ODT *ODT:* 0.125, 0.25, 0.5, 1, 2, oral-disint
    Klonopin *Tab:* 0.5*, 1, 2 mg

➤ *diazepam* (D)(IV)(G)
    Diastat *Rectal gel delivery system:* 2.5 mg
    Diastat AcuDial *Rectal gel delivery system:* 10, 20 mg
    Valium *Tab:* 2*, 5*, 10*mg
    Valium Injectable *Vial:* 5 mg/ml (10 ml); *Amp:* 5 mg/ml (2 ml); *Prefilled
    syringe:* 5 mg/ml (5 ml)
    Valium Intensol *Conc oral soln:* 5 mg/ml (30 ml w. dropper) (alcohol 19%)
    Valium Oral Solution *Oral soln:* 5 mg/5 ml (500 ml) (winter green-spice)

➤ *divalproex sodium* (D)(G)
    Depakene *Cap:* 250 mg; *Syr:* 250 mg/5 ml (16 oz)
    Depakote *Tab:* 125, 250, 500 mg
    Depakote ER *Tab:* 250, 500 mg ext-rel
    Depakote Sprinkle *Cap:* 125 mg

➤ *eslicarbazepine* (C)
    Aptiom *Tab:* 200*, 400, 600*, 800*mg

➤ *felbamate* (C)(G)
    Felbatol *Tab:* 400*, 600*mg
    Felbatol Oral Suspension *Oral susp:* 600 mg/5 ml (4, 8, 32 oz)
    Peganone *Tab:* 250, 500 mg

➤ *bapentin* (C)
    Horizant *Tab:* 300, 600 ext-rel
    Neurontin (G) *Cap:* 100, 300, 400 mg; *Tab:* 600*, 800*mg
    Neurontin Oral Solution *Oral soln:* 250 mg/5 ml (480 ml) (strawberry-anise)

➤ *lacosamide* (C)(V)(G)
    Vimpat *Tab:* 50, 100, 150, 200 mg; *Oral soln:* 10 mg/ml (200, 465 ml); *Vial:*
    10 mg/ml soln for IV infusion, single-use (20 ml)

(*continued*)

(continued)

▷ **lamotrigine** (C)(G)
Lamictal *Tab:* 25*, 100*, 150*, 200*mg
Lamictal Chewable Dispersible Tab *Chew tab:* 2, 5, 25, 50 mg (black current)
Lamictal ODT *ODT:* 25, 50, 100, 200 mg oral-disint
Lamictal XR *Tab:* 25, 50, 100, 200, 250, 300 mg ext-rel

▷ **levetiracetam** (C)(G)
Elepsia *Tab:* 1000, 1500 mg ext-rel
Keppra *Tab:* 250*, 500*, 750*, 1000*mg
Keppra Oral Solution *Oral soln:* 100 mg/ml (16 oz) (grape) (dye-free)
Keppra XR *Tab:* 500, 750 mg ext-rel
Levitiracetam IV *Premixed:* 500, 1,000, 1,500 mg for IV infusion (100 ml)
Roweepra *Tab:* 250, 500, 750 mg; 1 gm

▷ **mephobarbital** (D)(II)
Mebaral *Tab:* 32, 50, 100 mg

▷ **methsuximide** (C)
Celontin Kapseals *Cap:* 150, 300 mg

▷ **oxcarbazepine** (C)(G)
Trileptal *Tab:* 150, 300, 600 mg; *Oral susp:* 300 mg/5 ml (lemon) (alcohol)
Oxtellar XR *Tab:* 150, 300, 600 mg ext-rel

▷ **perampanel** (C)(III)
Fycompa *Tab:* 2, 4, 6, 8, 10, 12 mg
Fycompa Oral Suspension *Oral susp:* 0.5 mg/ml (340 ml w. dosing syringe)

▷ **phenytoin** (D)(G), *primidone* (D)(G)
Dilantin *Cap:* 30, 100 mg ext-rel
Dilantin Infatabs *Chew tab:* 50 mg
Dilantin Oral Suspension *Oral susp:* 125 mg/5 ml (237 ml) (alcohol 6%)
Phenytek *Cap:* 200, 300 mg ext-rel

▷ **pregabalin** (C)(V)
Lyrica *Cap:* 25, 50, 75, 100, 200, 225, 300 mg
Lyrica CR *Tab:* 82.5, 165, 330 mg ext-rel
Lyrica Oral Solution *Oral soln:* 20 mg/ml

▷ **primidone** (C)
Mysoline *Tab:* 50*, 250*mg
Mysoline Oral Solution *Oral susp:* 250 mg/5 ml (8 oz)

▷ **rufinamide** (C)(G)
Banzel *Tab:* 200*, 400*mg
Banzel Oral Solution *Susp:* 40 mg/ml (orange) (lactose-free, gluten-free, dye-free)

▷ **tiagabine** (C)(G)
Gabitril *Tab:* 2, 4, 12, 16 mg

▷ **topiramate** (D)(G)
Topamax *Tab:* 25, 50, 100, 200 mg

(continued)

(*continued*)

> **Topamax Sprinkle Caps** *Cap:* 15, 25, 50 mg
> **Trokendi XR** *Cap:* 25, 50, 100, 200 mg ext-rel
> **Qudexy** *Tab:* 25, 50, 100, 150, 200 mg ext-rel
> **Qudexy XR** *Cap:* 25, 50, 100, 150, 200 mg ext-rel

▷ *vigabatrin* (C)(G)
   Sabril *Tab:* 500 mg
   Sabril for Oral Solution 500 mg/pkt pwdr for reconstitution

▷ *zonisamide* (C)
   Zonegran *Cap:* 25, 50, 100 mg

APPENDIX S. ANTI-HIV DRUGS

ANTI-HIV DRUGS WITH DOSE FORMS

▷ **Aptivus** (C) *tipranavir*
   Gel cap: 250 mg (alcohol); *Oral soln:* 100 mg/ml (95 ml w. dosing syringe)
   (Vit E 116 IU/ml) (buttermint-butter, toffee)

Comment: *valganciclovir* is indicated for the treatment of AIDS-related
cytomegalovirus (CMV) retinitis.

▷ **Atripla** (D) *efavirenz+emtricitabine+tenofovir disoproxil*
   Tab: efa 600 mg+emtri 200 mg+teno diso 300 mg

▷ **Combivir** (C)(G) *lamivudine+zidovudine*
   Tab: aba+lami 150+zido 300 mg

▷ **Complera** (B) *emtricitabine+tenofovir disoproxil*
   Tab: emtri 200 mg+teno diso 300 mg+rilpiv 25 mg

▷ **Crixivan** (C) *indinavir sulfate*
   Cap: 100, 200, 333, 400 mg

▷ **Cytovene** (C)(G) *ganciclovir*
   Cap: 250, 500 mg; *Vial:* 50 mg/ml single-dose (500 mg, 10 ml)

▷ **Descovy** (D) *emtricitabine+tenofovir alafenamide+rilpivirine*
   Tab: emtri 200 mg+teno ala 25 mg

▷ **Edurant** (B) *rilpivirine*
   Tab: 25 mg

▷ **Emtriva** (B) *emtricitabine*
   Cap: 200 mg; *Oral soln:* 10 mg/ml (170 ml) (cotton candy)

▷ **Epivir** (C)(G) *lamivudine*
   Tab: 150*, 300*mg; *Oral soln:* 10 mg/ml (240 ml) (strawberry-banana) (sucrose 3
   gm/15 ml)

▷ **Epzicom** (B) *abacavir sulfate+lamivudine*
   Tab: aba 600 mg+lami 300 mg

(*continued*)

(continued)

▷ **Evotaz (B)** *atazanavir+cobicistat*
  Tab: ataz 300+cobi 150 mg

▷ **Fortovase (B)** *aquinavir*
  Soft gel cap: 200 mg

▷ **Fuzeon (B)** *enfuvirtide*
  Vial: 90 mg/ml pwdr for SC inj after reconstitution (1 ml, 60 vials/kit)
  (preservative-free)

▷ **Genvoya (B)** *elvitegravir+cobicistat+emtricitabine+tenofovir alafenamide (TAF)*
  Tab: elv 150 mg+cob 150 mg+emtri 200 mg+teno alafen 10 mg

▷ **Intelence (C)** *etravirine*
  Tab: 25*, 100, 200 mg

▷ **Invirase (B)** *saquinavir mesylate*
  Hard gel cap: 200 mg

▷ **Isentress (C)** *raltegravir (potassium)*
  Tab: 400 mg film-coat; *Chew tab:* 25, 100*mg (orange-banana) (phenylalanine);
  Oral susp: 100 mg/pkt pwdr for oral susp (banana)

▷ **Kaletra (C)** *lopinavir plus ritonavir*
  Cap: lopin 100 mg+riton 25 mg, *lopin* 200 mg+riton 50 mg; *Oral soln:* lopin 80
  mg+riton 20 mg per ml (160 ml w. dose cup) (cotton candy) (alcohol 42%)
  Hard gel cap: 200 mg

▷ **Lexiva (C)(G)** *fosamprenavir*
  Tab: 700 mg; *Oral soln:* 50 mg/ml (grape, bubble gum) (peppermint)

▷ **Norvir (B)** *ritonavir*
  Soft gel cap: 100 mg (alcohol); *Oral soln:* 80 mg/ml (8 oz) (peppermint-caramel)
  (alcohol)

▷ **Odefsey (D)** *emtricitabine+rilpivirine+tenofovir alafenamide*
  Tab: emtri 200 mg+rilpiv 25 mg+tenof alafen 25 mg

▷ **Prezcobix (B)** *darunavir+cobicistat*
  Tab: daru 800+cobi 150 mg

▷ **Prezista (C)(G)** *darunavir*
  Tab: 75, 150, 600, 800 mg; *Oral susp:* 100 mg/ml (200 ml) (strawberry cream)

▷ **Rescriptor (C)** *delavirdine mesylate*
  Tab: 100, 200 mg

▷ **Retrovir (C)(G)** *zidovudine*
  Tab: 300 mg; *Cap:* 100 mg; *Syr:* 50 mg/5 ml (240 ml) (strawberry); *Vial:* 10 mg/ml
  (20 ml vial for IV infusion) (preservative-free)

▷ **Reyataz (B)** *atazanavir*
  Cap: 100, 150, 200, 300 mg

(continued)

(*continued*)

▷ Selzentry (B) *maraviroc*
  Tab: 150, 300 mg

▷ Stribild (B) *elvitegravir+cobicistat+emtricitabine+tenofovir disoproxil fumarate*
  Tab: elv 150 mg+cob 150 mg+emtri 200 mg+teno diso fumar 300 mg

▷ Sustiva (C) *efavirenz*
  Tab: 75, 150, 600, 800 mg; *Cap:* 50, 200 mg

▷ Tivicay (B) *dolutegravir*
  Tab: 50 mg

▷ Triumeq (C) *abacavir sulfate+dilutegravir+lamivudine*
  Tab: aba 600 mg+dilu 50 mg+lami 300 mg

▷ Trizivir (C)(G) *abacavir sulfate+lamivudine+zidovudine*
  Tab: aba 300 mg+lami 150 mg+zido 300 mg

▷ Truvada (B)(G) *emtricitabine+tenofovir disoproxil fumarate*
  Tab: emt 100 mg+teno 150 mg, 133 mg+teno 200 mg, emt 167 mg+teno 250 mg,
  emt 200 mg+teno 300 mg

▷ Valcyte (C)(G) *valganciclovir*
  Tab: 450 mg

▷ Videx EC (C)(G) *didanosine*
  Cap: 125, 200, 250, 400 mg ent-coat del-rel; *Chew tab:* 25, 50, 100, 150, 200 mg
  (mandarin orange; buffered with calcium carbonate and magnesium hydroxide)
  (phenylalanine); *Pwdr for oral soln:* 2, 4 gm (120, 240 ml)

▷ Videx Pediatric Pwdr for Oral Solution (C) *didanosine*
  Pwdr for oral soln: 2, 4 gm (120, 240 ml)

▷ Viracept (B) *nelfinavir mesylate*
  Tab: 250, 625 mg; *Pwdr for oral soln:* 50 mg/gm (144 gm) (phenylalanine)

▷ Viramune (C)(G) *nevirapine*
  Tab: 200*mg; *Oral susp:* 50 mg/5 ml (240 ml)

▷ Viramune XR (C) *nevirapine*
  Tab: 100, 400 mg ext-rel

▷ Viread (C) *tenofovir disoproxil fumarate*
  Tab: 150, 200, 250, 300 mg; *Oral pwdr:* 40 mg/1 gm pwdr (60 gm w. dosing scoop)

▷ Vistide (C) *cidofovir*
  Inj: 75 mg/ml (5 ml vials for IV infusion) (preservative free)

Comment: *cidofovir* is indicated for the treatment of AIDS-related *cytomegalo-virus*
(CMV) retinitis.

▷ Vitekta (C) *elvitegravir*
  Inj: 75 mg/ml (5 ml vials for IV infusion) (preservative free)

(*continued*)

(*continued*)

> Comment: *cidofovir* is indicated for the treatment of AIDS-related cytomegalovirus (CMV) retinitis.

▷ **Zerit (C)(G)** *stavudine*
  Cap: 15, 20, 30, 40 mg; *Oral soln:* 1 mg/ml pwdr for reconstitution (200 ml) (fruit) (dye-free)

▷ **Ziagen (C)(G)** *abacavir sulfate*
  Tab: 300*mg; *Oral soln:* 20 mg/ml (240 ml) (strawberry-banana) (parabens, propylene glycol)

○ APPENDIX T. COUMADIN (WARFARIN)

T.1. COUMADIN TITRATION AND DOSE FORMS

> ▷ *warfarin* **(X)(G)** dosage initially 2-5 mg/day; usual maintenance 2-10 mg/day; adjust dosage to maintain INR in therapeutic range:
> *Venous thrombosis:* 2.0-3.0
> *Atrial fibrillation:* 2.0-3.0
> *Post MI:* 2.5-3.5
> *Mechanical and bioprosthetic heart valves:* 2.0-3.0 for 12 weeks after valve insertion, then 2.5-3.5 long-term
> *Pediatric:* not recommended <18 years
> **Coumadin** *Tab:* 1*, 2*, 2.5*, 3*, 4*, 5*, 6*, 7.5*, 10*mg
> **Coumadin for Injection** *Vial:* 2 mg/ml (2.5 ml)
> Comment: **Coumadin for Injection** is for peripheral IV administration only.

T.2. COUMADIN OVER-ANTICOAGULATION REVERSAL

> ▷ *phytonadione (vitamin K)* **(G)** 2.5-10 mg PO <u>or</u> IM; max 25 mg
> **AquaMEPHYTON** *Vial:* 1 mg/0.5 ml (0.5 ml); 10 mg/ml (1, 2.5, 5 ml)
> **Mephyton** *Tab:* 5 mg

T.3. AGENTS THAT INHIBIT COUMADIN'S ANTICOAGULATION EFFECTS

Increase Metabolism	Decrease Absorption	Other Mechanism(s)
azathioprine	azathioprine	coenzyme Q10
carbamazepine	cholestyramine	estrogen
dicloxacillin	colestipol	griseofulvin
ethanol	sucralfate	oral contraceptives
griseofulvin		ritonavir
nafcillin		spironolactone

(*continued*)

(*continued*)

Increase Metabolism	Decrease Absorption	Other Mechanism(s)
pentobarbital phenobarbital phenytoin primidone rifabutin rifampin		trazodone vitamin C (high dose) vitamin K

APPENDIX U. LOW MOLECULAR WEIGHT HEPARINS

Comment: Administer by subcutaneous injection *only*, in the abdomen, and rotate sites. Avoid concomitant drugs that affect hemostasis (e.g., oral anticoagulants and platelet aggregation inhibitors, including **aspirin**, NSAIDs, **dipyridamole**, **sulfinpyrazone**, **ticlopidine**). Not recommended <18 years-of-age.

LOW MOLECULAR WEIGHT HEPARINS WITH DOSE FORMS

▷ *ardeparin* (C)
  Normiflo *Soln for inj:* 5,000 anti-Factor Xa U/0.5 ml; 10,000 anti-Factor Xa U/0.5 ml (sulfites, parabens)

▷ *dalteparin* (B)
  Fragmin *Prefilled syringe:* 2500 IU/0.2 ml, 5000 IU/0.2 ml (10/box) (preservative-free); *Multi-dose vial:* 1,000 IU/ml (95,000 IU, 9.5 ml) (benzyl alcohol)

▷ *danaparoid* (B)
  Orgaran *Amp:* 750 anti-Xa units/0.6 ml (0.6 ml, 10/box); *Prefilled syringe:* 750 anti-Xa units/0.6 ml (0.6 ml, 10/box) (sulfites)

▷ *enoxaparin* (B)(G)
  Lovenox *Prefilled syringe:* 30 mg/0.3 ml, 40 mg/0.4 ml, 60 mg/0.6 ml, 80 mg/0.8 ml (100 mg/ml) (preservative-free); *Vial:* 100 mg/ml (3 ml)

▷ *tinzaparin* (B)
  Innohep *Vial:* 20,000 *anti-Factor Xa* IU/ml (2 ml) (sulfites, benzyl alcohol)

APPENDIX V. FACTOR XA INHIBITORS

FACTOR XA INHIBITOR DOSE FORMS AND THERAPY

▷ *apixaban* (C) 5 mg bid; reduce to 2.5 mg bid if any two of the following: ≥80 years, ≤60 kg, serum Cr ≥1.5
  Pediatric: not recommended
  Eliquis *Tab:* 2.5, 5 mg
Comment: Eloquis is indicated to reduce the risk of stroke and systemic embolism in patients with nonvalvular atrial fibrillation (NVAF).

(*continued*)

(continued)

▷ **betrixaban** *Recommended dose:* is an initial single dose of 160 mg, followed by 80 mg once daily, taken at the same time each day with food;
Recommended duration of treatment: 35 to 42 days; reduce dose with severe renal impairment or with P-glycoprotein (P-gp) inhibitors
Pediatrics: not established
 Bevyxxa *Cap:* 40, 80 mg
Comment: Bevyxxa is indicated for the prophylaxis of venous thromboembolism (VTE) in adults who are hospitalized for acute mental illness and at risk for thromboembolic complications due to moderate or severe restricted mobility and other VTE risk factors. There are no data with the use of **betrixaban** in pregnancy, but treatment is likely to increase the risk of hemorrhage during pregnancy and delivery. No data are available regarding the presence of **betrixaban** or its metabolites in human milk or the effects of the drug on the breastfed infant.

▷ **edoxaban** (**C**) transition to and from **Savaysa**; assess CrCl prior to initiation:
NVAF CrCl >50 mL/min: 60 mg once daily; *CrCl 15-50 mL/min:* 30 mg once daily
DVT/PE CrCl >50 mL/min: 60 mg once daily following initial parental anticoagulant; *CrCl 15-50 mL/min, <60 kg, or concomitant Pgp inhibitors:* 30 mg once daily
Pediatric: not established
 Savaysa *Tab:* 15, 30, 60 mg
Comment: Savaysa is indicated to reduce the risk of stroke and systemic embolism in patients with nonvalvular atrial fibrillation (NVAF), treatment of DVT and pulmonary embolism (PE) following 5-10 days of initial therapy with parenteral anticoagulant. Not for use in persons with NVAF with CrCl >95 mL/min.

▷ **fondaparinux** (**B**) Administer SC; administer first dose no earlier than 6-8 hours after hemostasis is achieved, start warfarin usually within 72 hours of last dose of *fondaparinux*
Post-op: 2.5 mg once daily x 5-9 days
Hip/Knee Replacement: once daily x 11 days
Hip Fracture: once daily x 32 days
Abdominal Surgery: once daily x 10 days
Prophylaxis: do not use <50 kg
Treatment: once daily for at least 5 days until INR=2-3 (usually 5-9 days); max 26 days; <50 kg: 5 mg; 50-100 kg: 7.5 mg; >100 kg: 10 mg
Pediatric: not established
 Arixtra *Soln for SC inj:* 2.5 mg/0.5 ml, 5 mg/0.4 ml, 7.5 mg/0.6 ml, 10 mg/0.8 ml *prefilled syringe* (10/box) (preservative-free)

▷ **prasugrel** (**B**)(**G**) *Loading dose:* 60 mg once in a single-dose; *Maintenance:* 10 mg once daily; *<60 kg:* consider 5 mg once daily; take with aspirin 75-325 mg once daily
Pediatric: not recommended
 Effient *Tab:* 5, 10 mg
Comment: Effient is indicated to reduce the risk of thrombotic cardiovascular events in persons with acute coronary syndrome (ACS) who are to be managed with percutaneous coronary intervention (PCI) including unstable angina, non-ST elevation myocardial infarction (NSTEMI) and STEMI. Do not use if active pathological bleeding (e.g., peptic ulcer, intracranial hemorrhage), prior TIA or stroke, or if patient likely to undergo urgent CABG. Discontinue 7 days before surgery and if TIA or stroke occurs.

(continued)

(continued)

> ▷ **rivaroxaban** (C) take with food
> *Treatment of DVT* or *PE:* 15 mg twice daily for the first 21 days; then 20 mg once daily
> *Reduction in risk of DVT* or *PE recurrence:* 20 mg once daily with the evening meal; *CrCl <30 mL/min:* avoid
> *Prophylaxis of DVT:* take 6-10 hours after surgery when hemostasis established, then 10-20 mg once daily with the evening meal; *CrCl 30-50 mL/min:* 10 mg; *CrCl <30 mL/min:* avoid; discontinue if acute renal failure develops; monitor closely for blood loss
> *Hip:* treat for 35 days; *Knee:* treat for 12 days
> *Nonvalvular AF:* take once daily with the evening meal; *CrCl >50 mL/min:* 20 mg; *CrCl 15-50 mL/min:* 15 mg; *CrCl >15 mL/min:* avoid
> *Pediatric:* not recommended
> **Xarelto** *Cap:* 10, 15, 20 mg
> **Comment:** **Xarelto** is indicated to reduce the risk of stroke and systemic embolism in nonvalvular atrial fibrillation (AF), to treat deep vein thrombosis (DVT) and pulmonary embolism (PE), to reduce the risk of recurrence of DVT and/or PE following 6 months treatment for DVT and/or PE, and prophylaxis of DVT which may lead to PE in patients undergoing knee or hip replacement surgery. **Xarelto** eliminates the need for bridging with heparin or low molecular heparin; no need for routine monitoring of INR or other coagulation parameters; no need for dose adjustments for age, weight, or gender; no known dietary restrictions. Switching from **warfarin** or other anticoagulant, see mfr pkg insert.

 APPENDIX W. DIRECT THROMBIN INHIBITORS

DIRECT THROMBIN INHIBITOR DOSING AND DOSE FORMS

> ▷ **aspirin** (D) single dose once daily
> *Pediatric:* not established
> **Durlaza** *Cap:* 162.5 mg 24-hr ext-rel (30, 90/bottle)
> ▷ **dabigatran etexilate mesylate** (C) swallow whole; *CrCl >30 mL/min:* 150 mg bid; *CrCl 15-30 mL/min:* 75 mg twice daily; *CrCl <15 mL/min:* not recommended
> *Pediatric:* not recommended
> **Pradaxa** *Cap:* 75, 150 mg
> **Comment:** **Pradaxa** is indicated to reduce the risk of stroke and systemic embolism in nonvalvular AF, DVT prophylaxis, PE prophylaxis in patients who have undergone hip replacement surgery, treatment of DVT and PE in patients who have been treated with a parenteral anticoagulant for 5-10 days, and to reduce the risk of recurrent DVT and PE in patients who have been previously treated. **Pradaxa** is contraindicated in patients with a mechanical prosthetic heart valve and not recommended with a bioprosthetic heart valve. Presently there is only one reversal agent for this drug class. *idarucizumab* (**Praxbind**) is a specific reversal agent for *dabigatran* (**Pradaxa**). It is a humanized monoclonal antibody fragment (Fab) that binds to dabigatran and its acylglucuronide metabolites with higher affinity than the binding affinity of dabigatran to thrombin, neutralizing its anticoagulant effects. [See **Pradaxa** reversal agent, *idarucizumab* (**Praxbind**) at the end of this appendix].

(continued)

(*continued*)

> ➤ **desirudin** *(recombinant hirudin)* **(C)** 15 mg SC every 12 hours, preferably in the
> abdomen <u>or</u> thigh, starting up to 5-15 minutes before surgery (after induction of
> regional block anesthesia, if used); may continue for 9-12 days post-op; *CrCl <60
> mL/min:* reduce dose (see mfr pkg insert)
> *Pediatric:* not recommended
> **Iprivask** *Pwdr for SC inj after reconstitution:* 15 mg/single-use vial (10/box)
> (preservative-free, diluent contains mannitol)
>
> **Comment:** **Iprivask** is indicated for DVT prophylaxis in patients undergoing hip
> replacement surgery. It is not interchangeable with other hirudins.
>
> ### IDARUCIZUMAB REVERSAL AGENT: HUMANIZED MONOCLONAL–ANTIBODY
> ### FRAGMENT (FAB)
>
> ➤ **idarucizumab** **(NE)** administer 5 gm (2 vials) IV drip <u>or</u> push; administer within 1
> hour of removal from vial
> *Pediatric:* not established
> **Praxbind** *Vial:* 2.5 g/50 ml, single-use (preservative-free)
>
> **Comment:** Presently, there is inadequate human and animal data to assess risk of
> **idarucizumab** (**Praxbind**) use in pregnancy. Risk/benefit should be considered prior
> to use.

 APPENDIX X. PLATELET AGGREGATION INHIBITORS

PLATELET AGGREGATION INHIBITOR DOSING AND DOSE FORMS

> ➤ **cilostazol** **(B)** 100 mg bid
> *Pediatric:* not recommended
> **Pletal** *Tab:* 50, 100 mg
>
> **Comment:** **Pletal** is an antiplatelet/vasodilator (PDE III inhibitor)
>
> ➤ **clopidogrel** **(B)** 75 mg once daily
> *Pediatric:* not recommended
> **Plavix** *Tab:* 75, 300 mg
>
> **Comment:** **Plavix** is indicated for the reduction of atherosclerotic events in recent
> MI <u>or</u> stroke, established PAD, non-ST-segment elevation acute coronary syndrome
> (unstable angina/non-STEMI), <u>or</u> STEMI.
>
> ➤ **dipyridamole** **(B)(G)** 75-100 mg qid
> *Pediatric:* not recommended
> **Persantine** *Tab:* 25, 50, 75 mg
>
> **Comment:** **dipyridamole** is indicated as an adjunct to oral anticoagulants after cardiac
> valve replacement surgery to prevent thromboembolism.
>
> ➤ **dipyridamole+aspirin** **(B)(G)** swallow whole; one cap bid
> *Pediatric:* not recommended
> **Aggrenox** *Cap: dipyr* 200 mg+*asa* 25 mg

(*continued*)

(*continued*)

▷ *pentoxifylline* (C) [hemorrheologic (xanthine)]
  Pediatric: not recommended
    Trental *Tab:* 400 mg sust-rel

▷ *prasugrel* (C)(G)
  Pediatric: not recommended
    Effient *Tab:* 5, 10 mg

Comment: **Effient** is indicated to reduce the risk of cardiovascular events in patients with acute coronary syndrome (ACS) who are to be managed with percutaneous coronary intervention (unstable angina <u>or</u> non-STEMI), and STEMI when managed with either primary <u>or</u> delayed PCI.

▷ *ticagrelor* (C) initiate 180 mg loading dose once in a single dose with *aspirin* 325 mg loading dose in a single dose; maintenance 90 mg twice daily with *aspirin* 75-100 mg once daily; ACS patients may start *ticagrelor* after a loading dose of *clopidogrel*
    Brilinta *Tab:* 90 mg

Comment: **Brilinta** is indicated to reduce the risk of cardiovascular events in patients with acute coronary syndrome (ACS) (unstable angina, Non-ST elevation (NSTEMI), myocardial infarction, <u>or</u> STEMI).

▷ *ticlopidine* (B) 250 mg bid
  Pediatric: not recommended
    Ticlid *Tab:* 250 mg

Comment: **Ticlid** is indicated to reduce the risk of thrombotic stroke in selected patients intolerant of *aspirin*.

APPENDIX Y. PROTEASE-ACTIVATED RECEPTOR-1 (PAR-1) INHIBITOR

PROTEASE-ACTIVATED RECEPTOR-1 (PAR-1) INHIBITOR DOSING AND DOSE FORM

▷ *vorapaxar* (B) administer 2.08 mg once daily; use with *aspirin* <u>or</u> *clopidogrel*
  Pediatric: <12 years: not established; ≥12 years: same as adult
    Zontivity *Tab:* 2.08 mg (equivalent to 2.5 mg vorapaxar sulfate)

Comment: **Zontivity** is indicated to reduce thrombotic cardiovascular events in patients with a history of myocardial infarction <u>or</u> with peripheral arterial disease (PAD). Contraindicated with active pathological bleeding (e.g., peptic ulcer, intra-cranial hemorrhage), prior TIA <u>or</u> stroke. Not recommended with severe hepatic impairment.

APPENDIX Z. PRESCRIPTION PRENATAL VITAMINS

Comment: It is recommended that prenatal vitamins be started at least 3 months prior to conception to improve preconception nutritional status, and continued throughout pregnancy and the postnatal period, in lactating and nonlactating women, and throughout the childbearing years.

(*continued*)

(*continued*)

▷ **CitraNatal 90 DHA** take 1 tab* and 1 DHA cap daily
Tab: thiamine 3 mg, riboflavin 3.4 mg, niacinamide 20 mg, pyridoxine HCL 20 mg, folic acid 1 mg, Vit C 120 mg, Vit D3 400 IU, Vit E 30 IU, calcium (as citrate) 160 mg, copper (as oxide) 2 mg, iodine (as potassium iodide) 150 mcg, iron (as carbonyl) 90 mg, zinc (as oxide) 25 mg, docusate sodium 50 mg
Cap: docosahexaenoic acid (DHA) 300 mg

▷ **CitraNatal Assure** take 1 tab and 1 DHA cap daily
Tab: thiamine 3 mg, riboflavin 3.4 mg, niacinamide 20 mg, pyridoxine HCL 25 mg, folic acid 1 mg, Vit C 120 mg, Vit D3 400 IU, Vit E 30 IU, calcium (as citrate) 125 mg, copper (as oxide) 2 mg, iodine (as potassium oxide) 150 mcg, iron (as carbonyl and ferrous gluconate) 35 mg, zinc (as oxide) 25 mg, docusate sodium 50 mg
Cap: docosahexaenoic acid (DHA) 300 mg

▷ **CitraNatal B-Calm** take 1 tab every 8 hours; begin with tab #1.
Tab: pyridoxine HCL 25 mg, folic acid 1 mg, Vit C 120 mg, Vit D3 400 IU, calcium (as citrate) 120 mg, iron (as carbonyl) 20 mg
Tab: pyridoxine 25 mg
Comment: **Citranatal B-Calm** may be used as an adjunct treatment to help minimize pregnancy-related nausea and vomiting.

▷ **CitraNatal DHA** take 1 tab and 1 DHA cap daily
Tab: thiamine 3 mg, riboflavin 3.4 mg, niacinamide 20 mg, pyridoxine HCL 20 mg, folic acid 1 mg, Vit C 120 mg, Vit D3 400 IU, Vit E 30 IU, calcium (as citrate) 125 mg, copper (as oxide) 2 mg, iodine (as potassium oxide) 150 mcg, iron (as carbonyl and gluconate) 27 mg, zinc (as oxide) 25 mg, docusate sodium 50 mg
Cap: docosahexaenoic acid (DHA) 250 mg

▷ **CitraNatal Harmony** take 1 gelcap daily
Gelcap: pyridoxine HCL 25 mg, folic acid 1 mg, Vit D3 400 IU, Vit E 30 IU, calcium (as citrate) 104 mg, iron (as carbonyl and ferrous fumarate) 27 mg, docusate sodium 50 mg, docosahexaenoic acid (DHA) 260 mg

▷ **CitraNatal Rx** take 1 tab* and 1 DHA cap daily
Tab: thiamine 3 mg, riboflavin 3.4 mg, niacinamide 20 mg, pyridoxine HCL 20 mg, folic acid 1 mg, Vit C 120 mg, Vit D3 400 IU, Vit E 30 IU, calcium (as citrate) 125 mg, copper (as oxide) 2 mg, iodine (as potassium iodide) 150 mcg, iron (as carbonyl and gluconate) 27 mg, zinc (as oxide) 25 mg, docusate sodium 50 mg

▷ **Duet DHA Balanced** take 1 tab and 1 gelcap daily
Tab: Vit A (as beta carotene) 2800 IU, thiamine 1.5 mg, riboflavin 2 mg, niacinamide 20 mg, pyridoxine HCL 50 mg, Vit B12 12 mcg, folic acid 1 mg, Vit C 120 mg, Vit D3 640 IU, Vit E 15 IU, calcium (as carbonate) 215 mg, iron (as polysaccharide iron complex and sodium iron EDTA, Ferrazone) 25 mg, copper (as oxide) 1.8 mg, magnesium (as oxide) 25 mg, zinc (as oxide) 25 mg, iodine (as potassium iodide) 210 mcg, selenium 65 mcg, choline (as bartrate) 55 mg
Gelcap: omega 3 fatty acids 267 mg (includes docosahexaenoic acid [DHA], eicosapentaenoic acid [EPA], alpha-linolenic acid [ALA], docasapentaeoic acid [DPA]) (gelatin, gluten-free)

▷ **Duet DHA Complete** take 1 tab and 1 gelcap daily
Tab: Vit A (as beta carotene) 3000 IU, thiamine 1.8 mg, riboflavin 4 mg, niacinamide 20 mg, pyridoxine HCL 50 mg, Vit B12 12 mcg, folic acid 1 mg, Vit C 120 mg,

(*continued*)

Vit D3 800 IU, Vit E 3 mg, calcium (as carbonate) 230 mg, iron (as polysaccharide iron complex and sodium iron EDTA, ferrazone) 27 mg, copper (as oxide) 2 mg, magnesium (as oxide) 25 mg, zinc (as oxide) 25 mg, iodine 220 mcg
Gelcap: omega 3 fatty acids ≥430 mg (as docosahexaenoic acid (DHA) ≥295 mg, as other omega 3 fatty acids ≥135 mg (eicosapentaenoic acid (EPA), docasapentae-noic acid (DHA) (gluten-free)

▷ **Natachew** take 1 chew tab daily
Chew tab: Vit A 1000 IU (as beta carotene), thiamine 2 mg, riboflavin 3 mg, nia-cinamide 20 mg, pyridoxine HCL 10 mg, B12 12 mcg, folic acid 1 mg, Vit C 120 mg, Vit D3 400 IU, Vit E 11 IU, iron (as ferrous fumarate) 29 mg (wildberry)

▷ **Natafort** take 1 tab daily
Tab: Vit A 1000 IU (as acetate and beta carotene), thiamine 2 mg, riboflavin 3 mg, niacinamide 20 mg, pyridoxine HCL 10 mg, B12 12 mcg, folic acid 1 mg, Vit C 120 mg, Vit D3 400 IU, Vit E 11 IU, iron (as carbonyl and sulfate) 60 mg

▷ **Neevo DHA** take 1 cap daily
Cap: l-methylfolate (as Metafolin) 1.3 mg, thiamin 1.4 mg, riboflavin 1.4 mg, niacinamide 18 mg, pyridoxine HCL 25 mg, B12 1 mg, Vit C 85 mg, Vit D3, 5 mcg, Vit E 15 IU, calcium (as carbonate) 110 mg, iron (ferrous fumarate) 27 mg, iodine (as potassium iodide) 220 mcg, magnesium (as oxide) 60 mg, docosahexaenoic acid (DHA, vegetarian source (algal oil) 581.92 mg (soy, gelatin, sorbitol, glycerin)

Comment: **Neevo DHA** is indicated as a nutritional supplement during pregnancy, and the prenatal and postnatal periods, in women with dietary needs for the biologically active form of folate, who are at risk for hyperhomocysteinemia, impaired folic acid absorption, and/or impaired folic acid metabolism due to 667C >T mutations in the MTHFR gene.

▷ **Nexa Plus** take 1 cap daily
Cap: pyridoxine HCL 25 mg, folic acid 1.25 mg, Vit C 28 mg, Vit D3 800 IU, Vit E 30 IU, biotin 250 mcg, calcium (as carbonate [158 mg]+docusate calcium [2 mg]) 160 mg, iron (as ferrous fumarate) 29 mg, docosahexaenoic acid (DHA, plant-based source [algal oil]) 350 mg (soy)

▷ **Nexa Select** take 1 softgel cap daily
Softgel cap: pyridoxine HCL 25 mg, folic acid 1.25 mg, Vit C 28 mg, Vit D3 800 IU, Vit E 30 IU, calcium (as phosphate) 160 mg, iron (as ferrous fumarate) 29 mg, docosahexaenoic acid (DHA) plant-based source (algal oil) 325 mg, docusate sodium 55 mg (soy)

▷ **Prenate AM** take 1 tab daily
Tab: pyridoxine HCL 75 mg, folate (as folic acid 400 mcg+Quatrefolic 1.1 mg [equivalent to 600 mcg folic acid]) 1 mg, Vit B12 12 mcg, calcium (as carbonate) 200 mg, ginger extract 500 mg, lingon-berry 25 mg

▷ **Prenate Chewable** take 1 chew tab daily
Chew tab: pyridoxine HCL 10 mg, Vit B12 125 mcg, calcium (as carbonate) 500 mg, Vit D3 300 IU, biotin 280 mcg, boron amino acid chelate 250 mcg, folate (as Quatrefolic) 1 mg, magnesium (as oxide) 50 mg, blueberry extract 25 mg (Dutch chocolate)

(*continued*)

(*continued*)

▷ **Prenate DHA** take 1 gel cap daily
Gelcap: pyridoxine HCL 26 mg, folate (as folic acid) 400 mcg+Quatrefolic 1.1 mg [equivalent to 600 mcg folic acid]) 1 mg, Vit B12 13 mcg, Vit C 90 mg, Vit D3 220 IU, Vit E 10 IU, calcium (as carbonate) 145 mg, iron (as ferrous fumarate) 28 mg, magnesium (as oxide) 50 mg, docosahexaenoic acid (DHA) 300 mg (fish oil, soy, gelatin)

▷ **Prenate Elite** take 1 gel cap daily
Gelcap: Vit A (as beta-carotene) 2600 IU, thiamine 3 mg, riboflavin 3.5 mg, pyridoxine HCl 21 mg, niacinamide 21 mg, pantothenic acid 6 mg, folate (as folic acid 400 mcg+Quatrefolic 1.1 mg [equivalent to 600 mcg folic acid]) 1 mg, Vit B12 13 mcg, Vit C 75 mg, Vit D3 450 IU, Vit E 10 IU, biotin 330 mcg, calcium (as carbonate) 100 mg, iron (as ferrous fumarate) 27 mg, magnesium (as oxide) 25 mg, copper (as oxide) 1.5 mg, iodine 150 mcg, iron (as ferrous fumarate) 26 mg, zinc (as oxide) 15 mg

▷ **Prenate Enhance** take 1 gel cap daily
Gelcap: pyridoxine HCL 25 mg, folate (as folic acid 400 mcg+Quatrefolic 1.1 mg [equivalent to 600 mcg folic acid]) 1 mg, Vit B12 12 mcg, Vit C 85 mg, Vit D3 1000 IU, Vit E 10 IU, biotin 500 mcg, calcium (as carbonate+Formical) 155 mg, iodine (as potassium) 150 mcg, iron (as ferrous fumarate) 28 mg, magnesium (as oxide) 50 mg, docosahexaenoicacid (DHA) 400 mg (soy, gelatin)

▷ **Prenate Essential** take 1 gel cap daily
Gelcap: pyridoxine HCL 26 mg, folate (as folic acid 400 mcg+Quatrefolic 1.1 mg [equivalent to 600 mcg folic acid]) 1 mg, Vit B12 13 mcg, Vit C 90 mg, Vit D3 220 IU, Vit E 10 IU, biotin 280 mcg, calcium (as carbonate) 145 mg, iodine (as potassium iodide) 150 mcg, iron (as ferrous fumarate) 29 mg, magnesium (as oxide) 50 mg, docosahexaenoic acid (DHA) 300 mg, eicosapentaenoic acid (EPA) 40 mg (fish oil, soy, gelatin)

▷ **Prenate Mini** take 1 gel cap daily
Gelcap: pyridoxine HCL 26 mg, folate (as folic acid) 400 mcg+Quatrefolic 1.1 mg [equivalent to 600 mcg folic acid]) 1 mg, Vit B12 13 mcg, Vit C 60 mg, Vit D3 220 IU, Vit E 10 IU, calcium (as carbonate) 100 mg, iron (as carbonyl iron) 29 mg, iodine (as potassium iodide) 150 mcg, biotin 280 mcg, magnesium (as oxide) 25 mg, docosahexaenoic acid (DHA) 300 mg, blueberry extract 25 mg (fish oil, soy, gelatin)

▷ **Prenate Restore** take 1 gel cap daily
Gelcap: pyridoxine HCL 25 mg, folate (as folic acid 400 mcg+Quatrefolic 1.1 mg [equivalent to 600 mcg folic acid]) 1 mg, Vit B12 12 mcg, Vit C 85 mg, Vit D3 1000 IU, Vit E 10 IU, biotin 500 mcg, calcium (as carbonate+Formical) 155 mg, iron (as ferrous fumarate) 27 mg, magnesium (as oxide) 45 mg, docosahexaenoic acid (DHA) 400 mg, *Bacillus coagulans* 150 million CFU (as lactospore) 10 mg (soy, gelatin)

▷ **Prenexa** take 1 gel cap daily
Gelcap: pyridoxine HCL 25 mg, folic acid 1.25 mg, Vit C 28 mg, Vit D3 400 IU, Vit E 30 IU, calcium (as phosphate) 160 mg, iron (as ferrous fumarate) 27 mg, docosahexaenoic acid (DHA) plant-based source (algal oil) 300 mg, docusate sodium 55 mg (soy)

APPENDIX AA. DRUGS FOR THE MANAGEMENT OF ALLERGY, COUGH, AND COLD SYMPTOMS

Comment: Oral prescription drugs for the management of allergy symptoms, cough, and symptoms of the common cold are listed in alphabetical order by brand name.

LEGEND

acriv	*acrivastine*
benzo	*benzonatate*
brom	*brompheniramine*
carb	*carbinoxamine*
carbeta	*carbetapentane*
chlor	*chlorpheniramine*
cod	*codeine*
cypro	*cyproheptadine*
deslorat	*desloratadine*
dexchlo	*dexchlorpheniramine*
dextro	*dextromethorphan*
diphen	*diphenhydramine*
hydrox	*hydroxyzine*
guaiac	*potassium guaiacolsulfonate*
guaif	*guaifenesin*
homat	*homatropine*
hydro	*hydrocodone*
hydrox	*hydroxyzine*
levocetir	*levocetirizine*
meth	*methscopolamine*
phenyle	*phenylephrine*
prometh	*promethazine*
pseud	*pseudoephedrine*
pyril	*pyrilamine tannate*

▷ **Allerex (C)** 1 AM tab in the morning and 1 PM tab in the evening prn
  Pediatric: <12 years: not recommended; ≥12 years: same as adult
  AM tab: meth 2.5 mg+pseud 120 mg ext-rel; *PM tab:* meth 2.5 mg+chlor 8 mg+phenyle 10 mg* ext-rel (*Dose Pack 20:* 10 AM tabs+10 PM tabs; *Dose Pack 60:* 30 AM tabs+30 PM tabs)

▷ **Allures-D (C)** 1 tab q 12 hours prn
  Pediatric: <12 years: not recommended; ≥12 years: same as adult
  Tab: meth 2.5 mg+pseud 120 mg ext-rel

▷ **Allerex DF (C)** 1 AM tab in the morning and 1 PM tab in the evening prn
  Pediatric: <12 years: not recommended; ≥12 years: same as adult
  AM tab: meth 2.5 mg+chlor 4 mg; *PM tab:* meth 2.5 mg+chlor 8 mg* (*Dose Pack 20:* 10 AM tabs+10 PM tabs; *Dose Pack 60:* 30 AM tabs+30 PM tabs)

(*continued*)

▷ **Allerex PE (C)** 1 AM tab in the morning and 1 PM tab in the evening prn
Pediatric: <12 years: not recommended; ≥12 years: same as adult
AM tab: meth 2.5 mg+phenyle 40 mg/*PM tab:* meth 8 mg+phenyle 10 mg* (*Dose Pack 20:* 10 AM tabs+10 PM tabs; *Dose Pack 60:* 30 AM tabs+30 PM tabs)

▷ **Allerex Suspension (C)** 15 ml q 12 hours prn
Pediatric: <6 years: not recommended; 6-12 years: 2.5-5 ml q 12 hours prn; >12 years: same as adult
Susp: chlor 3 mg+phenyle 7.5 mg ext-rel (raspberry)

▷ **Atarax (B)(G)** 25 mg tid <u>or</u> qid prn
Pediatric: <2 years: not recommended; 2-6 years: 6.25 mg q 4-6 hours prn; 6-12 years: 12.5-25 mg q 4-6 hours prn; >12 years: same as adult
Tab: hydrox 10, 25, 50, 100 mg; *Syr:* hydrox 10 mg/5 ml (alcohol 0.5%)

▷ **Bromfed DM (C)(G)** 2 tsp q 4 hours prn: max 6 doses/day
Pediatric: <2 years: not recommended; 2-6 years: 2 tsp q 4 hours prn; 6-12 years: 1 tsp q 4 hours prn; max 6 doses/day; >12 years: same as adult
Susp: brom 2 mg+pseudo 30 mg+dextro 10 mg per 5 ml (butterscotch; alcohol 0.95%)

▷ **Bromfed DM Sugar-Free (C)(G)** 2 tsp q 4 hours prn: max 6 doses/day
Pediatric: <2 years: not recommended; 2-6 years: 1/2 tsp q 4 hours prn; 6-12 years: 1 tsp q 4 hours prn; >12 years: same as adult
max 6 doses/day
Susp: brom 2 mg+pseudo 30 mg+dextro 10 mg per 5 ml (butterscotch) (alcohol 0.95%)

▷ **Clarinex (C)** 1 tab daily prn
Pediatric: <6 years: not recommended; ≥6 years: 1/2-1 tab once daily
Tab: deslorat 5 mg

▷ **Clarinex RediTabs (C)** 5 mg daily prn
Pediatric: <6 years: not recommended; 6-12 years: 2.5 mg once daily; >12 years: same as adult
ODT: deslorat 2.5, 5 mg (tutti-frutti) (phenylalanine)

▷ **Clarinex Syrup (C)** 1 tab daily prn
Pediatric: <6 months: not recommended; 6-11 months: 1 mg (2 ml) daily prn; 1-5 years: 1.25 mg (2.5 ml) daily prn; 6-11 years: 2.5 mg (5 ml) daily prn; ≥11 years: 5 mg (10 ml) daily prn
Tab: deslorat 0.5 mg per ml (4 oz) (tutti-frutti) (phenylalanine)

▷ **Duratuss AC 12 (C)** 1-2 tsp q 12 hours prn
Pediatric: <2 years: not recommended; 2-6 years: 1/2 tsp q 12 hrs prn; 6-12 years: 1 tsp q 12 hours prn; >12 years: same as adult
Susp: diphen 12.5 mg+dextro 15 mg+phenyle 15 mg per 5 ml (strawberry banana) (sugar-free, alcohol-free, phenylalanine)

▷ **Duratuss DM (C)** 1 tsp q 4 hours prn
Pediatric: <2 years: not recommended; 2-6 years: 1/4 tsp q 4 hrs prn; >6 years: 1/2 tsp q 4 hours prn
Susp: dextro 25 mg+guaif 225 mg per 5 ml (grape) (sugar-free, alcohol-free)

▷ **Duratuss DM 12 (C)** 1-2 tsp q 12 hours prn; max 6 tabs/day
Pediatric: <2 years: not recommended; 2-6 years: 1/2 tsp q 12 hrs prn; >6 years: 1/2-1 tsp q 12 hours prn; >6 years: same as adult
Susp: dextro 15 mg+guaif 225 mg per 5 ml (grape) (sugar-free, alcohol-free)

(*continued*)

(*continued*)

▷ **Flowtuss Oral Solution (C)(II)(G)** 1-2 tsp q 4-6 hours prn; max 6 tsp/24 hours
   Pediatric: <6 years: not recommended; 6-12 years: 1/2 tsp q 4-6 hours prn; max
   15 ml/day; >12 years: same as adult
   Oral soln: hydro 2.5 mg+guaif 200 mg per 5 ml (black raspberry)
Comment: *hydrocodone* is known to be excreted in human milk.
▷ **Hycodan (C)(III)** 1 tab q 4-6 hours prn; max 6 tabs/day
   Pediatric: <6 years: not recommended; 6-12 years: 1/2 tab q 4-6 hours prn; max
   3 tabs/day; >12 years: same as adult
   Tab: hydro 5 mg+homat 1.5 mg
Comment: *hydrocodone* is known to be excreted in human milk.
▷ **Hycodan Syrup (C)(II)(G)** 1 tsp q 4-6 hours prn
   Pediatric: <6 years: not recommended; 6-12 years: 1/2 tsp q 4-6 hours prn; max
   15 ml/day; >12 years: same as adult
   Syr: hydro 5 mg+homat 1.5 mg per 5 ml
Comment: *hydrocodone* is known to be excreted in human milk.
▷ **Hycofenix Oral Solution (C)(II)** 1 tsp q 4-6 hours prn
   Pediatric: <6 years: not recommended; 6-12 years: 1/2 tsp q 4-6 hours prn; max
   15 ml/day; >12 years: same as adult
   Oral soln: hydro 2.5 mg+pseudo 30 mg+quaf 200 mg per 5 ml (black raspberry)
Comment: *hydrocodone* is known to be excreted in human milk.
▷ **Obredon Oral Solution (C)(II)** 10 ml q 4-6 hours prn cough; max 60 ml/day
   Pediatric: <18 years: not recommended; >18 years: same as adult
   Oral soln: hydro 2.5 mg+guaif 200 mg per 5 ml
Comment: **Obredon** is indicated only for short term treatment of cough due to the
common cold. **Obredon** is not indicated for persistent or chronic cough such as
occurs with smoking, asthma, chronic bronchitis, or emphysema, or where cough
is accompanied by excessive phlegm. Use with caution in patients with diabetes,
thyroid disease, Addison's disease, BPH or urethral stricture, and asthma. **Obredon** is
contraindicated with paralytic ileus, anticholinergics, TCAs, and within 14 days of an
MAOI. *hydrocodone* is known to be excreted in human milk. There is no FDA-approved
generic form of *hydrocodone+guaifenesin.*
▷ **Palgic (C)** 4 mg daily prn; max 24 mg/day in divided doses 6-8 hours apart
   Pediatric: <2 year: not recommended; 2-3 years: 2 mg tid or qid prn or 0.2-0.4 mg/kg/
   day divided tid or qid; 3-6 years: 2-4 mg daily prn or 0.2-0.4 mg/kg/day divided tid or
   qid; >6 years: same as adult
   Tab: carb 4*mg; *Syr:* carb 4 mg per 5 ml (bubble gum)
▷ **Periactin (B)(G)** initially 4 mg tid prn, then adjust as needed; usual range 12-16 mg/
   day; max 32 mg/day
   Pediatric: <2 years: not recommended; 2-6 years: 2 mg 2-3 times/day: max
   12 mg daily; 7-14 years: 4 mg 2-3 times/day: max 16 mg daily; >14 years: same as
   adult
   Tab: cypro 4*mg; *Syr:* cypro 2 mg per 5 ml
▷ **Prolex-DH (C)(III)** 1-1½ tsp qid prn
   Pediatric: <3 years: not recommended; 3-6 years: 1/4-1/2 tsp qid prn; 6-12 years: 1/2-
   1 tsp qid prn; >12 years: same as adult
   Liq: hydro 4.5 mg+pot guaiac 300 mg per 5 ml (tropical fruit punch) (alcohol-free,
   sugar-free)
▷ **Phenergan (C)(G)** 25 mg po or rectally tid ac and HS prn
   Pediatric: <2 years: not recommended; 2-12 years: 0.5 mg/lb or 6.25-25 mg po or
   rectally tid; ≥12 years: same as adult

(*continued*)

(*continued*)

Tab: prometh 12.5*, 25*, 50 mg; *Syr:* prometh 6.25 mg per 5 ml; *Syr fortis:* prometh 25 mg per 5 ml; *Rectal supp:* prometh 12.5, 25, 50 mg

▷ **Promethazine DM (C)(V)(G)** 1 tsp q 4-6 hours prn
Pediatric: <6 years: not recommended; 6-12 years: 1/2-1 tsp q 4-6 hours prn; >12 years: same as adult
Syr: prometh 6.25 mg+dextro 15 mg per 5 ml (alcohol 7%)
Comment: Contraindicated with asthma.

▷ **Promethazine VC (C)(V)(G)** 1 tsp q 4-6 hours prn; max 30 ml/day
Pediatric: 2-6 years: 1.25 ml q 4-6 hours prn; max 7.5 ml/day; 6-12 years: 2.5 ml q 4-6 hours prn; max 15 ml/day; >12 years: same as adult
Syr: prometh 6.25 mg+phenyle 5 mg per 5 ml (alcohol 7%)
Comment: Contraindicated with asthma.

▷ **Promethazine VC w. Codeine (C)(V)(G)** 1 tsp q 4-6 hours prn; max 30 ml/day
Pediatric: <6 years: not recommended; 6-12 years: 1/2-1 tsp q 4-6 hours prn; max 30 ml/day; >12 years: same as adult
Syr: prometh 6.25 mg+phenyle 5 mg+cod 10 mg per 5 ml (alcohol 7%)
Comment: *codeine* is known to be excreted in breast milk. <12 years: not recommended; 12-<18 years: use extreme caution; not recommended for children and adolescents with asthma or other chronic breathing problem. The FDA and the European Medicines Agency (EMA) are investigating the safety of using *codeine*-containing medications to treat pain, cough and colds, in children 12-<18 years because of the potential for serious side effects, including slowed or difficult breathing.

▷ **Promethazine w. Codeine (C)(V)(G)** 1 tsp q 4-6 hours prn
Pediatric: <6 years: not recommended; 6-12 years: 1/2-1 tsp q 4-6 hours prn; >12 years: same as adult
Liq: prometh 6.25 mg+cod 10 mg per 5 ml (alcohol 7%)
Comment: *codeine* is known to be excreted in breast milk. <12 years: not recommended; 12-<18 years: use extreme caution; not recommended for children and adolescents with asthma or other chronic breathing problem. The FDA and the European Medicines Agency (EMA) are investigating the safety of using *codeine*-containing medications to treat pain, cough and colds, in children 12-<18 years because of the potential for serious side effects, including slowed or difficult breathing.

▷ **Rynatan (C)** 1-2 tabs q 12 hours prn
Pediatric: not recommended
Tab: chlor 9 mg+phenyle 25 mg

▷ **Rynatan Pediatric Suspension (C)**
Pediatric: <2 years: not recommended; 2-6 years: 1/2-1 tsp q 12 hours prn; 6-12 years: 1-2 tsp q 12 hours prn; >12 years: same as adult
Susp: chlor 4.5 mg+phenyle 5 mg

▷ **Ryneze (C)** 1 tab q 12 hours prn
Pediatric: <6 years: not recommended; 6-12 years: 1/2 tab q 12 hours prn; >12 years: same as adult
Tab: chlor 8 mg+meth 2.5 mg

▷ **Robitussin AC (C)(III)(G)** 2 tsp q 4 hours prn; max 60 ml/day
Pediatric: <2 years: not recommended; 2-6 years: 1/4-1/2 tsp q 4 hours prn; 6-12 years: 1 tsp q 4 hours prn; >12 years: same as adult
Liq: cod 10 mg+guaif 100 mg per 5 ml

▷ **Rondec Syrup (C)(G)** 1 tsp qid prn; max 30 ml/day
Pediatric: <2 years: not recommended; 2-6 years: 1/4 tsp q 4-6 hours prn; max 7.5 ml/day; 6-12 years: 1/2 tsp q 4-6 hours prn; max 15 ml/day; ≥12 years: same as adult
Syr: phenyle 12.5 mg+chlor 4 mg per 5 ml (bubblegum) (sugar-free, alcohol-free)

(*continued*)

(*continued*)

▷ **Semprex-D (B)** 1 cap q 4-6 hours prn; max 4 doses/day
Pediatric: <12 years: not recommended; ≥12 years: same as adult
    Cap: acriv 8 mg+pseud 60 mg
▷ **Tanafed DMX (C)(G)** 2-4 tsp q 12 hours prn
Pediatric: <2 years: not recommended; 2-6 years: 1/2-1 tsp q 12 hours prn; 6-12 years: 1-2 tsp q 12 hours prn; >12 years: same as adult
    Susp: dexchlor 2.5 mg+pseud 75 mg+dextro 25 mg per 5 ml (cotton candy) (alcohol-free)
▷ **Tessalon Caps (C)** 100-200 mg tid prn; max 600 mg/day
Pediatric: <10 years: not recommended; ≥10 years: same as adult
    Cap: benzo 200 mg
Comment: Swallow whole. Do not suck or chew.
▷ **Tessalon Perles (C)** 100-200 mg tid prn; max 600 mg/day
Pediatric: <10 years: not recommended; ≥10 years: same as adult
    Perles: benzo 100 mg
Comment: Swallow whole. Do not suck or chew.
▷ **Tussi-12 D Tablets (C)** 1-2 tabs q 12 hours prn
Pediatric: <6 years: use susp; 6-11 years: 1/2-1 tab q 12 hours prn; >11 years: same as adult
    Tab: carbeta 60 mg+pyril 40 mg+phenyle 10*mg
▷ **Tussi-12 DS (C)** 1-2 tsp q 12 hours prn
Pediatric: <2 years: individualize; 2-6 years: 1/2-1 tsp q 12 hours prn; 6-12 years: 1-2 tsp q 12 hours prn; >12 years: same as adult
    Liq: carbeta 30 mg+pyril 30 mg+phenyle 5 mg per 5 ml (strawberry-currant) (tartrazine)
▷ **TussiCaps 5 mg/4 mg (C)(III)** 2 caps q 12 hours prn; max 4 caps/day
Pediatric: <6 years: not recommended; 6-12 years: 1 cap q 12 hours prn; max 2 caps/day; >12 years: same as adult
    Cap: hydro 5 mg+chlor 4 mg ext-rel (alcohol)
▷ **TussiCaps 10 mg/8 mg (C)(III)** 1 cap q 12 hours prn; max 2 caps/day
Pediatric: <12 years: not recommended; >12 years: same as adult
    Cap: hydro 10 mg+chlor 8 mg ext-rel (alcohol)
▷ **Tussionex (C)(III)** 1 tsp q 12 hours prn
Pediatric: <6 years: not recommended; 6-12 years: 1/2 tsp q 12 hours prn; >12 years: same as adult
    Susp: hydro 10 mg+chlor 8 mg per 5 ml ext-rel
▷ **Tussi-Organidin DM NR Liquid (C)(III)** 5 ml q 4 hours prn; max 40 ml/day
Pediatric: <6 months: not recommended; 6-23 months: 0.6 ml q 4 hours prn; max 3.7 ml/day; 2-5 years: 1.25 ml q 4 hours prn; max 7.5 ml/day; 6-12 years: 2.5 ml q 4 hours prn; max 15 ml/day; ≥12 years: same as adult
    Liq: dextro 10 mg+guaif 300 mg per 5 ml (grape) (sugar-free, alcohol-free)
▷ **Tussi-Organidin NR (C)(V)** 1 tsp q 4 hours prn; max 40 ml/day
Pediatric: <2 years: not recommended; 2 years: 1.5 ml q 4-6 hours prn; max 6 ml/day; 3 years: 1.75 ml q 4-6 hours prn; max 7 ml/day; 4 years: 2 ml q 4-6 hours prn; max 8 ml/day; 5 years: 2.25 ml q 4-6 hours prn; max 9 ml/day; 6-11 years: 2.5 ml q 4 hours prn; max 20 ml/day; ≥12 years: same as adult
    Liq: cod 10 mg+guaif 300 mg per 5 ml (grape) (sugar-free, alcohol-free)
▷ **Tuzistra XR (C)(III)** 1-2 tsp q 12 hours prn; max 20 ml/day
Pediatric: <18 years: not recommended; ≥18 years: same as adult
    Liq: cod 14.7 mg+chlor 2.8 mg per 5 ml (cherry)

(*continued*)

(continued)

▷ **Vistaril (C)(G)** 25 mg tid <u>or</u> qid prn
  Pediatric: <6 years: 50 mg/day prn; 6-12 years: 50-100 mg daily prn; >12 years: same as adult
    Cap: hydrox 25, 50, 100 mg; *Susp:* hydrox 25 mg/5 ml (lemon)
▷ **Xyzal, Xyzal Oral Solution (B)** 2.5-5 mg in the evening prn
  CrCl 30-50 mL/min: 2.5 mg every other day
  CrCl 10-30 mL/min: 2.5 mg twice weekly
  CrCl <10 mL/min <u>or</u> hemodialysis: contraindicated
  Pediatric: <6 months: not recommended; 6 months-6 years: max 1.25 mg once daily in the PM prn; 6-12 years: max 2.5 mg once daily in the PM prn; >12 years: same as adult
    Tab: levocetir 5*mg film-coat; *Oral soln:* levocetir 0.5 mg/ml (150 ml)

APPENDIX BB. SYSTEMIC ANTI-INFECTIVES

Comment:
- Adverse effects of aminoglycosides include nephrotoxicity and ototoxicity.
- Use cephalosporins with caution in persons with penicillin allergy due to potential cross allergy.
- Sulfonamides are contraindicated with sulfa allergy and G6PD deficiency. A high fluid intake is indicated during sulfonamide therapy.
- Tetracyclines should be taken on an empty stomach to facilitate absorption. Tetracyclines should not be taken with milk.
- Tetracyclines are contraindicated during pregnancy and breastfeeding, and in children <8 years of age, due to the risk of developing tooth enamel discoloration.
- Systemic quinolones and fluoroquinolones are contraindicated in pregnancy and children <18 years of age due to the risk of joint dysplasia.

Anti-infectives by Class With Dose Forms		
Generic Name	**Brand Name**	**Dose Form/Volume**
Amebicides		
chloroquine phosphate **(C)(G)**	**Aralen**	*Tab:* 500 mg
chloroquine phosphate+ primaquine phosphate **(C)(G)**	Aralen Phosphate+ Primaquine Phosphate	*Tab:* chlor 300 mg+prim 45 mg
iodoquinol **(C)**	**Yodoxin**	*Tab:* 210, 650 mg
metronidazole **(not for use in 1st; B in 2nd, 3rd)(G)**	**Flagyl**	*Tab:* 250*, 500*mg
	Flagyl 375	*Cap:* 375 mg
	Flagyl ER	*Tab:* 750 mg ext-rel
tinidazole **(C)**	**Tindamax**	*Tab:* 250*, 500*mg
Aminoglycosides		
amikacin **(C)(G)**	**Amikin**	*Vial:* 500 mg, 1 gm (2 ml)

(continued)

(continued)

Anti-infectives by Class With Dose Forms		
Generic Name	**Brand Name**	**Dose Form/Volume**
gentamicin (C)(G)	**Garamycin**	*Vial:* 20, 80 mg/2 ml
streptomycin (D)(G)	**Streptomycin**	*Amp:* 1 gm/2.5 ml or 400 mg/ml (2.5 ml)
Antifungals		
atovaquone (C)	**Mepron**	*Susp:* 750 mg/5ml (210 ml)
clotrimazole (B)(G)	**Mycelex Troche**	10 mg (70, 40/bottle)
fluconazole (C)(G)	**Diflucan**	*Tab:* 50, 100, 150, 200 mg; *Oral susp:* 10, 40 mg/ml (35 ml) (orange)
griseofulvin, microsize (C)	**Grifulvin V**	*Tab:* 250, 500 mg; *Oral susp:* 125 mg/ 5 ml (120 ml) (alcohol 0.02%)
	Gris-PEG	*Tab:* 125, 250 mg
itraconazole (C)	**Sporanox**	*Cap:* 100 mg; *Soln:* 10 mg/ml (150 ml); *Pulse Pack:* 100 mg caps (7/pck)
ketoconazole (C)(G)	**Nizoral**	*Tab:* 200 mg
nystatin (C)(G)	**Mycostatin**	*Pastille:* 200,000 units/pastille (30 pastilles/pck); *Oral susp:* 100,000 units/ ml (60 ml w. dropper)
terbinafine (B)(G)	**Lamisil**	*Tab:* 250 mg
voriconazole (D)(G)	**Vfend**	*Tab:* 50, 200 mg
Antihelmintics		
albendazole (C)(G)	**Albenza**	*Tab:* 200 mg
ivermectin (C)(G)	**Stromectol**	*Tab:* 3 mg
mebendazole (C)(G)	**Emverm, Vermox**	*Chew tab:* 100 mg
pyrantel pamoate (C)(G)	**Antiminth** **Pin-X**	*Cap:* 180 mg; *Liq:* 50 mg/ml (30 ml); 144 mg/ml (30 ml); *Oral susp:* 50 mg/ml (30 ml) (caramel) (sodium benzoate, tartrazine-free)
thiabendazole (C) (G)	**Mintezol** (currently not available in the United States)	*Chew tab:* 500*mg (orange); *Oral susp:* 500 mg/5 ml (120 ml) (orange)
Antimalarials		
atorvaquone (C)	**Mepron**	*Susp:* 750 mg/5 ml
atovaquone+ proguanil (C)	**Malarone**	*Tab:* atov 250 mg+proq 100 mg
	Malarone Pediatric	*Tab:* atov 62.5 mg+proq 25 mg

(continued)

(continued)

Anti-infectives by Class With Dose Forms		
Generic Name	Brand Name	Dose Form/Volume
chloroquine (C)(G)	Aralen	*Tab:* 500 mg; *Amp:* 50 mg/ml (5 ml)
doxycycline (D)(G)	Acticlate	*Tab:* 75, 150**mg
	Adoxa	*Tab:* 50, 75, 100, 150 mg ent-coat
	Doryx	*Cap:* 100 mg; *Tab:* 50, 75, 100, 150, 200 mg
	Doxsteric	*Tab:* 50 mg del-rel
	Monodox	*Cap:* 50, 75, 100 mg
	Oracea	*Cap:* 40 mg del-rel
	Vibramycin	*Cap:* 50, 100 mg; *Syr:* 50 mg/5 ml (raspberry-apple) (sulfites); *Oral susp:* 25 mg/5 ml (raspberry)
	Vibra-Tab	*Tab:* 100 mg film-coat
hydroxychloroquine (C)(G)	Plaquenil	*Tab:* 200 mg
mefloquine (C)	Lariam	*Tab:* 250 mg
minocycline (D)(G)	Dynacin	*Cap:* 50, 100 mg
	Minocin	*Cap:* 50, 75, 100 mg; *Oral susp:* 50 mg/5 ml (60 ml) (custard) (sulfites, alcohol 5%)
	Minolira	*Tab:* 105, 135 mg ext-rel
	Solodyn	*Tab:* 55, 65, 80, 105, 115 mg ext-rel
Antiprotozoal/Antibacterials		
quinine sulfate (C)(G)	Qualaquin	*Cap:* 324 mg
metronidazole (**not for use in 1st; B in 2nd, 3rd**)(G)	Flagyl, Protostat	*Tab:* 250*, 500*mg
	Flagyl 375	*Cap:* 375 mg
	Flagyl ER	*Tab:* 750 mg ext-rel
nitazoxanide (C)(G)	Alinia	*Tab:* 500 mg; *Oral susp:* 100 mg/5 ml (60 ml) (strawberry)
tinidazole (C)	Tindamax	*Tab:* 250*, 500*mg

(continued)

(*continued*)

Anti-infectives by Class With Dose Forms		
Generic Name	Brand Name	Dose Form/Volume
Antituberculars		
ethambutol (EMB) (B)(G)	**Myambutol**	*Tab:* 100, 400*mg
isoniazid (INH) (C)(G)	*generic only*	*Tab:* 100, 300*mg; *Syr:* 50 mg/5 ml; *Inj:* 100 mg/ml
pyrazinamide (PZA) (C)	*generic only*	*Tab:* 500*mg
rifampin (C)(G)	**Priftin**	*Tab:* 150 mg
	Rifadin	*Cap:* 150, 300 mg
Rifampin+isoniazid (C)	**Rifamate**	*Cap:* rif 300 mg+iso 150 mg
rifampin+isoniazid+ pyrazinamide (C)	**Rifater**	*Tab:* rif 120 mg+iso 50 mg+pyr 300 mg
Antivirals (*for HIV-specific antiviral drugs see page 586*)		
acyclovir (C)(G)	**Zovirax**	*Cap:* 200 mg; *Tab:* 400, 800 mg; *Oral susp:* 200 mg/5 ml (banana)
amantadine (C)(G)	**Symmetrel**	*Tab:* 100 mg; *Syr:* 50 mg/5ml (16 oz) (raspberry)
famciclovir (B)	**Famvir**	*Tab:* 125, 250, 500 mg
lamivudine (C)	**Epivir-HBV**	*Tab:* 100 mg; *Oral soln:* 5 mg/ml (240 ml) (strawberry-banana)
oseltamivir (C)	**Tamiflu**	*Cap:* 75 mg
rimantadine (C)	**Flumadine**	*Tab:* 100 mg
valacyclovir (B)	**Valtrex**	*Tab:* 500 mg; 1 gm
zanamivir	**Relenza**	*Tab:* lami 150+zido 300 mg
Cephalosporins		
1st Generation Cephalosporins		
cefadroxil (B)	**Duricef**	*Cap:* 500 mg; *Tab:* 1 gm; *Oral susp:*250 mg/5 ml (100 ml); 500 mg/5 ml (75, 100 ml) (orange-pineapple)
cefazolin (B)	**Ancef, Zolicef**	*Vial:* 500 mg; 1, 10 gm

(*continued*)

(continued)

Anti-infectives by Class With Dose Forms		
Generic Name	**Brand Name**	**Dose Form/Volume**
cephalexin (B)	Keflex	*Cap:* 250, 333, 500, 750 mg; *Oral susp:* 125, 250 mg/5 ml (100, 200 ml)
2nd Generation Cephalosporins		
cefaclor (B)(G)	generic only	*Tab:* 500 mg; *Cap:* 250, 500 mg; *Susp:* 125 mg/5 ml (75, 150 ml) (strawberry); 187 mg/5 ml (50, 100 ml) (strawberry); 250 mg/5 ml (75, 150 ml) (strawberry); 375 mg/5 ml (50, 100 ml) (strawberry)
cefaclor ext-rel (B) (G)	Cefaclor Extended Release	*Tab:* 375, 500 mg ext-rel
cefamandole (B)	Mandol	*Vial:* 1, 2 gm
cefotetan (B)	Cefotan	*Vial:* 1, 2 gm
cefoxitin (B)	Mefoxin	*Vial:* 1, 2 gm
cefprozil (B)	Cefzil	*Tab:* 250, 500 mg; *Oral susp:* 125, 250 mg/5 ml (50, 75, 100 ml) (bubble gum) (phenylalanine)
ceftaroline (B)	Teflaro	*Vial:* 400, 600 mg
cefuroxime sodium (B)(G)	Zinacef	*Vial:* 750 mg; 1.5 gm
loracarbef (B)	Lorabid	*Pulvule:* 200, 400 mg; *Oral susp:* 100 mg/5 ml (50, 100 ml); 200 mg/5 ml (50, 75, 100 ml) (strawberry bubble gum)
3rd Generation Cephalosporins		
cefoperazone (B)	Cefobid	*Vial:* 1, 2 gm pwdr for reconstitution
cefotaxime (B)	Claforan	*Vial:* 500 mg; 1, 2 gm pwdr for reconstitution
cefpodoxime (B)	Vantin	*Tab:* 100, 200 mg; *Oral susp:* 50, 100 mg/5 ml (50, 75, 100 ml) (lemon creme)
ceftazidime (B)	Ceptaz	*Vial:* 1, 2 gm pwdr for reconstitution
	Fortaz	*Vial:* 500 mg; 1, 2 gm pwdr for reconstitution
	Tazicef	*Vial:* 1, 2 gm pwdr for reconstitution
	Tazidime	*Vial:* 1, 2 gm pwdr for reconstitution

(continued)

(*continued*)

Anti-infectives by Class With Dose Forms		
Generic Name	Brand Name	Dose Form/Volume
Ceftazidime/ avibactam (B)	Avycaz	*Vial:* 2.5 gm pwdr for reconstitution
ceftibuten (B)	Cedax	*Cap:* 400 mg; *Oral susp:* 90 mg/5 ml (30, 60, 90, 120 ml); 180 mg/5 ml (30, 60, 120 ml) (cherry)
3rd/4th Generation Cephalosporins		
cefdinir (B)	Omnicef	*Cap:* 300 mg; *Oral susp:* 125 mg/5 ml (60, 100 ml) (strawberry)
cefditoren pivoxil (C)	Spectracef	*Tab:* 200 mg
cefepime (B)	Maxipime	*Vial:* 1 gm pwdr for reconstitution
cefixime (B)(G)	Suprax	*Tab/Cap:* 400 mg; *Oral Susp:* 100 mg/5 ml (50, 75, 100 ml) (strawberry)
ceftaroline (B)	Teflaro	*Vial:* 400, 600 mg
ceftriaxone (B)(G)	Rocephin	*Vial:* 250, 500 mg; 1, 2 gm
cytolozane+ tazobactam (B)	Zerbaxa	*Vial:* 1.5 gm pwdr for reconstitution
Penicillins		
amoxicillin (B)(G)	Amoxil	*Cap:* 250, 500 mg; *Tab:* 500, 875* mg; *Chew tab:* 125, 200, 250, 400 mg (cherry-banana-peppermint) (phenylalanine); *Oral susp:*125, 250 mg/ml (80, 100, 150 ml) (bubble gum); 200, 400 mg/5 ml (50, 75, 100 ml) (bubble gum); *Oral drops:* 50 mg/ml (30 ml) (bubble gum)
	Moxatag	*Tab:* 775 mg ext-rel
	Trimox	*Cap:* 250, 500 mg; *Oral susp:* 125, 250 mg/5ml (80, 100, 150 ml) (raspberry-strawberry)

(*continued*)

(*continued*)

Anti-infectives by Class With Dose Forms		
Generic Name	Brand Name	Dose Form/Volume
amoxicillin+ clavulanate (B)(G)	**Augmentin**	*Tab:* 250, 500, 875 mg; *Chew tab:* 125, 250 mg (lemon lime); 200, 400 mg (cherry-banana; phenylalanine); *Oral susp:* 125 mg/5 ml (banana), 250 mg/5 ml (orange) (75, 100, 150 ml); 200, 400 mg/5 ml (50, 75, 100 ml) (orange)
	Augmentin ES-600	*Oral susp:* 600 mg/5 ml (50, 75, 100, 125, 150, 200 ml) (strawberry cream) (phenylalanine)
	Augmentin XR	*Tab:* 1000*mg ext-rel
ampicillin (B)(G)	**Omnipen**	*Cap:* 250, 500 mg; *Oral susp:* 125, 250 mg/ml (100, 150, 200 ml)
	Principen	*Cap:* 250, 500 mg; *Syr:* 125, 250 mg/5 ml
ampicillin+ sulbactam (B)(G)	**Unasyn**	*Vial:* 1.5, 3 gm
carbenicillin (B)	**Geocillin**	*Tab:* 382 mg film-coat
dicloxacillin (B)(G)	**Dynapen**	*Cap:* 125, 250, 500 mg; *Oral susp:* 62.5 mg/5 ml (80, 100, 200 ml)
ertapenem (B)	**Invanz**	*Vial:* 1 gm pwdr for reconstitution
meropenem (B)(G)	**Merrem**	*Vial:* 500 mg; 1 gm pwdr for reconstitution (sodium 3.92 mEq/gm)
penicillin g benzathine (B)(G)	**Bicillin LA, Bicillin C-R**	*Cartridge-needle unit:* 600,000 million units (1 ml); 1.2 million units (2 ml); 2.4 million units (4 ml)
	Permapen	*Prefilled syringe:* 1.2 million units
penicillin g potassium (B)(G)	*generic only*	*Vial:* 5, 20 MU pwdr for reconstitution; *Premixed bag:* 1, 2, 3 MU (50 ml)
penicillin g procaine (B)(G)	*generic only*	*Prefilled syringe:* 1.2 million units
penicillin v potassium (B)(G)	**Pen-Vee K**	*Tab:* 250, 500 mg; *Oral soln:* 125 mg/5 ml (100, 200 ml); 250 mg/5 ml (100, 150, 200 ml)

(*continued*)

(*continued*)

Anti-infectives by Class With Dose Forms		
Generic Name	Brand Name	Dose Form/Volume
piperacillin+ tazobactam (B)(G)	**Zosyn**	*Vial:* 2, 3, 4 gm pwdr for reconstitution
Quinolone and Fluoroquinolones		
1st Generation Quinolone		
enoxacin (C)	**Penetrex**	*Tab:* 200, 400 mg
1st Generation Fluoroquinolones		
ciprofloxacin (C)(G)	**Cipro**	*Tab:* 250, 500, 750 mg; *Oral susp:* 250, 500 mg/5 ml (100 ml) (strawberry); *IV conc:* 10 mg/ml after dilution (20, 40 ml); *Premixed bag:* 2 mg/ml (100, 200 ml)
	Cipro XR	*Tab:* 500, 1000 mg ext-rel
	ProQuin XR	*Tab:* 500 mg ext-rel
lomefloxacin (C)	**Maxaquin**	*Tab:* 400 mg
norfloxacin (C)(G)	**Noroxin**	*Tab:* 400 mg
ofloxacin (C)(G)	**Floxin**	*Tab:* 200, 300, 400 mg
lomefloxacin (C)	**Floxin**	*Tab:* 200, 300, 400 mg
3rd Generation Fluoroquinolone		
levofloxacin (C)(G)	**Levaquin**	*Tab:* 250, 500, 750 mg
4th Generation Fluoroquinolone		
delafloxacin (C)	**Baxdela**	*Tab:* 400 mg; *Vial:* 300 mg pwdr for reconstitution
gemifloxacin (C)(G)	**Factive**	*Tab:* 320*mg
moxifloxacin (C)(G)	**Avelox**	*Tab:* 400 mg
Ketolide		
telithromycin (C)	**Ketek**	*Tab:* 300, 400 mg
Macrolides		
azithromycin (B)	**Zithromax**	*Tab:* 250, 500, 600 mg; *Granules:* 1 gm/ pck for reconstitution (cherry-banana)
	ZithPed Syr	*Oral susp:* 100 mg/5 ml, (15 ml); 200 mg/5 ml (15, 22.5, 30 ml) (cherry)

(*continued*)

(*continued*)

Anti-infectives by Class With Dose Forms		
Generic Name	Brand Name	Dose Form/Volume
	Zithromax Tri-Pak	*Tab:* 3 x 500 mg tabs/pck
	Zithromax Z-Pak	*Tab:* 6 x 250 mg tabs/pck
	Zmax	*Granules:* 2 gm/pkt for reconstitution (cherry-banana)
clarithromycin (C) (G)	**Biaxin**	*Tab:* 250, 500 mg; *Oral susp:* 125, 250 mg/5 ml (50, 100 ml) (fruit punch)
	Biaxin XL	*Tab:* 500 mg ext-rel
dirithromycin (C) (G)	*generic only*	*Tab:* 250 mg
erythromycin base (B)(G)	**Ery-Tab**	*Tab:* 250, 333, 500 mg ent-coat
	PCE	*Tab:* 333, 500 mg
erythromycin estolate (B)(G)	**Ilosone**	*Pulvule:* 250 mg; *Tab:* 500 mg; *Liq:* 125, 250 mg/5 ml (100 ml)
erythromycin ethylsuccinate (B) (G)	**E.E.S.**	*Tab:* 400 mg; *Oral susp:* 200 mg/5 ml (100, 200 ml) (cherry); 200, 400 mg/5 ml (100 ml) (fruit)
erythromycin ethylsuccinate (B) (G)	**EryPed**	*Oral susp:* 200 mg/5 ml (100, 200 ml) (fruit); 400 mg/5 ml (60, 100, 200 ml) (banana); *Oral drops:* 200, 400 mg/5 ml (50 ml) (fruit); *Chew tab:* 200 mg (fruit)
erythromycin stearate (B)(G)	**Erythrocin**	*Film tab:* 250, 500 mg
Macrolide+Sulfonamide		
erythromycin ethylsuccinate+ sulfisoxazole (C)(G)	**Pediazole**	*Oral susp:* eryth 200 mg+sulf 600 mg per 5 ml (100, 150, 200 ml) (strawberry-banana)
Sulfonamides		
sulfamethoxazole (B/D)(G)	**Gantrisin Pediatric**	*Oral susp:* 500 mg/5 ml; *Syr:* 500 mg/5 ml

(*continued*)

(*continued*)

Anti-infectives by Class With Dose Forms		
Generic Name	Brand Name	Dose Form/Volume
trimethoprim (C) (G)	**Primsol**	*Oral soln:* 50 mg/5 ml (bubble gum) (dye-free, alcohol-free)
	Trimpex	*Tab:* 100 mg
	Proloprim	*Tab:* 100, 200 mg
trimethoprim+ sulfamethoxazole (C)(G)	**Bactrim, Septra**	*Tab:* trim 80 mg+sulfa 400 mg*
	Bactrim DS, Septra DS	*Tab:* trim 160 mg+sulfa 800 mg*; *Oral susp:* trim 40 mg+sulfa 200 mg per 5 ml (100 ml) (cherry) (alcohol 0.3%)
Tetracyclines		
demeclocycline (D)	**Declomycin**	*Tab:* 300 mg
doxycycline (D)(G)	**Adoxa**	*Tab:* 50, 100 mg ent-coat
	Doryx	*Cap:* 100 mg
	Monodox	*Cap:* 50, 100 mg
doxycycline (D)(G)	**Vibramycin**	*Cap:* 50, 100 mg; *Syr:* 50 mg/5 ml; (raspberry) (sulfites); *Oral susp:* 25 mg/5 ml (raspberry-apple); *IV conc:* doxy 100 mg+asc acid 480 mg after dilution; doxy 200 mg+asc acid 960 mg after dilution
	Vibra-Tab	*Tab:* 100 mg film-coat
minocycline (D)(G)	**Dynacin**	*Cap:* 50, 100 mg
	Minocin	*Cap:* 50, 100 mg; *Oral susp:* 50 mg/5 ml (60 ml) (custard) (sulfites, alcohol 5%); *Vial:* 100 mg soln for inj
	Minolira	*Tab:* 105, 135 mg ext-rel
tetracycline (D)(G)	**Achromycin V**	*Cap:* 250, 500 mg
	Sumycin	*Tab:* 250, 500 mg; *Oral susp:* 125 mg/5 ml (fruit) (sulfites)
Unclassified/Miscellaneous		
aztreonam (B)	**Cayston**	*Vial:* 75 mg pwdr for reconstitution (preservative-free)
chloramphenicol (C)(G)	**Chloromycetin**	*Vial:* 1 gm

(*continued*)

(*continued*)

Anti-infectives by Class With Dose Forms		
Generic Name	Brand Name	Dose Form/Volume
clindamycin (B)(G)	Cleocin	*Cap:* 75 (tartrazine), 150 (tartrazine), 300 mg; *Oral susp:* 75 mg/5 ml (100 ml) (cherry); *Vial:* 150 mg/ml (2, 4 ml) (benzyl alcohol)
dalbavancin (C)	Dalvance	*Vial:* 500 mg pwdr for reconstitution (preservative-free)
daptomycin (B)(G)	Cubicin	*Vial:* 500 mg pwdr for reconstitution
doripenem (B)	Doribax	*Vial:* 500 mg pwdr for reconstitution
fosfomycin (B)	Monurol	*Sachet:* 3 gm single-dose (mandarin orange; sucrose)
imipenem+ cilastatin (C)(G)	Primaxin	*Vial:* imip 500 mg+cila 500 mg; imip 750 mg+cila 750 mg pwdr for reconstitution
lincomycin (B)(G)	Lincocin	*Vial:* 300 mg/ml (10 ml)
linezolid (C)(G)	Zyvox	*Tab:* 400, 600 mg; *Oral susp:* 100 mg/5 ml (orange) (phenylalanine); *IV:* 2 mg ml (100, 200, 300 ml)
meropenem (B)	Merrem	*Vial:* 500 mg; 1 gm (sodium 3.92 mEq/gm)
meropenem+ vaborbactam	Vabomere	*Vial:* mero 1 gm+vabor 1 gm pwdr for reconstitution, single-dose
nitrofurantoin (B) (G)	Furadantin	*Oral susp:* 25 mg/5 ml (60 ml)
	Macrobid	*Cap:* 100 mg
	Macrodantin	*Cap:* 25, 50, 100 mg
quinupristin+ dalfopristin (B)	Synercid	*Vial:* quin 150 mg+dalfo 350 mg, quin 180 mg+dalfo 420 mg single-dose
tygecycline (D)(G)	Tygacil	*Vial:* 50 mg pwdr for reconstitution
rifaximin (C)	Xifaxan	*Tab:* 200, 550 mg
telavancin (C)	Vibativ	*Vial:* 250, 750 mg pwdr for reconstitution (preservative-free)
vancomycin (C)(G)	Vancocin	*Cap:* 125, 250 mg; *Vial:* 500 mg, 1 gm pwdr for reconstitution

APPENDIX CC.1. *ACYCLOVIR* (ZOVIRAX SUSPENSION)

Weight

Pounds	15	20	25	30	35	40	45	50	55	60	65	70
Kilograms	6.8	9	11.4	13.6	15.9	18.2	20.5	22.7	25	27.3	29.5	31.8

Single Dose (ml)/Frequency/Strength/5-Day Volume (ml)

	15	20	25	30	35	40	45	50	55	60	65	70
20 mg/kg/d ml/dose qid	3.5	4.5	5.5	6.5	8	9	10	11.5	12.5	13.5	14.5	16
mg/5 ml	200	200	200	200	200	200	200	200	200	200	200	200
Volume (ml)	70	90	110	130	160	180	200	230	250	270	290	320

Zovirax Oral Suspension <2 years: not recommended; >2 years, <40 kg: 20 mg/kg dosed qid x 5 days; ≥2 years, >40 kg: 800 mg dosed qid x 5 days; *Oral susp:* 200 mg/5 ml (banana).

APPENDIX CC.2. *AMANTADINE* (SYMMETREL SYRUP)

Weight

Pounds	15	20	25	30	35	40	45	50	55	60	65	70
Kilograms	6.8	9	11.4	13.6	15.9	18.2	20.5	22.7	25	27.3	29.5	31.8

Single Dose (ml)/Frequency/Strength/10-Day Volume (ml)

	15	20	25	30	35	40	45	50	55	60	65	70
4 mg/kg/d ml/dose bid	3	4	5	6	7	8	9	10	11	12	13	14
mg/5 ml	50	50	50	50	50	50	50	50	50	50	50	50
Volume (ml)	30	40	50	60	70	80	90	100	110	120	130	140
8 mg/lb/d ml/dose bid	6	8	10	12								
mg/5 ml	50	50	50	50								
Volume (ml)	60	80	100	60								

Symmetrel Suspension (C)(G) Symmetrel <1 year: not recommended; 1-8 years: max 150 mg/day; 9-12 years: 100 mg bid; >12 years: 100 mg bid or 200 mg once daily; *Syr*: 50 mg/5 ml (raspberry).

APPENDIX CC.3. *AMOXICILLIN* (AMOXIL SUSPENSION, TRIMOX SUSPENSION)

Weight

Pounds	15	20	25	30	35	40	45	50	55	60	65	70
Kilograms	6.8	9	11.4	13.6	15.9	18.2	20.5	22.7	25	27.3	29.5	31.8
Single Dose (ml)/Frequency/Strength/10-Day Volume (ml)												
20 mg/kg/d ml/dose tid	2	2.5	3	3.5	4	5	5.5	6	7	7.5	8	9
mg/5 ml	125	125	125	125	125	125	125	125	125	125	125	125
Volume (ml)	60	75	90	105	120	150	165	180	210	225	240	270
30 mg/kg/d ml/dose tid	3	3.5	2.5	3	3	3.5	4	4.5	5	5.5	6	6.5
mg/5 ml	125	125	250	250	250	250	250	250	250	250	250	250
Volume (ml)	90	105	75	90	90	105	120	135	150	165	180	195
40 mg/kg/d ml/dose bid	5	7	4.5	5	6	7	8	9	10	11	12	13
mg/5 ml	125	125	250	250	250	250	250	250	250	250	250	250
Volume (ml)	100	140	90	100	120	140	160	180	200	220	240	250
45 mg/kg/d ml/dose bid	4	2.5	3	4	4.5	5	6	6.5	7	7.5	8.5	9

(continued)

APPENDIX CC.3: *AMOXICILLIN* (AMOXIL SUSPENSION, TRIMOX SUSPENSION) (*continued*)

mg/5 ml	200	400	400	400	400	400	400	400	400	400	400	400
Volume (ml)	80	50	60	80	90	100	120	130	140	150	170	180
90 mg/kg/d ml/dose bid	8	5	6	7	9	10	12	13	14	15	17	18
mg/5 ml	200	400	400	400	400	400	400	400	400	400	400	400
Volume (ml)	160	100	120	140	180	200	240	260	280	300	340	360

<40 kg (88 lb): 20-30 mg/kg/day in 3 divided doses or 40-90 mg/kg/day in 2 divided doses; >40 kg: same as adult.

Amoxil Suspension (B)(G) 125, 250 mg/5 ml (80, 100, 150 ml) (strawberry); 200, 400 mg/5 ml (50, 75, 100 ml) (bubble gum).

Trimox Suspension (B)(G) 125, 250 mg/5 ml (80, 100, 150 ml) (raspberry-strawberry).

APPENDIX CC.4. AMOXICILLIN+CLAVULANATE (AUGMENTIN SUSPENSION)

Weight												
Pounds	15	20	25	30	35	40	45	50	55	60	65	70
Kilograms	6.8	9	11.4	13.6	15.9	18.2	20.5	22.7	25	27.3	29.5	31.8
Single Dose (ml)/Frequency/Strength/10-Day Volume (ml)												
40 mg/kg/d ml/dose bid	5.5	7	4.5	5.5	6.5	7	8	9	10	11	12	13
mg/5 ml	125	125	250	250	250	250	250	250	250	250	250	250
Volume (ml)	110	140	90	110	130	140	160	180	200	220	240	260
45 mg/kg/d ml/dose bid	3	4	5	6	7	8	9	10	11.5	12.5	13.5	14.5
mg/5 ml	250	250	250	250	250	250	250	250	250	250	250	250
Volume (ml)	60	80	100	120	140	160	180	200	230	250	270	290
45 mg/kg/d ml/dose bid	4	2.5	3	4	4.5	5	6	6.5	7	7.5	8.5	9
mg/5 ml	200	400	400	400	400	400	400	400	400	400	400	400
Volume (ml)	80	50	60	80	90	100	120	130	140	150	170	180
90 mg/kg/d ml/dose bid	4	5	6.5	8	9	10	11.5	13	14	15.5	16.5	18
mg/5 ml	400	400	400	400	400	400	400	400	400	400	400	400
Volume (ml)	80	100	130	160	180	200	240	260	280	300	340	360

Augmentin Suspension (B)(G) 40–45 mg/kg/day divided tid or 90 mg/kg/day divided bid; 125 mg/5 ml (75, 100, 150 ml) (banana), 250 mg/5 ml (75, 100, 150 ml) (orange); 200, 400 mg/5 ml (50, 75, 100 ml) (orange-raspberry) (phenylalanine).

APPENDIX CC.5. *AMOXICILLIN+CLAVULANATE* (AUGMENTIN ES 600 SUSPENSION)

Weight

Pounds	15	20	25	30	35	40	45	50	55	60	65	70
Kilograms	6.8	9	11.4	13.6	15.9	18.2	20.5	22.7	25	27.3	29.5	31.8

Single Dose (ml)/Frequency/Strength/10-Day Volume (ml)

	15	20	25	30	35	40	45	50	55	60	65	70
40 mg/kg/d ml/dose bid	1	1.5	2	2	2.5	3	3.5	4	4	4.5	5	5
mg/5 ml	600	600	600	600	600	600	600	600	600	600	600	600
Volume (ml)	30	40	40	40	50	60	70	80	80	90	100	100
45 mg/kg/d ml/dose bid	1.25	1.5	2	2.5	3	3.5	4	4.5	5	5	5.5	6
mg/5 ml	600	600	600	600	600	600	600	600	600	600	600	600
Volume (ml)	25	30	40	50	60	70	80	90	100	100	110	120
90 mg/kg/d ml/dose bid	2.5	3.5	4	5	6	7	8	8.5	9.5	10	11	12
mg/5 ml	600	600	600	600	600	600	600	600	600	600	600	600
Volume (ml)	50	70	80	100	120	140	160	170	190	200	220	240

Augmentin ES 600 Suspension (B) <3 months: not recommended; ≥3 months, <40 kg: 90 mg/kg/day in 2 divided doses; ≥40 kg: not recommended; 600 mg/5 ml (50, 75, 100, 125, 150, 200 ml) (strawberry cream) (phenylalanine).

APPENDIX CC.6. *AMPICILLIN* (OMNIPEN SUSPENSION, PRINCIPEN SUSPENSION)

Weight

Pounds	15	20	25	30	35	40	45	50	55	60	65	70
Kilograms	6.8	9	11.4	13.6	15.9	18.2	20.5	22.7	25	27.3	29.5	31.8

Single Dose (ml)/Frequency/Strength/10-Day Volume (ml)

	15	20	25	30	35	40	45	50	55	60	65	70
50 mg/kg/d ml/dose q6h	3.5	4.5	3	3.5	4	4.5						
mg/5 ml	125	125	250	250	250	250						
Volume (ml)	140	180	120	140	160	180						
100 mg/kg/d ml/dose q6h	3.5	4.5	6	7	8	9						
mg/5 ml	250	250	250	250	250	250						
Volume (ml)	140	180	240	280	320	360						

Omnipen Suspension, Principen Suspension (B)(G) >20 kg: 250–500 mg q 6 h 125, 250 mg/5 ml (100, 150, 200 ml) (fruit).

APPENDIX CC.7. *AZITHROMYCIN* (ZITHROMAX SUSPENSION, ZMAX SUSPENSION)

Weight								
Pounds	11	22	33	44	55	66	77	88
Kilograms	5	10	15	20	25	30	35	40
Single Dose (ml)/Frequency/Strength/Volume (ml)								
3 Day Regimen								
10 mg/kg qd	2.5	5	7.5	5	6	7.5	9	10
mg/5 ml	100	100	100	200	200	200	200	200
Volume (ml)	7.5	15	22.5	15	18	22.5	27	30
5 Day Regimen								
10 mg/kg qd								
Day 1	2.5	5	7.5	5	6	7.5	7.5	10
Days 2–5	1.25	2.5	4	2.5	3	4	4	5
Volume (ml)	10	15	23.5	15	18	23.5	23.5	30

Zithromax ES 600 Suspension (B)(G) 100 mg/5 ml (15 ml), 200 mg/5 ml (15, 22.5, 30 ml) (cherry-vanilla-banana).

APPENDIX CC.8. *CEFACLOR* (CECLOR SUSPENSION)

Weight												
Pounds	15	20	25	30	35	40	45	50	55	60	65	70
Kilograms	6.8	9	11.4	13.6	15.9	18.2	20.5	22.7	25	27.3	29.5	31.8
Single Dose (ml)/Frequency/Strength/10-Day Volume (ml)												
20 mg/kg/d ml/dose tid	2	2.5	3	3.5	4	5	5.5	6	7	7.5	8	8.5
mg/5 ml	125	125	125	125	125	125	125	125	125	125	125	125
Volume (ml)	60	75	90	105	120	150	165	180	210	225	240	255
20 mg/kg/d ml/dose tid	1.5	1.5	2	2.5	3	3	4	4	4.5	5	5.5	6
mg/5 ml	187	187	187	187	187	187	187	187	187	187	187	187
Volume (ml)	45	45	60	75	90	90	105	120	135	150	165	180
40 mg/kg/d ml/dose tid	2	2.5	3	3.5	4	5	5.5	6	6.5	7	8	8.5
mg/5 ml	250	250	250	250	250	250	250	250	250	250	250	250
Volume (ml)	60	75	90	105	120	150	165	180	195	210	240	255
40 mg/kg/d ml/dose tid	1.5	1.5	2	2.5	3	3	3.5	4	4.5	5	5	5.5
mg/5 ml	375	375	375	375	375	375	375	375	375	375	375	375
Volume (ml)	45	45	60	75	90	90	105	120	135	150	150	165

Ceclor Suspension (B) <6 months: not recommended; 125, 250 mg/5 ml (75, 150 ml) (strawberry); 187, 375 mg/5 ml (50, 100 ml) (strawberry).

APPENDIX CC.9. *CEFADROXIL* (DURICEF SUSPENSION)

Weight												
Pounds	15	20	25	30	35	40	45	50	55	60	65	70
Kilograms	6.8	9	11.4	13.6	15.9	18.2	20.5	22.7	25	27.3	29.5	31.8
Single Dose (ml)/Frequency/Strength/10-Day Volume (ml)												
30 mg/kg/d ml/dose bid	2	3	3.5	4	5	5.5	6	7	7.5	8	9	9.5
mg/5 ml	250	250	250	250	250	250	250	250	250	250	250	250
Volume (ml)	40	60	75	80	100	110	120	140	150	160	180	190
30 mg/kg/d ml/dose qd	2	3	3.5	4	5	5.5	6	7	7.5	8	9	9.5
mg/5 ml	500	500	500	500	500	500	500	500	500	500	500	500
Volume (ml)	20	30	35	40	50	55	60	70	75	80	90	95

Duricef Suspension (B) 250 mg/5 ml (100 ml) (orange-pineapple); 500 mg/5 ml (75, 100 ml) (orange-pineapple).

APPENDIX CC.10. *CEFDINIR* (OMNICEF SUSPENSION)

Weight

Pounds	15	20	25	30	35	40	45	50	55	60	65	70
Kilograms	6.8	9	11.4	13.6	15.9	18.2	20.5	22.7	25	27.3	29.5	31.8

Single Dose (ml)/Frequency/Strength/10-Day Volume (ml)

	15	20	25	30	35	40	45	50	55	60	65	70
7 mg/kg/d ml/dose bid	2	2.5	3	4	4.5	5	6	6.5	7	7.5	8	9
mg/5 ml	125	125	125	125	125	125	125	125	125	125	125	125
Volume (ml)	40	50	60	80	90	100	120	130	140	150	160	180
14 mg/kg ml/dose bid	4	5	6	8	9	10	12	13	14	15	16	18
mg/5 ml	125	125	125	125	125	125	125	125	125	125	125	125
Volume (ml)	40	50	60	80	90	100	120	130	140	150	160	180

Omnicef Suspension (B) <6 months: not recommended; 125 mg/5 ml (60, 100 ml) (strawberry).

APPENDIX CC.11. *CEFIXIME* (SUPRAX ORAL SUSPENSION)

Weight

Pounds	15	20	25	30	35	40	45	50	55	60	65	70
Kilograms	6.8	9	11.4	13.6	15.9	18.2	20.5	22.7	25	27.3	29.5	31.8
Single Dose (ml)/Frequency/Strength/10-Day Volume (ml)												
8 mg/kg/d ml/dose bid	1.3	1.8	2.2	2.5	3.1	3.5	4	4.5	5	5.5	6	6.5
mg/5 ml	100	100	100	100	100	100	100	100	100	100	100	100
8 mg/kg/d ml/dose qd	2.7	3.6	4.5	5.5	6.3	7.2	8.2	9	10	11	12	13
mg/5 ml	100	100	100	100	100	100	100	100	100	100	100	100
Volume (ml)	27	36	45	55	65	70	80	90	100	110	120	130

Supra Oral Suspension (B)(G) <6 months: not recommended; 100 mg/5 ml (50, 75, 100 ml) (strawberry).

APPENDIX CC.12. CEFPODOXIME PROXETIL (VANTIN SUSPENSION)

Weight

Pounds	15	20	25	30	35	40	45	50	55	60	65	70
Kilograms	6.8	9	11.4	13.6	15.9	18.2	20.5	22.7	25	27.3	29.5	31.8

Single Dose (ml)/Frequency/Strength/10-Day Volume (ml)

	15	20	25	30	35	40	45	50	55	60	65	70
5 mg/kg/d ml/dose bid	3.5	4.5	5.5	7	8	9	10	11	12.5	13.5	15	16
mg/5 ml	50	50	50	50	50	50	50	50	50	50	50	50
Volume (ml)	70	90	110	140	160	180	200	220	250	270	300	320
5 mg/kg/d ml/dose bid	2	2	3	3.5	4	4.5	5	5.5	6	7	7.5	8
mg/5 ml	100	100	100	100	100	100	100	100	100	100	100	100
Volume (ml)	40	40	60	70	80	90	100	110	120	140	150	160

Vantin Suspension (B) <2 months: not recommended; 50, 100 mg/5 ml (50, 75, 100 ml) (lemon-crème).

APPENDIX CC.13. *CEFPROZIL* (CEFZIL SUSPENSION)

Weight

Pounds	15	20	25	30	35	40	45	50	55	60	65	70
Kilograms	6.8	9	11.4	13.6	15.9	18.2	20.5	22.7	25	27.3	29.5	31.8

Single Dose (ml)/Frequency/Strength/10-Day Volume (ml)

	15	20	25	30	35	40	45	50	55	60	65	70
7.5 mg/kg/d ml/dose bid	2	3	3.5	4	5	5.5	6	7	7.5	4	4.5	5
mg/5 ml	125	125	125	125	125	125	125	125	125	250	250	250
Volume (ml)	40	60	70	80	100	110	120	140	150	80	90	100
15 mg/kg/d ml/dose bid	2	3	3.5	4	5	5	6	7	7.5	8	9	9.5
mg/5 ml	250	250	250	250	250	250	250	250	250	250	250	250
Volume (ml)	40	60	70	80	100	100	120	140	150	160	180	190
20 mg/kg/d ml/dose qd	3	3.5	4.5	5.5	6.5	7	8	9	10	11	12	13
mg/5 ml	250	250	250	250	250	250	250	250	250	250	250	250
Volume (ml)	60	70	90	110	130	140	160	180	200	220	240	260

Cefzil Suspension (B) ≤6 months: not recommended; 2-12 years: 7.5-20 mg/kg bid >12 years: same as adult, 250-500 mg bid or 500 mg once daily; 125, 250 mg/5 ml (50, 75, 100 ml) (bubble gum) (phenylalanine).

APPENDIX CC.14. *CEFTIBUTEN* (CEDAX SUSPENSION)

Weight

Pounds	15	20	25	30	35	40	45	50	55	60	65	70
Kilograms	6.8	9	11.4	13.6	15.9	18.2	20.5	22.7	25	27.3	29.5	31.8

Single Dose (ml)/Frequency/Strength/10-Day Volume (ml)

9 mg/kg/d ml/dose qd	3.5	4.5	6	7	8	9	10	11.5	12.5	13.5	15	16
mg/5 ml	90	90	90	90	90	90	90	90	90	90	90	90
Volume (ml)	35	45	60	70	80	90	100	115	125	135	150	160
9 mg/kg/d ml/dose qd	1.75	2.3	3	3.5	4	4.5	5	5.4	6.2	6.6	7.5	8
mg/5 ml	180	180	180	180	180	180	180	180	180	180	180	180
Volume (ml)	20	25	30	35	40	45	50	55	60	65	70	80

Cefzil Suspension (B) 90 mg/5 ml (30, 60, 90, 120 ml) (cherry); 180 mg/5 ml (30, 60, 120 ml) (cherry).

APPENDIX CC.15. *CEPHALEXIN* (KEFLEX SUSPENSION)

Weight												
Pounds	15	20	25	30	35	40	45	50	55	60	65	70
Kilograms	6.8	9	11.4	13.6	15.9	18.2	20.5	22.7	25	27.3	29.5	31.8
Single Dose (ml)/Frequency/Strength/10-Day Volume (ml)												
25 mg/kg/d ml/dose tid	1	1.5	2	2	3	3	3.5	4	4	4.5	5	5
mg/5 ml	125	125	125	125	125	125	125	125	125	125	125	125
Volume (ml)	30	45	60	60	90	90	105	120	120	135	150	150
25 mg/kg/d ml/dose qid	1	1	1.5	2	2	2.5	2.5	3	3	3.5	4	4
mg/5 ml	250	250	250	250	250	250	250	250	250	250	250	250
Volume (ml)	40	40	60	80	80	100	100	120	120	140	160	160
50 mg/kg/d ml/dose tid	2	3	4	4.5	5	6	7	7.5	8	9	10	10.5
mg/5 ml	250	250	250	250	250	250	250	250	250	250	250	250
Volume (ml)	60	90	120	135	150	180	210	225	240	270	300	315
50 mg/kg/d ml/dose qid	2	2	3	3.5	4	4.5	5	6	6	7	7.5	8
mg/5 ml	250	250	250	250	250	250	250	250	250	250	250	250
Volume (ml)	80	80	120	140	160	180	200	240	240	280	300	320

Keflex Suspension (B)(G) <2 months: not recommended; 125, 250 mg/5 ml (100, 200 ml) (strawberry).

APPENDIX CC.16. *CLARITHROMYCIN* (BIAXIN SUSPENSION)

Weight

Pounds	15	20	25	30	35	40	45	50	55	60	65	70
Kilograms	6.8	9	11.4	13.6	15.9	18.2	20.5	22.7	25	27.3	29.5	31.8

Single Dose (ml)/Frequency/Strength/10-Day Volume (ml)

7.5 mg/kg/d ml/dose bid	2	3	3.5	4	5	5.5	6	7	7.5	8	9	10
mg/5 ml	125	125	125	125	125	125	125	125	125	125	125	125
Volume (ml)	40	60	70	80	100	110	120	140	150	160	180	200
7.5 mg/kg/d ml/dose bid	1	1.5	2	2	2.5	3	3	3.5	4	4	4.5	5
mg/5 ml	250	250	250	250	250	250	250	250	250	250	250	250
Volume (ml)	20	30	40	40	50	60	60	70	80	80	90	100

Biaxin Suspension (B) <6 months: not recommended; 125, 250 mg/5 ml (50, 100 ml) (fruit-punch).

APPENDIX CC.17. *CLINDAMYCIN* (CLEOCIN PEDIATRIC GRANULES)

Weight

Pounds	15	20	25	30	35	40	45	50	55	60	65	70
Kilograms	6.8	9	11.4	13.6	15.9	18.2	20.5	22.7	25	27.3	29.5	31.8

Single Dose (ml)/Frequency/Strength/10-Day Volume (ml)

	15	20	25	30	35	40	45	50	55	60	65	70
8 mg/kg/d ml/dose tid	1	1.5	2	2.5	3	3	3.5	4	4.5	5	5	5.5
mg/5 ml	75	75	75	75	75	75	75	75	75	75	75	75
Volume (ml)	30	45	60	75	90	90	105	120	135	150	150	165
16 mg/kg/d ml/dose tid	2.5	3	4	5	5.5	6.5	7	8	9	9.5	10.5	11
mg/5 ml	75	75	75	75	75	75	75	75	75	75	75	75
Volume (ml)	75	90	120	150	165	105	210	240	270	285	315	330

Cleocin Pediatric Granules (B)(G) 75 mg/5 ml (100 ml) (cherry).

APPENDIX CC.18. *DICLOXACILLIN* (DYNAPEN SUSPENSION)

Weight												
Pounds	15	20	25	30	35	40	45	50	55	60	65	70
Kilograms	6.8	9	11.4	13.6	15.9	18.2	20.5	22.7	25	27.3	29.5	31.8
Single Dose (ml)/Frequency/Strength/10-Day Volume (ml)												
12.5 mg/kg/d ml/dose qid	2	2.5	3	3.5	4	4.5	5	6	6	7	7.5	8
mg/5 ml	62.5	62.5	62.5	62.5	62.5	62.5	62.5	62.5	62.5	62.5	62.5	62.5
Volume (ml)	80	100	120	140	160	180	200	240	240	280	300	320
25 mg/kg/d ml/dose qid	3.5	4.5	6	7	8	9	10	11.5	12.5	13.5	15	16
mg/5 ml	62.5	62.5	62.5	62.5	62.5	62.5	62.5	62.5	62.5	62.5	62.5	62.5
Volume (ml)	140	180	240	280	320	360	400	460	500	540	600	640

Dynapen Suspension (B)(G) 6.25 mg/5 ml (80, 100 ml) (raspberry-strawberry).

APPENDIX CC.19. *DOXYCYCLINE* (VIBRAMYCIN SYRUP/SUSPENSION)

Weight

Pounds	15	20	25	30	35	40	45	50	55	60	65	70
Kilograms	6.8	9	11.4	13.6	15.9	18.2	20.5	22.7	25	27.3	29.5	31.8

Single Dose (ml)/Frequency/Strength/10-Day Volume (ml)

	15	20	25	30	35	40	45	50	55	60	65	70
1 mg/lb/d ml/dose qd	1.5	2	2.5	3	3.5	4	4.5	5	5.5	6	6.5	7
50 mg/5 ml	50	50	50	50	50	50	50	50	50	50	50	50
Volume (ml)	15	20	25	30	35	40	45	50	55	60	65	70
1 mg/lb/d ml/dose qd	3	4	5	6	7	8	9	10	11	12	13	14
25 mg/5 ml	25	25	25	25	25	25	25	25	25	25	25	25
Volume (ml)	30	40	50	60	70	80	90	100	110	120	130	140

Vibramycin Syrup (B)(G) <8 years: not recommended; double dose first day; 50 mg/5 ml (80, 100, ml) (raspberry-apple) (sulfites).

Vibramycin Suspension (B)(G) <8 years: not recommended; double dose first day; 25 mg/5 ml (80, 100, ml) (raspberry).

APPENDIX CC.20. ERYTHROMYCIN ESTOLATE (ILOSONE SUSPENSION)

Weight												
Pounds	15	20	25	30	35	40	45	50	55	60	65	70
Kilograms	6.8	9	11.4	13.6	15.9	18.2	20.5	22.7	25	27.3	29.5	31.8
Dose/Volume (10 days) in ml												
10 mg/kg/d ml/dose bid	3	3.5	4.5	5.5	6	7	8	9	10	5.5	6	6.5
mg/5 ml	125	125	125	125	125	125	125	125	125	250	250	250
Volume (ml)	60	70	90	110	120	140	160	180	200	110	120	130
15 mg/kg/d ml/dose bid	4	5.5	7	8	9.5	5.5	6	7	7.5	8	9	9.5
mg/5 ml	125	125	125	125	125	250	250	250	250	250	250	250
Volume (ml)	80	110	140	160	190	110	120	140	150	160	180	190
20 mg/kg/d ml/dose bid	3	3.5	4.5	5.5	6.5	7	8	9	10	11	12	13
mg/5 ml	250	250	250	250	250	250	250	250	250	250	250	250
Volume (ml)	60	70	90	110	120	140	160	180	200	220	240	260
25 mg/kg/d ml/dose bid	3.5	4.5	5.5	7	8	9	10	11.5	12.5	13.5	15	16
mg/5 ml	250	250	250	250	250	250	250	250	250	250	250	250
Volume (ml)	70	90	110	140	160	180	200	230	250	280	300	320

Ilosone Suspension (B)(G) 125, 250 mg/5 ml (100 ml).

APPENDIX CC.21. *ERYTHROMYCIN ETHYLSUCCINATE* (E.E.S. SUSPENSION, ERY-PED DROPS/SUSPENSION)

Weight

Pounds	15	20	25	30	35	40	45	50	55	60	65	70
Kilograms	6.8	9	11.4	13.6	15.9	18.2	20.5	22.7	25	27.3	29.5	31.8

Single Dose (ml)/Frequency/Strength/10-Day Volume (ml)

	15	20	25	30	35	40	45	50	55	60	65	70
30 mg/kg/d ml/dose qid	1.5	2	2	2.5	3	3.5	4	4	4.5	5	5.5	6
mg/5 ml	200	200	200	200	200	200	200	200	200	200	200	200
Volume (ml)	60	80	80	100	120	140	160	160	180	200	220	240
30 mg/kg/d ml/dose qid			1	1.5	1.5	2	2	2	2.5	2.5	3	3
mg/5 ml			400	400	400	400	400	400	400	400	400	
Volume (ml)			60	60	80	80	80	100	100	120	120	
50 mg/kg/d ml/dose qid	2	3	3.5	4.5	5	5.5	6.5	7	8	8.5	9	10
mg/5 ml	200	200	200	200	200	200	200	200	200	200	200	200
Volume (ml)	80	120	140	180	200	220	260	280	320	340	360	400

(continued)

APPENDIX CC.21: *ERYTHROMYCIN ETHYLSUCCINATE* (E.E.S. SUSPENSION, ERY-PED DROPS/SUSPENSION) *(continued)*

50 mg/kg/d ml/dose qid	1	1.5	2	2	2.5	3	3	3.5	4	4.5	4.5	5
mg/5 ml	400	400	400	400	400	400	400	400	400	400	400	400
Volume (ml)	40	60	80	80	100	120	140	140	160	180	180	200

Ery-Ped Drops/Suspension (B)(G) 200 mg/5 ml (100, 200 ml) (fruit); 400 mg/5 ml (60, 100, 200 ml) (banana); Oral drops: 200, 400 mg/5 ml (50 ml) (fruit).

E.E.S. Suspension (B)(G) 200 mg/5 ml, 400 mg/5 ml (100 ml) (fruit).

E.E.S. Granules (B)(G) 200 mg/5 ml (100, 200 ml) (cherry).

APPENDIX CC.22. *ERYTHROMYCIN+SULFAMETHOXAZOLE* (ERYZOLE, PEDIAZOLE)

Weight

Pounds	15	20	25	30	35	40	45	50	55	60	65	70
Kilograms	6.8	9	11.4	13.6	15.9	18.2	20.5	22.7	25	27.3	29.5	31.8

Single Dose (ml)/Frequency/Strength/10-Day Volume (ml)

10 mg/kg/d ml/dose bid	3	4	5	6	6.5	7.5	8.5	9.5	10	11	12	13.5
mg/5 ml	200	200	200	200	200	200	200	200	200	200	200	200
Volume (ml)	90	120	150	180	200	225	255	285	300	330	360	400

Eryzole (C)(G) <2 months: not recommended; *eryth* 200 mg/*sulf* 600 mg/5 ml (100, 150, 200, 250 ml).

Pediazole (C)(G) <2 months: not recommended; *eryth* 200 mg/*sulf* 600 mg/5 ml (100, 150, 200 ml) (strawberry-banana).

APPENDIX CC.23. *FLUCONAZOLE* (DIFLUCAN SUSPENSION)

Weight

Pounds	15	20	25	30	35	40	45	50	55	60	65	70
Kilograms	6.8	9	11.4	13.6	15.9	18.2	20.5	22.7	25	27.3	29.5	31.8

Single Dose (ml)/Frequency/Strength/21-Day Volume (ml)

3 mg/kg/d ml/dose qd	2	3	3.5	4	5	5.5	6	7	7.5	8	9	9.5
mg/ml	10	10	10	10	10	10	10	10	10	10	10	10
Volume (ml)	44	66	77	88	110	121	132	154	165	176	198	209
6 mg/kg/d ml/dose qd	4	5.5	2	2	2.5	3	3	3.5	4	4	4.5	5
mg/ml	10	10	40	40	40	40	40	40	40	40	40	40
Volume (ml)	88	121	44	44	55	66	66	77	88	88	99	110

Diflucan Suspension (B)(G) double-dose first day; 10, 40 mg/5 ml (35 ml) (orange).

APPENDIX CC.24. FURAZOLIDONE (FUROXONE LIQUID)

Weight												
Pounds	15	20	25	30	35	40	45	50	55	60	65	70
Kilograms	6.8	9	11.4	13.6	15.9	18.2	20.5	22.7	25	27.3	29.5	31.8
Single Dose (ml)/Frequency/Strength/7-Day Volume (ml)												
5 mg/kg/d ml/dose qid	2.5	3.5	4	5	6	7	8	8.5	9.5	10	11	12
mg/15 ml	50	50	50	50	50	50	50	50	50	50	50	50
Vol	100	140	160	200	240	280	320	340	380	400	440	480

Furoxone Liquid (C)(G) double-dose first day; 50 mg/15 ml (35 ml).

APPENDIX CC.25. *GRISEOFULVIN, MICROSIZE* (GRIFULVIN V SUSPENSION)

Weight												
Pounds	15	20	25	30	35	40	45	50	55	60	65	70
Kilograms	6.8	9	11.4	13.6	15.9	18.2	20.5	22.7	25	27.3	29.5	31.8
Single Dose (ml)/Frequency/Strength/30-Day Volume (ml)												
5 mg/lb/d ml/dose day	3	4	5	6	7	8	9	10	11	12	13	14
mg/5 ml	125	125	125	125	125	125	125	125	125	125	125	125
Volume (ml)	90	120	150	180	210	240	270	300	330	360	390	420

Grifulvin V Suspension (C)(G) double-dose first day; 125 mg/5 ml (120 ml) (orange) (alcohol 0.02%).

APPENDIX CC.26. *ITRACONAZOLE* (SPORANOX SOLUTION)

Weight												
Pounds	15	20	25	30	35	40	45	50	55	60	65	70
Kilograms	6.8	9	11.4	13.6	15.9	18.2	20.5	22.7	25	27.3	29.5	31.8
Single Dose (ml)/Frequency/Strength/7-Day Volume (ml)												
5 mg/kg/d ml/dose qd	3.5	4.5	6	7	8	9	10	11.5	12.5	14	15	16
mg/ml	10	10	10	10	10	10	10	10	10	10	10	10
Volume (ml)	25	32	42	49	56	63	70	71	88	98	105	112

Sporanox V Solution (C)(G) double-dose first day; 10 mg/ml (150 ml) (cherry-caramel).

APPENDIX CC.27. LORACARBEF (LORABID SUSPENSION)

Weight

	15	20	25	30	35	40	45	50	55	60	65	70
Pounds	15	20	25	30	35	40	45	50	55	60	65	70
Kilograms	6.8	9	11.4	13.6	15.9	18.2	20.5	22.7	25	27.3	29.5	31.8

Single Dose (ml)/Frequency/Strength/10-Day Volume (ml)

	15	20	25	30	35	40	45	50	55	60	65	70
15 mg/kg/d ml/dose bid	2.5	3.5	4	5	3	3.5	4	4	5	5	5.5	6
mg/5 ml	100	100	100	100	200	200	200	200	200	200	200	200
Volume (ml)	50	70	80	100	60	70	80	80	100	100	110	120
30 mg/kg/d ml/dose bid	2.5	3.5	4	5	6	7	8	8.5	9.5	10	11	12
mg/5 ml	200	200	200	200	200	200	200	200	200	200	200	200
Volume (ml)	50	70	80	100	120	140	160	170	190	200	220	240

Lorabid Suspension (B) 100 mg/5 ml (50, 100 ml) (strawberry bubble gum); 200 mg/5 ml (50, 75, 100 ml) (strawberry bubble gum).

APPENDIX CC.28. *NITROFURANTOIN* (FURADANTIN SUSPENSION)

Weight												
Pounds	15	20	25	30	35	40	45	50	55	60	65	70
Kilograms	6.8	9	11.4	13.6	15.9	18.2	20.5	22.7	25	27.3	29.5	31.8
Single Dose (ml)/Frequency/Strength/10-Day Volume (ml)												
5 mg/kg ml/dose qid	1.5	2.5	3	3.5	4	4.5	5	5.5	6	7	7.5	8
mg/5 ml	25	25	25	25	25	25	25	25	25	25	25	25
Volume (ml)	60	100	120	140	160	190	200	220	240	280	300	320

Furadantin Suspension (B)(G) 25 mg/5 ml (60 ml).

APPENDIX CC.29. PENICILLIN V POTASSIUM (PEN-VEE K SOLUTION, VEETIDS SOLUTION)

Weight

Pounds	15	20	25	30	35	40	45	50	55	60	65	70
Kilograms	6.8	9	11.4	13.6	15.9	18.2	20.5	22.7	25	27.3	29.5	31.8

Single Dose (ml)/Frequency/Strength/10-Day Volume (ml)

	15	20	25	30	35	40	45	50	55	60	65	70
25 mg/kg/d ml/dose qid	2	2.5	3	3.5	4	4.5	5	5.5	6	7	7.5	8
mg/5 ml	125	125	125	125	125	125	125	125	125	125	125	125
Volume (ml)	80	90	120	140	160	180	200	220	240	280	300	320
25 mg/kg/d ml/dose qid	1	1	1.5	2	2	2.5	2.5	3	3	3.5	4	4
mg/5 ml	250	250	250	250	250	250	250	250	250	250	250	250
Volume (ml)	40	40	60	80	80	100	100	120	120	140	160	160
50 mg/kg/d ml/dose qid	2	2.5	3	3.5	4	4.5	5	6	6.5	7	7.5	8
mg/5 ml	250	250	250	250	250	250	250	250	250	250	250	250
Volume (ml)	80	100	120	140	160	180	200	240	260	280	300	320

Pen-Vee K Solution (B)(G) 125 mg/5 ml (100, 200 ml), 250 mg/5 ml (100, 150, 200 ml).

Veetids Solution (B)(G) 125, 250 mg/5 ml (100, 200 ml).

APPENDIX CC.30. *RIMANTADINE* (FLUMADINE SYRUP)

Weight												
Pounds	15	20	25	30	35	40	45	50	55	60	65	70
Kilograms	6.8	9	11.4	13.6	15.9	18.2	20.5	22.7	25	27.3	29.5	31.8
Single Dose (ml)/Frequency/Strength/10-Day Volume (ml)												
5 mg/kg/d ml/dose qd	3.5	4.5	6	7	8	9	10	11.5	12.5	13.5	15	16
mg/5 ml	50	50	50	50	50	50	50	50	50	50	50	50
Volume (ml)	35	45	60	70	80	90	100	115	125	135	150	160

Flumadine Syrup (B) >10 years: same as adult; 50 mg/5 ml (2, 8, 16 oz) (raspberry).

APPENDIX CC.31. *TETRACYCLINE* (SUMYCIN SUSPENSION)

Weight												
Pounds	15	20	25	30	35	40	45	50	55	60	65	70
Kilograms	6.8	9	11.4	13.6	15.9	18.2	20.5	22.7	25	27.3	29.5	31.8
Single Dose (ml)/Frequency/Strength/10-Day Volume (ml)												
25 mg/kg/d ml/dose qid	1.5	2.5	3	3.5	4	4.5	5	6	6.5	7	7.5	8
mg/5 ml	125	125	125	125	125	125	125	125	125	125	125	125
Volume (ml)	60	100	120	140	160	180	200	240	260	280	300	320
50 mg/kg/d ml/dose qid	3.5	4.5	6	7	8	9	10	11.5	12.5	13.5	15	16
mg/5 ml	125	125	125	125	125	125	125	125	125	125	125	125
Volume (ml)	140	180	240	280	320	360	400	460	500	540	600	640

Sumycin Suspension (D)(G) <8 years: not recommended; 125 mg/5 ml (100, 200 ml) (fruit) (sulfites).

APPENDIX CC.32. *TRIMETHOPRIM* (PRIMSOL SUSPENSION)

Weight

Pounds	15	20	25	30	35	40	45	50	55	60	65	70
Kilograms	6.8	9	11.4	13.6	15.9	18.2	20.5	22.7	25	27.3	29.5	31.8

Single Dose (ml)/Frequency/Strength/10-Day Volume (ml)

	15	20	25	30	35	40	45	50	55	60	65	70
5 mg/kg/d ml/dose bid	3.5	4.5	6	7	8	9	10	11.5	12.5	13.5	15	16
mg/5 ml	50	50	50	50	50	50	50	50	50	50	50	50
Volume (ml)	70	90	120	140	160	180	200	230	250	270	300	320

Primsol Suspension (C)(G) 50 mg/5 ml (50 mg/5 ml) (bubble gum) (dye-free, alcohol-free).

APPENDIX CC.33. *TRIMETHOPRIM+SULFAMETHOXAZOLE* (BACTRIM SUSPENSION, SEPTRA SUSPENSION)

Weight

Pounds	15	20	25	30	35	40	45	50	55	60	65	70
Kilograms	6.8	9	11.4	13.6	15.9	18.2	20.5	22.7	25	27.3	29.5	31.8

Single Dose (ml)/Frequency/Strength/10-Day Volume (ml)

	15	20	25	30	35	40	45	50	55	60	65	70
10 mg/kg/d ml/dose bid	2	2	3	3.5	4	4.5	5	5.5	6	7	7.5	8
mg/5 ml	200	200	200	200	200	200	200	200	200	200	200	200
Volume (ml)	40	40	60	70	80	90	100	110	120	140	150	160
20 mg/kg/d ml/dose bid	4	4	6	7	8	9	10	11	12	14	15	16
mg/5 ml	200	200	200	200	200	200	200	200	200	200	200	200
Volume (ml)	80	80	120	140	160	180	200	220	240	280	300	320

Bactrim Pediatric Suspension, Septra Pediatric Suspension (C)(G) trim 40 mg/sulfa 200 mg/5 ml (100 ml) (cherry) (alcohol 0.3%).

APPENDIX CC.34. *VANCOMYCIN* (VANCOCIN SUSPENSION)

Weight												
Pounds	15	20	25	30	35	40	45	50	55	60	65	70
Kilograms	6.8	9	11.4	13.6	15.9	18.2	20.5	22.7	25	27.3	29.5	31.8
Single Dose (ml)/Frequency/Strength/10-Day Volume (ml)												
40 mg/kg/d ml/dose tid	2	2.5	3	3.5	4.5	5	5.5	6	7	7.5	8	8.5
mg/5 ml	250	250	250	250	250	250	250	250	250	250	250	250
Volume (ml)	60	75	90	105	135	150	165	180	210	225	240	255
40 mg/kg/d ml/dose qid	1.5	2	2.5	3	3	3.5	4	4.5	5	5.5	6	6.5
mg/5 ml	250	250	250	250	250	250	250	250	250	250	250	250
Volume (ml)	60	80	100	120	120	140	160	180	200	220	240	260
40 mg/kg/d ml/dose tid	1	1	1.5	2	2	2.5	3	3	3.5	3.5	4	4
mg/6 ml	500	500	500	500	500	500	500	500	500	500	500	500
Volume (ml)	30	30	45	60	60	75	90	90	105	105	120	120
40 mg/kg/d ml/dose qid	1	1	1.5	1.5	1.5	2	2	2.5	2.5	3	3	3.5
mg/6 ml	500	500	500	500	500	500	500	500	500	500	500	500
Volume (ml)	40	40	60	60	60	80	80	100	100	120	120	140

Vancomycin Suspension (C)(G).

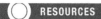
2017 ACC/AHA/AAPA/ABC/ACPM/AGS/APhA/ASH/ASPC/NMA/PCNA Guideline for the Prevention, Detection, Evaluation, and Management of High Blood Pressure in Adults: A report of the American College of Cardiology/ American Heart Association Task Force on Clinical Practice Guidelines
http://hyper.ahajournals.org/content/hypertensionaha/early/2017/11/10/ HYP.0000000000000065.full.pdf

ACR Guidelines on Prevention & Treatment of Glucocorticoid-induced Osteoporosis [press release, June 7, 2017]. Atlanta, GA: American College of Rheumatology
https://www.rheumatology.org/About-Us/Newsroom/Press-Releases/ID/812/ACR-Releases-Guideline-on-Prevention-Treatment-of-Glucocorticoid-Induced-Osteoporosis

Advance for Nurse Practitioners
http://nurse-practitioners.advanceweb.com

Advanced Practice Education Associates
www.apea.com

Ake, J. A., Schuetz, A., Pegu, P., Wieczorek, L., Eller, M. A., Kibuuka, H., . . . Robb, M. L. (2017). Safety and immunogenicity of PENNVAX-G DNA prime administered by biojector 2000 or CELLECTRA electroporation device with modified vaccinia Ankara-CMDR boost. *The Journal of Infectious Diseases*, *216*(9), 1080–1090. doi:10.1093/infdis/ jix456

American Academy of Dermatology
https://www.aad.org/home

American Academy of Pediatrics (AAP)
http://aapexperience.org

American Association of Nurse Practitioners
www.aanp.org

American College of Cardiology. Then and now: ATP III vs. IV: Comparison of ATP III and ACC/AHA guidelines.
http://www.acc.org/latest-in-cardiology/articles/2014/07/18/16/03/then-and-now-atp-iii-vs-iv

American Diabetes Association (ADA), Professional Diabetes Resources Online.
http://professional.diabetes.org/content/clinical-practice-recommendations/?loc=rp-slabnav

American Diabetes Association. (2018). Children and adolescents: Standards of medical care in diabetes—2018. *Diabetes Care*, *41*(Suppl 1), S126–S136. doi.org/10.2337/dc18-S012

American Diabetes Association. (2018). Management of diabetes in pregnancy: Standards of medical care in diabetes—2018. *Diabetes Care*, *41*(Suppl 1), S137–S143. doi.org/10.2337/ dc18-S013

American Diabetes Association. (2018). Microvascular Complications and Foot Care: Standards of Medical Care in Diabetes—2018. *Diabetes Care*, *41*(Suppl 1), S105-S118. doi. org/10.2337/dc18-S010

American Diabetes Association. (2018). Older adults: Standards of medical care in diabetes—2018. *Diabetes Care, 41*(Suppl 1), S119–S125. doi.org/10.2337/dc18-S011

American Diabetes Association. (2018). Pharmacologic approaches to glycemic treatment: Standards of medical care in diabetes—2018. *Diabetes Care, 41*(Suppl 1), S73–S85. doi.org/10.2337/dc18-S008

American Diabetes Association. (2018). Summary of revisions: Standards of medical care in diabetes—2018. *Diabetes Care, 41*(Suppl 1), S4–S6. doi.org/10.2337/dc18-Srev01

American Family Physician
http://www.aafp.org/online/en/home.html

American Geriatrics Society 2015 updated Beers Criteria for potentially inappropriate medication use in older adults. *Journal of the American Geriatrics Society, 63*(11), 2227–2246

American Headache Society
www.americanheadachesociety.org

American Pain Society
http://americanpainsociety.org

American Pharmacists Association. (2015). *Pediatric and neonatal dosage handbook: A universal resource for clinicians treating pediatric and neonatal patients* (22nd ed.). Hudson, OH: Lexicomp.

American Trypanosomiasis Centers for Disease Control and Prevention. *Parasites— American Trypanosomiasis (also known as Chagas disease). Resources for health professionals.*

Anderson, E., Fantus, R. J., & Haddadin, R. I. (2017). Diagnosis and management of herpes zoster ophthalmicus. *Disease-a-Month, 63*(2), 38–44.

Andorf, S., Purington, N., Block, W. M., Long, A. J., Tupa, D., Brittain, E., . . . Chinthrajah, R. S. Anti-IgE treatment with oral immunotherapy in multi-food allergic participants: A double-blind, randomised, controlled trial [published online December 12, 2017]. *Lancet Gastroenterology Hepatology, 3*(2), 85–94 doi:10.1016/S2468-1253(17)30392-8

Aronow, W. S. Initiation of antihypertensive therapy. Presented at: American Heart Association (AHA) Scientific Sessions 2017; November 11-15, 2017; Anaheim, CA. http://www.abstractsonline.com/pp8/ - !/4412/presentation/55060

ATP III and ACC/AHA Guidelines
http://www.acc.org/latest-in-cardiology/articles/2014/07/18/16/03/then-and-now-atp-iii-vs-iv

Auron, M, & Raissouni, N. (2015). Adrenal insufficiency. *Pediatric Review, 36*(3), 92–102.

Belknap, R, Holland, D, Feng P, et al. Self-administered versus directly observed once-weekly isoniazid and rifapentine treatment of latent tuberculosis infection: A randomized trial. [Published online ahead of print November 7, 2017]. Annals of Internal Medicine. doi:10.7326/M17-1150

Bosworth, T. (2017) *Testosterone deficiency treatment recommendation.*
    https://www.medpagetoday.com/resource-center/hypogonadism/treatment-
    recommendations/a/64511

Brody, A. A., Gibson, B., Tresner-Kirsch, D., Kramer, H., Thraen, I., Coarr, M. E., & Rupper,
    R. (2016). High prevalence of medication discrepancies between home health referrals
    and Centers for Medicare and Medicaid Services home health certification and plan
    of care and their potential to affect safety of vulnerable elderly adults. *Journal of the
    American Geriatrics Society, 64*(11), e166–e170.

Brunk, D. Learn 'four Ds' approach to heart failure in diabetes. Clinician Reviews [Posted
    online January 28, 2018]. https://www.mdedge.com/clinicalendocrinologynews/
    article/157198/diabetes/learn-four-ds-approach-heart-failure-diabetes

Canestaro, W. J., Forrester, S. H., Raghu, G., Ho, L., & Devine, B. E. (2016). Drug treatment of
    idiopathic pulmonary fibrosis: Systematic review and network meta-analysis. *Chest, 149,*
    756–766.

CDC 2015 Sexually Transmitted Diseases Treatment Guidelines
    http://www.cdc.gov/std/tg2015/default.htm

CDC Guidelines for Conception in HIV Positive Women Stress the Use of PrEP in Sexual
    Partners
    https://www.medpagetoday.com/resource-centers/contemporary-hiv-prevention/
    cdc-guide-lines-conception-hiv-positive-women-stress-use-prep-sexual-
    partners/775?xid=NL_MPT_MPT_HIV_2017-09-26&eun=g766320d0r

CDC Guideline for Prescribing Opioids for Chronic Pain—United States. (2016).
    https://jamanetwork.com/learning/article-quiz/10.1001/jama.2016.1464#qundefined

CDC: Morbidity and Mortality Weekly Report (MMWR)
    http://www.cdc.gov/mmwr/mmwr_wk.html

CDC Provider Information Sheet–PrEP during conception, pregnancy, and breast-feeding
    information for clinicians counseling patients about PrEP use during conception,
    pregnancy, and breastfeeding
    https://www.cdc.gov/hiv/pdf/prep_gl_clinician_factsheet_pregnancy_english.pdf

Centers for Disease Control and Prevention. (2017). Recommended Immunization Schedule
    for Children and Adolescents Aged 18 Years or Younger, United States.
    https://www.cdc.gov/vaccines/schedules/downloads/child/0-18yrs-child-combined-
    schedule.pdf

Centers for Disease Control and Prevention
    www.cdc.gov

Centers for Disease Control and Prevention. (2017). *Adult Immunization Schedule by Medical
    and other Indications*
    http://www.cdc.gov/vaccines/schedules/hcp/imz/adult-conditions.html

Centers for Disease Control and Prevention. (2016). *Diphtheria, Tetanus, and Pertussis
    Vaccine Recommendations.*
    http://www.cdc.gov/vaccines/vpd/dtap-tdap-td/hcp/recommendations.htm

Centers for Disease Control and Prevention. (2016). *Facts About ADHD*
www.cdc.gov/ncbddd/adhd/facts.html

Centers for Disease Control and Prevention. (2016). *Pneumococcal vaccination: summary of who and when to vaccinate*
http://www.cdc.gov/vaccines/vpd/pneumo/hcp/who-when-to-vaccinate.html

Chang, A., Martins, K. A. O., Encinales, L., Reid, S. P., Acuña, M., & Encinales, C., . . . Firestein, G. S. (2017). A cross-sectional analysis of chikungunya arthritis patients 22 months post-infection demonstrates no detectable viral persistence in synovial fluid. *Arthritis Rheumatology*. doi:10.1002/art.40383

Chang, A., Encinales, L., Porras, A., Pachecho, N., Reid, S. P., Martins, K. A. O., . . . Simon, G. L. (2017). Frequency of chronic joint pain following chikungunya infection: A Colombian cohort study. *Arthritis Rheumatology*, doi:10.1002/art.40384

Chow, A. W., Benninger, M. S., Brook, I., Brozek, J. L., Goldstein, E. J., Hicks, L. A., . . . Infectious Disease Society of America. (2012). IDSA clinical practice guideline for acute and bacterial rhinosinusitis in children and adults. *Clinical Infectious Diseases, 54*(8), e72–e112.

Chutka, D. S., Takahashi, P. Y., & Hoel, R. W. (2004). Inappropriate medications for elderly patients. Mayo Clinic Proceedings. 79(1), 122–139.

Clinician Reviews
http://www.clinicianreviews.com

Cohen, J. D., Li, L., Wang, Y., Thoburn, C., Afsari, B., Danilova, L., . . . Papadopoulos, N. (2018). Detection and localization of surgically resectable cancers with a multi-analyte blood test. *Science*, eaar3247. doi:10.1126/science.aar3247

Coker, T. J., & Dierfeldt, D. M. (2016). Acute bacterial prostatitis: Diagnosis and management. *American Family Physician, 93*(2), 114–120.

Consultant 360
http://www.consultant360.com/home

Daily Med: NIH. US Library of Medicine
https://dailymed.nlm.nih.gov/dailymed/index.cfm

Davis, M. C., Miller, B. J., Kalsi, J. K., Birkner, T., & Mathis, M. V. (2017). Efficient trial design—FDA approval of valbenazine for tardive dyskinesia. *New England Journal of Medicine, 376*, 2503–2506.

Dhadwal, G., & Kirchhof, M. G. The risks and benefits of cannabis in the dermatology clinic. [Published online ahead of print October 23, 2017]. *Journal of Cutaneous Medicine and Surgery*. doi:10.1177/1203475417738971

Dietrich, E. A., & Davis, K. (2017). Antibiotics for acute bacterial prostatitis: Which agent, and for how long? *Consultant, 57*(9), 564–565.

Domino, F. J., Baldor, R. A., Golding, J., & Stephens, M. B. (2016). *The 5-minute clinical consult standard 2016*. Philadelphia, PA: Wolters Kluwer.

Dowell, D., Haegerich, T. M., & Chou, R. (2016). CDC guidelines for prescribing opi-oids for chronic pain. *Journal of the American Medical Association, 315*(15), 1624–1645. doi:10.1001/jama.2016.1464

DRUGS.COM
www.drugs.com

DRUGS.COM: Drugs Interaction Checker
https://www.drugs.com/drug_interactions.php

DRUGS at FDA: FDA Approved Drug Products
http://www.accessdata.fda.gov/scripts/cder/drugsatfda/index.cfm

Emer, J. J., Bernardo, S. G., Kovalerchik, O., & Ahmad, M. (2013). Urticaria multiforme. *The Journal of Clinical and Aesthetic Dermatology, 6*(31), 34–39.

eMPR: Monthly Prescribing Reference (new FDA approved products, new generics, new drug withdrawals, safety alerts)
http://www.empr.com

Endocrinology on the comprehensive type 2 diabetes management algorithm —2017 executive summary. (2017). *Endocrine Practice, 23*(2), 207–238. doi:10.4158/ep161682.cs

Engorn, B., & Flerlage, J. (Eds.). (2015). The Harriet Lane handbook: A handbook for pediatric house officers (20th ed.). Philadelphia, PA: Elsevier.
https://online.epocrates.com/drugs

FDA News Release: FDA Approves Drug to Treat Duchenne Muscular Dystrophy. (2017)
https://www.fda.gov/NewsEvents/Newsroom/PressAnnouncements/ucm540945.htm

FDA: Recalls, Market Withdrawals, and Safety Alerts
http://www.fda.gov/Safety/Recalls/default.htm

Fleming, J. E., & Lockwood, S. (2017). Cannabinoid hyperemesis syndrome. *Federal Practitioner, 34*(10), 33–36.

Flynn, J. T., Kaelber, D. C., Baker-Smith, C. M., Blowey, D., Carroll, A. E., Daniels, S. R., . . . Subcommittee On Screening And Management Of High Blood Pressure In Children. (2017). Clinical practice guideline for screening and management of high blood pressure in children and adolescents. [Published online ahead of print August 22, 2017]. *Pediatrics, 140*(3), e20171904.

Freedberg, D. E., Kim, L. S., & Yang, Y.-X. (2017). The risks and benefits of long-term use of proton pump inhibitors: Expert review and best practice advice from the American Gastroenterological Association. *Gastroenterology, 152*(4), 706–715. doi:10.1053/j.gastro.2017.01.031

Garber, A. J., Abrahamson, M. J., Barzilay, J. I., Blonde, L., Bloomgarden, Z. T., Bush, M. A., . . . Umpierrez, G. E. (2017). Consensus statement by the American Association of Clinical Endocrinologists and American College of Endocrinology on the comprehensive type 2 diabetes management algorithm – 2017 executive summary. *Endocrine Practice, 23*(2), 207–238. doi:10.4158/ep161682.cs

Gilbert, D. N., Chambers, H. F., Eliopoulos, G. M., Gilbert, D. N., Chambers, H. F., Eliopoulos, S. M., & Pavia, A. (2016). *The Sanford guide to antimicrobial therapy, 2016* (46th ed.). Sperryville, VA: Antimicrobial Therapy.

Gordon, C., Amissah-Arthur, M. B., Gayed, M., Brown, S., Bruce, I. N., D'Cruz D., . . . British Society for Rheumatology Standards, Audit and Guidelines Working Group. (2017). The British Society for Rheumatology guideline for the management of systemic lupus erythematosus in adults: Executive Summary. *Rheumatology (Oxford)*. doi:10.1093/rheumatology/kex291. [Epub ahead of print]

Gordon, C., Amissah-Arthur, M. B., Gayed, M., Brown, S., Bruce, I. N., D'Cruz D., . . . British Society for Rheumatology Standards, Audit and Guidelines Working Group. The British Society for Rheumatology guideline for the management of systemic lupus erythematosus in adults. *Rheumatology (Oxford)*. 2017 Oct 6. doi:10.1093/rheumatology/kex286

Greenhawt, M., Turner, P. J., & Kelso, J. M. (2018). Allergy experts set the record straight on flu shots for patients with egg sensitivity. *Annals of Allergy, Asthma & Immunology, 120*(1), 49–52. doi:10.1016/j.anai.2017.10.020

Groot, N., de Graaff, N., Avcin, T., Bader-Meunier, B., Brogan, P., Dolezalova, P., . . . Beresford, M. W. (2017). European evidence-based recommendations for diagnosis and treatment of childhood-onset systemic lupus erythematosus [cSLE]: The [Single Hub and Access point for paediatric Rheumatology in Europe] SHARE initiative. *Annals of the Rheumatic Diseases, 76*(11), 1788–1796. doi:10.1136/annrheumdis-2016-210960

Groot, N., de Graeff, N., Marks, S. D., Brogan, P., Avcin, T., Bader-Meunier, B., . . . Kamphuis, S. (2017). European evidence-based recommendations for the diagnosis and treatment of childhood-onset lupus nephritis [cLN]: The SHARE initiative. *Recommendation*. doi. org/10.1136/annrheumdis-2017-211898

Guidelines updated for thyroid disease in pregnancy and postpartum. (2017). *American Journal of Nursing, 4*(117), 16.

Hanania, N. Omalizumab helps asthma COPD overlap patients, presented at the 2017 CHEST Annual Meeting in Toronto, Canada, as reported by Beck, DL, in November 10, 2017, *Family Practice News* http://www.mdedge.com/familypracticenews/article/151778/copd/omalizumab-helps-asthma-copd-overlap-patients?channel=41038&utm_source=News_FPN_eNL_111617_F&utm_medium=email&utm_content=Omalizumab for asthma COPD overlap patients

Handbook of Antimicrobial Therapy (20th ed.). (2015). New Rochelle, NY: The Medical Letter

Harrison's Infectious Diseases (3rd ed.). (2016). New York, NY: McGraw Hill Education

Huang, A. R., Mallet, L., Rochefort, C. M. (2012). Medication-related falls in the elderly: Causative factors and preventive strategies. *Drugs & Aging. 29*(5), 359–376.

International Diabetes Federation (IDF) Clinical Practice Guidelines http://www.idf.org/guidelines

Inzucchi, S. E., Iliev, H., Pfarr, E., & Zinman, B. Empagliflozin and assessment of lower-limb amputations in the EMPA-REG OUTCOME Trial [published online November 13, 2017]. *Diabetes Cares, 41*(1), e4–e5. doi:10.2337/dc17-1551

James, P. A., Oparil, S, Carter, B. L, Cushman, W. C., Dennison-Himmelfarb, C., Handler, J., . . . Ortiz, E. (2014). Evidence-based guidelines for the management of high blood pressure in adults: Report from the panel members appointed to the eighth joint national committee (JNC 8). *Journal of the American Medical Association, 311*(5), 507–520.

Jarrett, J. B., & Moss, D. Oral agent offers relief from generalized hyperhidrosis–An inexpensive and well-tolerated anticholinergic reduces sweating in patients with localized—and generalized—hyperhidrosis. *Clinician Reviews.* July 2017 [posted online] https://www.mdedge.com/sites/default/files/Document/June-2017/CR02707024.PDF

JNC 8 Guideline Summary. *Pharmacist's Letter/Prescriber's Letter* https://www.scribd.com/doc/290772273/JNC-8-guideline-summary

Journal of the American Academy of Nurse Practitioners https://www.aanp.org/publications/jaanp

Journal of the American Medical Association (JAMA) Internal Medicine http://archinte.jamanetwork.com/journal.aspx

Journal of the American Geriatrics Society http://onlinelibrary.wiley.com/journal/10.1111/(ISSN)1532–5415

Justesen, K., & Prasad, S. (2016). On-demand pill protocol protects against HIV. *Clinician Reviews, 26*(9), 18–19, 22.

Kasper, D. L., & Fauci, A. S. (2017). Listeria monocytogenes infections. In: *Harrison's Infectious Diseases (3rd ed.).* New York, NY: McGraw Hill Education

Khera, M., Adaikan, G., Buvat, J, Carrier, S., El-Meliegy, A., Hatzimouratidis, K., . . (2016). Diagnosis and treatment of testosterone deficiency: Recommendations from the Fourth International Consultation for Sexual Medicine (ICSM 2015). *The Journal of Sexual Medicine, 13*, 1787–1804.

Kim, D. K., Riley, L. E., Harriman, K. H., Hunter, P., & Bridges, C. B. (2017). Advisory Committee on Immunization Practices recommended immunization schedule for adults aged 19 years or older—United States, 2017. *Morbidity and Mortality Weekly Report, 66*, 136–138. doi:10.15585/mmwr.mm6605e2

Kumar, S., Yegneswaran, B., & Pitchumoni, C. S. (2017). Preventing the adverse effects of glucocorticoids: A reminder. *Consultant, 57*(12), 726–728.

Langer, R., Simon, J. A., Pines, A., Lobo, R. A., Hodis, H. N., Pickar, J. H., . . . Utian, W. H. (2017). Menopausal hormone therapy for primary prevention: Why the USPSTF is wrong. *The North American Menopause Society, 24*(10), 1101–1112. doi:10.1097/GME.0000000000000983

Leach, M. Z. (November 7, 2017). First UK guidelines for adults with lupus. *Rheumatology Network* http://www.rheumatologynetwork.com/article/first-uk-guidelines-adults-lupus

Lieberthal, A. S., Carroll, A. E., Chonmaitree, T., Ganiats, T. G., Hoberman, A., Jackson, M. A., & Tunkel, D. E. (2013). *The diagnosis and management of acute otitis media. Pediatrics, 131*(3), e964–e999.

Lortscher, D, Admani, S, Satur, N, & Eichenfield, LF. (2016). Hormonal contraceptives and acne: a retrospective analysis of 2147 patients. *J Drugs Dermatol, 15*(6), 670–674. http://jddonline.com/articles/dermatology/S1545961616P0670X

Mallick, J., Devi, L., & Malik, P. K., & Mallick J. (2016). Update on normal tension glaucoma. *Journal of Ophthalmic and Vision Research, 11*(2), 204–208. doi:10.4103/2008-322X.183914

Manchikanti, L., Kaye, A. M., Knezevic, N. N., McAnally, H., Slavin, K., Trescot, A. M., . . . Hirsch, J. A. (2017). Responsible, safe, and effective prescription of opioids for chronic non-cancer pain: American Society of Interventional Pain Physicians (ASIPP) guidelines. *Pain Physician, 20*(2S), S3–S92.

Mandell, G. L., Bennett, J. E., & Dolin, R. (Eds.). (2014). *Principles and practices of infectious diseases* (8th ed.). Philadelphia, PA: Elsevier Churchill Livingstone.

Mandell, L. A., Wunderink, R. G., Anzueto, A., Bartlett, J. G., Campbell, G. D., Dean, N. C., . . . American Thoracic Society. (2007). Infectious diseases society of America/American Thoracic Society consensus guidelines on the management of community-acquired pneumonia in adults. *Clinical Infectious Diseases, 44*(Suppl 2), S27–S72. https://enp-network.s3.amazonaws.com/NPA_Long_Island/pdf/Pneumonia.pdf

McDonald, J., & Mattingly, J (2016). Chagas disease: Creeping into family practice in the United States. *Clinician Reviews, 26*(11), 38–45.

McLean, A. J., & Le Couteur, D. G. (2004). Aging biology and geriatric clinical pharmacology. *Pharmacological Reviews, 56*(2), 63–84.

McMillan, J. A., Lee, C. K. K., Siberry, G. K., & Carroll, K. (2013). *The Harriet Lane handbook of pediatric antimicrobial therapy.* Philadelphia, PA: Elsevier Saunders.

McNeill, C., Sisson, W., & Jarrett, A. (2017). Listerosis: A resurfacing menace. *International Journal of Nursing Practice, 13*(10), 647–654.

MDedge: Family Practice News
https://www.mdedge.com/familypracticenews/

MedlinePlus
https://www.nlm.nih.gov/medlineplus/ency/article/000165.htm

MedPage Today
http://www.medpagetoday.com

Medscape
http://www.medscape.com

Medscape: Drug Interaction Checker
http://reference.medscape.com/drug-interactionchecker?src=wnl_drugguide_170410_mscpref &uac=123859AY&impID=1324737&faf=1

Merel, S. E., & Paauw, D. S. (2017). Common drug side effects and drug-drug interactions in elderly adults in primary care. *Journal of the American Geriatrics Society, 65*(7), 1578–1585.

Miller, G. E., Sarpong, E. M., Davidoff, A. J., Yang, E. Y., Brandt, N. J., Fick, D. M. (2016). Determinants of potentially inappropriate medication use among community-dwelling older adults. *Health Services Research, 52*(4), 1534–1549.

Molina, J. M., Capitant, C., Spire, B., Pialoux, G., Cotte, L., Charreau, I., . . . ANRS IPERGAY Study Group. (2015). On-demand preexposure prophylaxis in men at high risk for HIV-1 infection. *The New England Journal of Medicine, 373*, 2237–2246.

Monaco, K. HRT benefits outweigh risks for certain menopausal women—Menopause Society statement aims to clear up confusion https://www.medpagetoday.com/Endocrinology/Menopause/66158?xid=NL_MPT_IRXHealthWomen_2017-12-27&eun=g766320d0r

Morales, A., Bebb, R. A., Manoo, P., Assimakopoulos, P., Axler, J., Collier, C., . . . Lee, J. (2015). Appendix 1 (as supplied by the authors): Full-text guidelines Multidisciplinary Canadian Clinical Practice Guideline on the diagnosis and management of testosterone deficiency syndrome in adult males. http://www.cmaj.ca/content/suppl/2015/10/26/cmaj.150033.DC1/15-0033-1-at.pdf

National Academy of Medicine http://nam.edu

National Cholesterol Education Program Expert Panel on Detection, Evaluation, and Treatment of High Blood Cholesterol in Adults (Adult Treatment Panel IV, 2012) http://circ.ahajournals.org/content/circulationaha/106/25/3143.full.pdf

National Heart Lung and Blood Institute (NHLBI) http://www.nhlbi.nih.gov

National Institute of Diabetes and Digestive and Kidney Diseases. Adrenal Insufficiency and Addison's Disease. http://www.nidk.nih.gov/health-infromation/health-topics/endocrine/adren [Accessed May 31, 2016]

New England Journal of Medicine (NEJM) Journal Watch General Medicine http://www.jwatch.org/general-medicine

Ní Chróinín, D., Neto, H. M., Xiao, D., Sandhu, A., Brazel, C., Farnham, N., . . . Beveridge, A. (2016). Potentially inappropriate medications (PIMs) in older hospital in-patients: Prevalence, contribution to hospital admission and documentation of rationale for continuation. *Australasian Journal on Ageing, 35*(4), 262–265.

Ostergaard, L., Vesikari, T., Absalon, J., Beeslaar, J., Ward, B. J., . . . B1971009 and B1971016 Trial Investigators. A bivalent meningococcal B vaccine in adolescents and young adults [published online December 14, 2017]. *The New England Journal of Medicine, 35*(4), 262–265. doi:10.1111/ ajag.12312

Paz-Bailey, G, et al . Zika virus persistence in body fluids, final report in body fluids: Final report. ASTMH 2017. Paper presented at the 66th Annual Meeting of the American Society of Tropical Medicine and Hygiene, November 5–9, Baltimore, MD.

Pharmacist's Letter www.pharmacistsletter.com

Physician's Desk Reference (PDR)
    http://www.pdr.net

PLR Requirements for Prescribing Information
    https://www.fda.gov/Drugs/GuidanceComplianceRegulatoryInformation/
    LawsActsandRules/ucm084159.htm

Pregnancy and Lactation Labeling Final Rule (PLLR)
    https://www.drugs.com/pregnancy-categories.html

Prescriber's Letter
    http://prescribersletter.therapeuticresearch.com/pl/sample.
    aspx?cs=&s=PRL&AspxAutoDetectCookieSupport=1

Psychopharmacology
    http://link.springer.com/journal/213

Reference for Interpretation of Hepatitis C Virus (HCV) Test Results
    www.cdc.gov/hepatitis

Robinson, C. L., Romero, J. R., Kempe, A., & Pellegrini, C. (2017). Advisory committee
    on immunization practices recommended immunization schedule for children and
    adolescents aged 18 years or younger—United States, 2017. *MMWR. Morbidity and
    Mortality Weekly Report, 66*(5), 134–135. doi:10.15585/mmwr. mm6605e1

Rosenberg, E, et al . (2017, November 5–9). *Prevalence and incidence of Zika virus infection
    among household contacts of Zika patients, Puerto Rico, 2016-2017. ASTMH 2017* . Paper
    presented at the 66th Annual Meeting of the American Society of Tropical Medicine and
    Hygiene, Baltimore, MD

RxLIST
    http://www.rxlist.com/script/main/hp.asp

RxLIST: Drugs A-Z
    http://www.rxlist.com/drugs/alpha_a.htm

Sáez-Llorens, X., Tricou, V., Yu, D., Rivera, L., Jimeno, J., Villarreal, A. C., … Wallace, D.
    (2018). Immunogenicity and safety of one versus two doses of tetravalent dengue vaccine
    in healthy children aged 2–17 years in Asia and Latin America: 18-month interim data
    from a phase 2, randomised, placebo-controlled study. *The Lancet Infectious Diseases,
    18*(2), 162–170. doi:10.1016/s1473-3099(17)30632-1

Sanford Guide Web Edition
    https://webedition.sanfordguide.com

Saunders, K. H., Shukla, A. P., Igel, L. I., & Aronne, L. J. (2017). Obesity: When to consider
    medication. *The Journal of Family Practice, 66*(10), 608–616.
    http://www.mdedge.com/sites/default/files/Document/September-2017/JFP06610608.
    PDF

Schaeffer, A. J., & Nicolle, L. E. (2016). Urinary tract infections in older men. *The New
    England Journal of Medicine. 374*(6), 562–571.

Schwartz, S. R., Magit, A. E., Rosenfeld, R. M., Ballachanda, B. B., Hackell, J. M., Krouse, H. J., . . . Cunningham, E. R. (2017). Clinical practice guideline (update): Earwax (cerumen impaction). *Otolaryngology Head Neck Surgery, 156*(1S), S1–S29.

Solutions for Safer ER/LA Opioid Prescribing in a New Era of Health Care. American Nurses Credentialing Center, Post Graduate Institute of Medicine www.cmeuniversity.com

Sterling, T. R., Villarino, M. E., Borisov, A. S., Shang, N., Gordin, F., Bliven-Sizemore, E., . . . TB trials consortium PREVENT TB study team. (2011). Three months of rifapentine and isoniazid for latent tuberculosis infection. *The New England Journal of Medicine, 365,* 2155–2166. doi:10.1056/NEJMoa1104875

Stone, N. J., Robinson, J. G., Lichtenstein, A. H., Bairey Merz, C. N., Blum, C. B., Eckel, R. H., . . . American College of Cardiology/American Heart Association Task Force on Practice Guidelines. (2014). 2013 ACC/AHA guideline on the treatment of blood cholesterol to reduce atherosclerotic cardiovascular risk in adults: A report of the American College of Cardiology/American Heart Association Task Force on Practice Guidelines. *Circulation, 129*(25 suppl 2), S1–S45.

Sun, T., Liu, J., & Zhao, D. W. (2016). Efficacy of N-Acetylcysteine in idiopathic pulmonary fibrosis. *Medicine, 95*(19), e3629. doi:10.1097/md.0000000000003629

Taipale, H., Mittendorfer-Rutz, E., Alexanderson, K., Majak, M., Mehtälä, J., Hoti, F., . . . Tiihonen, J. Antipsychotics and mortality in a nationwide cohort of 29,823 patients with schizophrenia [published online December 20, 2017]. *Schizophrenia Research, pii: S0920–9964*(17), 30762–30764. doi:10.1016/j.schres.2017.12.010

Taketomo, C. K., Hodding, J. H., & Kraus, D. M. (2015). *Pediatric and neonatal dosage handbook: A universal resource for clinicians treating pediatric and neonatal patients* (22nd ed.). Wolters Kluwer.

Tebas, P., Roberts, C. C., Muthumani, K., Reuschel, E. L., Kudchodkar, S. B., Zaidi, F. I., . . . Maslow, J. N. (2017). Safety and Immunogenicity of an Anti–Zika Virus DNA Vaccine—Preliminary Report. *New England Journal of Medicine.* doi:10.1056/nejmoa1708120

The 2017 hormone therapy position statement of The North American Menopause Society. (2017). *Menopause: The North American Menopause Society.* doi:10.1097/GME.0000000000000921

The American Congress of Obstetrics and Gynecology (ACOG) http://www.acog.org

The American Geriatrics Society http://www.americangeriatrics.org

The JAMA Network.com www.jamanetwork.com

The Journal for Nurse Practitioners www.elsevier.com/locate/tjnp

The Medical Letter on Drugs and Therapeutics http://secure.medicalletter.org

The Nurse Practitioner Journal
www.tnpj.com

Third Report of the National Cholesterol Education Program (NCEP) Expert Panel on Detection, Evaluation, and Treatment of High Blood Cholesterol in Adults (Adult Treatment Panel III) Final Report.
http://www.ncbi.nlm.nih.gov/pubmed/12485966

Tomaselli, G. F., Mahaffey, K. W., Cuker, A., Dobesh, P. P., Doherty, J. U., Eikelboom, J. W., … Wiggins, B. S. (2017). 2017 ACC Expert Consensus Decision Pathway on Management of Bleeding in Patients on Oral Anticoagulants. *Journal of the American College of Cardiology, 70*(24), 3042–3067. doi:10.1016/j.jacc.2017.09.1085

Sun, T., Liu, J., & Zhao, D. W. (2016). Efficacy of N-Acetylcysteine in Idiopathic Pulmonary Fibrosis. Medicine, 95(19), e3629. doi:10.1097/md.0000000000003629

Tricou, V, et al. *Progress in development of Takeda's tetravalent dengue vaccine. ASTMH 2017.* Paper presented at the 2017 American Society of Tropical Medicine & Hygiene

Updated CDC guidance: Superbugs threaten hospital patients. *Medscape Education Clinical Briefs.* (2016, March 31)
http://www.medscape.org/viewarticle/859361?nlid=105320_2713&src=wnl_cmemp_160523_mscpedu_nurs&impID=1106718&faf=1

UpToDate.com
http://www.uptodate.com

U.S. Pharmacist Weekly Newsletter
http://www.uspharmacist.com

Vail, B. Chapter 36: Diabetes Mellitus. In: South-Paul, JE, Matheny, SE, & Lewis, EL. (2015). *Current Diagnosis & Treatment: Family Medicine (4th ed.).* New York, NY: McGraw-Hill Education

Vogt, C. (2017, November 14). New AHA/ACC guidelines lower high BP threshold. Consultant360
https://www.consultant360.com/exclusives/new-ahaacc-guidelines-lower- high-bp-threshold

Vrcek, I., Choudhury, E., & Durairaj, V. (2017). Herpes zoster ophthalmicus: A review for the internist. *The American Journal of Medicine, 130*(1), 21–26.

Wald, E. R., Applegate, K. E., Bordley, C., Darrow, D. H., Glode, M. P., Marcy, S. M., . . . American Academy of Pediatrics. (2013). Clinical practice guidelines for the diagnosis and management of acute bacterial sinusitis in children 1 to 18 years. *Pediatrics, 132*(1), e262–280.

Wallace, D. V., Dykewicz, M. S., Oppenheimer, J., Portnoy, J. M., & Lang, D. M. (2017). Pharmacologic Treatment of Seasonal Allergic Rhinitis: Synopsis of Guidance From the 2017 Joint Task Force on Practice Parameters. Annals of Internal Medicine, 167(12), 876. doi:10.7326/m17-2203

Watkins, S. L., Glantz, S. A., & Chaffee, B. W. (2018). Association of Noncigarette Tobacco Product Use With Future Cigarette Smoking Among Youth in the Population Assessment of Tobacco and Health (PATH) Study, 2013-2015. *JAMA Pediatrics, 172*(2), 181. doi:10.1001/jamapediatrics.2017.4173

Watson, T., Hickok, J., Fraker, S., Korwek, K., Poland, R. E., & Septimus, E. (2017). Evaluating the risk factors for hospital-onset Clostridium difficile infections in a large healthcare system. Clinical Infectious Diseases. doi:10.1093/cid/cix1112

WebMD: Drugs and Medications A to Z. Latest Drug News
http://www.webmd.com/drugs

Wimmer, B. C., Cross, A. J., Jokanovic, N., Wiese, M. D., George, J., Johnell, K., . . . Bell, J. S. (2016). Clinical Outcomes Associated with Medication Regimen Complexity in Older People: A Systematic Review. *Journal of the American Geriatrics Society, 65*(4), 747–753. doi:10.1111/jgs.14682

Wong, J., Marr, P., Kwan, D., Meiyappan, S., & Adcock, L. (2014). Identification of inappropriate medication use in elderly patients with frequent emergency department visits. *Canadian Pharmacists Journal/Revue Des Pharmaciens Du Canada, 147*(4), 248–256. doi:10.1177/1715163514536522

World Health Organization. Growing antibiotic resistance forces updates to recommended treatments for sexually transmitted infections. August 30 2016
http://www.who.int/mediacentre/news/releases/2016/antibiotics-sexual-infections/en

World Health Organization. (2016). WHO Guidelines for the Treatment of *Chlamydia trachomatis*
http://www.who.int/reproductivehealth/publications/rtis/chlamydia-treatment-guidelines/en

World Health Organization. (2016). WHO Guidelines for the Treatment of *Neisseria gonorrhoeae.*
http://www.who.int/reproductivehealth/publications/rtis/gonorrhoea-treatment-guidelines/en

World Health Organization. WHO Guidelines for the Treatment of *Treponema pallidum* (Syphilis)—2016
http://www.who.int/reproductivehealth/publications/rtis/syphilis-treatment-guidelines/en

World Health Organization. (2017, March). WHO Model List of Essential Medicines (20th list). Geneva, Switzerland: Author
http://www.who.int/medicines/publications/essentialmedicines/20th_EML2017.pdf?ua=1

World Health Organization. (2017, March). WHO Model List of Essential Medicines for Children (6th list). Geneva, Switzerland: Author
http://www.who.int/medicines/publications/essentialmedicines/6th_EMLc2017.pdf?ua=1

World Health Organization. (2017, June 6). WHO updates essential medicines list with new advice on use of antibiotics, and adds medicines for hepatitis C, HIV, tuberculosis and cancer. Geneva, Switzerland: Author
http://www.who.int/mediacentre/news/releases/2017/essential-medicines-list/en

Xie, Y., Bowe, B., Li, T., Xian, H., Yan, Y., & Al-Aly, Z. Long-term kidney outcomes among users of proton pump inhibitors without intervening acute kidney injury [published online february 22, 2017]. *Kidney International, 91*(6), 1482–1494. Dx.doi.org/10.1016/j.kint.2016.12.021

Yılmaz, D, Heper, Y, & Gözler, L. (2017). Effect of the use of buzzy during phlebotomy on pain and individual satisfaction in blood donors. *Pain Management Nursing, 18*(4), 260–267.

Yoon, I.-K., & Thomas, S. J. (2017). Encouraging results but questions remain for dengue vaccine. *The Lancet Infectious Diseases, 18*(2), 125–126doi:10.1016/S1473-3099(17)30634-5

Zarrabi, H., Khalkhali, M., Hamidi, A., Ahmadi, R., & Zavarmousavi, P. (2016). Clinical features, course and treatment of methamphetamine-induced psychosis in psychiatric inpatients. *BMC Psychiatry, 16*, 44. doi:10.1186/s12888-016-0745-5

See **Appendix A** for descriptions of FDA pregnancy categories
See **Appendix B** for descriptions of controlled drug categories
∗ no assigned pregnancy category

Drug	Pg. Nos.	Preg. Cat.	DEA Sched.
abacavir, Ziagen	225, 589	C	
abaloparatide, Tymlos	259, 335	C	
A/B Otic, *antipyrine+benzocaine+glycerin*	338, 342	C	
abatacept, **Orencia**	409, 421	C	
Abilify, *aripiprazole*	52, 122, 300, 582	C	
Abreva, *docosanol*	217	∗	
Abstral, *fentanyl citrate sublingual tablet*	355	C	
acamprosate, **Campral**	10	C	
Acanya, *clindamycin+benzoyl peroxide gel*	5, 172	C	
acarbose, **Precose**	487	B	
Accolate, *zafirlukast*	34, 425	B	
Accuneb, *albuterol*	30	C	
Accupril, *quinapril*	199, 242	D	
Accuretic, *quinapril+hydrochlorothiazide*	247	D	
Accutane, *isotretinoin, retinoic acid*	8	X	
acebutolol, **Sectral**	238, 574	B	
Aceon, *perindopril*	242	D	
Acetadote, *acetylcysteine*	3	B	
acetaminophen, **Feverall, Ofirmev, Panadol, Tempra, Tylenol**	165–166, 344, 513	B	
acetazolamide, **Diamox, Diamox Sequels**	182–183	C	

Drug	Pg. Nos.	Preg. Cat.	DEA Sched.
Adderall, Adderall XR, *dextroamphetamine saccharate+dextroamphetamine sulfate+amphetamine aspartate+amphetamine sulfate*	41, 312	C	II
Adempas, *riociguat*	411, 412	X	
adenovir dipivoxil, **Hepsera**	207	C	
Adipex-P, *phentermine*	315	C	IV
Apidra, *insulin glulisine (rDNA origin)*	482	C	
Adlyxin, *lixisenatide*	492	C	
Admelog, Admelog Solostar, *insulin lispro*	482	*	
Adoxa, *doxycycline*	4, 6, 22, 54, 55, 60, 73, 84, 89, 90, 160, 184, 189, 220, 288, 290, 366, 380, 397, 430, 436, 445, 505, 509, 605	D	
Adrenaclick, *epinephrine*	15, 448	C	
Advair HFA, Advair DisKus, *fluticasone propionate+salmeterol*	36	C	
Advanced Relief Visine, *tetrahydrozoline+polyethylene glycol 400+povidone+dextran 70*	96	*	
Advicor, *lovastatin+niacin-er*	149, 255	X	
Advil, *ibuprofen*	167	B/D	
Adzenya XR-ODT, *amphetamine sulfate*	41	C	II
Afeditab CR, *nifedipine*	244	C	
AeroBid, Aerobid M, *flunisolide*	33, 572	C	
Aggrenox, *dipyridamole+aspirin*	593	D	
Akineton, *biperiden hydrochloride, biperiden lactate*	363	C	
Akynzeo, *netupitant+ palonosetron*	301	C	
Alamast, *pemirolast*	95	C	
alcaftadine, **Lastacaft**	95	B	
Alaway, *ketotifen fumarate*	95	C	

Drug	Pg. Nos.	Preg. Cat.	DEA Sched.
alosetron, **Lotronex**	278	B	
Aloxi, *palonosetron*	72, 81, 313, 325	B	
Alphagan P, *brimonidine*	180	B	
alprazolam, **Niravam, Xanax, Xanax XR**	24, 359	D	IV
alprostadil for injection, **Edex**	161	X	
alprostadil urethral suppository, **Muse**	161	X	
Alrex, *loteprednol etabonate*	94, 164	C	
Alsuma Injectable, *sumatriptan*	192	C	
Altace, *ramipril*	199, 242	D	
Altavera, *ethinyl estradiol+ levonorgestrel*	549	X	
ALTernaGEL, *aluminum hydroxide*	173	C	
Atelvia, *risedronate (as sodium)*	335, 343	C	
Altoprev, *lovastatin*	146	X	
aluminum hydroxide, **ALTernaGEL, Amphojel**	173–174	C	
Alunbrig, *brigatinib*	576	*	
Alupent, *metaproterenol*	31–32, 38	C	
Alvesco, *ciclesonide*	32	C	
amantadine, **Symmetrel**	48, 361, 606, 615	C	
Amaryl, *glimepiride*	487	C	
Ambien, Ambien CR, *zolpidem tartrate*	28, 170, 272	B	IV
ambrisentan, **Letairis**	411	X	
ambrosia artemisiifolia 12 amb a, **Ragwitek**	424	C	
Amerge, *naratriptan*	192	C	
Americaine, Americaine Otic, *benzocaine*	338, 342	C	
Amevive, *alefacept*	402	B	
amikacin, **Amikin**	603	C	
Amikin, *amikacin*	603	C	
amiloride, **Midamor**	201, 240	B	
amiodarone, **Cordarone**	573	D	

Drug	Pg. Nos.	Preg. Cat.	DEA Sched.
Azulfidine, Azulfidine EN-Tabs, *sulfasalazine*	108, 418, 454, 502	B/D	
Babylax, *glycerin suppository*	104, 156	C	
bacillus athracis immune globulin intravenous (human), Anthrasil	21	*	
bacitracin, Bacitracin Ophthalmic	96	C	
Bacitracin Ophthalmic, *bacitracin*	96	C	
baclofen, Lioresal	307, 457, 476	C	
Bactrim, Bactrim DS, *sulfamethoxazole+trimethoprim*	57, 62, 73–74, 111, 140, 142, 189–190, 339, 341, 372, 381, 382, 384, 398, 399, 413, 432, 437, 442, 498, 510–511, 612, 648	C	
Bactroban, *mupirocin*	263, 443, 524	B	
Balacet, *propoxyphene napsilate+ acetaminophen*	353	C	IV
balsalazide, Colazal	500	B	
Balziva, *ethinyl estradiol+ norethindrone*	550	X	
Banzel, *rufinamide*	585	C	
Baraclude, *entecavir*	207	C	
Basaglar, *insulin glargine (recombinant)*	483	C	
basiliximab, Simulect	440	B	
Bavencio, *avelumab*	576	*	
Baxdela, *delafloxacin*	75–76, 610	*	
Bayer, *aspirin*	166	D	
becaplermin, Regranex Gel	499	C	
beclomethasone dipropionate, Beconase AQ, QNASL, Qvar	32, 385, 425, 571	C	
Beconase AQ, *beclomethasone dipropionate*	385, 425	C	
bedaquiline, Sirturo	478	B	
Belbuca, *buprenorphine*	321	C	III
Belsomra, *suvorexant*	272, 314	*	IV

Drug	Pg. Nos.	Preg. Cat.	DEA Sched.
Cardene, Cardene SR, *nicardipine*	18, 244	C	
Cardizem, Cardizem CD, Cardizem LA, *diltiazem*	19, 194, 243	C	
Cardura, Cardura XL, *doxazosin*	48, 245, 268	C	
carfilzomib, **Kyprolis**	578	∗	
cariprazine, **Vraylar**	52, 582	∗	
carisoprodol, **Soma**	307–309, 457, 458	C	
Carmol 40, *urea cream*	443	C	
Carnexiv, *carbamazepine*	51, 584	D	
carteolol, **Ocupress**	181	C	
Cartia XT, *diltiazem*	18, 243	C	
carvedilol, **Coreg**	200, 239	C	
Casodex, *bicalutamide*	577	X	
Cataflam, *diclofenac potassium*	150, 563	C	
Catapres, Catapres-TTS, *clonidine*	44, 245, 392	C	
Cayston, *aztreonam*	612	B	
Cedax, *ceftibuten*	60, 340, 374, 441, 472, 608, 628	B	
cefaclor, **Cefaclor Extended Release**	59, 74, 264, 292-293, 338, 340, 374, 379, 441, 444, 471, 508, 524, 607, 622	B	
Cefaclor Extended Release, *cefaclor*	59, 74, 264, 292-293, 338, 340, 374, 379, 441, 444, 471, 508, 524, 607, 622	B	
cefadroxil, **Duricef, Ultracef**	59, 264, 374, 433, 444, 471, 508, 524, 606, 623	B	
cefazolin, **Ancef, Kefzol**	46, 606	B	
cefdinir, **Omnicef**	59, 340, 374, 379, 441, 444, 471, 524, 608, 624	B	
cefditoren pivoxil, **Spectracef**	59, 374, 444, 472, 608	C	
cefepime, **Maxipime**	608	B	
cefixime, **Suprax**	59, 340, 374, 436, 441, 472, 498, 508, 608, 625	B	
Cefizox, *ceftizoxime*	185	B	
Cefobid, *cefoperazone*	607	B	

Drug	Pg. Nos.	Preg. Cat.	DEA Sched.
Clenia, *sulfacetamide+sulfur*	4, 131	C	
Cleocin, Cleocin T, Cleocin Vaginal Cream, Cleocin Vaginal Ovules, *clindamycin*	5, 46, 47, 55, 117, 172, 221, 293, 364, 433, 613, 631	B	
clevidipine butyrate, **Cleviprex**	243	C	
Cleviprex, *clevidipine butyrate*	243	C	
Climara, *estradiol transdermal system*	296, 299, 332	X	
Climara Pro, *estradiol+ levonorgestrel*	297, 332	X	
clindamycin, **Clindets, Cleocin, Cleocin T, Cleocin Vaginal Cream, Cleocin Vaginal Ovules, Evoclin Foam**	5, 46, 47, 55, 117, 172, 221, 293, 364, 433, 613, 631	B	
Clindets, *clindamycin*	172	B	
Clinoril, *sulindac*	565	D	
clobazam, **Onfi**	584	C	IV
clobetasol propionate, **Clobex Shampoo, Clobex Spray, Cormax, Olux, Temovate**	568	C	
Clobex Shampoo, Clobex Spray, *clobetasol propionate*	568	C	
clomipramine, **Anafranil**	158, 317, 475	C	
clonazepam, **Klonopin**	24–25, 360, 477, 584	C	IV
clonidine, **Catapres, Catapres-TTS, Kapvay, Nexiclon, Nexi-clon XR**	44, 245, 392	C	
clopidogrel, **Plavix**	371, 593	B	
clorazepate, **Tranxene**	9, 25, 360	C	IV
Clorpres, *clonidine+ chlorthalidone*	252	C	
clotrimazole, **Gyne-Lotrimin, Gyne-Lotrimin-3, Lotrimin, Mycelex G, Mycelex G Vaginal, Mycelex Troche**	66, 67, 69–70, 136, 463, 464, 466, 468, 604	B	
clozapine, **Clozaril, Fazaclo, Versacloz**	582	B	
Clozaril, *clozapine*	582	B	
coal tar, **Scytera, T/Gel**	131, 376, 402–403	C	
codeine sulfate	346	C	III
Cogentin, *benztropine*	363	C	
Cognex, *tacrine*	12	C	

Drug	Pg. Nos.	Preg. Cat.	DEA Sched.
Coreg, *carvedilol*	200, 239	C	
Corgard, *nadolol*	19, 194, 238	C	
Cormax, *clobetasol propionate*	568	C	
Cortane-B Otic, *hydrocortisone+ chloroxylenol+pramoxine*	337	C	
Cortef, *hydrocortisone*	569, 570	C	
Cotempla XR-ODT, methylphenidate	43	✱	
Cortenema, *hydrocortisone*	500	C	
Cortifoam, *hydrocortisone*	500	C	
Cortisporin Cream, Cortisporin Ophthalmic, Cortisporin Otic, *polymyxin b+neomycin+ hydrocortisone*	99, 337–338, 342	C	
Cortisporin Ointment, *polymyxin b+bacitracin zinc+neomycin+ hydrocortisone*	99	C	
Corzide, *nadolol+ bendroflumethiazide*	249	C	
Cosopt, *dorzolamide+timolol*	182	C	
Cotazym, Cotazym S, *pancrelipase*	163, 356	C	
Coumadin, *warfarin*	371, 589	D	
Covera-HS, *verapamil*	18, 194, 244	C	
Cozaar, *losartan*	242	D	
Creon, *pancrelipase*	162–163, 356	C	
Crestor, *rosuvastatin*	146, 254	X	
crisaborole, **Eucrisa**	122	✱	
Crixivan, *indinavir*	229, 586	C	
crofelemer, **Fulyzaq, Mytesi**	137, 139	C	
Crolom, *cromolyn sodium*	94, 282	B	
cromolyn sodium, **Children's NasalCrom, Crolom, Intal, Nasal Crom**	34, 94, 282, 426	B	
crotamiton, **Eurax**	433	C	
Cryselle, *ethinyl estradiol+ norgestrel*	550	X	
Cubicin, *daptomycin*	613	B	
Cuprimine, *penicillamine*	418, 454, 512	D	

Drug	Pg. Nos.	Preg. Cat.	DEA Sched.
Daralex, *daratumumab*	577	*	
daratumumab, Daralex	577	*	
darbepoetin alpha, Aranesp	15–16	C	
darifenacin, Enablex	266	C	
darunavir, Prezista	228, 587	B	
Daytrana, *methylphenidate*	43	C	II
Daypro, *oxaprozin*	565	C	
DDAVP Nasal Spray, *desmopressin*	158, 266	B	
Debrox, *carbamide peroxide*	77	A	
Decadron, Decadron LA, *dexamethasone*	570	C	
deferasirox, Exjade, Jadenu, Jadenu Sprinkle	276	B	
delafloxacin, Baxdela	75–76, 610	*	
delavirdine mesylate, Rescriptor	226, 587	C	
Deltasone, *prednisone*	48, 570	C	
Delzicol, *mesalamine*	107–108, 500–501	B	
Demadex, *torsemide*	153, 201, 240	B	
Demerol, *meperidine*	348	D	II
Demulen 1/35-21, Demulen 1/50-21, Demulen 1/35-28, Demulen 1/50-28, *ethinyl estradiol+ethynodiol diacetate*	550	X	
Denavir, *penciclovir*	218	B	
denosumab, Xgeva, Prolia	336	C	
Depakene, *valproic acid*	477	D	
Depakote, *divalproex*	51, 196, 476, 477, 584	D	
Depen, *penicillamine*	418, 454, 512	D	
Depo-Medrol, *methylprednisolone*	571	C	
Depo-Provera, Depo-SubQ, *medroxyprogesterone*	157, 299, 558	X	
Derma-Smoothe/FS, *fluocinolone acetonide*	123, 131, 399 527, 567	C	
Dermatop, *prednicarbate*	567	C	
Descovy, emtricitabine+tenofovir alafenamide	230, 586	*	

Drug	Pg. Nos.	Preg. Cat.	DEA Sched.
Duavee, *conjugated estrogens+ bazedoxifene*	298, 332	X	
Duet DHA Balanced, Duet DHA Complete, *prenatal vitamins*	595	A	
Duexis, *ibuprofen+famotidine*	564	B/D	
dulaglutide, **Trulicity**	491	C	
Dulcolax, *bisacodyl*	103, 156	B	
Dulera, *mometasone+formoterol*	37	C	
duloxetine, **Cymbalta**	27, 119, 168, 369, 392	C	
DuoFilm, *salicylic acid*	520	∗	
DuoNeb, *ipratropium+albuterol*	35	C	
Duragesic, *fentanyl transdermal system*	354	C	II
Duramorph PF, *morphine sulfate*	350	C	II
Duratuss AC, *diphenhydramine+ dextromethorphan+ phenylephrine*	599	C	
Durezol, *difluprednate*	164, 344	C	
Duricef, *cefadroxil*	59, 264, 374, 433, 444, 471, 508, 524, 606, 623	B	
Durlaza, *aspirin*	592	D	
durvalumab, **Imfinzi**	578	∗	
dutasteride, **Avodart**	49	X	
Dutoprol, *metoprolol succinate+ ext-rel hydrochlorothiazide*	248	C	
Duzallo, *allopurinol+lesinurad*	187	∗	
Dyazide, *triamterene+ hydrochlorothiazide*	153, 202, 241	B	
Dymista, *azelastine+ fluticasone propionate*	427	C	
Dynacin, *minocycline*	4, 6, 22, 23, 29, 221, 288, 291, 446, 510, 605, 612	D	
DynaCirc, DynaCirc CR, *isradipine*	243	C	
Dyrenium, *triamterene*	152, 240	B	
Ecallantide, **Kalbitor**	214	C	
echothiophate, **Phospholine Iodide**	181	C	

Drug	Pg. Nos.	Preg. Cat.	DEA Sched.
Elimite, *permethrin*	432	B	
Eliquis, *apixaban*	590	C	
ella, *ulipristal*	518, 560	X	
Elmiron, *pentosan polysulfate sodium*	274	B	
Elocon, *mometasone furoate*	567	C	
Emadine, *emedastine difumarate*	94	C	
Embeda, *morphine+naltrexone*	350	C	II
emedastine difumarate, Emadine	94	C	
Emend, *aprepitant*	71, 80, 326	B	
Emetrol, *phosphorated carbohydrated solution*	173	*	
emicizumab-kxwh, Hemlibra	204	*	
empagliflozin, Glyxambi	493	C	
Emsam, *selegiline*	121, 394	C	
emtricitabine, Emtriva	225, 586	B	
Emtriva, *emtricitabine*	225, 586	B	
Emverm, *mebendazole*	221, 376, 431, 461, 473, 523, 604	C	
Enablex, *darifenacin*	266	C	
enalapril, Epaned, Vasotec	199, 241	D	
enasidenib, Idhifa	578		
Enbrel, *etanercept*	404, 408, 418–419	B	
Endari, *l-glutamine*	439, 577	*	
Enduronyl, Enduronyl Forte, *methyclothiazide+deserpidine*	151, 201, 239, 241	B	
enfuvirtide, Fuzeon	230, 587	B	
Enjuvia, *estrogens (conjugated)*	298	X	
enoxaparin, Lovenox	590	B	
Enpresse, *ethinyl estradiol+levonorgestrel*	550	X	
Enstilar, *calcipotriene+ betamethasone*	401	C	
entacapone, Comtan	363	C	

Drug	Pg. Nos.	Preg. Cat.	DEA Sched.
entecavir, Baraclude	207	C	
Entocort EC, *budesonide*	108, 499	C	
Entresto, *sacubitril+valsartan*	200	D	
Entyvio, *vedolizumab*	111, 503	B	
Epaned, *enalapril*	199, 241	D	
Epanova, *omega 3-acid ethyl esters*	144, 253	*	
Epclusa, *sofosbuvir+velpatasvir*	210	*	
Epiduo Gel, Epiduo Forte Gel, *adapalene+benzoyl peroxide*	7	C	
Epi-E-Zpen, *epinephrine*	15, 448	C	
epinastine, Elestat	95	C	
epinephrine, Adrenaclick, Adrenalin, Auvi-Q, Epi-E-Zpen, EpiPen, EpiPen Jr, Symjepi, Twinject	15, 448	C	
EpiPen, EpiPen Jr, *epinephrine*	15, 448	C	
Epivir, Epivir-HBV, *lamivudine, 3TC*	207, 226, 586, 606	C	
eplerenone, Inspra	200, 245	B	
Epogen, *epoetin alpha*	16	C	
epoetin alpha, Epogen, Procrit	16	C	
eprosartan, Teveten	242	D	
Epzicom, *abacavir+lamivudine*	230, 586	C	
Equagesic, *meprobamate+aspirin*	308, 458	D	IV
Equetro, *carbamazepine*	51, 584	D	
ergoloid, Hydergine, Hydergine LC, Hydergine Liquid	13	C	
erlotinib, Tarceva	580	D	
Errin, *norethindrone*	558	X	
Ertaczo, *sertaconazole*	467	C	
ertapenem, Invanz	380, 511, 609	B	
EryPed, *erythromycin ethylsuccinate*	6, 57, 60, 73, 76, 79, 84, 89, 90, 100, 101, 117, 141, 162, 189, 221, 265, 290, 319, 364, 372, 375, 377, 383, 445, 472, 505, 525, 611, 635–636	B	

Drug	Pg. Nos.	Preg. Cat.	DEA Sched.
Ery-Tab, *erythromycin base*	6, 56, 73, 76, 79, 84, 89, 100, 101, 117, 141, 162, 189, 220, 264, 290, 293, 319, 364, 372, 375, 377, 380, 382, 445, 472, 505, 525, 611	B	
Erythrocin, *erythromycin stearate*	611	B	
erythromycin base, Ery-Tab, PCE	6, 56, 73, 76, 79, 84, 89, 100, 101, 117, 141, 162, 189, 220, 264, 290, 293, 319, 364, 372, 375, 377, 380, 382, 445, 472, 505, 525, 611	B	
erythromycin ethylsuccinate, E.E.S., EryPed	6, 57, 60, 73, 76, 79, 84, 89, 90, 100, 101, 117, 141, 162, 189, 221, 265, 290, 319, 364, 372, 375, 378, 383, 445, 472, 505, 525, 611, 635–636	B	
erythromycin gluceptate, Ilotycin	57, 97, 319, 449	B	
erythromycin stearate, Erythrocin	611	B	
escitalopram, Lexapro	26, 118, 358	C	
Esclim, *estradiol transdermal system*	296, 299	X	
Esidrix, *hydrochlorothiazide*	151, 201, 239, 512	B	
Esimil, *guanethidine monosulfate+hydrochlorothiazide*	249	B	
esomeprazole, Nexium	177, 367, 528	B	
estazolam, ProSom	272	X	IV
Estrace, Estrace Vaginal Cream, *estradiol*	40, 296–298, 332	X	
Estraderm, *estradiol*	299, 332	X	
estradiol, Minivelle, Vagifem, Vivelle, Vivelle Dot, Yuvafem	40, 151, 296–299, 332	X	
Estrasorb, *estradiol*	298	X	
Estratest, Estratest HS, *esterified estrogens+methyltestosterone*	297	X	
Estring, *estradiol vaginal ring*	296	X	

Drug	Pg. Nos.	Preg. Cat.	DEA Sched.
Flomax, *tamsulosin*	48, 268, 513	B	
Flonase Allergy Relief, *fluticasone propionate*	386, 426	C	
Florone, *diflorasone diacetate*	568	C	
Flovent HFA, *fluticasone propionate*	33, 572	C	
Floxin, Floxin Otic Solution, *ofloxacin*	61, 85, 160, 337, 341, 381, 398, 437, 446, 498, 505, 510, 526, 610	C	
Fluad, *influenza virus vaccine w. adjuvant*	269	B	
Fluarix, *influenza virus vaccine*	269	B	
Fluarix Quadrivalent, *influenza virus vaccine*	269	B	
Flublok, *influenza virus vaccine*	269	B	
Flucelvax, *influenza virus vaccine*	270	C	
fluconazole, **Diflucan**	66–67, 70, 604, 638	C	
Flu-Immune, *influenza virus vaccine*	270	C	
FluLaval, *influenza virus vaccine*	270	C	
Flumadine, *rimantadine*	606, 645	C	
flunisolide, **AeroBid, AeroBid M, Nasalide, Nasarel**	33, 386, 426, 572	C	
fluocinonide, **Lidex, Lidex-E, Vanos**	568, 569	C	
fluocinolone acetonide, **Capex Shampoo, Derma-Smoothe/FS, Synalar**	123, 131, 399, 527, 566, 567	C	
fluoride, **Luride**	170–171	∗	
fluorometholone, **FML, FML Forte, FML S.O.P. Ointment**	93	C	
fluorometholone acetate, **Flarex**	94	C	
Fluoroplex, *fluorouracil, 5-fluorouracil, 5-FU*	9	D	
fluorouracil, 5-fluorouracil, 5-FU, **Adrucil, Efudex, Fluoroplex**	9	D	
fluoxetine, **Prozac, Prozac Weekly, Sarafem**	26, 65, 118, 195–196, 317, 358, 396, 475	C	
fluoxymesterone, **Halotestin**	459	X	

Drug	Pg. Nos.	Preg. Cat.	DEA Sched.
fluphenazine decanoate, **Prolixin Decanoate**	301, 582, 583	C	
fluphenazine hydrochoride, **Prolixin**	301	C	
flurandrenolide, **Cordran, Cordran SP, Cordran Tape**	567–569,	C	
flurazepam, **Dalmane**	169, 272	X	IV
flurbiprofen, **Ansaid**	563	B	
Flushield, *influenza virus vaccine*	270	C	
flutamide, **Eulexin**	577	D	
fluticasone furoate, **Veramyst**	386, 426	C	
fluticasone propionate, **ArmorAir, Children's Flonase Allergy Relief, Cutivate, Flonase Allergy Relief, Flovent, Flovent HFA, Xhance**	33, 386, 426, 567	C	
fluvastatin, **Lescol**	146, 254	X	
Fluzone, *influenza virus vaccine*	270	C	
FML Liquifilm, *fluorometholone*	93	C	
FML-S, *sulfacetamide sodium+ fluorometholone*	99	C	
Focalin, Focalin XR, *dexmethylphenidate*	42, 312	C	II
fondaparinux, **Arixtra**	591	B	
Foradil Aerolizer, *formoterol fumarate*	35	C	
Forfivo XL, *bupropion hydrochloride*	44–45, 121, 469–470, 582	C	
formoterol, **Foradil Aerolizer, Perforomist**	35	C	
Fortamet, *metformin*	446	B	
Fortaz, *ceftazidime*	607	B	
Forteo, *teriparatide*	259, 335	C	
Fortesta, *testosterone*	460	X	III
Fortical, *calcitonin-salmon*	333	C	
Fortovase, *saquinavir*	229, 587	B	
Fosamax, *alendronate*	334, 342	C	
Fosamax Plus D, *alendronate+ calcium*	334, 343	C	

Drug	Pg. Nos.	Preg. Cat.	DEA Sched.
Helidac Therapy, *bismuth subsalicylate+metronidazole+ tetracycline*	203	D	
Hemlibra, *emicizumab-kxwh*	204	*	
heparin	590	C	
Hepsera, *adenovir dipivoxil*	207	C	
Herplex, *idoxuridine*	282	C	
hexachlorophene, PhisoHex	443	C	
Hiprex, *methenamine hippurate*	511	C	
Horizant, *gabapentin enacarbil*	133, 169, 387, 414	C	
HMS, *medrysone*	94	C	
Humalog, Humalog KwikPen, *insulin lispro*	482	B	
Humalog Mix 75/25, Humalog Mix 50/50, *insulin lispro protamine+insulin lispro*	485	B	
Humatin, *paromomycin*	14	C	
Humatrope, *somatropin*	190	C	
Humira, *adalimumab*	109, 403–404, 408, 418, 502	B	
Humulin 70/30, Humulin 50/50, *insulin isophane suspension+insulin regular*	485	B	
Humulin L, Iletin II Lente, *insulin zinc suspension (lente)*	484	B	
Humulin N, *insulin zinc isophane suspension*	484	B	
Humulin R, Humulin R U-500, *insulin regular*	482	B	
Humulin U, *insulin extended zinc suspension (ultralente)*	484	B	
Hyal, *sodium hyaluronate*	330	B	
Hyalgan, *sodium hyaluronate*	330, 422	B	
Hycet, *hydrocodone bitartrate+ acetaminophen*	347	C	II
Hycodan, Hycodan Syrup, *hydrocodone+homatropine*	600	C	II

Drug	Pg. Nos.	Preg. Cat.	DEA Sched.
Hydergine, Hydergine LC, Hydergine Liquid, *ergoloid*	13	C	
hydralazine	20, 246	C	
Hydrea, *hydroxyurea*	439, 577	D	
hydrochlorothiazide, **Esidrix, Microzide**	151, 201, 239, 512	B	
hydrocodone bitartrate, **Hysingla ER, Vantrela ER, Zohydro ER**	347	C	II
hydrocortisone, **Anusol-HC, Cortaid, Cortef, Cortifoam, Hydrocortone, Hytone, Proctocort, Texacort**	205, 499, 566, 569, 570	C	
hydrocortisone acetate, **U-Cort**	566	C	
hydrocortisone butyrate, **Locoid**	567	C	
hydrocortisone phosphate, **Hydrocortone Phosphate**	571	C	
hydrocortisone probutate, **Pandel**	567	C	
hydrocortisone retention enema, **Cortenema**	500	C	
hydrocortisone sodium succinate, **Solu-Cortef**	570	C	
hydrocortisone valerate, **Westcort**	567	C	
Hydrocortone, *hydrocortisone*	569, 570	C	
Hydrocortone Phosphate, *hydrocortisone phosphate*	571	C	
hydroflumethiazide, **Saluron**	151	B	
hydromorphone, Dilaudid, Dilaudid HP, Exalgo, Paladone	348	C	II
hydroquinone, Lustra, Lustra AF	236, 293, 519	C	
hydroxychloroquine, Plaquenil	292, 417, 455, 605	C	
hydroxypropyl cellulose, **Lacrisert**	142	*	
hydroxypropyl methylcellulose, **Bion Tears, GenTeal Mild**	142	*	
hydroxyurea, **Droxia, Hydrea, Siklos**	438–439, 577	D	
hydroxyzine, **Atarax, Vistaril**	11, 23, 82, 125, 128, 130, 359, 424, 428, 517, 599	C	
hyoscyamine, **Anaspaz, Levbid, Levsin, Levsinex Timecaps, NuLev**	106, 266, 273, 278, 506	C	

Drug	Pg. Nos.	Preg. Cat.	DEA Sched.
Hypotears, *hydroxypropyl cellulose*	142	✱	
HyQvia, *recombinant human hyaluronidase (human normal immunoglobulin)*	397	C	
Hysingla ER, *hydrocodone bitartrate*	347	C	
Hytone, *hydrocortisone*	566	C	
Hytrin, *terazosin*	48, 245, 268	C	
Hyzaar, *losartan/ hydrochlorothiazide*	247	D	
ibandronate (as monosodium monohydrate), **Boniva**	334, 343	C	
Ibrance, *palbociclib*	577	✱	
Ibudone, *hydrocodone+ ibuprofen*	348	D	II
ibuprofen, **Advil, Caldolor, Motrin, PediaCare Fever Drops, PediaProfen**	166–167, 344, 513	D	
icatibant, **Firazyr**	214	C	
icosapent ethyl, **Vascepa**	144, 253	✱	
idarucizumab, **Praxbind**	593	✱	
Ifixi, infliximab-qbtx	110, 331, 405, 409, 420, 503	B	
Iletin II Lente, *insulin zinc suspension (lente)*	484	B	
Iletin II NPH, *insulin isophane suspension*	484	B	
Iletin II Regular, *insulin regular*	482	B	
iloperidone, **Fanapt**	583	C	
Ilotycin, *erythromycin gluceptate*	57, 97, 319, 449	B	
imatinib mesylate, **Gleevec**	577	D	
imbrutinib, **Imbruvica**	577	✱	
Imbruvica, *imbrutinib*	577	✱	
Imdur, *isosorbide mononitrate*	19	B	
Imfinzi, *durvalumab*	578	✱	
imipramine, **Tofranil, Tofranil PM**	120, 134, 158, 185, 195, 198, 275, 279, 318, 359, 388, 390, 393, 477	C	
imiquimod, **Aldara, Zyclara**	9, 521	B	

Drug	Pg. Nos.	Preg. Cat.	DEA Sched.
ivermectin, **Sklice, Soolantra, Stromectol**	3, 221, 364, 461, 473, 604	C	
Jadenu, Jadenu Sprinkle, *deferasirox*	276	∗	
Jalyn, *dutasteride+tamsulosin*	49	X	
Janumet, Janumet XR, *sitagliptin+metformin*	496	B	
Januvia, *sitagliptin*	495	B	
Jenest-21, Jenest-28, *ethinyl estradiol+norethindrone*	551	X	
Jentadueto, Jentadueto XR, *linagliptin+metformin*	496	B	
Jolessa, *ethinyl estradiol+ levonorgestrel*	551, 557	X	
Jublia, *efinaconazole*	318	C	
Junel 1/20, Junel 1.5/30, *ethinyl estradiol+norethindrone*	551	X	
Junel Fe 1/20, Junel Fe 1.5/30, *ethinyl estradiol+norethindrone*	551	X	
Juvisync, *sitagliptin+simvastatin*	497	X	
Juxtapid, *lomitapide mesylate*	145	X	
Kadian, *morphine sulfate*	350	C	II
Kalbitor, *ecallantide*		C	
Kaletra, *lopinavir+ritonavir*	223, 224, 231, 587	C	
Kaopectate, *kaolin/pectin*	137	C	
Kapvay, *clonidine*	44, 245, 392	C	
Kariva, *ethinyl estradiol+ desogestrel*	551	X	
Kayexalate, *sodium polystyrene sulfonate*	235	C	
K-Dur, *potassium chloride*	258	C	
Keflex, *cephalexin*	46, 60, 75, 78, 101, 160, 184, 293, 319, 340, 364, 374, 413, 433, 444, 472, 509, 525, 607, 629	B	
Kefzol, *cefazolin*	46	B	
Kelnor, *ethinyl estradiol+ ethynodiol diacetate*	551	X	

Drug	Pg. Nos.	Preg. Cat.	DEA Sched.
Kemadrin, *procyclidine*	363	C	
Kenalog, Kenalog E, *triamcinolone*	29	C	
Kenalog Injectable, Kenalog Lotion, Kenalog Ointment, Kenalog Spray, *triamcinolone acetonide*	566–568	C	
Keppra, Keppra Oral Solution, Keppra XR, *levetiracetam*	585	C	
Keratol 40, *urea cream*	443	C	
Kerlone, *betaxolol*	238	C	
Kerydin, *tavaborole*	318	C	
Ketek, *telithromycin*	61, 381, 610	C	
ketoconazole, **Extina, Nizoral, Xolegel**	68, 131, 136, 462, 463, 464, 466–468, 604	C	
ketorolac tromethamine, **Acular, Acular PF, Sprix, Toradol**	96, 164, 564	C	
ketoprofen fumarate, **Alaway, Zaditor**	95	C	
Keytruda, *pembrolizumab*	578	∗	
Kineret, *anakinra*	420	B	
Kisquali, *ribociclib*	578	∗	
Kisqali Femara Co-Pack, *ribociclib+letrozole*	578	∗	
Klaron, *sulfacetamide*	4, 6	C	
Klonopin, *clonazepam*	24–25, 360, 477, 584	C	IV
Klotrix, *potassium chloride*	258	A	
Kombiglyze XR, *saxagliptin+ metformin*	496	B	
Konsyl, *calcium polycarbophil*	102	C	
Kristalose, *lactulose*	103	B	
Krystexxa, *pegloticase*	186	C	
K-Tab, *potassium chloride*	258	C	
Imfinzi, *durvalumab*	578	C	
Kyleena, *levonorgestrel*	559	X	
Kynamro, *mipomersen*	145	B	
Kyprolis, *carfilzomib*	578	∗	
Kytril, *granisetron*	72, 80, 325	B	

Drug	Pg. Nos.	Preg. Cat.	DEA Sched.
labetalol, Normodyne, Trandate	239	C	
lacosamide, Vimpat	584	C	V
Lacri-Lube, Lacri-Lube NP, *petrolatum+mineral oil*	143	✳	
Lacrisert, *hydroxypropyl cellulose*	142	✳	
Lactaid Drops, Lactaid Extra, Lactaid Fast ACT, Lactaid Original, Lactaid Ultra, *lactase*	283	✳	
lactase, Lactaid Drops, Lactaid Extra, Lactaid Fast ACT, Lactaid Original, Lactaid Ultra	283	✳	
lactulose, Kristalose	103	B	
Lamictal, Lamictal XR, *lamotrigine*	51, 585	C	
Lamisil, Lamisil AT, *terbinafine*	318, 463, 465, 467, 468, 604	B	
lamivudine, 3TC, Epivir, Epivir-HBV	207, 226, 586, 606	C	
lamotrigine, Lamictal, Lamictal XR	51, 585	C	
Lanoxicaps, *digoxin*	202	C	
Lanoxin, *digoxin*	202	C	
lansoprazole, Prevacid, Prevacid Suspension, Prevacid SoluTab, Prevacid 24HR	177, 367, 528	B	
lanthanum, Fosrenol	236	C	
Lantus, *insulin glargine (recombinant)*	483	C	
Lariam, *mefloquine*	292, 455, 605	C	
Lartuvo, *olaratumab*	578	✳	
Lasix, *furosemide*	152, 201, 240	C	
Lastacaft, *alcaftadine*	95	B	
latanoprost, Xalatan	182	C	
Latisse, *bimatoprost*	262,	✳	
Latuda, *lurasidone*	53, 583	B	
Lazanda Nasal Spray, *fentanyl nasal spray*	355, 515	C	II
Leena, *ethinyl estradiol+ norethindrone*	551	X	
leflunomide, Arava	417, 454	X	

Drug	Pg. Nos.	Preg. Cat.	DEA Sched.
Mavik, *trandolapril*	199, 242	D	
Mavyret, *glecaprevir+pibrentasvir*	209	*	
Maxair, Maxair Autohaler, *pirbuterol*	32	C	
Maxalt, Maxalt-MLT, *rizatriptan*	192	C	
Maxaquin, *lomefloxacin*	509, 610	C	
Maxidex Ophthalmic, *dexamethasone*	93	C	
Maxidone, *hydrocodone+ acetaminophen*	347	C	II
Maxipime, *cefepime*	608	B	
Maxitrol, *neomycin+polymyxin b+dexamethasone sodium phosphate*	99	C	
Maxzide, *triamterene/ hydrochlorothiazide*	153, 202, 241	C	
Mebaral, *mephobarbital*	585	D	II
mebendazole, **Emverm Vermox**	221, 376, 431, 461, 473, 523, 604	C	
mecasermin, **Increlex**	190	B	
meclizine, **Antivert, Bonine, Dramamine II, Zentrip**	283, 294, 302, 519	B	
meclofenamate	564	B/D	
Medihaler-ISO, *isoproterenol*	31	B	
Medrol, Medrol Dosepak, *methylprednisolone*	569, 571	C	
medroxyprogesterone, **Depo-Provera**	157, 299, 558	X	
medrysone, **HMS**	94	C	
mefenamic acid, **Ponstel**	150, 564	C	
mefloquine, **Lariam**	292, 455, 605	C	
Mefoxin, *cefoxitin*	56, 185, 365, 607	B	
Megace, Megace ES, *megestrol*	20, 579	D	
megestrol, **Megace, Megace ES**	20, 579	D	
meglitinide, **Prandin**	488	C	
Mekinist, *trametinib*	579	*	
melphalan, **Alkeran**	576	D	
Mellaril, *thioridazine*	114, 115, 302, 583	C	

Drug	Pg. Nos.	Preg. Cat.	DEA Sched.
miltefosine, Impavido	285	D	
Minipress, *prazosin*	245, 268, 392	C	
Minivelle, *estradiol transdermal system*	299, 332	X	
Minizide, *prazosin+polythiazide*	249	C	
Minocin, *minocycline*	4, 6, 22, 23, 29, 221, 288, 291, 446, 510, 605, 612	D	
minocycline, Dynacin, Minocin, Minolira, Solodyn	4, 6, 22, 23, 29, 221, 288, 291, 446, 510, 605, 612	D	
Minolira, *minocycline*	6, 605, 612	✻	
minoxidil, Loniten, Rogaine	47–48, 246	C	
mipomersen, Kynamro	145	B	
mirabegron, Myrbetriq	266	C	
MiraLax, *polyethylene glycol*	103	C	
Mirapex, Mirapex ER, *pramipexole dihydrochloride*	361, 414	C	
Mircette, *ethinyl estradiol+ desogestrel diacetate*	553	X	
Mirena, *levonorgestrel IUD*	559	X	
mirtazapine, Remeron, Remeron Soltab	122, 393	C	
misoprostol, Cytotec	368, 562	X	
Mitigare, *colchicine*	186	C	
Mobic, *meloxicam*	150, 188, 310, 330, 407, 417, 564	C	
modafinil, Provigil	311, 446, 447	C	
Modicon, *ethinyl estradiol+ norethindrone*	553	X	
Moduretic, *amiloride+ hydrochlorothiazide*	153, 202, 241	B	
moexipril, Univasc	242	D	
mometasone furoate, Elocon, Asmanex Twisthaler	33, 386, 567, 572	C	
mometasone furoate monohydrate, Nasonex	386, 426	C	

Drug	Pg. Nos.	Preg. Cat.	DEA Sched.
Mylanta, Mylanta DS, *aluminum hydroxide+magnesium hydroxide+simethicone*	174	C	
Mylicon, *simethicone*	91, 107, 170, 278	C	
Myrbetriq, *mirabegron*	266	C	
Mysoline, *primidone*	585	D	
Mytesi, *crofelemer*	137, 139	C	
MyWay, *levonorgestrel*	560	X	
nabilone, **Cesamet**	81	C	
nadolol, **Corgard**	19, 194, 238	C	
nafarelin, **Synarel**	157	X	
nafcillin	589	B	
naftifine, **Naftin**	463, 465, 466	B	
Naftin, *naftifine*	463, 465, 466	B	
nalbuphine, **Nubain**	355	B	
Nalfon, *fenoprofen*	563	B/D	
nalidixic acid, **NegGram**	510	B	
nalmefene, **Revex**	326	B	
naloxegol, **Movantik**	324	C	
naloxone, **Narcan, Narcan Nasal Spray**	326	B	
naltrexone, **ReVia, Vivitrol**	321	C	
Namenda Oral Solution, Namenda XR, *memantine*	13	B	
naphazoline, **Vasocon-A**	95	C	
Naphcon A, *naphazoline+ pheniramine*	96	C	
Naprelan, *naproxen*	167	B	
Naprosyn, *naproxen*	167, 565	B	
naproxen, **Aleve, Anaprox, Anaprox DS, EC-Naprosyn, Naprelan, Naprosyn**	167	B	
naratriptan, **Amerge**	192	C	
Narcan, Narcan Nasal Spray, *naloxone*	326	B	
Nardil, *phenelzine*	121, 393	C	

Drug	Pg. Nos.	Preg. Cat.	DEA Sched.
Nasacort, Nasacort AQ, *triamcinolone acetonide*	387, 426	C	
NasalCrom, *cromolyn sodium*	426	B	
Nasalide, *flunisolide*	386, 426	C	
Nasarel, *flunisolide*	426	C	
Nascobal Gel, Nascobal Nasal Spray *cyanocobalamin, vitamin b-12*	17	C	
Nasonex, *mometasone furoate monohydrate*	386, 426	C	
Natachew, Natafort, *prenatal vitamins*	596	A	
Natacyn, *natamycin*	101	C	
natalizumab, **Tysabri**	110, 306	C	
natamycin, **Natacyn**	101	C	
Natazia, *estradiol valerate+ dienogest*	553	X	
nateglinide, **Starlix**	488	C	
Natesto, testosterone	460	X	III
nebivolol, **Bystolic**	238	C	
Necon 0.5/35-21, Necon 0.5/35-28, Necon 1/35-21, Necon 1/35-28, Necon 10/11-21, Necon 10/11-28, *ethinyl estradiol+ norethindrone*	553	X	
Necon 1/50-21, Necon 1/50-28, *mestranol+norethindrone*	553	X	
nedocromil, **Alocril, Tilade**	34, 95	B	
Neevo, Neevo DHA, *prenatal vitamins*	596	A	
nefozodone, **Serzone**	193	C	
NegGram, *nalidixic acid*	510	B	
nelarabine, **Arranon**	576	D	
nelfinavir, **Viracept**	229, 588	B	
Nelova 1/50-21, Nelova 1/50-28, *ethinyl estradiol+mestranol*	554	X	
Nelova 0.5/35-21, Nelova 0.5/35-28, Nelova 1/35-21, Nelova 1/35-28, Nelova 10/11-21, Nelova 10/11-28, *ethinyl estradiol+norethindrone*	554	X	
Nembutal, *pentobarbital*	272	D	II

Drug	Pg. Nos.	Preg. Cat.	DEA Sched.
Neoral, *cyclosporine*	142, 402	C	
Neosporin Ointment, Neosporin Ophthalmic Ointment, *neomycin+polymyxin b+ bacitracin zinc*	57, 450	C	
nepafenac, **Nevanac**	96, 164, 344	C	
Neptazane, *methazolamide*	183	C	
netarsudil, **Rhopressa**	182	C	
Neupro Transdermal Patch, *rotigotine*	362, 415	C	
neratinib, **Nerlynx**	549	∗	
Neurontin, *gabapentin*	133, 168–169, 387, 414	C	
Nevanac, *nepafenac*	96, 164, 344	C	
nevirapine, **Viramune**	227, 588	C	
Nexavar, *sorafenib*	579	D	
Nexiclon, Nexiclon XR, *clonidine*	44, 245, 392	C	
Nexa Plus, Nexa Select, *prenatal vitamins*	596	A	
Nexium, *esomeprazole*	177, 367, 528	B	
Nexplanon, *etonogestrel*	559	X	
niacin, **Niaspan, Slo-Niacin**	148, 254	C	
Niaspan, *niacin*	148, 254	C	
nicardipine, **Cardene, Cardene SR**	18, 244	C	
Nicoderm, Nicoderm CQ, *nicotine transdermal system*	470	D	
Nicorette Gum, *nicotine polacrilex*	470	X	
Nicorette Mini Lozenge, *nicotine polacrilex*	470	X	
nicotine nasal spray, **Nicotrol NS**	470–471	D	
nicotine transdermal system, **Habitrol, Nicoderm, Nicoderm CQ, Nicotrol, Nicotrol Step-down Patch, ProStep**	470	D	
nicotine polacrilex, **Nicorette Gum, Nicorette Mini Lozenge**	470	X	
Nicotrol, Nicotrol Step-down Patch *nicotine transdermal system*	470	D	
Nicotrol NS, *nicotine nasal spray*	471	D	

Drug	Pg. Nos.	Preg. Cat.	DEA Sched.
Norinyl 1+50-21, Norinyl 1/50-28, *mestranol+ norethindrone*	554	X	
Normiflo, *ardeparin*	590	C	
Normodyne, *labetalol*	239	C	
Noroxin, *norfloxacin*	185, 398, 510, 610	C	
Norpace, Norpace CR, *disopyramide*	574	C	
Norplant, *levonorgestrel*	559	X	
Norpramin, *desipramine*	120, 134, 158, 198, 388, 390, 477	C	
Nor-QD, *norethindrone*	558	*	
Northera, *droxidopa*	260	C	
Nortrel 0.5/35, Nortrel 1/35, *ethinyl estradiol+norethindrone*	554	X	
nortriptyline, **Pamelor**	120, 134, 158, 195, 198, 279, 388, 390, 393, 396, 478	D	
Norvasc, *amlodipine*	18, 243	C	
Norvir, *ritonavir*	229, 587	B	
Novolin 70/30, *insulin isophane suspension+insulin regular*	485	B	
Novolin L, *insulin zinc suspension (lente)*	484	B	
Novolin N, *insulin isophane suspension (lente)*	484	B	
Novolin R, *insulin regular*	482	B	
NovoLog, *insulin aspart*	482	C	
Noxafil, *posaconazole*	30, 67, 68, 70	C	
Nubain, *nalbuphine*	355	B	
Nucala, *mepolizumab*	38, 39, 159	*	
Nucynta, Nucynta ER, *tapentadol*	370–371	C	II
Nudexta, *dextromethorphan+ quinidine*	306, 363, 400	C	
NuLev, *hyoscyamine*	107, 267, 274, 278, 507	C	
Nulojix, *belatacept*		*	
Numorphan, *oxymorphone*	352	C	II

Drug	Pg. Nos.	Preg. Cat.	DEA Sched.
Ovral-21, Ovral-28, *ethinyl estradiol+norgestrel*	555	X	
Ovrette, *norgestrel*	558	X	
oxaprozin, **Daypro**	565	C	
oxazepam	10, 24, 360	D	IV
oxcarbazepine, **Trileptal, Oxtellar XR**	585	C	
Oxaydo, *oxycodone*	351	B	II
Oxecta, *oxycodone*	351	B	II
oxiconazole, **Oxistat**	463, 465, 467, 468	B	
Oxistat, *oxiconazole*	463, 465, 467, 468	B	
Oxsoralen, Oxsoralen Ultra, *methoxsalen*	519	C	
Oxtellar XR, *oxcarbazepine*	585	C	
oxybutynin, **Ditropan, Ditropan XL, GelniQUE, Oxytrol**	234, 267, 274	B	
oxycodone, **Oxaydo, Oxecta, OxyContin, OxyFast, OxyIR, Roxicodone, RoxyBond, Xtampza**	350–351	B	II
OxyContin, *oxycodone controlled-release*	351	B	II
OxyFast, *oxycodone immediate-release*	351	B	II
OxyIR, *oxycodone*	351	B	II
oxymetazoline, **Afrin, Visine L-R**	92, 95	C	
oxymorphone, **Numorphan, Opana**	352	C	II
Oxytrol, *oxybutynon*	234, 267, 274	B	
Ozempic, *semaglutide*	492	*	
palbociclib, **Ibrance**	577	*	
Palgic, *carbinoxamine*	600	C	
paliperidone, **Invega, Invega Sustenna**	583	C	
palivizumab, **Synagis**	414	*	
palonosetron, **Aloxi**	72, 81, 313, 325	B	
Pamelor, *nortriptyline*	120, 134, 158, 195, 198, 279, 388, 390, 393, 396, 478	D	

Drug	Pg. Nos.	Preg. Cat.	DEA Sched.
Pediapred, *prednisolone sodium phosphate*	570	C	
PediaProfen, *ibuprofen*	166	B/D	
Pediazole, *erythromycin ethylsuccinate+sulfisoxazole*	341, 611, 637	C	
PediOtic, *neomycin+ polymyxin b+hydrocortisone*	342	C	
Pegasys, *peginterferon alpha-2a*	208	C	
peginesatide, **Omontys**	16	C	
peginterferon alpha-2a, **Pegasys**	208	C	
peginterferon alfa-2b, **Peg-Intron**	209	C	
Peg-Intron, *peginterferon alfa-2b*	209	C	
pegloticase, **Krystexxa**	186	C	
pegvisomant, **Somavert**	8	B	
pembrolizumab, **Keytruda**	578	✱	
pemirolast, **Alamast**	95	C	
pemoline, **Cylert**	44, 313	B	
penbutolol, **Levatol**	238	C	
penciclovir, **Denavir**	218	B	
penicillamine, **Cuprimine, Depen**	418, 454, 512	D	
penicillin g benzathine, **Bicillin, Bicillin L-A, Permapen**	265, 375, 434, 451, 609	B	
penicillin v potassium, **Pen-Vee K**	46, 55, 56, 77, 117, 162, 265, 375, 434, 473, 609, 644	B	
Penlac Nail Laquer, *ciclopirox topical solution*	318	✱	
Pennsaid, *diclofenac sodium*	345, 406, 563	C	
pentazocine, **Talwin**	353	C	IV
pentobarbital, **Nembutal**	272	D	II
pentosan polysulfate sodium, **Elmiron**	274	B	
pentoxifylline, **Trental**	371, 594	C	
Pen-Vee K, *penicillin v potassium*	46, 55, 56, 77, 117, 162, 265, 375, 434, 473, 609, 644	B	

Drug	Pg. Nos.	Preg. Cat.	DEA Sched.
Premarin, Premarin Vaginal Cream, *estrogens (conjugated)*	14, 40, 296, 298, 332	X	
Premphase, Prempro, *estrogens (conjugated)+* *medroxyprogesterone*	297	X	
prenatal vitamins, **Citranatal 90 DHA, Citranatal Assure, Citranatal B-Calm, Citranatal DHA, Citranatal Harmony, Citranatal Rx, Duet DHA Balanced, Duet DHA Complete, Natachew, Natafort, Neevo, Neevo DHA, Nexa Plus, Nexa Select, Pre-nate AM, Prenate Chewable, Prenate DHA, Prenate Elite, Prenate Enhance, Prenate Essential, Prenate Restore, Prenate Mini, Prenexa**	594–597	A	
Prenate AM, Prenate Chewable, Prenate DHA, Prenate Elite, Prenate Enhance, Prenate Essential, Prenate Restore, Prenate Mini, *prenatal vitamins*	594–597	A	
Prenexa, *prenatal vitamins*	597	A	
Preparation H Cream, *petrolatum+shark liver oil+* *phenylephrine*	205	C	
Preparation H Ointment, *petrolatum/ glycerin+shark liveroil+phenylephrine*	205	C	
Preparation H Suppository, *petrolatum+cocoa butter+* *phenylephrine*	205	C	
Prepopik, *sodium picosulfate+ magnesium oxide+citric acid*	91	*	
Prestalia, *perindopril arginine+ amlodipine*	250	D	
Prevacid, Prevacid Suspension, Prevacid SoluTab, Prevacid 24 HR, *lansoprazole*	177, 367, 528	B	
Preven, *ethinyl estradiol+ levonorgestrel*	560	X	
Previfem, *ethinyl estradiol+ norgestimate*	555	X	
Prevlite, *cholestyramine*	86, 87	C	

Drug	Pg. Nos.	Preg. Cat.	DEA Sched.
ribavirin, **Copegus, Rebetol, Ribasphere RibaPak, Virazole**	208	X	
Ribasphere RibaPak, *ribavirin*	208	X	
ribociclib, Kisquali	578	✱	
RID, *pyrethrins*	365	C	
Ridaura, *auranofin*	417, 453	C	
Rifadin, *rifampin*	478, 606	C	
Rifamate, *rifampin+isoniazid*	478, 606	C	
rifampin, **Rifadin**	478, 606	C	
rifapentine, **Priftin**	478, 606	C	
Rifater, *rifampin+isoniazid+ pyrazinamide*	478, 606	C	
rifaximin, **Xifaxan**	140, 613	C	
rilpivirine, **Edurant**	227, 586	B	
rimantadine, **Flumadine**	606, 645	C	
rimexolone, **Vexol**	94	C	
riociguat, **Adempas**	411, 412	X	
Riomet, *metformin*	488	B	
risedronate (as sodium), **Actonel, Alteva**	334–335, 343	C	
Risperdal Consta, Risperdal M-Tab, *risperidone*	53, 114, 115, 392, 583	C	
risperidone, **Risperdal Consta, Risperdal M-Tab**	53, 114, 115, 392, 583	C	
Ritalin, Ritalin SR, *methylphenidate*	42, 43, 312–313	C	II
ritonavir, **Norvir**	229, 587	B	
Rituxan Hycela, *rituximab+ hyaluronidase*	579	✱	
rivaroxaban, **Xarelto**	592	C	
rivastigmine, **Exelon**	12	B	
rizatriptan, **Maxalt, Maxalt-MLT**	192	C	
Robaxin, *methocarbamol*	308, 457	C	
Robinul, *glycopyrrolate*	368	B	
Robitussin AC, *codeine+ guaifenesin*	601	C	III

Drug	Pg. Nos.	Preg. Cat.	DEA Sched.
Sabril, *vigabatrin*	586	C	
sacubitril+valsartan, **Entresto**	200	D	
Safyral, *ethinyl estradiol+ drospirenone+levomefolate*	555	X	
Saizen, *somatropin*	191	C	
salicylic acid, **DuoFilm, Keralyt Gel**	520, 521	*	
salmeterol, **Serevent, Serevent Diskus**	35–36, 62	C	
Saluron, *hydroflumethiazide*	151	B	
Salutensin, *reserpine+ hydroflumethiazide*	252	C	
Sumavel DosePro, *sumatriptan*	192	C	
Sanctura, Sanctura XR, *trospium chloride*	268	C	
Sancuso, *granisetron*	72, 80, 325	B	
Sansert, *methysergide maleate*	196	X	
Saphris, *asenapine*	52, 582	C	
saquinavir, **Fortovase**	229, 587	B	
saquinavir mesylate, **Invirase**	229, 587	B	
Sarafem, *fluoxetine*	396	C	
Savaysa, *edoxaban*	591	C	
Savella, *milnacipran*	168	C	
saxagliptin, **Onglyza**	495	B	
Scopace, *scopolamine*	303, 519	C	
scopolamine, **Scopace, Transderm-Scop**	283, 294, 303, 519	C	
Scytera, *coal tar*	131, 376, 403	C	
Seasonale, *ethinyl estradiol+ levonorgestrel*	557	X	
Seasonique, *ethinyl estradiol+ levonorgestrel*	557	X	
Sectral, *acebutolol*	238, 574	B	
Seebri Neohaler, *glycopyrrolate*	65, 155	C	
Segluromet, *ertugliflozen+ metformin*	494	C	
selegiline, **Emsam, Zelapar**	121, 363, 394	C	

Drug	Pg. Nos.	Preg. Cat.	DEA Sched.
selenium sulfide, Selsun, Selsun Blue, Selsun Gold	131, 468	C	
selexipag, Uptravi	410	*	
Selsun, Selsun Blue, Selsun Gold, *selenium sulfide*	131, 468	C	
Selzentry, *maraviroc*	230, 588	B	
semaglutide, Ozempic	492	*	
Semprex, *acrivastine+pseudoephedrine*	602	C	
Septra, Septra DS, *sulfamethoxazole+trimethoprim*	57, 62, 73–74, 111, 140, 142, 189–190, 339, 341, 372, 381, 382, 384, 398, 399, 413, 432, 437, 442, 498, 510–511, 612, 648	C	
Serentil, *mesoridazine*	114, 115, 302	C	
Serevent Diskus, *salmeterol*	36, 62	C	
serolimus, Rapamune	328	C	
Seroquel, Seroquel XR, *quetiapine fumarate*	53, 114, 115, 302, 583	B	
Serostim, *somatropin*	191	C	
sertaconazole, Ertaczo	467	C	
sertraline, Zoloft	26, 119, 317, 358, 391, 396, 475	C	
Serzone, *nefozodone*	193	C	
sevelamer, Renagel, Renvela	236	C	
Shingrix, *zoster vaccine recombinant, adjuvanted*	218	*	
Signifor LAR, *pasireotide*	8	C	
Siklos, *hydroxyurea*	439	D	
sildenafil, Revatio, Viagra	161, 411–412	B	
Silenor, *doxepin*	273	C	
Siliq, brodalumab	403	B	
silodosin, Rapaflo	48, 268	B	
Silvadene, *silver sulfadiazine*	66, 218, 219, 450	B	
silver sulfadiazine, Silvadene	66, 218, 219, 450	B	

Drug	Pg. Nos.	Preg. Cat.	DEA Sched.
tacrolimus, **Protopic**	126, 389, 400	C	
tadalafil, **Adcirca, Cialis**	49, 161, 412	B	
tafluprost, **Zioptan**	182	C	
Tagamet, Tagamet HB, *cimetidine*	175, 366	B	
Tagrisso, osimertinib	580	✳	
Talwin, *pentazocine*	352–353	C	IV
Talwin-NX, *pentazocine/ naloxone*	353, 355	C	
Tamiflu, *oseltamivir*	270, 606	C	
tamoxifen citrate, **Nolvadex**	579	D	
tamsulosin, **Flomax**	48, 268, 513	B	
Tanafed DMX, *dexchlorpheniramine+ pseudoephedrine+ dextromethorphan*	602	C	
tapentadol, **Nucynta, Nucynta ER**	370	C	II
Tapazole, *methimazole*	252	D	
Tarceva, *erlotinib*	580	D	
Tarina, *ethinyl estradiol+ norethindrone*	556	X	
Tarka, *trandolapril+verapamil*	250	D	
Tasigna, *nilotinib*	580	✳	
Tasmar, *tolcapone*	363	C	
tavaborole, **Kerydin**	318	C	
Taytulla, *estradiol+ norethindrone*	556	X	
tazarotene, **Avage, Tazorac**	7, 172, 236, 285, 402, 519, 526	X	
Tazicef, *ceftazidime*	607	B	
Tazidime, *ceftazidime*	607	B	
Tazorac, *tazarotene*	7, 172, 236, 285, 402, 519, 526	X	
Tecentriq, *atezolizumab*	580	D	
Tecfidera, *dimethyl fumarate*	303	C	
Teczem, *enalapril+diltiazem*	250	D	
tedizolid, **Sivextro**	77, 381	C	
Teflaro, *ceftaroline fosamil*	75, 264, 379, 607, 608	B	

Drug	Pg. Nos.	Preg. Cat.	DEA Sched.
Tegretol, Tegretol XR, *carbamazepine*	51, 476, 584	D	
Tekamlo, *aliskiren+amlodipine*	250–251	D	
Tekturna, *aliskiren*	246	D	
Tekturna HCT, *aliskiren+ hydrochlorothiazide*	250	D	
telavancin, Vibativ	613	C	
telbivudine, Tyzeka	207	C	
telithromycin, Ketek	61, 381, 610	C	
telmisartan, Micardis	242	D	
telotristat ethyl, Xermelo	72, 138	∗	
temazepam, Restoril	272	X	IV
Temovate, *clobetasol propionate*	568	C	
Tenex, *guanfacine*	245	B	
tenofovir alafenamide (AF), Vemlidy	207	B	
tenofovir disoproxil fumarate, Viread	226, 588	B	
Tenoretic, *atenolol+ chlorthalidone*	248	D	
Tenormin, *atenolol*	19, 193, 238, 575	D	
Terazol, Terazol 3, Terazol 7, *terconazole*	70	C	
terazosin, Hytrin	48, 245, 268	C	
terbinafine, Lamisil, Lamisil AT	318, 463, 465, 467, 468, 604	B	
terbutaline	32	B	
terconazole, Terazol, Terazol 3, Terazol 7	70	C	
teriflunomide, Aubagio	304	X	
teriparatide, Forteo	259, 335	C	
Tessalon Caps, Tessalon Perles, *benzonatate*	602	C	
testosterone, Androderm, AndroGel, Axiron, Fortesta, Natesto, Striant, Testim, Testostoderm, Testostoderm TTS	459–460	X	III
Testred, *methyltestosterone*	459	X	III
tetracaine	561	C	

Drug	Pg. Nos.	Preg. Cat.	DEA Sched.
trametinib, Mekinist	579	*	
Trandate, *labetalol*	239	C	
trandolapril, **Mavik**	199, 242	D	
tranexamic acid, **Lysteda**	299	B	
Transderm-Nitro, *nitroglycerin*	20	C	
Transderm-Scop, *scopolamine*	283, 294, 303, 519	C	
Tranxene, *clorazepate*	9, 25, 360	C	IV
tranylcypromine, **Parnate**	121	C	
Travatan, Travatan Z, *travoprost*	182	C	
travoprost, **Travatan, Travatan Z**	182	C	
trazodone, **Oleptro**	122, 393	C	
Trelegy Ellipta, *fluticasone furoate+umeclidinium+vilanterol*	64, 156	*	
Trental, *pentoxifylline*	371, 594	C	
treprostinil, **Orenitram**	412	B	
Tresiba, *insulin degludec (insulin analog)*	484	C	
tretinoin, **Atralin, Avita, Renova, Retin-A, Retin-A Micro Gel, Tretin-X**	7, 172, 237, 285, 519, 526	C	
Tretin-X, *tretinoin*	7, 172, 526	C	
Trexall, *methotrexate*	282, 384, 418, 454	X	
Treximet, *sumatriptan+ naproxen sodium*	193	C/D	
triamcinolone, **Aristocort, Kenalog-E**	29, 570, 571	C	
triamcinolone acetonide, **Azmacort, Kenacort, Kenalog Injectable, Kenalog Lotion, Kenalog Ointment, Kenalog Spray, Nasacort, Nasacort AQ, Oralone, Triact**	29, 387, 426, 566–568, 570, 571	C	
triamcinolone diacetate, **Aristocort Forte**	570, 571	C	
triamterene, **Dyrenium**	152, 240	C	
triazolam, **Halcion**	169, 272	X	IV
Tribenzor, *olmesartan medoxomil+amlodipine+ hydrochlorothiazide*	251	D	
TriCor, *fenofibrate*	147, 253	C	

Drug	Pg. Nos.	Preg. Cat.	DEA Sched.
Videx, Videx EC, *didanosine*	225, 588	B	
Viekira XR, Viekira Pak, *ombitasvir+paritaprevir+ ritonavir+dasabuvir*	210	B	
vigabatrin, **Sabril**	586	C	
Vigamox, *moxifloxacin*	97	C	
Viibryd, *vilazodone*	119–120	C	
vilazodone, **Viibryd**	119–120	C	
Vimovo, *naproxen+esomeprazole*	188, 310, 329, 407, 416, 565	D	
Vimpat, *lacosamide*	584	C	V
Viokace, *pancrelipase*	163, 357	C	
Vira-A, *vidarabine*	282	C	
Viracept, *nelfinavir*	229, 588	B	
Viramune, *nevirapine*	227, 588	C	
Virazole, *ribavirin*	208	X	
Viread, *tenofovir disoproxil fumarate*	226, 588	B	
Viroptic, *trifluridine*	102, 282	C	
Visine, *tetrahydrozoline*	143	*	
Visine L-R, *oxymetazoline*	95	*	
Visine AC, *tetrahydrozoline+zinc sulfate*	96	*	
Visken, *pindolol*	238	B	
Vistaril, *hydroxyzine*	11, 23, 82, 125, 128, 130, 359, 424, 428, 517, 603	C	
Vistide, *cidofovir*	415, 588	C	
vitamin b-12, cyanocobalamin, **Calomist, Nascobal Gel, Nascobal Nasal Spray**	17	C	
Vivactil, *protriptyline*	120, 134, 159, 279, 388, 390, 478	C	
Vivelle, Vivelle Dot, *estradiol transdermal system*	40, 151, 296–299, 332	X	
Vivitrol, *naltrexone*	321	C	
Vivlodex, *meloxicam*	150, 188, 310, 330, 407, 417, 564	C	

Drug	Pg. Nos.	Preg. Cat.	DEA Sched.
Voltaren, Voltaren Ophthalmic Solution, Voltaren-XR, *diclofenac sodium*	8–9, 310, 311, 329, 345, 406, 407, 416, 563	C	
voriconazole, **Vfend**	30, 66, 604	D	
Vosevi, *sofobuvir+velpatasvir+ voxilaprevir*	**211**	✱	
Vospire ER, *albuterol*	37	C	
Vraylar, *cariprazine*	52, 582	✱	
Vytorin, *ezetimibe+simvastatin*	147	X	
Vyvanse, *lisdexamfetamine*	42, 50	C	II
Vyxeos, *daunorubicin+cytarabine*	580	✱	
warfarin, **Coumadin**	371, 589	D	
WelChol, *colesevelam*	86, 87, 148, 497	B	
Wellbutrin, Wellbutrin SR, Wellbutrin XL, *bupropion hydrochloride*	44–45, 121, 469–470, 582	C	
Westcort, *hydrocortisone valerate*	567	C	
witch hazel, **Tucks**	205	✱	
Xalatan, *latanoprost*	182	C	
Xanax, Xanax XR, *alprazolam*	24, 360	D	IV
Xarelto, *rivaroxaban*	592	C	
Xartemis XR, *oxycodone+ acetaminophen*	352	C	II
Xeljanz, Xeljanz XR, *tofacitinib*	417	C	
Xeloda, *capecitabine*	580	D	
Xenical, *orlistat*	314	B	
Xermelo, *telotristat ethyl*	72, 138	✱	
Xhance, *fluticasone propionate*	386	✱	
Xifaxan, *rifaximin*	140, 613	C	
Xiron, *bromfenac*	95	C	
Xodol, *hydrocodone+ acetaminophen*	348	C	II
Xolair, *omalizumab*	11–12, 34, 39, 40, 518	B	
Xolegel, *ketoconazole*	131	C	
Xopenex, *levalbuterol*	31	C	
Xtampza, *oxycodone*	351	B	II

Drug	Pg. Nos.	Preg. Cat.	DEA Sched.
Xtoro, *finafloxacin*	337	C	
Xultophy, *insulin degludec+ liraglutide*	486, 492	C	
Xylocaine Injectable, Xylocaine Viscous Solution, *lidocaine*	29, 215, 561, 562	B	
Xyrem, *sodium oxybate*	311	B	
Xyzal Allergy 24HR, *levocetirizine*	124, 127, 130, 423, 429, 516 603	B	
Yasmin, *ethinyl estradiol+ drospirenone*	557	X	
Yaz, *ethinyl estradiol+ drospirenone*	395, 557	X	
Yescarta, *axicabtagene*	581	*	
Yodoxin, *diiodohydroxyquin, iodoquinol*	603	C	
Yosprala, *esomeprazole+aspirin*	528	D	
Yuvafem, *estradiol*	40, 151, 296–299, 332	X	
Zaditor, *ketotifen*	95	C	
zafirlukast, Accolate	34, 425	B	
zaleplon, Sonata	169, 271	C	IV
Zamicet, *hydrocodone+ acetaminophen*	348	C	II
Zanaflex, *tizanidine*	308, 458	C	
zanamivir for inhalation, Relenza	270, 606	B	
Zantac, Zantac Chewable Tablets, Zantac Efferdose, *ranitidine*	176, 367	B	
Zaroxolyn, *metolazone*	153, 202, 240	B	
zdu, zidovudine, Retrovir	226, 587	C	
Zebeta, *bisoprolol fumarate*	238	C	
Zebutal, *butalbital+ acetaminophen+caffeine*	197, 346	C	II
Zegerid, *omeprazole+sodium bicarbonate*	178	B	
Zejula, *niraparib*	581	*	
Zelapar, *selegiline*	363	C	
Zembrace SymTouch, *sumatriptan*	192	C	
Zemplar, *paricalcitol*	236, 257	C	